# International Public Health
## Diseases, Programs, Systems, and Policies

*Edited by*

**Michael H. Merson, MD**
Dean of Public Health
Professor and Chairperson
Department of Epidemiology and Public Health
Yale University School of Medicine
New Haven, Connecticut

**Robert E. Black, MD, MPH**
Professor and Chair
Department of International Health
School of Hygiene and Public Health
Johns Hopkins University
Baltimore, Maryland

**Anne J. Mills, MA, DHSA, PhD**
Professor
Department of Public Health and Policy
London School of Hygiene and Tropical Medicine
London, United Kingdom

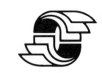

AN ASPEN PUBLICATION®
Aspen Publishers, Inc.
Gaithersburg, Maryland
2001

The author has made every effort to ensure the accuracy of the information herein. However, appropriate information sources should be consulted, especially for new or unfamiliar procedures. It is the responsibility of every practitioner to evaluate the appropriateness of a particular opinion in the context of actual clinical situations and with due considerations to new developments. The author, editors, and the publisher cannot be held responsible for any typographical or other errors found in this book.

Library of Congress Cataloging-in-Publication Data

International public health: diseases, programs, systems, and policies/edited by Michael H. Merson, Robert E. Black, Anne J. Mills.
p.  cm.
Includes bibliographical references and index.
ISBN 0-8342-1228-5
1. World health. 2. Public health—International cooperation. I. Merson, Michael H. II. Black, Robert E. III. Mills, Anne J.
RA441.I578 2000
362.1—dc21
00-058301

Orders: (800) 638-8437
Customer Service: (800) 234-1660

**About Aspen Publishers** • For more than 40 years, Aspen has been a leading professional publisher in a variety of disciplines. Aspen's vast information resources are available in both print and electronic formats. We are committed to providing the highest quality information available in the most appropriate format for our customers. Visit Aspen's Internet site for more information resources, directories, articles, and a searchable version of Aspen's full catalog, including the most recent publications:
**www.aspenpublishers.com**
**Aspen Publishers, Inc.** • The hallmark of quality in publishing
Member of the worldwide Wolters Kluwer group.


Editorial Services: Denise Hawkins Coursey
Library of Congress Catalog Card Number: 00-058301
ISBN: 0-8342-1228-5


*Printed in the United States of America*
1  2  3  4  5

# Contents

# Contributors

**Sir George Alleyne**
Director
Pan American Health Organization
World Health Organization
Washington, DC

**Robert E. Black, MD, MPH**
Professor and Chair
Department of International Health
School of Hygiene and Public Health
Johns Hopkins University
Baltimore, Maryland

**David E. Bloom, MA, PhD**
Professor of Economics and Demography
School of Public Health
Harvard University
Boston, Massachusetts

**Kent Buse, PhD, MSc**
Assistant Professor of Public Health
Division of Global Health
Department of Epidemiology and Public Health
Yale University School of Medicine
New Haven, Connecticut

**Benjamin Caballero, MD, PhD**
Professor and Director
Center for Human Nutrition
School of Hygiene and Public Health
Johns Hopkins University
Baltimore, Maryland

**Alex Cohen, PhD**
Instructor in Social Medicine
Department of Social Medicine
Harvard Medical School
Boston, Massachusetts

**Leon Eisenberg, MD**
Maude and Lillian Presley Professor of Medical
    Anthropology, Emeritus
Department of Social Medicine
Harvard Medical School
Boston, Massachusetts

**Adnan Ali Hyder, MD, MPH, PhD**
Assistant Scientist and International Health
    Consultant
Department of International Health
Johns Hopkins University
Baltimore, Maryland

**Dean T. Jamison, PhD**
Professor of Public Health and Professor of
    Education
Director
Program on International Health, Education,
    and Environment
University of California, Los Angeles
Los Angeles, California

**Ilona Kickbusch, PhD, MA**
Professor of Public Health
Head, Division of Global Health
Department of Epidemiology and Public Health
Yale University School of Medicine
New Haven, Connecticut

**Tord Kjellström, MB, MMechEng, MedDr**
Professor of Environmental Health
Director
New Zealand Environmental and Occupational
    Health Research Center
Department of Community Health
The University of Auckland
Auckland, New Zealand

**Matthew T. McKenna, MD, MPH**
Chief
Epidemiology and Health Services Research
    Branch
Division of Cancer Prevention and Control
National Center for Chronic Disease Prevention
    and Health Promotion
Atlanta, Georgia

**Anthony J. McMichael, MB, PhD**
Professor of Epidemiology
Department of Epidemiology and Population
    Health
London School of Hygiene and Tropical
    Medicine
London, United Kingdom

**David V. McQueen, ScD, MA**
Associate Director for Global Health Promotion
National Center for Chronic Disease Prevention
    and Health Promotion
Office of the Director
Centers for Disease Control and Prevention
Atlanta, Georgia

**Jane Menken, PhD**
Professor of Sociology
University of Colorado at Boulder
Boulder, Colorado

**Michael H. Merson, MD**
Dean of Public Health
Professor and Chairperson
Department of Epidemiology and Public Health
Yale University School of Medicine
New Haven, Connecticut

**Anne J. Mills, MA, DHSA, PhD**
Professor
Department of Public Health and Policy
London School of Hygiene and Tropical
    Medicine
London, United Kingdom

**Richard H. Morrow, MD, MPH, FACP**
Professor
Department of International Health
School of Hygiene and Public Health
Johns Hopkins University
Baltimore, Maryland

**Christina R. Phares, MPH**
Division of Epidemiology
University of California, Berkeley School of
    Public Health
Berkeley, California

**M. Omar Rahman, DSc, MPH, MD**
Associate Professor of Epidemiology and
    Demography
Department of Population and International
    Health
Harvard School of Public Health
Boston, Massachusetts

**M. Kent Ranson, MD, MPH**
Doctoral Student
Department of Public Health and Policy
London School of Hygiene and Tropical
    Medicine
London, United Kingdom

**Arthur L. Reingold, MD**
Professor and Head
Division of Epidemiology
University of California, Berkeley School of
    Public Health
Berkeley, California

**William A. Reinke, MBA, PhD**
Professor
Department of International Health
School of Hygiene and Public Health
Johns Hopkins University
Baltimore, Maryland

**Jennifer Prah Ruger, PhD, MA, MSc**
Health Economist
World Bank
Washington, DC

**Susan C. Scrimshaw, PhD**
Dean
School of Public Health
Professor of Community Health Sciences and
  Anthropology
University of Illinois at Chicago
Chicago, Illinois

**David A. Sleet, PhD**
Associate Director for Science
Division of Unintentional Injury Prevention
National Center for Injury Prevention and
  Control
Centers for Disease Control and Prevention
Atlanta, Georgia

**Kirk R. Smith, PhD, MPH**
Professor
Environmental Health Sciences
University of California, Berkeley
Berkeley, California

**Michael J. Toole, BMedSc, MB BS,
  DiplTropMedHygiene**
Associate Professor
Monash and Deakin Universities
Head, International Health Unit
MacFarlane Burnet Centre for Medical
  Research
Melbourne, Australia

**Ronald J. Waldman, MD, MPH**
Professor of Clinical Public Health
Director
Program on Forced Migration and Health
Center for Population and Family Health
Joseph L. Mailman School of Public Health
Columbia University
New York, New York

**Gill Walt, PhD**
Reader in Health Policy
Department of Public Health and Policy
London School of Hygiene and Tropical
  Medicine
London, United Kingdom

**Mitchell G. Weiss, MD, PhD**
Professor and Head of Discipline
Department of Public Health and Epidemiology
Swiss Tropical Institute and University of Basel
Basel, Switzerland

**Keith P. West, Jr., DrPH, MPH, RD**
Professor
Division of Human Nutrition
School of Hygiene and Public Health
Johns Hopkins University
Baltimore, Maryland

**Anthony B. Zwi, MBBCh, MSc, PhD,
  FFPHM**
Head, Health Policy Unit
Senior Lecturer in Health Policy and
  Epidemiology
Health Policy Unit
London School of Hygiene and Tropical
  Medicine
London, United Kingdom

# Foreword

Increasingly, nations around the world are recognizing that in matters of global policy, it is not enough to be concerned with the health status of their own population. As we continue to evolve into a global community, one nation's public health concern becomes the concern of all nations. At the same time, we err if we believe that the nation state will somehow abrogate the responsibility for dealing with health (The nation-state is dead, 1996). This new text, *International Public Health,* is a timely and valuable resource not only for students engaged in a formal course of study, but also for those who are already working in this field. The title accurately conveys the wide range of issues that are addressed, and the international approach implies not only the recognition of the geographical dispersion of public health issues, but also the arrangements nations make to deal with them.

Historically, international health represented the efforts by strong, industrialized nations to assist lower income ones. It reflected an approach that was predominantly missionary and altruistic in character. International health courses were popular among students for providing academic content as well as preparation for opportunities to work in other countries and fulfill a very basic and laudable desire to help those perceived as being less fortunate. Today, it is an area of global concern, where genuine cooperation occurs among nation states. Many public health issues have come to be seen as affecting all nations, and self-interest, if nothing else, prompts acceptance of the fact that, at least in health, we are indeed our brothers' keepers. Various factors have dictated that the risks affecting nations are no longer restricted to the infectious diseases, and a new range of health threats that go beyond national boundaries has emerged (Jamison, Frenk, & Knaul, 1998).

This book is an important contribution to the field because it is among the first to emphasize health issues that affect populations around the globe. It deals with public health—the international dimensions of public health. There can be no disciplinary purity in this field, as the care for the public's health involves an ever-increasing number of skills that go beyond those that are traditionally medical. We now find epidemiologists, anthropologists, lawyers, economists, sociologists, management scientists, and molecular biologists making a contribution to the public's health. It is thus refreshing to see the range of disciplines and high level of expertise that are represented in this book.

It is not only the state of health and health outcomes that concerns us, but also whether national and international action have taken into account the major social and cultural determinants of that health. I am pleased that this text devotes its first chapter to the subject of measurement. I foresee that at both local and global levels, increasing attention will need to be given not only to the actual state of health, but also to the differences in health status within and between nations. There are increasing disparities in health status that are unfair, unnecessary, and are therefore believed to represent inequities. Equity has become a major issue in international public health that goes beyond the natural sympathy for those whose situation is worse than others. The disparities in health that result in inequities can be a cause of social instability and lead to the loss or diminution of the cohesion that societies need to function optimally (Fukuyama, 1995).

The international approach to public health means that we must support joint actions by nations to promote, protect, or restore the health of the public. My experience has been that nations, either through their formal representatives or the various institutions they have established, can work together to improve health. For example, the successes achieved by national immunization programs would not have been possible except through the decisive, collective action of many nations.

International action in public health has often been focused on the need to address health problems that derive from global health risks, and there are many. The spread of disease through causative agents found in persons, insect vectors, or food is the most striking example and was one of the first to spur international action. It has taken on new and frightening twists with the emergence of antibiotic resistance and the transfer of resistant strains across geographic boundaries. Prescription practices that lead to the development of antibiotic resistance in one country will indubitably have effects in other countries (World Health Organization, 1997).

The ready spread of information with its central role in the many faces of globalization can itself constitute or contribute to a global health risk. The spread of advertising from one country to another may lead to the adoption of unhealthy practices, as we have seen in the case of tobacco. Less attention is paid to the spread of information about health services and their capabilities, but much of the clamor for more ad-

vanced restorative health technologies that result in increases in health expenditure derives from expectations created by images from the more industrialized societies.

Is it possible to construct international arrangements to counter or reduce such global health risks?

The possibility of effective and successful international efforts in health, as in every other field, depends essentially on three factors. First, there must be mutuality of interests. Nations will not cooperate unless they perceive that some benefit accrues to them, and to seek it otherwise is to lean toward coercion as a mechanism for ensuring compliance. Next, there has to be specificity of action. The general idea of international solidarity has to be followed by the identification of a specific issue around which solidarity can be built. Finally, there must be sufficient resources and adequate planning to address the issue, or the proposed international cooperation is likely to remain at the level of rhetoric. To this end, this book serves as a superior text for students because it provides a comprehensive analysis of international public health issues that will assist them in making sound planning and management decisions.

There is no doubt that attention to the international dimensions of public health will increase because, as has been shown in this book, many of our current and future dominant health problems will be global or at least multinational or international in nature. Accordingly, the health of people everywhere will indeed be seen and appreciated as a public good that is to be enjoyed for its own sake. However, when public health is dealt with internationally, it can be instrumental in creating more understanding among the nations of the world and contribute significantly to human development.

*Sir George Alleyne*
Director
Pan American Health Organization
World Health Organization
Washington, DC

## REFERENCES

Fukuyama, F. (1995). *Trust: The social virtues and the creation of prosperity*. New York: The Free Press.

Jamison, D.T., Frenk, J., & Knaul, F. (1998). International collective action in health: Objectives, functions and rationale. *Lancet, 351,* 514–517.

The nation-state is dead. Long live the nation-state. (December 23, 1995–January 5, 1996). *The Economist*, 15–18.

World Health Organization. (1997). Monitoring and management of bacterial resistance to antimicrobial agents: A World Health Organization Symposium. Geneva, Switzerland, 29 November–2 December, 1995. *Clinical Infectious Diseases, 24* (Suppl.1), S1–176.

# Introduction

*Michael H. Merson, Robert E. Black, and Anne J. Mills*

The three of us are privileged to be faculty at schools that provide graduate education to students who plan to enter or have already begun careers in public health. Many of them wish to learn about the public health problems and challenges facing low- and middle-income countries, often referred to as developing countries. Most are committed to teaching, to public health practice or administration, or to undertaking research in these countries or in international settings. This textbook is written for these students and those who teach and mentor them. In this introduction, we define international public health, provide a brief history of the field, and summarize the many challenges currently before it. We then explain how we put this textbook together and how we think it can best be used.

## WHAT IS INTERNATIONAL PUBLIC HEALTH?

The term *public health* evokes different ideas and images. One is often asked: Is it a profession, a discipline, or a system? Is it concerned primarily with the health care of the poor? Does it mean working in an urban clinic, or providing clean water and sanitation? C.-E.A. Winslow (1920), often regarded as the founder of modern public health in the United States, 80 years ago defined public health as:

the science and art of *preventing* disease, prolonging life and promoting

physical health and efficiency through organized *community* efforts for the sanitation of the environment, the control of communicable infections, the *education* of the individual in personal hygiene, the *organization* of medical and nursing *services* for the early diagnosis and preventive treatment of disease, and the development of the *social machinery* which will ensure to every individual a standard of living adequate for the maintenance of health; organizing these benefits in such a fashion as to enable every citizen to realize his *birthright* of health and longevity.

The unique features of public health (Exhibit I–1) were aptly defined in 1994 by an Essential Public Health Services Working Group of the Core Public Health Functions Steering Committee of the United States Public Health Service and further elaborated upon by Turnock (1997). Its most distinguishing feature is its focus on prevention. This can mean prevention of illness, deaths, hospital admissions, days lost from school or work, or consumption of unnecessary human or fiscal resources. Unfortunately, prevention efforts are often difficult; their successes are often not visible and most programs lack sufficient priority and resources to achieve their maximum impact. In all countries, much greater attention and budgets are directed toward

**Exhibit I–1** Selected Unique Features of Public Health

- use of prevention as a prime intervention strategy
- grounded in a broad array of sciences
- basis in social justice philosophy
- link with government and public policy

the provision of medical care, including the purchase of drugs.

One of the most unique characteristics of public health is its grounding in a multitude of sciences. These include the quantitative sciences of epidemiology and biostatistics; the biological sciences concerned with humans, microorganisms, and vectors; and the social and behavioral sciences, including economics, psychology, anthropology, and sociology. The latter have received more attention in recent years, as greater importance has been placed on defining and directing prevention efforts toward the economic, social, and behavioral determinants of illness and not only at individuals deemed at high risk for a particular public health problem (Ashton & Seymour, 1988). A similar growth in those trained in the managerial sciences in public health stems from the current debates on the organization and financing of health services in countries rich and poor. No doubt that in the future, with the human genome now fully cloned, public health efforts will need to apply the recent advances in genetics toward prevention of illness and disease, while being sure to protect the confidentiality rights of individuals. It is evident that the multidisciplinary and interdisciplinary nature of public health requires partnerships among those with diverse experiences and perspectives.

Social justice is the main pillar of public health. Its basic tenet is that the knowledge obtained on how to ensure a healthy population must be extended equally to all groups in any society, even when the burden of disease and ill health within that society is distributed unequally. Often this fair distribution of benefits is impeded by differences in gender, social class, ethnicity, and race. A critical challenge for public health is overcoming those barriers that prevent the application of the broad array of available prevention approaches and tools.

Although many public health activities are carried out by nongovernmental organizations (NGOs) and the private sector, governments play a crucial role in at least two ways. First, they design and implement public policies that bear upon social and environmental conditions, such as employment, housing, and pollution control. Second, they provide specific programs and services, usually to populations with greatest disadvantage, in an effort to ensure equity in access and in health status. Because of its link to government and its social justice underpinnings, public health is a profession that often stimulates political debate and controversy: witness the difficulties in obtaining government support in almost all countries for needle exchange programs, despite their proven efficacy in reducing the transmission of the human immunodeficiency virus (HIV) (Hurley, Jolley, & Kaldor, 1997).

One is often asked to explain the differences between public health and medicine (Exhibit I–2). These have been nicely summarized by Feinberg (1994). Those working in public health are concerned with the health of populations, have a public service ethic tempered by concerns for the individual, and place their emphasis on health promotion and disease prevention. Those working in medicine are more interested in the well-being of individuals, have a personal service ethic conditioned by awareness of social responsibilities, and focus their efforts on disease diagnosis and treatment of patients. Those working in public health require knowledge and input from many sectors—health, environment, social welfare, and education (to name but a few)—whereas those practicing medicine rely primarily on the services of the health care system. Of course these differences are not always so sharp, and efforts are underway around the world to enhance collaboration between public health and medicine. Nevertheless,

**Exhibit I–2** Some Differences between Public Health and Medicine

| Public Health | Medicine |
|---|---|
| • primary focus on population | • primary focus on individual |
| • public service ethic, tempered by concerns for the individual | • personal service ethic, conditioned by awareness of social responsibilities |
| • emphasis on health promotion and disease prevention | • emphasis on diagnosis and treatment; care for the whole patient |
| • reliance on many sectors | • reliance on health care system |

they help to illustrate what is meant by public health.

We define international public health as the application of the principles of public health to health problems and challenges that transcend national boundaries and to the complex array of global and local forces that affect them. Today, these global forces include urbanization, migration, and an explosion in information technology and expanding global markets. Most of the attention in international public health is focused on low- and middle-income countries, which have the greatest mortality and morbidity and inadequate health systems to meet the needs of their most vulnerable populations. Improving the health status of these populations requires an understanding of their social, cultural, and economic characteristics. In the study of international public health, much can be learned by comparing the approaches used by different countries in addressing their main public health problems.

What are some of the problems and issues that today's student of international public health needs to understand?

- the main causes of mortality and morbidity in the world today and also in the future, in view of the demographic transition facing many countries
- the cultural diversity of population groups within countries and regions, their values, belief systems, and responses to illness and death
- the causes and consequences of human population growth and the effects of reproductive health programs on women and children
- the complex relationship between nutritional status and disease patterns, including the importance of specific micronutrient deficiencies
- the main infectious agents and vectors, and the social, economic, behavioral, and environmental factors responsible for the major communicable and noncommunicable diseases
- the various approaches to the design, financing, organization, and management of preventive and curative services in the public and private sectors in countries with diverse economies and resources
- the appropriate responses to complex humanitarian emergencies, especially those that involve large displacements of populations within a country and between neighboring countries
- the importance of health for the economic development of a nation and productivity of its population, and the reciprocal impact of development, as reflected by such factors as educational levels and economic growth, on health status
- the roles of national, regional, international, and intergovernmental development agencies, as well as nongovernmental and private voluntary agencies

This textbook contains chapters dedicated to these and related topics. More detail will be provided about these later, after first offering a brief history of international public health and a summary of the main challenges facing those seeking careers in this field today.

## A BRIEF HISTORY OF INTERNATIONAL PUBLIC HEALTH

The history of international public health can be viewed as a history of how populations experience health and illness; how social, economic, and political systems create the possibilities for healthy or unhealthy lives; how societies create the preconditions for the production and transmission of disease; and how people, both as individuals and as social groups, attempt to promote their own health or avoid illness (Rosen, 1993). A number of authors have documented this history (Arnold, 1988; Basch, 1999; Leff & Leff, 1957; Rosen, 1993; Winslow & Hallock, 1949). A brief history is presented here primarily to provide a perspective for the challenges that face us today (Exhibit I–3).

It is difficult to select a date for the origins of the field of public health. Some would begin with Hippocrates, whose book *Airs, Waters and Places*, published around 400 BC, was the first systematic effort to present the causal relations between environmental factors and disease and to offer a theoretical basis for an understanding of endemic and epidemic diseases. Others would cite the introduction by the Romans of public sanitation and an organized water supply system in the first century. Many would select the bu-

Exhibit I–3 A Summarized History of International Public Health

| | |
|---|---|
| 400 BC | Hippocrates presents causal relation between environment and disease |
| First Century AD | Romans introduce public sanitation and organized water supply system |
| Fourteenth century | "Black Death" epidemic leads to quarantine and cordon sanitaire |
| Middle Ages | Colonial expansion spreads infectious diseases around the world |
| 1750–1850 | Industrial Revolution results in extensive health and social improvements in cities in Europe and United States |
| 1850–1910 | Great expansion in knowledge about the causes and modes of transmission of communicable diseases |
| 1910–1945 | Reductions in child mortality; establishment of schools of public health and international foundations and intergovernmental agencies interested in public health |
| 1945–1990 | Creation of World Bank and other UN agencies; WHO eradicates smallpox; HIV/AIDS epidemic begins; Alma Ata Conference gives emphasis to primary health care; UNICEF leads efforts for universal childhood immunization; greater attention to chronic diseases |
| 1990–2000 | Priority given to health sector reform, cost-effectiveness, public-private partnerships in health, and use of information and communications technologies |

bonic plague (or "Black Death") epidemic of the fourteenth century, which began in Central Asia, was carried on ships to Constantinople, Genoa, and other European ports, and then spread to the interior, killing 25 million persons in Europe alone. Believing that plague was introduced by ships, port cities like Venice and Marseilles adopted a 40-day quarantine period for entering vessels and established a "cordon sanitaire," an approach that was to be used to control other infectious diseases in subsequent centuries.

The Middle Ages was also the period when many cities in Europe, particularly through guilds, took an active part in founding hospitals and other institutions to provide medical care and social assistance. It was also a time when many European countries expanded their horizons abroad, exploring and colonizing new lands. They brought some diseases with them (for example, influenza, measles, and smallpox), and those that settled were forced to confront diseases that had never been seen in Europe (such as syphilis, dysentery, malaria, and sleeping sickness). European explorers would also bring new pathogens from one part of Africa to another or from one area of the globe to another (for example, from Africa to North America through the slave trade). On long voyages, however, the greatest enemy of the sailor was often scurvy, until 1875 when the British government issued its famous order that all men-of-war should carry a supply of lemon juice.

The Age of Enlightenment (1750–1830) was a pivotal period in the evolution of international public health. It was a time of social action in relation to health, as reflected by the new interest taken in health problems of specific groups. During this period, rapid advances in technology led to the development of factories. In England and elsewhere, this was paralleled by expansion of the coal mines. The Industrial Revolution had arrived. As a result, the populations of cities of England and other industrialized nations grew enormously, creating many unsanitary conditions that caused outbreaks of cholera and other epidemic diseases that resulted in high rates of child mortality. Near the end of this period

significant efforts were made to address these problems. Improvements were made in urban water supplies and sewerage, municipal hospitals arose throughout cities in Europe and the East Coast of the United States, laws were enacted limiting the work of children, and data on deaths and births began in many places to be systematically collected.

However, as industrialization continued, more efforts to protect the health of the public were needed. These occurred first in England, often regarded as the first modern industrial country, through the efforts of Edwin Chadwick. Beginning in 1832, he headed up the royal Poor Law Commission, which undertook an extensive survey of health and sanitation conditions throughout the country. The work of this commission eventually led in 1848 to the Public Health Act, which created a General Board of Health that was empowered to appoint local boards of health and medical officers of health to deal effectively with public health problems. The impact of these developments was felt throughout Europe and especially in the United States, where it stimulated creation of health departments in many cities and states.

It was in fact cholera, which in the first half of the nineteenth century spread in waves from South Asia to the Middle East and then to Europe and the United States, that did the most to stimulate the formal internationalization of public health. The policy of "cordon sanitaire," applied by many European nations in an effort to control the disease, had become a major influence on trade, necessitating an international agreement. In 1851 the First International Sanitary Conference was convened in Paris to discuss the role of quarantine in the control of cholera, as well as plague and yellow fever, which were causing epidemics throughout Europe. Although no real agreement was reached, the conference laid the foundations for international cooperation in health.

The main development in international public health in the latter part of the nineteenth century was the enormous growth of knowledge in the area of microbiology, as exemplified by Louis

Pasteur's proof of the germ theory of disease, by Robert Koch's discovery of the tubercle bacillus, and by Walter Reed's demonstration of the role of the mosquito in transmitting yellow fever. Between 1880 and 1910, the etiological cause and means of transmission of most communicable diseases were discovered in laboratories in North America and Europe. This was paralleled by related discoveries in the sciences of physiology, metabolism, endocrinology, and nutrition. Dramatic decreases soon were seen in child and adult mortality through improvement in social and economic conditions, discovery of vaccines, and implementation of programs in health education. The way was now clear for the development of public health administration, based on a scientific understanding of the elements involved in transmission of communicable diseases.

The first 2 decades of the twentieth century witnessed the establishment of three formal intergovernmental public health bodies: the International Sanitary Bureau to serve nations in the Western hemisphere (in 1904); L'office Internationale d'Hygiene Public in Paris concerned with prevention and control of the main quarantinable diseases (in 1909); and the League of Nations Health Office (LNHO) in Geneva, which provided assistance to member states on technical matters related to health (in 1920). In 1926 the LNHO started publication of the *Weekly Epidemiological Record,* which has continued until this present day as the weekly publication of the World Health Organization (WHO). It also established many scientific and technical commissions, issued reports on the status of many infectious and chronic diseases, and sent its staff around the world to assist national governments in dealing with their health problems.

In North America and countries in Europe the explosion of scientific knowledge in the latter part of the nineteenth century and the belief that it could solve social problems stimulated medical schools, such as Johns Hopkins University, to establish schools of public health. In France public subscriptions helped to fund the Institut Pasteur (in honor of Louis Pasteur) in Paris,

which subsequently developed a network of institutes throughout the francophone world that produced sera and vaccines and conducted research on a wide variety of tropical diseases. Another significant development during this period was the founding of the Rockefeller Foundation (in 1909) and its International Health Commission (in 1913). During its 38 years of operation, the commission cooperated with many governments in campaigns against endemic diseases, such as hookworm, malaria, and yellow fever. The foundation also provided essential financial support to help establish medical schools in China, Thailand, and elsewhere, and later supported international health programs in a number of American and European schools of medicine and public health. All these developments were paralleled by the development and strengthening of competencies in public health among the militaries in the United States and the countries of Europe, stimulated in great part by the buildup to and realities of World War I. Following the war, there was increasing recognition that much of ill health in the "colonial world" was not easily solvable with medical interventions and was intractably bound up with problems of malnutrition and poverty.

Most historians would date the beginning of our current era of international public health with the end of World War II. The need to reconstruct the economies of America and countries of Western Europe, and the rapid emergence of newly independent countries in Africa and Asia, led to the establishment of many new intergovernmental organizations. The United Nations Monetary and Financial Conference, held in Bretton Woods, New Hampshire, and attended by representatives from 43 countries, led to the establishment of the International Bank for Reconstruction and Development (or World Bank) and the International Monetary Fund. The former initially lent money to countries only at prevailing market interest rates, but beginning in 1960 also provided loans to poorer countries at much lower interest rates and with far better terms through its International Development Association. It was not until the early 1980s that the World Bank began to accelerate greatly its provisions of loans to countries for programs in health and education, but by the end of the decade these loans were the greatest source of "foreign assistance" to low- and middle-income countries. In the decade after World War II, many other United Nations organizations (for example, the United Nations Children's Fund, or UNICEF) and specialized agencies (such as WHO) were formed to assist countries in strengthening their health and other social sectors. In addition, most of the wealthier industrialized countries established agencies or bureaus that funded bilateral projects in specific low- and middle-income countries. For the former major colonial powers, such assistance was often given mostly to their former colonies.

Many of the international public health efforts in the 1960s and 1970s were dedicated to the control of specific diseases. A global effort to control malaria was hampered by a number of operational and technical difficulties, including the vector's increasing resistance to insecticides and the parasite's resistance to available antimalaria drugs. However, the campaign to eradicate smallpox led by WHO successfully eliminated the disease in 1981, and it stimulated the establishment of the Expanded Program on Immunization, which focused on the delivery of effective vaccines to infants. Also, during the 1970s two large international research programs were initiated under the cosponsorship of various United Nations agencies: the Special Program for Research on Human Reproduction (focusing on development and testing of new contraceptive technologies) and the Tropical Disease Research Program (providing support for the development of better means of diagnosis, treatment, and prevention of six tropical diseases, including malaria). Greater attention also was given to the chronic diseases, such as cardiovascular and cerebrovascular diseases and cancer.

In 1978 WHO organized a conference in Alma Ata in the former Soviet Union that gave priority to the delivery of primary health care services and the goal of Health for All by the Year 2000.

Rather than focusing only on control of specific diseases, this conference called for international public health efforts to strengthen the capacities of low- and middle-income countries to extend their health services to populations with poor access to prevention and care. The concerns of tropical medicine, which were concentrated on the infectious diseases of warm climates, were being replaced by an emphasis on the provision of health services to reduce morbidity and premature mortality in resource-poor settings (DeCock, Lucas, Mabey, & Parry, 1995). Given the limited financial and management capacities of many governments, increased attention was paid to the role of NGOs in providing these services. As a result, many mission hospitals, particularly in sub-Saharan Africa, expanded their activities in their local communities, the number of local NGOs began to increase, and a number of international NGOs (for example, Save the Children, Oxfam, and more recently Médecins sans Frontières) greatly expanded their services, often with support of bilateral agencies. Disease-specific efforts, most notably UNICEF's Child Survival Program with its acronym GOBI (growth charts, oral rehydration, breastfeeding, immunization) and its goal of Universal Childhood Immunization by the Year 1990, was seen by many as a program that both focused on specific health problems and provided an excellent means of strengthening health systems.

The one new and unexpected development was the arrival of the HIV/AIDS epidemic. By the time a simple laboratory test to detect HIV was discovered in 1985, more than 2 million persons in sub-Saharan Africa had been infected. In 1987 WHO formed the Global Program on AIDS, which within 2 years became the largest international public health effort ever established, with an annual budget of $90 million and 500 staff working in Geneva and in more than 80 low- and middle-income countries and regions. In 1995, with some 20 million persons, mostly living in these countries, now infected with HIV, and with the understanding that the epidemic could only be brought under control through a true multisectoral effort, the program was transformed into a joint effort of six UN agencies that became known as UNAIDS. Despite the continuing efforts of UN and bilateral aid agencies, many international and local NGOs, and national governments, the epidemic continues to expand and now promises to be the most devastating global epidemic since the plague epidemic of the Middle Ages.

In the last decade of the twentieth century, changes well beyond the health sector have had a marked impact on its style of operation. Major shifts in political and economic ideologies have led to a reconsideration of the role of governments and how they should finance and deliver public services. Much greater attention has been given to focusing more narrowly government's role and to making greater use of the private sector. Indeed, international public health in the last decade of the twentieth century can be characterized by emphases on health sector reform, cost-effectiveness as an important principle in the choice of interventions in the public sector, and public-private partnerships in health, paralleled by a rapid expansion of information and communications technologies.

Although rising incomes have been known for a long time to improve health status, during the past decade there has been increased attention to the importance of a healthy population for economic development. Participation of sectors other than the health sector is now viewed as essential for achieving a healthy population. More and more countries, experiencing the demographic transition from societies where most persons are young to societies with rapidly increasing numbers of middle aged and older adults, have had to provide preventive and care services that address health problems of both the poor and wealthy nations simultaneously. Witness the fact that India now has the largest middle class in the world with high rates of cardiovascular and other noncommunicable diseases. Not surprisingly, issues around equity in the availability of drugs and vaccines and in access to other technological advances, and around the ethics of international research, have

gained greater attention. Healthy populations are now viewed as essential for domestic security as well as economic development. The challenges of international public health have never been greater.

## CURRENT CHALLENGES IN INTERNATIONAL PUBLIC HEALTH

We have witnessed major improvements in the health of populations the past century, with the pace of change increasing rapidly in low- and middle-income countries since the Bretton Woods Conference. Public health, and more broadly an improved understanding of how social, behavioral, economic, and environmental factors influence the health of populations, has contributed to these improvements to an extent far greater than access to medical care. However, these improvements have not been universal. For example, at the turn of the twenty-first century:

- More than 10 million children below age 5 die each year from preventable causes; 70% of these are due to pneumonia, diarrhea, malaria, malnutrition, and measles.
- More than 150 million married women want to space or limit childbearing, but do not have access to modern contraceptives.
- Nearly 600,000 women die annually from complications of pregnancy and childbirth, and another 18 million suffer pregnancy-related health problems that can be permanently disabling.
- Each year 13 million persons die from infectious diseases, most of which are preventable or curable; half of these deaths are in adults and are due to tuberculosis, malaria, or HIV/AIDS.

There is a broad consensus that poverty is the most important underlying cause of preventable death, disease, and disability. Unfortunately, more people live in poverty today than 20 years ago. Literacy, access to housing, safe water, sanitation, food supplies, and urbanization are determinants of health status that interact with poverty. Economic globalization, driven by increasing world trade, greater openness of national economies to world markets, and the vast expansion of information technology, has contributed to uneven economic growth, increased economic inequality, and concerns about subordination of human and labor rights (Ahmad, 1999).

It is within this context that the 1999 WHO *World Health Report* laid out the four major challenges (Exhibit I–4) that must be addressed in order to improve the world's health (WHO, 1999). These are:

- *Reduction of the burden of excess mortality and morbidity among the poor, by focusing more on interventions that can achieve the greatest health gain possible within prevailing resource limits.* This means giving attention to diseases that disproportionally affect the poor, such as tuberculosis, malaria, and HIV/AIDS; reduction of maternal mortality; improvement of maternal and childhood nutrition; and extending the coverage of immunization programs. The resources of both public and private sectors are needed for these efforts.

**Exhibit I–4** Four Current Challenges To Improve World Health

1. reduction of excess mortality and morbidity among the poor
2. countering threats to health resulting from economic crises, unhealthy environments, and risky behavior
3. development of more effective health systems that can improve health status, reduce health inequities, enhance responsiveness to legitimate expectations, and increase efficiency
4. investing in research and development directed toward diseases of the poor

- *Countering potential threats to health resulting from economic crises, unhealthy environments, and risky behaviors.* As an example, 80% of all smokers today live in low- and middle-income countries. Promotion of healthy lifestyles is the key strategy for risk reduction: cleaner air and water and injury prevention are also important. An essential component of this strategy is to ensure that females, as well as males, increase their educational attainment.

- *Development of more effective health systems that can improve health status, reduce health inequities, enhance responsiveness to legitimate expectations, and increase efficiency.* The financing challenge is to identify appropriate sources of funding to meet consumer demands in a way that protects those less able to pay. Governments need to create an appropriate regulatory environment, while they seek to diversify the sources of service provision and to select, with advice and input from consumers, those health programs that will be supported with public funds. Consumers must also be provided with more knowledge about how they can improve their own health. At the global level, there is a need to improve the capacities of international organizations to provide humanitarian assistance and to respond to complex emergencies, which are often beyond the capabilities of individual governments.

- *Investments in research and development directed toward diseases that overwhelmingly affect the poor.* This requires the creation of incentives for the private sector, such as tax credits to stimulate their undertaking of such research, often through public-private partnership arrangements. Policy research is also needed, for example, to learn more about the reasons for the gaps in health status between countries and the best policies and actions to reduce inequities in health and access to health services, including the appropriate roles of government and nongovernmental bodies.

Meeting these challenges will require new forms of international and intersectorial cooperation between UN agencies with an established health role, other international bodies such as the World Trade Organization, regional bodies such as the European Union, bilateral agencies, NGOs, foundations, and the private sector, including pharmaceutical companies. It also must include the new philanthropists in international health—Bill and Melinda Gates, George Soros, and Ted Turner—who bring not only significant amounts of funds into the global system but also a new, more informal and personal style of operations. Ensuring the ideal formation and effective functioning of this "global health system" will itself be an enormous challenge for the next decade of international public health.

## USE AND CONTENT OF THIS TEXTBOOK

This textbook has been prepared with these challenges foremost in our mind. Its focus is on diseases, programs, health systems, and health policies in low- and middle-income (or developing) countries, making reference to and using examples from the United States, Western Europe, and other high-income countries as appropriate.* The individual chapters present much information on health problems and issues that transcend national boundaries and are of concern to many nations.

Our intent has been, first and foremost, to provide a textbook for graduate students in various disciplines who are studying international public health. Given its broad range of content, the book as a whole may serve as the main source for an introductory course on international public health. Alternatively, some chapters (or parts of chapters) can be used in courses dedicated to more specific subjects and topics. Students who use the textbook in this way will hopefully be stimulated to explore other chap-

ters once they read the ones they have been assigned. We believe the textbook can also be a useful reference for those already working in the field of international public health in government agencies, as well as those employed by international health and development agencies, NGOs, or the private sector.

Because of the many dynamic areas and subjects we wanted to cover, we have chosen to prepare an edited textbook. We selected content experts for each chapter rather than presuming to have the expertise to write the entire book ourselves. We recognize that an edited textbook has its shortcomings, such as some inconsistency in style and presentation and occasional overlap in chapter contents. We have done our best to limit these, and hope the reader will agree that those that remain are a small price to pay for fulfilling our goal of providing the reader with the highest quality content.

Another consequence of the dynamic nature of international public health is the occasional difficulty in providing the most up-to-date epidemiologic information on all causes of mortality and morbidity. One obvious example of this is the rapidly evolving HIV/AIDS situation in Africa and Asia. To assist the reader in obtaining this information, we have provided references in various chapters, including Internet resources.

The textbook has 14 chapters. The first two chapters set the background. Chapter 1 reviews the importance of using quantitative indicators for decision making in health. It presents the latest developments in the measurement of health status and disease burden, including the increasing use of composite measures of health that combine the effects of disease-specific morbidity and mortality on populations. It then summarizes current estimates and future trends in selected countries and regions, as well as of the global burden of disease. Chapter 2 examines the social, cultural, and behavioral parameters that are essential to understanding public health efforts. It does this by describing key concepts in the field of anthropology, particularly as they relate to health belief systems and types of heal-

---

*A classification of countries can be found on the World Bank Website: http://www.worldbank.org/data/databytopic/class.htm.

ers around the world, and by presenting key theories of health behavior that are relevant to behavior change. The importance of combining qualitative and quantitative methodologies in measuring and assessing health status and programs is emphasized.

The next three chapters are devoted to the three greatest public health challenges traditionally faced by low-income countries—reproductive health, infectious diseases, and nutrition.

Reproductive health has long been addressed primarily through family planning programs directly intended to reduce fertility. Chapter 3 presents more current views of reproductive health that broaden this concept to include empowerment of women in decisions about health and fertility. It provides information on population growth and demographic changes around the world and reviews how women control their fertility and indexes of the effects of various social and biological determinants of fertility. It then examines the role of family planning programs in the reduction of fertility and unwanted pregnancies and, lastly, considers the influence of fertility patterns on the health of children and women.

Collectively, the infectious diseases have undoubtedly been the most important causes of premature mortality and morbidity in low- and middle-income countries. Chapter 4 presents the descriptive epidemiological features and available prevention and control strategies for communicable diseases that are of greatest public health significance in these countries today. These include the vaccine-preventable diseases; diarrhea and acute respiratory infections in children; tuberculosis, malaria, and other parasitic diseases; and HIV/AIDS and other sexually transmitted diseases in adults. Examples of successful programs using one or more of available control approaches—preventing exposure, immunization, drug prophylaxis, and treatment— are described, as are the challenges and obstacles that confront low- and middle-income countries in successfully controlling these diseases.

Nutritional concerns in low- and middle-income countries are largely ones of deprivation and hunger, leading to nutritional deficiencies and ensuing health consequences. Chapter 5 focuses on several spheres of nutrition that are of utmost concern in these countries as we enter the twenty-first century. These include undernutrition and its components of protein malnutrition and micronutrient deficiencies (particularly vitamin A, iron, iodine, and zinc); the role of breastfeeding and complementary feeding in infants and young children; and diverse nutritional problems in adults, ranging from undernutrition among older adults to overnutrition in more affluent segments of the populations of rapidly developing countries.

The book's subsequent three chapters address public health priorities that have been associated with higher income countries but are gaining importance in resource-poor countries as they become more developed economically and their populations live longer and progress through the demographic transition. These are chronic diseases and injury, mental health, and environmental health.

Chronic diseases, frequently called "noncommunicable" or "degenerative diseases," are generally characterized by a long latency period, prolonged course of illness, noncontagious origin, functional impairment or disability, and incurability. Many of the consequences of serious injury have chronic disease characteristics. Chapter 6 provides an overview of chronic diseases and injury in low- and middle-income countries, with particular attention given to such problems as cardiovascular diseases, stroke, cancer, and diabetes. The descriptive epidemiology of these diseases, the behavior risk factors that serve as determinants of these diseases, and the main approaches used to prevent chronic diseases and injuries are presented.

It is only recently that mental health has received appropriate attention commensurate with its great importance in low- and middle-income countries. Chapter 7 reviews what is known about the epidemiology of suicide and key categories of mental disorders, particularly mood and anxiety disorders, schizophrenia, and substance abuse. It further examines the impact of cultural beliefs on the diagnosis of these disorders and the impact of major social changes, such as urbanization and migration, on mental health. Lastly, the chapter reviews the status of limited national efforts to date in resource-limited countries to launch programs to prevent mental illness and promote mental health.

Chapter 8 provides a comprehensive review of environmental health issues and problems in low- and middle-income countries. It begins with a summary of conceptual and methodological issues that comprise the important area of risk assessment and monitoring, and then reviews the profiles of environmental health hazards within the household (for example, water and sanitation), in the workplace (for example, on farms, in mines and factories), in the community (for example, outdoor air pollution), and at regional and global levels. The latter includes such controversial topics as climate change, ozone depletion, and biodiversity. The chapter concludes with a discussion of the issues and projects that bear on the future of environmental health research and policy.

Chapter 9 focuses on the public health challenges that characterize complex humanitarian emergencies (CHEs). These conflicts occur within and across state boundaries, have political antecedents, are protracted in duration, and are embedded in existing social, political, economic, and cultural structures and cleavages. In 1997 there were an estimated 30 million internally displaced persons and 23 million refugees seeking asylum across international borders, the vast majority fleeing conflict zones. The chapter considers the impact of CHEs on populations and health systems and reviews the technical interventions that are available to alleviate suffering and limit their adverse effects on populations. Attention is drawn to the importance of an effective and efficient early response in influencing the long-term survival of populations and health systems and the nature of any postconflict society that is established.

The next two chapters are concerned with the development and implementation of effective health systems, which have a crucial influence on the ability of countries to address their disease burden and improve the health of their populations. Chapter 10 focuses on the design of health systems considered largely from an economic perspective. It provides a conceptual map of the health system along with its key elements; addresses the fundamental and often controversial question as to the role of the state; and then considers the key functions of any health system, which include regulation, financing, resource allocation, and provision. It concludes by reviewing current trends in health system reform. Four country examples are used throughout the chapter to illustrate key differences in health systems across the world.

As multipurpose and multidisciplinary endeavors, health systems require coordination among numerous individuals and units. Thus they require effective and efficient management. Chapter 11 is dedicated to this topic. It provides an understanding of important management concepts, principles, and methods, citing requisites and examples of their successful application. Subjects included are organizational structure and relations, human and physical resources management, and financial management, including resource allocation and cost analysis. A final section presents some commonly used management methods, such as situation analysis, decision analysis, and survey methods.

Health and health systems interrelate with a nation's economy in two main ways. The first, as noted earlier, comprises the bidirectional relationships between health status and national income and development. For example, health affects income through its impact on labor productivity, saving rates, and age structure, while a higher income improves health by increasing the capacity to produce food and to have adequate housing and education, and through incentives for fertility limitation. The second concerns linkages between health care delivery institutions, health financing (including insurance) policies, and economic outcomes. Chapter 12 reviews information available on both these challenging and closely related topics that are critical to government policy makers seeking the best ways to improve the quality of life of their populations, particularly in those countries that carry the heaviest burden of disease and poverty.

Chapter 13 presents the current state of affairs regarding global cooperation in international public health. It begins by explaining why countries seek this cooperation, the processes by which it occurs, and the institutions and actors involved. The remaining part reviews the important shift that has taken place in the overall framework of international cooperation since the establishment of the United Nations system in the late 1940s, from one characterized by vertical relationships between states and international and intergovernmental organizations, to one of horizontal, cooperative participation among nation states, UN agencies, the private sector, and NGOs. This shift has great significance for the formation of future international public health policies and programs.

The final chapter provides a review of the main global influences and responses that are affecting global health at the start of the twenty-first century. It begins with a brief overview of the phenomenon of globalization and its impact on public health. It details how today's transnational forces are affecting global susceptibility to communicable and noncommunicable diseases, and the ability of the international community to respond to them. It then elaborates on how the horizontal relationships among the main participants in international public health, as described in the previous chapter, are seeking a new approach to global health governance that will best meet the new health challenges resulting from globalization. Finally, it concludes with a 10-step proposal to reorient public health policy, practice, and research in the coming decades.

The reader will note that there are many case studies presented in exhibits scattered throughout the text. These have been written to provide concrete examples and illustrations of key points and concepts covered in each chapter. At the conclusion of each chapter there is a list of questions that can help course instructors stimulate classroom discussions around important issues covered in the chapter. The editors recognize that the book could include separate chapters on additional topics—maternal and child health, women's health, health and human rights, and demography, to name but a few. We have opted instead to provide in-depth information on the core subjects that were selected, although we did our best to cover some aspects of all of the above subjects in one or more of the chapters.

In many ways, international public health is at an important crossroad. Its greatest challenge is to confront global forces, while at the same time promoting local, evidence-based, cost-effective, public health programs that deal with disease-specific problems and more general issues, such as poverty and gender inequality (Beaglehole & Bonita, 1998). Public health-related research is essential to gain a better understanding of the determinants of illness and of innovative approaches to prevention and care, and to find means of improving the efficiency and coverage of health systems. Whether as a practitioner, policy maker, or researcher, international public health professionals can make an enormous difference by being well-trained in their discipline and being highly sensitive to the beliefs, culture, and value systems of the populations with whom they collaborate or serve. We hope this textbook will aid in this process.

**REFERENCES**

Ahmad, K. (1999, September). World Bank predicts development for next century. *Lancet, 354,* 1005.

Arnold, D. (1988). Introduction: Disease, medicine and empire. In D. Arnold (Ed.), *Imperial medicine and indigenous societies* (pp. 1–26). Manchester, England: Manchester University Press.

Ashton, J., & Seymour, H. (1988). *The new public health: The Liverpool experience*. Philadelphia: Open University Press.

Basch, P.F. (1999). *Textbook of international health* (2nd ed.). New York: Oxford University Press.

Beaglehole, R., & Bonita, R. (1998, February). Public health at the crossroads: Which way forward? *Lancet, 351,* 590–592.

DeCock, K.M., Lucas, S.B., Mabey, D., & Parry, E. (1995, September). Tropical medicine for the 21st century. *British Medical Journal, 311,* 860–862.

Feinberg, H.V. (1994). Ethical approaches to health and development. In K. Aoki (Ed.), *Ethical dilemmas in health and development* (pp. 3–13). Tokyo: Japan Science Society Press.

Hurley, S.F., Jolley, D.J., & Kaldor, J.M. (1997). Effectiveness of needle-exchange programmes for prevention of HIV infection. *Lancet, 349,* 1797–1800.

Leff, S., & Leff, V. (1957). *From witchcraft to world health.* New York: Macmillan.

Rosen, G. (1993). *A history of public health* (Expanded Ed.). Baltimore, MD: Johns Hopkins University Press.

Turnock, B.J. (1997). *Public health: What it is and how it works*. Gaithersburg, MD: Aspen Publishers, Inc.

Winslow, C.-E.A. (1920, March). The untilled fields of public health. *Modern Medicine, 2,* 3, 183–191.

Winslow, C.-E.A., & Hallock, G.T. (1949). *Health through the ages*. New York: Metropolitan Life Insurance Company.

World Health Organization. (1999). *The world health report.* Message from the director-general (pp. viii–xi). Geneva, Switzerland: Author.

# Acknowledgments

This book is a collaborative effort of 31 authors around the world. Many people helped us bring it into being. Principal among these is Lisa Rollins, the Project Manager from the Department of Epidemiology and Public Health at Yale, who helped ensure that everyone met the many production deadlines, served as liaison to all constituents, and coordinated our activities with the Publisher.

We would also like to thank the co-editors' assistants, Nicola Lord (London School of Hygiene and Tropical Medicine) and Barbara Ewing (Johns Hopkins School of Hygiene and Public Health), who assisted in meeting the deadlines and facilitating communications with the editors.

Additionally, we are grateful for the assistance of Deanna Fryer (Yale) in organizing the many chapters as they arrived and for arranging our international conference calls, and of Diane Griffin (Johns Hopkins) for her persistence in following up with the various authors.

# CHAPTER 1

# Disease Burden Measurement and Trends

*Adnan Ali Hyder and Richard H. Morrow*

Agreement on definitions is fundamental to understanding and discussing issues of health and disease. The next steps are knowing how to measure and track changes in the health of populations in time and place, understanding underlying causal factors, and assessing what kinds of health and social programs will provide the greatest gains for healthy life.

In its 1948 charter the World Health Organization (WHO) defined health as not the absence of disease, but rather in positive terms as "a state of complete physical, mental and social well-being and not merely the absence of disease or infirmity." Although this is an important ideological conceptualization, it has not been operationally useful. For most practical purposes, objectives of health programs are more readily defined in terms of prevention or treatment of disease.

Disease has been defined in many ways. For example, distinctions may be made between sickness and illness, but for purposes of defining and measuring disease burden a general definition will be used here. Disease is anything that an individual (or population) experiences that causes, literally, "dis-ease," that is, anything that leads to discomfort, pain, distress of all sorts, disability of any kind, and death, constitutes disease from whatever cause, including injuries or psychiatric disabilities.

It is also important to be able to diagnose and classify specific diseases to the extent that such classification aids in determining which health intervention programs would be most useful. Thus understanding the pathogenesis of the disease process and defining disease are critical measures for understanding and classifying "causes" in order to determine the most effective prevention and treatment strategies for reducing the effects of a disease or risk factor. Just as the purpose of diagnosis of a disease in an individual patient is to provide the right treatment, the major purpose of working through a burden of disease analysis in a population is to provide the basis for the most effective mix of health and social program interventions.

This chapter emphasizes some of the latest developments in measurement of population health status and disease burden. These include the increasing use of summary, composite measures of health that combine the mortality and morbidity effects of diseases into a single indicator; results of the *Global Burden of Disease* study; and developments in the measurement of disability and risk factors (Murray & Lopez, 1996a). The more traditional approaches to measuring health are widely available in other public health textbooks and will be used for illustrative and comparative purposes here.

This chapter has four sections, beginning with this introduction. The second discusses the reasons for and approaches to measuring disease burden, the reasons for using quantitative indicators, and the importance of using data for decision making in health. The third section is a critical review of methods for composite measures combining mortality and morbidity effects of diseases on populations at national and regional levels. It also explores the potential utility of these measures and discusses their limitations and implications. The fourth section demonstrates the application of these methods for measurement of health status and assessment of global health trends. It reviews current estimates and future trends of selected countries and regions, as well as the global burden of disease.

## REASONS AND APPROACHES FOR MEASURING HEALTH AND DISEASE

### Rationale

The many reasons for obtaining health-related information all hinge on the need for data to guide efforts toward reducing the consequences of disease and enhancing the benefits of good health. These include the need to identify which interventions would have the greatest effect, to identify emerging trends and anticipate future needs, to assist in determining priorities for expenditures, to provide information for education to the public, and to help in setting health research agendas. The primary information requirement is for understanding and assessing the health status of a population and its changes with time.

In recent years much has been made of the importance of evidence-based decisions in health. There is little reason to doubt that evidence is better than intuition, but that depends upon how the evidence is used. In this chapter we examine evidence—the facts of health and disease—and demonstrate how to assemble this evidence so that it can best be used in assisting better decisions concerning health and disease.

A well-documented example of the relationship between decision making and data can be seen in an assessment of the health status in Ghana in the mid-1970s, as illustrated in Exhibit 1–1. This case illustrates how able people with good intentions made decisions using established health system approaches, but good evidence that was also being gathered at the same time was ignored. A major reason for

the failure to use available evidence was that it was not put forward in a form helpful to decision makers. The Health Planning Unit of the Ghana Ministry of Health developed a quantitative method for assessing the health impact of different diseases and for assisting in determining priorities for allocation of resources to alternative health programs. They used available data that were put in terms that had meaning for the decision makers—the gain in healthy life per dollar expended. This method was the first use of combining morbidity and mortality into a common composite indicator that could examine the gains in total healthy life per dollar expended on alternate health programs. At that time, the Ghana Ministry of Health had just developed the 1977–1981 5-year plan with assistance from the Ghana Medical School. The plan called for expanding and extending the existing hospital and health center services. However, when the evidence was examined, an alternative community-based primary health care strategy that required equivalent expenditures was found to provide 20 times as much healthy life per dollar. This finding greatly strengthened the rationale for introducing a community-based primary health system in place of the hospital-centered system.

### Measuring Health and Disease

The relative importance (burden) of different diseases in a population depends upon their frequency (incidence or prevalence) and severity (the mortality and extent of serious morbidity).

#### Counting Disease

The first task in measuring disease in a population is to count its occurrence. Counting disease frequency can be done in several ways and it is important to understand what these different methods of counting actually mean. The most useful way depends upon the nature of the disease and the purpose for which it is being counted. There are three commonly used measures of disease occurrence: cumulative incidence, incidence density, and prevalence.

**Exhibit 1–1**  Assessing a Health System with Data

Assessment of the health status in Ghana in the late 1970s indicated that despite the remarkable increase in resources going into the health sector, the general health status of the population was still low. In the previous 10 years there had been little or no improvement in the infant mortality rate, the maternal mortality rate, or in the rate of communicable disease. That situation is strikingly illustrated in the first graphic, which refers to the health care dilemma in Ghana at that time. It shows how the financial resources of the nation were being allocated in reverse proportion to the numbers of people in need.

The health system of Ghana could be likened to a pyramid, with the teaching hospital in Accra at the top (second graphic) and a network of health posts and dressing stations at the bottom. This was a system based on service delivery points (that is, facilities). It focused attention on buildings rather than on the health services for the people. Such an emphasis on facilities creates false "needs" among the people for more facilities. Good health becomes synonymous with the provision of a doctor and a hospital rather than the enjoyment of a disease-free environment.

Health information allows for such assessments that play a vital role in health planning and policy development.

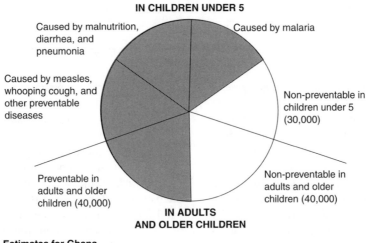

**Estimates for Ghana**

| | | |
|---|---|---|
| Total deaths | 200,000 | |
| Deaths in children under 5 | 120,000 | |
| Preventable deaths in these children | | 90,000 |
| Deaths in adults and older children | 80,000 | |
| Preventable deaths in these adults and older children | | 40,000 |
| Total preventable deaths | | 130,000 |

"Preventable deaths" are those that can be prevented through adequate primary care at a cost that Ghana can afford.

*continues*

**Exhibit 1–1** continued

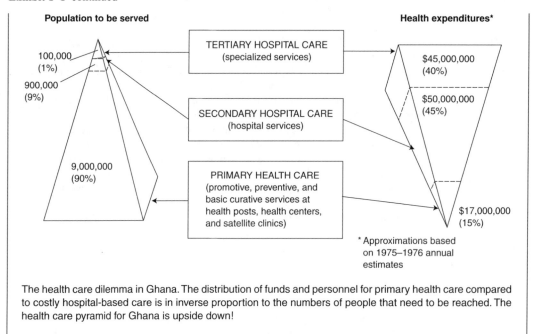

The health care dilemma in Ghana. The distribution of funds and personnel for primary health care compared to costly hospital-based care is in inverse proportion to the numbers of people that need to be reached. The health care pyramid for Ghana is upside down!

*Cumulative incidence,* or *incidence proportion,* is the number of new cases of a disease that occur in a population at risk for developing the disease during a specified period of time. It is the proportion of people who develop new disease in a specific period of time. For this to have meaning there are three necessary components: a definition of the onset of the event, a defined population, and a particular period of time. The critical point is *new cases* of disease—the disease develops in a person who did not have the disease previously. The numerator is the number of new cases of disease (the event) and the denominator is the number of people at risk for developing the disease. Everyone included in the denominator must have the potential to become part of the group that is counted in the numerator. For example, to calculate the incidence of prostate cancer, the denominator must include only men, because women are not at risk for developing prostate cancer. The third component is the period of time. Any time unit can be used as long as all those counted in the denominator

are followed for a comparable period with those who are counted as new cases in the numerator.

*Incidence density,* or often simply *incidence rate,* is the occurrence of new cases of disease per unit of person-time. This directly incorporates time into the denominator and is generally the most useful measure of disease frequency, often expressed as new events per person-year or per 1,000 person-years. Incidence is a measure of events (that is, transition from a nondiseased to a diseased state) and can be considered a measure of risk. This risk can be looked at in any population group, defined by age, sex, place, time, sociodemographic characteristics, occupation, or by exposure to a toxin or any suspected causal factor.

*Prevalence* is a measure of present status rather than of newly occurring disease. It measures the proportion of people who have defined disease at a specific time. Thus it is a composite measure made up of two factors—the incidence of the disease that has occurred in the past and continues to the present or to some specified point in time. That is, prevalence equals incidence rate of the disease multiplied by the average duration of the disease. For most chronic diseases, prevalence rates are more commonly available than are incidence rates.

### Severity of Disease

To understand the burden of disease in a population, it is important to consider not only the frequency of the disease, but also its severity as indicated by the morbidity and premature mortality that it causes. Premature mortality is defined as death before the expectation of life had the disease not occurred. Morbidity is a statement of the extent of disability that a person suffers as a consequence of the disease over time and can be measured by a number of indicators, as discussed below.

## Mortality

Traditionally, mortality has been the most important indicator of the health status of a population. John Graunt developed the first known systematic collection of data on mortality with the *Bills of Mortality* in the early 1600s in London. He described the age pattern of deaths, categorized them by "cause" as understood at the time, and demonstrated variation from place to place and from year to year. Mortality rates according to age, sex, place, and cause continue as central information about a population's health status and a crucial input for understanding and measuring the burden of disease. For example, infant and maternal mortality rates are considered leading indicators of the health situation in any region or country. Considerable literature exists on the use of mortality to indicate health status and its application to national and subnational levels (Murray & Chen, 1992); paradigms such as the demographic transition are based largely on the decline of mortality in the under-fives (Mosley et al., 1993; Omran, 1971).

Both the *fact* of death by age, sex, and place, which is required by law in most countries through *death registration*, and *cause* of death, as required by law in many through *death certifi-*

*cation*, provide essential information. Although death is a cardinal event and generally the most widely available kind of health information, in many of the low-income countries the fact of death, let alone cause of death, frequently is still not reliably available.

In industrialized countries vital statistics (that is, the registration of births and deaths, usually by age, sex, and place) are routinely collected and highly reliable. In most middle-income countries their reliability and completeness have been steadily improving and often are fairly satisfactory. In the low-income countries, as in most of Africa, however, the collection of vital statistics remains highly incomplete, although improving. An analysis of death registration in the *Global Burden of Disease* study showed that only two of eight world regions had complete vital registration systems for 1990 (Murray & Lopez, 1996a). But even in these countries increasing use of household survey methods provides estimates, at least, of the under-five mortality.

However, obtaining information about cause of death remains poorly done even in most middle-income countries; most information depends upon special surveys or studies of select populations and under specific circumstances. Verbal autopsies have been used increasingly for judging likely cause of death in under-five children. These can be quite useful for a few selected causes of death, such as neonatal tetanus and severe diarrhea, but it has been found that sensitivity and specificity are limited for many diseases whose symptoms are variable and quite nonspecific (such as malaria).

Age-specific mortality profiles are a prerequisite for a burden of disease analysis. Although extensive work has been done to document and analyze child mortality in developing countries, little has been done for adult mortality (Feachem & Kjellstrom, 1992). Developing countries have higher rates of adult mortality than the market economy nations (Murray & Chen, 1992), and mortality rates are higher for both women and men at every age when compared to the industrialized world. In Africa the enormous increase in AIDS deaths in young and middle-age women and men may further augment these analyses.

The major deficiencies in empirical cause-specific mortality data in developing countries pose a challenge to assessing overall national mortality patterns. Preston (1976) analyzed life tables for 43 national populations, including 9 developing countries, to develop cause-specific mortality profiles. The pattern of cause-specific mortality changes at different levels of total mortality, with a general trend of decreasing infectious and parasitic disease cause-specific mortality with declining total mortality. Indeed, mortality from these communicable causes was a major reason for the difference between high- and low-mortality populations (Murray & Chen, 1992). The relationship between total mortality and cause-specific mortality is important because it allows an estimation of cause-of-death structure based on the total mortality profile. In-depth investigation of multicountry data sets reveals that the broad groups of diseases had a strong relationship; specific causes had a less reliable pattern (Murray & Chen, 1992).

The cause-of-death certification system based on the WHO–International Classification of Diseases (ICD) has been widely used for hospital in-patient records and their analyses in many countries (Murray & Chen, 1992). As would be expected, wide variations in the reliability of these analyses occur because of variations in the training and expertise of people coding cause of death, as well the supervision and feedback provided. But there have been steady improvements in many countries and these kinds of analyses provide some of the best information available on outcomes of major causes of serious morbidity.

Mortality can be expressed in two important quantitative measures. The *mortality rate* is a form of incidence and is expressed as number of deaths per person-time, in a defined population in a defined time period. The numerator can be total deaths, age- or sex-specific deaths, or cause-specific deaths; the denominator is the number of persons at risk of dying in the stated category as defined earlier for incidence. The *case-fatality ratio* is the proportion of those with a given disease who die of that disease (at any time unless specified). The mortality rate is equal to the case fatality ratio multiplied by the incidence rate of the disease in the population.

The distinction between the *proportion* of deaths attributable to a set of causes versus the *probability* of death from these causes is important to understand. For example, the probability of death from noncommunicable causes (indeed from virtually all causes) is higher in low- and middle-income regions than in the industrialized world. However, the proportion of deaths attributable to these chronic causes is less than those attributed to infectious causes. The risk of death and the rates of death by these causes do not increase; rather, the proportion of attributable deaths increases as the communicable proportion declines with development. For example, in 1990 the risk of dying from cancer was 50% greater in low- and middle-income countries than in industrialized countries, even though it accounted for a much smaller proportion of total deaths.

## Mortality Transitions

The term *demographic transition* was first used by F.W. Notestein in 1945 to describe the changes in birth and death rates that historically have accompanied the shift from a traditional to a modern society (Exhibit 1–2) (see also Chapter 3). With modernization (a complex term indicating social and economic development), sharp declines in mortality have been followed by a reduction in fertility, although usually lagging by years or decades. The term *transition* refers to the shift from a stable high stationary stage of population in which very high birth rates are balanced by very high death rates and with little or no population growth. As a society undergoes modernization, there is a transition with falling mortality, especially in the under-five age group, but with continuing high birth rates leading to explosive population growth. Birth rates then tend to drop and a new low stationary stage is reached in which birth and death rates are low and balance continues. The end results are a striking change in the age structure of the population with a decreased proportion of children and an aging population. These changes are reflected in changes in the population age distributions as shifts from a wide-based pyramid, reflecting larger numbers in the younger age groups, to a narrow base, nearly rectangular configuration, with nearly equal percentages in each age group (Exhibit 1–2).

Historically, all countries that have undergone modernization with a marked drop in under-five mortality have had rapid population growth. Until recently this population growth was followed by falling fertility rates in virtually all such countries, but the reasons for the drop are not entirely clear. Maurice King has pointed to a potential major problem that may arise, termed the "demographic trap," in which fertility rates do not drop. This situation would lead to the classic Malthusian scenario in which massive starvation and epidemic diseases overtake the population. King points out that there is no guarantee that there will be a drop in birth rate in all countries undergoing modernization and that changes in fertility depend very much upon social and cultural characteristics.

In 1971 Omran described the underlying reasons for the demographic transition and used the term *epidemiologic transition* to explain the changing causal factors of disease that accounted for the dramatic drop in under-five mortality, which was largely due to reduction in malnutrition and communicable diseases. In the *Global Burden of Disease* study diseases were categorized into three groups: Group I (diseases characteristic of the developing world), Group II (diseases characteristic of the technically advanced countries), and Group III (injuries of all kinds). Those in Group I mainly are affected in the epidemiologic transition leading to an overall decline in mortality and a relative shift toward the Group II disease pattern (see Chapter 6).

It is important to note that although high rates of maternal mortality are characteristic of the developing world (and this is included in Group I), reductions of maternal mortality occur in a different timeframe from that of under-five mortality. Reductions in maternal mortality require a much better developed infrastructure, including ready availability of surgical and blood transfusion capacity plus improved communication and transportation systems. Thus drops in maternal

---

**Exhibit 1–2** The Demographic and Epidemiologic Transitions

Changes in the pattern of disease proceed in two steps. The first is the demographic transition, when mortality from infectious disease declines and, partly as a result of declining fertility and differential rates of decline among causes of death, the second is the epidemiologic transition. The population grows older, and noninfectious diseases become the main causes of ill health. Health patterns in the developing world over the next three decades will be profoundly influenced by both these transitions.

It is commonly assumed that when a country is going through its demographic transition, the changes in its health indicators are primarily a function of declines in mortality. In fact, both the age structure and the cause-of-death structure are strongly influenced by the rapid decline in fertility. When fertility is high, the age structure of a population is heavily skewed toward the young, irrespective of the level of mortality. Because birth rates remain high and larger numbers of women enter the reproductive ages every year, the base of the population is continually expanding. When birth rates start to fall rapidly, the absolute number of babies born each year may remain unchanged or even decline. The graphs that follow show the shape of the age structure of the population that begins to be transformed from a broad-based triangle into a rectangle, or even into a pear shape with a more pronounced narrowing of the base.

*continues*

**Exhibit 1–2** continued

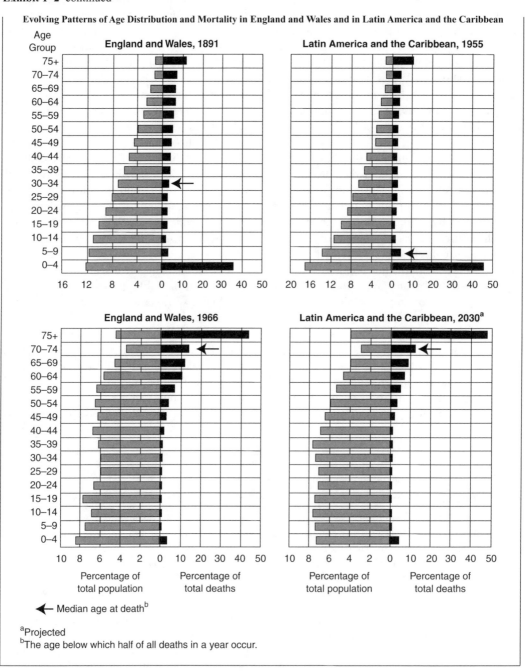

Evolving Patterns of Age Distribution and Mortality in England and Wales and in Latin America and the Caribbean

Percentage of total population    Percentage of total deaths

Percentage of total population    Percentage of total deaths

← Median age at death[b]

[a]Projected
[b]The age below which half of all deaths in a year occur.

mortality occur much further along the road toward economic development, and changes occur only after shifts in the under-five mortality have been seen (see Chapter 3).

Major changes in the patterns and causes of injury are also likely to occur with modernization. In particular, road traffic injuries tend to increase as countries go through the stage of development in which there is great increase in vehicles and speeds at which they are operated before improved roads and law enforcement take place. There may also be important shifts in the nature of violence and toward whom it is directed related to crime patterns, civil unrest, ethnic conflicts, and intrafamily tensions. Thus the shifting injury patterns must also be examined as transitions of mortality are studies over time in countries.

## Morbidity

Measures of mortality have been the principal indicators of health status for a long time. Their relative ease of observation, presence of data, and history of use make them suitable for assessing health status and consequent changes. However, the problem with mortality-based indicators is that they "note the dead and ignore the living" (Kaplan, 1990). Morbidity, on the other hand, usually has been measured using hospital records and outpatient registers from clinics. Measurements of morbidity are much more problematic than either frequency or mortality since there is no clearly defined endpoint, such as death provides. In addition, there are several components of morbidity that need to be assessed—duration, severity, and consequences.

Hospital inpatient discharge records when they are based upon good clinical evidence and coded by staff well trained in coding procedures can provide high-quality data on the major causes of morbidity serious enough to require hospitalization. They can provide good cause of death data for those hospitalized, and some sense of outcome status of those with serious conditions. Hospital data are generally improving in quality, especially in middle-income countries and in selected sentinel, usually tertiary care, teaching hospitals in some poor countries. Such information is highly biased because of the highly skewed distribution of those using such hospitals, but in many situations it is possible to have a good understanding of those biases and make appropriate adjustments in order to draw useful conclusions.

Generally, outpatient records in most of the world are highly deficient in terms of diagnosis and often provide only the patient's chief complaint and probably the treatment dispensed. The main value of most such records is limited to establishing the fact of using a facility. There are usually strong biases in the use of outpatient facilities, including access factors (distance and cost of use), nature and severity of the disease problem, and opportunity for alternate services.

Visits to health care facilities, functional disability (measures of activity less than usual), and time spent away from work (absenteeism, work days lost) have been used to assess the magnitude of morbidity from various conditions. A common approach to evaluating morbidity in a population has been the assessment of the impact on social roles or functional performance, such as days missed from work or spent in bed (Kaplan, 1990). There is considerable literature on a wide variety of instruments used to measure such functional capacity, especially in clinical medical literature, that is not directly useful for population-based morbidity assessment.

Data about morbidity presented in the literature are often based on self-perceived or observed assessments, and frequently from survey-based interview information. The perception of morbidity and its reporting, the observation of morbidity and its impact, and other factors are responsible for the wide variation between reported and measured prevalence of conditions (Murray & Chen, 1992). This has resulted in an underestimation of the presence and impact of morbidity in both low- and middle-income and industrialized nations. This situation also underscores the variation in morbidity data that often has been interpreted to indicate that wealthy individuals and low mortality populations tend to *report* higher rates of morbidity (Murray & Lopez, 1996a).

Concepts that give separate identity to disease, illness, and sickness have been in the literature for half a century from the description of the sick role in 1929 to development of a disability framework in the 1960s. This framework considered *disease* as an organic level disorder confined to the individual, *illness* as a subjective state of dysfunction from the disorder at the individual level, and *sickness* as a social dysfunction within a society that goes beyond the individual. These are analogous terms to the classification developed in 1980 by the World Health Organization. The two are not synonymous, and the WHO system has been more widely used recently.

The International Classification of Impairments, Disabilities, and Handicaps (ICIDH) was developed by the WHO to classify nonfatal health outcomes. This assessment was based on a progression from disease to handicap and is analogous to the ICD series. ICIDH categories include *impairment*—loss or abnormality of psychological, physiological, or anatomical structure or function; *disability*—restriction or lack of ability to perform an activity considered normal; and *handicap*—disadvantage from a disability or impairment, for a given individual based on the inability to fulfill a normal role as defined by age, sex, or sociocultural factors. These distinctions clarify more than just processes and help define the contribution of medical services, rehabilitation facilities, and social welfare to the reduction of sickness.

Monitoring of the consequences of diseases, evaluation of use of services, and standardization of a classification and indexing system were originally conceived to be the main objectives of the ICIDH. Since its creation the ICIDH classification has also been used to generate indicators for disability such as impairment-, disability-, and handicap-free life expectancies as mentioned in the next section. These in turn have been used to estimate "health-adjusted life expectancies" using severity and preference weights for time spent in states of less-than-perfect health.

### Data for Decisions

In the collection and assessment of information, the level of precision required is an impor-

tant feature. This level of precision needs to be guided by the purpose of collecting the information. The ultimate reason for data is to guide decision making—to make it better and more efficient at helping reduce the burden of disease on populations. The level of precision depends on the decisions to be taken such that even gross estimations can sometimes be helpful. This may be disconcerting to some people, but the time, person, and monetary cost of further precision needs to be justified by its potential impact on decision making. Low- and middle-income countries with their scarce resources need timely and appropriate information to plan and implement health interventions that maximize the health of their populations. Methods, indicators, and assessments of disease must support and contribute to this primary purpose of health systems.

## METHODS AND INDICATORS OF DISEASE BURDEN

This section focuses on various approaches used for composite measures that combine mortality and morbidity into one number for measuring the burden of disease and examines methodological issues and the value choices that are incorporated into such methods. In doing so this chapter helps clarify the origins of the methods used in burden of disease measurement, document the numerous types of indicators, and set the ground for the contribution of the methods to analysis of trends. A number of indicators and methods have been reviewed, and the general format followed is an explanation of the indicator, brief background, its advantages and limitations, and utility in the current health care arena. Aspects of mortality and morbidity that are specifically related to construction of composite indicators are included in this section. The issues involved in the measurement of disability have been reviewed separately, as are the values and social preference choices, which are common to many indicators.

## Rationale for Composite Measures

Rationing of health care resources is a fact of life everywhere; choices as how best to use resources for health must be made (World Bank, 1993; Hyder, 1998). The global scarcity of resources is reflected in the health sector, especially in the low- and middle-income nations (Evans, Hall, & Warford, 1981; World Bank, 1993). The realities in low- and middle-income countries make the issue of choice that much starker; it becomes even more important than in industrialized countries to choose carefully how to optimize health expenditures to obtain the most health in the most equitable fashion from these expenditures. Important tools under development to assist in making better choices for health spending are based on measures of the effectiveness of health interventions to improve health status in relation to their cost.

No country has sufficient resources to meet all the health needs of its population, and low- and middle-income countries have resources only to deal with a few of their most urgent problems. In many low- and middle-income nations this shortage of resources has been aggravated by the combined reduction in expenditures allocated to health and increasing health care costs. Further, most low-income countries have made poor use of what resources they do expend on health, often putting the bulk of expenditures into tertiary health care. At the same time, the demand for health care is rising rapidly everywhere, compelling virtually all countries to reform their health systems.

Many kinds of questions are being asked regarding the role of resource allocation in the provision of health services. What policies are best suited to deal with competing health needs? What is the most economically efficient way to finance such programs? What are the optimal organizational and management models to meet the objectives of these programs? Answers to these questions need formulation to assess the health and economic policies unique to each country (see Chapter 10).

The process for health policy formulation is poorly delineated in most low- and middle-income countries, but a limited number of discrete factors largely determine the allocation of health resources. The most common is the pattern of expenditure in last year's budget. Other major influences include requirements of international agencies to meet their mandated health priorities and the perceived burden of disease by policy makers. The well-educated and politically powerful community of specialist doctors and hospital administrators has traditionally influenced the major share of health resource allocation. In the absence of relevant disease burden and intervention data, tertiary curative care has attracted the major share of health funds.

In most sectors decisions on resource allocation are based on perceived value for money, but the health sector has had no coherent basis for determining the comparative value of different health outcomes. If one is to make decisions about whether to put money into programs that reduce mortality in under-fives, as compared to those that reduce disabling conditions in adults, there is a need to have a common denominator.

In the past 20 years, and especially in this past decade, work has been carried out to develop composite indicators combining morbidity and mortality into a single measure that may serve as a common denominator for such purposes. Such an indicator represents the amount of healthy lifetime lost due to a disease from both disability and premature death. The common unit of measure is time lost from healthy life. For a given health budget one would want to see maximum healthy life gain per unit expenditure. An important tool for achieving optimal efficiency in health spending would be one that provided a measure of cost-effectiveness of health interventions or the ratio of costs to health benefits. The composite indicators described in this chapter (such as *healthy life year* [HeaLy]) can be used as a measure of the effectiveness of a broad range of health interventions and directly feed into cost-effectiveness calculations. Money can then be allocated to the interventions that produce the largest gain in healthy life for the dollar amount spent for that intervention.

The information in this chapter represents the continuing initiative of health professionals to develop a more rational methodology for the allocation of health resources. The emphasis of such efforts is on the systematic analysis of information and use in the context of health, especially evaluating strategies for improving health. Health information responsibilities in low- and middle-income countries are widely scattered over many government ministries and departments and are often not computerized. Public and private, academic and nongovernment sources may have their own health data tucked away in files and drawers, with only a small portion published in local or international journals. Application of any method in this environment is challenging.

In countries where appropriate data do not exist and the information is unpublished, decisions are made without reference to evidence. Efforts to measure burden of disease may stimulate attempts to evaluate current data and to develop methods of obtaining the information needed for their determination. Actions based on policies derived from evidence will be more convincing and should help to focus on those interventions (and essential support systems) that will optimally reduce the disease burden given available resources. Increased focus on the major health problems facing low- and middle-income nations is in line with calls for essential national health research. Such an approach emphasizes the importance of relevant national research in the decision-making process and supports the appropriate development of health systems incorporating responsible decision making in countries.

In recent years, a number of approaches to measuring health status by use of composite indicators have been developed (Ghana Health Assessment Team, 1981; Morrow, 1984; World Bank, 1993; Murray & Lopez, 1994, 1996a, 1996b; Hyder, Rotllant, & Morrow, 1998). Such burden of disease methods and indicators can assist in

- prioritizing health services
- making explicit and transparent the assumptions used for allocating health resources
- identifying at-risk groups
- evaluating health interventions and programs
- focusing attention on the key information to be collected by data systems
- setting health research priorities

The most important reason for attempting to capture the complex mix of incommensurate consequences resulting from disease into a single number is the need to weigh the benefits of health interventions against their costs. Costs of health programs are expressed in a unidimensional measure, such as U.S. dollars; therefore, the benefits to be achieved from their expenditure must also be so expressed. *Healthy life time* is a unidimensional measure that can be used to compress health benefits and losses into the single time dimension. An explicit, objective, quantitative approach should enable better budgetary decisions and permit resource allocation in the health sector to be undertaken in a more effective and equitable fashion.

It is important to keep in mind that a composite indicator is simply a tool to be used to assist decision makers in resource allocation. Like any tool, it can be misused. Conclusions that are reached on the basis of the use of these indicators must be carefully examined and looked at from all viewpoints. Not only are there problems of trying to put so many dimensions together, which inevitably leads to distortion, but there are serious issues concerning reliability and validity of information upon which these are based. Thus all the problems determining cause of death and counting the number of diseases and assessing the extent of disability from a condition will lead to great uncertainties when they are added and multiplied together. The development of a single indicator with a specific number provides deceptive substantiality to what may be made up of fragile data. Continuing vigilance in how data are obtained, compiled, and used is critical, and those responsible for using the tool must have a clear technical understanding of what is behind the numbers and what underlying assumptions and limitations are associated with these approaches. But with all these caveats, alternative approaches to improved decision making leave even more to be desired.

## Aspects of Mortality

Discussion of mortality has been presented earlier in detail, and the same issues apply to its use in burden of disease measurement. It is also reviewed under the sections on specific indicators. Mortality is expected at an age defined by the expectation of life at birth; when it occurs prior to that age it is considered a premature event. The contribution of premature mortality in terms of time lost is used in composite indicators.

Traditional indicators of mortality have been the standard for assessing health status. Child mortality under the age of 5 years is considered a sensitive indicator of overall health of nations, especially women and children. For example, the United Nations Children's Fund (UNICEF) publishes an annual global report that includes a ranking of nations based on this indicator (United Nations Children's Fund, 1999). These indicators have the added advantage of having been studied for their relationships with other indicators of social and economic development of nations. Gross national product (GNP) per capita, for example, is an indicator of national wealth, and the relationship between this variable and child mortality has been studied. In general, the higher the level of economic development, the lower the rate of child mortality. However, there are always exceptions and these need to be examined carefully. For example, Sri Lanka and the Indian state of Kerala are both low-income regions that have low mortality rates. These examples demonstrate that the relationship between mortality and poverty is complex and needs in-depth investigation. To improve the health of nations, absolute poverty as well as the disparities within societies are impediments to empowerment of the poor and needy, especially women and children.

## Aspects of Morbidity

Measurements of morbidity are much more challenging than those of mortality. If all the various forms of disability are to be compared with mortality, they must be measured in an equivalent manner for use in health assessments. To do so, measurement of disability must attempt to quantify the duration and severity of this complex phenomenon. A defined process is needed that rates the severity of disability as compared to mortality, measures the duration of time spent in a disabled state, and converts disability from various causes into a common scale. General measures of disability without regard to cause (often carried out by special surveys) are useful to determine the proportion of the population that is disabled and unable to carry out normal activities.

In general, three components need to be assessed. The first component is the *case disability ratio* (CDR), which is the proportion of those who are diagnosed with the disease who have disability. For most diseases that are diagnosed clinically the CDR will be 1. However, when the diagnosis is based upon, for example, infection rather than disease (such as tuberculosis) or upon a genetic marker rather than the physical manifestation (such as sickle trait), the CDR is likely to be less than 1.

The second component is the *extent* of disability—how incapacitated the person is as a result of the disease. The extent of disability is expressed from 0, which means no disability, to 1, which is equivalent to death. The assessment of extent can be quite subjective, particularly since there are so many different types and dimensions of disability. A number of methods have been tried to achieve comparability and obtain consensus concerning the measurement of the severity component. Generally, for most conditions a reasonable degree of consensus can be reached within broad categories (for example, 25% disabled as compared to 50%), but efforts to go to much finer distinctions have been equivocal. Except for high prevalence chronic conditions, there may be little need to become more refined for purposes of health program decisions.

The third component is the *duration* of the disability. The duration is generally counted from onset until cure and recovery or death. Sometimes there is continuing permanent disability after the acute phase is completed and thus the duration would be life expectation from the time of onset.

### Measuring Disability

There is substantial literature investigating the expressed preferences of individuals for different health states. Measurement of individual preferences for health states has been done by a variety of methods and has yielded results that have been interpreted as indicative of severity (Torrence, 1986; Kaplan, 1990). This literature has also attempted to make the duration of time spent in the health state mutually exclusive to the preference for that state. Factors affecting such a system of preference elicitation include the type of respondent, the type of instrument used to measure the response, and other factors, such as the time from entry into the disabled state. Individuals who are in a particular state, healthy individuals, health care providers, caretakers, and family members have all been interviewed in studies. Adaptation, conditioning, development of special skills, and vocational training can all change the response of individuals over time within a particular health state and thus affect the value of that state to the individual.

Mechanisms for asking a cross section of people about the value of their health state exist, but using them and generalizing results to the whole population have limitations. People may be excluded from the group involved, may be unwilling or unable to participate in such an investigative process, and those excluded may be the ones most afflicted by a disability. Healthy people may have different valuations for health states than people who are in those states, and even the latter may change their response depending on the time and adaptive processes. The reference point (the subject) from which quality of life can be measured has been considered a *static* reference as assumed in many instruments that measure quality of life. The point of reference changes according to theories of change associated with adaptation, coping, expectancy, optimism, and other phenomena causing results of health-related quality of life to vary. As presented in de Querville's hypothesis, the value placed on a year of life by a paraplegic soon after entering that health state would be different from that obtained after several years of adjustment to that state. Such factors affect the results both at one point of measurement and repeated measurements over time.

Instruments used to extract such preferences involve visual and interview techniques (Torrence, 1986; Murray & Lopez, 1996a). The situation of two alternative scenarios is often presented to the subject and the point of indifference sought (as in the standard gamble techniques.) Despite the development of literature on such methods, there is no consensus or standard method. The particular context used for asking questions, and variable reliability and validity of such studies, make this work challenging.

### Attributes of Disability

Estimates of the duration of disability are derived from current information on diseases, as are the proportion of cases disabled by cause. The duration of disability, as opposed to severity or extent, can be measured objectively.

The reduction of different types of disability—physical, functional, mental, social—and the variations in perception of their severity to a single measure is a great challenge. Composite measures attempt to compare the severity of a disabled state to that of either complete health or death (totally disabled). Severity of disability scales have been developed by group consensus using community surveys (Kaplan, 1990), a mixture of community and expert groups (Ghana Health Assessment Team, 1981), and experts only (World Bank, 1993). These scales usually compare perfect health states to death on a scale of 0 to 1 (Table 1–1).

In Murray and Lopez's *Global Burden of Disease 1990* study, the disability severity estimates were based on available data from similar or geographically close regions and expert opinion. Twenty-two indicator conditions were selected and used to construct seven disability classes (Table 1–1). Outcomes from all other health conditions were categorized within these seven classes, sometimes with special categories for treated and untreated groups. Critical review, internal consistency checks, and other reviews have been used to improve the quality of data used. Omission of disabilities from rare diseases and short-term disabilities is unlikely to have introduced significant bias. Major psychiatric conditions receive a high score in these systems and have emerged as an important source of disability worldwide.

The results of the *Global Burden of Disease* study have placed an appropriate focus on the loss of healthy life from mental disorders, which is substantiated by other work. The *WHO Collaborative Study on Psychological Problems in General Health Care* provides a perspective on

the impact of mental illness as functional disability and its cross-cultural presence. Using standard questionnaires this study of 14 countries found that psychopathology was consistently associated with increased disability, after adjusting for physical disability, with a dose-response relationship. The results were consistent across cultures and centers indicating a leading role of psychological disorders in the production of disability, irrespective of the socioeconomic features at play.

Murray and Lopez (1994) have supported the notion that it is better to make an informed estimate regarding the flow of disability from a condition than not to make it, since the latter leaves out the disability-related effects of disease completely. The latter choice makes the situation falsely appear as one in which disability is of no importance, while in fact the cumulative impact of disability from even acute, short-term events such as diarrhea is also significant. This argument makes the attempt to capture dis-

**Table 1–1** Disability Classification Systems

*Ghana Health Assessment Team, 1981*

| Class | Severity | Example(s) |
|---|---|---|
| 1 | 0 | normal health |
| 2 | 0.01–0.25 | loss of one limb |
| 3 | 0.26–0.50 | loss of two limbs |
| 4 | 0.51–0.75 | loss of three limbs |
| 5 | 0.76–0.99 | loss of four limbs |
| 6 | 1.00 | equivalent to death |

*Global Burden of Disease Study, 1990*

| Disability Class | Severity Weight | Indicator Conditions |
|---|---|---|
| 1 | 0.00–0.02 | Vitiligo, height, weight |
| 2 | 0.02–0.12 | Acute watery diarrhea, sore throat, severe anemia |
| 3 | 0.12–0.24 | Radius fracture, infertility, erectile dysfunction, rheumatoid arthritis, angina |
| 4 | 0.24–0.36 | Below-knee amputation, deafness |
| 5 | 0.36–0.50 | Rectovaginal fistula, major mental retardation, Down syndrome |
| 6 | 0.50–0.70 | Major depression, blindness, paraplegia |
| 7 | 0.70–1.00 | Psychosis, dementia, migraine, quadriplegia |

ability in national burden of disease profiles very important.

## Composite Indicators

Measures of health status that combine mortality and morbidity (composite indicators) have utility in enabling comparisons within and across populations. They can estimate the quantitative health benefits from interventions and serve as tools to assist in the allocation of resources. The development of such measures entails two major processes: the measurement of life, including losses of time from premature mortality and disability; and the valuing of life, which incorporates issues of duration, age, extent of future life, productivity, dependency, and equity (Morrow & Bryant, 1995). The purpose of developing such measures and the need for refining them become clear if the following objectives are to be achieved:

- the use of such methods at the country level for evaluating the impact of diseases
- their use in the allocation of resources within the health sector
- the generation of more relevant and useful data for policy makers

Precursors of composite indicators have been in the literature for many decades and generally were developed to assist prioritization of health issues. Usually these were based on the measurement of losses of time, losses of productive time, income forgone, or other costs incurred as a result of diseases. The earlier indicators were used to estimate time loss from health outcomes and convert this to a dollar value to give an overall loss estimate in dollars. This measure was more of an economic measure than a disease-burden measure with a focus on productive time lost. Since both costs and benefits can be obtained in dollar terms, this measure can be used for cost benefit type of analysis.

The measurement of health-related quality of life has also been in the medical and clinical research literature for decades. *Health-related quality of life* refers to how well an individual

functions in daily life and the perception of well-being. Various domains of quality have been defined, such as health perception, functional status, and opportunity, and several instruments have been developed to evaluate them. There are disease-specific and general instruments, and these abound in fields dealing with chronic disabled states such as psychiatry, neurology, and counseling. These scales are often dependent on self-reported information, although some incorporate observational data as well. There has been repeated concern and work on their reliability and validity. However, these measures are not discussed further, since they do not directly relate to the development of composite indicators, have been primarily used in clinical assessments, and there are hundreds of such instruments but no accepted standard.

Six composite indicators for burden of disease assessment that are generally accepted and used are reviewed below. A summary is presented at the end of the section.

### Potential Years of Life Lost

This indicator is the simplest formulation measuring the gap between current loss of life and what could be achieved under optimal health interventions. The indicator, potential years of life lost (PYLL), is based on the notion that the death of an individual at the age of 5 represents a greater loss than the death of an individual at the age of 55. This concept is applied using a predefined potential to life that has varied in the literature from 55 to 85 years (Ghana Health Assessment Team, 1981; World Bank, 1993). This measure simply sums the years of life lost between age at actual death compared to this potential across the whole population. Thus it measures the total number of years lost through the failure of individuals to live the years they were expected to live.

Murray has developed a classification of this basic measure depending on the potential limit to life used (Table 1–2). The use of arbitrary cutoff potential yields the PYLL, while use of life expectancies converts the indicator to measures that overcome the problem of ignoring deaths above a potential limit. *Period expected years* use *local* mortality patterns as a potential, which both underestimates the potential life expectation of a community and will undergo change over time as mortality declines. *Cohort-based* data, if available, can be used in situations where the mortality rates are expected to undergo change over time. Both of these measures may have little value for intercountry comparisons since the mortality potential can vary considerably, resulting in major differences. The use of a *standard* potential is a useful alternative and has facilitated national comparisons in the *Global Burden of Disease* study (Murray & Lopez, 1996a).

Limitations of the PYLL approach include not counting deaths at or above the potential such that if 65 years (as used by the Centers for Disease Control and Prevention in the United States) is the selected potential, then deaths above 65 do not count. Moreover, if the effects of health interventions are being analyzed, then benefits in the 65+ age group will also not be counted. This potential limit will affect the total years gained from an intervention since simply using a higher defined limit will yield a greater loss. Morbidity and disability are not considered in this indicator, making it of limited use to an overall burden of disease analysis.

### Days of Life Lost

The approach of the Ghana Health Assessment Team (1981) to measure *days of healthy life lost* (DHLL) forms the foundation of new approaches. The development of a nonmonetary measure of health benefit together with a method useful for health planning was demonstrated by the team using *days of healthy life lost per1,000 population per year* as an index. The Ghana study is a landmark work in the development of composite indicators (Exhibit 1–1).

The Ghana Ministry of Health Planning Unit developed the healthy life approach specifically for use in resource allocation decisions (Morrow & Bryant, 1995). The DHLL index was based on the estimation of incidence, case fatality, case disability, average ages of onset and duration,

and the local expectation of life for more than 50 disease categories modified from the ICD used in Ghana at the time. These variables were used to estimate the days of life lost to premature mortality, temporary disability, and permanent disability from each disease. Summed over the whole population and based on rates per 1,000 gave the final values used in the results (Table 1–3). The data were based on a variety of sources, including a recent census with a one-year postcensus follow-up that provided age-, sex-, and place-specific mortality rates and an analysis of death certificates. The results were used for evaluation of the relative importance of diseases and a review of the major preventive and treatment interventions that assisted in the development of a new district-based primary health care approach for the health system (Ghana Health Assessment Team, 1981; Morrow, 1984).

Ghana life tables based on the census were used to determine the expectation of life at each age and loss from premature death from each disease. Disability, estimated for the main disease categories, was added in for each, and a composite indicator developed for complete disease assessment. The estimation of disability to the level of detail was impressive, although based on expert opinion for most diseases. Each year of life at whatever age it was lived was valued equally. Discounting and possible approaches to adding in social or economic productivity values were discussed for consideration in the future, but they were not included in the analysis. The value of sensitivity analysis and the importance of making all assumptions and data sources open and transparent were emphasized. Later these results were used to demonstrate the effects of using different values in these choices (Barnum, 1987).

Days of healthy life, though clearly far ahead of other literature at that time, had some limitations. The extent of disability, divided into temporary, permanent, and prior to death for each disease, was based largely on clinical experience supplemented by a number of special studies carried out by Ghana medical school faculty.

**Table 1–2** Formulations of "Years of Life Lost" Measures

| Symbol | Name | Formula | Range | Source of Potential | Example |
|--------|------|---------|-------|---------------------|---------|
| PYLL | potential | $\Sigma\, d_x\,(L-x)$ | L, x = 0 | arbitrary | PYLL |
| PEYLL | period expected | $\Sigma\, d_x\, e_x$ | l, x = 0 | local period life expectancy | DLL |
| CEYLL | cohort expected | $\Sigma\, d_x\, e^c_x$ | l, x = 0 | local cohort life expectancy | DALY |
| SEYLL | standard expected | $\Sigma\, d_x\, e^*_x$ | l, x = 0 | model life table | HeaLY |

*Note:* x = age; $e_x$ = period life expectancy at age x; l = last age to which people survive; $d_x$ = number of deaths at age x; L = selected potential; c = cohort = based expectation of life; $e^*$ = expectation based on some model/ideal standard; PYLL = potential years of life lost; PEYLL = period expected years of life lost; DLL = days of life lost; CEYLL = cohort expected years of life lost; SEYLL = standard expected years of life lost; DALY = disability-adjusted life years; HeaLY = healthy life years.

The ability to measure and evaluate such disability would be great progress, but it was not present at that time in Ghana and is not routinely available for most diseases in low- and middle-income regions. The method of assessing disability severity by community and expert-based consensus demonstrates one way in which this can be done as a participatory process. The use of nonexperts was clearly useful, especially in cases such as infertility, where the physical dysfunction may not define the eventual social disability. The variability of the data used for different diseases was accepted and sensitivity analysis presented to demonstrate the effect of differing assumptions. Some of the estimates used had high variability, but the objective of using them was clear and the level of precision required dependent on the decision-making process. The participatory process undertaken and the political support to conduct the exercise were essential for its success.

### Quality-Adjusted Life Year

The *quality-adjusted life year* (QALY) indicator has been used in industrialized countries to assist health care decision making, particularly for assessing individual preference for different nonfatal health outcomes that might result from a choice of specific interventions. The QALY indicator was introduced in 1976 under the guid-

ing principle of selecting between alternative health interventions based on how an "informed individual" would choose (Zeckhauser & Shephard, 1976). The attempt was to reduce outputs from different interventions to a comparable, single unit for ease of decision making.

It is a measure that relies on weighting the different range of possible health states and the duration of time spent in each state to compute their equivalency with healthy life. Assigning weights is a subjective exercise incorporating the opinions of individuals and the community. The following attributes are common to most forms of QALYs:

- is used as a measure in cost-effectiveness
- uses discounting, usually 3 to 5% per annum
- defines health states between perfect health and death and measures preference weights for each state; *death is 0 and perfect health is 1*
- is used to explore choice between alternative health states
- is based primarily on an individual perspective

As such the QALY was not originally developed as an indicator of disease burden in a population but rather as a differentiating indicator for individual choices. It was used for as-

**Table 1–3** Healthy Days of Life: The Ghana Health Assessment Team Approach

| Symbol | Description | Units |
|--------|-------------|-------|
| Ao | average ages of onset and death | years |
| E(Ao) | expectation of life at age of onset from Ghana life table, 1968 | years |
| C | case fatality rate | % |
| Dod | severity of disablement in those who die of the disease; 0 = none, 100 = death | % |
| Q | proportion of diseased who do not die but are permanently disabled | % |
| D | extent of disablement in those permanently disabled from disease | % |
| t | average duration of temporary disablement in those who neither die nor are permanently disabled by disease * extent of disablement in those temporarily disabled | days * % |
| L1 | $(C/100) * [E(Ao) - (Ad - Ao)] * 365.25$ | days of life lost from premature deaths |
| L2 | $(C/100) * (Ad - Ao) * (Dod/100) * 365.25$ | days of life lost from disability before death |
| L3 | $(Q/100) * E(Ao) * (D/100) * 365.25$ | days of life lost from chronic disability |
| L4 | $[(100 - C - Q) / 100] * +$ | days of life lost from acute disability |
| L | L1 + L2 + L3 + L4 | average days of life lost from disease by each person |
| I | annual incidence of disease | /1,000 population/year |
| R | L * I | days of life lost by community attributable to disease |

*Note:* * = multiply.

sessment of individual preferences for different health outcomes from alternative interventions (Morrow & Bryant, 1995). But the idea has generated many alternative formulations and methods for assessment and has been put to a variety of purposes.

There is a voluminous literature on the various alternative methods to generate QALYs and their use in health care (Kaplan, 1990; Nord, 1993). A central notion behind the QALY was the realization that a year of life spent in one health state may be preferred over a year spent in another. Measures that focus on quantity of life *exclusively* fail to reflect these types of value choices. Thus comparing time spent in a health state with the value given to that state forms the basis of comparing outcomes from treatment options, for example. This choice and perceived quality of life is then captured in the measure and used to determine choices in health care. The community needs to be asked about the relative value of such preferences with an appropriate instrument, scale of measurement, and process (Nord, 1993).

QALYs have been developed under various methods, one of them being maximizing utility based on utilitarian theories for individual choices and has been extensively discussed in the literature. Another version of QALYs is based on the measurement of benefits from interventions on a common scale, which stems from combining 8 degrees of disability and 4 levels of distress to categorize patients in one of 29 possible health states. Each one of these was valued, compared to others, and QALYs were derived by summing the time and value product for the progress of an individual through these states as treatment is given. The nature of this construct easily allows the use of QALYs for individual decision making with potential for application in policy decisions.

QALYs have been used to help in the allocation of resources between alternative health interventions under the rubric of cost-utility analysis (Torrence, 1986; Kaplan, 1990; Nord, 1992). *Cost-utility analysis* has been defined as a spe-

cial form of cost-effectiveness analysis with a common unit of measure, the QALY, for gains by alternative health interventions (Torrence, 1986). Interventions can be ranked in terms of *cost per QALY* and money allocated to those that have the lowest result. Torrence indicates that such an approach is also more compatible and acceptable to health policy makers, while explicitly incorporating values for different health states (Exhibit 1–3).

Use of QALYs involves the aggregation of information over all individuals and expands the sum of individual choices to become the collective choice. This leads to the *aggregation problem*, which may be illustrated with the help of an example. Suppose there are two interventions, C and D, where C generates an extra 3 QALYs per person treated, while D generates an extra 1 QALY per person treated. If C costs twice as much as D per treatment, the cost per QALY calculation clearly favors C at the single person level. At the aggregate level, however, the lower cost of D allows twice as many persons to be treated and increases the probability of treatment. Overall, the majority of the population may have a higher probability of some, although lower, benefit with D and thus this option may be selected at the population level. This limitation of QALYs stems from its individual oriented perspective and is not found in other composite indicators that have been designed for application at the population level (see DALYs or HeaLYs, below).

Decisions based on QALYs may neglect factors considered important for policy making but not measured by the individual level scale. This includes the impact of an afflicted person on family members, the positive or negative consequences, and change in quality of life of other people. Another limitation is that the distribution of QALYs gained by interventions is not part of the measurement. The aggregate benefit determines the decision to implement an intervention, while the distributive element of that benefit does not play a role. This criticism is common to other measures of disease burden as well.

**Exhibit 1–3** Oregon: Application of the Quality Adjusted Life Year

The best known application of the QALY method occurred in the state of Oregon. In 1988 Oregon faced a budgetary shortfall for its Medicaid program, and coverage for organ transplants was denied. This began a series of "experiments" in which the decision-making process was analyzed using QALYs for the distribution of treatment options among people. The Oregon Plan used the QALY approach to develop 709 condition-treatment pairs, in the attempt to rank treatments according to the QALY per dollar to be gained (Morrow & Bryant, 1995).

The end result was a list that ranked dental diseases and their treatment higher than some life-saving procedures. Such inconsistencies together with objections raised by groups advocating for the disabled gave rise to several major revisions of the rankings.

The attempt in Oregon suffered from several technical and political problems reviewed elsewhere (Nord 1993). The lack of success in developing a satisfactory list of services based on the QALY has been ascribed to the unjustified use of a quality of well-being scale. This caused the ranking of many simple conditions and their treatment much lower than the public desired. Although unsuccessful in Oregon, such a method may have the potential to be converted to a population-based approach.

### Health Expectancies

Health expectancy indices combine the mortality experience of a population with the disability and handicap experience. Mortality is captured by using a life table method, while the disability component is expressed by additions of prevalence of various disabilities within the life table method (Sullivan, 1971). This indicator allows an assessment of the proportion of life spent in disabled states such as the expectation of life at birth of disability. When compared to the total expectation of life, this translates to an appreciation of the magnitude of the total disability burden in a population. Comparison of the various methods and specific indicators is available in the literature (Robine, 1994).

For example, a population may have a life expectancy at birth of $x$ years for males, and a disability-free life expectancy of $y$ years (less than $x$). This means that $x-y$ gives the *disabled life expectancy* at birth or the average number of years expected with disability at birth; $x-y/x$ would then give the proportion of total expected life lived with disability (or $1-[x-y/x]$ as proportion disability-free). This method assumes that disability prevalence rates and mortality rates remain relatively constant over the time consideration. These disability-free life expectancies can be distributed by age or sex and provide estimates for targeting a particular group to investigate the causes of disability.

Health expectancies focus on measures of life expectation, which themselves are derived from period or cohort data. They measure the gap between current and ideal levels, which is the basis for some of the other indicators considered in this section. This means that this measure uses current estimates of disability prevalence rates as applied to current mortality (in life tables) to judge the health status of the population. Health expectancies are uniquely disability focused, but there is no unified severity scale for application such that the extent of the handicap can be further rated from mild to severe, although the difference between impairment and handicap is clear. Similarly, they have been criticized as lacking discriminatory powers between disability states and do not take the transition between states and preferences for such movement into account, although these issues have since been integrated into some versions of this measure (Robine, 1994).

As originally designed, this measure does not relate to specific diseases but rather to the type and nature of the outcome or disability. The lack of correlation between a condition or disease entity and the measure makes it less valuable for resource allocation. Use of health expectancies in cost-effectiveness calculations is in the early stages as well.

### Disability-Adjusted Life Year

The *disability-adjusted life year* (DALY) was developed to enable condition and country-based comparisons of disease burden and facilitate health care decision making. It first appeared in the World Development Report of 1993 (World Bank, 1993) and set the stage for discussion and exploration into composite measures. Since then a number of comprehensive publications about DALYs have appeared and more are expected under the results of the *Global Burden of Disease* study (Murray & Lopez, 1994, 1996a; Murray & Lopez, 1999). Although the volume of literature has increased, the number of pieces with contribution to the methods used in DALYs have been few (Anand & Ranaan-Eliya, 1996; Hyder et al., 1998). Frequent reference to this measure will be found throughout this chapter and an introduction is provided here.

The DALY is a composite indicator of disease burden that measures the impact of both mortality and morbidity on populations. The loss of life from premature deaths is assessed by evaluating all deaths in a year and using them to estimate *years of life lost* (YLL) for each disease category. Life lost from disability is estimated using *years of life lived with disability* (YLD) based on the incidence of diseases and disability information.* The combination of YLLs and YLDs gives DALYs and, for example, these have been estimated for both sexes, five age groups, and eight regions of the world in the *Global Burden of Disease* study for the year 1990 (Murray & Lopez, 1996a).

---

*For formulas or other details see Chapter 1 of Murray & Lopez, 1996a.

The DALY calculation uses the age distribution of deaths by cause for a year to estimate standard expected years of life for each disease (see PYLL above). The loss of life is obtained by comparison with a model life table based on very low levels of mortality *reflecting high life expectation at birth of more than 80 years* (Coale & Guo, 1989). This loss of life from premature mortality depends upon accurate recording of deaths in any year and reflects current mortality experience. Thus the starting premise of this approach is a good death registration and cause of death recording system in a country.

For disability, the DALY method uses estimates of incidence, duration, and severity to calculate the time lived with disability across age groups. This information is based on the expectation of a proportion of cases in most conditions experiencing some form of disability over time. The onset of this disability, an estimate of severity at each stage, and the period of time spent in each stage are estimated to generate YLDs. A description of the severity scale used in the DALYs has been given above in the section on measurement of disability (see Table 1–1).

Once the years of life lost to mortality and morbidity have been estimated, they are discounted at 3% per annum. This social time preference has been used for most estimates, while at the same time DALY results discounted at 0% are now available. The DALYs are age-weighted, which means that each year of life has been given a different value according to an exponential curve (World Bank, 1993). This has caused the most concern for other health professionals and in the *Global Burden of Disease* study results now can be obtained with no age weighting (all years equally valued). It has been argued that age weighting of DALYs does not affect the final result, but this has been challenged (Anand & Ranaan-Eliya, 1996; Barendregt, Bonneux, & Van Der Maas, 1996; Barker & Green, 1996; Hyder, 1998).

The calculation for DALYs can be expressed in the form of an integral that was first published in the World Bank literature (Murray & Lopez,

1994). This single equation incorporating all technical and value choices has the advantage of multiple computations; comparative need was served well by this standardized process, but national and local priority setting under these computations have been questioned (Morrow & Bryant, 1995; Bobadilla, 1998; Hyder, 1998). The combination of social preference values with measurement of healthy life in the same equation may be useful for intercountry comparison at the global level, but the value system and weighting may change for country estimations.

DALYs have been called a "type of QALY," although there are several differences (Murray & Lopez, 1996a). DALYs can provide a measure of effectiveness of interventions, as do the QALYs, but DALYs have a population perspective. More important, DALYs assess the burden of disease by measuring the gap between current and ideal health conditions. This notion of measuring the gap is critical for a healthy life approach. In order to make mortality and morbidity comparable, standard preference weights for life expectation, discounting, and value of life lived at different ages have been applied over a vast range of conditions. Thus each condition is compared in terms of the extent of disability, with death as 1 and perfect health as 0 (in QALYs this scale is reversed). Instead of local data, global information for major population groups has been developed and in the *Global Burden of Disease* work the whole process has been standardized extensively to enable global comparisons.

In the process of the *Global Burden of Disease* study, the use of several different sources for estimates prompted the investigators to develop tools for internal consistency checks (including software). Checks for consistency between estimates of incidence, fatality, remission, and general mortality rates for diseases were used. These are based on the movement of susceptible people as they become cases and then either revert back to health by being cured or suffer from general or cause-specific mortality.

This is a further build-up of the relationship between incidence and prevalence using instantaneous rates or measures of density and may be used to evaluate data.

### Healthy Life Year

The *healthy life year* (HeaLY) is a composite measure that combines the amount of healthy life lost due to morbidity plus that attributed to premature mortality and is based on modifications from the Ghana work discussed above (Hyder, 1998). The HeaLY can be applied to population groups in order to determine the impact of a particular disease or disease group, to work out the effects of an intervention or package of interventions, or to compare areas, populations, or socioeconomic groups.

The HeaLY approach focuses on knowledge of the pathogenesis and natural history of disease (Last, 1995) as the conceptual framework for assessing morbidity and mortality and for interpreting the effects of various interventions (Figure 1–1). For the purpose of estimating healthy life lost or gained, disease has been defined in the clinical sense to designate an individual who has symptoms or signs of, literally, *dis-ease*. With some exceptions, those with infection or some biological characteristic such as AS hemoglobin are considered healthy unless they have specific identifiable symptoms or signs. Preclinical or subclinical disease is not generally counted. However, the diagnostic criteria for some conditions such as hypertension, HIV infection, or onchocerciasis (diagnosed by skin snip) include individuals without signs or symptoms. Such criteria (for example, indicators of infection, high blood pressure, or genetic markers) are appropriate when they serve as the basis for intervention programs. Interventions may also be directed at reducing identifiable risk factors such as tobacco smoking or risky sexual behavior. To the extent that risk reduction can be translated into disease reduction, the approach to measuring the benefits and costs of a risk reduction intervention program remains the same.

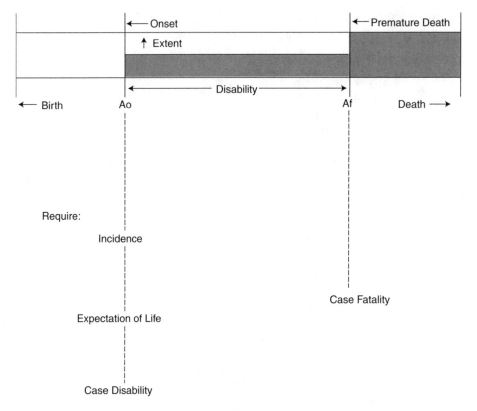

Note: Ao = average age at onset; Af = average age at death.

**Figure 1–1** Conceptual Basis of the HeaLY Method: The Disability-Death Model

The onset of disease usually will be dated from the start of symptoms or signs, as determined by the individual afflicted, a family member, and a medical practitioner or as the result of a lab test. There are several different patterns of disease evolution; Figure 1–2 illustrates healthy life lost from disability and from premature death due to typical cases of cirrhosis, polio, and multiple sclerosis in terms of onset, extent and duration of disability, and termination. The conclusion of the disease process depends on a host of factors, from correct diagnosis to appropriate treatment. The possible outcomes include clinical recovery or the complete disappearance of clinical signs and symptoms, and premature death or death primarily as a result of the disease. The latter includes death directly caused by the disease and death

that is indirectly brought upon by the disease as a result of disability. Termination of a disease state may also be marked by recovery followed by progression to another disease.

The definition of variables and formula to calculate HeaLYs are described below and summarized in Table 1–4. Each disease will have a distribution of ages at which onset or death may occur, but for most diseases the *average age* will provide a satisfactory approximation. In view of the limitations of data, this is the starting assumption for the application of the HeaLY method to countries. However, like other choices in this method, if data or sensitivity testing indicate that the average age is not satisfactory, then estimations may be based on age distributions. Similarly, if the natural history of a disease is different in different age groups, then the disease

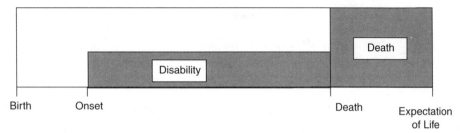

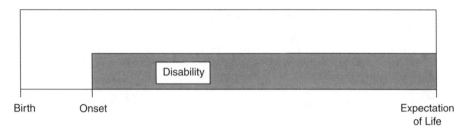

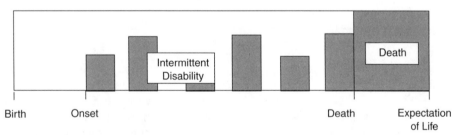

**Figure 1–2** Different Patterns of Healthy Life Lost

can be specifically classified by age (for example, neonatal tetanus as compared to adult tetanus, and childhood pneumonia as compared to adult pneumonia), in which case the diseases in the under-five age group may be considered sufficiently different with defined interventions, making them worthy of separate consideration.

In recurrent diseases or diseases with multiple episodes (for example, diarrhea), age at onset denotes the average age at first episode. For some diseases, such as malaria, which is characterized by recurrent episodes, and schistosomiasis, in which reinfection occurs at frequent intervals, it may be useful to view them as single lifetime diseases. For example, malaria in Africa may be considered for each individual as a single, lifelong disease with chronic, usually asymptomatic parasitemia but having intermittent severe clinical attacks with high mortality in late infancy and early childhood while immunity

**Table 1–4** Variables for Estimating Healthy Life Years (HeaLY)

| Sign | Explanation | Expression |
|---|---|---|
| I | incidence rate per 1,000 population per year | /1,000/year |
| Ao | average age at onset | years |
| Af | average age at death | years |
| E(Ao) | expectation of life at age of onset | years |
| E(Af) | expectation of life at age of death | years |
| CFR | case fatality ratio: proportion of those developing the disease who die from the disease | 0.00–1.00 |
| CDR | case disability ratio: proportion of those developing the disease who have disability from the disease | 0.00–1.00 |
| De | extent of disability (from none to complete disability equivalent to death) | 0.00–1.00 |
| Dt | average duration of disability for those disabled by the disease; a composite of temporary and permanent disability based on the proportion of cases in each category | years |
| HeaLY | healthy life years lost per 1,000 population per year: = I * {[CFR*{E(Ao)–[Af – Ao]}] + [CDR*De*Dt]} | HeaLYs per 1,000 per year |

is being acquired, followed by recurring, mild clinical episodes with virtually no mortality after age 10.

The expectation of life in HeaLYs (like DALYs) has been based upon normative expectations of what should be achieved under optimal circumstances. This is approximated by women in Japan demonstrating the highest global expectation of life. The expectation has been taken from female estimates of regional, low mortality Coale and Demeney model life tables (Coale & Demeney, 1983). The West model representing the most general mortality pattern, with an expectation of life at birth of 82.5 years for females (level 26), has been used for the HeaLY method (Coale & Guo, 1989).

The definition of disease (*dis-ease*) makes the value of case disability ratio 1.00 by default

since all cases are disabled (to varying degrees and duration) if they have been labeled as diseased. However, there are some diseases such as sickle cell trait and genetic traits where all cases may not be considered diseased by definition, and these need to be noted. The average duration of disability in years is important since disability can be either temporary or permanent. If the disability is temporary, then Dt is the duration of that disability until recovery (Table 1–4). If the disability is permanent and the disease does not affect life expectation, then Dt is the expectation of life at age of onset of disease [Dt = E(Ao)]. On the other hand, if the disability is permanent and the disease does reduce life expectation, then Dt is the expectation of life at age of onset reduced by the difference between ages of fatality and onset [Dt = E(Ao) – (Af –

Ao)]. For permanent disability therefore Dt = {CFR * [E(Ao) – [Af – Ao]]} + {[1 – CFR] * E(Ao)}, which marks the onset of disease as the point of reference as stated above and includes periods of disability prior to death as well.

A disability severity scale (Table 1–1) was developed largely by expert opinion and a group consensus process by the Ghana Health Assessment Team (1981). Team members in collaboration with the Ministry of Health, community members, and clinicians from the University of Ghana Medical School scored disability for specific diseases in terms of severity into broad categories of 25% each, with 0.00 for no disability to 1.00 for disability equivalent to death. For example, the scale ranks the loss of one limb as 0.25 disabled and the loss of two limbs as 0.50 disabled. These scores represent an estimate of the *average* disability suffered by typical cases of the specific disease over its course. The Ghana scale is simple, and similar types of scales may be developed in countries interested in doing burden of disease studies.

The healthy life years lost from premature death and from disability are added and expressed as the total years of life lost due to death and disability from a specific disease per 1,000 population per year. These effects are cumulated for all the new cases from the time of onset and include events that may happen many years later. These are all attributed to the year in which disease onset occurred. This is analogous to a "prospective" view of the event (disease onset) and its consequences as cases are "followed" over time.

The healthy life lost attributable to the incident cases in a given year includes the stream of life lost due to premature death and disability in future years as well as that in the current year. The health status of a population is determined by the amount of healthy life it achieves as a proportion of the total amount that the people could achieve under optimum conditions. A cohort of 1,000 newborns with an expectation of life of 82.5 years has the potential of 82,500 years of healthy life. In a steady state, a random sample of 1,000 from such a population has the po-

tential of 41,250 years of healthy life (Morrow & Bryant, 1995; Hyder, 1998). Each year this population would experience events leading to 1,000 years of healthy life lost attributable to mortality, with a distribution of age at death equivalent to that which leads to a life expectation of 82.5. Any disease that leads to disability or to death earlier than that set by this age-at-death distribution would increase the amount of healthy life lost beyond this *minimum*. Discounting future life or adding productivity, dependency, or age weighting would affect these denominator numbers.

HeaLYs measure the *gap* between the current situation in a country with that of an ideal or standard, as defined by the selected expectation of life. In recent work the standard used is based on the life expectation approximated in Japan. Thus if exactly the same method was used to estimate the HeaLY losses for females in Japan, they would amount to 0 per 1,000 people for loss due to mortality; only that due to disability would be counted. In other words, since the population under study is the ideal, and assuming stability of the population, constancy of mortality rates, and no disability, there would be no gap to measure. This does not mean that the population is not having a loss of healthy life but only the minimum as defined by the structure of the population and the expectation of life, as described above. Any country that is experiencing losses greater than this minimum, either as a result of excess mortality or disability, will have a gap to be measured and that is what the HeaLYs register.

### Summary

Exhibit 1–4 presents a summary of important characteristics of composite indicators reviewed above. As indicated, most of the indicators measure both mortality and morbidity as originally developed and nearly all are based on a population perspective (with the exception of the QALY). Exhibit 1–5 also summarizes these measures using a recently proposed classification system.

## Data for Composite Measures

### *Types of Data*

Data needs for estimating the burden of disease in a region or country are extensive and have been a source of concern (Anand & Ranaan-Eliya, 1996; Barker & Green, 1996; Bobadilla, 1998). Brief descriptions of the types of data required are given below and available data need to be carefully reviewed and optimally utilized.

*Demographic Data.* Population data are integral to the burden of disease estimation for both denominators and consistency checks. In a national setting, a recent census is useful for providing accurate population counts by age and sex. Particularly useful, when there is inadequate death registration, is to have a one-year postcensus follow-up on a sample of enumeration areas in order to obtain robust age, sex, and place mortality. The age-sex distribution of the population is critical and often is a major factor that determines the nature of the disease burden. A good vital registration system (defined as greater than 90% coverage) is a major asset by providing birth and death numbers. Adjustments to such types of data may have to be made depending on the quality of information available. Underreporting, age misreporting, and other bias in data may have to be addressed prior to use in burden of disease estimation.

---

Exhibit 1–4 Indicators of Disease Burden: Selected Attributes

### Attributes

1. Measures consequence of premature mortality
2. Measures consequence of disability
3. Applicable to the population level
4. Appropriate for cause specific analysis
5. May be disaggregated by age, gender, regions
6. Applicable for global, regional, national analysis

*Mortality.* Mortality data are required for any burden of disease analysis, and good estimates of death rates are useful in estimating other parameters. Age, sex, and place mortality rates greatly assist the analysis by defining the contribution of mortality as currently experienced. They may also serve as an essential framework that puts constraints on estimates from a wide variety of special studies that fill important information gaps but may be incomplete or biased in the populations covered. Reporting errors, such as underreporting of deaths and reporting of age at death, need to be carefully examined. Information has to be evaluated for deficiencies in the under-five years and older ages. For the youngest ages, the probabilities of deaths in the first year ($1q0$) and in the next four years ($4q1$) provide better estimates of the risk of death than the overall mortality rates. Methods like the Brass method for indirect estimates of mortality provide good ways to evaluate age-specific mortality data for potential errors.

Cause of death data are required for all ages, and this presents a challenge for many reasons even before the validity of such a record is questioned. Cause of death recording can be difficult to obtain, especially for deaths that do not occur in health care facilities. If available, the cause classification may not be updated, ICD-based, or based on a mixture of diseases and symptoms. The cause of death classification system may have age-related variation such that young adult deaths may be better recorded than those in the oldest ages. Such challenges are expected in low- and middle-income parts of the world and a fair assessment of other information, such as mortality surveys using postmortem interviews to determine cause of death and hospital registers, may assist in defining causes of deaths. If such data are not available, extrapolation from older data or other regions may have to be done and the assumptions noted.

*Morbidity.* Meaningful data on disability are more challenging to find and interpret and may not be readily available. Most of this information may be institution-based or restricted to one or

**Exhibit 1–5** Summary Measures of Population Health

Summary measures of population health refer to composite indicators that attempt to capture a wide array of health outcomes in a single measure. Recently, the World Health Organization has suggested a topology of such measures based on a simple survivorship curve (see below). For example, the curve in the diagram is a survivorship curve of a hypothetical population that demonstrates the proportion (y-axis) of an initial birth cohort that remains alive at any age (x-axis). The area under the curve (A+B) represents total life expectancy at birth. A part of this life is spent in full health, which is defined by area A, while a part of it is spent with some disability, as defined by area B. On the other hand, the border at the right is a survivorship function for a population that lives to the maximum potential and dies. Area C indicates the gap between the ideal survivorship and the real-life expectancy curve of the hypothetical population.

Summary measures that take into account the proportion of life lived in full health (A) and the proportion lived with disability (B) are known as *health expectancies*, such as disability-free life expectancy and health-adjusted life expectancy. Health expectancies assign lower weights to life lived in less than full health on a scale of 0 to 1, in which full health is rated 1.

Summary measures that quantify the difference between the actual health of a population and some stated norm or ideal are known as *health gaps*, such as disability-adjusted life years (DALYs) and healthy life years (HeaLYs). These account for the difference defined by area C and some proportion of the life lived with disability (area B) at a lower weight than full health. Health gaps assign weights to life lived with disability on a scale of 0 to 1, where 1 denotes complete disability equivalent to death.

In other words:

Health Expectancies = Area A + function of area B

Health Gaps = Area C + function of area B

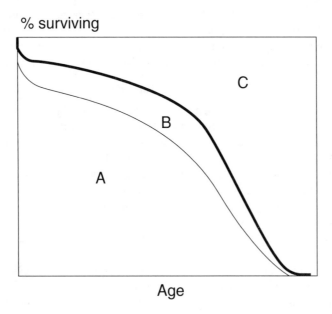

two sources, such as hospital inpatient and clinic outpatient records. Representativeness of small studies and the range and types of morbidity covered in any survey need careful evaluation. National disability surveys or regional studies conducted for the evaluation of disabled people may be available. These are useful in providing some estimates of the prevalence of serious disabilities and their age and sex spectrum. However, the linkage between disability and disease is often not available, and thus attributing one type of disability to several causes becomes difficult. For example, the attribution of proportions of blindness to diabetes, hypertension, injuries, trachoma, and cataracts can be challenging since all these conditions can lead to blindness. Cross-checking disability and disease also allows errors like double counting of disabled people to be revealed.

Information on the duration of disability may be found in specialized studies and the experience of institutions. The severity of disability will have to be rated on a scale and the types of methods used in the literature have been described earlier. This is the type of data that has to be constructed *de novo,* although the scales used in Ghana, the *Global Burden of Disease,* and the Dutch studies may be applied as a basis to make estimates. The process used to construct a severity scale, the type of people participating, and the nature of the condition all may affect the final scale.

***Risk Factors.*** A risk factor-based burden of disease analysis can be useful for assisting in policy decisions concerning approaches to interventions. Smoking, alcohol, hypertension, and malnutrition are risk factors for a variety of health outcomes and there are specific interventions that may help reduce their prevalence (see Exhibit 1–6). These risk factors pose a number of challenges; some may be both an outcome and a risk factor (hypertension), while others are difficult to measure (violence), and yet others lead to many outcomes (smoking and alcohol). Retaining the linkage becomes difficult, and the

disease portion attributable to one factor may be difficult to estimate. Relationship such as:

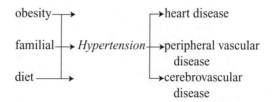

needs careful evaluation if the burden from heart disease is to be attributed to hypertension, since there are other causes of heart disease. Similarly, the reduction in heart disease by an intervention for hypertension will only affect that defined portion and no more, although it may also affect all the other diseases caused by hypertension (such as cerebrovascular diseases).

Since the ultimate aim of such methods is to assist in the allocation of resources, the link between condition and potential interventions needs to be maintained. The effectiveness of interventions will be determined on their ability to reduce the healthy life lost (or "gain" back the healthy life). Thus for the evaluation of an intervention that reduces hypertension, the HeaLY losses from hypertension are required. HeaLY losses from headache (some of which may be caused by hypertension) will not be suitable. This specificity is dependent both on the data available and the objectives of the exercise.

### Variables

The types of data described above need to be processed in the form of specific disease-based estimates. The key variables are defined in Table 1–4. One of the most important is the incidence rate of a disease expressed per 1,000 general population per year. This variable plays a central role in the natural history of disease concept, and it is only when reductions in incidence are achieved that the entire morbidity and mortality burden from a disease is prevented. Although incidence is a basic epidemiologic indicator, it is usually not found in routine data collection systems. Special studies, prospective

**Exhibit 1–6** The Burden of Disease from Risk Factors: Malnutrition

The impact of diseases on populations can be measured in various forms, including mortality, morbidity, and loss of healthy life. The same indicators can be used to assess the impact of risk factors for ill health. An evaluation of such risk factors is even more critical to preventive public health, especially if they are amenable to cost-effective interventions. Since risk factors eventually lead to the whole range of effects that they can cause, either directly or through disease processes, it is important to capture all these effects as well. Composite indicators that combine measurements of the mortality and disability impact of conditions are therefore attractive for such use.

Malnutrition represents a major threat to child health globally. This composite entity is both a disease and a risk factor. The contribution of malnutrition to child ill health and mortality has focused on either the direct impact on premature death (malnutrition as a cause of death) or direct effect on specific conditions (malnutrition as a complicating factor). Holistic assessments of malnutrition have been attempted in this decade with estimations of the impact of malnutrition as an associated cause of death for overall mortality in children (Pelletier, 1994).

The World Bank's *World Development Report 1993: Investing in Health* estimated that only 2.4%

of global *disability-adjusted life years* (DALY) could be attributed to protein-energy malnutrition. This assessment attributed the combined burden from premature mortality and disability to one cause of death, for more than 100 causes of death.

Further analysis of the same global data in the *Global Burden of Disease Study 1990* estimated the burden of risk factors (smoking, alcohol, etc.). This estimated that 16% of the total DALYs lost in the world in 1990 were due to malnutrition. These estimations were based on malnutrition as a physiological state, with weight for age parameters from national surveys as the input data, using the assumption of intermediate time lag from exposure to burden. They did not evaluate any other anthropometric measures of malnutrition and did not include any micronutrient deficiencies.

Composite measures have been used recently to further develop methods for analyzing risk factors. These methods are based on theoretical distributions of a risk factor for a population in the absence and presence of interventions. The latter scenarios are used to define distributions, which can be theoretically, feasibly, and effectively realized; this is referred to as *counterfactual* analysis. It is intended that these methods will be used for a global risk factor analysis for the year 2000, which will include an analysis for malnutrition.

---

surveys, and continuous follow-up work allow estimation of incidence for various diseases. Since prevalence is often the most common measure of frequency found in health information systems and surveys, the relationship between these variables helps in the estimation of incidence.

Age is required in various formats. Age at onset is when disease onset occurs in a population; age at fatality denotes the age at death as a result of the disease. The case fatality ratio is the proportion of those developing the disease that die from it at any time. It is expressed as a decimal between 0.00 (for nonfatal conditions)

and 1.00 (for universally lethal conditions such as AIDS).

The expectation of life at age of onset is the average number of years the individual is expected to live beyond the average age of onset of disease. Expectation of life at fatality is the average number of years the individual would have lived beyond the average age at death without the disease.

The case disability ratio is a quantitative assessment of the morbidity experienced by cases and is expressed as a decimal between 0.00 (for no case being disabled) and 1.00 (for all cases becoming disabled). The average duration of disability in years is important, and disability severity scales have been described earlier.

### Checking Data

Data used for generation of indicators need to be evaluated for validity, reliability, and consistency, using qualitative and quantitative criteria determined *a priori*. For example, large population-based studies may be given preference over smaller sample-based work if both were available and quality of data comparable. Better conclusions may be possible by cross-checking with different sources of data. Community-based studies, which may be fairly representative of the population but have limited diagnosis, may be combined with hospital-based work in which diagnosis may be valid but would be from a biased population sample. There can be other simple checks for data quality, such as the ones described below.

***Comparison of Total Numbers.*** Cross-checks need to be done to compare total numbers. It is essential to check that the number of deaths in a year in a region are the same as the sum of all deaths from all causes in the same region. Similarly, program-based data can be compared to data from other sources to ensure better estimates of causes of death. The comparison of totals allows one to work within a frame of mortality and avoids double counting of one death. However, it does not assist in the distribution of deaths within that frame.

***Relationship between Variables.*** Checks based on the epidemiologic relationship between parameters refer to the application of simple, yet vital, relationships such as:

- Prevalence (point) = incidence x average duration of disease
- Cause mortality rate = incidence x case fatality rate

These checks allow estimates from different sources to be compared for internal consistency. These relationships can also be used to derive one of the estimates in the equations when the others are known.

***Sensitivity Analysis.*** Sensitivity analysis is a useful tool to use to determine whether more precise data are required for purposes of a particular decision. A one-way sensitivity analysis (Petiti, 1994) evaluates the effect of manipulating one variable at a time on the dependent variable. The outcome is often most sensitive to one or more variables, making their precision important in the estimation. Two and higher sensitivity analyses may be carried out and are more difficult to interpret.

## Methodological Issues in Composite Indicators

### Expectation of Life

The potential to life (or end point) needed to measure years of life lost to disease can be determined arbitrarily, such as the 65 years in PYLL, or based on the expectation of life. Measures based on the latter have the choice of using local or model life tables to estimate the expectation of life. National and local life tables are based on the mortality and fertility experiences of the population. On the other hand, a model life table is based on expected mortality schedules and can be selected for a lower mortality level than the country currently experiences. This allows a comparison with a situation that may be considered worth achieving and forms the basis of national health planning.

Model life tables in common use are the United Nations model life tables and the Coale and Demeney life tables (1983). The latter have been revised (Coale & Guo, 1989) and have been used in the *Global Burden of Disease* study (Murray & Lopez, 1996a). The West model life table does not refer to any geographical entity and is considered to represent a widespread general mortality pattern. Level 26 has expanded the female life expectancy to 82.5 years, which is actually experienced by women in Japan and therefore represents a level that is achievable.

This issue of which expectation of life to use and the implications on estimates has largely been discussed in the literature with respect to

DALYs. National life tables have the advantage of bearing a real mortality schedule on the analysis, although the mortality profile of regions may change with time (Bobadilla, 1998). Model life tables, especially those with lower mortality schedules, have the advantage of defining a potential target, but they may cause overestimation of the disease burden (Anand & Ranaan-Eliya, 1996). This may have a greater effect on noncommunicable diseases than other diseases. The impact of the choice of life table in a burden of disease analysis needs to be determined by the objective of the exercise and implications for the results can be explored in each situation.

### Discounting

Individuals and groups of people view future losses and benefits a little differently than present ones. An immediate loss or benefit is viewed differently from those in the future, depending on the time of occurrence, and is recognized as a *time preference*. Using this view, economists have argued that the present value of these future costs, losses, or benefits is the appropriate measure of the events involved. Estimating this present value is known as *discounting*.

Discounting is the process by which an arithmetic stream of costs (or benefits or losses) is converted to a continuously depreciating amount. This concept has been applied in the health sector since both the benefits and losses in health often occur in the future. An intervention today may not produce immediate benefits (such as in immunization) or it may result in benefits being sustained over a long time (such as in supplementary nutrition). Using the same approach, the present value of these future benefits is less than the simple arithmetic sum of these benefits. Thus a healthy life year in the present has greater intrinsic value to an individual or community than one in the future. Preference for immediate consumption, and the inevitability and randomness of death, contribute to this choice for immediate benefits. The impact of using discounting and different discount rates at the population level needs to be explored with each study.

The rate at which society is supposed to discount has been referred to as the *social discount rate* (SDR), which is a numeric reflection of societal values about inter-temporal allocation of current resources. These rates are considered to be lower than the rates of return available in the private sector. Discounting has been justified on the grounds that as a community, people value remote events and health benefits less than more recent ones. Remote events are also less likely (lower probability) to occur, resulting in the uncertainty of benefits, and the probability of survival declines with time, meaning that there is a probability that the person will not be alive at some later point in time to enjoy future benefits when they occur.

There is no consensus regarding the choice of a discount rate in health. But it is clear that the higher the discount rate, the lower the present value of given money or benefit stream. It is important to note that the absence of a discount rate does not mean there is no discounting. Rather, it represents a choice for a 0% per annum discount rate and may be far from social consensus (Barnum, 1987). The choice for a 0% discount rate would also need justification, and it may be better to present a range of rates in any calculation.

Discounting has been opposed in health on the arguments that demonstrate the variation in personal discount rates, that rates have been extracted using tools that are only an approximation at best, and that people may be more willing to invest collectively than individually for their welfare in the future compared to the present. There are other ethical and moral criticisms to the use of discounting. The apparent simplicity of discounting is deceiving, and major philosophical issues are at stake. It has been recommended that authors should be explicit about the use of discounting and specific on the methods used and their effect on results.

### Age Weighting

Age weighting refers to the valuing of a year of life according to the age at which it is lived. The valuing of a year of life equally, irrespective of age, has been considered egalitarian (Busschbach, Hesing, & de Charro, 1993; Morrow & Bryant, 1995). On the other hand, the absence of a measure of utility has been questioned since it may not represent the real preferences of people. These arguments have led to a discussion of age-related valuing of life.

Age-related valuing has been explained by showing that individuals value their own life lived at different ages differently. These values have been reported in the literature for decades and recent studies have found them to be consistent across different aged respondents (Busschbach et al., 1993). Murray reports a body of literature indicating that studies in many countries reveal a preference to save younger lives as compared to older ones. The results were true for people of all ages (Busschbach et al., 1993) and thus seem to indicate a wider principle. Moreover, the absence of age weighting has been taken to indicate a discrimination against the young adult ages since they are thought to contribute more to society in several ways.

Economic arguments in terms of productivity have been put forward for valuing life at some ages more than others. Although there have been claims that human life cannot be expressed in economic terms, this claim often only results in *implicit* valuations. Barnum has argued for adding productivity to the valuing of human life, stating that it has been ignored in health policy, is easily quantifiable, and does not ignore the welfare of children since the whole population is dependent on adult productivity for quality and sustenance (Barnum, 1987). Such economic appraisal of human life is often based on the net transfer of resources from the "producers" to the "consumers" and the consequent interdependence of people.

Developers of this economic approach have broadened the concept to include nonmonetary production, such as contribution to social and psychological development of the society. There are more responsibilities for other people at some ages, and people are seen as more valuable to overall society at these ages. These factors

have also been used to develop age weights for composite indicators such that younger adults receive a higher value than others. It has been suggested that at the individual level, younger ages are also considered more valuable because of the potential to grow and develop personally at that age (Busschbach et al., 1993).

QALYs as defined by Torrence (1986) and HeaLYs both use an egalitarian approach of valuing an extra year of life at any age equally. Thus another year of life at age 20, 40, and 70 is valued equally. This has been suggested as the method that avoids valuing life at any age (avoiding imposition of a particular value) and yet retains that choice for local areas (Morrow & Bryant, 1995; Hyder, 1998). The original formulation of DALY uses an exponential function to capture age weights such that a year of life at age 25 is valued more than a year of life at ages 5 and 65 (Murray & Lopez, 1994). Such methods are not the only way to aggregate over populations, and other systems of valuing may be found in the literature.

### Disease Groups: Classification

Murray and Chen (1992) introduced a disease group system based on the WHO–ICD classification system. Group I comprises communicable, infectious, maternal, perinatal, and nutritional diseases and thus combines a set of causes that have been viewed separately in traditional literature. These decline at rates faster than overall mortality rates as socioeconomic conditions improve, and a relatively small share of deaths in the developed world falls in this category. Group II, with noncommunicable and chronic diseases, excludes injuries. Group III, comprising injuries and accidents, represents the most variable group and is often independent of all the other categories.

The distribution of the disease burden between these three groups is one indicator of the type of disease burden and the level of epidemiological transition in a country (Exhibit 1–2). The Group I:II ratios vary from 1:1 in the developing world to 1:2 in Latin America, 1:5 in China, and

1:17 in the developed world (Murray & Lopez, 1994). Group III comprises 5–15% of the total burden, indicative of the global presence of injuries as a cause of death and disability. It is important to distinguish between the proportion of deaths attributed to these groups as opposed to the risk of dying from these groups. For example, the proportion of deaths attributable to Group II causes increases as one moves from high- to low-mortality countries (or to an older age structure of the population). However, the risks and rates of those diseases often do not change, leading to a misconception regarding the interpretation of such effects (Murray & Chen, 1992).

**Implementing a Burden of Disease Study**

A brief description of generic steps to be taken for a national burden of disease study is given below. This will need modification (either reduction or further detail) depending on the country and availability of data (Exhibit 1–7). It is to be noted that the process of this application entails many more steps, such as participation by the country, formation of a team of officials, conduct of a cost-effectiveness exercise to improve allocative efficiency within the health sector, and improvements in the health information system. The description of these is beyond the scope of this chapter.

The steps required for a burden of disease estimation for a country include those listed below. They may be carried out simultaneously or in some sequence, depending on the specific national situation.

- Assessing the demographic information with population counts (census), births and deaths, with age and sex breakdown; geographical (urban/rural) distributions and socioeconomic status information may be useful additions
- Collecting cause of death information for all deaths in a year by age and sex, according to the WHO—International Classification of Disease system

- Defining disability by cause/disease and the developing of a severity scale using expert and community input
- Collating information by disease from all sources and assessing reliability/validity; using expert opinion when needed for defining variables for a spreadsheet
- Defining social preferences such as age weighting, discounting, valuing life, and expectation of life and deciding on their usage
- Estimating healthy life lost for each disease condition and by disease groups
- Performing a sensitivity analysis to check robustness of results and to seek critical variables
- Considering other variations, including assessment of losses by risk factors, regional/age/sex breakdowns, and future projections
- Reviewing policy implications on overall mortality and morbidity in the country, and for each cause; feeding into cost-effectiveness analysis and further research
- Including other modifications as appropriate to the country setting

These steps summarize the essentials of applying the burden of disease methods to a country. A very important consideration in this process is time. The national studies in Mexico and the state of Andhra Pradesh in India have taken upwards of three years with two to three full-time people. The conduct of such studies must be timely for use by policy makers and useful for resource allocation decisions. The precision and comprehensive nature of the study would need to be balanced by the timely need for results.

**COMPARISONS AND TRENDS IN DISEASE BURDEN**

Using data to compare and assess trends is a critical reason for the generation of information. This comparative analysis may include global, regional, and national comparisons at one point in time. In addition, comparisons over time either between countries and regions or of

**Exhibit 1–7** The Burden of Disease in Pakistan, 1990

Pakistan is a developing country in South Asia that had a population of 112 million in 1990. A study was undertaken to estimate the burden of disease in Pakistan attributable to 1990 and calculate the loss of healthy life from a spectrum of common conditions. Nearly 200 data sources were evaluated, including national surveys, population-based studies, sentinel survey systems, and disease-specific studies.

Overall, 456 discounted HeaLYs per 1,000 people were lost due to new cases of diseases in 1990, and diarrhea and pneumonia in children caused the greatest loss of healthy life. Sixty-three percent of healthy life was lost from premature mortality while 37 percent was lost due to disability. Hypertension and injuries were the leading causes of healthy life lost from disability. Nearly half the healthy life is lost in the 0–5 age group, demonstrating a great burden on the initial years in the country.

The burden of disease in Pakistan is dominated by communicable diseases. The impact of non-communicable diseases is clear on a review of the top conditions responsible for loss of healthy life from both premature mortality and disability, and this can be expected to increase. Injuries need to be recognized as a public health problem in the country. The loss of healthy life in Pakistan is comparable to the Middle Eastern Crescent (which includes Pakistan) in the *Global Burden of Disease 1990* study (Murray & Lopez, 1996a). According to these estimates, Pakistan fares better than countries in sub-Saharan Africa but worse than those in Latin America.

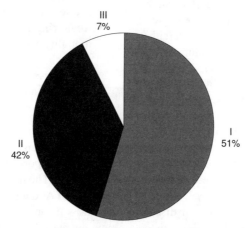

*Loss of Healthy Life in Pakistan: Top 10 Conditions for 1990*

| Premature Mortality Only | | Disability Only | |
|---|---|---|---|
| Rank | Disease | Rank | Disease |
| 1 | Diarrhea | 1 | Hypertension |
| 2 | Childhood pneumonia | 2 | Injuries |
| 3 | Tuberculosis | 3 | Eye diseases |
| 4 | Rheumatic heart disease | 4 | Malnutrition |
| 5 | Chronic liver disease | 5 | Birth diseases |
| 6 | Congenital malformations | 6 | Congenital malformations |
| 7 | Birth diseases | 7 | Dental diseases |
| 8 | Ischemic heart disease | 8 | Ischemic heart disease |
| 9 | Child septicemia | 9 | Adult female anemia |
| 10 | Other respiratory | 10 | Mental retardation |

the same region serve a useful purpose. This section of the chapter illustrates the use and application of data to assess health status in countries and compare it across time and geographical boundaries.

## Comparative Disease Burden Assessments

This section reviews a number of country-based burden of disease studies completed in the 1990s (Exhibit 1–7). Most of these were conducted under the auspices of the World Bank with national counterparts. Not only do the explicit objectives for these studies differ, but there are also implicit agendas within the design and conduct of these studies making their comparison challenging. This review presents 15 studies (Exhibit 1–8) involving 19 countries on 4 continents, including Central Asia and the newly independent states.

The multicountry review presented here will not individually list the types of factors that may compromise either the analysis or result of such studies. Lack of information, poor use of methods, absence of consistency checks, and excessive reliance on expert opinion are common limitations in these studies. It is important to state that the lack of disease data, lack of reliable data, and the lack of population-based data are the major limiting factors for all such work. The absence of data cannot be corrected unless special efforts are instituted for appropriate and valid, community-based collection of data. Such data collection needs to be scientific but also relevant to national or regional needs and decisions. The cost of collecting more data must be justified for the further development of that region and play a role in health care resource allocation decisions to gain back healthy life lost from diseases.

### Comparing Disease Burdens

*Loss of Healthy Life.* The absolute loss of healthy life varies greatly in countries with a range from 21,000 to 17 million DALYs. Absolute losses are difficult to compare, but the coun-

**Exhibit 1–8** Countries with Burden of Disease Studies

| Africa | Europe |
|---|---|
| • Eritrea[a] | • Estonia |
| • Ethiopia[a] | • Georgia |
| • Guinea | • Russia |
| • Kenya[a] | **Latin America** |
| • Mauritius | |
| • Tanzania[a] | • Chile |
| • Uganda[a] | • Colombia |
| **Asia** | • Jamaica |
| • Andhra Pradesh[c] | • Mexico |
| • Sri Lanka | • Uruguay |
| • Turkmenistan[b] | |
| • Uzbekistan[b] | |

[a] countries included in a joint "East Africa" study
[b] Central Asian republics
[c] state of Andhra Pradesh in India

tries show some similarities when the DALY rates per 1,000 population are compared (Table 1–5). Most of the Latin American nations fall in the 140–160 DALY per 1,000 range. The lower counts of the Central Asian nations are reflective more of incomplete data and mortality-restricted analysis, rather than a real absence of diseases. Guinea, Sri Lanka, and Andhra Pradesh, India, are high-burden settings as expected, whereas Mauritius is far lower, compatible with its middle-income and more industrialized status.

*Male-Female Ratio.* The sex distribution of absolute DALY losses indicates a surprisingly uniform 60:40 ratio of male:female proportions (Table 1–5). In none of the countries is the female burden higher, despite the variation in the methods and measures as noted above, and the ratio approximates equality best in Andhra Pradesh. This result is reflective of a higher overall *lifetime disease burden* on the male species. In addition, factors such as underreporting of information with respect to females or undercounting of the contribution from female causes of healthy life lost may play a role. However, this is also con-

**Table 1–5** National Comparisons of the Burden of Disease

| Country | Total (%) | | | Total Rate (/1,000) | Units Used; Study Year |
| | Male | Female | All (100%) | | |
|---|---|---|---|---|---|
| Guinea | NA | NA | 3,157,636 | 535 | YLL only; 1992 |
| Mauritius | 79,133 (60) | 53,680 (40) | 132,813 | 121 | DALY; 1993 |
| Sri Lanka | NA | NA | 21,413 | 214 | DALY; 1994 |
| Andhra Pradesh, India | 9,159,640 (52) | 8,497,874 (48) | 17,657,514 | 344 | DALY; 1991 |
| Georgia | 242,658 (60) | 164,914 (40) | 407,572 | 74 | YLL only; 1990 |
| Estonia | 85,183 (57) | 64,459 (43) | 149,642 | 94 | DALY; 1993 |
| Uzbekistan | 1,225,031 (57) | 925,265 (43) | 2,150,296 | 103 | YLL only; 1990 |
| Turkmenistan | NA | NA | 458,955 | 104 | DALY; 1993 |
| Russia | NA | NA | 2,900,000 | 19.5 | Person-years; 1993 |
| Jamaica | 168,756 (58) | 121,244 (42) | 290,000 | 116 | DALY; 1990 |
| Mexico | 7,600,000 (59) | 5,300,000 (41) | 12,800,000 | 154 | DALY; 1991 |
| Columbia | 3,713,982 (65) | 2,033,160 (35) | 5,747,142 | 161 | DALY; 1994 |
| Uruguay | 240,679 (55) | 192,707 (45) | 433,386 | 140 | DALY; 1992 |

*Note:* (/1000) = per 1,000 population per year; YLL = years of life lost; DALY = disability-adjusted life years; NA = data not available.

sistent with a higher female life expectancy in most countries of the world, as compared to the male life expectancy at birth—what has been termed the "biological female advantage."

*Age Pattern.* An examination of the age distribution of the national burdens (Table 1–6) reveals wide variation, which seems to be stratified by levels of development. Guinea, Andhra Pradesh, and Uzbekistan—all considered developing nations—have the highest proportion of their burden in the first 5 years of life, followed by a smaller peak in the productive years. Presumably, a smaller number of people in the oldest ages contribute to a lower burden in those ages. Most of the other countries have the working ages (15–44 years) reporting the highest burden, with smaller proportions in both the youngest and oldest age groups. These patterns reflect a consistently high burden in the early years in all the countries studied with an increasing shift to the working and older ages with increasing development.

*Disease Groups.* Another way to assess these results is to evaluate the distribution based on the disease groups proposed by the *Global Burden of Disease* study (World Bank, 1993; Murray & Lopez, 1994). Table 1–7 shows the percentage distribution of the burden based on Group I (communicable, infectious, maternal, and perinatal), Group II (noncommunicable, chronic), and Group III (injuries and accidents). There is great variation in the portions allocated to these groups, with Group I being allocated 12–70% of the burden. The picture clarifies when the countries are stratified by GNP per capita as a measure of development, and an important trend can be seen in Table 1–7. As income rises, the proportion of the burden attributable to Group I causes decreases, while that of Group II increases. The effect is progressive, although countries like Turkmenistan (middle income) still retain a high Group I burden. This is consistent with the notion of epidemiological transition and the change in disease profile with development of nations.

**Table 1–6** Age Distribution of Disease Burden

| Country | Disease Burden by Age Group in Years (%) | | | | |
|---|---|---|---|---|---|
| | *<5* | *5–14* | *15–44* | *45–59* | *60+* |
| Guinea | 60 | 13 | 17 | 5 | 5 |
| Mauritius | 15 | 4 | 38 | 19 | 24 |
| Andhra Pradesh | 38 | 8 | 28 | 13 | 13 |
| Georgia | 5 | 1 | 23 | 24 | 47 |
| Uzbekistan | 55 | 5 | 15 | 12 | 13 |
| Jamaica | 15 | 8 | 41 | 13 | 23 |
| Mexico | 33 | 8 | 32 | 12 | 15 |
| Colombia | 22 | 9 | 47 | 11 | 11 |
| Uruguay | 14 | 3 | 22 | 18 | 43 |

What is also interesting is that the portion attributable to Group III remains relatively stable over the income range. Intentional and unintentional injuries are still responsible for 5–20% of the disease burden in any setting. This suggests that although the nature and type of injuries may change, the relative importance of this condition does not. Injuries contribute significantly to premature death and disability in low- and middle-income countries, and their proportionate contribution increases as socioeconomic development proceeds. The primary causes within this category also tend to change with development, although causes such as road traffic crashes are ubiquitous. This is very significant for health policy formulation in low- and mid-

**Table 1–7** Distribution of Disease Burden within Countries

| Country | Disease Burden in Disease Categories (of 100%) | | |
|---|---|---|---|
| | *Group I* | *Group II* | *Group III* |
| Low-income nations (GNP per capita $635 or less)* | | | |
| Andhra Pradesh | 54 | 30 | 16 |
| Guinea | 70 | 23 | 7 |
| Lower medium-income nations (GNP per capita >$635–<$2,555) | | | |
| Colombia | 22 | 39 | 39 |
| Jamaica | 16 | 60 | 24 |
| Turkmenistan | 51 | 45 | 4 |
| Uzbekistan | 46 | 40 | 14 |
| Upper medium-income nations (>$2,555–<$7,911) | | | |
| Mauritius | 16 | 74 | 10 |
| Mexico | 32 | 48 | 20 |
| Uruguay | 12 | 73 | 15 |

*Note:* Disease classification system—Group I: communicable, infectious, maternal, and perinatal; Group II: noncommunicable and chronic; Group III: injuries and accidents.
*GNP per capita from the World Bank, 1991.

dle-income countries and in the industrialized world.

***Health Status Comparisons.*** Mortality and morbidity alone have been used for decades for such international comparisons. Child mortality under the age of five years is considered a sensitive indicator of overall health of nations, especially women and children. UNICEF publishes an annual global report including a ranking of nations based on this indicator (Table 1–8). GNP per capita is an indicator of national wealth, and the relationship between these variables does not follow an expected sequence of the country with the lowest GNP per capita having the worst indicators of health. As Table 1–8 indicates, countries that have relatively higher per capita income can have poor indicators of health service accessibility (coverage of tetanus toxoid vaccination for pregnant women) and health impact (prevalence of anemia in pregnant women). For example, Pakistan has a per capita GNP that is higher than Bhutan, but it has 13% less coverage for vaccination of pregnant women. These examples demonstrate that the relationship between health and poverty is complex and needs in-depth investigation. To improve the health of nations, absolute poverty as well as the disparities within societies are impediments to empowerment of the poor and needy, especially women and children.

Evaluation of the disease burden in low- and middle-income nations reveals the persistence of infectious, childhood, and maternal conditions. These and other conditions of childhood predominate in the low- and middle-income countries, and their impact is severe on the poor. Cost-effective interventions, such as immunization, exist for these conditions, and yet effective delivery has not been achieved. UNICEF reports that half the world's poor are children. They are paying an excessively high price for the failures of adults, while diseases and wars continue to threaten the lives of millions of children. It is estimated that more babies are being born into poverty than ever before. Poverty means that a child born in Malawi or Uganda will likely live only half as long as one born in Sweden or Singapore. It also means that one in three babies born in Niger or Sierra Leone will not live to see his or her fifth birthday.

In 1999 UNICEF reported a new *risk index* for children in countries worldwide. This proposed index was developed with the intent of measuring children's welfare in a new manner. This national index measures countries on a scale of 0 to 100 and is based on the following factors: mortality rate of children under five; percentage of children who are moderately or severely underweight; access to primary schooling; risks from armed conflict; and risks from HIV/AIDS. The developed nations—United States, Australia, New Zealand, and Japan—are in the lowest risk index; whereas the poorest nations of Angola, Sierra Leone, and Afghanistan are in the highest risk category. As a continent, Africa is in the highest risk category. This index does not consider other factors that impinge on child welfare, such as child labor, sexual exploitation, and lack of family support. However, the collation of traditional indicators of child and national health (such as child mortality) with issues of access (to primary education) and emerging threats (HIV) makes for an innovative approach to measuring the suffering linked to poverty and bringing it to the attention of the global community.

## Global Assessments of Disease Burden

Information regarding health and disease for all countries of the world can be collated to provide a picture of global health status. In addition, global health assessments may be done as a separate activity, and such data can then be disaggregated into regional information. Global assessments serve to highlight the major challenges facing the world community, and trends in such assessments indicate progress, if any, in improving the health of people worldwide. Such information is critical to the work of organizations such as WHO and UNICEF in their efforts to combat ill health and disease worldwide.

**Table 1–8** Health Status Indicators and National Income for Selected Developing Nations

| Country | Ranking by Child Mortality (<5 years) | Life Expectation (years) | Stunted Children <5 years(%) | Among Pregnant Women | | GNP per Capita (U.S. dollars) |
| --- | --- | --- | --- | --- | --- | --- |
| | | | | Coverage of Tetanus Vaccination (%) | Prevalence of Anemia (%) | |
| Niger | 1 | 48 | 40 | 19 | 41 | 200 |
| Sierra Leone | 2 | 37 | — | 11 | — | 200 |
| Angola | 3 | 47 | 53 | 53 | — | 270 |
| Afghanistan | 4 | 45 | 52 | 3 | 29 | 250 |
| Mongolia | 27 | 66 | 22 | — | 45 | 360 |
| Pakistan | 33 | 64 | — | 57 | 37 | 480 |
| Bhutan | 39 | 53 | 56 | 70 | — | 390 |
| Nicaragua | 71 | 68 | 24 | 95 | 36 | 380 |
| Peru | 72 | 68 | 26 | 57 | 53 | 2,420 |
| Guatemala | 74 | 67 | 50 | 38 | 39 | 1,470 |

This section will highlight results of a global exercise for assessment of the disease burden, recent evaluations, and projections for the future.

### The Global Burden of Disease 1990 Study

The *Global Burden of Disease 1990* study was an intensive work that presented estimates for mortality, disability, and DALYs by cause for eight regions of the world. A review of this literature has been summarized below based on the work of Murray and Lopez (1994, 1996a, 1996b), the World Bank (1993), and Mosley, Jamison, Bobadilla, and Meashem (1993). Demographic estimates of deaths in 1990 by age and sex form the basis of this work in addition to assessment of disability for evaluation of the disease burden using DALYs. The results presented were based on a variety of sources, including vital registrations systems, sample registration, special studies, surveys, and expert opinion.

***Premature Mortality.*** Globally, in 1990, ischemic heart disease, cerebrovascular disease, and respiratory infections were the top three *causes of death*, while 10 causes accounted for 52% of deaths worldwide. One death in 10 was from injuries, with road traffic accidents included in the top 10 causes of deaths. The developing world accounted for 98% of all deaths in children, 83% of deaths in persons 15–59 years, and 59% of deaths in persons 70+ years. Of all deaths in the developing world, 32% were in children. Thus an inordinate proportion of the mortality burden at the beginning of the last decade was in developing countries, even at adult and older ages.

Table 1–9 shows the differences in the 10 leading causes of deaths for 1990 between the developed and the developing world. The presence of perinatal conditions, tuberculosis, measles, and malaria in the developing world is indicative of the high impact of these conditions on premature mortality. These conditions are absent from the top 10 causes in the developed world, reflecting the success in combating these infectious and perinatal conditions. It is important to note that noncommunicable diseases such as ischemic heart disease were already prominent causes of premature death in the developing world in 1990. In addition, road traffic injuries appear on both lists, indicating the high burden from this cause of injuries that needs to be monitored.

***Disability.*** The *Global Burden of Disease 1990* study also evaluated the contribution of conditions to *disability* in the world. Leading causes of disability in 1990 worldwide are shown in Table 1–10. Neuropsychiatric conditions dominate the causes of disability represented by 4 of the top 10 conditions. However, a diverse spectrum of conditions, such as iron deficiency, congenital anomalies, and osteoarthritis, also appear on the list. This has been a unique contribution of the *Global Burden of Disease* work for placing nonfatal health outcomes in the center of international health policy in recent years. The important, and yet often ignored, impact of these conditions is obvious once estimates such as these are presented.

***Disease Burden.*** Based on the estimation of deaths and disability presented above, the global disease burden for 1990 was estimated using *disability-adjusted life years* (DALYs, section 3.4). Leading causes of the global burden of 1990 (Table 1–11) indicate the impact of those conditions affecting the developing world. The top 10 list is a mixture of the unfinished agenda of communicable and perinatal conditions, noncommunicable diseases, and road traffic injuries. This situation highlights the challenge facing the global health community as it continues to fight the infectious diseases, improving the response to chronic conditions, and preparing to meet the increasing impact of injuries, all at the same time.

The proportion of healthy life lost from premature mortality as compared to the total disease burden (from mortality and disability) can be compared between regions. The contribution of premature mortality to the disease burden in four regions of the world—sub-Sa-

**Table 1–9** Leading Causes of Deaths in Developed and Developing Regions, 1990

| *Developed Regions* | | *Developing Regions* | |
|---|---|---|---|
| *Rank* | *Cause* | *Rank* | *Cause* |
| 1 | ischemic heart disease | 1 | lower respiratory infections |
| 2 | cerebrovascular disease | 2 | ischemic heart disease |
| 3 | cancer of trachea/bronchus/lung | 3 | cerebrovascular disease |
| 4 | lower respiratory infections | 4 | diarrheal diseases |
| 5 | chronic obstructive pulmonary diseases | 5 | perinatal conditions |
| 6 | cancer of rectum and colon | 6 | tuberculosis |
| 7 | cancer of stomach | 7 | chronic obstructive pulmonary diseases |
| 8 | road traffic accidents | 8 | measles |
| 9 | self-inflicted injuries | 9 | malaria |
| 10 | diabetes mellitus | 10 | road traffic accidents |

haran Africa, Middle Eastern Crescent, India, and Pakistan—is shown in Figure 1–3. All regions depicted demonstrate that the proportion of healthy life lost attributable to premature mortality only is within the 64–75% range (this excludes the contribution of disability to the disease burden). Pakistan is on the lower side, while sub-Saharan Africa forms the higher end of the spectrum. Such analysis reflects the persisting high burden from diseases that directly causes death at ages much prior to the expected duration of life in these regions.

**Table 1–10** Leading Causes of Disability Losses Globally, 1990

| *Rank* | *Cause* |
|---|---|
| 1 | unipolar major depression |
| 2 | iron deficiency anemia |
| 3 | falls |
| 4 | alcohol use |
| 5 | chronic obstructive pulmonary diseases |
| 6 | bipolar disorders |
| 7 | congenital anomalies |
| 8 | osteoarthritis |
| 9 | schizophrenia |
| 10 | obsessive-compulsive disorders |

*Note:* Disability losses are defined by years of life lived with disability—YLDs.

***Age and Disease Distributions.*** The age distribution of healthy life losses from premature mortality (YLL) in three developing regions—Middle Eastern Crescent, sub-Saharan Africa, and Pakistan—are compared for 1990 in Figure 1–4. In all three regions 60% of the overall burden is in the 0–5 age group, while there is a decreasing trend for all age groups beyond these years. What is interesting is that losses for Africa are higher than the Middle East and Pakistan in the next two age groups of 5–14 and 15–29 years. Beyond the 30–44 age group, losses for Pakistan are highest and Africa lowest. This crossover at 30–44 is again indicative of changing disease patterns, with the influx of chronic

**Table 1–11** Leading Causes of Global Burden of Disease, 1990

| *Rank* | *Cause* |
|---|---|
| 1 | lower respiratory conditions |
| 2 | diarrheal diseases |
| 3 | perinatal conditions |
| 4 | unipolar major depression |
| 5 | ischemic heart disease |
| 6 | cerebrovascular diseases |
| 7 | tuberculosis |
| 8 | measles |
| 9 | road traffic accidents |
| 10 | congenital anomalies |

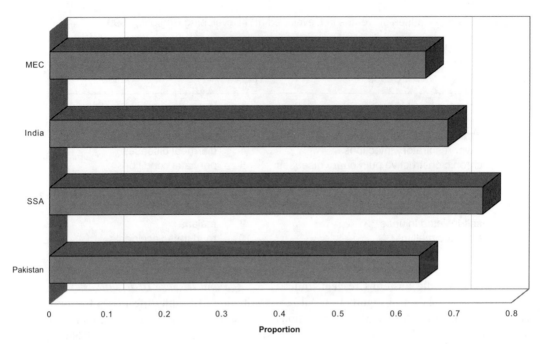

*Note:* MEC = Middle Eastern Crescent; SSA = sub-Saharan Africa.

**Figure 1–3** Proportion of Total Healthy Life Lost Attributable to Premature Mortality Only, 1990

conditions and their age effects even within the developing world.

This situation can also be seen using the disease groups first defined in the *World Development Report 1993,* which have been described above (see "Methodological Issues in Composite Indicators"). Figure 1–5 presents the distribution of the global burden in 1990 by the groups and demonstrates the nearly equal impact of infectious (Group I) and chronic diseases (Group II). Comparable figures for loss of healthy life in Pakistan, the Middle Eastern Crescent, and developing countries as a whole are presented in Figure 1–6. This indicates the high losses from Group I diseases as may have been expected in these developing regions. It is important to note that noncommunicable diseases represent a considerable portion of the disease burden in 1990. In addition, injuries are a small though significant proportion in all regions, and that may not have been expected.

The analyses above again indicate that the subregions within the developing world (such as the Middle East and Pakistan) are in a different stage of the epidemiological transition, as compared to sub-Saharan Africa (or Ghana—Exhibit 1–9). The influx of chronic diseases has added another layer of problems in the former regions, while the burden of communicable diseases has not yet been eradicated. This "double burden" is a major challenge for the health systems in these nations. In addition, the scarcity of resources in many of these countries makes the situation even more critical, and it becomes imperative to define interventions that are cost effective and able to reduce the burden represented above.

***Risk Factors.*** Ten risk factors were also evaluated in the *Global Burden of Disease* study for 1990. Table 1–12 shows the contribution of these risk factors as a proportion of the global disease burden. The attribution of the burden to these risk factors ranges from 16% for malnutrition to 0.5% for air pollution. Malnutrition as a risk factor is of critical importance in child health across the world. In this assessment, only child-

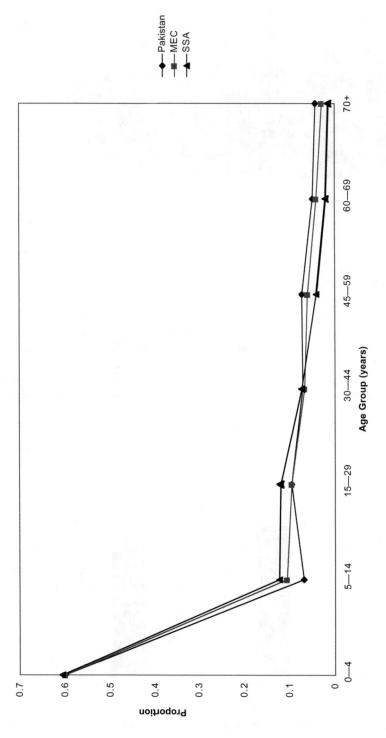

*Note:* MEC = Middle Eastern Crescent; SSA = sub-Saharan Africa.

**Figure 1-4** Age Distribution of Healthy Life Lost from Premature Mortality Only, 1990

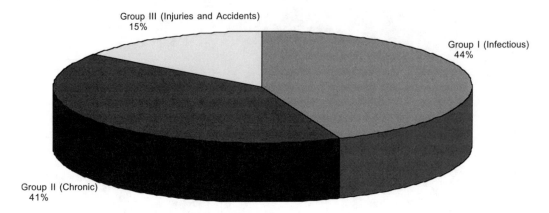

**Figure 1–5** *Global Burden of Disease 1990* by Disease Groups

hood malnutrition was considered. Tobacco and illicit drugs affect a wide range of age groups and manifest their negative health consequences over time. Unsafe sex is also pertinent to a wide age range and yet can have immediate as well as longer term health consequences. In the era of HIV/AIDS, this is a important risk factor to monitor.

This attempt was the first time such a study for risk factors had been attempted at the global level, and a greater inspection of the methodology is required for a better understanding of these estimates. For example, consideration of hypertension was based on a physiological state; air pollution was considered an exposure; and both disease and injury outcomes were counted for alcoholism. Other differences in the measure of exposure, reference distributions, and time lag between exposure and burden require that such results need to be carefully studied and im-

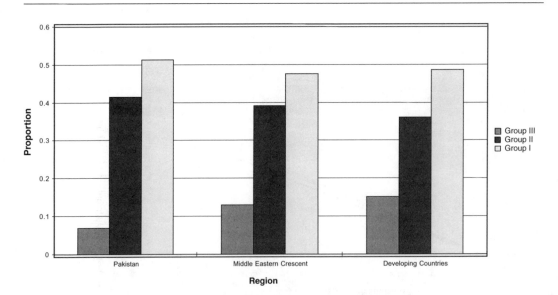

**Figure 1–6** Proportion of Disease Burden by Disease Groups in Selected Regions, 1990

**Exhibit 1–9** The Historical Burden of Disease in Ghana

The application of burden of disease methods to a secondary data set from Ghana is demonstrated in this case study. Ghana, a West African nation, was the site of the first extensive effort at constructing a composite indicator with the work of the Ghana Health Assessment Team (1981). The data for this case study have been taken from the comprehensive information gathered at that time and reflect the health status of the population as it was in 1976–1981 with the health system in operation. It was estimated that health services of a modern, Western nature were available and made use of by about 30% of the population overall.

With the expectation of life and duration of disability discounted (3% per annum), the burden of disease in Ghana for 1981 was 595 HeaLYs per 1,000. Malaria and measles caused the greatest loss of healthy life. The World Bank (1993) introduced disease groups: Group I—communicable, infectious, maternal, and perinatal diseases; Group II—chronic and noncommunicable; and Group III—accidents and injuries. Regrouping the Ghana data revealed discounted HeaLY losses per 1,000 per year of 417 for Group I, 148 for Group II, and 30 for Group III. Comparable numbers for DALYs from the *Global Burden of Disease 1990* study for sub-Saharan Africa are 409, 111, and 54 per 1,000 population respectively. The distribution of disease burden did not change in that part of the world during the 1980s.

Infectious diseases dominated the loss of healthy life in Ghana with 70% of the burden due to Group I causes. The presence of a small but significant burden of Group II conditions is indicative of the impact of chronic disorders, even in 1981. The place of injuries as the seventh leading cause of HeaLY loss in Ghana and comprising 5% of the total burden is about half that of SSA—a consequence of less violence and war. The significance of intentional and unintentional injuries and their impact on health and health care is clearly demonstrated by the use of composite measures.

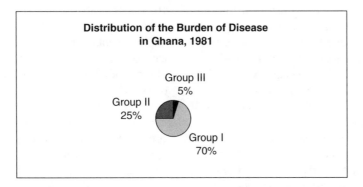

Distribution of the Burden of Disease
in Ghana, 1981

Group III 5%
Group II 25%
Group I 70%

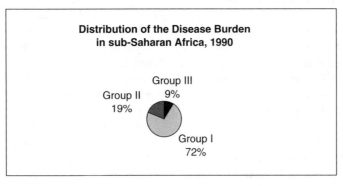

Distribution of the Disease Burden
in sub-Saharan Africa, 1990

Group III 9%
Group II 19%
Group I 72%

**Table 1–12** Global Burden of Disease from Risk Factors, 1990

| Risk Factor | Percentage Total DALYs* |
|---|---|
| Malnutrition | 15.9 |
| Poor water supply sanitation | 6.8 |
| Personal and domestic | |
|    hygiene | 3.5 |
|    Unsafe sex | 2.6 |
|    Tobacco | 3.5 |
|    Alcohol | 2.7 |
|    Occupation | 1.4 |
|    Hypertension | 1.0 |
|    Physical inactivity | 0.6 |
|    Illicit drugs | 0.5 |

*Percentage of total global 1.3 billion DALYs in 1990.

**Table 1–13** Leading Causes of Global Mortality, 1998

| Rank | Condition |
|---|---|
| 1 | ischemic heart disease |
| 2 | cerebrovascular disease |
| 3 | acute lower respiratory infection |
| 4 | HIV/AIDS |
| 5 | chronic obstructive pulmonary disease |
| 6 | diarrheal disease |
| 7 | perinatal condition |
| 8 | tuberculosis |
| 9 | cancer of trachea/bronchus/lung |
| 10 | road traffic accidents |

proved. The assessment of the burden of disease from risk factors is the subject of current global explorations led by WHO.

***The Current Global Burden of Disease: 1998.*** The global burden as assessed for 1990 set the precedent for a regular monitoring of the mortality and morbidity impact of diseases on the world. This process has now been adopted by WHO, and annual updates are expected. The latest results available at the time of writing are for 1998 and reflect the current status of ill health in the world.

Table 1–13 shows the leading causes of global deaths in 1998. A comparison with 1990 (Table 1–10) reveals that the top two conditions and a few others remain the same. However, HIV/AIDS has moved up in ranking over the past 8 years, indicating the growing mortality impact of this disease in the 1990s. During the same time, measles disappeared from the top 10 list reflecting global efforts to curb this childhood condition. Road traffic crashes remain in the top 10 as a major contributor to the global disease burden from injuries.

According to the World Health Organization, 1.38 billion DALYs were lost globally due to premature mortality and disability in 1998. More than half of these may be attributed to losses in males, although the percentages are close in both genders (Figure 1–7). The leading causes of the global burden in 1998 are shown in Table 1–14. The list is similar to the 1990 list (Table 1–11) with the notable addition of HIV/AIDS and malaria, and the disappearance of tuberculosis and congenital malformations from the top 10. The persistent, and in some cases resurgent, impact of malaria, together with methodological improvements in measuring the malaria burden, have contributed to making this age-old scourge of man a current global challenge. Unipolar depression remains important (see Chapter 7).

WHO has categorized member states by income levels into high-, middle-, and low-income nations. Most developing countries fall in the latter two categories, whereas industrialized nations comprise the first category. The population of the world in 1998 was slightly more than 5 billion people, with 85% in the low- and middle-income nations (Figure 1–8). As may be expected, more than 90% of the global burden can be located in the low- and middle-income nations. This indicates the great double challenge faced by the majority of the people in the world—they are poor and they are unhealthy. This relationship between ill health and poverty has long been recognized and has been the object of much research and inquiry. This is a complex, multi-causal, and interdependent relationship that involves a spectrum of factors

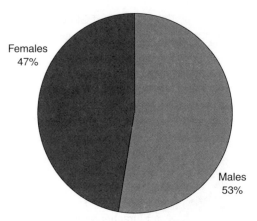

Note: 100% = 1.38 billion DALYs lost in 1998.

**Figure 1–7** Global Burden of Disease 1998 by Gender

in the health, social, educational, cultural, political, and economic sectors of life.

### Future Projections

Future projections of data have been attempted with the intent of providing some basis for health planning. This is a challenging task that requires further data manipulations and the use of assumptions. These assumptions must predict the changes of disease prevalence and incidence over time, effect of interventions, and other factors. As a result, all projections are estimates with substantial variations and highly dependent on the data used to derive them.

The *Global Burden of Disease* study for 1990 also attempted to project the global burden in the future to the year 2020. These were based on projected changes in the expectation of life, age structure of the global community, disease profiles based on current states, and other relevant parameters (Murray & Lopez, 1996a). In addition, the projections were guided by forecasts for income per capita, human capital, and smoking intensity. The interested reader may look up the relevant references for details.

The results of this exercise reveal the leading causes of projected global burden of disease for 2020, as shown in Table 1–15. The domination of chronic diseases is obvious, although respi-

ratory conditions still appear to be important. Injuries from road traffic crashes are projected to become the third leading cause of the global disease burden. It is interesting to note that the mortality and disability consequences of wars make it the eighth leading cause of projected global disease burden. In addition, the lower ranking of HIV in the list compared to the 1998 profile (Table 1–14) is reflecting the assumptions that interventions for this condition will succeed in reducing the burden in the intervening decades. This may or may not hold true, and other assumptions may be used to project a different scenario for the future.

The growing importance of noncommunicable diseases may be a global phenomenon, and their impact on low- and middle-income countries and regions needs to be assessed. Table 1–15 also shows the projected leading causes of the disease burden in the developing world only for 2020. Here again, four of the top five conditions are chronic diseases and injuries. However, unlike the list for the world, the persistent burden of respiratory infections and diarrheal diseases is evident. The situation for the future in the low- and middle-income world is likely to be one where the "triple burden" of persistent communicable diseases, prevalent noncommunicable conditions, and increasing injuries will present a serious challenge to the

**Table 1–14** Leading Causes of Global Burden of Disease (DALYs), 1998

| Rank | Condition |
| --- | --- |
| 1 | acute lower respiratory infection |
| 2 | perinatal conditions |
| 3 | diarrheal diseases |
| 4 | HIV/AIDS |
| 5 | unipolar major depression |
| 6 | ischemic heart disease |
| 7 | cerebrovascular disease |
| 8 | malaria |
| 9 | road traffic accidents |
| 10 | measles |

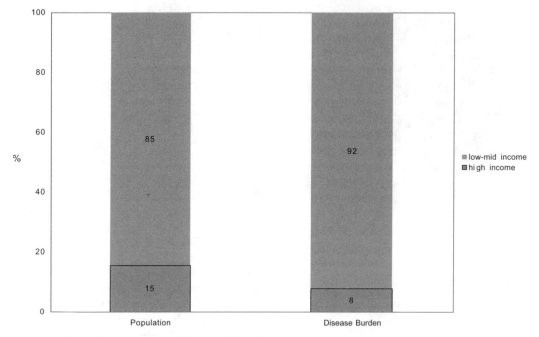

*Note:* Total Global Disease Burden for 1998 = 1.38 billion DALYs.

**Figure 1–8** Global Burden of Disease, 1998, by Income Level of Countries

global community. An appropriate current response in global health becomes that much more important in view of these future projections.

## CONCLUSION

The health of populations is of fundamental importance to international public health. One of the foremost steps in the pursuit of health improvement is the measurement of ill health. This process of measurement defines the magnitude of problems, causal factors, potential solutions, and impact of interventions. Measuring the impact of diseases on populations in terms of mortality, morbidity, and other composite indicators is an essential prerequisite to determining effective ways to reduce the burden of illness.

The burden of disease can be measured by using indicators of mortality alone, such as infant mortality rates. Nonfatal health outcomes of disease must also be considered, and indicators such as days away from work have been used. The combination of both premature mortality and disability impact of diseases will allow for an overall assessment. Such composite indicators use time to measure the loss of healthy life in populations. There are many versions of such indicators, and they need to be understood prior to their use for decision making in health.

Trends in disease burden offer important clues to the success of health programs and for the development of new interventions. At the same time, they reflect other nonhealth factors that are important to the production or maintenance of health in populations. Similarly, inter-country and inter-regional comparisons allow for the measurement of progress between nations and highlight inequalities in health status and opportunities. Such trends can be studied with respect to social, economic, educational, and other factors as well.

Health systems across the world are being affected by changes in disease profiles and population dynamics. These systems must develop the

**Table 1–15** Projected Leading Causes of Disease Burden in 2020

| | *Global* | | *Developing Regions Only* |
|---|---|---|---|
| *Rank* | *Cause* | *Rank* | *Cause* |
| 1 | ischemic heart disease | 1 | unipolar major depression |
| 2 | unipolar major depression | 2 | road traffic injuries |
| 3 | road traffic accidents | 3 | ischemic heart disease |
| 4 | cerebrovascular disease | 4 | chronic obstructive pulmonary diseases |
| 5 | chronic pulmonary obstructive diseases | 5 | cerebrovascular disease |
| 6 | lower respiratory infections | 6 | tuberculosis |
| 7 | tuberculosis | 7 | lower respiratory infections |
| 8 | war | 8 | war |
| 9 | diarrheal diseases | 9 | diarrheal diseases |
| 10 | HIV | 10 | HIV |

capacity to respond to such changes effectively, within the resources of each nation. The decisions taken in this respect must be based on evidence about the patterns of diseases and their impact. Collection of good data, which is both useful for decision making and timely, is a challenge for the global health community. It remains an imperative, however, if there is to be further and equitable global health development.

## DISCUSSION QUESTIONS

1. What is the primary purpose of a health system in a country? How can data help achieve this purpose?
2. What are the essential elements of health information and what types of data are required to assess ill health?
3. What are the relative strengths and weaknesses of composite indicators compared to more traditional indicators of disease burden?
4. In your country, what would be the most appropriate set of indicators to assess the impact of diseases on the population? Why?

**REFERENCES**

Anand, S., & Ranaan-Eliya. (1996). *Disability adjusted life years: A critical review.* Working Paper No. 95–06. Harvard Center for Population and Development Studies.

Barendregt, J.J., Bonneux, L., & Van Der Maas, P.J. (1996). DALYs: The age weights on balance. *Bulletin of the World Health Organization, 74,* 439–443.

Barker, C., & Green, A. (1996). Opening the debate on DALYs. *Health Policy and Planning, 11*(2), 179–183.

Barnum, H. (1987). Evaluating healthy days of life gained from health projects. *Social Science and Medicine, 24,* 833–841.

Bobadilla, J.L. (1998). *Searching for essential health services in low and middle income countries.* Washington, DC: Inter-American Development Bank.

Busschbach, J.J.V., Hesing, D.J., & de Charro, F.T. (1993). The utility of health at different stages of life: A qualitative approach. *Social Science and Medicine, 37*(2), 153–158.

Coale, A.J., & Demeney, P. (1983). *Regional model life tables and stable populations*. New York: Academic Press.

Coale, A.J., & Guo, G. (1989). Revised regional model life tables at a very low levels of mortality. *Population Index, 55*, 613–643.

Evans, J.R., Hall, K.L., & Warford, J. (1981). Health care in the developing world: Problems of scarcity and choice. *New England Journal of Medicine, 305*, 1117–1127.

Feachem, R.G.A., & Kjellstrom, T. (Eds.). (1992). *The health of adults in the developing world*. New York: Oxford University Press.

Ghana Health Assessment Team. (1981). A quantitative method for assessing the health impact of different diseases in less developed countries. *International Journal of Epidemiology, 10*, 73–80.

Hyder, A.A. (1998). *Measuring the burden of disease: Introducing healthy life years*. Doctoral dissertation, Johns Hopkins University, Baltimore, MD.

Hyder, A.A., Rotllant, G., & Morrow, R.H. (1998). Measuring the burden of disease: Healthy life years. *American Journal of Public Health, 88*, 196–202.

Kaplan, R.M. (1990). The General Health Policy Model: An integrated approach. In B. Spilker (Ed.), *Quality of life assessment in clinical trials*. New York: Raven Press.

Last, J.M. (Ed.). (1995). *A dictionary of epidemiology* (3rd ed.). New York: Oxford University Press.

Morrow, R.H. (1984). The application of a quantitative approach to the assessment of the relative importance of vector and soil transmitted diseases in Ghana. *Social Science and Medicine, 19*, 1039–1049.

Morrow, R.H., & Bryant, J.H. (1995). Health policy approaches to measuring and valuing human life: Conceptual and ethical issues. *American Journal of Public Health, 85*, 1356–1360.

Mosley, H.W., Jamison, D.T., Bobadilla, J.L., & Meashem, A. (Eds.). (1993). *Disease control priorities in the developing world*. New York: Oxford University Press.

Murray, C.J.L., & Chen, L.C. (1992). Understanding morbidity change. *Population and Development Review, 18*(3), 481–503.

Murray, C.J.L., & Lopez, A.D. (1994). *Global comparative assessments in the health sector*. Geneva, Switzerland: World Health Organization.

Murray, C.J.L., & Lopez, A.D. (Eds.). (1996a). *The global burden of disease 1990*. Geneva, Switzerland: World Health Organization.

Murray, C.J.L., & Lopez, A.D. (Eds.). (1996b). *Global health statistics 1990*. Geneva, Switzerland: World Health Organization.

Murray, C.L.J. & Lopez, A.D. (1999). On the comparable quantification of health risks: lessons from the Global Burden of Disease study. *Epidemiology, 10*, 594–605.

Nord, E. (1992). Methods for quality adjustment of life years. *Social Science and Medicine, 34*, 559–569.

Nord, E. (1993). Unjustified use of the quality of well being scale in priority setting in Oregon. *Health Policy 24*, 45–53.

Omran, A. (1971). The epidemiologic transition: A theory of the epidemiology of population change. *Milbank Memorial Fund Quarterly, 49*, 509–538.

Pelletier, D.L. (1994). The relationship between child anthropometry and mortality in developing countries: implications for policy, programs, and future research. *Journal of Nutrition, 124*, 20475–20815.

Petiti, D.B. (1994). *Meta-analysis, decision analysis and cost-effectiveness analysis: Methods for quantitative synthesis in medicine*. New York: Oxford University Press.

Preston, S.H. (1976). *Mortality patterns in national populations*. New York: Academic Press.

Robine, J.M. (1994). *Disability free life expectancy trends in France: 1981–1991: International comparisons*. In C. Mathers et al. (Eds.), *Advances in health expectancies*. Canberra, Australia: Australian Institute of Health and Welfare.

Sullivan, D.F. (1971). A single index of mortality and morbidity. *HSMHA Health Reports, 86*, 347–354.

Torrence, G.W. (1986). Measurement of health state utilities for economic appraisal: A review. *Journal of Health Economics, 5*, 1–30.

United Nations Children's Fund. (1999). *Annual report, 1999*. New York: UNICEF.

World Bank. (1993). *World development report 1993: Investing in health*. New York: Oxford University Press.

World Health Organization. (1980). *International classification of impairments, disabilities and handicaps: A manual of classification relating to the consequences of disease*. Geneva, Switzerland: Author.

Zeckhauser, R., & Shephard, D. (1976). Where now for saving lives? *Law and Contemporary Problems, 40*(b), 5–45.

# CHAPTER 2

# Culture, Behavior, and Health

*Susan C. Scrimshaw*

"If you wish to help a community improve its health, you must learn to think like the people of that community. Before asking a group of people to assume new health habits, it is wise to ascertain the existing habits, how these habits are linked to one another, what functions they perform, and what they mean to those who practice them" (Paul, 1955).

People around the world have beliefs and behaviors related to health and illness that stem from cultural forces and individual experiences and perceptions. A 16-country study of community perceptions of health, illness, and primary health care found that in all 42 communities studied, people used *both* the Western biomedical system and indigenous practices, including indigenous practitioners. Also, there were discrepancies between services the governmental agencies said existed in the community and what was really available. Due to positive experiences with alternative healing systems, and shortcomings in the Western biomedical system, people relied on both (Scrimshaw, 1992). Experience

has shown that health programs that fail to recognize and work with indigenous beliefs and practices also fail to reach their goals. Similarly, research to plan and evaluate health programs must take cultural beliefs and behaviors into account if researchers expect to understand why programs are not working, and what to do about it.

This chapter draws on the social sciences, particularly anthropology, psychology, and sociology, to examine the cultural and behavioral parameters that are essential to understanding international health efforts. It begins with some key concepts from the field of anthropology and the subfield of medical anthropology. It continues with lists and brief descriptions of types of health belief systems and types of healers around the world. Next, some key theories of health behavior and behavioral and cultural change are described and discussed. Methodological issues are then presented, followed by a case study of AIDS in Africa. The chapter concludes with a summary of how all these areas need to be considered in international health efforts.

*Acknowledgments:* I would like to thank Carolyn Cline for assistance in editing and preparing the bibliography, Pamela Ippoliti for editorial assistance, Susan Levy for providing key examples from intervention literature, and Isabel Martinez for assistance with the literature search, for helpful comments on the chapter and, in particular, for preparing the case study on AIDS. I am also grateful to Carole Chrvala for sharing notes on the various intervention theories.

## BASIC CONCEPTS FROM MEDICAL ANTHROPOLOGY

Health and illness are defined, labeled, evaluated, and acted upon in the context of culture. Culture is defined as "that complex whole which includes knowledge, belief, art, morals, law, custom, and any other capabilities acquired by man as a member of society" (Tylor, 1871). Medical anthropologists observe different cultures and their perspectives on disease and illness by looking at the biological and the ecological aspects of disease, the cultural perspectives, and the ways in which cultures approach prevention and treatment.

To understand the cultural context of health, it is essential to work with several key concepts. First, the concepts of *insider* and *outsider* perspectives are useful for examining when we are seeing things from our point of view and when we are trying to understand someone else's view of things. *Insider (emic* in anthropological terminology) shows the culture as viewed from within. It refers to the meaning that people attach to things from their cultural perspective. For example, the view that worms (ascaris) in children are normal and are caused by eating sweets is the perspective within some cultures. The *outsider* perspective (*etic* in anthropology) refers to the same thing as seen from the outside. Rather than meaning, it conveys a structural approach, or something as seen without understanding its meaning for a culture. It can also convey an outsider's meaning attached to the same phenomenon: for example, that ascaris is contracted through eggs ingested by contact with contaminated soil or foods contaminated by contact with that soil. The eggs get into the soil through fecal wastes from infected individuals. The concepts of *insider* and *outsider* perspectives allow us to look at health, illness, and prevention and treatment systems from several perspectives; to analyze the differences between these perspectives; and to develop approaches that will work within a cultural context.

To continue the example, in Guatemalan villages where these beliefs prevailed, researchers learned that mothers believed that worms were normal and were not a problem unless they became agitated. In their view, worms live in a bag or sac in the stomach and are fine while so confined. Agitated worms get out and appear in the feces or may be coughed up. Mothers also believed that worms are more likely to become agitated during the rainy season because the

thunder and lightning frightened them. From an outsider perspective, this makes sense, as sanitation is more likely to break down in the rainy season, so there is more chance of infection and more diarrheal disease, which will reveal the worms. The dilemma for the health workers was to get the mothers to accept deworming medication for their children, because most of the time worms were perceived as normal. If the health workers tried to tell the mothers that their beliefs were wrong, the mothers would reason that the health workers did not understand illness in a Guatemalan village and would reject their proposal. The compromise was to suggest that the children be dewormed just before the rainy season, in order to avoid the problem of agitated worms. It worked.[*]

The *insider-outsider* concept leads to another set of concepts. *Disease* is the outsider, usually the Western biomedical definition. It refers to an undesirable deviation from a measurable norm. Deviations in temperature, white cell count, red cell count, bone density, and many others are seen as indicators of disease. *Illness* on the other hand, means "not feeling well." Thus it is a subjective, insider view. This sets up some immediate dissonances between the two views. It is possible to have an undesirable deviation from a Western biomedical norm and to feel fine. Hypertension, early stages of cancer, HIV infection, and early stages of diabetes are all instances where people may feel well but have a disease. This means that health care providers must communicate the need for behaviors to "fix" something that people may not realize is wrong.

It is also possible for someone to feel ill and for the Western biomedical system not to identify a disease. When this occurs, there is a tendency for Western trained health care providers to say that nothing is wrong or that it is a "psychosomatic" problem. Although both of these can be the case, there are several other expla-

---

[*]I am indebted to Elena Hurtado of Guatemala for this example.

nations for this occurrence. One possibility is that Western biomedical science has not yet figured out how to measure something. Several recent examples of this include AIDS, generalized anxiety attacks, and chronic fatigue syndrome. All of these were labeled psychosomatic at one time and now have measurable deviations from a biological norm. Similarly, painful menstruation used to be labeled "subconscious rejection of femininity," but it is now associated with elevated prostaglandin levels and can be helped by a prostaglandin inhibitor.

Another possibility is something that anthropologists have called "culture bound syndromes" (Hughes, 1990), but this might be better described as "culturally defined syndromes." Culturally defined syndromes are an insider way of describing and attributing a set of symptoms. They often refer to symptoms of a mental or psychological problem, but a physiological disease may exist, posing a challenge to the health practitioner. For example, Rubel (1984) found that an illness called *susto*, or fright, in Mexico corresponded with symptoms of tuberculosis in adults. If people were told there was no such thing as *susto* and that they, in fact, had tuberculosis, they rejected the diagnosis and the treatment on the grounds that the doctors obviously knew nothing about *susto*. This was complicated by the fact that tuberculosis was viewed as serious and stigmatizing. The solution was to discuss the symptoms with people and mention that Western biomedicine has a treatment for those symptoms (Rubel et al., 1984). *Susto* may also be used to describe other sets of symptoms, for example, those of diarrheal disease in children (Scrimshaw & Hurtado, 1988).

With culturally defined syndromes, it is essential for an outsider to ask about the symptoms associated with the illness and to proceed with diagnosis and treatment on the basis of those symptoms. This is good practice in any event, because people often make a distinction between the cause of a disease or illness and its symptoms. Even if the perceived cause is inconsistent with the Western biomedical system, a disease can be diagnosed and treated based on the symptoms without challenging people's beliefs about the cause.

The term *Western biomedical system* is used throughout this chapter because a term like *modern medicine* would deny the fact that there are other medical systems, such as Chinese and Ayurvedic medicine, that have modern forms. *Indigenous medical system* is used to refer to an insider—within the cultural system. Thus the Western biomedical system is an indigenous medical system in some countries, but it still may exist side by side with other indigenous systems, even in the United States and western Europe. In most of the world, the Western biomedical system now coexists with, and often dominates, local or indigenous systems. Because of this, and because of class differences, physicians and policy makers in a country may not accept or even be aware of the extent to which indigenous systems exist and their importance. Also, many countries contain multiple cultures and languages. The cross-cultural principles discussed in this chapter may be just as important to work within a country as to work in multiple countries or cultures.

Another key concept from medical anthropology is that of *ethnocentrism*. Ethnocentric refers to seeing your own culture as "best." This is a natural tendency, because the survival and perpetuation of a culture depend on teaching children to accept it and on its members feeling that it is a good thing. In the context of cross-cultural understanding, ethnocentrism poses a barrier if people approach a culture with the attitude that it is inferior. *Cultural relativism* in anthropology refers to the idea that each culture has developed its own ways of solving the problems of how to live together; how to obtain the essentials of life, such as food and shelter; how to explain phenomena; and so on. No one way is "better" or "worse"; they are just different. This works well for classic anthropology but is a challenge when international health is considered. What if a behavior is "wrong" from an epidemiologic perspective? How does one distinguish between a "dangerous" behavior (for example, using an HIV-contaminated needle, swimming in a river with snails known to carry schistosomiasis, ingesting a powder with lead in it as part of a healing ritual) and behaviors that are merely different and therefore seem odd? For example, Bolivian peasants used very fine clay in a drink believed to be good for digestion and stomach ailments. Health workers succeeded in discouraging this practice in some communities because "eating dirt" seemed like a bad thing. The health workers then found themselves faced with increased caries and other symptoms of calcium deficiency. Upon analysis, the clay was a key source of calcium for these communities. In addition, we use clay in Western biomedicine, but we color it pink or give it a mint flavor and put it in a bottle.

Thus there is a delicate balance between being judgmental without good reason and introducing behavior change because there is real harm from existing behaviors. In general, it is best to leave harmless practices alone and focus on understanding and changing harmful behaviors. This is harder than it seems, because the concept of cultural relativism also applies to perceptions of quality of life. A culture in which people believe in reincarnation may approach death with more equanimity and may not adopt drastic procedures, which only briefly prolong life. In some cultures, loss of a body organ is viewed as impeding the ability to go to an afterlife or the next life, and such surgery may be refused. It is important in international public health for cultural outsiders to be cautious about statements about what is good for someone else.

The concept of holism is also useful in looking at health and disease cross-culturally. Holism is an approach used by anthropologists that looks at the broad context of whatever phenomenon is being studied. Holism involves staying alert for unexpected influences, because you never know what may have a bearing on the program you are trying to implement. For public health, this is crucial because there may be diverse factors influencing health and health behavior.

One classic example of this is the detective work that went into discovering the etiology of the New Guinea degenerative nerve disease, Kuru. Epidemiologists could not figure out how people contracted the disease, which appeared to have a long incubation period and to be more frequent in women and children than in men. Many hypotheses were advanced, including inheritance (genetic), infection (bacterial, parasitic), and psychosomatic.

By the early 1960s the most accepted of the prevailing hypotheses was that it was genetically transmitted. Yet this did not explain the sex differences in infection rates in adults but not in children, nor how such a lethal gene could persist. Working with Gadjusek of the National Institutes of Health (NIH), cultural anthropologists Glasse and Lindenbaum used in-depth ethnographic interviews to establish that Kuru was relatively new to that region of New Guinea, as was the practice of cannibalism. Women and children were more likely to engage in the ritual consumption of dead relatives as a way of paying tribute to them, which was culturally less acceptable for men. Also, this tissue was cooked, but women, who did the cooking, and children, who were around during cooking, were more likely to eat it when it was partially cooked and therefore still infectious. Lindenbaum and Glasse suggested the disease was transmitted by cannibalism. In order to confirm their hypothesis, Gadjusek's team inoculated chimpanzees with brain material from women who had died of Kuru and the animals developed the disease. The disease was found to be a slow virus, transmitted through the ingestion of brain tissue. Since then, the practice of cannibalism has declined and the disease has now virtually disappeared (Gadjusek, Gibbs, & Alpers, 1967: Lindenbaum, 1971).

## CULTURAL VIEWS OF HEALTH, ILLNESS, AND HEALERS

Cultures vary in their definitions of health and of illness. A condition that is endemic in a population may be seen as normal and may not be defined as illness. Ascaris in young children has already been mentioned as a perceived "normal" condition in many populations. Similarly, malaria is seen as normal in some parts of Africa, because everyone has it or has had it. In Egypt, where schistosomiasis was common and affected the blood vessels around the bladder, blood in the urine was referred to as "male menstruation" and was seen as normal. These definitions may also vary by age and by gender. In most cultures, symptoms such as fever in children are seen as more serious than in adults. Men may deny symptoms more than women in some cultures, but women may do the same in others. Often, adult denial of symptoms is due to the need to continue working.

Sociologist Talcott Parsons (1948) first discussed the concept of the *sick role*, wherein an individual must "agree" to be considered ill and to take actions (or allow others to take actions) to define the state of his or her health, discover a remedy, and do what is necessary to become well. Individuals who adopt the sick role neglect their usual duties, may indulge in dependent behaviors, and seek treatment to get well. By adopting the sick role, they are viewed as having "permission" to be exempted from usual obligations, but they are also under an obligation to try to restore health. The process of seeking to remain healthy or to restore health will be discussed later.

## Belief Systems

Exhibit 2–1 depicts types of insider cultural explanations of disease causation. It is based on the literature and is an attempt to be as comprehensive as possible for cultures around the world. It is important to note that the exhibit consists of generalizations about culture-specific health beliefs and behaviors and that generalizations cannot be assumed to apply to every individual from a given culture. We can learn about the hot/cold balance system of Latinos, Asians, and Middle Easterners, but the details of the system will vary from country to country, village to village, and individual to individual. When someone walks in the door of a clinic, you cannot know if he or she as an individual

adheres to the beliefs described for his or her culture and what shape the individual's belief system takes. This makes the task both easier and harder. It means a practitioner working with a Mexican population does not have to memorize which foods are hot and which are cold in Mexico, but the practitioner does need to know that the hot-cold belief system is important in Mexican culture.

The beliefs are classified into various categories, which are discussed below. The categories are used for diagnosis and treatment and for explaining the etiology or origin of the illness. Often, multiple categories are used. For example, emotions may be seen as causing a "hot" illness.

### Body Balances

Under body balances, the concept of "hot" and "cold" is one of the most pervasive around the world. It is particularly important in Asian, Latin American, and Mediterranean cultures. Hot and cold beliefs are part of what is referred to as "humoral medicine," which is thought to have derived from Greek, Arabic, and East Indian pre-Christian traditions (Foster, 1953; Weller, 1983; Logan, 1972). This concept of opposites (such as hot and cold, wet and dry) also may have developed independently in other cultures (Rubel & Haas, 1990). For example, in the Chinese medical tradition, hot is referred to as "yin" and cold as "yang" (Topley, 1976). In the hot and cold belief system, a healthy body is seen as in balance between the two. Illness may be brought on by violating the balance, such as washing the hair too soon after childbirth (cold may enter the body, which is still "hot" from the birth), eating hot/heavy foods at night, or breastfeeding while upset (the milk will be hot from the emotions and make the baby ill). It should be noted that hot does not always refer to temperature. Often foods such as beef and pork are classified as hot regardless of temperature, whereas fish may be seen as cold regardless of temperature. When illness has been diagnosed, the system is used to attempt to restore balance. Thus in Central America some diarrheas in chil-

Exhibit 2–1 Types of Insider Cultural Explanations of Disease Causation

- **Body Balances**
  - Temperature: Hot, cold
  - Energy
  - Blood: Loss of blood; properties of blood reflect imbalance; pollution from menstrual blood
  - Dislocation: Fallen fontanel
  - Organs: Swollen stomach; heart; uterus; liver; umbilicus; others
  - Incompatibility of horoscopes
- **Emotional**
  - Fright
  - Sorrow
  - Envy
  - Stress
- **Weather**
  - Winds
  - Change of weather
  - Seasonal disbalance
- **Vectors or Organisms**
  - Worms
  - Flies
  - Parasites
  - Germs
- **Supernatural**
  - Bewitching
  - Demons
  - Spirit possession
  - Evil eye
  - Offending god or gods
  - Soul loss
- **Food**
  - Properties: Hot, cold, heavy (rich), light
  - Spoiled foods
  - Dirty foods
  - Sweets
  - Raw foods
  - Combining the "wrong" foods (incompatible foods)
  - Mud
- **Sexual**
  - Sex with forbidden person
  - Overindulgence in sex
- **Heredity**
- **Old Age**

dren are viewed as hot, and protein-rich "hot" foods such as meats are withheld, aggravating the malnutrition that may be present and may be exacerbated by the diarrheal disease (Scrimshaw & Hurtado, 1988). There is extensive literature on the topic of hot and cold illness classifications and treatments for many of the world's cultures.

Energy balance is particularly important in Chinese medicine, where it is referred to as "chi." When the balance is disturbed, there are internal problems of homeostasis. Foods (often following the hot/cold theories) and acupuncture are among the strategies used to restore balance (Topley, 1976).

Blood beliefs include the concept that blood is irreplaceable, and loss of blood, even small amounts, is a major risk. Adams (1955) describes a nutritional research project in a Guatemalan village where this belief inhibited the researcher's ability to obtain blood samples until the phlebotomists were instructed to draw as little blood as possible. Also, villagers were told that the blood would be examined to see if it was "sick" or "well" (another belief about blood) and they would be informed and given medicines if it were sick, which in fact did occur.

Menstrual blood is regarded as dangerous, especially to men, in many cultures, and elaborate precautions are taken to avoid contamination (Buckley & Gottlieb, 1988). As with the Guatemalan example, blood may have many properties that both diagnose and explain illness. Bad blood is seen as causing scabies in south India (Beals, 1976, p. 189). Haitians have a particularly elaborate blood belief system, which includes concepts such as *mauvais sang* (literally, bad blood, which is when blood rises in the body and is dirty), *saisissement* (rapid heartbeat and cool blood, due to trauma), and *faiblesses* (too little blood). Blood may also be seen as "opposites," such as clean-unclean, sweet-normal, bitter-normal, high-normal, heavy-weak, clotted-thin, quiet-turbulent (C. Scott, personal communication, 1976). It is easy to see how these concepts could be used in a current program to prevent HIV infection in a Haitian community, because the culture already has ways of describing problems with blood.

Dislocation of body parts may occur with organs, but also with a physical aspect, such as the fontanel or "soft spot" in a baby's head where the bones have not yet come together in the first year or so to allow for growth. From the outsider perspective, a depression in this spot can be indicative of dehydration, often due to diarrheal disease, but from the insider perspective it is referred to as a cause of the disease (*caida de mollera*) in Mexico and Central America.

Many cultures associate illness with problems in specific organs. Good and Good (1981) talk about the importance of the heart for both Chinese and Iranian cultures. They discuss a case in which problems with cardiac medication were wrongly diagnosed for a Chinese woman who kept complaining about pain in her heart. In fact, she was referring to her grief over the loss of her son. The Hmong of Laos link many problems to the liver, referring to "ugly liver," "difficult liver," "broken liver," "short liver," "murmuring liver," and "rotten liver." These are said to refer to mental and emotional problems, and so are idiomatic rather than literal (O'Connor, 1995, p. 92).

Topley (1976) mentions incompatibility of horoscopes between mother and child in Chinese explanations for some children's illnesses.

### Emotional

Illnesses of emotional origin are important in many cultures. Sorrow (as in the case of the Chinese woman above), envy, fright, and stress are seen as causing illnesses. In a Bolivian village in 1965 a young girl's smallpox infection was attributed to her sorrow over the death of her father.

Envy can cause illness because people with envy could cast the "evil eye" on someone they envy, even unwittingly, or the envious person can become ill from the emotion (Reichel-Dolmatoff & Reichel-Dolmatoff, 1961). Fright, called *susto* in Latin America, has already been mentioned. In addition to the case of tuberculosis in adults discussed previously, it is a common explanation for illness in children. It is also mentioned for Chinese culture (Topley, 1976).

### Weather

Everything from the change of seasons to unusual variations within seasons (too warm, too cold, too wet, too dry) can be blamed for causing illness. Winds, such as the Santa Ana in California or the Scirocco in the North African desert, are also implicated.

### Vectors or Organisms

Vectors or organisms are blamed for illness in some cultures and represent a blend of Western biomedical and indigenous concepts. "Germs" is a catchall category, as is "parasites." Worms are seen as causing diarrhea, whereas flies are seen as causing illness and, sometimes, as carrying germs.

### Supernatural

The supernatural is another frequently viewed source of illness, especially in Africa and Asia, but certainly not confined to those regions. In fact, the evil eye is a widespread concept, where someone can deliberately or unwittingly bring on illness by looking at someone with envy, malice, or too hot a gaze. In cultures where most people have dark eyes, strangers with light eyes are seen as dangerous. In Latin America, a light-eyed person who admires a child can risk bringing evil eye to that child, but can counter it by touching the child. In other cultures, touching the child can be unlucky, so it is important to learn about local customs. Frequently, amulets and other protective devices, such as small eyes of glass, red hats, and a red string around the wrist, are worn to prevent evil eye. These objects can be viewed as an opportunity to discuss preventative health measures, because they are an indication that people are thinking about prevention.

Bewitching is deliberate malice, either done by the individual who wishes someone ill (literally) or by a practitioner at someone else's request. Bewitching can be countered by another practitioner or by specific measures taken by an individual. In some regions of Africa epidemics are blamed on "too many witches," and people disperse to get away from them, thus reducing the critical population density, which had sustained the epidemic (Alland, 1970).

Belief in soul loss is widespread throughout the world. Soul loss can be caused by things such as fright, bewitching, evil eye, and demons. It can occur in adults and children. Soul loss is serious and can lead to death. It must be treated through rituals to retrieve the soul. In Bolivia a village priest complained that his attempt to visit a sick child was thwarted when the family would not allow him to enter the house. The family later reported that an indigenous healer was performing a curing ritual at the time, and the soul was flying around the house as they were trying to persuade it to reenter the child. Opening the door to the priest would have allowed the soul to escape. The child's symptoms were those of severe malnutrition.

Spirit possession is also worldwide and is found frequently in African and Asian cultures. Writing about a village in South India, Beals (1976) mentions spirit possession in a daughter-in-law whose symptoms were refusing to work and speaking insultingly to her mother-in-law. He suggests that spirit possession is a "culturally sanctioned means of psychological release for oppressed daughters-in-law" (p. 188). Freed and Freed (1967) discuss similar cases for other parts of India. In Haiti spirit possession is seen as a mark of favor by the spirits and is sought. One of the drawbacks, however, is that the possessing spirits object to the presence of foreign objects in the body, so some women do not want to use intrauterine devices.

Demons are viewed as causing illness in Chinese culture, while offending God or gods is a problem in others (Topley, 1976). In South India epidemic diseases such as chickenpox and cholera (and, formerly, smallpox) are believed to be caused by disease goddesses. They bring the diseases to punish communities that become sinful (Beals, 1976, p. 187). The concept of punishment from God is seen in a case study from Mexico, where onchocerciasis (river blindness), which is caused by a parasite transmitted by the bite of a fly that lives near streams, is often thought to be due to sins committed either by the victim or relatives of the victim. These transgressions against God are punished by God closing the victim's eyes (Gwaltney, 1970).

### Food

Food can cause illness through its role in the hot and cold belief system, through spoiled foods, dirty foods, raw foods, and combining the wrong foods. Sweets are implicated as a cause of worms in children, and children who eat mud or dirt may get ill. Foods may also cause problems if eaten at the wrong time of day, such as "heavy" foods at night. There is an extensive literature on food beliefs and practices worldwide, which has important implications for public health practice.

### Sexual

In Ecuador in the early 1970s children's illnesses were sometime blamed on affairs between one of the child's parents and a *compadre* or *comadre*—one of the child's godparents (Scrimshaw, 1974). Such a relationship was viewed as incestuous and dangerous to the child. In India sex is sometimes viewed as weakening to the man, so overindulgence is considered a cause of weakness. To return to the concept of blood beliefs, it is thought that 30 drops of blood are needed to make one drop of semen, thus weakening a man.

### Heredity and Old Age

Heredity is sometimes blamed for illness, early death, or some types of death. Similarly, old age may be the simple explanation given for illness or death.

**Exhibit 2–2** Taxonomy of Diarrhea

| | Mother's milk | | Food | Tooth Eruption | Fallen Fontanel, Fallen Stomach | Evil Eye | Stomach Worms | Cold Enters Stomach | Dysentery |
|---|---|---|---|---|---|---|---|---|---|
| **CAUSE** | Hot: Physical activity, Hot foods, Pregnancy | Emotional: Anger, Sadness, Fright | Bad food, Excess, Does not eat on time, Quality (Hot / Cold) | | Fallen stomach; Fallen fontanel | | | From feet; From head | |
| **SYMPTOMS** (All types have watery and frequent stools) | | Very dangerous | Flatulence, feeling of fullness | Tooth eruption | Green with mucus; Sunken fontanel; vomiting; green in color | Fever | Worms | White in color | Blood in stools, "urgency"; color is red or black |
| **TREATMENT** | Not breastfeeding when hot; Mother changes diet; Breastfeeding stops | Home, drugstore, Injectionist, witch, spiritist | Home, folk curer | None | Folk curer | Folk curer | Drugstore, home, folk curer | Folk curer | Home, drugstore, health post |

## Illness in Various Forms

Exhibit 2–2 illustrates the way in which some of these beliefs are used to explain a particular illness, diarrheal disease in Central America. It is typical of the way in which an illness may be seen as having different forms, or manifestations, with different etiologies. It is also typical of the way in which several different explanations may be used for one set of symptoms.

In this case, Exhibit 2–2 and Figure 2–1, the diagram of treatments, were key in expanding the orientation of the Central American diarrheal disease program. The program had intended to focus the distribution of oral rehydration solutions (ORS) in the clinics, but the insider perception was that you usually only take a child to the clinic for the worst form of diarrhea, dysentery. Instead, the most common treatment consisted of fluids in the form of herbal teas or sodas with medicines added. Often, storekeepers and pharmacists were consulted. It made sense to provide the ORS at stores and pharmacies as well as at clinics, so that all diarrheas were more likely to be treated (Scrimshaw & Hurtado, 1988).

In a related situation, Kendall, Foote, and Martorell (1983) found that, when the government of Honduras did not include indigenous or "folk" terminology for diarrheal disease in their mass media messages regarding oral rehydration, people did not use ORS for diarrheas attributed to indigenously defined causes.

## Healers

Exhibit 2–3 lists types of healers. This list includes types ranging from indigenous to Western biomedical. Pluralistic healers are those who mix the two traditions, although some Western biomedical healers and those from other medical systems may also mix traditions in their practices.

As with the types of explanations of disease, the types of healers listed here are found in different combinations in different cultures. There is always more than one type of healer available to a community, even if members have to travel to seek care. The 16-country study of health-seeking behavior described earlier found that in *all* communities people used more than one healing tradition, and usually more than one type of healer (Scrimshaw, 1992). The process of diagnosing illness and seeking a cure has been referred to as *patterns of resort* rather than the older term *hierarchy of resort* (Scrimshaw & Hurtado, 1987). This is because people may zigzag from one practitioner to another, crossing from type to type of healer and not always starting with the simplest and cheapest, but with the one they can best afford and who they feel will be most effective, given the severity of the problem. Even middle- and upper-class individuals, who can afford Western biomedical care, may also use other types of practitioners and practices.

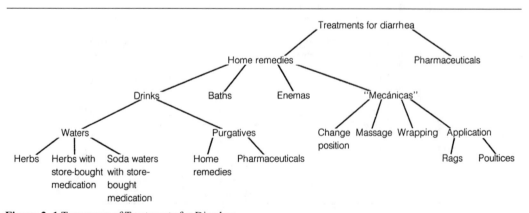

**Figure 2–1** Taxonomy of Treatments for Diarrhea

**Exhibit 2–3** Types of Healers

**Indigenous**
- Midwives
- Shamans
- Curers
- Spiritualists
- Witches
- Sorcerers
- Priests
- Diviners
- Herbalists
- Bonesetters

**Pluralistic**
- Injectionists
- Indigenous health workers
- Western trained birth attendants
- Traditional chemists/herbalists
- Storekeepers and vendors

**Western Biomedical**
- Pharmacists
- Nurse-midwives
- Nurses
- Nurse practitioners
- Physicians
- Dentists
- Other health professionals

**Other Medical Systems**
- Chinese medical system
    - practitioners
    - chemists/herbalists
    - acupuncturists
- Ayurvedic practitioners
- Taoist priests

Indigenous practitioners are usually of the culture and follow traditional practices. Today they often mix elements of Western biomedicine and other traditional systems. In many instances, they are "called" to their profession through dreams, omens, or an illness, which usually can only be cured by their agreement to become a practitioner. Most learn through apprenticeship to other healers, but some are taught by dreams. Often they will take courses in Western practices in programs such as those developed to train "barefoot doctors" or community-based health promoters. In some instances, they must conceal their role as traditional healer from those running the training programs. The incorporation of some Western biomedical knowledge and skills often enhances a practitioner's prestige in the community.

Some indigenous practitioners charge for their services, but many do not, accepting gifts instead. In a few traditions (including some Chinese), practitioners are paid as long as family members are well, but they are not paid for illness treatment. The duty of the practitioner in those cases is to keep people well, which argues for the acceptability of prevention programs in those cultures.

For the most part, indigenous practitioners do "good" or healing. Some can do both good and ill (for example, shamans, sorcerers, and witches in many cultures). A few practice only evil or negative rituals (some shamans, sorcerers, and witches). Their work must then be countered by someone who does "good" magic. The power of belief is such that if individuals believe they have been bewitched, they may need a counteractive ritual, even if the Western biomedical system detects and treats a specific disease. In Guayaquil, Ecuador, one woman believed she had been *maleada* (cursed) by a woman who was jealous of her and this was making her and her children ill. A *curandera* (curer) was brought in to do a *limpia* (ritual cleansing) of the house and family to remove the curse (Scrimshaw, 1974).

The importance of the power of belief is not confined only to bewitching. One anthropologist working with a Haitian population discovered that a Haitian burn patient made no progress until she went to a *Houngan* (voodoo priest) on the patient's behalf and had the appropriate healing ritual conducted (J. Halifax-Groff, personal communication, 1976).

In some cultures healers are seen as diagnosticians, while others do the treatment (Alland,

1970). Other healers may do both, but refer some kinds of illness to other practitioners. In Haiti both midwives and voodoo priests refer some cases to the Western biomedical system. Healers who combine healing practices or who combine the ability to do both diagnosis and treatment are viewed as more powerful than other types. Topley (1976) discusses this for Hong Kong and notes that Taoist priest healers are particularly respected. They are seen as both priest and doctor and "claim to combine the ethics of Confucianism, the hygiene and meditation of Taoism, and the prayers and self-cultivation of the Buddhist monk."

Pluralistic healers combine Western biomedical and indigenous practices. Injectionists will give an injection of antibiotics, vitamins, or other drugs purchased at pharmacies or stores. Sometimes these injections are suggested by the pharmacist or storekeeper; other times they are self-prescribed. Because antibiotics were so dramatic in curing infections when Western biomedicine was first introduced in many cultures, injections are seen as conveying greater healing than the same substance taken orally. Thus many antibiotics now available orally and vitamins are injected. In today's environment this increases the risk of contracting HIV or hepatitis.

Traditional chemists and herbalists, as well as storekeepers and vendors (many communities are too small to have a pharmacy), sell Western biomedical medications, including those that require a prescription in the United States and western Europe. While prescriptions may be "legally" required in many countries, the laws are not rigorously enforced. This is also true for pharmacies, which are very important, sometimes the most important, sources of diagnosis and treatment in many communities around the world.

Western biomedical practitioners are an important source of care, but they may also be expensive or hard to access from remote areas. As mentioned earlier, if an individual believes that an illness is due to a cause explained by the indigenous system and a Western biomedical practitioner denies that cause, the individual

may not return to that practitioner but seek help elsewhere.

As noted, there are other medical systems with long traditions, systematic ways of training practitioners, and well-established diagnostic and treatment procedures. Until recently Western biomedical practitioners totally rejected both these and indigenous systems, often failing to recognize how many practices and medicines Western biomedicine derived from other systems (for example, quinine, digitalis, many anesthetics, aspirin, and estrogen). Elements of these systems that were derided in the past, such as acupuncture, have now found their way into Western biomedical practice and are being "legitimized" by Western research.

## THEORIES OF HEALTH BEHAVIOR AND BEHAVIOR CHANGE

The fields of sociology, psychology, and anthropology have developed many theories to explain health beliefs and behaviors and behavior change. Some theories developed by sociologists and psychologists in the United States were developed first for U.S. populations and only later applied internationally. Others were developed with international and multicultural populations in mind from the beginning. Only a few of the many theories of health and illness beliefs and behavior are listed below, but they are ones that have been quite influential in general or are ones applicable for international work in particular.

### Health Belief Model

The health belief model suggests that decision making about health behaviors is influenced by four basic premises—perceived susceptibility to the illness, perceived severity of the illness, perceived benefits of the prevention behavior, perceived barriers to that behavior—as well as other variables, such as sociodemographic factors (Rosenstock, Strecher, & Becker, 1974). In general, people are seen as weighing perceived susceptibility (how likely they are to get the disease) and perceived severity (how serious the disease is) against their belief in the benefits and effectiveness of the prevention behavior they must undertake and the costs of that behavior in terms of barriers such as time, money, and aggravation. The more serious the disease is believed to be, and the more effective the prevention, the more likely people are to incur the costs of engaging in the prevention behavior. This model has been extensively studied, critiqued, modified, and expanded to explain people's responses to symptoms and compliance with health care regimens for diagnosed illnesses. One concern has been that this model does not work as well for chronic problems or habitual behaviors because people learn to manage their behaviors or the health care system. Also, it has been accused of failing to take environmental and social forces into account, which in turn increases the potential for blaming the individual. The difficulty in quantifying the model for research and evaluation purposes is also a problem.

Work by Bandura led to the inclusion of self-efficacy in the model. Self-efficacy has been defined as "the conviction that one can successfully execute the behavior required to produce the desired outcome" (Bandura, 1977, 1989). The concept of locus of control, or belief in the ability to control one's life, also has been used with this model. In one recent example, a comparison of migrant Yugoslavian and Swedish diabetic females revealed stronger locus of control in the Swedes and more passivity toward self-care in the Yugoslavs, who also have a lower self-efficacy that the authors attribute to the different political systems in the two countries—collectivism in Yugoslavia, individualism in Sweden (Hjelm, Nyberg, Isacsson, & Apelqvist, 1999).

The value of the four basic premises of the health belief model has held up well under scrutiny. Perceived barriers have the strongest predictive value of the four dimensions, followed by perceived susceptibility and perceived benefits. Perceived susceptibility is most frequently associated with compliance with health screening exams. Perceived severity of risk has been noted to have a weaker predictive value for protective health behaviors while it is strongly associated with sick-role behaviors.

In *Medical Choice in a Mexican Village*, Young (1981) describes a health decision-making process very similar to that found in the health belief model. In choosing between home remedies, pharmacy or store, indigenous healer or doctor, the villagers weigh the perceived severity of the illness, the potential efficacy of the cure to be sought, the cost (money, time, and so on) of the cure and their own resources to seek treatment and pay the cost as they make their decision. The simplest, least costly treatment is always the first choice, but the severity of illness and efficacy issues may force a more costly option. Other studies of health-seeking behavior have found similar patterns throughout the world.

**Theory of Reasoned Action**

The theory of reasoned action was first proposed by Ajzen and Fishbein (1972) to predict an individual's intention to engage in a behavior in a specific time and place. The theory was intended to explain virtually all behaviors over which people have the ability to exert self-control. There are five basic constructs that precede the performance of a behavior. These are behavioral intent, attitudes, beliefs and evaluations of behavioral outcomes, subjective norms, and normative beliefs. Behavioral intent is seen as the immediate predictor of behavior. Factors that influence behavioral choices are mediated through this variable. In order to maximize the predictive ability of an intention to perform a specific behavior, the measurement of the intent must closely reflect the measurement of the behavior. Thus measurement of the intention to begin to take oral contraceptives must include questions about the date a woman plans to visit a clinic and which clinic she plans to attend. The failure to address action, target, context, and time in the measurement of behavioral intention will undermine the predictive value of the model.

In a recent test of this theory in the prediction of condom use intentions in a national sample of young people in England, measures of past behavior were the best predictors of intentions and attenuated the effects of attitude and subjective norms (Sutton, McVey, & Glanz, 1999).

## Diffusion of Health Innovations Model

The diffusion of health innovations model proposes that communication is essential for social change, and that diffusion is the process by which an innovation is communicated through certain channels over time among members of a social system (Rogers, 1983; Rogers & Shoemaker, 1972). An innovation is an idea, practice, service, or other object that is perceived as new by an individual or group.

Ideally, the development of a diffusion strategy for a specific health behavior change goal will proceed through six stages. These include:

- recognition of a problem or need
- conduct of basic and applied research to address the specific problem
- the development of strategies and materials that will put the innovative concept into a form that will meet the needs of the target population
- commercialization of the innovation, which will involve production, marketing, and distribution efforts
- diffusion and adoption of the innovation
- consequences associated with adoption of the innovation

According to classic diffusion theory, a population targeted by an intervention to promote acceptance of an innovation is comprised of six groups: innovators, early adopters, early majority, late majority, late adopters, and laggards. The rapidity and extent to which health innovations are adopted by a target population are mediated by a number of factors, including relative advantage, compatibility, complexity, communicability, observability, trialability, cost efficiency, time, commitment, risk and uncertainty, reversibility, modifiability, and emergence. Relative advantage refers to the extent to which a health innovation is better (faster, cheaper, more beneficial) than an existing behavior or practice. Antibiotics were quickly accepted in most of the world because they were dramatically faster and more effective than traditional practices. Compatibility is the degree to which the innovation is congruent with the target population's existing set of practices and values. Polgar and Marshall (1976) point out that injectable contraceptives were acceptable in the village in India where Marshall worked because injections were viewed so positively due to the success of antibiotics. The degree to which an innovation is easy to incorporate into existing health regimens may also affect rates of diffusion. Iodized salt is easier to use, because salt is already a habit, than taking an iodine pill. Health innovations are also more likely to be adopted quickly and by larger numbers of individuals if the innovation itself can be easily communicated.

The concept of trialability involves the ease of trying out a new behavior. For example, it is easier to try a condom than to be fitted for a diaphragm. Observability refers to role models, such as village leaders volunteering to be the first in a vaccination campaign. A health innovation is also more likely to be adopted if it is seen as cost efficient. A famous case study of water boiling in a Peruvian town demonstrated that the cost in time and energy of gathering wood and making a fire to boil the water far outweighed any perceived benefits, so water boiling was seldom adopted (Wellin, 1955). Successful health innovations are likely to be those that do not require expenditure of lots of additional time, energy, or other resources.

One of the overall messages regarding communicating health education and promotion stated by Rogers (1973) is that mass media and interpersonal communication channels should be *used in conjunction.* Implementing both methods is of particular importance in developing countries, especially in rural communities. He emphasizes that mass media deliver information to a large population to add knowledge, although interpersonal contacts are needed to persuade people to adopt new behaviors (thereby using the knowledge function, the persuasion function, and the innovation-decision process). In Rogers's work and other work cited by him, "family planning diffusion is almost entirely via interpersonal channels" (p. 263). Five examples in different countries, including India, Taiwan, and Hong Kong, are presented where interpersonal channels were the primary source for family planning information and were the motivating factors to seeking services.

The limitations to mass media in this area include

- *Limited exposure:* In less developed countries, smaller audiences have access to mass media (radio is the most common mass media tool) and illiteracy is also a barrier.
- *Message irrelevancy:* The content of mass media messages may be of no practical use for many rural and "nonelite" populations. Often instrumental information— "how to"—is not included in the messages (for example, information on where to receive services or on the positive and negative consequences of adapting a particular health behavior).
- *Low credibility:* For people to accept and believe the messages being diffused, trustworthiness needs to exist between the "sender" and receiver. Often radio and TV stations are a government monopoly and may be considered as government propaganda by the receivers. Radio and TV in Nigeria, Pakistan, and other African and Asian countries are controlled by the government (Rogers, 1973).

The diffusion of innovations model focuses solely on the processes and determinants of adoption of a new behavior and does not help to understand or explain the maintenance of behavior change. Many health behaviors require permanent or long-term changes. Also, it is important to understand if a new behavior is being conducted appropriately, consistently, or at all. One example is the story of condom use, which was demonstrated by unrolling the condom over a banana. Women who became pregnant while they reported using condoms had been faithfully putting them on bananas.

## PRECEDE Model

The PRECEDE model of health promotion was first proposed by Green, Kreuter, Deeds, and Partridge in 1980. PRECEDE is an acronym for "predisposing, reinforcing, and enabling causes in educational diagnosis and evaluation." This model focuses on communities rather than individuals as the primary units of change. This approach incorporates specific recommendations for evaluating the effectiveness of interventions and provides a highly focused target for the intervention.

The framework of the PRECEDE model outlines progression through seven phases. Phase One, also known as social diagnosis, relies on the assessment of the general problems of concern that have a negative impact on overall quality of life for members of the target population. Those populations might include patients, health care providers, family caregivers, lay health workers, or consumers of health care. During Phase One there is an emphasis on identification of social problems encountered by the target population. This provides an important opportunity to involve the community. Community participation in and acceptance of programs greatly increase their likelihood of success.

Phase Two focuses on epidemiologic diagnosis. Activities associated with Phase Three focus on the identification of nonbehavioral (and often nonmodifiable) causes and behavioral causes of the priority health problem. Phase Four of the model is identified as educational diagnosis and consists of activities to identify predisposing, reinforcing, and enabling factors associated with the target health behavior. At Phase Five intervention planners must decide which of the factors are to be addressed by various aspects of the intervention. Phase Six is administrative diagnosis and refers to the development and implementation of the intervention program. Viable intervention strategies suggested by Green and colleagues (1980) include group lectures, individual instruction, mass media messages, audiovisual aids, programmed learning, educational television, skill development workshops, simulations, role playing, educational games, peer group discussions, behavior modification, modeling, and community development. The seventh and final phase is focused on evaluation, which begins during each of the preceding six phases and ranges from simple process evaluation to impact and outcome evaluation.

## Transtheoretical Model

Theories around the concept of stages of change have been evolving since the early 1950s. Currently the most widely accepted stage change model is the transtheoretical model of behavior change developed by Prochaska, DiClemente, and Norcross (1992). This model has four core constructs: (1) stages of change, (2) decisional balance, (3) self-efficacy, and (4) processes of change. Interventions relying on this model are expected to include all four constructs in the development of strategies to communicate, promote, and maintain behavior change.

The stages of change include several steps. The first is *precontemplation*, which refers to individuals who have no intention to take action within the next six months. The *contemplation* stage refers to those who express an intention to take some action to change a negative health behavior or adopt a positive one within the next six months. The *preparation* stage refers to the intent to make a change within the next 30 days. The *action* stage is defined as the demonstration of an overt behavior change for an interval of less than six months. In the fifth stage, *maintenance*, a person will have sustained a change for at least six months.

Decisional balance is an assessment of the costs and benefits of changing, which will vary with the stage of change. Self-efficacy is divided into two concepts. The first is *confidence* that one can engage in the new behavior. Second, the *temptation* aspect of self-efficacy refers to factors that can tempt one to engage in unhealthy behaviors across different settings.

The fourth construct of the transtheoretical model deals with the process of change. This includes 10 factors that can impact the progression of individuals from the precontemplation to the maintenance stages.

## Explanatory Models

Explanatory models were initially proposed by physician-anthropologist Kleinman (1980, 1986, 1988). They differ from some of the theories described earlier in this section in that they are designed for multicultural settings. They include models such as the meaning-centered approach to staff-patient negotiation described by Good and Good (1981). These models focus on individual interactions between physician or other staff and patients, but the concepts, such as Kleinman's negotiation model, have proved useful for research and for behavioral interventions for larger populations.

Exhibit 2–4 adapts and summarizes concepts from Good and Good's description of the meaning-centered approach. The approach involves mutual interpretations across systems of meaning. The interpretive goal is understanding the patient's perspective. The underlying premise is that disorders vary profoundly in their psychodynamics, cultural influences in interpretation, behavioral expression, severity, and duration. As noted earlier, it is difficult to provide "codes" to culture and symptoms due to factors such as individual variation, groups assimilating or changing, and groups adding beliefs and behaviors from other cultures. For example, *espiritismo* (spiritism) was strongest in the Puerto Rican groups in the United States, but it has now been adopted by other cultures of Latin American origin as well. Instead of trying to provide "formulas" for understanding health and illness belief systems for different cultures, the focus is on meaning of symptoms. The medical encounter is seen as involving the interpretation of symptoms and other relevant information. The suggestions in the "Actions" section can be used

**Exhibit 2–4** Meaning-Centered Approach to Clinical Practice

**Primary Principles**

Groups vary in the specificity of their medical complaints.

Groups vary in their style of medical complaining.

Groups vary in the nature of their anxiety about the meaning of symptoms.

Groups vary in their focus on organ systems.

Groups vary in their response to therapeutic strategies.

Human illness is fundamentally semantic or meaningful (it may have a biological base, but is a human experience).

**Corollary**

Clinical practice is inherently interpretive.

**Actions**

Practitioners must
- elicit patients' requests, questions, etc.
- elicit and decode patients' semantic networks
- distinguish disease and illness and develop plans for managing problems
- elicit explanatory models of patients and families, analyze conflict with biomedical models, and negotiate alternatives

both to explain insider/outsider views to health providers and to give them tools to work with individual patients or populations. (See Chapter 7 for further explanation of insider and outsider perspectives.)

**Other Theories**

A number of other theories can be useful in looking at culture and behavior. These include multiattribute utility theory, which predicts behavior directly from an individual's evaluation of the consequences or outcomes associated with both performing and not performing a given behavior. Some, such as social learning theory, have been criticized by anthropologists who argue against the notion that people are like a "black box" into which you can pour information and expect a specific behavior change.

**METHODOLOGIES FOR UNDERSTANDING CULTURE AND BEHAVIOR**

Many of the research methodologies developed in the United States did not translate easily, literally, or figuratively to international settings. Differences in linguistic nuances, in the meanings of words and concepts, in what people would reveal to a stranger, and in what they would reveal to someone from their community all complicated the application of the quantitative methodologies used by sociologists, psychologists, and epidemiologists. The realization of these problems came about gradually, through failed projects; missed interpretations; and, particularly, once AIDS appeared. As a disease whose only prevention is still behavioral, with many hidden or taboo behaviors involved, AIDS brought out the need for qualitative research and for research conducted by individuals from the cultures being studied. The field of international public health has now moved from an almost exclusively quantitative orientation to the recognition that we have a toolbox of methodologies. Some may be more valuable than others for some situations or questions; other times, a mix of several methodologies may offer the best approach. These methodologies derive from epidemiology, survey research, psychology, anthropology, marketing, and other fields. The biggest disagreement has been over the relative value of quantitative and qualitative methods.

The debate on the scientific value of qualitative versus quantitative research is well summarized by Pelto and Pelto (1978). They define science as the "accumulation of systematic and reliable knowledge about an aspect of the universe, carried out by empirical observation and interpreted in terms of the interrelating of concepts referable to empirical observations" (p. 22). The Peltos add that "if the 'personal factor' in anthropology makes it automatically unscientific, then much of medical science, psychology, geography, and significant parts of all disciplines (including chemistry and physics) are unscientific" (p. 23).

In fact, scientific research is not truly objective but is governed by the cultural framework and theoretical orientation of the researcher. One example is the past tendency of biomedical researchers in the United States to focus on adult men for many health problems that also occur in women (such as heart disease). The earlier example of Kuru demonstrates the limitations of cultural bias.

The methodological concepts of validity and reliability provide a common foundation for the integration of quantitative and qualitative techniques. Validity refers to the accuracy of scientific measurement, "the degree to which scientific observations measure what they purport to measure" (Pelto & Pelto, 1978, p. 33). For example, in Spanish Harlem in New York City the question "*¿sabe como evitar los hijos?*" (do you know how to avoid [having] children?) elicited responses on contraceptive methods and was used as the first in a series of questions on family planning. By not using family planning terminology at the outset, the study was able to avoid biasing respondents (Scrimshaw & Pasquariella, 1970). The same phrase in Ecuador, however, produced reactions like, "I would never take out [abort] a child!" If the New York questionnaire had been applied in Ecuador without testing it through semistructured ethnographic interviews, the same words would have produced answers to what was in fact a different question (Scrimshaw, 1974). Qualitative methods often provide greater validity than quantitative methods because they rely on multiple data sources, including direct observation of behavior and multiple contacts with people over time. Thus they can be used to increase the validity of survey research. Reliability refers to replicability: the extent to which scientific observations can be repeated and the same results obtained. In general, this is best accomplished through survey research or other quantitative means. Surveys can test hypotheses and examine questions generated through qualitative data. Qualitative methods may help us *discover* a behavior or how to ask questions about it, while quantitative data can tell us how extensive the behavior is in a population and what other variables are associated with it.

Murray (1976) describes just such a discovery during qualitative research in a Haitian community, where the simple question—"Are you pregnant?"—had two meanings. Women could be pregnant with *gros ventre* (big belly) or could be pregnant and in *perdition*. Perdition meant a state where a woman was pregnant, but the baby was "stuck" in utero and refused to grow. Perdition was attributed to causes such as "cold," spirits, or ancestors. Women may be in perdition for years, and may be separated, divorced, or widowed, but the pregnancy is attributed to her partner when it commenced. Murray then included questions about perdition in a subsequent survey, which revealed that it was apparently a cultural way of making infertility or subfecundity socially acceptable, as many women in perdition fell into these categories.

Surveys are effective tools for collecting data from a large sample, particularly when the distribution of a variable in a population is needed (for example, the percentage of women who obtain prenatal care) or when rarely occurring events (for example, neonatal deaths) must be assessed. Surveys are also used to record people's answers to questions about their behavior, motivations, perception of an event, and similar topics. Although surveys are carefully designed to collect data in the most objective manner possible, they often suffer inaccuracies based on respondents' perceptions of their own behavior or their desire to please the interviewer with their answers. Surveys also can have difficulty uncovering motives (that is, why individuals behave as they do), and they are not apt to uncover behaviors, which may be consciously or unconsciously concealed.

In "Truths and Untruths in Village Haiti: An Experiment in Third World Survey Research," Chen and Murray (1976) describe some of these problems. The traditional anthropological approach involves one person or a small team in a research site for at least a year. This is done in part to take into account the changes in people's lifestyles with the changes in seasons, activities, available food, and so on. Also, the anthropologist often needs time to learn a language or dialect and learn enough about the culture to provide a context for questions and observations. More recently a subset of anthropological tools (ethnographic interview, participant observation, conversation, and observation) plus the market researchers' tool of focus groups have been combined in a rapid anthropological assessment process known as Rapid Assessment Procedures (RAP) (Scrimshaw & Hurtado, 1987; Scrimshaw, Carballo, Ramos, & Blair, 1991; Scrimshaw, Carballo, Carael, Ramos, & Parker, 1992).

The RAP evolved around the same time as Rapid Rural Appraisal was developed by rural sociologists (Chambers, 1992). Both methods made listening to community voices easier for program planners and health care providers and became a frequently used tool for program development and evaluation. RAPs have been developed for many topics, including AIDS, women's health, diarrheal disease, seizure disorders, and water and health.

A final comment on methodology is that as the social sciences are increasingly combining methodologies and sharing each other's tools, it is also important to share theoretical approaches. Where methodology is concerned, this leads to using multilevel approaches to research, in which environment, biological factors, cognitive issues, societal and cultural context, and political and economic forces all can contribute to the analyses. This should take place at least to the extent that an examination is made of data one step above and one step below the phenomenon being explained (Rubenstein, Scrimshaw, & Morrissey, 2000).

---

*This case study was developed by Isabel Martinez, MPH.

## Case Study: The Slim Disease—HIV/AIDS in Sub-Saharan Africa*

AIDS changed the way in which epidemiologic and behavioral research could be conducted and health interventions designed and carried out. This case study illustrates virtually all the topics covered in this chapter.

### Epidemiology

In 1999 worldwide 33.6 million adults and children were living with HIV/AIDS. Of these millions, 70% of the world's HIV-positive cases are in Africa where an estimated 14.7 million people have already died from AIDS. Sub-Saharan Africa has been hit hardest, with an estimated 23.3 million people with HIV/AIDS. The virus has spread throughout the African population at alarming rates. HIV prevalence among pregnant women has risen to between 15–30% in some provinces in South Africa alone (United Nations, 1999b).

Unlike the West, where AIDS has been largely associated with gay men and injecting drug users, in Africa the most common transmission is through heterosexual sex. A husband often infects his wife through his involvement with other partners. A pregnant, HIV-positive woman may transmit the virus to her fetus through the placenta or breastfeeding. Rural communities are not immune to HIV and AIDS, considering that the majority of the population lives in nonurban settings (Hunt, 1989; Salopek, 2000).

Generally, AIDS patients in Africa suffer from intestinal infections, skin disease, tuberculosis, herpes zoster, and meningitis. In the industrialized countries, AIDS is associated with Karposi's sarcoma (a skin cancer), meningitis, and pneumonia. So why does the same disease spread so differently from one region of the world to another? History, politics, economics, and cultural and social environments influence the course of a disease in a society. In the case of Africa, traditional family, social, and environmental structures were disrupted by European colonization, which imposed changes. Even after countries became independent from Europe, political, ecological, and economic structures remained disrupted and often unstable. Many of these factors contribute to an environment in which AIDS easily took hold (Akeroyd, 1997; Bond, Kreniske, Susser, & Vincent, 1997; Hunt, 1989). These factors and their association with the AIDS pandemic are described below. In addition to illustrating the relationship between cultural norms, prevention and health care access, and disease, the following demonstrates the profound relationship between the general sociocultural, political, physical, and economic environment and health.

### Risk of AIDS Associated with Migratory Labor

The integral family structure of the African culture has been broken up by the migratory labor system in eastern, central, and southern Africa. The migratory labor system is historically part of the regions' industrial development and colonization by European powers. These large industries, including mining, railroad work, plantation work, and primary production facilities like oil refineries, "absorbed" massive labor from rural areas. Men typically left their homes and traveled outside their communities to work sites for long periods of time. This system has not only kept families apart, but has also increased the numbers of sex partners—thus giving rise to the prevalence of sexually transmitted infections (STIs) and later AIDS. In many African cultures, regular sex is believed essential to health. Men in the migratory labor system have sex with prostitutes close to their work sites, become infected, and eventually return home and infect their wives, whose babies may in turn become infected (Hunt, 1989; Salopek, 2000).

### War

Almost half of the world's current 27 violent conflicts are in Africa. A country at war faces the weakness of its political system, and the situation intensifies the impact of the AIDS epidemic. Several populations become more vulnerable to HIV/AIDS during wartime, including those affected by food emergencies and scarcity, displaced persons, and refugees. Women are especially at risk. They are six times more likely to contract HIV in refugee camps than populations outside. Women are victims of rape as a weapon of war by the enemy side. Armed forces and the commercial sex workers they interact with are also affected by the epidemic (UNAIDS, 1999; Akeroyd, 1997; Carballo & Siem, 1996).

### Gender Roles and Cultural Traditions

African women's struggle with the AIDS pandemic has been depicted often in the literature (Salopek; 2000; UNAIDS, 1999; Hunt, 1989; Akeroyd, 1997; Carballo & Siem, 1996; Messersmith, 1991). The risk to women from husbands or partners returning from work in other areas has already been discussed. Another risk—sex work or prostitution by women as a means of survival—is now almost a death sentence considering the great risk of contracting HIV/AIDS. There are many reasons why some African women find the need for themselves to engage in sex work, though studies have linked the reasons to a political economy context. Sex in exchange for favors, material goods, or money is conducted in all socioeconomic levels, from female entrepreneurs in foreign trade having to use sexual ploys to ensure business to impoverished young women needing money to support themselves and their families. The women typically travel outside their community or country into urban areas and locations where tourists vacation. As mentioned earlier, prostitution also takes place in the surrounding communities near labor camps and vacation areas. Even if women in sex work are knowledgeable about preventing HIV infection through use of condoms, cost, availability, and resistance of some males to use them raise barriers for their safety and play a part in further transmission of the disease (Akeroyd, 1997; Messersmith, 1991).

Other cultural factors that place young women at greater risk for HIV infection include a superstition in some areas that having sex with a virgin will cure an HIV-infected man, and the practice of female circumcision. In both these circumstances, the risk of contracting HIV through sex or infected surgical instruments increases for adolescents (Salopek, 2000; Akeroyd, 1997).

These and additional cultural factors have contributed to the fact that for the first time in the history of the epidemic, more women than men are infected (Akeroyd, 1997; Hunt, 1989; Messersmith, 1991; Salopek, 2000).

### Additional Cultural Beliefs

Secrecy regarding HIV/AIDS is common within regions of the sub-Saharan culture. Denying that AIDS is affecting one's community or that one is infected increases chances of transmitting the virus because preventative actions are not taken (Akeroyd, 1997; Salopek, 2000; UNAIDS, 1999; United Nations, 1999d). Preventative actions go beyond preventing sexual transmission to concerns about transmission during treatment of ill individuals and during funeral practices.

In some parts of Africa AIDS is referred to as the "slim disease" because of the wasting away that occurs as a result of the infections. Because of this belief, men prefer sex with plump women, believing that they are not infected. AIDS is called "whiteman's disease" in Gabon and "that other thing" in Zimbabwe. HIV and AIDS are a source of shame and denial in the culture. AIDS is also considered a punishment for overindulgence of the body. One sangoma, or faith healer, who has helped revive an ancient Zulu custom of virginity testing of young girls, supported her belief in reviving this custom, saying, "We have adopted too many Western things without thinking, and we lost respect for our bodies. This has allowed things like AIDS to come torture us" (Akeroyd, 1997; Hunt, 1989; Salopek, 2000; UNAIDS, 1999).

### Social and Economic Impacts

Two of the gravest social and economic consequences of the AIDS epidemic in sub-Saharan Africa include millions of orphaned children and a stifled economy for almost an entire continent. About half of HIV infections occur before the age of 25 and most of those afflicted die before 35. This tragedy has left more than 10 million orphans in Africa—90% of the world's AIDS orphans. Because this disease strikes people during their most productive years, the growth and development of Africa's economy is being threatened because infected people eventually become too weak to work, then die. This affliction has left many of Africa's traditionally prosperous industries, such as farming, mining, and oil, extremely vulnerable because of lack of healthy workers and AIDS-related cost of workers' medical care. These social and economic crises may threaten political stability in many African countries and weaken the health of the population. The AIDS epidemic in Africa will eventually have an impact on many parts of the world if the problem is not controlled. The increase of travel nationally and internationally has aided the spread of diseases. In addition, if the problems associated with the transmission of HIV/AIDS are not addressed, they will get worse, more threatening, and more expensive to control (Bartholet, 2000; Bond et al., 1997; Carballo & Siem, 1996; Hunt, 1989; *Newsweek,* 2000; Salopek, 2000; UNAIDS, 1999).

### Barriers to Prevention or Treatment of HIV/AIDS

Many barriers to prevention of HIV/AIDS exist in Africa. These include lack of financial resources and allocating funds to projects that might be less crucial than those related to health. For example, a foreign country funded a multimillion dollar hospital in Zambia, while the rural clinics where the majority of the population live are often not even stocked with aspirin. Treatment of HIV/AIDS with current Western therapies is so expensive that many countries cannot afford it, and negotiating with pharmaceutical companies for less expensive supplies has not always been successful (Bartholet, 2000; Salopek, 2000).

Changing people's health behavior and addressing cultural beliefs has also been a tough challenge in prevention. Promoting safe sex, the use of contraception, and abstaining from some cultural rituals can be perceived as changing traditional gender roles for both men and women and can go against some religious values that are part of the core for some communities. The need to hide or look away from the problem of HIV/AIDS stems from the disgrace attached to the disease, which makes it difficult for people even to discuss it, much less be tested. The stigma of HIV/AIDS needs to be removed in order for prevention efforts to be accepted by the people (Akeroyd, 1997; Bartholet, 2000; *Newsweek*, 2000; Salopek, 2000; UNAIDS, 1999; United Nations, 1999).

One project in Ghana used both the health belief model and social learning theory to examine the determinants of condom use to prevent HIV infection among youth. The authors of the study found that perceived barriers significantly interacted with perceived susceptibility and self-efficacy. Youth who perceived a high level of susceptibility to HIV infection and a low level of barriers to condom use were almost six times as likely to have used condoms at last intercourse. A high level of perceived self-efficacy and a low level of perceived barriers increased the likelihood of use three times (Adih & Alexander, 1999).

### Prevention Efforts by Community and Governmental Agencies and NGOs

Uganda and Senegal have received much recognition for controlling the spread of HIV/AIDS. Both of these countries have reduced their infection rate through aggressive public education and condom promotion campaigns, expanded treatment programs for other sexually transmitted infections, and mobilization of non-governmental organizations (NGOs). The current president of Uganda has worked to reduce the stigma for people with HIV/AIDS. Senegal reacted quickly to the threat of disease starting in the early 1990s. A survey of its citizens regarding sexual behavior, knowledge, and attitudes was conducted followed by public education campaigns. Health officials believe the education efforts surrounding AIDS have contributed to women choosing to remain virgins longer

and an increase of condom use among sex workers and men and women who have casual sex. A decrease of STIs in sex workers and pregnant women was also noted (*Newsweek*, 2000; UNAIDS, 1999; United Nations, 1999a).

The theory of self-efficacy has proved useful in addressing AIDS. For example, one study in South Africa found that knowledge of risk and its prevention was important, but not sufficient. The authors stress the need to improve personal autonomy in decision making about sexual behavior and condom use for both men and women through skills development programs that promote self-efficacy (Reddy, Meyer-Weitz, van den Borne, & Kok, 1999).

International health and development organizations have joined in the fight against AIDS in Africa. The United Nations and its specialized agencies have major programs assisting countries and communities in prevention efforts, including joining forces to accelerate the development of experimental vaccines. Academic institutions have also teamed up with local community and church organizations to create prevention projects and help organize the communities to reach more of the public. These efforts have assisted in empowering many volunteers, mostly women, to motivate others in their communities through education and increasing women's negotiation skills for safe sex or condom use (Msiza-Makhubu, 1997; United Nations, 1999d; World Health Organization, 1997).

There is also a growing movement of doctors in Africa working with traditional healers to do outreach and education on AIDS. As discussed earlier, traditional healers have better access to many populations. People seek their help because of tradition and lack of adequate health care (Associated Press, 2000; Green, 1994).

The individual behaviors that place people at risk are part of a larger root cause of the problem in Africa, including colonialism, big industry's design of mass labor migration, poverty, gender inequalities, and war. Ideal prevention and intervention strategies must address health behavior changes as well as economic and community development in Africa (Akeroyd, 1997; Bond et al., 1997; Tylor, 1871; United Nations, 1999c, 1999d; World Health Organization, 1997).

## CONCLUSION

This has been a brief exploration of cultural and behavioral issues for international public health. Anthropology, sociology, and psychology have much greater depth in both method and theory than can be described in this chapter. There is a rich and extensive literature on health beliefs and behaviors, environmental and biological contexts, health systems, and programmatic successes and failures. It is essential to take these factors into account in considering international public health work. A program must consider structural factors, such as setting, hours, child care, and ambience, as well as factors of content, such as culturally acceptable services, which includes providers who treat patients with respect and understanding. Research and preventive services regarding health beliefs and behaviors must accept and integrate concepts different from those of Western biomedicine, of middle- or upper-class health care providers, or of health care providers from an ethnic or cultural group that is different from their patients. This demands the ability inherent in some of the anthropological methods and approaches discussed earlier: the ability to "get into someone's head" and understand things from an insider perspective. There is nothing like the experience of spending time with people, in their own homes or community, and striving to reach that insider understanding.

---

### DISCUSSION QUESTIONS

1. What prevention strategies would you develop for the prevention of AIDS if you were the minister of health of a sub-Saharan country? What would be your strategies if you were a community leader? Would these strategies differ? If yes, how? How would you address some of the cultural beliefs or traditions associated with HIV/AIDS mentioned in the case study?
2. If you were entering a community to introduce a health program, who would you talk to? What would you ask? Why?
3. What is the hot/cold illness belief system? Why is it important? How would you incorporate it into a maternal and child health program?
4. Many people believe that healers such as midwives and shamans are called to their profession by a greater spiritual power. What significance does this have for official health programs around the world? How should they address this belief?
5. If an indigenous practice seems peculiar to you, but does no apparent harm, what should you do?
6. How could you learn what people in a community really believe about health and illness?

---

### REFERENCES

Adams, R.N. (1955). A nutritional research program in Guatemala. In B.D. Paul (Ed.), *Health, culture, & community* (pp. 435–458). New York: Russell Sage Foundation.

Adih, W.K., & Alexander, C.S. (1999). Determinants of condom use to prevent HIV infection among youth in Ghana. *Journal of Adolescent Health, 24*(1), 63–72.

Ajzen, I., & Fishbein, M. (1972). Attitudes and normative beliefs as factors influencing behavioral intentions. *Journal of Personality and Social Psychology, 21*(1), 1–9.

Akeroyd, A.V. (1997). Sociocultural aspects of AIDS in Africa: Occupational and gender issues. In G.C. Bond, J. Kreniske, I. Susser, & J. Vincent (Eds.), *AIDS in Africa and the Caribbean.* Boulder, CO: Westview Press.

Alland, A. (1970). *Adaptation in cultural evolution: An approach to medical anthropology.* New York: Columbia University Press.

Associated Press. (2000, February 8). Conference stress uses for traditional healers in AIDS battle. InteliHealth (*www.intelihealth.com/IH/ihtIH/EMIHc000/333/333/268121.html*).

Bandura, A. (1977). *Social learning theory.* Englewood Cliffs, NJ: Prentice Hall.

Bandura, A. (1989). Human agency in social cognitive theory. *American Psychologist, 44,* 1175–1184.

Bartholet, J. (2000, January 17). The plague years. *Newsweek.*

Beals, A.R. (1976). Strategies of resort to curers in south India. In C. Leslie (Ed.), *Asian medical systems: A comparative study* (pp. 184–200). Berkeley, CA: University of California Press.

Bond, G.C., Kreniske. J., Susser, I., & Vincent, J. (1997). The anthropology of AIDS in Africa and the Caribbean. In G.C. Bond, J. Kreniske, I. Susser, & J. Vincent (Eds.), *AIDS in Africa and the Caribbean* (pp. 3–9). Boulder, CO: Westview Press.

Buckley, T., & Gottlieb, A. (Eds.). (1988). *Blood magic.* Berkeley, CA: University of California Press.

Carballo, M., & Siem, H. (1996). Migration, migration policy and AIDS. In M. Knipe & R. Rector (Eds.), *Crossing borders: Migration, ethnicity and AIDS* (pp. 31–48). London: Taylor and Francis.

Chambers, R. (1992). Rapid but relaxed and particularly rural appraisal: Towards applications in health and nutrition. In N.S. Scrimshaw & G.R. Gleason (Eds.), *Rapid assessment procedures: Qualitative methodologies for planning and evaluation of health related programmes* (pp. 295–305). Boston: International Nutrition Foundation for Developing Countries.

Chen, K-H., & Murray, G.F. (1976). Truths and untruths in village Haiti: An experiment in third world survey research. In J.F. Marshall & S. Polgar (Eds.), *Culture, natality, and family planning* (pp. 241–262). Chapel Hill, NC: Carolina Population Center.

Foster, G.M. (1953). Relationships between Spanish and Spanish-American folk medicine. *Journal of American Folklore, 66,* 201–17.

Freed, S.A., & Freed, R.S. (1967). Spirit possession as illness in a north Indian village. In J. Middleton (Ed.), *Magic, witchcraft, and curing* (pp. 295–320). Garden City, NY: Natural History Press.

Gadjusek, D.C., Gibbs, C.J., & Alpers, M. (1967). Transmission and passage of experimental "Kuru" to chimpanzees. *Science, 155,* 212–214.

Good, B.J., & Good, M.J.D. (1981). The meaning of symptoms: A cultural hermeneutic model for clinical practice. In L. Eisenberg & A. Kleinman (Eds.), *The relevance of social science for medicine* (pp. 165–196). Dordrecht, Holland: Reidel.

Green, E. (1994). *AIDS and STDs in Africa: Bridging the gap between traditional healing and modern medicine.* Boulder, CO: Westview Press.

Green, L., Kreuter, M., Deeds, S., & Partridge, K. (1980). *Health education planning: A diagnostic approach.* Palo Alto, CA: Mayfield.

Gwaltney, J.L. (1970). *The thrice shy.* New York: Columbia University Press.

Hjelm, K., Nyberg, P., Isacsson, A., & Apelqvist, J. (1999). Beliefs about health and illness essential for self-care practice: A comparison of migrant Yugoslavian and Swedish diabetic females. *Journal of Advanced Nursing, 30*(5), 1147–1159.

Hughes, C. (1990). Ethnopsychiatry. In T.M. Johnson & C.E. Sargent (Eds.), *Medical anthropology: Contemporary theory and method.* New York: Praeger Publishers.

Hunt, C.W. (1989). Migration labor and sexually transmitted diseases: AIDS in Africa. *Journal of Health in Social Science Behavior, 30,* 353–373.

Kendall, C., Foote, D., & Martorell, R. (1983). Anthropology, communications, and health: The mass media and health practices program in Honduras. *Human Organization, 42,* 353–360.

Kleinman, A. (1980). *Patients and healers in the context of culture.* Berkeley, CA: University of California Press.

Kleinman, A. (1986). *Social origins of distress and disease.* New Haven, CT: Yale University Press.

Kleinman, A. (1988). *The illness narratives.* New York: Basic Books.

Lindenbaum, S. (1971). Sorcery and structure in fore society. *Oceania, 41,* 277–287.

Logan, M.H. (1972). Humoral folk medicine: A potential aid in controlling pellagra in Mexico. *Ethnomedizin, 4,* 397–410.

Messersmith, L.J. (1991). *The women of good times and Baba's Place: The multi-dimensionality of the lives of commercial sex workers in Bamako, Mali.* Doctoral dissertation. Los Angeles: University of California at Los Angeles.

Msiza-Makhubu, S.B. (1997). *Peer education and support for AIDS prevention among women in South Africa.* Doctoral dissertation. Chicago: University of Illinois at Chicago.

Murray, G.F. (1976). Women in perdition: Ritual fertility control in Haiti. In J.F. Marshall & S. Polgar (Eds.), *Culture, natality, and family planning* (pp. 59–78). Chapel Hill, NC: Carolina Population Center.

*Newsweek U.S. Edition: International.* (2000, January 17). Africa matters: Interview with U.S. ambassador to the United Nations, Richard Holbrooke.

O'Connor, B. (1995). *Healing traditions.* Philadelphia: University of Pennsylvania Press.

Parsons, T. (1948). Illness and the role of the physician. In C. Kluckholm & H. Murray (Eds.), *Personality in nature, society, and culture.* New York: Alfred A. Knopf.

Paul, B.D. (Ed.). (1955). *Health, culture, & community.* New York: Russell Sage Foundation.

Pelto, P.J., & Pelto, G.H. (1978). *Anthropological research: The structure of inquiry.* New York: Cambridge University Press.

Polgar, S., & Marshall, J.F. (1976). The search for culturally acceptable fertility regulating methods. In J.F. Marshall & S. Polgar (Eds.), *Culture, natality, and family planning* (pp. 204–218). Chapel Hill, NC: Carolina Population Center.

Prochaska, J., DiClemente, C., & Norcross, J. (1992). In search of how people change: Applications to addictive behaviors. *American Psychologist, 47,* 1102–1104.

Reddy, P., Meyer-Weitz, A., van den Borne, B., & Kok, G. (1999). STD-related knowledge, beliefs and attitudes of Xhosa-speaking patients attending STD primary health-care clinics in South Africa. *International Journal of Sexually Transmitted Diseases and AIDS, 10*(6), 392–400.

Reichel-Dolmatoff, G., & Reichel-Dolmatoff, A. (1961). *The people of Aritama.* London: Routledge and Kegan Paul, Ltd.

Rogers, E.M. (1973). *Communication strategies for family planning.* New York: Free Press.

Rogers, E.M. (1983). *Diffusion of innovations* (3rd ed.). New York: Free Press.

Rogers, E.M., & Shoemaker, F.F. (1972). *Communication of innovations* (2nd ed.). New York: Free Press.

Rosenstock, I., Strecher, V., & Becker, M. (1974). Social learning theory and the health belief model. *Health Education Monograph, 2,* 328–386.

Rubel, A.J., & Haas, M.R. (1990). Ethnomedicine. In T.M. Johnson & C.D. Sargent (Eds.), *Medical anthropology, contemporary theory and method.* New York: Praeger Publishers, 115–131.

Rubel, A.J., O'Nell, C.W., & Collado-Ardon, R. (1984). *Susto: a folk illness.* Berkeley, CA: University of California Press.

Rubenstein, R.A., Scrimshaw, S.C., & Morrissey, S. (2000). Classification and process in sociomedical understanding towards a multilevel view of sociomedical methodology. In G.L. Albrecht, R. Fitzpatrick, & S.C. Scrimshaw (Eds.), *The handbook of social studies in health & medicine* (pp. 36–49). London: Sage Publications.

Salopek, P. (2000, January 10). We die lying to ourselves. *Chicago Tribune.*

Scrimshaw, S.C. (1974). *Culture, environment, and family size: A study of urban in-migrants in Guayaquil, Ecuador.* Doctoral dissertation. New York: Columbia University.

Scrimshaw, S.C.M. (1992). Adaptation of anthropological methodologies to rapid assessment of nutrition and primary health care. In N.S. Scrimshaw & G.R. Gleason (Eds.), *Rapid assessment procedures: Qualitative methodologies for planning and evaluation of health related programmes* (pp. 25–49). Boston: International Nutrition Foundation for Developing Countries.

Scrimshaw, S.C.M., Carballo, M., Carael, M., Ramos, L., & Parker, R.G. (1992). *HIV/AIDS rapid assessment procedures: Rapid anthropological approaches for studying AIDS related beliefs, attitudes and behaviours.* Monograph. Tokyo: United Nations University.

Scrimshaw, S.C.M., Carballo, M., Ramos, L., & Blair, B.A. (1991). The AIDS rapid anthropological assessment procedures: A tool for health education planning and evaluation. *Health Education Quarterly, 18*(1), 111–123.

Scrimshaw, S.C., & Hurtado, E. (1987). *Rapid assessment procedures for nutrition and primary health care: Anthropological approaches to improving program effectiveness (RAP).* Tokyo: United Nations University.

Scrimshaw, S.C., & Hurtado, E. (1988). Anthropological involvement in the Central American diarrheal disease control project. *Social Science and Medicine, 27*(1), 97–105.

Scrimshaw, S.C., & Pasquariella, B.G. (1970). Obstacles to sterilization in one community. *Family Planning Perspectives, 2*(4), 40–42.

Sutton, S., McVey, D., & Glanz, A. (1999). A comparative test of the theory of reasoned action and the theory of planned behavior in the prediction of condom use intentions in a national sample of English young people. *Health Psychology, 18*(1), 72–81.

Thao, X. (1986). Hmong perception of illness and traditional ways of healing. In G.L. Hendricks, B.T. Downing & A. Deinard (Eds.), *The Hmong in transition* (pp. 365–378). New York: Center for Migration Studies of New York and Southeast Asian Refugee Studies Project of the University of Minnesota.

Topley, M. (1976). Chinese traditional etiology and methods of cure in Hong Kong. In C. Leslie (Ed.), *Asian medical systems: A comparative study* (pp. 243–265). Berkeley, CA: University of California Press.

Tylor, E.B. (1871). *Primitive culture.* London: J. Murray.

UNAIDS. (1999). AIDS epidemic update: December 1999. Geneva, Switzerland: World Health Organization.

United Nations. (1999a). Acting early to prevent AIDS: The case of Senegal. UNAIDS.

United Nations. (May 6–8, 1999b). HIV/AIDS in Africa: Socio-economic impact and response. Joint conference of African ministers of finance and ministers of economic development and planning, Addis-Abada, Ethiopia (http://www.unaids.org/publications/graphics/addis/sld001.htm).

United Nations. (June 1999c). Sexual behavioral change for HIV: Where have the theories taken us? *UNAIDS,* 199.27E (English original, text by Rachel King.)

United Nations, Wellcome Trust Centre for the Epidemiology of Infectious Disease. (1999d). Trends in HIV incidence and prevalence: Natural course of the epidemic or results of behavioral change? *UNAIDS.*

Weller, S.C. (1983). New data on intracultural variability: The hot-cold concept of medicine and illness. *Human Organization, 42,* 249–257.

Wellin, E. (1955). Water boiling in a Peruvian town. In B.D. Paul (Ed.), *Health, culture, & community* (pp. 71–103). New York: Russell Sage Foundation.

World Health Organization (1997). *Women and HIV/AIDS prevention training manual: Peer education program, a global approach.* Collaborating Centre for International Nursing Development in Primary Health Care Research, Geneva, Switzerland: Author.

Young, C.J. (1981). *Medical choice in a Mexican village.* New Brunswick, NJ: Rutgers University Press.

# CHAPTER 3

# Reproductive Health

*Jane Menken and M. Omar Rahman*

Reproductive health in the low- and middle-income countries has long been addressed primarily through family planning and maternal and child health programs, and through programs to prevent and treat sexually transmitted infections (STIs) and their consequences. It has been tied to policy concerns about population growth as well as health. In 1994 the United Nations sponsored the third decennial International Conference on Population and Development (ICPD) in Cairo. The previous two conferences had emphasized family planning and economic development, respectively, as the major focus of population policy—policy that was intended to reduce fertility and, thereby, population growth. The rationale for support of family planning programs included both the right of individuals to control their own fertility and the belief that reduced fertility would lead to reduced population growth, which would have benefits for individuals, nations, and the world. For the first time, in 1994, women's health advocates, many from nongovernmental organizations (NGOs), played a major role in the ICPD and brought to the fore issues of reproductive health that went beyond family planning. They called for a fundamental redefinition of population policy that focused on the status of women and gave "prominence to reproductive health and the empowerment of women while downplaying the demographic rationale for population policy" (McIntosh & Finkle, 1995, p. 223).

The 1994 ICPD adopted a Programme of Action that included the following as its definition of reproductive health:

Reproductive health is a state of complete physical, mental and social well being, and not merely the absence of disease or infirmity, in all matters relating to the reproductive system and its processes. Reproductive health therefore implies that people are able to have a satisfying and safe sex life and that they have the capability to reproduce and the freedom to decide if, when, and how often to do so. Implicit in this last condition are the right of men and women to be informed and to have access to safe, effective, affordable and acceptable methods of family planning of their choice, as well as other methods of their choice for the regulation of fertility which are not against the law, and the right of access to appropriate health-care services that enable women to go safely through pregnancy and childbirth and provide couples with the best chance of having a healthy infant. It also includes sexual health, the purpose of which is the enhancement of life and personal relations, and not merely counseling and care related to reproduction and sexually transmitted diseases (United Nations, 1994).

This vision of reproductive health has, not unexpectedly, proved controversial and has not been achieved to the extent hoped for by its

79

proponents (*New York Times*, 1999a, 1999c). A less controversial and more limited version guided the 1997 U.S. National Academy of Sciences report on reproductive health:

1. Every sex act should be free of coercion and infection.
2. Every pregnancy should be intended.
3. Every birth should be healthy for both mother and child (Tsui, Wasserheit, & Haaga, 1997).

Even so, no country has met these more limited goals, and the problems are greatest in the low- and middle-income countries.

In this chapter, both the older and the newer views of family planning and reproductive health are emphasized. Since Chapter 4 includes sexually transmitted infections (STIs) and HIV/AIDS, these crucial aspects of reproductive health are only briefly mentioned here. In the section on demographic trends, the focus is on population growth and change and the transitions underway around the world from situations of high fertility and high mortality to those of low fertility and low mortality. How people control their fertility and indexes of the effects of various fertility determinants on overall fertility in a range of countries are then considered. In the third section family planning programs and their role in reduction of fertility and unintended pregnancy are examined. The next two sections consider the role of fertility patterns in the health of children and women. In the final section brief recommendations for future research and programs are presented.

## DEMOGRAPHIC TRENDS AND FERTILITY DETERMINANTS

### History of Population Growth

In order to understand the context of the concerns about population and reproductive health in the world today, it is instructive to review the history of population growth and its associated impacts. Figure 3–1 shows the growth of population and, in particular, the extraordinary changes of the past 200 years. World population reached 1 billion just after 1800. By the turn of the twentieth century it had reached 1.6 billion and before 1930 had surpassed 2 billion. It had taken less than 125 years to add the second billion people, compared to the long sweep of history needed to reach the first billion. Population passed the 3 billion mark in 1960. Each additional billion has taken less time to add, so that, in late 1999, population reached 6 billion. The population has doubled since 1960, adding 3 billion people in only about 40 years (U.S. Bureau of the Census, 1999; Weeks, 1999, table 1.1 and figure 1.1). The majority of this expansion has taken place in the low- and middle-income regions of Asia, Africa, Latin America, and Oceania (see Figure 3–2), which accounted for 80% of the world's population in 1998, compared to 68% at mid-century. Their share of world population is expected to continue increasing, reaching 87% in the middle of the twenty-first century (United Nations, 1998). The encouraging news is that the rate at which the world's population is growing has declined continuously since about 1960 (Figure 3–3), although the absolute *number* of people added in each decade has continued to increase. Only after 2000 is that number expected to begin to decline. Population growth rates are declining in most of the low- and middle-income countries, but at an uneven pace, with some countries and regions experiencing much more rapid change than others. China is a particularly prominent example; its growth rate was 2.1% in 1960, increased to 2.6 in 1965, and has steadily dropped to below 1% by 1995. The United Nations estimates that world population in the middle of the twenty-first century will be between 7 and 11 billion people. By that time, the growth rate will be well under 1% but will not yet have achieved the no-growth stable situation. Because of reduced fertility and increased life expectancy, the 2050 population will have more people over 60 than children under 15. Currently 10% are over 60 and 30% under 15, and world population will continue to age, so that 22% are expected to be over 60 in 2050, while only 20% will be under 15 (United Nations, 1998).

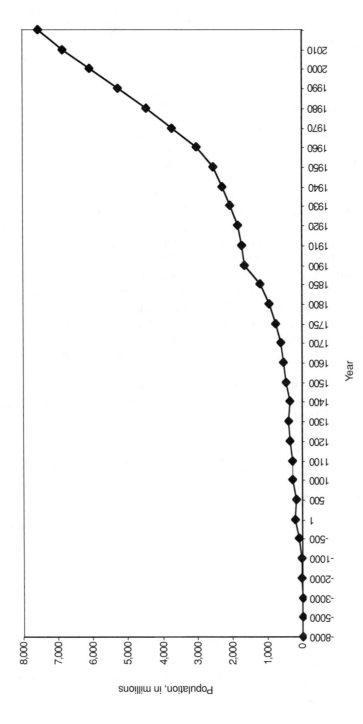

**Figure 3–1** The Growth of Population and, in Particular, the Extraordinary Changes of the Past 200 Years

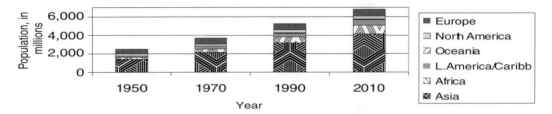

**Figure 3–2** Population Size by Continent, 1950–2010

## The Demographic Transition

What explains the historic experience of low initial growth followed by an explosive increase and, finally, a steady decline in growth? The classical theory of demographic transition proposed by Notestein (1953) and others postulated that all societies initially started off with high fertility and high mortality. At some point in societal development, mortality rates fell due to public health advances, while fertility rates remained high. This combination resulted in explosive population growth, with birth rates far exceeding death rates, until at some point birth rates also started to decline and a new equilibrium was reached at low fertility and low mortality levels. Until fairly recently, the classic theory of demographic transition held sway, and all societies were supposed to go through it in a lock-step manner. In the early to mid-1970s, however, an international team of researchers participated in the Princeton University Euro-

pean Fertility Project and carefully examined the historic fertility decline in Europe. They came to the somewhat surprising conclusion that the process of demographic transition was quite varied and did not always follow the path suggested by classical theory (Coale & Watkins, 1986). Under that scenario, a certain level of socioeconomic development was required for the initial mortality decline, which was followed, at some later point, by fertility decline. Instead, the project found that mortality decline took place in different societies at different levels of development and that there was no specific threshold of mortality above which fertility decline would not take place. The current consensus about demographic transition is that there is no specific sequence in which fertility and mortality decline. They can decline together or one before the other. Further, there are no specific thresholds of development required for either process to begin. Finally, the interval between a high fertility and high mortality regime and a subse-

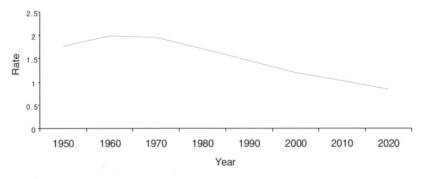

**Figure 3–3** World Population Growth Rate, 1950–2020

quent low fertility and low mortality regime is also not fixed and can vary considerably. The experience of the low- and middle-income world has borne out this new consensus. Demographic transitions have taken place at different rates in different places and with different sequences; a common thread, however, is that the transition has often been considerably more rapid than the European or North American historical record.

Population growth rates and fertility and mortality for different parts of the world since the mid-twentieth century are shown in Table 3–1 and for the specific case of Bangladesh in Exhibit 3–1. Growth rates are given as percent change in population per year for the five years subsequent to the specified date. When a population stops changing in size, it becomes *stationary* and its growth rate is zero. The *total fertility rate* (TFR) is the number of children women would bear, on average, if they lived to the end of the reproductive period under the childbearing pattern of a particular year (for example, if they had, at age 15, the birth rate of 15-year-olds in 1970; at age 16, the birth rate of 16-year-olds in 1970; and so on). Life expectancy at birth is the average number of years people would live if their entire life were spent under the mortality conditions of a particular year (for example, if they experienced the infant mortality of 1970, the death rate at age 1 of 1970, and so on). The numbers resulting from these examples would be the 1970 TFR and the 1970 life expectancy. A TFR of about 2.1 is usually referred to as *replacement level* fertility. If, over the long run, women have about that number of children on average, the population will become stationary, neither growing nor declining. Women will be contributing to the next generation one child for themselves and one for their partner, and a bit more for girls who were born but did not survive to reproduce.

As shown in Table 3–1, life expectancy has risen continuously over the latter half of the twentieth century. The exceptions are the countries of Africa hardest hit by AIDS, where disease is wiping out all earlier gain. The 1998 UN projections for the nine countries with adult HIV prevalence of 10% or more (Botswana, Kenya, Malawi, Mozambique, Namibia, Rwanda, South Africa, Zambia, and Zimbabwe) estimate that average life expectancy will be 17 years less by 2010 than it would have been in the absence of AIDS (United Nations, 1998, p. 4). Much of the increase in every country in life expectancy is due to improvements in infant and child survival; by contrast, the HIV-related declines are primarily the result of increased adult mortality.

TFR had declined by 1970 in all parts of the world with the exception of Africa. That decline was, in less industrialized regions, overwhelmed by increases in life expectancy, so that their growth rates—and their population growth—increased. But fertility continued to fall, and to do so sufficiently to counteract the continuing increase in life expectancy. This fertility transition is serving to bring growth rates down in all low- and middle-income regions today. HIV/AIDS may be contributing to recent decline in fertility in the hardest hit parts of the world; there is mounting evidence that infected women have reduced fecundity. The changes in population growth rate, total fertility rate, and life expectancy are illustrated in Exhibit 3–1, which provides information for Bangladesh from 1950 to 1995.

In order to understand the different types of fertility transitions that have taken place, the determinants of fertility and fertility change in different contexts need to be understood. There is an extensive literature that examines the impact of socioeconomic factors on desired family size (for example, Bankole & Westoff, 1995; Bulatao & Lee, 1983; Rutstein, 1998). Much of the discussion centers on the costs and benefits of children and the notion that couples desire additional children as long as the benefits are greater than the costs. These benefits and costs are, in turn, determined by a range of factors, some of which are *structural* (for example, wages, rates of return on investments, opportunity costs) and some of which are *attitudinal* (changes in values and expectations). Improvements in the educational status of women, for example, are thought to decrease desired family

**Table 3–1** Population Growth Rate, Total Fertility Rate, and Life Expectancy for Regions of the World, by Time Period

| Region | Year | | | |
|---|---|---|---|---|
| | 1950 | 1970 | 1990 | 2010[a] |
| World | | | | |
|   Growth Rate | 1.77 | 1.95 | 1.46 | 1.03 |
|   TFR | 4.99 | 4.48 | 2.93 | 2.35 |
|   Life Expectancy | 46.5 | 58.0 | 64.1 | 69.2 |
| Less Developed Regions | | | | |
|   Growth Rate | 2.04 | 2.37 | 1.75 | 1.23 |
|   TFR | 6.16 | 5.43 | 3.27 | 2.48 |
|   Life Expectancy | 40.9 | 54.7 | 61.9 | 67.6 |
| More Developed Regions | | | | |
|   Growth Rate | 1.21 | 0.79 | 0.41 | 0.10 |
|   TFR | 2.77 | 2.11 | 1.68 | 1.65 |
|   Life Expectancy | 66.6 | 71.2 | 74.1 | 77.3 |
| Asia | | | | |
|   Growth Rate | 1.91 | 2.28 | 1.55 | 1.00 |
|   TFR | 5.91 | 5.09 | 2.85 | 2.18 |
|   Life Expectancy | 41.3 | 56.3 | 64.5 | 70.8 |
| Africa | | | | |
|   Growth Rate | 2.15 | 2.56 | 2.51 | 2.04 |
|   TFR | 6.58 | 6.60 | 5.47 | 3.80 |
|   Life Expectancy | 37.8 | 46.1 | 51.1 | 56.1 |
| Latin America & Caribbean | | | | |
|   Growth Rate | 2.66 | 2.45 | 1.72 | 1.18 |
|   TFR | 5.89 | 5.03 | 2.97 | 2.28 |
|   Life Expectancy | 51.4 | 60.9 | 68.1 | 72.5 |
| Oceania | | | | |
|   Growth Rate | 2.21 | 2.09 | 1.51 | 1.09 |
|   TFR | 3.85 | 3.21 | 2.50 | 1.09 |
|   Life Expectancy | 60.9 | 66.6 | 72.9 | 76.4 |
| Northern America | | | | |
|   Growth Rate | 1.70 | 1.01 | 1.02 | 0.66 |
|   TFR | 3.47 | 2.01 | 2.02 | 1.88 |
|   Life Expectancy | 69.0 | 71.5 | 75.9 | 78.9 |
| Europe | | | | |
|   Growth Rate | 1.00 | 0.60 | 0.16 | −0.14 |
|   TFR | 2.57 | 2.14 | 1.57 | 1.54 |
|   Life Expectancy | 66.2 | 70.8 | 72.6 | 75.9 |

*Notes:* Growth rate (percentage per year), total fertility rate, and life expectancy are for the subsequent 5-year period (for example, 1950–1955). Life expectancy is for both sexes combined.

[a]Figures for 2010 are from the medium-variant projection.

size because they increase the potential wages that women can earn and thus raise the opportunity costs of childbearing and childrearing. Education may, in addition, lead to attitudinal change about quantity-quality tradeoffs in numbers of children (for example, having fewer chil-

**Exhibit 3–1**  Demographic Change in Bangladesh

Bangladesh will be used as a case study through-out this chapter for a number of reasons. First, it has experienced high population growth rates that were the result of continuing high fertility during a period when mortality was declining. At midcentury, life expectancy was under 40 years for both men and women and, in fact, was higher for males until the early 1990s. By that time, almost 20 years had been added to life expectancy, which was 55.6 years for both sexes. Second, in the last quarter of the twentieth century, total fertility in Bangladesh dropped remarkably, from a rate of about 7 in 1970–1975 to 3.4 in the early 1990s, and 3.3 (not shown) for the mid-1990s. As a con-sequence of the decline in mortality, the growth rate rose from 1.7% at midcentury to 2.8% for 1975–1980. The subsequent fertility decline caused the growth rate to decline to 1.6% for 1990–1995. Growth at this level, continued over many years, leads to a population doubling in size in only 43 years. And, finally, the Bangladesh fertility decline was accomplished in the context of a strong family planning program. In addition, there were unusual systematic research efforts that were intended to improve the design of the program and delivery of services that were ap-propriate to the specific context of Bangladesh.

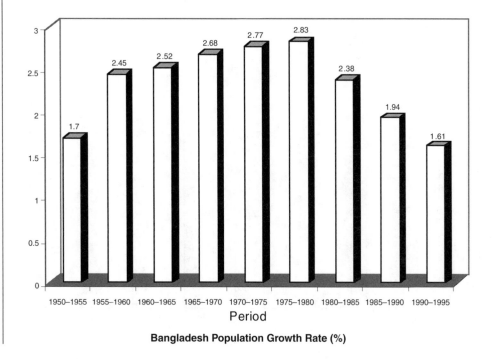

**Bangladesh Population Growth Rate (%)**

*continues*

**Exhibit 3–1** continued

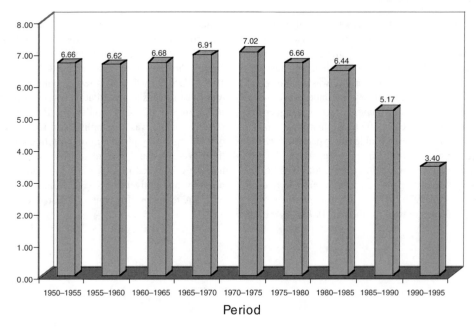

**Total Fertility Rate (per Woman)**

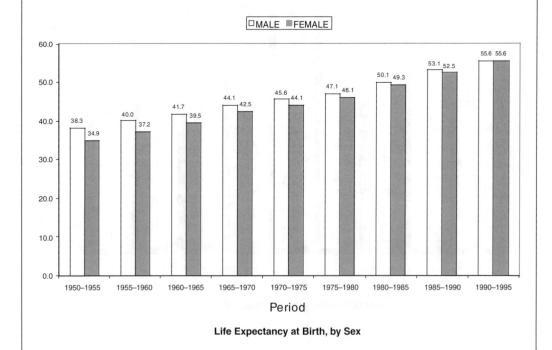

**Life Expectancy at Birth, by Sex**

dren so that greater investment in the education of each child is feasible).

Implicit in this theoretical framework is the idea that couples weigh a variety of alternatives, with childbearing being just one of the possible behavioral choices available. Another structural factor is increasing landlessness, which decreases the benefits of the labor provided by children and thereby tends to reduce family size. More recent research emphasizes attitudinal change. It posits that values and expectations can change as a result of outside influences. Thus exposure to messages in which small families are treated as a marker for modernity may motivate couples to reduce their desired family sizes, even in the absence of any changes in the structural costs and benefits of children. This remains a controversial topic.

Although this chapter focuses on low- and middle-income countries—in almost none of which fertility has declined to replacement level—it is worth noting that the industrialized world, especially Europe, is concerned about its low fertility and population decline. For Europe as a whole, TFR declined below 1.9 before 1980 and has continued to decline. It is expected that the entire continent will have a negative growth rate for 2000 (United Nations, 1998). Understanding what maintains below replacement fertility and what causes it to increase is an important issue for the industrialized world.

## How Do People Control Their Fertility?

In addition to considering *why* people control their fertility, *how* people actually do so must be understood as well. It is useful first to consider the *proximate determinants* that lead to variation in fertility in the absence of deliberate family planning (Bongaarts, 1978; Bongaarts & Potter, 1983; Menken & Kuhn, 1996; Sheps & Menken, 1973). These proximate determinants can be divided into those that affect the *reproductive span* and those that influence the *intervals between successive births* within that span. As shown in Figure 3–4, the *effective reproductive span* exists within boundaries set by both the *bio-*

*logical* and the *social reproductive spans*. The former, the *biological span*, is the time during which a woman is capable of childbearing because she has the biological capacity to ovulate and to carry a pregnancy to a live birth. It is usually marked by menarche and menopause, but first ovulation may occur well after menarche and last ovulation precedes menopause. However, in no society do women devote their full biological span to reproduction. Were they to do so, according to Bongaarts (1978), women who survive to sterility would bear more than 15 children on average. This figure is well beyond the maximum ever recorded for any population. Every society has social controls on initiation and cessation of sexual activity. Entry into sexual activity will be referred to as *marriage* and cessation as *marriage dissolution*. These terms are used as social markers rather than representing legal ceremonies and arrangements of the state. Specifically, marriage dissolution can occur through breakup of the relationship or through widowhood. The *social reproductive span* is, therefore, the interval between initiation and cessation of sexual activity. The *effective reproductive span* is the overlap of the biological and the social spans. It begins with the later of menarche and marriage and ends with the earliest of sterility, death, and cessation of sexual activity. In many societies, this effective reproductive span is interrupted by time between successive unions or by temporary separation of spouses. Within the effective reproductive span, the pace of childbearing is determined by the lengths of the successive intervals between births (B1, B2, and so on in Figure 3–4). *Birth intervals* in the absence of deliberate family planning will be discussed first. The birth interval may be divided into several segments:

- the postpartum period after a birth until both *ovulation* and *sexual relations* resume
- the *time to conception*
- *additional time* due to fetal loss through spontaneous abortion
- the *pregnancy leading to the next live birth*

### Fertility in the Absence of Contraception and Induced Abortion

The postpartum period ends when both ovulation and intercourse have resumed. It is largely determined by the duration and intensity of breastfeeding and by postpartum prohibitions against intercourse by a nursing mother. Women who do not breastfeed usually menstruate for the first time about two months after the birth (Salber, Feinleib, & MacMahon, 1966), whereas frequent, intense breastfeeding can postpone average time of ovulation to more than 20 months (Wood, Lai, Johnson, Campbell, & Maslar, 1985). Some populations, particularly in sub-Saharan Africa, have traditionally had prohibitions against intercourse that can increase the postpartum period beyond the resumption of ovulation, but these practices are rare outside this region and their observance is believed to be decreasing. Therefore, breastfeeding not only provides the child with nourishment but also, depending on the pattern of suckling, can postpone the return of ovulation for many months.

Breastfeeding exerts this effect through a maternal response to suckling that suppresses the secretion of gonadotrophins. The classic studies of McNeilly (1996) and his coworkers have shown, for women in Edinburgh, that if the frequency of suckling is maintained above five times a day and the duration is maintained above 65 minutes a day, amenorrhea will often be the consequence. Others have found that nightfeeds are particularly important in maintaining amenorrhea (Jones, 1988). In addition, demographic studies suggest that the duration of lactational amenorrhea increases with the age of the woman (Wood, 1994). The effects of breastfeeding patterns are so important that they are the major factor in explaining differences in fertility among populations in which no family planning was practiced.

The time to conception depends upon the monthly probability of conception in the absence of birth control and can vary among populations, by age and according to the frequency and pattern of intercourse. The monthly probability of conception, known as *fecundability*,

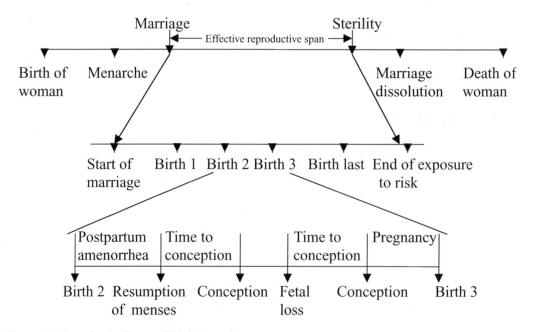

**Figure 3–4** Reproductive Span and Birth Intervals

is extremely difficult to measure, and available estimates differ in part because of the methods used to determine that a conception has occurred. If early fetal loss occurs before the woman is aware she is pregnant, then the estimates of conception are biased downward. According to Wood (1994), the best recent study of early fetal loss is by Wilcox et al. (1988), who followed a group of women aged 20–35 and collected blood and urine samples regularly. There were 198 pregnancies detected by assays of these samples; 43, or about 22%, were lost before the woman realized she was pregnant and before clinical diagnosis. Usually, however, fecundability has been measured by accepting a woman's report of her pregnancy. This measure of *apparent* fecundability has yielded values that range from about 0.1 to 0.3 for relatively young women (Menken, 1975; Wood, 1994). The average waiting time to conception is the inverse of fecundability, so that this time is, for younger women, 3–10 months. In many cases, fecundability has been estimated from reported waiting times to conception using a variety of mathematical models (some of which are summarized by Wood, 1994).

Fecundability depends in part on a couple's frequency and pattern of intercourse, which determines the likelihood that coitus will occur during the woman's fertile period. Both those wishing to conceive a wanted child and those hoping to avoid pregnancy without the use of hormonal or barrier contraceptives depend on knowledge of the woman's cycle to time their sexual activity and thereby change their probability of conception. Fecundability declines with age, although there is increasing evidence that the decline does not take place until the late 30s, on average, if patterns of intercourse remain unchanged. Lactation has a fertility-reducing effect even after a woman has resumed menstruation and ovulation (John, Menken, & Chowdhury, 1987; Wood, 1994). Apparently, continued suckling beyond ovulation reduces fecundability through a response that interferes with the functioning of the corpus luteum. Although fertilization can occur, the corpus luteum

may not produce sufficient progesterone for the pregnancy to continue (McNeilly, 1996).

Spontaneous abortion occurs frequently; the observed rate, as already described, depends upon how early the pregnancy is detected. From the time conceptions are *recognizable* by virtue of late menses, about 24% end in spontaneous abortion (French & Bierman, 1962). Even higher proportions of fertilized ova do not lead to live births. Wilcox et al. (1988), in the study cited earlier in which urine specimens were collected from which early pregnancy could be detected, found that 31% of the pregnancies ended in fetal loss. Rates of spontaneous abortion increase with the age of the woman (Wood, 1994). The time added to the birth interval by a recognized fetal loss is the sum of the time from pregnancy to the next ovulation (usually estimated to be just more than three months on average, since the vast majority of spontaneous abortions occur very early in pregnancy) plus the time to the next conception. There is little evidence of great variation among populations in the rates of spontaneous abortion.

Gestation leading to a live birth does not vary much, usually lasting between 35 and 40 weeks, with little variation between population groups (Wood, 1994). In some populations with outstanding care of premature infants, gestation may be somewhat shorter on average, but we know of no good data demonstrating a decline in the average duration of gestation.

A crosscutting issue is that of infertility and sterility. There is concern, especially in parts of Africa, that infertility and early sterility are affecting fertility. The effect may be through absolute sterility that causes the effective reproductive span to end early, or through decreased fecundability or increased risk of spontaneous abortion (Larsen, 1993, 1995, 1996). In most cases, however, the concern is with early sterility, much of which is believed to be due to STIs.

Thus the main reasons that populations not practicing family planning vary in fertility are differences in the effective reproductive span and the duration of the postpartum period, with variation in time to conception playing a lesser role.

### Deliberate Control of Fertility

People can deliberately reduce their fertility (1) by reducing the effective reproductive span through postponement of marriage, interrupted marriage, or sterilization that ends reproductive capacity early; (2) by use of contraception (which increases the time to conception); and (3) by induced abortion (which increases the time added to the birth interval by pregnancies that do not lead to a live birth). Family planning programs can promote both the motivation to reduce fertility and the means to do so. Many governments encourage or enforce later marriage explicitly through changes in the legal age of marriage and implicitly through programs that foster female education. Family planning programs have traditionally focused on education regarding methods of fertility control, motivation to reduce the number of wanted children, and provision of family planning methods. These methods include (1) promotion of breastfeeding, both for the health of the infant and to prolong the postpartum period; (2) contraception, intended to prolong the time to conception; and, except where there is opposition for religious reasons, (3) abortion, which increases the time added to the birth interval.

Although specific family planning methods will be discussed in greater detail below, it seems appropriate to consider two important general issues here: (1) Why is it that populations in which the desired number of children is low still have high proportions of unintended births? and (2) Why is reliance on abortion an inefficient approach to family planning?

Contraception, even when highly effective, may still not prevent all unintended pregnancies. A simple calculation makes this problem clear. Suppose a woman is using a highly effective method, one that reduces her probability of conceiving to about .001 per month. She begins using it at age 30 and wants no more children before she reaches menopause at age 45. We can calculate the probability that she has no pregnancy in each of 13 lunar months over the next 15 years—or 195 lunar months. The probability of succeeding (not getting pregnant) is .999 each month. The probability of not getting pregnant in 195 months is $.999^{.195}$, which equals .38. In other words, she only has a 38% chance of avoiding pregnancy for 15 years. Among women like her, 62% will have at least one unintended pregnancy in that time period. For this reason, even women who are serious users of contraception are at high risk of unintended pregnancy. Family planning program and health planners, in developing their programs, usually emphasize unmet need for contraception or problems in the use of various methods. They, however, also need to be aware that even perfectly used contraception with low monthly or annual failure rates carries with it this high long-term risk of unintended pregnancy.

The second point concerns induced abortion. In a population that relies primarily on induced abortion to reduce fertility, if a woman becomes pregnant unintentionally, she may choose to have an abortion. About three months after conception, she again begins ovulating and is capable of conceiving. Suppose her time to conception averages 10 months. Then 13 months after the first abortion, she is again pregnant and must have another abortion if she is not to have an unwanted birth. And 13 months later, again an abortion, and so on. Preventing a birth for 15 years may require that many abortions. It is, therefore, not surprising that many women in Eastern European countries that relied primarily on abortion reported numbers of abortions in the double digits. Women in the former Soviet Union, for example, are believed to have six or more abortions on average over the course of their lifetime (David, 1992). Abortion, is, however, extremely effective as a backup to effective contraception. A woman who has an abortion and subsequently uses extremely effective contraception is unlikely to have more than one or two unintended pregnancies—but our previous analysis shows that she may have one or two.

For these reasons, it is not surprising that sterilization, the one method that has a failure rate near zero, is so widely selected by women and couples who want no additional children. In the United States in 1995 it was the modal method selected by couples where the woman was over 30 (Weeks, 1999).

### The Effect on Fertility of the Proximate Determinants: Bongaarts's Indexes

Bongaarts (1978) developed a set of indexes to measure the effect on fertility of some of these proximate determinants. They are based on the assumption that there is some maximum potential fertility, *TF*, for women. This figure is usually estimated to be just over 15 children.

$C_i$ **The index of postpartum infecundity** varies from 0 to 1. It represents the proportion of potential fertility, *TF*, remaining when the average postpartum period of the population of interest is taken into account. Therefore, $C_i = 1$ if the population does not breastfeed at all. The *fertility reducing* effect of postpartum infecundity is $(1-C_i)$.

$C_A$ **The index of abortion** is the proportion of *TF*, *after postpartum infecundity is first taken into account*, remaining when the effect of induced abortion in reducing live births is taken into account. Spontaneous abortions are included in the original estimate of *TF*, since they are treated as a purely biological occurrence. Few countries have sufficient information available on abortion to make reasonable estimates of $C_A$, so it usually must be disregarded in application.

$C_C$ **The index of contraception** is the proportion of *TF*, after the effects of postpartum infecundity and induced abortion are taken into account, remaining after contraceptive use is considered; and, finally,

$C_m$ **The index of marriage** is the proportion of *TF*, after the first three factors are considered, remaining when the particular marriage or sexual union pattern is taken into account.

Thus, in the Bongaarts decomposition of the Total Fertility Rate,

$$TFR = TF \times C_i \times C_A \times C_C \times C_m.$$

It should be noted that both $C_C$ and $C_m$ contain adjustments for infertility or sterility. In the first, the adjustment takes into account infertility and sterility and assumes no use of contraception by infertile and sterile couples. In the second, there is a weighting factor, in that nonmarriage has a greater effect on fertility reduction when the woman is young; for example, the effect of nonmarriage is much greater for a 25-year-old than a 42-year-old.

Table 3–2 presents these indexes, except for $C_A$, which is assumed to be 1.0 because of lack of data, for a number of populations around 1970 and for several historical populations (Bongaarts & Potter, 1983). The major impact of breastfeeding can be seen through the values of the index $C_i$ in countries that, at the period in question, used little contraception. All the South and East Asian countries, as well as Kenya, have indexes that do not exceed 0.67; thus their potential fertility is reduced by at least one-third by long postpartum periods. In fact, the long breastfeeding practiced in Bangladesh and Indonesia at that period reduced their fertility to only about half its potential. In Europe the demographic transition to low levels of fertility was caused, to a great extent, by late marriage and a relatively high degree of nonmarriage. The index of marriage is far lower, on average, for the industrialized countries around 1970 than for the low- and middle-income countries. But two historical populations shown had indexes of marriage under .45, indicating that nonmarriage reduced their potential fertility by at least 55%. By 1970 fertility in the industrialized countries shown was reduced by contraceptive use to no more than 30% of its potential level.

Thus, in industrialized countries, breastfeeding has little effect on fertility, but nonmarriage

**Table 3–2** Estimates of Total Fertility Rate and Bongaarts's Proximate Determinants Indexes

| Region (Year) | Total Fertility Rate TFR | Index of Postpartum Infecundity $C_i$ | Index of Marriage $C_m$ | Index of Contraception $C_C$ |
|---|---|---|---|---|
| **Low- and Middle-Income Countries** | | | | |
| Bangladesh (1975) | 6.34 | .54 | .85 | .90 |
| Colombia (1976) | 4.57 | .84 | .58 | .61 |
| Dominican Republic (1975) | 5.85 | .61 | .60 | 1.0 |
| Indonesia (1976) | 4.69 | .58 | .71 | .75 |
| Jordan (1976) | 7.41 | .80 | .74 | .81 |
| Kenya (1976) | 8.02 | .67 | .77 | 1.0 |
| Korea (1970) | 3.97 | .66 | .58 | .68 |
| Lebanon (1976) | 4.77 | .78 | .58 | .69 |
| Sri Lanka (1975) | 3.53 | .61 | .51 | .74 |
| Syria (1973) | 7.00 | .73 | .73 | .86 |
| Thailand (1975) | 4.70 | .66 | .63 | .74 |
| **Industrialized Countries** | | | | |
| Denmark (1970) | 1.78 | .93 | .55 | .23 |
| France (1972) | 2.21 | .93 | .52 | .30 |
| Hungary (1966) | 1.80 | .93 | .62 | .21 |
| United Kingdom (1967) | 2.38 | .93 | .61 | .27 |
| United States (1967) | 2.34 | .93 | .63 | .26 |
| **Historical Populations** | | | | |
| Bavarian Villages (1700–1850) | 4.45 | .85 | .37 | .91 |
| Grafenhausen (1700–1850) | 4.74 | .67 | .44 | 1.0 |
| Hutterites | 9.50 | .82 | .73 | 1.0 |
| Quebec (1700–1730) | 8.00 | .81 | .63 | 1.0 |

*Note:* Each index represents the proportion of potential fertility remaining after the particular factor is taken into account in the order: postpartum infecundity, marriage, and contraceptive use.

and use of contraception reduce the TFR to relatively low levels. In the 1970s contraceptive use had little impact on fertility in the low- and middle income countries shown in Table 3–2, including Bangladesh, for which additional information is given in Exhibit 3–2; lower fertility was achieved in some of these countries through long-term breastfeeding. Populations that had high TFRs achieved them through a combination of high indexes of marriage and breastfeeding and little or no contraception.

### More Recent Estimates of the Effects of Proximate Determinants: Stover's Revision of the Bongaarts's Indexes

The indexes of the effects of the proximate determinants on fertility have been revised a number of times by Bongaarts and others in order to take advantage of newly available, more detailed and reliable data and substitute more realistic assumptions. Stover's (1998) reformulation, for example, drops the original indexes

**Exhibit 3–2** Proximate Determinants of Fertility in Bangladesh

As shown in Table 3–2, fertility in Bangladesh was estimated to be about 6.3 in 1975. (This estimate differs somewhat from the United Nations figure given in Exhibit 3–1 for the same period due to different data sources used.) This high fertility was due to the combination of almost universal marriage for women of reproductive age ($C_m$ = .85) and little fertility control within marriage ($C_C$ = .90). Fertility could, however, have been much higher but for prolonged amenorrhea, which is related to the long breastfeeding practiced in this country. Total fertility was just over half (.54) of what it would have been if women had not breastfed at all. In fact, relative to the other countries with little contraceptive use and high proportions married, Bangladesh fertility was quite low.

Some early family planning programs specifically targeted women who had just delivered a baby. The rationale was that a woman would be more likely, at that point in her life, to be thinking about whether she wanted more children and, if she did, whether she would prefer to postpone the next birth. One of the lessons from the study of proximate determinants in Bangladesh and elsewhere is that contraceptive use in the postpartum period simply overlaps with a woman's natural immunity to conception and therefore fails to provide any additional protection against unintended pregnancy. This finding has been used by program designers in thinking about how best to use their scarce resources.

of marriage and contraceptive use ($C_m$ and $C_C$). Instead, more recent data permit him to treat infertility, sterility, and sexual activity more directly than was possible earlier (Table 3–3). He includes three new indexes:

$C_x$ **The index of sexual activity** depends on the reported proportion of women in the population who are sexually active. Its interpretation is, therefore, the proportion of potential fertility remaining after celibacy is taken into account.

$C_f$ **The index of infecundity** reflects the effect on fertility of infecundity among sexually active women and is simply 1-*inf*, where *inf* is the proportion that reports that they believe themselves infecund.

$C_u$ **The index of contraceptive use** reflects actual contraceptive use by women who believe themselves to be fecund and who are not experiencing postpartum amenorrhea.

Thus, the fertility reducing effect of the proximate determinants is given by

$$C_x \times C_i \times C_a \times C_u \times C_f$$

where, again, the index of abortion can rarely be estimated.

These results show that the two main factors producing lower fertility in Latin America are relatively low participation in sexual activity and relatively high contraceptive use. By contrast, in most countries of Africa there is much higher participation in sexual activity and low use of contraception. Fertility would be even higher were it not for the effects of postpartum infecundity, which reduces fertility by at least 40% in the countries represented here. What is striking is the documentation of the rather large impact on overall fertility (about 20%) in some countries due to infertility among sexually active women.

**FAMILY PLANNING PROGRAMS**

A fundamental rationale for family planning programs is to reduce unintended fertility because of its negative health and welfare consequences and because control of their fertility has been recognized as a human right for women and

**Table 3–3** Estimates of Total Fertility Rate and Bongaarts's Revised Proximate Determinants Indexes

| Region (Year) | Total Fertility Rate | Index of Sexual Activity $C_x$ | Index of Postpartum Infecundity $C_i$ | Index of Infecundity $C_f$ | Index of Contraceptive Use $C_u$ |
|---|---|---|---|---|---|
| **Africa** | | | | | |
| Burkina Faso (1993) | 6.9 | .66 | .49 | .88 | .94 |
| Cameroon (1991) | 5.8 | .69 | .57 | .81 | .84 |
| Ghana (1993) | 5.5 | .64 | .55 | .86 | .81 |
| Madagascar (1992) | 6.1 | .71 | .61 | .83 | .89 |
| Namibia (1992) | 5.4 | .59 | .59 | .86 | .70 |
| Niger (1992) | 7.4 | .86 | .58 | .78 | 1.0 |
| Nigeria (1990) | 6.0 | .73 | .53 | .80 | .93 |
| Rwanda (1992) | 6.2 | .60 | .56 | .85 | .86 |
| Senegal (1993) | 6.0 | .63 | .56 | .81 | .93 |
| Zambia (1992) | 6.5 | .69 | .60 | .86 | .90 |
| **Latin America and the Caribbean** | | | | | |
| Brazil (1991) | 3.7 | .59 | .83 | .88 | .39 |
| Colombia (1990) | 2.9 | .53 | .77 | .89 | .36 |
| Dominican Republic (1991) | 3.3 | .54 | .81 | .88 | .41 |
| Paraguay (1990) | 4.7 | .49 | .76 | .86 | .47 |
| Peru (1992) | 3.5 | .55 | .68 | .89 | .53 |

couples. Over the past 50 years, societal changes have occurred that include reduced infant mortality, increased urbanization, improved education for women, increased economic opportunities, and the dissemination and adoption of modern ideas about small families. The response by couples in the low- and middle-income countries has been accelerated change in expectations about both the number and timing of births (Bongaarts, 1983; Freedman, 1987). Programs that subsidized the cost of family planning services were found in 155 countries in 1997 (Gelbard, Haub, & Kent, 1999). In Bangladesh, for example, high proportions report wanting no more children (see Exhibit 3–3). However, in part due to the lack of available, accessible, and effective contraception, there has been a growing gap between observed and desired fertility that, in turn, has led to an increase in unintended fertility (Bankole & Westoff, 1995; Bulatao, 1998). In Bangladesh it has been estimated that

18% of women expressing desire to control their fertility have not been able to meet this need (see Exhibit 3–3).

**Unintended Fertility**

A number of definitional issues underlie estimates of unintended fertility and its distribution. In general, data on unintended fertility come from representative population surveys in which one of two measurement approaches, direct or indirect, has been taken.

The direct approach is to ask women who are pregnant at the time of the survey or have had at least one birth in the five years prior to the survey whether each of those births (including the outcome of the current pregnancy) was intended or unintended. A birth can be classified as unintended either because it exceeds the woman's reported desired number of births or because it came too early but is still within the

**Exhibit 3–3** Desired Family Size and Unmet Need for Contraception in Bangladesh

One rationale for family planning programs was that couples who wanted to have fewer children were unable to do so either because they lacked knowledge of the means of fertility control or access to those means, through lack of supplies or services. Even in the earliest surveys carried out in Bangladesh, a high proportion of married women reported they wanted no more children. In 1969, 44% reported they did not want to have another child. This proportion had risen only slightly by the early 1980s, but by 1996 nearly 58% reported wanting no more (Cleland, Phillips, Amin, & Kamal, 1994). Remarkably, the proportion wanting to stop at two or three children has risen more than 20 percentage points in just 13 years.

In the most recent survey (1996), when asked their ideal number of children, women under 30 and women with 2 or fewer children report 2.1–2.4 children as ideal, while those 30–49 or with 3+ children respond with 2.4–3.0 on average. Yet, before the inception of well-run family planning programs, among the barriers to achieving this low fertility were the economic costs of access to services, including the cost of transportation, and supplies; the social costs, both of travel by women whose mobility was traditionally constrained; the psychic costs of use in a society that offered little social or familial support for low fertility; and the health costs of side effects, whether subjective or objective, from contraceptive use.

These barriers have been overcome to the extent that 50% of married women of reproductive age are current contraceptive users; yet the 1994 data in Table 3–8 show that for 18%, their need was still unmet.

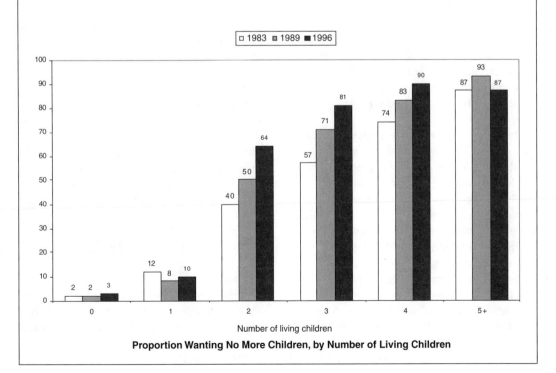

Proportion Wanting No More Children, by Number of Living Children

desired number of births. The latter are often called *mistimed births,* while the former are referred to as *unwanted* (Tsui et al., 1997). Unfortunately usage of these terms is not completely consistent; some authors include mistimed births as part of their estimates of unwanted births, while others count only those births that exceed the desired family size as unwanted (Brown & Eisenberg, 1995).

The indirect approach to unintended fertility does not focus on the intendedness of specific births. Instead, women are asked about their ideal family size if they could start all over again. The answers are then averaged for a population, leading to an estimate of the desired TFR. Alternatively, the desired TFR is calculated from the observed births that do not exceed each woman's reported ideal fertility. In a final step, the gap between observed and desired TFRs is transformed into an estimate of the proportion unwanted among all births (Bongaarts, 1990; Cochrane & Sai, 1993).

The major weakness of the direct approach is that women may be reluctant to classify specific births as unwanted, leading to artificially low estimates of unwanted births. The major weakness of the indirect approach is that it asks a hypothetical question, which may not be particularly meaningful. On the other hand, it avoids the problem of mothers' unwillingness to classify a specific birth as unwanted (Bongaarts, 1991; Tsui et al., 1997).

Both methods have been criticized because they rely exclusively on mothers' intentions and not the intentions of other family members, most importantly fathers, to gauge unintended fertility. It has been argued that the intentions of the mother, especially in many low- and middle-income countries, may not accurately reflect the desirability of a birth. Evidence suggests that intergenerational differences in family size goals (that is, preferences of grandparents versus parents) may be more pronounced than interspousal differences (Caldwell, 1986; Mason & Taj, 1987). Ultimately the justification for relying on the stated preferences of the mother in determining desired family size and unintended

or unwanted births stems from the fact that the mother is the person most responsible for the birth and child care (Tsui et al., 1997).

Demographic and Health Surveys (DHS) have been fielded in more than 50 low- and middle-income countries from 1984 to mid-1999.[*] They are intended to provide comparable information on a variety of subjects related to health and fertility issues. Data from selected DHS surveys show, using the direct method of gauging unwanted births (that is, those exceeding the desired family size), that roughly 15–25% of births are unwanted, with the percentage varying considerably by region (Table 3–4). Sub-Saharan Africa has the lowest proportion of unwanted births (the median percent unwanted for countries in this region is 5%, so that one-half of all countries in the region have 5% or less of births classified as unwanted). North Africa and the Middle East have the highest percent unwanted (the median is 25%). The lowest proportion of unwanted births is in countries with the highest observed TFRs—only 16% of births were unwanted in countries where the TFR is greater than 6. The highest percentages unwanted, roughly about one-third, are in countries with TFRs between 4 and 6. Finally, in low fertility countries where the TFR is below 4 births per woman, around 25% of births are unwanted (Bongaarts, 1990, 1997a).

It is worth noting that this evidence suggests that increases in contraception prevalence rates do not necessarily cause a decline in the proportion of unwanted births and, in fact, may initially be associated with an increase in the proportion of unwanted births. This scenario can happen if desired fertility rates drop faster than the compensating rises in contraceptive prevalence rates and in the use of methods of fertility control so effective that unintended births rarely occur. Thus when couples have high fertility desires, it is difficult to exceed those desires, so nearly all children are wanted. As desired fertility falls, use and effective use of contraception or abortion may not increase quickly enough to avoid

---

[*]Data provided from www.macroint.com/dhs/.

**Table 3–4** Percent Unwanted of Most Recent Birth or Current Pregnancy in Countries with Recent DHS Surveys, by Region

| Region | TFR 1985–1990 | Unwanted Births (%) | | | | |
|---|---|---|---|---|---|---|
| | | Minimum Value | 25th Percentile | 50th Percentile | 75th Percentile | Maximum Value |
| Sub-Saharan Africa | 6.32 | 2 | 4 | 5 | 8 | 22 |
| North Africa and the Middle East | 4.48[a] | 4 | 16 | 25 | 28 | 35 |
| Asia | 3.39 | 9 | 12 | 14 | 15 | 22 |
| Latin America and Caribbean | 3.35 | 10 | 13 | 17 | 35 | 42 |

[a]Calculated from United Nations 1999 for countries with Demographic and Health Surveys arround 1990.

unwanted births. Finally, at low levels of fertility, women want so few children that after the birth of the last wanted child they face preventing pregnancy for many years, during which an unwanted pregnancy and birth can, and frequently do, occur.

With regard to mistimed births, DHS data suggest that roughly 20% of births in the industrialized world are mistimed, that is, they come too early. There are no apparent regional differences in mistimed births and no clear association between contraceptive prevalence and the proportion of mistimed births. Thus, even in a region like sub-Saharan Africa, with very low unwanted fertility, there is still considerable mistimed fertility. This finding suggests that there is a need for contraception to delay first births and control spacing of subsequent births even though there may be little demand for contraception to control the number of births (Bankole & Westoff, 1995).

## Consequences of Unintended Pregnancies and Births

Aside from helping individual couples fulfill their desires and expectations, why should we care about unintended pregnancies and births and, moreover, try to reduce them? A compelling public health reason is their negative consequences. Unintended pregnancies increase the lifetime risk of maternal mortality simply by increasing the number of pregnancies (Koenig, Phillips, Campbell, & D'Souza, 1988). This topic is covered in greater detail in the next section. Unintended pregnancies can lead to unsafe abortion, poor infant health, and lower investment in the child.

### Abortion

In many cases, unintended pregnancies are terminated by abortions, frequently are conducted illegally under unhygienic conditions, and pose significant health risks to the mother. The legal status of abortion and, consequently, access to safe abortion services are highly variable. Roughly 50% of women in the low- and middle-income countries have access to legal abortions. This number is, however, heavily influenced by the fact that abortion is legal in China and India. Outside China and India, 19% of women live in countries where abortion is almost always legal, 52% in countries where it is selectively legal, and 28% in countries where it is always illegal (Henshaw & Morrow, 1990; Population Reference Bureau, 1995). Although data are incomplete, it is estimated that in 1987 there were 26–31 million legal abortions and 10–22 million illegal abortions worldwide (Henshaw & Morrow, 1990). Even where abortion is legal, access is limited, there are poor systems of referral, and services often are of poor quality. For example, despite the fact that manual vacuum extraction is much safer, the most frequently used method for abortion in most countries is dilatation and curettage, which has significant associated morbidity. The World Health Organization (WHO) estimates that there are about 20 million unsafe abortions, that is, those not attended by a trained health professional; these abortions result in about 69,000 deaths in the industrialized world (WHO, 1994a).

Some countries that already have low fertility have relied heavily on legal abortion to achieve low fertility. In those areas, improved access to contraception could help prevent unintended pregnancies. In Hungary, for example, contraceptive use has increased over the past 30 years, with a concomitant reduction in abortion. Similar evidence of a decline in abortion with expansion of contraceptive availability exists for Russia, Kazakhstan, and Korea (DaVanzo & Adamson, 1998).

Another abortion-related issue is the recent rise in the male-to-female sex ratio at birth in Southeast Asia. Data from a number of countries including China and Korea show that the sex ratio at birth is unusually high compared to the expected ratio of 1.06 male births to every female birth, and is steadily increasing. Rising sex ratios at birth suggest that selective abortion of female fetuses may be increasing (Larsen, Chung, & Das Gupta, 1998; Westley, 1995). This practice is embedded in the context of strong societal preferences for male children and declining family size desires, which increase the incentives to have the desired family composition as well as the desired number of children. The recent availability of modern technology has provided the means to actualize these preferences. There are, basically, three different ways of determining the sex of a fetus: chorionic villi sampling, amniocentesis, and ultrasound. Ultrasound is the safest and cheapest method, but only works reliably around five to six months into the pregnancy (that is, the end of the second trimester). It is widely available in rural areas in India, China, and other parts of East Asia. Despite strong legal sanctions against sex-selective abortion, the availability of relatively cheap ultrasound technology has promoted this practice,

leading to deleterious consequences for women and children.

### Consequences for Infant Health

Unintended births are risky for infant health, as they are concentrated in demographically high-risk categories (Tables 3–5 through 3–7), that is, the proportion unintended is much higher in births to young mothers and older mothers, higher parity mothers (where parity is the number of births a woman has had), and following a short birth interval (National Research Council, 1989). Why these demographic characteristics are associated with high risks for infant health is discussed in greater detail below. But unwanted births have higher mortality even when the pregnancy fits into otherwise demographically low-risk categories (mothers aged 24–29 and parity 2–4).

### Human Capital Investments

In addition to deleterious health consequences for the mother and the index child, unintended births have spillover and long-term cumulative effects by reducing human capital investments (that is, allocation of resources for education and health) in the family as a whole. A number of studies in low- and middle-income countries have shown that older children, especially girls, suffer disproportionately in terms of lower educational attainment and health status as family size increases—the latter being a proxy for unwanted births (Bledsoe & Cohen, 1993; Desai, 1995; Frenzen & Hogan, 1982; Lloyd, 1994). Note that cross-sectional associations between large family sizes and lower health and educational attainments need to be interpreted cautiously due to the possibility that parents who choose to have large families may also choose to invest differently in different children (Knodel, Chamrathrithirong, & Debavalya, 1987). There is, however, some evidence, from a family planning quasi-experiment in which villages were assigned different levels of family planning services, that part of the relationship between large family sizes and low human capital investments is causal (Foster & Roy, 1996).

**Table 3–5** Percent Unintended of Most Recent Birth or Current Pregnancy by Mother's Age: Selected Countries

| Country (Year) | Mother's Age | | |
| --- | --- | --- | --- |
| | *<20* | *20–34* | *35+* |
| Bolivia (1993) | 41.5 | 53.9 | 74.0 |
| Colombia (1986) | 34.9 | 48.3 | 60.5 |
| Egypt (1988) | 13.9 | 41.3 | 75.0 |
| Kenya (1993) | 61.2 | 55.3 | 65.4 |
| Nigeria (1990) | 13.7 | 12.5 | 21.6 |
| Philippines (1993) | 37.6 | 46.4 | 58.2 |
| Tanzania (1991) | 22.7 | 26.1 | 31.7 |
| Thailand (1987) | 28.3 | 38.4 | 47.2 |

**Table 3–6** Percent Unintended of Most Recent Birth or Current Pregnancy by Birth Order: Selected Countries

| Country (Year) | Birth Order | | |
| --- | --- | --- | --- |
| | *1* | *2–4* | *5+* |
| Bolivia (1993) | 32.7 | 50.1 | 78.6 |
| Colombia (1986) | 25.0 | 50.7 | 68.8 |
| Egypt (1988) | 3.8 | 39.5 | 67.2 |
| Kenya (1993) | 52.1 | 52.1 | 66.2 |
| Nigeria (1990) | 11.2 | 9.9 | 22.7 |
| Philippines (1993) | 22.3 | 47.4 | 63.6 |
| Tanzania (1991) | 18.7 | 25.0 | 39.5 |
| Thailand (1987) | 20.7 | 36.3 | 64.4 |

**Table 3–7** Percent Unintended of Recent Higher Order Birth or Current Pregnancy by Interval from Previous Birth to Conception: Selected Countries

| Country (Year) | Interval from Previous Birth to Conception | |
| --- | --- | --- |
| | *Birth Interval < 24 Months* | *Birth Interval ≥ 24 Months* |
| Bolivia (1993) | 68.4 | 60.1 |
| Colombia (1986) | 67.6 | 49.2 |
| Egypt (1988) | 54.0 | 50.2 |
| Kenya (1993) | 67.2 | 56.1 |
| Nigeria (1990) | 21.1 | 13.0 |
| Philippines (1993) | 62.1 | 49.3 |
| Tanzania (1991) | 33.5 | 27.5 |
| Thailand (1987) | 53.4 | 36.5 |

## Unmet Need for Contraception

A primary objective of family planning programs has been to reduce unintended births by addressing "the unmet need for contraception." This unmet need is conventionally estimated from representative population-based surveys of currently married women as the sum of the number of currently pregnant women who report that their pregnancy is unintended and the number of currently nonpregnant women who are not using contraception and would not like to have any more children or, at least, none in the next two years (Bankole & Westoff, 1995). On the basis of this definition, unmet need for contraception (Table 3–8) varies between 10–15% of married women in countries with high contraceptive prevalence rates (for example, Colombia, Indonesia, and Thailand) to about 35% of women in countries with low contraceptive prevalence rates (for example, countries in sub-Saharan Africa). For all low- and middle-income countries, the total number of women with unmet need is estimated at 150 million.

The above definition of "unmet need for contraception" has been criticized as an underestimate of actual need because it excludes both currently married women who are not pregnant and who are using inappropriate (because of health consequences or side effects) methods of contraception and sexually active women who are not currently married and who do not wish to become pregnant, at least in the next two years (Bongaarts, 1991; Dixon-Mueller & Germain, 1992; Pritchett, 1994a, 1994b).

Family planning programs have played an important role in reducing unmet need by making contraception physically accessible and financially affordable. Since the late 1950s, when the first national family planning programs in low- and middle-income countries began, there has been a significant increase in the prevalence of contraceptive use. This increase has played an important role in the significant reduction in fertility that has taken place especially over the past 3 decades in these regions, where the average number of births per couple has declined from more than six to fewer than three in the latter half of the twentieth century. Program success in improving contraceptive prevalence rates has, however, been somewhat uneven. It has depended on a number of factors, including a receptive social and family environment that accepts fertility control as legitimate behavior, a favorable political and bureaucratic climate, a management structure that pays close attention to both quality and quantity of services, and reliable sources of funding. Further, the programs that have succeeded have invested considerable resources in evaluation, research, and monitoring of services, and have had the flexibility to adapt to local conditions (Bongaarts, 1997; Bongaarts & Watkins, 1996; Bulatao, 1993, 1998; Freedman, 1987).

There has been a long-standing debate about the relative merits of "demand side" versus "supply side" interventions to reduce unmet need in contraception (Bongaarts, 1997; Pritchett, 1994a, 1994b). Demand-side proponents have argued that improvements in women's socioeconomic status are an essential and necessary prerequisite to the success of family planning programs. Thus educated women with higher status, compared to their less educated and lower status peers, are more likely to know about contraception and seek it out in order to actualize their latent fertility desires. Supply-side proponents, on the other hand, are described as positing that family planning programs, when properly managed, can increase access to and availability of contraception, even in the absence of changes in socioeconomic status of women. Thus they can lead to increased contraceptive prevalence rates and initiation of fertility decline. Table 3–9 shows that the onset of fertility decline is not dependent on any particular threshold in socioeconomic factors, such as levels of urbanization, female education, or infant mortality. Fertility decline appears to have started in a wide range of low- and middle-income countries at quite varied levels of socioeconomic status. Bangladesh is frequently cited as the best example of improved contraceptive prevalence rates and dramatic fertility decline

**Table 3–8** Unmet Need for Contraception for Married Women in Selected Countries

| Region (Year) | Percent with Unmet Need | Number of Women with Unmet Need (1000s) |
|---|---|---|
| **Africa** | | |
| Rwanda (1992) | 37 | 332 |
| Kenya (1993) | 36 | 1,101 |
| Ghana (1994) | 33 | 759 |
| Burkina Faso (1992–1993) | 33 | 522 |
| Tanzania (1991–1992) | 27 | 1,065 |
| Uganda (1988–1989) | 27 | 707 |
| Sudan (1989–1990) | 25 | 940 |
| Nigeria (1990) | 22 | 3,928 |
| Zimbabwe (1994) | 15 | 207 |
| **Asia** | | |
| Pakistan (1991–1992) | 32 | 5,738 |
| Nepal (1991) | 28 | 970 |
| Philippines (1993) | 26 | 2,512 |
| India (1992) | 20 | 31,005 |
| Bangladesh (1994) | 18 | 3,852 |
| Indonesia (1991) | 14 | 4,427 |
| Sri Lanka (1987) | 12 | 332 |
| Thailand (1987) | 11 | 999 |
| **Latin America and the Caribbean** | | |
| Guatemala (1987) | 29 | 382 |
| El Salvador (1985) | 26 | 182 |
| Mexico (1987) | 24 | 3,133 |
| Dominican Republic (1991) | 17 | 171 |
| Peru (1991–1992) | 16 | 471 |
| Brazil (1986) | 13 | 3,034 |
| Colombia (1990) | 12 | 545 |
| **Middle East Crescent** | | |
| Egypt (1992) | 22 | 1,818 |
| Jordan (1990) | 22 | 110 |
| Morocco (1992) | 20 | 650 |
| Tunisia (1988) | 20 | 217 |
| Turkey (1992) | 11 | 1,062 |

in the absence of socioeconomic improvements but in the presence of a well-run focused family planning program (Cleland et al., 1994), although the absence of socioeconomic change has recently come under question (Caldwell, Barkat-e-Khuda, Caldwell, Pieris, & Caldwell, 1999; Menken, Khan, & Williams, 1999). Although there appears to be no magic threshold of socioeconomic development for initiation of fertility decline, the decline is faster in countries with greater levels of socioeconomic development (Bongaarts & Watkins, 1996).

The demand-side versus supply-side debate is basically a false dichotomy. Neither development nor family planning programs are necessary prerequisites, nor is either sufficient to induce fertility decline (Ross & Mauldin, 1996). They work in complementary fashions, with the time scale of their respective impacts being very different. Investments in improving women's status and educational attainment certainly have an important impact in reducing unmet need, but it is a long-term impact. On the other hand, family planning programs can increase access to contraception in the short run and thus enhance knowledge about use and availability and address many of the negative myths about particular methods of contraception. Appropriately crafted and focused media campaigns, implemented as part of family planning programs, can also help legitimize contraception as an acceptable and desirable form of behavior. Moreover, it is important to note that access to the means to limit fertility in and of itself helps improve the status of women. Family planning programs work synergistically with improvements in socioeconomic status and are most effective when there is an informed, educated, empowered client base (Freedman, 1987). In summary, Bongaarts (1997b) estimates that about 40% of the fertility decline in the past three decades of the century in low- and middle-income countries (from a TFR of 6 to 3) can be attributed to family planning programs, and about 60% to changes in socioeconomic status, particularly for women.

### The Challenges Facing Family Planning

Despite significant family planning program success in reducing financial and logistic constraints to contraceptive access, there remains high unmet need for contraception. In recent studies by Bongaarts and Bruce (1995) and Casterline, Perez, and Biddlecom (1996), the major barriers to use of contraception appear to be: (1) lack of knowledge about contraception availability and use, (2) concerns about the deleteri-

ous health consequences of contraception, and (3) opposition from family and community to contraception use.

Given that physical access and financial constraints are not considered to be significant barriers to the use of contraception, the major challenges for family planning revolve around (1) improving the quality of services, particularly in the areas of information exchange and method choice; (2) integration with reproductive health services other than contraception; and (3) financial sustainability.

### Information Exchange

In upgrading the quality of family planning services, the major area of concern is information exchange between providers and clients. The fragmentary evidence that exists suggests that there frequently is inadequate information provided about the proper use of contraceptives, alternatives in the event of nonoptimal use, contraceptive side effects, and the appropriateness of the chosen method for women who have particular health problems (Winikoff, Elias, & Beattie, 1994). For example, quite a few women who are using oral birth control pills do not know that they can make up for a missed day by taking two the next day. Similarly, not enough women know that birth control pills should not be used if a woman is a smoker or has a heart condition (Trottier, Potter, Taylor, & Glover, 1994). In general, far fewer than 50% of women have meaningful knowledge about contraceptive methods (Bongaarts & Bruce, 1995). This lack of specific knowledge often leads to exaggerated notions of the health risks of contraception (Casterline et al., 1996). It is worth reiterating that contraception is, by and large, safe, especially when compared to the health risks deriving from an unplanned pregnancy. Ross and Frankenberg (1993) have estimated that the mortality risk of an unplanned, unwanted pregnancy is 20 times the risk of any modern contraceptive method and 10 times the risk of a properly performed abortion. Although the past two decades have witnessed great success in social marketing, whereby most women

**Table 3–9** Socioeconomic Indicators at the Start of Fertility Transition in Selected Countries

| Region | Start of Fertility Transition[a] | SNP per Capita[b] | Infant Mortality Rate | Female Secondary Enrollment | Percent Urban | Start of Population Program |
|---|---|---|---|---|---|---|
| **East Asia** | | | | | | |
| Indonesia | 1975 | 253 | 100 | 15 | 19 | 1968 |
| South Korea | 1960 | 550 | 70 | 14 | 28 | 1961 |
| Philippines | 1970 | 488 | 66 | 50 | 33 | 1970 |
| Thailand | 1970 | 471 | 73 | 15 | 13 | 1970 |
| **South Asia** | | | | | | |
| Bangladesh | 1975 | 138 | 138 | 11 | 9 | 1971 |
| India | 1965 | 218 | 150 | 13 | 19 | 1965 |
| Pakistan | 1985 | 304 | 113 | 8 | 30 | 1960 |
| Sri Lanka | 1965 | 216 | 63 | 35 | 20 | 1965 |
| **Latin America** | | | | | | |
| Brazil | 1965 | 889 | 104 | 16 | 50 | 1974 |
| Colombia | 1965 | 676 | 86 | 16 | 54 | 1970 |
| Costa Rica | 1965 | 1,109 | 72 | 25 | 38 | 1968 |
| Mexico | 1975 | 1,504 | 64 | 28 | 63 | 1974 |
| **Sub-Saharan Africa** | | | | | | |
| Botswana | 1980 | 721 | 63 | 22 | 15 | 1971 |
| Kenya | 1980 | 358 | 83 | 16 | 16 | 1967 |
| Zimbabwe | 1970 | 544 | 96 | 6 | 17 | 1968 |

[a]Fertility transitions are dated from initial declines of at least 0.7 point in total fertility over a 5-year period, following Bulatao and Elwan (1985).

[b]Constant 1987 U.S. dollars; these and other indicators are as of the fertility transition date.

are aware of the benefits of small families and the existence and availability of contraception, much more needs to be done to educate women about method choice and associated health risks and benefits.

Although concern about information exchange in family planning programs is long-standing, progress in addressing this problem is uneven. An issue that comes up repeatedly is whether there is a quality-quantity tradeoff. Program managers voice a common complaint that they have their hands full just providing physical access to contraceptives. Many feel they do not have the luxury of providing extensive information about contraception because of the time-intensive nature of this type of activity.

It is important to recognize that there actually is little contradiction or trade-off between paying attention to quality issues and achieving quantity targets for numbers of users. The two are integrally linked in several ways. First, the key steps needed to improve quality—such as attention to logistics, adequate supervision, motivation of workers at every level, real feedback to managers and supervisors, accountability for supplies and money—are exactly those steps needed to improve quantity. Second, family planning services are inseparable from information provision. In fact, provision of information is one of the key services that a family planning program can offer. Third, attention to quality will improve efficiency and will allow the addition of new users without new costs (Tsui et al., 1997).

### Contraceptive Use and Method Choice

Modern contraceptive methods are now so widely available in the low- and middle-income countries that about one-third of all couples outside of China and more than half of all couples in the industrialized world in which the woman is of reproductive age are users (Robey, Rutstein, & Morris, 1992). Table 3–10 shows the worldwide distribution of use according to method. In addition to demonstrating the great variation in use, the data are remarkable in that they show that, for much of the world, a high proportion of those couples using contraception are using sterilization—the one method that has almost zero risk of failure.

It is much harder to judge how much *choice* of method women in the low- and middle-income countries have, and how their array of choices has changed in recent years. With the exception of sub-Saharan Africa, where contraceptive prevalence rates are low, there was significant progress in overall method availability in most countries between 1982 and 1994 (Ross & Mauldin, 1996). In all 22 countries (with the exception of Nigeria) where DHS surveys were conducted between 1990–1993, at least half of all women had heard of at least one modern contraceptive method, and in 13 of these countries more than 90% of women knew of at least one contraceptive method (Curtis & Neitzel, 1996).

Of great concern is the fact that there has been relatively little innovation in contraceptive technology in the past 30 years, so that, in an era of increasing expectations for contraception, the menu of choices has not expanded greatly. This is largely a function of lack of funding (Harrison & Rosenfield, 1996; Tsui et al., 1997). In some situations, however, knowledge and use of existing technology have not been widely disseminated. One example is emergency contraception (the prevention of pregnancy through the use of contraceptive methods after unprotected sex), for which appropriate technologies (for example, a combination of oral contraceptive pills, progestin-only pills, and the copper T IUD)

have long been available but are not used by many women who could benefit from them (for example, victims of coercive sex) (International Planned Parenthood Foundation, 1995; Trussell, Ellertson, & Stewart, 1996).

### Political, Social, and Financial Constraints

While high unmet need is in part a function of specific management deficiencies in family planning programs, it is important to recognize that broader political and societal constraints also play a role. Kenney (1993) has identified the policies in a variety of countries that retard access to safe contraception. They include: (1) health and safety regulations that restrict choice of methods or providers (for example, the failure to approve oral contraceptives for use in Japan for more than 35 years, until June 1999 [Goto, Reich, & Aitken, 1999]— after the male impotence-relieving drug Viagra received endorsement early in 1999, within 6 months of application for approval [*New York Times*, 1999b]); (2) taxes and barriers to trade that affect importation of contraceptives; (3) regulation of advertising (usually due to concerns about modesty and privacy); and (4) restrictions on private sector involvement in family planning. In addition, law and policies in many countries restrict or forbid access to abortion.

In any discussion of family planning programs and their performance, the issue of financial sustainability is key. Family planning expenditures in low- and middle-income countries as a whole are estimated to be slightly under US$10 billion annually or roughly about $1–2 per person per year for the year 2000. In the past two decades, most of this expense has been paid for by national governments (50%) and individual households (20%), with international donor assistance accounting for only about 30% of the total. If donor assistance for family planning were to keep pace with the historical record of 30%, it would have had to rise substantially from its 1994 level of US$1.37 billion to US$3.0 billion in the year 2000. However, there has been a decline rather than an increase in funding

**Table 3–10** Percent Using Contraception, 1998: Married Couples[a] in which the Woman Is of Reproductive Age, by Region

| Region | Total | Sterilization | | Pill | IUD | Condom | Supply Methods[b] | Nonsupply Methods[c] |
|---|---|---|---|---|---|---|---|---|
| | | Female | Male | | | | | |
| **World** | 58 | 19 | 4 | 8 | 13 | 4 | 3 | 8 |
| **Low and Middle-Income Regions** | 55 | 21 | 4 | 6 | 14 | 2 | 2 | 5 |
| Africa | 20 | 2 | 0.1 | 7 | 4 | 1 | 2 | 4 |
| Asia | 60 | 24 | 5 | 5 | 17 | 3 | 2 | 4 |
| Latin America & Caribbean | 66 | 28 | 1 | 14 | 7 | 4 | 2 | 9 |
| Oceania | 29 | 9 | 0.2 | 5 | 1 | 1 | 6 | 7 |
| **Industrialized Regions** | 70 | 9 | 5 | 17 | 6 | 14 | 2 | 19 |
| Japan | 59 | 3 | 1 | 0.4 | 2 | 46 | 1 | 6 |
| Europe | 72 | 3 | 2 | 20 | 8 | 10 | 2 | 26 |
| Northern America | 71 | 24 | 14 | 15 | 1 | 10 | 4 | 3 |
| Australia/ New Zealand | 76 | 26 | 12 | 23 | 5 | 6 | 1 | 4 |

*Notes:* Most recent data available as of June 1998, pertaining approximately to 1993.

[a]Including, where possible, those in consensual unions.

[b]Other methods requiring supplies or medical services, including injectables, diaphragms, cervical caps, and spermicides.

[c]Including periodic abstinence or rhythm, withdrawal, douche, total sexual abstinence if practiced for contraceptive reasons, traditional methods, and other methods not separately reported.

over the past few years. In particular, the share of funding provided by the United States, by far the largest historical donor for family planning programs, has fallen by about 30%. In the coming decades, rising demand for contraception and increasing budget constraints will require that programs either mobilize more public resources or increase the cost of family planning services to the individual, so that more users can be accommodated (Bulatao, 1998).

### The Broader Effects of Family Planning Programs

Even before the 1994 International Conference on Population and Development in Cairo, concerns were expressed by women's groups and policy makers about the effects of family planning programs on the lives of individual women. Family planning programs have been criticized as exclusively concerned with reducing population growth. Studies in recent years have broadened research to include consideration of the effects of programs on quality of life for women. In particular, the Women's Studies Project (1999) found that family planning programs provided benefits to women:

• Most women and men are convinced that practicing family planning and having smaller families provide health and economic benefits.

- Family planning offers freedom from fear of unplanned pregnancy and can improve sexual life, partner relations and family well-being.
- Where jobs are available, family planning users are more likely than non-users to take advantage of work opportunities.
- Family planning helps women meet their practical needs and is necessary, but not sufficient, to help them meet their strategic needs. (Women's Studies Project, 1999, p. 2)

But the Project also found costs to women:

- Contraceptive side effects—real or perceived—are a serious concern for many women, more so than providers realize.
- When partners or others are opposed, practicing family planning can increase women's vulnerability.
- When women have smaller families, they may lose the security of traditional roles and face new and sometimes difficult challenges, including the burden of multiple responsibilities at home and work. (Women's Studies Project, 1999, p.2)

They also found the exclusion of men from most family planning programs affected the ability of women to take advantage of their services, since men play a dominant role in family planning decisions.

Most family planning programs have emphasized only the positive benefits of family planning; they are now being urged to pay attention to at least some of these broader considerations.

## A Broader Definition of Family Planning and Reproductive Health Programs

As discussed earlier, the 1994 ICPD brought about an international reevaluation of the conceptualization of family planning programs. They are now viewed as part of a larger rubric of more general reproductive health services and interventions, some of which are directly health related, while others are related indirectly. It is useful, however, to first consider conventional family planning programs.

## *Organization and Structure of Family Planning Programs*

While nearly all low- and middle-income countries have established infrastructure to deliver family planning services, their organization varies markedly. One exemplification, Bangladesh, is discussed in Exhibit 3–4. According to Tsui et al. (1997), successful performance is influenced by a focused commitment to achieving program objectives and access to adequate resources. At the national level, strong leadership, clearly formulated policies, explicit goals and objectives, and a clear agenda for meeting those goals can all contribute to the success of programs. In some countries, political commitment is evidenced by placing the family planning program under a national supervisory council or by establishing a separate ministry. Programs also need ways of assessing progress toward meeting their objectives. Indicators such as contraceptive prevalence, proportion of unwanted births, maternal mortality, pregnancy complications and their management, and actual fertility all provide information that, over time, can permit program evaluation. Therefore, one element of successful programs is the definition of result measures to be used and establishment of mechanisms for collecting the needed information. Caution is, however, in order. For example, goals that are defined in terms of targets, such as number of acceptors of particular methods in a given time, may lead workers to exert pressure on clients and reduce their options.

Family planning service programs have focused on a narrow set of goals—reducing unwanted fertility by providing access to the means of fertility control. Several models have been used for the design of programs. In the vertical model, family planning administration and service delivery are carried out by staff for whom this is their single function. In a second model, there is a separate family planning administration unit, but field staff at each level of the health care system can deliver a variety of linked services. In practice, the linkage between family planning and maternal and child health services has been the most common. Under the new

**Exhibit 3–4** The Bangladesh Family Planning Program

Family planning in Bangladesh can be traced to the private Family Planning Association created in 1953, before Bangladesh achieved its independence from Pakistan. By 1960 Pakistan had begun public sector programs, which Bangladesh continued after becoming a nation in 1971. The overall program has grown and changed over the years, but throughout there has been high-level political support and considerable funding from external donors. The program has emphasized provision of services, outreach activities at the village level, and mass communication through a variety of media.

As part of the early 1960s public sector programs, family planning services were offered in government health clinics as part of regular health services. A system of using village aides to provide education was established but abandoned after only 18 months for a variety of reasons, including poor training of the aides, complaints that their services were directed only to family planning and not to other health problems, inadequate resources, and poor supervision. It was followed by renewed efforts run by a new Family Planning Board independent of the Ministry of Health.

Their efforts in the late 1960s met with little success, primarily because of poor quality services provided by a program that had been instituted on a large scale, with little pilot testing and poor organization. The program emphasized the IUD, which was met with resistance by many concerned about side effects and problems with its use. It did not help that the program was seen by many as having been imposed on Bangladesh, then East Pakistan, by a government whose political support was declining.

In the aftermath of the war for independence, although the health and social sectors of the government were particularly negatively affected, it was felt that family planning was urgently needed. A large and complex program was established. A separate Population Wing was created within the Ministry of Health and Population to run the program. Thus health and family planning services were separated. At the local level, the primary health care staff was predominantly male. In a society where, because there can be little interaction between women and men who are not members of their families, male workers cannot provide maternal and child health services except for immunizations. This staffing was a legacy of early programs to combat smallpox, tuberculosis, and malaria; it was ill-suited to the new focus. By contrast, local family planning workers were women, although their supervisors were men. They go directly to households and offer family planning counseling and free supplies. They spend some time on maternal and child health, although they are not well trained for this purpose.

Over the years, the program has continued to be revised and expanded. In all cases, the elements of strong political support, strong financial support, and extensive administrative support have remained.

broader definition of reproductive health, it is expected that other types of services will be offered, so that the ways in which they are linked, both administratively and in provision of care, will have to be addressed.

Whatever model is followed, the program design involves decisions on which services will be offered and at which level of the health care system. Tsui et al. (1997) illustrate the possibilities as follows:

| Level | Interventions for prevention and management of unintended pregnancies |
|---|---|
| *Community* | Information, education, and communication programs |
| | Community-based distribution |
| | Social marketing of condoms, oral pills |
| *Health Post* | Counseling/screening for contraception |
| | Counseling and referral for menstrual regulation or abortion |
| | Provision of injectable contraceptives |

IUD insertions
Counseling and treatment of
contraceptive side effects

**Health Center**    Menstrual regulation/manual
vacuum aspiration abortion
Performing surgical
contraception on set days
Postabortion counseling and
contraception
Counseling and treatment of
contraceptive side effects

**District Hospital** Surgical contraception
Abortions through 20 weeks,
where indicated
Postabortion counseling and
contraception*

Their report concludes that the breadth and scope of the services to be delivered present a formidable challenge in design, execution, administration, and evaluation. Even if this challenge is met, a program can falter if inadequate resources are allocated to meet its needs for trained staff, equipment, and supplies. Additional demands will be placed on whatever system is in place if services related more generally to reproductive health are provided. Research on design and implementation can help improve family planning and reproductive health programs. Exhibit 3–5 illustrates the approach taken by Bangladesh in this regard.

### Additional Reproductive Health Care Services

Some reproductive health services are closely linked to contraception; it is likely that, without

*Source:* Reprinted with permission from A.O. Tsui, J.N. Wasserheit, and J.G. Haaga, eds., *Reproductive Health in Developing Countries. Expanding, Dimensions, Building Solutions.* Panel on Reproductive Health, Committee on Population, Commission on Behavioral and Social Sciences, and Education, Copyright 1997 by the National Research Council. Courtesy of the National Academy Press, Washington, D.C.

much added expense, they can be integrated into conventional family planning programs relatively easily. These may include pregnancy tests, Pap smears, and screening for STIs. The latter has been carried out, in many cases, only in the context of separate programs to treat STIs. That type of intervention misses the general population of women who may not realize that they are infected or know that they may pass their infection to their unborn or nursing children.

HIV/AIDS deserves special mention. The United Nations convened a conference in 1999 to assess progress since the 1994 ICPD. It concluded that the earlier conference had greatly underestimated the effects of HIV/AIDS on the populations of the low- and middle-income countries and called for specific programs and targets to reduce the spread of infection (*New York Times*, 1999c). Directly related to the family planning realm is their call for greater access to methods such as the female and male condoms that can reduce or prevent transmission of the virus.

Other desirable reproductive health interventions remain within the health realm, as can be seen in Exhibit 3–6, but require significant changes in staffing and significantly more financial resources. These include emergency obstetrics, general women's health services, abortion services where they are not already available, infertility services, and greatly expanded testing and counseling for HIV/AIDS. Some infertility services are already provided within the context of programs to reduce STIs, since these are a major cause of infertility and premature sterility (Tsui et al., 1997). But the others are generally lacking; however, without considerable expansion of the financial base for family planning and for the expanded reproductive health program, it is unlikely that these services can be provided in many of the low- and middle-income countries.

### Reproductive Health beyond Direct Health Care

Reproductive health interventions that go beyond the health care realm, while clearly valuable, are not linked in any obvious way to conventional family planning services. The

**Exhibit 3–5** Research To Improve the Family Planning Program in Bangladesh

How well does a family planning program work? Few experiments in applied research have been conducted to determine whether a particular design is effective in reaching the objectives of the program. The International Centre for Diarrhoeal Disease Research, Bangladesh (ICDDR,B) has carried out just these kinds of operations research experiments, which have served to improve the ways in which services are delivered within the Bangladesh family planning program.

An early effort, in 1975, was intended to test the hypothesis that there was latent demand for family planning. ICDDR,B maintains a field station in Matlab, approximately 40 km from the capital, Dhaka. A family planning program was introduced in roughly half of the area in which the center provided services, while people living in the remainder had access only to standard government or private services. Local women, mostly illiterate widows, were hired to visit households about every 90 days to offer oral contraception to women. Later, condoms were added to the offerings. The hypothesis was that couples wanted to reduce the fertility and would do so if only they were supplied with the means. Initial acceptance was good; prevalence of use rose in the early stage to almost 20% from its near-zero level prior to the program. But within less than nine months, it had dropped, so that the program area prevalence was only 6 percentage points higher than in the comparison area. Lessons learned: this type of demand-oriented program was inadequate in a situation where women and couples had little social support for contraceptive use. Rather, a system that addressed the noneconomic costs of use—whether social, psychological, or based on health concerns—was essential. In addition, there were problems with a daily pill regimen, and condoms were not popular. Analysis of the experiment through interviews with people in the community also demonstrated the importance of the characteristics of the family planning worker. Women who had little status in the community and who were past the reproductive age themselves did not have sufficient credibility to help others withstand the social costs of use. Improving access was simply not enough.

A subsequent experiment begun in 1978 tested better follow-up for users, an expanded set of method choices, employment of better educated younger women, and new management strategies. These were undertaken to ensure that there were regular visits and that problems were addressed rapidly. A new dual leadership system was introduced in which there was both technical (paramedical) and administrative supervision. The interval between visits was reduced to 14 days. Within a year, nearly one-third of women in the study area were users, while there was little change in the comparison area. Increases in contraceptive use continued so that by 1990 nearly 60% were users compared to only about 25% in the comparison area. Clearly, taking advantage of latent demand for contraception required that the program address the social costs of contraceptive use. It also demonstrated the value of providing service in the home.

In 1983 a new experiment was begun outside of Matlab, to see if lessons learned there could be applied within the government family planning program and without major additional resources or changes in administration. This pilot project was carried out in two areas. Because of the success of this Extension Project, the government changed the national program to increase female village workers, train them to provide injectable contraception within the home, and upgrade management to provide better support, both technical and supervisory, for local workers. In fact, one of the main lessons learned from these experiments was the need for careful supervision and support of workers. Another was the importance of designing a program for local cultural circumstances, in this case providing basic services in the home. Since these experiments, other projects have tested variations of the Extension Project model to see how much it could be altered and still achieve the objectives of increased use of family planning and reduced fertility.

The Extension Project, now known as the Operations Research Project, has, since the International Conference on Population and Development, initiated studies of how the family planning program can be expanded to provide a wide array of reproductive and other health services under what is termed the Essential Services Package.

**Exhibit 3–6** Strategies Used by the Bangladesh Family Planning and Reproductive Health Programs

According to Cleland et al. (1994), at least four sets of strategies have been implemented:
1. Strategies to improve the coverage and quality of services
   - Clinics, located within 5 miles of most couples, now provide free contraception and treatment of side effects.
   - Sterilization is offered without charge at all subdistrict hospitals and is carried out by well-trained personnel.
   - Related health services for children and women are provided either in the home or in clinics.
   - Community-based distribution of low-cost nonclinical contraceptives is provided through pharmacies and is well-publicized through various media.
2. Strategies to improve awareness and motivation
   - Mass media are used to provide extensive relevant information; family planning and reproductive health are openly discussed in public media.
   - Focused programs (for example, with religious leaders) are carried out to build awareness and consensus.
3. Strategies to foster village-based and household services
   - Outreach involves female workers who deliver services in the home. These services are now provided by both the government and nongovernmental organizations.
   - This strategy has been questioned in recent years by critics who say the time is past when women should be provided with services that encourage continued seclusion. They argue that the demand for family planning and reproductive health services is now so great that women will travel outside their homes to obtain these services and that this type of modernization is to be encouraged. In addition, issues of cost of maintaining the large cadre of home visitors is encouraging experimentation with less costly alternatives.
4. Strategies to foster community development and demand generation
   - These strategies have not been carried out within the family planning program itself but are directed toward improving the status of women. They include microcredit and other programs sponsored by local organizations, such as Grameen Bank and the Bangladesh Rural Advancement Committee, and government strategies to increase education of girls. In fact, education of women has increased substantially in recent years and, in many parts of Bangladesh, nearly all children, male and female, are obtaining at least several years of primary schooling.

As a final note, the Bangladesh effort is characterized by the use of research to help determine the design of programs. Ongoing studies at the International Centre for Diarrhoeal Disease Research, Bangladesh, now renamed the International Centre for Health and Population Research, include how the new Essential Services Package (which includes reproductive health, child survival, and curative care) can best be implemented within existing fixed service provision sites, how to meet the health needs of adolescents, strategies for improving prevention and management of reproductive tract and sexually transmitted infections (RTI/STI), and strategies for providing essential obstetric care.

Cairo agenda focused on improving the status of women. It called for interventions that affect overall status of women, such as income-generating activities for women and female education, and for sex education for youth, both male and female, to increase responsible sexual behavior. The 1999 follow-up conference reiterated and intensified these calls (*New York Times,* 1999c).

Others have called for programs that decrease violence against women. Violence in women's intimate relationships can lead to death through homicide or by driving the woman to suicide. A less drastic outcome is loss of control by women over their sexuality and, therefore, their sexual health. Another kind of violence against women is female genital mutilation, a practice that has been reported in more than 40 low- and middle-income countries and has followed immigrants from these areas to industrialized countries (Tsui et al., 1997).

### Can These Goals Be Achieved?

All parts of this new "beyond family planning" mandate are worthwhile. It is not clear, however, how this expansion, in the absence of clearly designated additional funds, will affect the ability of family planning programs to reach their objective of promoting safe contraception (Cleland et al., 1994; Finkle & Ness, 1985). In addition, there is concern that this expansion from family planning programs to reproductive health programs without additional funds will not only dilute what traditional family planning does reasonably well but will also not provide significant improvements in other areas (Bulatao, 1998; Mukaire, Kalikwani, Maggwa, & Kisubi, 1997; Twahir, Maggwa, & Askew, 1996).

In fact, the new agenda comes in an era when many industrialized countries are reducing their aid contributions. At Cairo, industrialized country donors pledged to provide $5.7 billion a year, but as of 1999 their contributions were only about $1.9 billion annually (*New York Times*, 1999a). Raising the political will as well as the funding for these new programs and for maintaining existing effective ones is perhaps the greatest challenge for reproductive health in the twenty-first century.

## IMPACT OF REPRODUCTIVE PATTERNS ON THE HEALTH OF CHILDREN

Over the past several decades, an impressive body of evidence has accumulated suggesting that certain kinds of reproductive patterns are injurious to infant and child health (Table 3–11). The risk factors are usually discussed as if they were completely independent. There are, however, a number of problematic issues in this approach to deleterious reproductive patterns. For example, many of the risk factors are integrally linked with one another and their independent effects are difficult to disentangle. Thus first births and young age of mothers are separately cited as risk factors, but young mothers usually are having their first birth. Similarly, children of high parity come from large families and are likely to have older mothers, yet all three are referred to individually.

### Parity and Child Health

First births are known to be more dangerous for the child than subsequent births. But the excess risk relative to births of order 2–4 is limited to the first year of life (and particularly to the neonatal period, where the odds ratios for mortality is 1.7). There appears to be no survival disadvantage after the first birthday (Hobcraft, 1987; Hobcraft, McDonald, & Rutstein, 1985). Moreover, excess risk for first-born children varies considerably across countries. It is not clear whether it is due to inadequate physiologic adjustment of first-time mothers to pregnancy (leading to lower intrauterine growth, shorter gestation, lower birthweight, a higher probability of birth trauma, higher risks of pregnancy-induced hypertension, higher prevalence of placental malaria in malaria-endemic areas, and so on), or due to the lack of experience of first-time mothers in care seeking and care taking. The latter is, of course, amenable to policy prescriptions that encourage first-time mothers to seek prenatal and postnatal care (Haaga, 1989; National Research Council, 1989).

Higher-order births may suffer due to poor maternal health as a result of cumulative exposure to previous pregnancies (Hobcraft et al., 1985; Pebley & Stupp, 1987). Mothers may suffer from inadequate recovery of their energy store after earlier pregnancies (maternal depletion hypothesis) and long-term cumulative effects of prior delivery-related injuries. Thus higher-order children (parity ≥5) may be at greater risk of poor intrauterine growth, greater trauma during birth, and, more generally, poorer health than lower-parity children (2–4). Although these mechanisms are plausible, the em-

**Table 3–11** Mechanisms by Which Reproductive Patterns Affect Child Health

| Reproductive Pattern | Mechanism through Which Child Health Is Affected |
| --- | --- |
| Firstborn children | First time mothers have a higher frequency of health problems during pregnancy and childbirth; parents have less experience with child care; poorer intrauterine growth |
| Higher-order children | Possible cumulative effect of earlier maternal reproductive injury—"maternal depletion" syndrome—leading to poorer intrauterine growth |
| Large families | Competition for limited resources, with some children (possibly disproportionately girls) losing out; possible spread of infection |
| Children born to very young mothers | Inadequate development of maternal reproductive system and incomplete maternal growth; young mothers less likely to know about and use prenatal and delivery care or provide good child care |
| Children born to older mothers | Greater risk of birth trauma; greater risk of genetic abnormalities |
| Short interbirth intervals | Inadequate maternal recovery time (maternal depletion); competition among similar-aged siblings for limited family resources; early termination of breastfeeding; low birthweight; increased exposure to infection from children of similar ages |
| Unwantedness | Neglect (conscious or unconscious); child born into a stressful situation |
| Maternal death or illness (e.g., chronic infection such as AIDS) | Early termination of breastfeeding; no maternal care; disease may be passed to child |
| Contraceptive use | Hormonal contraception may interrupt breastfeeding |

pirical evidence is variable and suggests that there is little additional risk that can be attributed to higher-order births, once short birth intervals are taken into account (Gubhaju, 1986; Hobcraft et al., 1985; National Research Council, 1989).

In addition to physiologic deficiencies, higher-order children may suffer deleterious consequences of competition for limited family resources. Thus they may get proportionately less food and less attention from their parents. This negative consequence of large families may not be limited only to higher-order births. If family resources are limited and there is no preference for specific children, all children may suffer as a result of large family sizes. There is, however, evidence that some children (particularly higher-order girls, and especially those with older sisters) suffer disproportionately from the impact

of large family size in specific social settings (Muhuri & Menken, 1997).

**Maternal Age**

Hobcraft (1987) found that children born to teenage mothers had significantly higher risks of dying than children born to mothers aged 25–34. This excess mortality risk was 1.2 for the neonatal period, 1.4 for the postneonatal period, 1.6 for toddlers, and 1.3 for children aged 2–5. There was, however, considerable variability among countries in excess mortality risk for children born to young mothers. Plausible explanations due to both physiological and social causes have been offered for the health disadvantage of children born to young mothers. They may be disadvantaged because maternal reproductive systems are inadequately developed (Aitken & Walls, 1986) or because young mothers lack experience and knowledge about prenatal and postnatal care (Geronimus, 1987). Unfortunately, there is little solid empirical evidence from low- and middle-income countries. It has been difficult to study possible competition between fetal growth and maternal development as underlying the excessive mortality of children born to young mothers in the low- and middle-income countries. Due to lack of reliable data on gynecological age (that is, age since menarche)—a particularly important concern because of delayed age at menarche in low- and middle-income countries (Foster, Menken, Chowdhury, & Trussell, 1987)—or chronological age below the age of 20, Haaga (1989) concluded that there was only weak evidence for this hypothesis. Studies that have addressed social causes (poor knowledge and use of prenatal care) have used socioeconomic status as a crude proxy for use of prenatal care services. In multivariate analyses, this measure fails to help explain the high risk of infants and children born to young mothers.

Children born to older mothers may suffer because of poorer maternal health due to age-related declines in physiologic function and a higher risk of genetic abnormalities (Hansen, 1986). However, there is little to suggest that this is a major risk factor in low- and middle-income countries.

## Short Birth Intervals

Short birth intervals, both prior and subsequent to the birth of a child, are probably the most consistent reproductive pattern identified as a risk factor for excess child mortality. Hobcraft (1987) reports that the excess mortality risk of children born less than 24 months after the preceding birth compared to those born 24 months or more after the preceding birth is 1.8 in the first year of life, 1.3 for toddlers (ages 1–2), and 1.3 for children aged 2–5. In terms of subsequent birth intervals, Hobcraft reports that

on average, across 34 countries, children whose birth was followed by a subsequent birth within less than 24 months had 2.2 times the risk of dying of children for whom the subsequent birth interval was longer. As is the case for other demographic risk factors, there is considerable variation between countries in risks related to short birth intervals.

There are a number of plausible explanations for the relationship between short prior and subsequent birth intervals (<24 months) and a child's risk of poor health and increased mortality. First, due to maternal depletion (resulting from inadequate recovery time from the nutritional burdens of breastfeeding and prior pregnancy [Merchant & Martorell, 1988]), those born after a short birth interval may suffer poorer intrauterine growth and possibly a higher risk of preterm birth. However, there is little empirical evidence to document to support this mechanism (Ferraz, Gray, Fleming, & Maria, 1988; National Research Council, 1989; Pebley & DaVanzo, 1988; Winikoff & Sullivan, 1987).

Second, children born before a short birth interval may suffer from premature cessation of breastfeeding, (which has been shown to be an important correlate of child survival in low- and middle-income countries [Palloni & Millman, 1986]), as the mother shifts her attention to the recent arrival. Studies that have controlled for the length of breastfeeding still show an association between short subsequent birth interval and high infant mortality (Pebley & Stupp, 1987). Thus premature termination of breastfeeding does not entirely explain this effect.

Third, children born in close proximity to one another may suffer from competition for limited family resources of time and food. The evidence for this type of competition is unclear and sometimes contradictory (DaVanzo, Butz, & Habicht, 1983; Palloni, 1985).

Fourth, close birth spacing may increase the likelihood of transmission of infectious diseases, such as diarrhea and measles, due to overcrowding and presence of children of similar ages (Aaby, Bukh, Lisse, & Smits, 1984). Finally, despite adequate controls for observable confounders in multivariate analyses, part of the relationship between short birth intervals (either preceding or following the index birth) and increased child mortality may be due to confounding from unobserved factors such as short gestational length or parental characteristics. Babies born before or after very short birth intervals are known to be at high risk for short gestational durations, which independently have been shown to increase child mortality dramatically (Miller, 1989; Pebley & Stupp, 1987).

In terms of unobserved parental characteristics, it is possible that women who are likely to have short birth intervals are inherently at higher risk for poorer child health outcomes than their peers who have longer birth intervals. This would lead to a spurious inference that short birth intervals are causally related to higher child mortality (Pebley & Stupp, 1987; Potter, 1988; Rosenzweig & Schultz, 1983).

## Unwanted Pregnancy and Birth

As discussed in the section on family planning programs, unwanted children have much higher risks of morbidity and mortality. They may suffer from both conscious and unconscious neglect, due to lower allocations of food, parental time and attention, and access to health care. In countries with strong son preference (usually associated with South and Southeast Asia), there is significant evidence for higher mortality for female children relative to their male siblings (Das Gupta, 1987; D'Souza & Chen, 1980; Muhuri & Menken, 1997; Muhuri & Preston, 1991). Moreover, as discussed previously, the recent rise in sex selective abortion in China and Southeast Asia (which has led to a disproportionately high male to female sex ratio at birth) is evidence of the high risk of mortality for unwanted female fetuses (Larsen et al., 1998; Tsui et al., 1997). The pattern of gender discrimination is, however, complex and nuanced and may vary by societal setting (Muhuri & Menken, 1997).

## Maternal Health

Maternal morbidity and mortality can have profoundly negative effects on child health, leading to high rates of morbidity and mortality. Population-based studies in South and Southeast Asia suggest that more than half of perinatal deaths (deaths in the first week of a child's life) are associated with poor maternal health and pregnancy and delivery-related complications (Fauveau, Wojtyniak, Mostafa, Sarder, & Chakraborty, 1990; National Statistics Office [Philippines] and Macro International, Inc., 1994). These deleterious consequences may result from a combination of physiologic processes (for example, cessation of breastfeeding following maternal morbidity and mortality; maternal fetal transmission of a variety of infectious agents, including HIV, toxoplasmosis, cytomegalovirus [CMV], rubella, hepatitis B virus, herpes simplex, syphilis, malaria, tuberculosis), emotional impacts, and lower levels of caregiving (National Research Council, 1989; Overall, 1987; Turner, Miller, & Moses, 1989; Weinbreck, et al., 1988). This is particularly a major concern in sub-Saharan Africa, where significant numbers of mothers are suffering from HIV and other STIs (National Research Council, 1989; Turner et al., 1989; Weinbreck et al., 1988).

## Methodological Concerns

The above-mentioned mechanisms by which specific reproductive patterns affect infant and child health are certainly plausible and suggestive. However, it is important to reiterate that the empirical evidence (in terms of the appropriateness of both data and statistical methods) supporting such mechanisms is variable and needs to be interpreted cautiously. Women have some control over their choices of reproductive patterns (that is, whether to have children early or late, whether to have shorter or longer birth intervals, and whether to have high parity births). Unobservable factors that are associated with both reproductive patterns and child health may be operating, and reverse causality may be a problem. Thus estimates of the impact of specific reproductive patterns on the risk of poor infant and child health may be overstated. For example, if women who choose to be young mothers are prone to behavior patterns that devalue prenatal and postnatal care, delaying childbirth for these women will not produce the salutary effects that the earlier discussion suggests. Similarly, there may be unobserved selection biases that operate so that a significant proportion of women who choose to have births at older ages, higher-parity births, and closely spaced births are intrinsically in better health (most likely because of higher socioeconomic status). If that is the case, then reducing higher parity births, increasing interbirth intervals, and reducing births to older women (>35) will not result in the degree of improvement that current studies suggest.

With regard to reverse causality, one example is the often-cited relationship between the mortality of an index child and a short subsequent birth interval. The inference is that a child is at a higher risk of death if the next-younger sibling arrives after only a short interval—presumably because the pregnancy and the arrival of a newborn cause early cessation of breastfeeding for the older child and a shift of other maternal resources. However, it is possible that the subsequent birth interval is short because the index child died or was ill and weaned earlier because of his or her existing health problems. Thus the direction of causation is not from the short subsequent birth interval to the death of the preceding child but, instead, in the reverse direction from the death of the preceding child to a short subsequent birth interval. While in principle there are statistical methods to deal with this kind of potential bidirectionality (Rosenzweig & Schultz, 1983; Schultz, 1984), in practice relatively few published studies have employed such sophisticated methods of analysis. In summary, because of these methodological concerns we should be careful not to overinterpret the evidence linking specific reproductive patterns and poor child health.

## Summary of the Impact of Reproductive Patterns on Child Mortality

Despite these caveats about overinterpretation and overestimation, it is instructive to consider the impact of specific deleterious reproductive patterns on infant and child mortality. The National Research Council (1989) has simulated the impact of various reproductive patterns on child mortality rates using data from 18 low- and middle-income countries, as reported by Hobcraft (1987). The simulations in Table 3–12 refer to death rates that would be observed in individual families with particular reproductive patterns; they assume the mortality risks associated with the specific reproductive pattern are causative. The data in Table 3–12 show that children of parity 2 and above are at much higher risk of mortality if they are born to teenage mothers than if the mothers are aged 20–34. Moreover, both teenage and nonteenage mothers can significantly reduce the risks of child mortality by adopting better spacing patterns (that is, birth intervals of 24 months or more). The best-case scenario for children of parity 2 and above is for those born to mothers between the ages of 20 and 34, whose older sibling has survived, and whose birth interval is 24 months or more. Only 67 of 1,000 such children fail to reach their second birthday. This is less than half the mortality risk of their peers born to teenage mothers whose birth intervals are less than 24 months. In the latter situation, 165 of 1,000 such children die before age two.

Other simulations show the deleterious consequences of increasing family size and birth intervals on the probability of a child surviving to his or her fifth birthday. The calculations were carried out under low, moderate, and high baseline child mortality rates (to take into account variation in overall mortality among populations). The baseline child mortality rates represent the probability of a child surviving to his

**Table 3–12** Estimated Risk of Dying (Deaths per 1,000 Births) Prior to Their Second Birthday for Second and Higher-Order Births to Women with Different Reproductive Patterns

| Age of Mother | Better Spacing Pattern | Poor Spacing Pattern |
|---|---|---|
| Teenage mothers | 92 | 165 |
| Mothers ages 20–34 | 67 | 120 |

Note: Better spacing pattern: birth intervals both proceeding and subsequent to this birth were 24 months and the older sibling survived; poor spacing pattern: birth intervals both preceding and subsequent to this birth were <24 months and the older sibling survived.

or her fifth birthday for children who have the lowest risk profile (that is, parity 2–3, preceding and subsequent birth intervals ≥24 months, and the older sibling survived). Thus, if the baseline child mortality rate is 150 deaths out of each 1,000 births, 15% of children who were parity 2–3, had long preceding and subsequent birth intervals (≥24 months), and whose older sibling survived would die before their fifth birthday. Mortality rates for specific combinations of parities below and above the baseline, of short and long intervals, and of survival of older sibling were estimated by Hobcraft. He then simulated the average number of children per 1,000 births who would die before their fifth birthday. Here only those where the older sibling survived is discussed. In terms of family size, small families were much better off than large families. Regardless of the baseline mortality rates or the closeness of birth spacing, the greater the family size, the higher the child mortality rates. In all cases, four-child families experienced fewer than half the deaths per 1,000 births of nine-child families. Similarly, families with long spacing experienced half or less the mortality per 1,000 births of families with consistently short spacing. Clearly the most beneficial scenario for children is that of well-spaced births and small overall family sizes.

## IMPACT OF REPRODUCTIVE PATTERNS ON THE HEALTH OF WOMEN

Pregnancy is one of the major health risks for women in the low- and middle-income coun-tries. Approximately 600,000 women die world-wide each year due to pregnancy-related causes, and the vast majority (98%) of these deaths is in the low- and middle-income countries (World Health Organization and UNICEF, 1996). Al-though these numbers are alarming, it is im-portant to recognize that there are 180 million pregnancies annually in the world, so that by and large reproduction is relatively safe for women. Maternal mortality risks are a fraction of infant mortality risks; for example, Bangladesh has both high infant mortality and very high mater-nal mortality risks, but the latter are roughly one-tenth of the former. The maternal mortality ratio is between 6–8 deaths per 1,000 childbirths, while the infant mortality rate (which has fallen considerably in the past decade) is about 80 infant deaths per 1,000 births (Demographic and Health Surveys, Macro International, Inc., 1998; Tsui et al., 1997).

## Definitions

In any discussion of maternal mortality, a number of potentially confusing definitional issues arises. The first is the definition of a ma-ternal death. A maternal death is usually defined as a death of a woman while pregnant or up to 42 days postdelivery from any cause (except ac-cidents). There has been some discussion as to whether this definition is overly restrictive (that is, leading to an undercount of maternal deaths) and should be expanded to include deaths up to 90 days postdelivery. In reality, data from a number of well conducted population-based studies using different postdelivery durations show that the majority of maternal deaths occur within 42 days postdelivery and about 40% occur within 24–48 hours of delivery. Furthermore, extending the definition to up to 90 days would result in only a marginal increase (6%) in the number of deaths classified as related to maternal causes (Egypt Ministry of Health, 1994; Fauveau, Koenig, Chakraborty, & Chowdhury, 1988).

The second issue is the measure of maternal mortality risk that should be used in comparing and contrasting the situation in different populations both geographically and across time. Maternal mortality risks are conventionally described using three distinct measures. It is important to understand and to think of them separately, as they are conceptually distinct.

The first measure is the *maternal mortality ratio*, which is defined as the ratio of the number of maternal deaths to the number of pregnancies. It is an indicator of the risk of dying that a woman faces for each pregnancy she undergoes. Although conceptually the denominator for such a risk measure should include all pregnancies, operationally, because of the difficulty of counting miscarriages and induced abortions, the denominator used is live births.

The second measure is the *maternal mortality rate,* which is defined as the number of maternal deaths divided by the number of women of reproductive age (that is, between ages 15–49). This is a composite measure that is the product of the maternal mortality ratio (deaths/births) and the birth rate in the reproductive age group (births/women between ages 15–49). The important point to note about the maternal mortality rate is that it can be modified by changing the frequency of pregnancies or births in the population without changing the risk of maternal death per pregnancy/birth. Although the maternal mortality ratio and the maternal mortality rate are conceptually distinct, they are often confused in the public health literature, with rates referring to ratios and vice versa. In this report, these two measures are carefully distinguished.

The third measure is the *lifetime risk of maternal mortality*. It is again a composite measure that takes into account not only the maternal mortality risk per pregnancy but also factors in the cumulative exposure to pregnancy that an individual woman experiences. The average cumulative exposure to pregnancy is usually taken to be the TFR for the population. It is an estimate of the number of births a woman in a particular society would have over her lifetime if she were to adhere to the current age-specific fertility rates in that population. The lifetime maternal mortality risk for a woman in the low- and middle-income countries was estimated by Tsui et al. (1997) to be 1:48. This estimate can be interpreted as follows: a woman in the low- and middle-income countries who (1) has the same total number of pregnancies over her lifetime as the current fertility norm (estimated to be 3.8 births) and (2) experiences at each pregnancy the same independent risk of maternal death as the current maternal mortality ratio (430 maternal deaths per 100,000 births) would have one chance in 48 of dying from pregnancy-related causes. Thus this lifetime risk captures both the risk of dying per pregnancy and the cumulative effect of exposure to multiple pregnancies.

## Maternal Mortality Risks

A major constraint with respect to investigating the magnitude of maternal mortality risks and its determinants is the lack of available and reliable population-based data. Even in low- and middle-income countries, many of which have high maternal mortality rates and ratios, maternal deaths are relatively rare. For example, in sub-Saharan Africa and South Asia, where maternal mortality ratios of 700 maternal deaths per 100,000 live births have been reported, one would need very large sample sizes to get reasonable estimates of maternal mortality risks and their accompanying determinants. A sample of 10,000 births (a large sample by any standards) would be expected to yield only 70 maternal deaths. In contrast, infant mortality rates in these settings are typically 15 times larger, and the same sample would yield 1,050 infant deaths. Therefore, estimates are presented only from the relatively few large-scale population-based studies of maternal mortality that have been conducted in low- and middle-income countries. They were carried out in Bangladesh (Alauddin, 1986; Chen, Gesche, Ahmed, Chowdhury, & Mosley, 1975; Fauveau et al., 1988; Khan, Jahan, & Begum, 1986; Koenig et al., 1988); Ethiopia (Kwast, Rochat, & Kidane-Mariam, 1986); Egypt (Egypt Ministry of Health, 1994; Fortney et al., 1985); and Jamaica (Walker, Ashley, McCaw, & Bernard, 1985).

There are huge disparities in maternal mortality among regions of the world. The disparity between the low- and middle-income countries and industrialized countries is much greater for maternal mortality (20 times higher risk of maternal death per pregnancy) than infant mortality (10 times higher risk of infant death per pregnancy). Lifetime risks of maternal mortality vary from 1:48 in the low- and middle-income countries to 1:1,800 in the industrialized countries (Table 3–13).

As is shown in Table 3–13, both the total number of pregnancies per woman and the individual risk of dying per pregnancy are much higher in the low- and middle-income countries

than the industrialized world. But it is the risk of dying per pregnancy that accounts for the vast majority of the difference in lifetime risk of maternal mortality. TFRs in the low- and middle-income countries are, on average, twice as high as in the industrialized countries (3.8 births per woman versus 1.8 births per woman). Maternal mortality ratios are, on average, 18 times higher (480 maternal deaths per 100,000 births in the low- and middle-income countries versus 27 maternal deaths per 100,000 births in the industrialized countries).

## Direct and Indirect Causes of Maternal Mortality and Morbidity

What does the mortality risk per pregnancy derive from? The causes of maternal mortality are conventionally divided into direct causes (those that occur only during pregnancy and the immediate postdelivery period) and indirect causes (those derived from conditions that precede, but are aggravated by, pregnancy, such as anemia, diabetes, malaria, tuberculosis, cardiac disease, hepatitis). In the low- and middle-income countries, direct causes account for 75–80% of maternal mortality and include, in approximate order of importance, hemorrhage, sepsis, hypertensive

**Table 3–13** TFR, Maternal Mortality Ratios, and Lifetime Risks by Region of the World in the 1990s

| Region | Total Fertility Rate (births per woman) | Maternal Mortality Ratio (deaths per 100,000 live births) | Maternal Deaths | |
|---|---|---|---|---|
| | | | Lifetime Risk | Deaths Per Year |
| World Total | 3.4 | 430 | 1 in 60 | 586,000 |
| Industrialized Countries | 1.8 | 27 | 1 in 1,800 | 4,000 |
| Low- and Middle-Income Countries | 3.8 | 480 | 1 in 48 | 582,000 |
| Africa | 6.0 | 870 | 1 in 16 | 235,000 |
| Asia | 3.4 | 390 | 1 in 65 | 323,000 |
| Latin America and the Caribbean | 3.3 | 190 | 1 in 130 | 23,000 |

disorders of pregnancy (eclampsia), complications of unsafe abortion, and obstructed or prolonged labor (Fauveau et al., 1988; World Health Organization, 1993c; World Health Organization and UNICEF, 1996). The vast majority of these maternal deaths can be attributed to three causes: hemorrhage, sepsis, and eclampsia. Attribution of cause of death is complicated by the fact that in most cases unsafe abortion and obstructed or prolonged labor eventually cause death via the proximate causes of hemorrhage or sepsis. There is variation in the order of importance of these causes in different studies from different parts of the world (Jamison, Mosley, Measham, & Bobadilla, 1993); this is partly due to real differences in the availability and use of obstetric care and partly due to differences in the quality of reporting. Thus, in countries that have poor access to obstetric care facilities, the proportion of deaths attributed to hemorrhage, sepsis, and abortion is proportionately larger. Differential reporting, particularly reluctance to attribute maternal deaths to abortion in countries where it is illegal, also artificially inflates the proportion of deaths attributed to hemorrhage and sepsis (Table 3–14).

The remaining 20–25% of maternal deaths can be attributed to illnesses aggravated by pregnancy (Jamison et al., 1993; World Health Organization, 1993b). Anemia hampers a woman's abilities to resist infection and to survive hemorrhage; it may increase the likelihood of her dying in childbirth by a factor of four (Chi, Agoestina, & Harbin, 1981). Hepatitis can cause hemorrhage or liver failure in pregnant women (Kwast & Stevens, 1987). Latent infections such as tuberculosis, malaria, or STIs can be activated or exacerbated during pregnancy and cause potentially severe complications for both mother and child (Jamison et al., 1993).

In keeping with the high rates of maternal mortality in the low- and middle-income countries, there are also high rates of maternal morbidity. It is estimated that between 30–40% of the approximately 180 million women who are pregnant annually in the world, or roughly 54 million women, report some kind of pregnancy-related morbidity annually (Koblinsky, Campbell, & Harlow, 1993; World Health Organization, 1993b). Of these, it is estimated that about 15 million a year develop relatively long-term disabilities deriving from complications from obstetric fistula or prolapse, uterine scarring, severe anemia, pelvic inflammatory disease, reproductive tract infections, as well as infertility (Tsui et al., 1997).

---

**Table 3–14** Major Causes of Maternal Deaths in Selected Countries, 1980–1985 (in percentages)

| Countries | Hemorrhage | Sepsis | Eclampsia | Abortion | Obstructed Labor/Ruptured Uterus | Other |
|---|---|---|---|---|---|---|
| United States | 10 | 8 | 17 | 6 | 3 | 56 |
| Cuba | 6 | 19 | 12 | 15 | — | 48 |
| Jamaica | 23 | 9 | 30 | 10 | 3 | 25 |
| Zambia (Lusaka) | 17 | 15 | 20 | 17 | — | 31 |
| Egypt (Menoufia) | 29 | 11 | 5 | 4 | — | 51 |
| Tanzania (four regions) | 18 | 15 | 3 | 17 | 6 | 41 |
| Ethiopia (Addis Ababa) | 6 | 2 | 6 | 25 | 4 | 57 |
| Bangladesh | 22 | 3 | 19 | 31 | 9 | 16 |
| Indonesia | 46 | 10 | 5 | 7 | — | 32 |
| India | 18 | 14 | 16 | 14 | 3 | 35 |

It is important to recognize that these figures are quite approximate, with significant variability from one country to another (Tsui et al., 1997). For example, Guatemalan women report one in five pregnancies as being complicated (Bailey, Szaszdi, & Scheiber, 1994), women in West Java report one in three pregnancies being complicated (Alisjahbana et al., 1995), and two of three pregnancies in Ghana had some complications (De Graft-Johnson, 1994). This variability stems at least in part from differences in study design and data quality. There have been relatively few population-based surveys. Moreover, many of the maternal morbidity data are based on self-reported symptoms that have been shown to have relatively low reliability and validity (Stewart & Festin, 1995). There are a few data sets with reliable information coming from the United States and Canada (Koblinsky et al., 1993; World Health Organization, 1994b), and from specific validation studies (Stewart & Festin, 1995). These data show that annually roughly 12–15% of women who are pregnant suffer life-threatening obstetric complications— that is, about 20 million women in the low- and middle-income countries (out of the approximately 150 million women giving birth annually). In contrast to the evidence on acute pregnancy related morbidity, little is known about the long-term chronic morbidity sequelae of pregnancy-related complications, which may significantly affect women's lives.

## Specific Causes of Pregnancy-Related Morbidity and Mortality

In the section below the focus is on some of the more prominent causes of pregnancy-related morbidity and mortality in the low- and middle-income countries.

### Obstructed and Prolonged Labor

Obstructed and prolonged labor leads to approximately 40,000 maternal deaths annually, with high proportions of survivors suffering from obstetric fistulas (see below) and their newborn often suffering from long-term sequelae

of anoxia. Predictive risk factors are not particularly reliable (Fortney, 1995; Maine, 1991), and monitoring during labor using a partograph is the only effective way to detect such problems (World Health Organization, 1994a). Figure 3–5 traces both the distal and proximal causes and consequences of obstructed labor, illustrating the interconnectedness of reproductive complications (Jamison et al., 1993, derived from Lettenmier, Liskin, Church, & Harris, 1988).

### Obstetric Fistula and Genital Prolapse

It is important to focus attention on these two conditions because of their severe consequences. An obstetric fistula is a passage or channel from the vaginal wall to either the rectum (recto-vaginal fistula) or the bladder (vesico-vaginal fistula). It is usually a result of a tear in the vaginal wall during complicated labor. Risk factors for obstetric fistulas include: young mother, stunted mother, mother who has complicated labor, and delivery in nonhospital settings with the help of traditional birth attendants (Lawson, 1992; Tahzib, 1983, 1985). Population-level estimates of obstetric fistulas are hard to come by, but fragmentary reports suggest that these are a significant cause of morbidity for pregnant women in low- and middle-income countries (Lawson, 1992; World Health Organization, 1991). The consequences of fistulas are severe, especially for young primiparas (women experiencing their first birth). The baby is often stillborn. The mother is incontinent of urine and feces. This condition is a source of enormous personal discomfort exacerbated by social stigma. In many cases it leads to divorce and social ostracism; these women are often barred from food preparation or even participating in prayer, due to lack of personal hygiene (Reed, Koblinsky, & Mosley, 2000).

Genital prolapse occurs when the vagina and uterus descend below their normal positions. It is usually a result of damage to supporting muscles and ligaments during childbirth and is most often associated with high parity. The condition is particularly uncomfortable for women who are squatting, which is the normal position

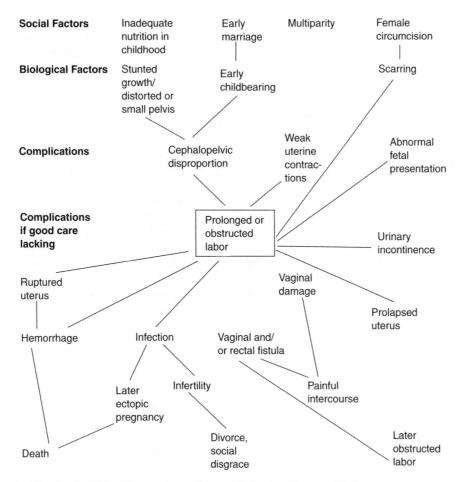

**Figure 3–5** Tracing the Web of Factors Anteceding and Following Obstructed Labor

for doing many chores in low- and middle-income countries. It can also lead to chronic backache, urinary problems, and pain during sexual intercourse. Subsequent pregnancies have a higher probability of fetal loss and further maternal morbidity.

While good estimates of these conditions are hard to come by, some reliable population studies suggest very high prevalence rates—as much as one-third of all pregnant women (Omran & Standley, 1981; Younis et al., 1993). The Giza study (Younis et al., 1993), which clinically validated reported prolapse, found that one-third

of women suffered from genital prolapse and also documented a relationship between genital prolapse and the risk of reproductive tract infections.

### Anemia

Approximately 50% of pregnant women around the world are estimated to be anemic (that is, have hemoglobin levels below 11g/dl). Dietary iron deficiency is the primary cause, followed by malaria, other parasitic diseases (schistosomiasis, hookworm), folate deficiency, AIDS, and sickle cell disease (Tsui et al., 1997).

In addition to its well-documented effects on pregnancy outcomes—prematurity, stillbirths, spontaneous abortions, and so on (Levin, Pollitt, Galloway, & McGuire, 1993)—anemia, even at fairly mild levels, has been implicated directly as contributing to maternal deaths (Harrison & Rossiter, 1985; United Nations, 1991). There is also some evidence that anemia predisposes women to higher risks of complications during pregnancy, including urinary tract infections, pyelonephritis, and pre-eclampsia (Kitay & Harbort, 1975). Anemia is also associated with reduced productivity and quality of life for women (Bothwell & Charllton, 1981).

The record of the impact of iron supplementation on reducing the prevalence of iron-deficiency anemia is not encouraging (Sloan, Jordan, & Winikoff, 1992). While a significant part of the failure to reduce anemia is due to inadequate efforts to provide iron supplementation, it is important to acknowledge that even in situations where there have been properly conducted supplementation trials, these programs by and large appear not to be very effective in reducing baseline anemia levels (Sood et al., 1975). This may be due to inadequacies of strategies that focus just on pregnant women. Long-term success in this effort probably involves the use of a multipronged strategy including iron supplementation schemes, efforts to raise household income, and efforts to reduce workload during pregnancy (Tsui et al., 1997). (See also Chapter 5.)

## Pregnancy-Related Hypertension

Both eclampsia and pre-eclampsia are significant causes of maternal morbidity but appear to be difficult to predict and prevent, although routine prenatal blood pressure measurements and urinalysis for proteinuria in the first prenatal visit continue to be recommended (Rooney, 1992; Stone et al., 1994). Women with moderate hypertension and proteinuria require appropriate follow-up. Treatment options and their effectiveness vary and no definitive conclusions or recommendations can be made. However, as a general rule, some combination of bed rest, antihypertensives, and anticonvulsants (especially magnesium sulfate for frank convulsions) provide some relief (Eclampsia Trial Collaborative Group, 1995; Rooney, 1992).

## Consequences for Infants

Pregnancy and delivery-related complications have important health consequences not only for mothers but also for infants, particularly in the perinatal period (that is, the first 7 days of birth/delivery). For most low- and middle-income countries, perinatal mortality rates range between 40 to 60 deaths per 1,000 births versus 10 per 1,000 for the industrialized countries (note that this ratio includes stillbirths in the denominator). As infant mortality rates drop, the proportion of infant deaths attributed to the perinatal period actually increases, since postneonatal deaths (those after the first 28 days of life and most sensitive to environmental contamination) are the first to drop. In general, perinatal deaths account for about 40% of infant deaths in most low- and middle-income countries, and an increasing percentage in industrialized countries.

Of the estimated 7.6 million perinatal deaths annually in low- and middle-income countries (World Health Organization, 1996), the vast majority are associated with maternal health problems during pregnancy and around delivery (Fauveau et al., 1990). Women who have inadequate nutritional status (including short stature, poor prepregnancy weight, inadequate weight gain during pregnancy, and anemia) or infections during pregnancy are more likely to have low birthweight babies (World Health Organization, 1993b). The single most important risk factor for perinatal mortality is low birthweight, with babies below 2,500 gms having 20–30 times the mortality risk of fetuses of normal weight. In addition to increasing the risk of perinatal mortality, there is also a substantial burden of long-term disability (cerebral palsy, seizures, severe learning disorders) for low birthweight babies who survive (Jamison et al., 1993; Tsui et al., 1997).

## High-Risk Pregnancies

For the sake of simplicity, the calculations of lifetime risk presented earlier assumed that the risk of maternal death per pregnancy is the same across women and across successive pregnancies within each woman. The reality is somewhat more complicated, with some types of pregnancies being riskier than others. These include pregnancies of first-time mothers, mothers with multiple previous pregnancies ($\geq 5$ pregnancies), very young and older mothers, and women already in poor health, and pregnancies that are terminated by unsafe abortions (National Research Council, 1989; Tsui et al., 1997). Table 3–15 summarizes the hypothesized mechanisms by which different reproductive patterns affect maternal health.

First pregnancies have a higher risk of maternal mortality than subsequent pregnancies (up to five) both in the industrialized and the low- and middle-income countries. Population-based data from Bangladesh (Koenig et al., 1988), Ethiopia (Kwast et al., 1986), and The Gambia (Greenwood et al., 1987) suggest that first pregnancies may be as much as three times riskier than later pregnancies.

The impact of young maternal age on maternal mortality is more difficult to evaluate because there are relatively few studies that have disaggregated the confounding effect of young maternal age and first pregnancy. Among those that have controlled confounding appropriately, the largest study to date looked at maternal mortality among 14,631 first births in rural Bangladesh (Koenig et al., 1988); it showed no age effect. However, other smaller studies from the same area (Chen et al., 1975), Indonesia (Chi et al., 1981), and Jamaica (Walker et al., 1985) have shown a higher mortality risk for mothers below age 20 compared to mothers 20–24. A further problem that makes interpretation difficult is that maternal age below 20 is not disaggregated into single years of age; in fact, the highest risk may be for young teenage mothers in the 15–17 year age group (Harrison & Rossiter, 1985).

The major causes of morbidity and mortality for young primigravidas (women pregnant for the first time) include a high risk of pregnancy-induced hypertension (World Health Organization, 1988), a high frequency of obstructed labor due to the pelvis being too small for the child's head to pass (Aitken & Walls, 1986), and a high incidence of placental malaria (MacGregor, Wilson, & Billewicz, 1983).

A number of studies have shown that women with 4 or more pregnancies have about 1.5 to 3 times the risk of maternal death as women of parities 2 and 3. In general, within each parity, older women, particularly those over 35, have higher risks of maternal death (Koenig et al., 1988; Chi et al., 1981; Walker et al., 1985). A major cause of maternal morbidity and mortality for older multiparous women is the higher risk of malpresentation (in which the fetus lies in a position other than the usual head first, as in a breech or transverse lie presentation). Malpresentation of the fetus may occur due to the flaccidity of the uterine wall from repeated stretching from successive pregnancies. It can lead to uterine rupture, hemorrhage associated with rupture, or infections resulting from unsuccessful attempts to deal with malpresentation. Another major cause of morbidity and mortality in older multiparous women is hemorrhage due to placental abnormalities, such as placenta previa (where the placenta overlies the cervical opening of the uterus) and abruptia placenta (where the placenta separates prematurely from the uterus prior to delivery of the baby) (Faundes, Fanjul, Henriquez, Mora, & Tognola, 1974).

There has been much talk about the possibility of a maternal depletion syndrome whereby multiple short birth intervals result in women not having enough time to recover their energy and nutritional levels, which in turn may lead to higher risks of maternal mortality (Jelliffe, 1976; Winikoff, 1983). However, no convincing evidence of this hypothesis has been presented (Koenig et al., 1988; National Research Council, 1989; Ronsman & Campbell, 1998). This could be due to the fact that intrinsically healthier women (in this case, women of higher socioeco-

**Table 3–15** Mechanisms by Which Reproductive Patterns Affect Maternal Health

| Reproductive Pattern | Mechanism through Which Maternal Health Is Affected |
|---|---|
| Number of pregnancies | Each pregnancy carries a risk of morbidity and mortality |
| First-time mothers | Higher risk than pregnancies 2–4 for obstructed labor, pregnancy induced hypertension, other obstetric complications due to initial adaptation to pregnancy |
| Higher order pregnancies | Higher risk for hemorrhage or uterine rupture due to cumulative toll of previous pregnancies and reproductive injuries |
| Pregnancy at very young maternal ages | Higher risk due to physiologically immature reproductive systems and reduced propensity for timely care seeking |
| Pregnancy at old maternal ages | Body in poorer condition for pregnancy and childbirth |
| Short interbirth intervals | Inadequate time to rebuild nutritional stores and regain energy levels |
| Unwanted pregnancies ending in unsafe abortions | Unsafe abortions increase exposure to injury, infection, hemorrhage, and death |
| Pregnancies for women already in poor health | Aggravated health condition |

nomic status) may be more likely to have multiple short birth intervals, whereas less healthy women may take longer to have subsequent births (Duffy & Menken, 1998).

Pregnancy is more dangerous for women who are already in poor health; the likelihood that a woman will die is increased if she has certain preexisting conditions such as malaria, hepatitis, anemia, sickle cell disease, and rheumatic heart disease (Koblinsky, 1995; Tsui et al., 1997; Morrow, Smetana, Sai, & Edgcomb, 1968; National Research Council, 1989; World Health Organization, 1993b).

Finally, unsafe abortions are a significant cause of maternal death in countries where abortion is not legal and regulated. Kwast et al. (1986) report that the primary cause of maternal mortality in Addis Ababa, Ethiopia, especially among primigravid, unmarried women is complications from illegal abortions. In Bangladesh, Koenig and colleagues (1988) reported that 18% of all maternal deaths in the Matlab surveillance area were from abortion complications (see the earlier discussion of abortion and its health consequences for women in the family planning program section).

## Mechanisms To Reduce Maternal Morbidity and Mortality in Low- and Middle-Income Countries

The major emphasis in the past few decades in low- and middle-income countries in reducing maternal morbidity and mortality has been on decreasing the total number of pregnancies per woman. As documented earlier, the total number of pregnancies per woman has fallen quite sharply in many parts of the low- and middle-income countries; this drop has contributed significantly to the decrease in the lifetime risk of maternal mortality by reducing cumulative exposure. For example, assume a constant maternal mortality ratio of 650 per 100,000. In Bangladesh, if the TFR had remained at its 1975 level of more than 7 instead of dropping to the 1998 level of 3.4, the lifetime risk of maternal mortality would have been 1:22 instead of the current estimate of 1:45.

In addition to the reduction in the TFR in low- and middle-income countries, there has been some progress in reducing high parity births (Table 3–16), births to older women (Table 3–17), and births following short intervals (that

**Table 3–16** Change in the Distribution of Birth Order over the Course of Fertility Decline and Percentage Decline in Total Fertility Rates for Selected Countries

| Country | Percentage of All Births of Order 1 | | Percentage of All Births of Order 5+ | | Percent Decline in Total Fertility Rate |
|---|---|---|---|---|---|
| | *1960s* | *1970s–1980* | *1960s* | *1970s–1980* | |
| Singapore | 23 | 44 | 33 | 2 | 65 |
| Hong Kong | 25 | 43 | 23 | 4 | 64 |
| Barbados | 22 | 40 | 35 | 10 | 54 |
| Mauritius | 18 | 36 | 36 | 11 | 52 |
| Costa Rica | 18 | 32 | 45 | 17 | 50 |
| Chile | 25 | 41 | 31 | 9 | 49 |
| Trinidad and Tobago | 19 | 32 | 37 | 19 | 43 |
| Puerto Rico | 27 | 32 | 27 | 10 | 42 |
| Panama | 21 | 29 | 35 | 22 | 42 |
| Malaysia | 12 | 26 | 41 | 22 | 42 |
| Fiji | 23 | 35 | 36 | 13 | 41 |

is, less than 24 months). Access to safe abortion has also increased (Tsui et al., 1997). An often overlooked benefit of fertility-reduction initiatives is their impact on reducing the frequency of unsafe abortions by providing access to effective contraception for those who want it (Bulatao, 1998; National Research Council, 1989).

Despite these positive efforts, there is a significant burden of maternal mortality that persists in low- and middle-income countries, despite the

**Table 3–17** Change in the Distribution of Births by Maternal Age in Selected Countries over the Course of Fertility Decline and Percent Decline in Total Fertility Rates between 1960 and 1980

| Country | Percentage of All Births to Women under Age 20 | | Percentage of All Births to Women Aged 35 and Older | | Percent Decline in Total Fertility Rate |
|---|---|---|---|---|---|
| | *1960s* | *1970s–1980* | *1960s* | *1970s–1980* | |
| Singapore | 8 | 4 | 14 | 5 | 65 |
| Hong Kong | 5 | 4 | 20 | 6 | 64 |
| Barbados | 21 | 25 | 15 | 6 | 54 |
| Mauritius | 13 | 14 | 15 | 7 | 52 |
| Costa Rica | 13 | 20 | 18 | 9 | 50 |
| Chile | 12 | 17 | 17 | 9 | 49 |
| Trinidad and Tobago | 17 | 19 | 11 | 8 | 43 |
| Puerto Rico | 18 | 18 | 11 | 7 | 42 |
| Panama | 18 | 20 | 11 | 9 | 42 |
| Malaysia | 11 | 7 | 14 | 13 | 42 |
| Fiji | 13 | 11 | 12 | 8 | 41 |

increase in the proportion of pregnancies that are in the demographically low-risk category (that is, parity 2–4 among mothers 24–29 with birth intervals ≥24 months). There are two reasons. First, the absolute risk of maternal death is still very high in these settings, even in the low-risk pregnancies. Second, some of the highest risk pregnancies, such as first pregnancies, are unavoidable.

In this regard, it is worth considering the following scenario. Bangladesh (with its very high risks of maternal mortality per pregnancy) experiences no change in the mortality risk per pregnancy but fertility declines to replacement levels (that is, each woman had just 2.1 births over her lifetime). Under these conditions, the lifetime risk of maternal mortality would still be 1 in 74—almost 24 times higher than the lifetime maternal mortality risk (1 in 1,800) of a woman in the industrialized countries. Even this scenario may be overly optimistic. Our calculation does not allow for any heterogeneity in maternal mortality risks across pregnancies. If first pregnancies are intrinsically more dangerous or if healthier women were the ones who had more pregnancies, simply reducing the number of births would not achieve the reduction in maternal mortality estimated above. Finally, a number of studies have shown that older women with more surviving sons have significantly lower mortality than their peers with fewer sons (Rahman, 1999; Rahman, Menken, & Foster, 1992). This research suggests that although increased numbers of pregnancies may expose a woman to considerable risk of morbidity and mortality, women in certain social settings (where family support is crucial) are actually better off when they are older if they have had higher fertility. These considerations lead to the conclusion that, in order to reduce maternal deaths significantly in low- and middle-income countries, an emphasis on reducing overall fertility levels and the frequency of high-risk pregnancies is unlikely to be sufficient. The emphasis has to be on reducing the mortality risk for every pregnancy as well.

## Obstetric Care

As pointed out above, the majority of maternal and perinatal mortality and morbidity stems from complications around the delivery process that are difficult to predict and avoid prenatally (National Statistics Office [Philippines] and Macro International, Inc., 1994; Maine, 1991; Thaddeus & Maine, 1994). Perhaps the most important benefit of prenatal care is in sensitizing the mother to warning signs of obstetric emergencies and the need to seek appropriate obstetric care when they occur (Tsui et al., 1997). It is instructive to review briefly what the basic acceptable package of obstetric care consists of. WHO uses the following criteria to assess the adequacy of obstetric care facilities (World Health Organization, 1995):

- the ability to carry out surgery, such as Caesarean section; removal of ectopic pregnancy
- treatment of infection, both orally and intravenously
- the ability to provide intravenous labor-inducing agents, such as oxytocin
- the ability to provide anesthesia, ranging from mild sedation, to epidural, to full general anesthesia
- the facilities for the medical treatment of shock, sepsis, anemia, and hypertensive disorders of pregnancy
- the ability to provide blood transfusions
- the ability to provide manual procedures, including vacuum extractions
- the ability to monitor labor
- the ability to provide safe abortion services
- the ability to provide special care for neonates

The historical record in the United States and Europe (Hogberg, Wall, & Brostroin, 1986; Loudon, 1991) and the more recent experience of specific low- and middle-income countries such as Sri Lanka show that the implementation even of only limited parts of the essential obstetric care package can result in major declines in maternal mortality. The maternal mortality ratio in Sri Lanka dropped dramatically from 555 per 100,000 births in the mid-1950s, to 239 in the 1960s, and to 95 in 1980 (World Health Organization, 1995). This was largely due to the expansion of health centers appropriately equipped for essential obstetric care and the increase in births attended by trained personnel.

For a variety of reasons (including cultural prohibitions and customs, lack of social mobility, lack of economic resources, lack of logistic resources, and lack of information), women in low- and middle-income countries for the most part do not use appropriate obstetric care services, with the most vulnerable group in this regard being rural, less educated, and poorer women (Govindasamy, Stewart, Rutstein, Boerma, & Sommerfelt, 1993). Only 37% of births in low- and middle-income countries take place in a health facility (World Health Organization, 1993a). The rest (some 55–60 million infants) are born with the help of traditional birth attendants, family members, or no assistance at all. It is interesting to note that prenatal care services are used significantly more than obstetric care services. In 39 of 43 countries covered by DHS surveys between 1985 and 1994, prenatal care coverage was significantly higher than delivery care from a trained provider (doctor, nurse, or midwife) (Macro International, 1994). These results need to be viewed with some caution, as prenatal care is self-reported and may include very low and episodic use of appropriate services. There is considerable variation in the DHS countries in use of both prenatal and maternal care services. South Asia (with the exception of Sri Lanka) has particularly low uses of prenatal care and maternal care services.

The failure to use appropriate maternal care services can be viewed as resulting from a multipart process that includes (1) deficiencies in identifying life-threatening medical complications that would benefit from obstetric care services; (2) constraints that prevent the use of obstetric services even when appropriate conditions for such use are identified (these may include lack of financial resources, transporta-

tion difficulties, other logistic problems); and (3) obstetric care facilities of such poor quality that they are ineffective in preventing obstetric complications and death, even when pregnant women come to such facilities (Thaddeus & Maine, 1994; Tsui et al., 1997). Each of these problems will be elaborated.

### Identification of Serious Medical Complications That Will Benefit from Obstetric Care

It is important to reiterate that most women in low- and middle-income countries deliver at home, far away from even rudimentary obstetric care facilities, and assisted for the most part by family members or traditional birth attendants. The ability to recognize a potentially life-threatening complication, and its need for specialized obstetric care (such as obstructed or prolonged labor, incipient hemorrhage, or other fetal distress) depends on appropriate education and sensitization of both family members and traditional birth attendants, with the former being perhaps the more important constituency.

A number of cultural factors affect recognition that obstetric complications can benefit from specific kinds of medical care. When a woman is bleeding, the need for obstetric intervention by trained medical personnel is better recognized. Other complications are, however, generally not viewed as benefiting from specialized obstetric care. In some cultures, complications are seen as determined by fate, with little that can be done to alter the course of events. In Indonesia, for example, malposition of the fetus is seen as the domain of traditional birth attendants, who deal with it with soothing massage whereby pregnant women maintain the inner calm considered necessary for correcting the baby's position (Ambaretnani, Hessler-Radelet, & Carlin, 1993). As a result, referral to obstetric care services is often significantly delayed. There are other instances in which, due to concerns about privacy and modesty, the home is perceived as the more natural and fitting place for birth than any health care facility. For the

Fulani and Hausa in Nigeria, pregnancy is seen as a shameful period with unpredictable outcome; thus no preparations are made for referral for obstetric services (Public Opinion Polls, 1993; Tsui et al., 1997).

It is clear from these examples that cultural sensitivities need to be taken into account when constructing appropriate educational messages that emphasize the identification of particularly serious obstetric risks and the need to refer them to health facilities with adequate obstetric care services. A purely technocratic approach, which focuses on modern systems of logic and evidence, may not be effective in bringing about changes in behavior. Much attention has been focused on training birth attendants, given that they are present in the majority of births in low- and middle-income countries. However, the evidence suggests that focusing on just training birth attendants leads to mixed results in terms of increased referrals for appropriate conditions. In urban and periurban areas there appears to be no impact, while there is some improvement in rural areas with low prevalence rates of use of maternal care services (Alisjahbana et al., 1995; Bailey et al., 1994). The consensus from a number of sources suggests that husbands and possibly other family members (mothers-in-law, mothers, and sisters) are the key people who should be targeted, as they are the final decision makers with regard to whether the woman will go to a modern health care facility (Alisjahbana et al., 1995; Center for Health Research, 1991; Bailey, Dominik, Janowitz, & Aaujo, 1991; Bower & Perez, 1993; Howard-Grabman, Seoane, & Davenport, 1994).

### Constraints Affecting Use of Obstetric Care Services Once Complications Are Identified

There are several concerns that affect the decision to use modern obstetric care services once a life-threatening complication is identified and the need for obstetric care is acknowledged. These include economic constraints (that is, not being able to afford the costs of such care, including transportation costs), logistic constraints (taking time off to accompany the patient to often distant care facilities), and quality concerns (attitude and treatment of health care providers) (Sundari, 1992; Thaddeus & Maine, 1994).

It is important to recognize that the economic costs of care include not only the nominal costs charged by the health care facility for delivery-related services, but also transportation costs (which are not insubstantial in many rural settings), costs of medications, and costs of housing. In many cultures family members need to accompany the patient, and this adds to transportation and housing costs. In addition to these direct costs, there is also the issue of opportunity costs or lost wages for the patient and particularly family members who accompany the patient. There is relatively little population-based data to estimate all the various components of costs that are incurred for a maternal delivery in a health care facility, but some reports suggest that costs may in fact be a barrier to the use of obstetric services. For example, data from three countries in Africa (Nigeria, Ghana, and Sierra Leone) show that there were declines in deliveries in seven referral sites from 1983 to 1989, paralleling increases in costs to patients for drugs and services (Prevention of Maternal Mortality Network, 1995). The impact of user fees on the use of obstetric care for complicated cases (as opposed to normal deliveries) has been inadequately investigated. The existing evidence shows a mixed response to the imposition of user fees, with use of modern medical facilities for obstetric complications being reduced to different degrees in different countries (Prevention of Maternal Mortality Network, 1995; Ambaretnani et al., 1993).

Clearly much more information needs to be collected to understand the changes in demand and use of obstetric care services with changes in costs of services. Special attention needs to be focused on getting data on the nonservice components of obstetric costs (that is, travel costs, opportunity costs, and so on).

Aside from economic costs, transportation constraints are a major factor in the low use of maternal care services. In most low- and middle-income countries advanced obstetric care (including surgical services with appropriate transfusion capabilities) is only available in a few health care facilities, often at a considerable distance from the patient. Transportation facilities are, for the most part, poorly developed and quite expensive. Thus problems need to be anticipated in advance to allow for enough time for the patient to reach the care facility. The degree to which lack of transportation is a major constraint to the use of modern obstetric services is not certain; the evidence is mixed. Data from rural Bangladesh suggest that relatively modest investments in transportation can have a significant impact on use of obstetric services, leading to reductions in maternal mortality (Fauveau, Stewart, Khan, & Chakraborty, 1991; Maine, Akalin, Chakraborty, de Francisco, & Strong, 1996). On the other hand, three different experiments that aimed at ensuring transport did not by themselves increase the use of obstetric services (Alisjahbana et al., 1995; Prevention of Maternal Mortality Network, 1995; Poedje et al., 1993; ).

Transportation concerns assume the patient has to be brought to the care facility. Another complementary approach is to bring the provider closer to the patient. There has been some limited success with posting certified midwives in health posts closer to the pregnant patient population, but such staffing may be difficult to sustain logistically and financially (Fauveau et al., 1991; Tsui et al., 1997).

Finally, the welcoming nature of the referral site and its flexibility in accommodating accompanying family members are often ignored but particularly important constraints to seeking modern obstetric care. Oftentimes, referral sites are perceived as impersonal and unfriendly and are passed over in favor of care from traditional birth attendants (Eades, Brace, Osei, & LaGuardia, 1993; Bailey et al., 1994).

### Quality of the Obstetric Care in the Care Facility

There is relatively little systematic data on the quality of health care services in obstetric care facilities. The few studies that exist suggest that the majority of obstetric care facilities in the low- and middle-income countries fall far short of minimal acceptable standards of care. Important indicators of quality include waiting time from admission to treatment, trends in numbers and rates of maternal and perinatal deaths, and trends in case fatality rates for all complications including Caesareans (O'Rourke, 1995; Prevention of Maternal Mortality Network, 1995).

Much of this problem can be traced to lack of adequate resources in terms of trained personnel, equipment, and bed capacity. For example, a UNICEF survey of three districts in India in 1993 found not only inadequate numbers of beds but also huge disparities in bed allocation between different levels of the health care system. The majority of beds were allocated to referral cites where a small minority of complicated births were managed. There were also major deficiencies in the availability of essential drugs and appropriately trained surgical and anesthesia professionals.

In addition to supply constraints, there are frequently also major deficiencies in the management of services and in provider attitudes. Triaging is not done systematically and very sick patients are often left waiting for much longer than medically desirable, while others with less severe problems are treated before them. Obstetric care is often ad hoc, with no consistent set of case management algorithms being followed. Nursing is often seriously below standard, and basic levels of hygiene are not adhered to, leading to considerable postoperative morbidity and mortality.

In a nationally representative study of 718 maternal deaths in Egypt in 1992 (Egypt Ministry of Health, 1994), avoidable factors (that is, those that could have been changed by either the health delivery system or the patient) were assessed by an expert panel. In about half the cases, the primary avoidable factor identified was poor management and diagnoses by health care professionals. For the rest, patient factors, particularly delay in seeking medical

care (or compliance with medical recommendations) were implicated. It is interesting to note
that the health professionals most cited for poor
quality of care were not traditional birth attendants or general practitioners but, in fact, obste-
tricians with supposedly appropriate training.
This sorry state of affairs is significantly related
to the lack of consistent management guidelines
for complicated obstetric cases.

Similar results have been reported from China
(World Health Organization, 1994b), where a
study of 1,173 maternal deaths in 1990 implicated deficiencies in the health care system as
the highest contributor (48%), followed by individual and family delays in using health care,
and transport problems. There appears to be a
clear rural/urban divide, with rural areas having
much higher frequency of problems that are
avoidable both from the point of view of the
health care system and from the point of view
of the patient.

Improvements in the quality of care require
a number of simultaneous initiatives. Governments must appropriately fund health care referral facilities so that they have adequate supplies
and equipment and are staffed by appropriate
specialists. There must be a clear chain of referral whereby trained birth attendants refer complicated obstetric cases to higher level facilities,
where specialist care is available. Efforts must
be made to follow consistent management protocols that are clearly articulated, and both birth
attendants and specialists must be trained to
adhere to them (Marshall & Buffington, 1991;
Scheiber, Meija, Koritz, Gonsalez, & Kwast,
1995). There has to be a monitoring system that
will provide regular audits of both process and
outcome indicators, such as waiting times and
case fatalities, and will be used in a continuous
process of review and upgrading (Egypt Ministry of Health, 1994).

If even some of these improvements in quality
of care are made, they will not only improve
outcomes for those women who reach the health
facility but will also increase the demand for
such services by pregnant women (Mantz &
Okong, 1994; O'Rourke, 1995).

## CONCLUSION

This chapter has outlined the need for reproductive health and family planning to help individual women and men and populations reduce
fertility and maintain reproductive health. Population growth rates are declining in much of the
world because people are reducing their fertility. The primary factors effecting this reduction
are early termination of the reproductive period
through sterilization, use of contraception to
reduce conception rates, and induced abortion.
Because of increased desire for smaller families, both unwanted fertility and unmet needs for
family planning and reproductive health services
exist in most of the low- and middle-income
countries. In order to meet this challenge, improvements are needed in the quality of family
planning services, especially in the areas of information exchange and method choice, integration of reproductive health services in addition
to contraceptive provision, and financial sustainability. Maternity care needs to be expanded so
that the sequelae of pregnancy and childbearing
can be reduced. Preventive services need to be
increased and targeted to those at greatest risk
of adverse outcomes. These include education
of both men and women regarding health and
sexuality and regarding family planning and the
prevention of STIs.

At the societal level, programs need to be supported to improve the status of women, whether
through education or through changes in laws and
culture to reduce violence. Although this may be
unfamiliar territory to public health professionals, the consequences for the health of women
and children make it essential that this broader
perspective become part of the health programs.

An overriding concern regarding continuing,
let alone expanded, funding remains. Many industrialized countries have reduced their aid
contributions; many low- and middle-income
countries are undergoing financial and health
crises. Part of the agenda for the future must be
research to determine cost-effective and effective programs that will address the reproductive
health needs of the twenty-first century.

## DISCUSSION QUESTIONS

1. Using the proximate determinants framework (originally proposed by Bongaarts and subsequently revised by Stover), discuss the relative impacts of contraception, breastfeeding, abortion, sexual activity, and infecundity on total fertility rates in Latin America versus Africa. What are the policy implications of these findings?

2. The 1994 Cairo ICPD substantially enlarged the scope of family planning to include a broader conception of women's health and development. Discuss the pros and cons of this expansion in the context of limited financial resources.

3. Discuss the impact of birth interval length, both prior and subsequent, on the health of children, taking into account methodological concerns about reverse causality. What are the implications for policy?

4. Consider the statement: "Family planning has only a limited role to play in reducing the risk of maternal mortality." Discuss whether you agree with this statement and elaborate on the policy implications of your analysis.

5. "Specific health technological inputs are a necessary but not sufficient determinant of significant improvements in reproductive health." Using the example of changes in women's status, discuss the validity of this proposition.

## REFERENCES

Aaby, P., Bukh, J., Lisse, I.M., & Smits, A.J. (1984). Overcrowding and intensive exposure as determinants of measles mortality. *American Journal of Epidemiology, 120*(1), 49–63.

Aitken, I.W., & Walls, B. (1986). Maternal height and cephalopelvic disproportion in Sierra Leone. *Tropical Doctor, 16*(3), 132–134.

Alauddin, M. (1986). Maternal mortality in rural Bangladesh: The Tangail district. *Studies in Family Planning, 17*(1), 13–21.

Alisjahbana, A.C., Williams, C., Dharmayanti, R., Hermawan, D., Kwast, B.E., & Koblinsky, M. (1995). An integrated village maternity service to improve referral patterns in a rural area in West Java. *International Journal of Gynecology and Obstetrics, 48 (supplement)*, s83–s94.

Ambaretnani, N.P., Hessler-Radelet, C., & Carlin, L.E. (1993). Qualitative research for the social marketing component of the Perinatal Regionalization Project, Tanjungsari, Java. MotherCare Working Paper #19, prepared for the U.S. Agency for International Development, Project #936–5966. Arlington, VA: John Snow, Inc.

Bailey, P.E., Dominik, R.C., Janowitz, B., & Aaujo, L. (1991). Obstetrica e mortalidade perinatal em uma area rural do nordeste Brasileiro. *Boletin de la Oficina Sanitaria Panamericana, 111*(4), 306–318.

Bailey, P.E., Szaszdi, J.A., & Scheiber, B. (1994). Analysis of the vital events reporting system of the Maternal and Neonatal Health Project: Quetzaltenango, Guatemala. MotherCare Working Paper #3, prepared for the U.S. Agency for International Development. Project #DPE-5966-Z-00–8083–00. Arlington, VA: John Snow, Inc.

Bankole, A., & Westoff, C.F. (1995). Childbearing attitudes and intentions. *DHS Comparative Studies*, no. 17. Calverton, MD: Macro International, Inc.

Bledsoe, C.H., & Cohen, B. (Eds.). (1993). Social dynamics of adolescent fertility in sub-Saharan Africa. Working Group on the Social Dynamics of Adolescent Fertility in Sub-Saharan Africa, Committee on Population, National Research Council. Washington, DC: National Academy Press.

Bongaarts, J. (1978). A framework for analyzing the proximate determinants of fertility. *Population and Development Review, 4,* 105–132.

Bongaarts, J. (1983). The proximate determinants of natural marital fertility. In R.A. Bulatao & R.D. Lee (Eds.), *Determinants of fertility in developing countries* (Vol. 1, pp. 103–108). New York: Academic Press.

Bongaarts, J. (1990). The measurement of unwanted fertility. *Population and Development Review, 16*(3), 487–506.

Bongaarts, J. (1991). Do reproductive intentions matter? *Demographic and Health Surveys World Conference, 1*, 223–248.

Bongaarts, J. (1997a). Trends in unwanted childbearing in the developing world. *Studies in Family Planning, 28*(4), 267–277.

Bongaarts, J. (1997b). The role of family planning programmes in contemporary fertility transitions. In G.W. Jones, R.M. Douglas, J.C. Caldwell, & R.M. D'Souza, (Eds.), *The continuing demographic transition* (pp. 422–443). New York and Oxford: Oxford University Press.

Bongaarts, J., & Bruce, J. (1995). The causes of unmet need for contraception and the social context of services. *Studies in Family Planning, 26*(2), 57–76.

Bongaarts, J., & Potter, R.G., Jr. (1983). *Fertility, biology, and behavior: An analysis of the proximate determinants.* New York: Academic Press.

Bongaarts, J., & Watkins, S.C. (1996). Social interactions and contemporary fertility transitions. *Population and Development Review, 22*(4), 639–682.

Bothwell, T.H., & Charllton, R. (1981). *Iron deficiency in women.* Washington, DC: International Nutrition Anemia Consultative Group.

Bower, B., & Perez, A. (1993). *Final project report: Cochabamba reproductive health project.* Report prepared for the U.S. Agency for International Development, MotherCare Project #5966-C-00–3038–00. Arlington, VA: John Snow, Inc.

Brown, S.S., & Eisenberg, L. (Eds.). (1995). *The best intentions: Unintended pregnancy and the well-being of children and families.* Committee on Unintended Pregnancy, Institute of Medicine. Washington, DC: National Academy Press.

Bulatao, R.A. (1993). Effectiveness and evolution in family planning programs. In *International population conference* (Vol. 1, pp. 189–200). Liege, Belgium: International Union for the Scientific Study of Population.

Bulatao, R.A. (1998). *The value of family planning programs in developing countries.* Santa Monica, CA: RAND.

Bulatao, R.A., & Lee, R. (Eds.). (1983). *Determinants of fertility in developing countries.* Vol. 1: *Supply and Demand for Children.* New York: Academic Press.

Caldwell, J.C. (1986). Routes to low mortality in poor countries. *Population and Development Review, 12*(2), 171–200.

Caldwell, J.C., Barkat-e-Khuda, Caldwell B., Pieris, I., & Caldwell, P. (1999). The Bangladesh fertility decline: An interpretation. *Population and Development Review, 25*(1), 67–84.

Casterline, J., Perez, A.E., & Biddlecom, A.E. (1996). Factors underlying unmet need for family planning in the Philippines. Research Division working paper no. 84. New York: Population Council.

Center for Health Research, Consultation and Education and MotherCare/John Snow, Inc. (1991). *Qualitative research on knowledge, attitudes, and practices related to women's reproductive health.* MotherCare Working Paper #9, prepared for the U.S. Agency for International Development. MotherCare Project #936–5966. Arlington, VA: John Snow, Inc.

Chen, L.C., Gesche, M.C., Ahmed, S., Chowdhury, A.I., & Mosley, W.H. (1975). Maternal mortality in Bangladesh. *Studies in Family Planning, 5*(11), 334–341.

Chi, L.C., Agoestina, T., & Harbin, J. (1981). Maternal mortality at twelve teaching hospitals in Indonesia—An epidemiologic analysis. *International Journal of Gynaecology and Obstetrics, 19*(4), 259–266.

Cleland, J., Phillips, J.F., Amin, S., & Kamal, G.M. (1994). *The determinants of reproductive change in Bangladesh.* Washington, DC: The World Bank.

Coale, A.J., & Watkins, S.C. (1986). *The decline of fertility in Europe.* Princeton, NJ: Princeton University Press.

Cochrane, S., & Sai, F. (1993). Excess fertility. In D.T. Jamison et al. (Eds.), *Disease control priorities in developing countries* (pp. 333–362). New York: Oxford University Press.

Curtis, S.L., & Neitzel, K. (1996). *Contraceptive knowledge, use, and sources.* DHS Comparative Studies No. 19. Columbia, MD: Institute for Resource Development.

Das Gupta, M. (1987). Selective discrimination against female children in rural Punjab. *Population and Development Review, 13*(1), 77–100.

DaVanzo, J., & Adamson, D.M. (1998). Family planning in developing countries: An unfinished success story. *Population Matters Issue Paper.* Santa Monica, CA: RAND.

DaVanzo, J., Butz, W.P., & Habicht, J.P. (1983). How biological and behavioral influences on mortality in Malaysia vary during the first year of life. *Population Studies, 37*(3), 381–402.

David, H.P. (1992). Abortion in Europe, 1920–91: A public health perspective. *Studies in Family Planning, 23*(1), 1–22.

De Graft-Johnson, J. (1994). Maternal morbidity in Ghana. Paper presented at the annual meeting of the Population Association of America, Miami, FL.

Demographic and Health Surveys, Macro International, Inc. (1998). Bangladesh demographic and health survey,

1996–1997. Bangladesh: National Institute of Population Research and Training; Mitra and Associates; Demographic and Health Surveys, Macro International, Inc.

Desai, S. (1995). When are children from large families disadvantaged? Evidence from cross-national analyses. *Population Studies, 49*, 195–210.

Dixon-Mueller, R., & Germain, A. (1992). Stalking the elusive "unmet need" for family planning. *Studies in Family Planning, 23*(5), 330–335.

D'Souza, S., & Chen, L.C. (1980). Sex differentials in mortality in rural Bangladesh. *Population and Development Review, 6*(2), 257–270.

Duffy, L., & Menken, J. (1998). Health, fertility, and socioeconomic status as predictors of survival and later health of women: A twenty-year prospective study in rural Bangladesh. Working Paper WP-98–11, Population Program, Institute of Behavioral Science, University of Colorado at Boulder.

Eades, C., Brace, C., Osei, L., & LaGuardia, K. (1993). Traditional birth attendants and maternal mortality in Ghana. *Social Science and Medicine, 36*(11), 1503–1507.

Eclampsia Trial Collaborative Group. (1995). Which anticonvulsant for women with eclampsia? Evidence from the Collaborative Eclampsia Trial. *Lancet, 345*, 1455–1463.

Egypt Ministry of Health. (1994). National maternal mortality study: Egypt, 1992–1993. Ministry of Health, Child Survival Project, Alexandria, Egypt.

Faundes, A., Fanjul, B., Henriquez, G., Mora, G., & Tognola, C. (1974). Influencia de la edad y de la paridad sobre algunos parametros de morbilidad materna y sobre la morbimortalidad fetal. *Revista Chile–a de Obstetrica y Ginecologia, 37*(1), 6–14.

Fauveau, V., Koenig, M., Chakraborty, J., & Chowdhury, A. (1988). Causes of maternal mortality in rural Bangladesh, 1976–1985. *Bulletin of the World Health Organization, 66*(5), 643–651.

Fauveau, V., Stewart, K., Khan, S.A., & Chakraborty, J. (1991). Effect on mortality of community-based maternity-care programme in rural Bangladesh. *Lancet, 338*, 1183–1186.

Fauveau, V., Wojtyniak, B., Mostafa, G., Sarder, A.M., & Chakraborty, J. (1990). Perinatal mortality in Matlab, Bangladesh: A community-based study. *International Journal of Epidemiology, 19*, 606–612.

Ferraz, E.M., Gray, R.H., Fleming, P.L., & Maria, T.M. (1988). Interpregnancy interval and low birthweight: Findings from a case-control study. *American Journal of Epidemiology, 128*, 1111–1116.

Finkle, J.L., & Ness, G.D. (1985). *Managing delivery systems—Identifying leverage points for improving family planning program performance.* Final report. Ann Arbor,

MI: Department of Population Planning and International Health, University of Michigan.

Fortney, J.A. (1995). Antenatal risk screening and scoring: A New Look. *International Journal of Gynecology and Obstetrics, 2* (supplement), s53–s58.

Fortney, J.A., Susanti, I., Gadalla, S., Saleh, S., Feldblum, P.J., & Potts, M. (1985, November). Maternal mortality in Indonesia and Egypt. WHO FHE/PMM/85.9.13. WHO Inter-regional Meeting on Prevention of Maternal Mortality, Geneva.

Foster, A., Menken, J., Chowdhury, A., & Trussell, J. (1987). Female reproductive development: A hazard model analysis. *Social Biology, 33*(3–4), 183–198.

Foster, A., & Roy, N. (1996). The dynamics of education and fertility: Evidence from a family planning experiment. Working Paper, Department of Economics, University of Pennsylvania.

Freedman, R. (1987). The contribution of social science research to population policy and family planning effectiveness. *Studies in Family Planning, 18*(2), 57–82.

French, F.E., & Bierman, J.M. (1962). Probabilities of fetal mortality. *Public Health Report, 77*, 835–847.

Frenzen, P.D., & Hogan, D.P. (1982). The impact of class, education, and health care on infant mortality in a developing society: The case of rural Thailand. *Demography, 19*, 391–408.

Gelbard, A., Haub, C., & Kent, M.M. (1999). World population beyond six billion. *Population Bulletin, 54*(1), 1–40.

Geronimus, A.T. (1987). On teenage childbearing and neonatal mortality in the United States. *Population and Development Review, 13*(2), 245–279.

Goto, A., Reich, M.R., & Aitken, I. (1999). Oral contraceptives and women's health in Japan. *Journal of the American Medical Association, 282*(22), 2173–2177.

Govindasamy, P., Stewart, K., Rutstein, S., Boerma, J., & Sommerfelt, A. (1993). High-risk births and maternity care. *Demographic and Health Surveys Comparative Studies,* No. 8. Columbia, MD: Macro International, Inc.

Greenwood, A.M., Greenwood, B.M., Bradley, A.K., Wiliams, K., Shenton, F.C., Tulloch, S., Byass, P., & Oldfield, F.S.J. (1987). A prospective survey of the outcome of pregnancy in a rural area in the Gambia. *Bulletin of the World Health Organization, 65*(5), 635–643.

Gubhaju, B. (1986). Effect of birth spacing on infant and child mortality in rural Nepal. *Journal of Biosocial Science, 18*(4), 435–447.

Haaga, J. (1989). Mechanisms for the association of maternal age, parity, and birth spacing with infant health. In A.M. Parnell (Ed.), *Contraceptive use and controlled fertility: Health issues for women and children.* Washington, DC: National Academy Press.

Hansen, J.P. (1986). Older maternal age and pregnancy outcome: A review of the literature. *Obstetrical and Gynecological Survey, 41,* 726–742.

Harrison, K.A., & Rossiter, L.A. (1985). Child-bearing, health and social priorities: A survey of 22,774 consecutive hospital births in Zaria, Northern Nigeria. *British Journal of Obstetrics and Gynecology, 5* (supplement), 1–119.

Harrison, P.F., & Rosenfield, A. (Eds.). (1996). *Contraceptive research and development: Looking to the future.* Committee on Contraceptive Research and Development, Institute of Medicine. Washington, DC: National Academy Press.

Henshaw, S., & Morrow, E. (1990). *Induced abortion: A world review, 1990 Supplement.* New York: Alan Guttmacher Institute.

Hobcraft, J.N. (1987, October). Does family planning save children's lives? Paper prepared for the International Conference on Better Health for Women and Children through Family Planning, Nairobi.

Hobcraft, J.N., McDonald, J.W., & Rutstein, S.O. (1985). Demographic determinants of infant and child mortality: A comparative analysis. *Population Studies, 39*(3), 363–385.

Hogberg, U., Wall, S., & Brostroin, G. (1986). The impact of early medical technology on maternal mortality in the late 19th century Sweden. *International Journal of Gynecology and Obstetrics, 24,* 251–261.

Howard-Grabman, L., Seoane, L.G., & Davenport, C.A. (1994). *The Warmi Project—A participatory approach to improve maternal and neonatal health: An implementor's manual.* MotherCare Project. Arlington, VA: John Snow, Inc.

International Planned Parenthood Foundation. (1995). *Consensus statement on emergency contraception.* London: Author.

Jamison, D.T., Mosley, W.H., Measham, A.R., & Bobadilla, J.L. (1993). Disease control priorities in developing countries. Published for the World Bank. New York: Oxford University Press.

Jelliffe, D.B. (1976). Maternal nutrition and lactation. In CIBA Foundation Symposium, Breastfeeding and the mother. Amsterdam: Excerpta Medica.

John, A.M., Menken, J., & Chowdhury, A. (1987). The effects of breastfeeding and nutrition on fecundability in rural Bangladesh: A hazards-model analysis. *Population Studies, 41*(3), 433–446.

Jones, R.E. (1988). A biobehavioral model for breastfeeding effects on return to menses postpartum in Javanese women. *Social Biology, 35,* 307–323.

Kenney, G.M. (1993). Assessing legal and regulatory reform in family planning: Manual on legal and regulatory reform. OPTIONS Projects Policy Paper No. 1. The Futures Group, Washington, DC.

Khan, A.R., Jahan, F.A., & Begum, S.F. (1986). Maternal mortality in rural Bangladesh: The Jamalpur District. *Studies in Family Planning, 17*(1), 7–12.

Kitay, D., & Harbort, R. (1975). Iron and folic acid deficiency in pregnancy. *Clinical Perinatalogy, 2,* 255–273.

Knodel, J., Chamrathrithirong, A., & Debavalya, N. (1987). *Thailand's reproductive revolution: Rapid fertility decline in a third world setting.* Madison, WI: University of Wisconsin Press.

Koblinsky, M.A. (1995). Beyond maternal mortality—Magnitude, interrelationship, and consequences of women's health, pregnancy-related complications and nutritional status on pregnancy outcomes. *International Journal of Gynecology and Obstetrics, 48* (supplement), 21–32.

Koblinsky, M.A., Campbell, O., & Harlow, S. (1993). Mother and more: A broader perspective on women's health. In M.A. Koblinsky, J. Timyan, & J. Gay (Eds.), *The health of women: A global perspective* (pp. 3–32). Boulder, CO: Westview Press.

Koenig, M.A., Phillips, J., Campbell, O., & D'Souza, S. (1988). Maternal mortality in Matlab, Bangladesh: 1976–1985. *Studies in Family Planning, 19*(2), 69–80.

Kwast, B.E., Rochat, R.W., & Kidane-Mariam, W. (1986). Maternal mortality in Addis Ababa, Ethiopia. *Studies in Family Planning, 17*(6), 288–301.

Kwast, B.E., & Stevens, J.A. (1987). Viral hepatitis as a major cause of maternal mortality in Addis Ababa, Ethiopia. *International Journal of Gynecology and Obstetrics, 25,* 99–106.

Larsen, U. (1993). Levels, age patterns and trends of sterility in selected countries south of the Sahara. International Population Conference, Montreal (Vol. 1). Liege, Belgium: International Union for the Scientific Study of Population.

Larsen, U. (1995). Trends in infertility in Cameroon and Nigeria. *International Family Planning Perspectives, 21*(4), 138–142.

Larsen, U. (1996). Childlessness, subfecundity and infertility in Tanzania. *Studies in Family Planning, 27*(1), 18–28.

Larsen, U., Chung, W., & Das Gupta, M. (1998). Fertility and son preference in Korea. *Population Studies, 52,* 3, 317–325.

Lawson, J. (1992). Vaginal fistulae. *Journal of the Royal Society of Medicine, 85,* 254–256.

Lettenmier, C., Liskin, L., Church, C.A., & Harris, J.A. (1988). Mothers' lives matter: Maternal health in the community. Population Reports, L, 7. Johns Hopkins University, Population Information Program, Baltimore.

Levin, H., Pollitt, E., Galloway, R., & McGuire, J. (1993). Micronutrient deficiency disorders. In D. Jamison, W.H. Mosley, A. Measham, & J.L. Bobadilla (Eds.), *Disease control priorities in developing countries.* New York: Oxford University Press.

Lloyd, C. (1994). Investing in the next generation: The implications of high fertility at the level of the family. In Robert Cassen (Ed.), *Population and development: Old debates, new conclusions* (pp. 181–202). New Brunswick, NJ: Transaction Publishers.

Loudon, I. (1991). On maternal and infant mortality 1900–1960. *Social History of Medicine, 4*(1), 29–73.

MacGregor, I.A., Wilson, M.E., & Billewicz, W.Z. (1983). Malaria infection of the placenta in the Gambia, West Africa: Its incidence and relationship to stillbirth, birthweight and placental weight. *Transactions of the Royal Society of Tropical Medicine and Hygiene, 77*(2), 232–244.

Macro International, Inc. (1994). Selected statistics from DHS. *Demographic and Health Surveys Newsletter, 6*(2).

Maine, D. (1991). Safe motherhood programs: Options and issues. Center for Population and Family Health, School of Public Health. New York: Columbia University.

Maine, D., Akalin, M.Z., Chakraborty, J., de Francisco, A., & Strong, M. (1996). Why did maternal mortality decline in Matlab? *Studies in Family Planning, 27,* 179–187.

Mantz, M.L., & Okong, P. (1994). *Evaluation report: Uganda life saving skills program for midwives, October-November, 1994.* Report prepared for the U.S. Agency for International Development. MotherCare Project #5966-C-00-3038-00. Arlington, VA: John Snow, Inc.

Marshall, M.A., & Buffington, S.T. (1991). *Life-saving skills manual for midwives* (2nd ed.). Washington, DC: American College of Nurse-Midwives.

Mason, K.O., & Taj, A.M. (1987). Differences between women's and men's reproductive goals in developing countries. *Population and Development Review, 13*(4), 611–638.

McIntosh, C.A., & Finkle, J.L. (1995). The Cairo conference on population and development: A new paradigm? *Population and Development Review, 21,* 223–260.

McNeilly, A. (1996). Breastfeeding and the suppression of fertility. *Food and Nutrition Bulletin, 17,* 340–345.

Menken, J. (1975). *Estimating fecundability.* Doctoral dissertation, Princeton University.

Menken, J., Khan, M.N., & Williams, J. (1999, March). The role of female education in the Bangladesh fertility decline. Paper presented at the annual meeting of the Population Association of America, New York.

Menken, J., & Kuhn, R. (1996). Demographic effects of breastfeeding: Fertility, mortality and population growth. *Food and Nutrition Bulletin, 17,* 349–361.

Merchant, K., & Martorell, R. (1988). Frequent reproductive cycling: Does it lead to nutritional depletion of mothers? *Progress in Food and Nutrition, 12,* 339–369.

Miller, J.E. (1989). Is the relationship between birth intervals and perinatal mortality spurious? Evidence from Hungary and Sweden. *Population Studies, 43*(3), 479–495.

Morrow, R.H., Jr., Smetana, H.F., Sai, F.T., & Edgcomb, J.H. (1968). Unusual features of viral hepatitis in Accra, Ghana. *Annals of Internal Medicine, 68*(6), 1250–1264.

Muhuri, P., & Menken, J. (1997). Adverse effects of next birth, gender, and family composition on child survival in rural Bangladesh. *Population Studies, 51,* 279–294.

Muhuri, P. & Preston, S.H. (1991). Effects of family composition on mortality differentials by sex among children in Matlab, Bangladesh. *Population and Development Review, 17*(3), 415–433.

Mukaire, J., Kalikwani, F., Maggwa, B.N., & Kisubi, W. (1997). *Integration of STI and HIV/AIDS services with MCH-FP services: A case study of the Busoga Diocese family life education program, Uganda.* Operations Research Technical Assistance, Africa Project II, Population Council, Nairobi.

National Research Council. (1989). *Contraception and reproduction: Health consequences for women and children in the developing world.* Committee on Population, Working Group on Healthy Consequences of Contraceptive Use and Controlled Fertility. Washington, DC: National Academy Press.

National Statistics Office (Philippines) and Macro International, Inc. (1994). Philippines National Safe Motherhood Survey, 1993. Calverton, MD: National Statistics Office and Macro International, Inc.

*New York Times.* (1999a, April 10). Population control measures to aid women are stumbling.

*New York Times.* (1999b, June 30). Insurance for VIAGRA spurs coverage for birth control.

*New York Times.* (1999c, July 3). Conference adopts plan on limiting population.

Notestein, F.W. (1953). Economic problems of population change. In *Proceedings of the Eighth International Conference of Agricultural Economics* (pp. 13–31). London: Oxford University Press.

Omran, A.R., & Standley, C.C. (Eds.). (1981). *Further studies on family formation patterns and health: An international collaborative study in Colombia, Egypt, Pakistan, and the Syrian Arab Republic.* Geneva, Switzerland: World Health Organization.

O'Rourke, K. (1995). The effect of hospital staff training on management of obstetrical patients referred by traditional birth attendants. *International Journal of Gynecology and Obstetrics, 48* (supplement), s95–s102.

Overall, J.C. (1987). Viral infections of the fetus and neonate. In R.D. Feigin & J.D. Cherry (Eds.), *Textbook of pediatric infectious diseases* (2nd ed., pp. 966–1007). Philadelphia: W.B. Saunders.

Palloni, A. (1985). Health conditions in Latin America and policies for mortality changes. In J. Vaillin & A. Lopez

(Eds.), *Health policy, social policy, and mortality prospects* (pp. 465–492). Liege, Belgium: Ordina Editions.

Palloni, A., & Millman, S. (1986). Effects of inter-birth intervals and breastfeeding on infant and early childhood mortality. *Population Studies, 40*(2), 215–236.

Pebley, A.R., & DaVanzo, J. (1988, April). Maternal depletion and child survival in Guatemala and Malaysia. Paper presented at the annual meeting of the Population Association of America, New Orleans.

Pebley, A.R., & Stupp, P.W. (1987). Reproductive patterns and child mortality in Guatemala. *Demography, 24*(1), 43–60.

Poedje, R., Setjalilakusuma, L., Abadi, A., Soegianto, B., Rihadi, S., Djaeli, A., & Budiarto, W. (1993). *Final project report: East Java safe motherhood study.* Report prepared for the U.S. Agency for International Development. MotherCare Project #936–5966. Arlington, VA: John Snow, Inc.

Population Reference Bureau. (1995). *Reproductive risk: A worldwide assessment of women's sexual and maternal health.* Washington, DC: Author.

Potter, J.E. (1988). Does family planning reduce infant mortality? *Population and Development Review, 14*(1), 179–187.

Prevention of Maternal Mortality Network. (1995). Situational analyses of emergency obstetric care: Examples from eleven operations research projects in West Africa. *Social Science and Medicine, 40* (supplement), 657–667.

Pritchett, L. (1994a). Desired fertility and the impact of population policies. *Population and Development Review, 20*(1), 1–55.

Pritchett, L. (1994b). The impact of population policies: Reply. *Population and Development Review, 20*(3), 621–630.

Public Opinion Polls. (1993). *MotherCare Nigeria Maternal Healthcare Project qualitative research.* MotherCare Working Paper #17B, prepared for the U.S. Agency for International Development. Project #936–5966. Arlington, VA: John Snow, Inc.

Rahman, O. (1999). Family matters. The impact of kin on elderly mortality in rural Bangladesh. *Population Studies, 53*, 2, 227–235.

Rahman, O., Menken, J., & Foster, A. (1992). Older widow mortality in rural Bangladesh. *Social Science and Medicine, 34*(1), 89–96.

Reed, H.E., Koblinsky, M.A., & Mosley, W.H. (Eds.). (2000). *The consequences of maternal morbidity and maternal mortality.* Committee on Population, Commission on Behavioral and Social Sciences and Education, National Research Council. Washington, DC: National Academy Press.

Robey, B.K., Rutstein, S.O., & Morris, L. (1992). The reproductive revolution: New survey findings. *Population Reports,* series M, no. 11.

Ronsman, C., & Campbell, O. (1998). Short birth intervals don't kill women: Evidence from Matlab, Bangladesh. *Studies in Family Planning, 29*(3), 282–290.

Rooney, C. (1992). *Antenatal care and maternal health: How effective is it? A review of the evidence.* WHO/MSM/92.4. Geneva, Switzerland: World Health Organization.

Rosenzweig, M.R., & Schultz, T.P. (1983). Estimating a household production function: Heterogeneity, the demand for health inputs, and their effects on birth weight. *Journal of Political Economy, 91*(5), 723–746.

Ross, J., & Frankenberg, E. (1993). *Findings from Two Decades of Family Planning Research.* New York: Population Council, 1993.

Ross, J.A., & Mauldin, W.P. (1996). Family planning programs: Efforts and results, 1972–1994. *Studies in Family Planning, 27*(3), 137–147.

Rutstein, S.O. (1998). Change in the desired number of children: A cross-country cohort analysis of levels and correlates of change. DHS Analytical Report, No. 9. Calverton, MD: Macro International, Inc.

Salber, E.J., Feinleib, M., & MacMahon, B. (1966). The duration of postpartum amenorrhea. *American Journal of Epidemiology, 82,* 347–358.

Scheiber, B.A., Mejia, M., Koritz, S., Gonsalez, C., & Kwast, B. (1995). *Medical audit of early neonatal deaths: INCAP: Quetzaltenango maternal and neonatal health project.* Technical Working Paper #1, prepared for the U.S. Agency for International Development. MotherCare Project #936–5966. Arlington, VA: John Snow, Inc.

Schultz, T.P. (1984). Studying the impact of household economic and community variables on child mortality. *Population and Development Review, 10* (supplement), 215–235.

Sheps, M.C., & Menken, J. (1973). *Mathematical models of conception and birth.* Chicago: University of Chicago Press.

Sloan, N.L., Jordan, E.A., & Winikoff, B. (1992). *Does iron supplementation make a difference?* MotherCare Working Paper #15, prepared for the U.S. Agency for International Development. MotherCare Project #936–5966. Arlington, VA: John Snow, Inc.

Sood, S.K., Ramachandran, K., Mathur, M., Gupta, K., Ramalingaswamy, V., Swarnabai, C., Ponniah, J., Mathan, V.I., & Baker, S.J. (1975). WHO sponsored collaborative studies on nutritional anemia in India. Part I: The effects of supplemental oral iron administration to pregnant women. *Quarterly Journal of Medicine, 174,* 241–258.

Stewart, M.K., & Festin, M. (1995). Validation study of women's reporting and recall of major obstetric complications treated at the Philippine General Hospital. *International Journal of Gynecology and Obstetrics, 48* (supplement), s53–s66.

Stone, J.L., Lockwood, C.J., Berkowitz, G., Alvarez, M., Lapinski, R., & Berkowitz, R. (1994). Risk factors for severe preeclampsia. *Obstetrics and Gynecology, 83,* 357–361.

Stover, J. (1998). Revising the proximate determinants of fertility framework: What have we learned in the past 20 years? *Studies in Family Planning, 29*(3), 255–267.

Sundari, T.K. (1992). The untold story: How the health care systems in developing countries contribute to maternal mortality. *International Journal of Health Service, 22*(3), 513–528.

Tahzib, F. (1983). Epidemiological determinants of vesicovaginal fistulae. *British Journal of Obstetric Gynaecology, 90,* 387–391.

Tahzib, F. (1985). Vesicovaginal fistula in Nigerian children. *Lancet, 2*(8467), 1291–1293.

Thaddeus, S., & Maine, D. (1994). Too far to walk: Maternal mortality in context. *Social Science and Medicine, 38*(8), 1091–1110.

Trottier, D.A., Potter, L.S., Taylor, B., & Glover, L.H. (1994). User characteristics and oral contraceptive compliance in Egypt. *Studies in Family Planning, 25*(4), 284–292.

Trussell, J., Ellertson, C., & Stewart, F. (1996). The effectiveness of the Yuzpe regimen of emergency contraception. *Family Planning Perspectives, 28*(2), 58–87.

Tsui, A.O., Wasserheit, J.N., & Haaga, J.G. (Eds.). (1997). *Reproductive health in developing countries, expanding dimensions, building solutions.* Panel on Reproductive Health, Committee on Population, Commission on Behavioral and Social Sciences and Education, National Research Council. Washington, DC: National Academy Press.

Turner, C.F., Miller, H.G., & Moses, L.E. (Eds.). (1989). *AIDS, sexual behavior, and intravenous drug use.* Committee on AIDS Research and the Behavioral, Social, and Statistical Sciences, Commission on Behavioral and Social Sciences and Education, National Research Council. Washington, DC: National Academy Press.

Twahir, A., Maggwa, B.N., & Askew, I. (1996). *Integration of STI and HIV/AIDS Services with MCH-FP services: A case study of the Mkomani clinic society in Mombasa, Kenya, Nairobi.* Operations Research Technical Assistance, Africa Project II. New York: Population Council.

United Nations. (1991). *Controlling iron deficiency.* Report based on an Administrative Committee on Coordination/Subcommittee on Nutrition workshop, Nutrition State-of-the-Art Series, Nutrition Policy Discussion, Paper No. 9. Geneva, Switzerland: Author.

United Nations. (1994). Programme of action of the 1994 International Conference on Population and Development. (A/CONF.171/13). Reprinted in *Population and Development Review, 21*(1), 187–213 and *21*(2), 437–461.

United Nations. (1998). *World population prospects: The 1998 Revision* (Vol. 1). ESA/P/WP.150. New York: Author.

U.S. Bureau of the Census. (1999). http://www.census.gov/ipc/www/worldpop.html.

Walker, G.J., Ashley, D.E., McCaw, A., & Bernard, G.W. (1985, November). *Maternal mortality in Jamaica: A confidential enquiry into all maternal deaths in Jamaica, 1981–1983.* WHO FHE/PMM/85.9.10. WHO Interregional Meeting on Prevention of Maternal Mortality, Geneva.

Weeks, J.R. (1999). *Population.* Belmont, CA: Wadsworth Publishing Co.

Weinbreck, P.V., Loustaud, F., Denis, B., Vidal, M., Mounier M., & DeLumley, L. (1988). Postnatal transmission of HIV infection. *The Lancet, 1,* 482.

Westley, S.B. (1995). Evidence mounts for sex-selective abortion in Asia. *Asia-Pacific Population and Policy,* No. 34. Honolulu, Hawaii: East-West Population Center.

Wilcox, A.J., Weinberg, C.R., O'Connor, J.F., Baird, D.D., Schlatter, J.P., Canfield, R.E., Armstrong, E.G., & Nisula, B.C. (1988). Incidence of early loss of pregnancy. *New England Journal of Medicine, 319,* 189–194.

Winikoff, B. (1983). The effect of birthspacing on child and maternal health. *Studies in Family Planning, 18*(3), 128–143.

Winikoff, B., Elias C., Beattie, K. (1994). Special issues of IUD use in resource-poor settings. In C.W. Bardin & D.R. Mishell, Jr. (Eds.), *Proceedings of the fourth international conference on IUDs* (pp. 230–238). New York: Population Council.

Winikoff, B., & Sullivan, M. (1987). Assessing the role of family planning in reducing maternal mortality. *Studies in Family Planning, 18*(3), 128–143.

Women's Studies Project. (1999). *The impact of family planning on women's lives.* Research Triangle Park, NC: Family Health International.

Wood, J.W. (1994). *Dynamics of human reproduction: Biology, biometry, demography.* New York: Aldine de Gruyter.

Wood, J.W., Lai, D., Johnson, P.L., Campbell, K.L., & Maslar, I.A. (1985). Lactation and birth spacing in Highland, New Guinea. *Journal of Biosocial Science,* supplement 9, 157–173.

World Health Organization (International Collaborative Study of Hypertensive Disorders of Pregnancy). (1988). Geographic variation in the incidence of hypertension in pregnancy. *American Journal of Obstetrics and Gynecology, 158*(1), 80–83.

World Health Organization. (1991). *Maternal mortality: A global factbook.* Geneva, Switzerland: Author.

World Health Organization. (1993a). *Coverage of maternity care: A tabulation of available information.* WHO/FHE/MSM/93.7. Geneva, Switzerland: Author.

World Health Organization. (1993b). *Making maternity care more accessible.* Press release No. 59. Geneva, Switzerland: Author.

World Health Organization. (1993c). The global burden of disease. Background paper prepared for the *World Development Report.* Geneva, Switzerland: Author.

World Health Organization. (1994a). *Maternal health and safe motherhood programme: Research progress report, 1987–1992.* WHO/FHE/MSM/94.18. Geneva, Switzerland: Author.

World Health Organization. (1994b). *The mother-baby package: Implementing safe motherhood in countries.* Document FRH/MSM/94.11. Geneva, Switzerland: Author.

World Health Organization. (1995). Essential or emergency obstetric care. *Safe Motherhood Newsletter, 18*(2), 1–2.

World Health Organization. (1996). *Perinatal mortality.* Document FRH/MSM/96.7. Geneva, Switzerland: Author.

World Health Organization & UNICEF. (1996). *Revised estimates of maternal mortality: A new approach by WHO and UNICEF.* Geneva, Switzerland: Author.

Younis, N., Khattab, H., Zurayk, H., el-Mouelhy, M., Fadle Amin, M., & Farag, A.M. (1993). A community study of gynecological and related morbidities in rural Egypt. *Studies in Family Planning, 24*(3), 175–186.

# CHAPTER 4

# Infectious Diseases

*Arthur L. Reingold and Christina R. Phares*

This chapter has as its focus the descriptive epidemiologic features of and available prevention and control strategies for the infectious diseases that currently are of public health significance in low- and middle-income countries. Because an in-depth discussion of these diseases cannot be covered in a single chapter, the emphasis is on how the epidemiologic features of a given disease and the relevant technological or resource limitations and cultural barriers have led to current approaches to prevention and control. Conceptually, these approaches include: preventing exposure to the infectious agent; making otherwise susceptible individuals or populations immune to the infectious agent; treating infected individuals or populations to prevent illness and transmission of the agent to others; and improving the timeliness and appropriateness of care of symptomatic individuals so as to minimize morbidity and mortality and, in some instances, also to reduce the likelihood of transmission to others. Examples of successful programs using one or more of these various conceptual approaches are discussed, as are the challenges and obstacles that confront low- and middle-income countries and their partners as they seek to reduce further the burden of disease caused by infectious agents.

*Acknowledgments:* The authors acknowledge Colin Garrett for his assistance in the preparation of this chapter.

## OVERVIEW

Collectively, infectious diseases have undoubtedly been the single most important contributors to human morbidity and mortality throughout history. Over the past 150 years, the mortality attributable to them has declined substantially in industrialized countries, and "chronic" diseases such as cardiovascular disease, cancer, stroke, chronic obstructive pulmonary disease, and diabetes mellitus have assumed prominence as the leading causes of death in these countries. Although there is uncertainty about the relative importance of various social, economic, environmental, and public health factors in this "epidemiologic transition," most of these reductions in mortality attributable to infectious diseases clearly preceded any advances in clinical medicine and public health that plausibly could have had an impact on the infectious diseases of public health significance of the time (for example, tuberculosis, rheumatic fever, scarlet fever, typhoid fever, and cholera). At present, only pneumonia, influenza, and human immunodeficiency virus (HIV)/acquired immunodeficiency syndrome (AIDS) rank among the top 10 causes of mortality in the United States.

The global burden of disease and epidemiologic transition are discussed in detail elsewhere in this book (see Chapter 1). While current projections suggest that acute infectious diseases will decrease substantially in their absolute and relative importance as causes of death and disability in low- and middle-income countries in the decades to come, it is clear that today they remain of great public health significance. According to a recent World Health Organization (WHO) report (1999), acute infectious diseases are, collectively, the leading cause of death among children and young adults, accounting for half of all deaths in low-income countries. In fact, in many countries the HIV/AIDS pandemic is reversing decades of progress in reducing mortality due to acute infectious diseases, with a resulting decrease in life expectancy. Further, it is now well-accepted that chronic infection contributes in important, if poorly understood, ways to the pathogenesis of a number of "chronic" diseases, including cervical cancer (in which human papilloma virus [HPV] plays a role), hepatic cancer and cirrhosis (in which hepatitis B virus [HBV] and probably hepatitis C virus [HCV] play a role), gastric cancer and peptic ulcer disease (in which *Helicobacter pylori* plays a role), and possibly cardiovascular disease (in which *Chlamydia pneumoniae* and perhaps other infectious agents may play a role). Hepatic cancer and cirrhosis due to HBV are the first vaccine preventable "chronic" diseases, and if current attempts to develop a vaccine against human papilloma virus are successful, cervical cancer may also become vaccine-preventable. Thus, for all of the above reasons, infectious diseases and their prevention and control will remain of major public health importance for low- and middle-income countries for the foreseeable future.

Underlying virtually every infectious disease of public health importance in low- and middle-income countries is the significant role played by poverty and its associated problems. For example, both obvious and more subtle forms of malnutrition and micronutrient deficiencies are associated with an increased risk of severe morbidity and mortality from a wide range of infectious diseases. At the same time, lack of education, poor access to clean drinking water, inability to dispose properly of human waste, household crowding, and lack of access to medical care—all manifestations of poverty—also contribute substantially.

However, low- and middle-income countries and the people living in them cannot be lumped together into a single group insofar as their risk of various infectious diseases is concerned. There are important geographic differences in their incidence and public health significance, due to differences in climate, the distribution of insect vectors, and variations in other environmental, social, and cultural factors. In addition, all low- and middle-income countries are not equally resource poor—they vary enormously in the resources that are available to provide clinical services (for example, oral rehydration therapy), mount public health programs (for example, vaccination programs), and reduce environmental sources of infection (for example, provide clean drinking water and adequate sanitation or control vector populations). Also, virtually all low- and middle-income countries include within them culturally, economically, and sometimes geographically diverse subpopulations with very different needs and resources, particularly with regard to infectious diseases. Given the diversity of the low- and middle-income countries and the infectious diseases that confront them, it will be possible in this chapter to discuss these diseases only selectively, using representative examples when appropriate.

## CONTROL OF INFECTIOUS DISEASES

The twentieth century saw an ever-increasing number of programs to prevent morbidity and mortality from specific infectious diseases in low- and middle-income countries. Strategies that have been employed have included various combinations of vector control (for example, for malaria, dengue, yellow fever, and onchocerciasis [river blindness]); vaccination (for example, for smallpox, measles, polio, neonatal tetanus, diphtheria, pertussis, tetanus, hepatitis B, meningococcal meningitis, and yellow fever); mass chemotherapy (for example, for hookworm, onchocerciasis, dracunculiasis [guinea worm], and sexually transmitted infections [STIs]); improved sanitation and access to clean water (for example, for diarrheal diseases); improved care-seeking and caregiving (for example, for diarrheal diseases, acute respiratory infections, and neonatal tetanus); and behavior change (for example, for HIV and other STIs, diarrheal diseases, and dracunculiasis), among others. The successful eradication of smallpox in the late 1970s through a combination of enhanced case finding, containment, and vaccination gave considerable impetus to attempts to control other infectious diseases (see Exhibit 4–1).

As the world health community has established goals for reducing morbidity and mortality from other infectious diseases, a variety of terms describing different levels of control have come into use. Organizations, such as WHO and its governing body, the World Health Assembly (WHA), have been careful to define their prevention goals vis-à-vis various diseases, and these are defined in appropriate sections of this chapter. A useful set of definitions of such terms was put forward at the Dahlem workshop on the Eradication of Infectious Diseases (Dowdle & Hopkins, 1998).

- *Control:* Reduction of disease incidence, prevalence, morbidity or mortality to a locally acceptable level as a result of deliberate efforts; continued intervention measures are required to maintain the reduction.
- *Elimination of disease:* Reduction to zero of the incidence of a specified disease in a defined geographic area as a result of deliberate efforts; continued intervention measures are required.
- *Elimination of infection:* Reduction to zero of the incidence of infection caused by a specific agent in a defined geographic area as a result of deliberate efforts; continued measures to prevent reestablishment of transmission are required.
- *Eradication:* Permanent reduction to zero of the worldwide incidence of infection caused by a specific agent as a result of deliberate efforts; intervention measures are no longer needed.
- *Extinction:* The specific infectious agent no longer exists in nature or in the laboratory.*

In the near term, extinction is possible only for smallpox, although concerns about its use as an agent of bio-terrorism have prevented the long-awaited destruction of the last known stocks of the virus. Eradication of other diseases, such as polio, measles, and Guinea worm, is considered theoretically possible using existing control methods and is being actively pursued (see below). However, for most of the infectious diseases responsible for the majority of morbidity and mortality in low- and middle-income countries at the turn of the twenty-first century, only their control is considered achievable in the foreseeable future (see Exhibit 4–2).

## CHILDHOOD VACCINE PREVENTABLE DISEASES: THE EXPANDED PROGRAM OF IMMUNIZATIONS

### Overview

Based on the success of the vaccination program mounted to control and then eradicate smallpox, WHO and various partner agencies launched the Expanded Program of Immunizations (EPI, or PEV in French) in 1974. At that time it was estimated that fewer than 5% of infants and children in low- and middle-income countries were receiving relatively inexpensive and highly effective vaccines that had been licensed and available for a number of years. There were many obstacles to vaccinating them, including the lack of demand for vaccines on the part of the community; the small number of sources of vaccines of adequate quality; the lack of the infrastructure needed to purchase, store, and distribute vaccines, some of which were temperature sensitive; a deficiency in the number of trained personnel to administer vaccination programs; and insufficient funds to purchase vaccines and vaccination supplies and equipment. Further, most countries lacked health information and surveillance systems to assess

*Source: The Eradication of Infectious Diseases: Report of the Dahlem Workshop on the Eradication of Infectious Diseases,* W.R. Dowdle and D.R. Hopkins, March 16–22. Copyright John Wiley & Sons Limited. Reproduced with permission.

**Exhibit 4–1** Smallpox Eradication

Most individuals who work in the area of international health consider the eradication of smallpox to have been the single most important contribution of public health in the twentieth century, and possibly the most significant accomplishment in the field of human health in recorded history. Although the ultimate eradication of smallpox through the use of vaccine was foreseen by Edward Jenner and President Thomas Jefferson at the beginning of the nineteenth century, it took more than 150 years for it to become a reality. Eradication of smallpox was possible because of several important features of the disease itself: technological advances in vaccine preparation and administration; development and application of a new approach to using the vaccine selectively rather than in mass campaigns; and a combination of international will and cooperation, strong leadership, and the focused effort of large numbers of health workers in multiple countries.

Features of smallpox that made it a candidate for eradication included its relatively inefficient transmission from person to person; the fact that individuals with smallpox were generally bedridden before the appearance of the rash, the stage in the illness when person-to-person transmission was most likely to occur; the fact that subclinical cases did not occur in unvaccinated individuals, and vaccinated individuals who developed mild smallpox did not efficiently transmit the virus; the lack of a carrier state; the presence of a single serotype of the virus; the marked seasonal fluctuation in cases; and the lack of a nonhuman reservoir for the virus in nature. Advances in vaccine development and delivery that were crucial to smallpox eradication included the development of a heat stable, freeze-dried vaccine and of two improved methods of delivering the vaccine—a bifurcated needle that was inexpensive, easy to use, and economical in its use of a small volume of vaccine; and jet injector guns that allowed a team to vaccinate more than 1,000 persons per hour.

However, despite the availability of a heat-stable smallpox vaccine and the means of vaccinating large numbers of persons, mass vaccination campaigns intended to render entire populations immune to smallpox were unsuccessful in eradicating the disease, even in countries that achieved vaccine coverage in the range of 80–95%. Smallpox virus continued to circulate among the remaining unvaccinated individuals, who were extremely difficult to identify and vaccinate. A delay in the arrival of sufficient vaccine to mount a mass campaign in Nigeria in 1966 led to the development of an alternative approach to preventing the spread of smallpox in an area: energetic case detection followed by isolation of all infected individuals and intense vaccination efforts focused on the area and population immediately surrounding a case. This approach, dubbed a "surveillance-containment" strategy, proved to be remarkably successful in eradicating smallpox once imaginative and locally acceptable approaches to detecting all suspected cases, isolating individuals with smallpox, and vaccinating those around them were implemented. Surveillance containment ultimately replaced mass campaigns, and global efforts to complete eradication of smallpox relying on this approach gained momentum.

It has been estimated that in 1967 as many as 10 to 15 million cases of smallpox occurred in 33 countries with endemic smallpox and 14 other countries with imported cases of smallpox. These countries, with a total population of more than 1.2 billion persons, included many of the poorest countries in the world and those presenting the greatest logistical barriers to mounting an effective eradication program. As a result of the efforts of dedicated public health workers in these countries and a small cadre of public health professionals from unaffected countries, the last case of smallpox not due to a laboratory accident had onset of a rash on October 26, 1977, in Somalia. On December 9, 1979, the World Health Organization's Global Commission for the Certification of Smallpox Eradication concluded that "smallpox eradication has been achieved throughout the world," a conclusion accepted by the World Health Assembly in May 1980.

**Exhibit 4–2** Levels of Control That Are Considered Achievable for Selected Infectious Diseases in the Foreseeable Future Using Currently Available Methods

| Extinction | Eradication | Elimination of Infection | Elimination of Disease | Control |
|---|---|---|---|---|
| • Smallpox | • Polio<br>• Measles<br>• Dracunculiaisis (Guinea worm) | • Onchocerciasis | • Rabies<br>• Trachoma | • Neonatal Tetanus<br>• Malaria<br>• Cholera<br>• Tuberculosis<br>• Schistosomiasis<br>• Diarrheal disease<br>• ARI<br>• AIDS<br>• STI<br>• Leprosy |

*Note:* ARI = acute respiratory infection; AIDS = acquired immunodeficiency syndrome; STI = sexually transmitted infection.

the burden of disease caused by various vaccine-preventable diseases or to evaluate the impact of a vaccination program. Remarkable progress since 1974 in correcting these problems has led to a realistic plan to eradicate polio worldwide; dramatic reductions in morbidity and mortality from measles and neonatal tetanus worldwide; and likely, but harder to demonstrate, reductions of a similar magnitude in morbidity and mortality from diphtheria and pertussis.

For the first 20 years or so of its existence, the EPI focused on diseases for which safe, effective, and inexpensive vaccines were available and could be given entirely during the first year of life. These included OPV (oral polio vaccine, a trivalent live vaccine against poliomyelitis), measles vaccine (a live vaccine), DPT (a three-component killed vaccine against diphtheria, pertussis, and tetanus), and BCG (bacillus Calmette-Guerin, a live vaccine against tuberculosis). Vaccination with tetanus toxoid (TT) was included for women of childbearing age to prevent neonatal tetanus in their newborn babies, even though the group being targeted for vaccination was not infants in the first year of life. Subsequently, it was recommended that vaccine against yellow fever be added in those countries where the disease is a threat. A vac-

cine against hepatitis B was then included after large quantities of relatively inexpensive vaccine became available. (See Table 4–1 for the current EPI schedule for infants.) Hepatitis B, yellow fever, and tuberculosis are discussed elsewhere in this chapter, so they will not be considered here.

**Poliomyelitis**

*Etiologic Agent, Clinical Features, and Characteristics of the Currently Available Vaccines*

Poliomyelitis (polio) is caused by any of the three known serotypes (1, 2, and 3) of poliovirus. Poliovirus is efficiently transmitted through the fecal-oral route. Ingestion of the virus leads to asymptomatic or mild, self-limited infection and shedding of the virus from the throat and gastrointestinal tract in the vast majority of those exposed. However, an estimated 1 in 100 to 1 in 850 infected persons develops symptomatic polio, with or without paralysis. Of those who develop paralysis, which primarily affects one or both legs, approximately 10% die acutely, 10–15% are left permanently unable to walk, and 10–15% are left lame (unable to walk nor-

**Table 4–1** Current Recommended Schedule of Vaccination under the Expanded Program of Immunizations

| Vaccine | Age at Vaccination |
|---|---|
| Bacillus Calmette-Guerin (BCG) | birth |
| Oral polio vaccine (OPV) | birth, 6, 10, and 14 weeks |
| Diphtheria-Pertussis-Tetanus (DPT) | 6, 10, and 14 weeks |
| Measles | 9 months |
| Hepatitis B[a] | scheme A: birth, 6, and 14 weeks |
|  | scheme B: 6, 10, and 14 weeks |
| Yellow fever[b] | 9 months |
| Tetanus Toxoid (TT) | 2 doses for women of childbearing age |

[a]Scheme A is recommended in countries where perinatal transmission of HBV is frequent (for example, Southeast Asia), and scheme B is recommended in countries where perinatal transmission is less frequent (for example, sub-Saharan Africa).

[b]In countries where yellow fever poses a risk.

mally). Treatment for polio is entirely supportive in nature. Before widespread vaccination, polio was the leading cause of lameness in low- and middle-income countries, and many of its victims remain a visible sign of the ravages of the disease and will need assistance long after acute cases of polio have been eradicated.

Killed, injectable polio vaccine (IPV) and live, oral polio vaccine (OPV) became available in the 1950s and 1960s, respectively. Both are safe and highly effective, and each has been used successfully to eradicate disease caused by wild-type poliovirus in industrialized countries. Although there are extremely rare cases of polio caused by the vaccine strain of the virus when OPV is given, WHO and other supporters of the EPI have always considered OPV to be preferable to IPV for routine use in low- and middle-income countries. Reasons for preferring OPV have included its extremely low cost (~$0.02/dose); its ease of administration; its ability to induce intestinal immunity that inhibits shedding of wild-type poliovirus; and its transmission to household and other close contacts through the fecal-oral route, providing repeated exposures to the vaccine and thus boosting immunity to polio in such contacts. However, for unclear reasons, the efficacy of OPV in low- and middle-income countries has consistently been found to be lower than that in industrialized

countries (~85% versus ~95% for the primary series) (Patriarca, Wright, & John, 1991).

### Descriptive Epidemiologic Features and Risk Factors

Before the widespread use of polio vaccine, polio was endemic in virtually all low- and middle-income countries, and most children were asymptomatically infected during the first few years of life. Symptomatic acute polio was similarly seen primarily in infants and young children. Based on surveys of the prevalence of lameness in school-age children, the annual incidence of symptomatic polio in low- and middle-income countries was estimated to be in the range of 20 to 40 per 100,000 total population (LaForce, Lichnevski, Keja, & Henderson, 1980). As oral polio vaccine came into widespread use and vaccine coverage increased, endemic infections with wild-type poliovirus decreased. However, vaccine coverage levels in the range of 40–80%, combined with a vaccine efficacy of ~85%, led to an accumulation of susceptible individuals and subsequent outbreaks in many countries with "good" EPIs (Sutter et al., 1991). In the early 1980s more than 50,000 cases of polio were being reported annually to WHO (Otten et al., 1992). By 1997 that number had been reduced by more than 90%.

## Current Approaches to Prevention and Control

In 1988 the WHA set a goal of interrupting polio transmission worldwide by the year 2000 and certifying that polio had been eradicated by 2005. The polio eradication effort is based on a combination of ongoing routine immunization of infants, annual national immunization days, and house-to-house "mop-up" campaigns to vaccinate those missed by these other approaches (Hull, Ward, Hull, Milstien, & de Quadros, 1994). In addition, sensitive surveillance for and laboratory testing of specimens from individuals with acute flaccid paralysis have been put into place to help identify cases of polio, thus allowing targeting of additional vaccination efforts and monitoring of the impact of the eradication program. The last confirmed case of paralytic polio caused by wild type poliovirus in the western hemisphere was detected in Peru in 1991. Polio eradication efforts in Asia have also been highly successful, but interruption of transmission of poliovirus throughout Asia by the end of 2000 is unlikely. Eradication efforts in Africa have faced even more formidable challenges, and although the number of cases of polio has been dramatically reduced, interruption of transmission of poliovirus in Africa cannot be achieved by the end of 2000 ("Progress toward Poliomyelitis Eradication," 1998). Global certification of polio eradication by the year 2005, however, is still envisioned.

## Measles

### Etiologic Agent, Clinical Features, and Vaccine Characteristics

Measles is caused by measles virus. Although there is some genotypic variation, all measles virus strains are considered to be of a single type. Measles virus is spread via the respiratory route and is transmitted extremely efficiently. It is highly infectious, and in the absence of vaccine-induced immunity, virtually every child can be expected to develop measles if the virus is circulating in the community. Measles is characterized initially by fever, cough, runny nose, and malaise, making it indistinguishable from many other viral respiratory infections for the first several days, during which the child is highly infectious. A characteristic rash then appears. Although most cases are self-limited, complications commonly include pneumonia, diarrhea, and ear infections. Less common complications include encephalitis and blindness. Measles is not amenable to antibiotic therapy, but treatment with vitamin A reduces the case fatality ratio (Hussey & Klein, 1990).

Before widespread use of measles vaccine, measles was consistently one of the leading causes of death among children worldwide, accounting for an estimated 20–30% of such deaths (Walsh, 1983). While the estimates of the case-fatality ratio for measles have varied from 1 to >30%, depending in part on whether the studies were community- or hospital-based, it is clear that the most potent predictors of mortality among children with measles are young age and malnutrition, particularly vitamin A deficiency (Markowitz et al., 1989). Furthermore, measles frequently leaves a child weakened and at increased risk of illness and death from other causes for a year or more after the acute episode.

Measles vaccine consists of a live, attenuated strain of the measles virus. It is safe, inexpensive, and highly effective when given to a child after circulating measles antibody acquired from the mother has disappeared. Because maternal antibody tends to disappear somewhat later and exposure to measles virus is substantially less common in industrialized countries, measles vaccine is typically given at 15 months of age in such countries. In low- and middle-income countries, the intensity of exposure to measles and the poorly understood more rapid decline in maternal antibodies combine to put infants at much greater risk of acquiring measles at a young age, when complications and death are more likely. As a result, measles vaccine is typically given at nine months of age in low- and middle-income countries.

### Descriptive Epidemiologic Features and Risk Factors

In the absence of vaccination, every child in an area where measles virus is circulating would be expected to contract measles. In the early 1980s an estimated 3 million children died annually of measles and its sequelae. By the mid-1990s, with an estimated 80% of the world's children vaccinated against measles, the estimated annual number of deaths attributable to measles worldwide was 1 million. The age at which an unvaccinated child develops measles is a function of when maternal antibodies disappear (generally at 6 to 12 months of age) and the intensity of exposure to measles virus in the community. Thus in crowded urban areas most unvaccinated children will develop measles between 6 months and five years of age, while in more sparsely populated, rural areas the age of acquisition of measles is older (Walsh, 1983). Family size, travel patterns, and types and locations of social interactions (for example, marketplaces) also influence the local epidemiologic features of measles. HIV infection appears to increase the risk of acquiring measles in infancy, presumably by decreasing the level of circulating maternal antibody in the infant.

### Current Approaches to Prevention and Control

Like smallpox, measles can, in theory, be completely eradicated because measles virus does not infect other species or live in the environment. However, because measles is more widespread and much more infectious than smallpox, and because there is substantial transmission of measles virus among infants below the age of routine vaccination, eradication of measles will be more difficult to achieve. Thus, rather than establish a goal of worldwide measles eradication, the WHA resolved in 1989 to reduce measles-related morbidity by 90% and measles-related mortality by 95% by the year 1995. As with polio, improved routine immunization of infants and mass campaigns targeting infants and children 9 months to 3–5 (or even up to 14) years of age are being undertaken as complementary strategies. Based on substantial success in reducing the incidence of measles and even interrupting measles virus transmission over large geographic areas for substantial periods of time, the 1994 Pan American Sanitary Conference made elimination of measles from the Western Hemisphere a goal for the year 2000 (Pan America Health Organization, 1994). With the target date in sight, measles virus transmission has been interrupted in most countries of the Americas, and a record low of 287 measles cases had been reported as of May 6, 2000, from only 8 of 46 countries and territories of WHO's Region of the Americas (that is, the Western Hemisphere). All these efforts to control and eventually eliminate measles through improving measles vaccine coverage have led to substantial reductions in measles morbidity and mortality, but it remains uncertain whether they will be sufficient to eliminate measles, particularly in Africa.

## Diphtheria

### Etiologic Agent, Clinical Features, and Vaccine Characteristics

Diphtheria is caused by the bacterium *Corynebacterium diphtheriae*. It is spread primarily via the respiratory route, although in low- and middle-income countries the organism is a common cause of ulcerative skin lesions and can be transmitted from such lesions. Diphtheria is a disease of the upper respiratory tract, manifested by fever, sore throat, an inflamed pharynx (and possibly nose and larynx), and a grayish membrane covering the inflamed mucosa. With involvement of the larynx, the airways can be blocked and death can result. The disease is toxin-mediated, and use of both antibiotics and diphtheria antitoxin (which is rarely, if ever, available in low- and middle-income countries) is beneficial in its treatment. The incidence of diphtheria and the morbidity and mortality attributable to it in low- and middle-income counries are largely unknown, but the disease is not believed to pose a major public health threat in such countries.

The diphtheria component of DPT vaccine is composed of inactivated diphtheria toxin adsorbed to aluminum salts. Two or more doses of DPT result in protection against diphtheria in 90–100% of those vaccinated.

### Descriptive Epidemiologic Features and Risk Factors

Although diphtheria is easier to diagnose than pertussis, it is likely that it is substantially underreported in many low- and middle-income countries. Thus the estimated 15,000–50,000 cases of diphtheria reported to WHO annually in the mid-1990s almost certainly do not reflect the actual burden of disease ("EPI Information System," 1998). Most cases of diphtheria occur in young children, primarily among those living in impoverished, crowded conditions. Lack of vaccination is undoubtedly the most important risk factor for developing or dying from diphtheria.

### Current Approaches to Prevention and Control

The current approach to reducing morbidity and mortality from diphtheria is to improve levels of vaccine coverage achieved through ongoing infant immunization programs (that is, the EPI) in various countries. Strategies for improving vaccine coverage include expanding the times when vaccinations are offered in clinics, reducing waiting times, and reducing the number of "missed opportunities" to vaccinate unvaccinated infants, among others. Because vaccination does not lead to elimination of carriage of *C. diphtheriae* from the naso-pharynx, ongoing control of diphtheria will require achieving and maintaining high levels of vaccine coverage among the target population.

## Pertussis

### Etiologic Agent, Clinical Features, and Vaccine Characteristics

Pertussis (whooping cough) is caused by the bacterium *Bordatella pertussis*. Like measles, pertussis is spread via the respiratory route and is highly contagious, particularly within a household and in crowded institutional settings. In classic cases of pertussis, nonspecific respiratory tract symptoms are followed by severe and protracted bouts of coughing that typically end with an inspiratory whooping sound. These bouts of coughing can persist for many weeks and be quite debilitating, even when complications such as pneumonia and neurologic damage do not develop. Antibiotic treatment has little or no impact on the natural course of the disease once symptoms have begun, but probably shortens the time an individual is infectious.

Pertussis is believed to be the cause of substantial morbidity and mortality in the absence of high levels of coverage with pertussis vaccine, but it is difficult to assess what proportion of respiratory infections and related deaths is due to pertussis. In part, this difficulty arises from the fact that many infants with pertussis never have the characteristic whoop seen in older children. Similarly, there is growing evidence that, in industrialized countries and presumably in low- and middle-income countries as well, *B. pertussis* is the cause of many cough illnesses in young adults that are never recognized as pertussis. Finally, the laboratory diagnosis of pertussis has been plagued by the insensitivity, nonspecificity, technical difficulty, and cost of the various diagnostic tests, making research studies difficult and routine surveillance extremely inaccurate.

Pertussis vaccines have, until quite recently, consisted of killed whole bacteria adsorbed to aluminum salts to make them more immunogenic. In most instances, pertussis vaccine is given to infants and young children as a part of DPT vaccine. When a full series of three doses is given, the efficacy of the pertussis component of DPT is in the range of 80%. Because whole-cell pertussis vaccine contains many bacterial products, it is the most reactogenic component of DPT and makes the vaccine the most reactogenic of those included in the EPI. Thus pain and tenderness at the injection site, with or without fever, is common after a DPT injection. More serious but rare complications of whole-cell pertussis vaccine (for example, encephalopathy) have been at the center of a protracted debate in many industrialized countries over its safety. Concern over these rare complications and attendant declines in vaccine acceptance have led to the development and licensure of acellular pertussis vaccines that are far less reactogenic and equally efficacious, but that are also far more expensive than whole-cell pertussis vaccine. Because of this large difference in cost, the EPI continues to use whole-cell pertussis vaccine in virtually all low- and middle-income countries.

### Descriptive Epidemiologic Features and Risk Factors

In the mid-1980s it was estimated that more than 600,000 children died of pertussis annually. The number of cases reported to WHO annually in the early 1980s was in the 1.5–2 million range; by 1997 the number was less than 200,000 ("EPI Information System," 1998). As noted above, any estimate of the burden of disease caused by pertussis is likely to underestimate the actual toll due to the difficulty of making the diagnosis. Limited studies suggest that most cases of pertussis in low- and middle-income countries occur in infancy and early childhood and that the highest case-fatality ratio is seen in infants. It is likely that poverty and the resultant crowding increase the risk of pertussis and that malnutrition increases the likelihood of dying among those who develop the disease, although lack of vaccination is undoubtedly the most important risk factor for developing or dying from pertussis at any age.

### Current Approaches to Prevention and Control

As is the case for diphtheria, the current approach to reducing morbidity and mortality from pertussis is to improve levels of vaccine coverage through the EPI and strategies for improved vaccine coverage. Because vaccination does not lead to elimination of carriage of *B. pertussis*, ongoing control of pertussis will require high levels of vaccine coverage among the target population.

## Tetanus

### Etiologic Agent, Clinical Features, and Vaccine Characteristics

Tetanus is caused by the toxin produced by the anaerobic bacterium *Clostridium tetani*. It is commonly found in the gastrointestinal tract of many domesticated animals (for example, cows, sheep, and goats). When deposited in the soil, *C. tetani* cells form spores that are highly resistant to heat and desiccation and remain viable for years or even decades. When these spores are introduced into a wound or other suitable environment, they sporulate and the bacterial cells reproduce, forming and releasing a highly potent neurotoxin as they grow. Symptoms produced by the neurotoxin include painful stiffening and spasms of the muscles, including those of the jaw (hence the name "lockjaw"), and, particularly in newborn infants, a resultant inability to suck or otherwise feed. Treatment of tetanus is largely supportive, even in the rare circumstance when tetanus antitoxin is available, and consists largely of giving muscle relaxants and fluids intravenously. However, even with supportive treatment, the case-fatality ratio is very high, particularly in infants with neonatal tetanus, of whom 80–90% will die.

The vaccine against tetanus, either in a single preparation or in DPT, is a toxoid—an inactivated form of tetanus toxin, adsorbed to aluminum salts. Tetanus toxoid is extremely safe and produces few reactions. The three doses of DPT given to infants and the two doses of TT given to women of childbearing age or pregnant women through the EPI produce immunity in 90–100% of those vaccinated.

### Descriptive Epidemiologic Features and Risk Factors

Whereas tetanus in adults is an avoidable and tragic illness, tetanus in newborn infants is a public health problem. Studies in the 1970s and 1980s showed that up to 60 newborn babies per 1,000 (6%) were developing neonatal tetanus in various low-income countries, primarily due to contamination of the umbilical stump, and that virtually all these babies died (Stanfield & Galazka, 1984). Deaths due to neonatal tetanus accounted for one-quarter to three-quarters of all neonatal deaths and up to one-quarter of infant mortality in these countries. In 1993 it was estimated that neonatal tetanus caused more than 500,000 deaths worldwide ("Expanded Programme on Immunization," 1994). Neonatal tetanus is more common in rural areas, particularly those where animal husbandry practices lead to substantial fecal contamination of the soil, and tends to be more common during the rainy season (Schofield, 1986). However, the key risk factors for neonatal tetanus clearly relate to where a delivery occurs, the level of training of the person assisting with the delivery, how the umbilical cord is cut, and the way the umbilical stump is treated. Because there is enormous diversity of cultural practices regarding how the cord is cut and what is placed on the umbilical stump (including mud, animal dung, clarified butter, and other nonsterile materials), the rate of and risk factors for neonatal tetanus vary substantially in different regions of the world (Stanfield & Galazka, 1984).

### Current Approaches to Prevention and Control

Because the *C. tetani* spores that cause neonatal tetanus are ubiquitous in soil and can persist there indefinitely, the organism itself cannot be eradicated. Neonatal tetanus, however, can be controlled or eliminated as a public health problem (defined as <1 case per 1,000 live births in each health district) by ensuring that a high proportion of women giving birth have received two doses of tetanus toxoid or that the delivery and subsequent cord care practices minimize the chances that *C. tetani* spores will be introduced. Studies such as those conducted in Egypt (see Figure 4–1) demonstrate clearly that immunization of women of reproductive age or of pregnant women has a dramatic impact on the risk of neonatal tetanus ("Progress toward Elimination of Neonatal Tetanus," 1996). Other studies suggest that training and equipping birth attendants so they can perform a "clean delivery"

("3 cleans"—delivery with clean hands, delivery on a clean surface, and use of clean instruments and dressings to cut and dress the umbilical cord) may be somewhat less effective at reducing the risk of neonatal tetanus, but have a greater impact on the risk of neonatal mortality from all causes combined. These two approaches can and have been used together. In recent years, the proportion of women giving birth in various geographic regions who have been adequately immunized with TT has increased substantially, but neonatal tetanus remains a problem in many low- and middle-income countries where many deliveries still occur at home.

### Obstacles to Prevention and Control

Despite Herculean efforts on the part of WHO, UNICEF, and others, it has remained difficult to achieve and maintain high levels of vaccine coverage in many countries, particularly in rural areas of the low-income countries. For a number of years there was substantial controversy about the relative merits of "vertical" approaches to vaccinating children (that is, mass campaigns) and "horizontal" approaches (that is, improving access to and use of primary care services that provided routine immunizations). Although the debate over vertical or horizontal programs continues in some health areas, it has largely been replaced with respect to vaccination of infants and children by a broad consensus that the two approaches can be complementary rather than conflicting. Thus attempts to strengthen routine infant (and pregnant woman) immunization programs in low- and middle-income countries around the world have proceeded in parallel with mass campaigns intended to hasten the eradication of polio and measles.

Further reduction or elimination of the childhood vaccine preventable diseases discussed in this section are contingent on the availability of sustained funding of and technical support for immunization programs, stimulation of increased demand for vaccination on the part of parents and communities, expanded access to immunization services, and effective surveil-

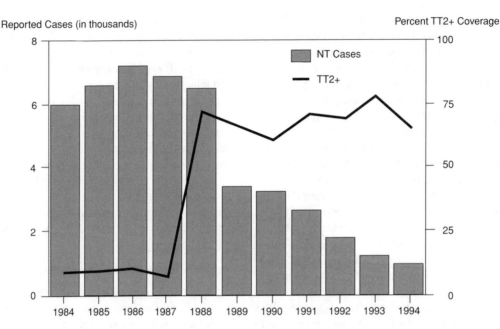

**Figure 4–1** Number of Reported Cases of Neonatal Tetanus (NT) and Percentage of Pregnant Women Receiving at Least Two Doses of Tetanus Toxoid (TT2+), by Year, in Egypt, 1984–1994

lance for these diseases. At the same time, there is a need to develop, test, and make available new and improved vaccines; to expand local production of existing vaccines in low- and middle-income countries; to ensure the potency and safety of the vaccines produced; and to ensure the availability and proper use of sterile injection equipment. For the past decade, the child vaccine initiative (CVI), a joint effort of WHO, UNICEF, the World Bank, and other agencies, supported and coordinated basic and operational research in all these areas, but it has recently been dismantled and replaced by a new interagency vaccine initiative entitled the Global Alliance for Vaccines and Immunizations (GAVI) (see Exhibit 4–3). In addition, the newly formed Bill and Melinda Gates Foundation is working to ensure the earliest possible incorporation of other vaccines into the EPI.

Assuming that worldwide polio eradication is successful, an important unanswered question is how long wild-type poliovirus can persist

in the environment and continue to circulate, requiring that high levels of vaccine coverage be sustained. At what point in the future will it be safe to discontinue use of polio vaccine, as was possible with smallpox, and how will we know when it is safe to do so (Dove & Racaniello, 1997)?

The inexplicable and unfortunate increase in all cause mortality seen in infants (primarily female infants) given experimental high titer measles vaccine at a young age has clearly set back efforts to develop a more potent measles vaccine (Aaby et al., 1994). Therefore, for the foreseeable future, efforts to eliminate measles will, of necessity, have to make use of the currently available vaccine. Important unanswered questions, therefore, relate to how best to use the currently available vaccine and what vaccination strategies or combinations of strategies will be most effective in interrupting transmission of this highly infectious agent, particularly in Africa. Although there is a clear need to sus-

**Exhibit 4–3** The Global Alliance for Vaccines and Immunizations

An estimated 2 million infants and children still die each year from diseases that can be prevented by currently available vaccines. Several million more infants and children die each year from tuberculosis, malaria, and AIDS, infectious diseases for which new vaccines are urgently needed.

Numerous obstacles, many of which are external to the public health and health care delivery systems, make it difficult to achieve and sustain high levels of coverage with existing vaccines in low- and middle-income countries. These obstacles include limited financial resources, insufficient numbers of trained health care workers, poor roads and other barriers to reaching remote parts of some countries, civil wars, and natural disasters, among others. Other barriers retard the development, testing, licensure, and ultimate availability of new vaccines, including the cost of the research and testing (and hence the eventual cost of new vaccines, particularly those requiring technological sophistication, such as conjugated vaccines)

and liability concerns on the part of potential manufacturers. Recognizing these problems and wishing to increase the speed with which current and new vaccines reach the world's children, a group of international agencies, including WHO, UNICEF, the World Bank, and others, launched the Global Alliance for Vaccines and Immunizations (GAVI) early in 2000. The mission of GAVI is "to fulfill the right of every child to be protected against vaccine-preventable diseases of public health concern." The initial activities of GAVI will focus on establishing a children's vaccine fund and on conducting an analysis of research and development gaps that impede the development and distribution of vaccines. Subsequently, it is expected that GAVI will work with multilateral and international agencies, vaccine manufacturers, foundations, and low- and middle-income countries to promote the rapid development of new vaccines and greater access to both current and new vaccines.

tain high levels of routine immunization against measles at or about nine months of age, the relative importance of various strategies for increasing population level immunity, such as periodic mass campaigns and routinely giving a second dose of measles vaccine at some time after the first birthday, remains to be determined. It is, at best, uncertain whether a new vaccine that is immunogenic at a younger age (in the face of circulating maternal antibodies) and that is safe can be developed and tested, or whether it is even needed in order to eliminate measles.

Historically, rubella vaccine has not been included in the EPI package of vaccines, even though it has been available for 30 years. In recent years, however, there has been growing recognition that congenital rubella syndrome is a problem in low- and middle-income countries, where an estimated 110,000 cases occur annually (Cutts & Vynnycky, 1999). While virtually all countries in the Americas now include rubella

vaccine in the EPI package, consideration needs to be given to using it routinely in Africa and Asia as well.

## ENTERIC INFECTIONS AND ACUTE RESPIRATORY INFECTIONS

Although it might seem odd to discuss enteric infections and acute respiratory infections (ARIs) together in one section, these seemingly disparate conditions have much in common. Each accounts for a substantial amount of childhood morbidity and mortality, as well as for a large proportion of outpatient visits and hospitalizations. Infants and young children almost uniformly experience multiple episodes of both types of illness, regardless of where they live. The identified risk factors for enteric infections and ARIs overlap substantially (for example, poverty, crowding, lack of parental education, malnutrition, low birthweight, and lack of breastfeeding), and most of these are difficult to change in the absence of major social change. Further, both enteric infections and ARIs are caused by a multitude of distinct microbial agents for most of which no vaccine currently exists or is likely to be available in the near future. As a result, the overall approach to minimizing morbidity and mortality from both enteric infections and ARIs has been virtually identical—to accept the fact that such infections and illnesses will occur while attempting to ensure that prompt and appropriate care is sought and given.

## Enteric Infections

### Overview

Enteric infections encompass those viral, bacterial, and parasitic infections of the gastrointestinal tract that are, with the exception of typhoid fever, generally manifested as diarrhea, either alone or in combination with fever, vomiting, and abdominal pain. Although most episodes of diarrheal disease are mild and self-limited, the loss of fluids and salts accompanying severe diarrhea can be life threatening. Also, not all episodes of diarrheal disease are self-limited— various studies suggest that anywhere from 3% to 23% of diarrheal illnesses in infants and young children persist for longer than two weeks (Black, 1993). Both self-limited and persistent diarrhea can have a substantial negative impact on the growth of a child, through malabsorption of nutrients and reduced intake due to vomiting, loss of appetite, and undesirable changes in feeding practices in response to diarrheal illness. Thus repeated episodes of diarrhea and persistent diarrhea often lead to malnutrition, which can, in turn, increase the likelihood of diarrhea persisting and producing a fatal outcome (El Samani, Willett, & Ware, 1988). It has been estimated that diarrheal disease has a more profound impact on the growth of children worldwide than any other infectious disease.

Cholera, while in a sense just one of many causes of watery diarrhea, is in many ways a disease unto itself. It can produce the most dra-matic fluid losses of any enteric infection and, in the absence of appropriate replacement of fluid and salts, can cause death within 24 to 48 hours of onset. Also, cholera epidemics and pandemics can produce enormous numbers of cases and large numbers of deaths, resulting in profound social disruption. As a result, cholera has been accorded a special status by public health officials and agencies (see Introduction).

Many episodes of diarrheal disease in children in low- and middle-income countries are accompanied by bloody stools or frank dysentery (abdominal cramps; painful, strained defecation; and frequent stools containing blood and mucous), which is usually the result of an invasive infection that produces local tissue damage and inflammation in the intestinal mucosa. Although the fluid loss that accompanies such episodes is generally not profound, life-threatening local intestinal and systemic complications can result. Damage to the intestinal mucosa can also lead to substantial losses of protein, resulting in growth retardation. The clinical management of such episodes poses a number of distinctive challenges (see below).

On average, children under the age of five in low- and middle-income countries experience two to three episodes of diarrhea a year. The burden of disease attributable to diarrheal diseases worldwide is enormous. Despite the impressive accomplishments of diarrheal disease control programs, it is estimated that children under 5 years collectively experience more than 1 billion episodes of diarrhea annually, and diarrheal disease is estimated to cause approximately 3.3 million deaths each year (Bern, Martines, de Zoysa, & Glass, 1992). Thus, like ARIs, diarrheal disease accounts for roughly 25% of all deaths among those less than five years of age.

Typhoid fever, which results from an enteric infection and which therefore shares many individual- and community-level risk factors with diarrheal disease, is not accompanied by diarrhea. Although it can be life threatening, typhoid fever has its most profound public health impact through its debilitating effects on school-age children, causing substantial morbidity and absenteeism from school and work (Medina & Yrarrazaval, 1983).

### Etiologic Agent

As noted above, diarrheal disease can be caused by a wide variety of viral, bacterial, and parasitic infections. In cases of endemic diarrheal disease, one or more etiologic agents can be identified in 70–80% of patients when state-of-the-art laboratory testing is performed. However, many of these agents can also be found in the stools of children who do not have diarrhea, and multiple infectious agents may be present in a child with diarrhea. Thus the presence of a given causative agent in a stool sample may not mean that it is the cause of that episode of diarrhea.

The above problems notwithstanding, the most important etiologic agents in young children in low- and middle-income countries are rotavirus, enterotoxigenic *Escherichia coli* (ETEC), shigella species, *Campylobacter jejuni*, and *Cryptosporidium parvum* (Black et al., 1980; Guerrant, Hughes, Lima, & Crane, 1990; Mølbak et al., 1994). Rotavirus is the single leading cause of nonbloody diarrhea in infants, whereas shigella species appear to be the leading cause of bloody diarrhea. Amebiasis (infection with *Entamoeba histolytica*), while frequently diagnosed, appears to be an extremely infrequent cause of bloody diarrhea in young children in low- and middle-income countries. *Vibrio cholerae* is the cause of a substantial fraction of cases of nonbloody diarrhea in endemic areas such as Bangladesh and India (Cholera Working Group, 1993; Nair et al., 1994); it is also the cause of large numbers of cases when epidemics of cholera occur in other regions, such as Africa and Latin America (Glass, Libel, & Brandling-Bennett, 1992; Goodgame & Greenough, 1975). Typhoid fever is caused by *Salmonella typhi*.

### Descriptive Epidemiologic Features and Risk Factors

Children experience the highest risk of diarrheal illness between 6 and 11 months of age and risk declines steadily thereafter (see Figure 4–2) (Bern et al., 1992). This age pattern is largely explained by the established risk factors for diarrheal disease and the likely sources of exposure to the causative agents. The risk of diarrheal disease in young infants is determined in large part by the feeding and hand-washing practices of the mother or other child care providers. Breast-feeding and lack of exposure to contaminated food, water, and other environmental sources are protective. As infants grow and become mobile, they begin to encounter numerous potential sources of infection with the agents of diarrheal disease, including contaminated water and weaning foods and human and animal waste that has not been disposed of properly. There is also evidence that uncontrolled fly populations can contribute to the risk of diarrheal illnesses, particularly those illnesses caused by etiologic agents requiring a small infectious dose (for example, shigella).

As noted, diarrheal disease and malnutrition are intricately intertwined in infants and young children. Although it is not clear that malnutrition is associated with an increased incidence of diarrheal disease, there is strong evidence that malnutrition increases the likelihood that a child with diarrhea will die or develop persistent diarrhea, and that diarrhea in turn has a negative impact on nutritional status and growth.

Unlike diarrheal disease, typhoid fever has long been thought to be a problem primarily in school-age children. However, infections with *S. typhi* clearly occur in infants and preschool-age children, and *S. typhi* infections in this younger age group may be substantially underascertained (Sinha et al., 1999). It has been estimated that there are more than 30 million new cases of typhoid fever worldwide each year. *S. typhi* infection is primarily acquired from contaminated food and water.

### Current Approaches to Prevention and Control

Unlike the case with ARIs (see below), a number of approaches to the primary prevention of diarrheal illness have been studied and

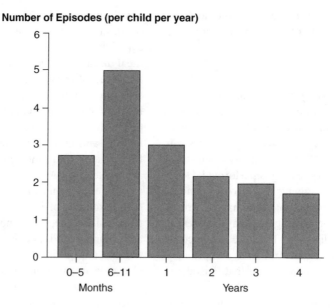

**Figure 4–2** Estimated Median Diarrheal Morbidity for Under-Five-Year-Olds, Based on the Results from 18 Studies in Developing Countries

found to be successful at lowering the rate of diarrheal illness in the community. These include providing communities with a protected source of clean drinking water, improving sanitation through the provision of latrines, promoting hand washing and other personal hygiene habits, reducing the fly population in the community, promoting breastfeeding and proper weaning practices, and various combinations of these interventions (Huttly, Morris, & Pisani, 1997). Although these various approaches have been shown to be effective in well-funded research studies, the feasibility of fostering and sustaining such improvements across large areas and populations is directly linked to the availability of the financial resources and to the political will to do so. In addition, such interventions can generally succeed only when the community is invested in making them work and when they are designed and introduced within a culturally acceptable framework (see Chapter 2).

In parallel with the testing of such primary prevention approaches to reduce the risk of diar-

rheal disease, there have been enormous efforts since the early 1980s to ensure that infants and children who develop diarrhea suffer a minimum of morbidity and mortality. These efforts have focused on prevention and early treatment of dehydration through proper case management in the home, maintenance of adequate nutritional intake to minimize the impact on growth, and appropriate treatment of infants and children who are brought to health facilities. Mothers and other caretakers of children are educated to use fluids available in the home to prevent dehydration, to use oral rehydration solutions (ORS) or cereal-based alternative solutions to prevent and treat dehydration, and to continue to breastfeed babies when they have diarrhea. ORS packets are now manufactured in many countries and widely distributed. At the same time, mothers and health care providers have been discouraged from using the wide range of largely ineffective, often expensive, and sometimes dangerous antimicrobial and antidiarrheal agents that are available. Care providers should reserve antimicrobial agents for the treatment of cholera and of dysentery suspected to be caused by shigella and to limit the use of intravenous fluids to those who are severely dehydrated. Although promoting and sustaining such changes in diverse countries and in the face of sometimes powerful cultural barriers requires a major effort, studies from Egypt and elsewhere suggest that morbidity and mortality from diarrheal disease have been reduced substantially by such efforts (El-Rafie et al., 1990).

Perhaps in part because of the emphasis given to primary prevention and proper case management for diarrheal disease, the role of vaccines in reducing morbidity and mortality from diarrhea has, until now, been quite limited. Vaccines against cholera and typhoid that represent substantial improvements over older vaccines are now available, and a vaccine against rotavirus was approved for use in the United States in 1999. However, the rotavirus vaccine was subsequently withdrawn in the United States because of an unacceptably high rate of significant adverse reactions. While a few countries in which typhoid fever is a major public health problem in school-age children have begun to use typhoid vaccine in this age group, there is continued debate about the proper role for vaccines against enteric infections and under what circumstances they should be given routinely in low- and middle-income countries (Keusch & Cash, 1997). The withdrawal of rotavirus vaccine in the United States makes its future availability and use difficult to predict in low- and middle-income countries (where the risks and benefits of using it may differ).

### Obstacles to Prevention and Control and Directions for Future Research

The greatest obstacle to reducing further the toll taken by diarrheal disease in low- and middle-income countries is the difficulty and expense of ensuring that everyone has regular access to clean, safe drinking water and to adequate sanitation. Although WHO at one point envisioned reaching this goal by 1990, it is now clear that the obstacles to doing so are immense and extraordinarily complex. Substantial investments will be needed simply to improve antiquated and increasingly inadequate water treatment and sewage treatment facilities in the rapidly expanding urban centers of many low- and middle-income countries. The problems associated with ensuring a safe drinking water supply and adequate sanitation in rural areas, although different, are equally challenging to overcome.

### Acute Respiratory Infections

#### Overview

Acute respiratory infections comprise infections of various parts of the respiratory tract, ranging from mild viral and bacterial infections of the upper respiratory tract (for example, the common cold, viral and group A streptococcal pharyngitis, and middle ear infections) to life-threatening infections of the lower respiratory tract (for example, bronchiolitis and pneumonia caused by a variety of bacterial and viral agents). Although upper respiratory tract infections globally cause substantial minor morbidity and economic loss through lost time at work, they rarely result in severe morbidity or in mortality. Interestingly, studies suggest that the incidence of upper respiratory tract infections, while varying with age and season, is remarkably similar in free-living populations throughout the world. Because they do not pose a major public health problem and because no effective interventions against them exist, upper respiratory tract infections will not be discussed further in this chapter, except for group A streptococcal pharyngitis, which can lead to rheumatic fever and is discussed below.

Lower respiratory tract infections, on the other hand, are the cause of enormous morbidity and of mortality, particularly among infants and young children living in low- and middle-income settings, even when those settings are within generally industrialized countries. In low- and middle-income countries, particularly those with good childhood immunization and oral rehydration therapy programs, lower respiratory tract infections in general, and pneumonias in particular, are typically one of, if not the leading cause of death among infants and children less than 5 years of age (Graham, 1990). It is estimated that approximately 2.6 million children less than 5 years of age die annually from pneumonia and other lower respiratory tract infections, most of them in low-income countries (Murray & Lopez, 1994). This estimate excludes deaths due to respiratory tract infections that are preventable with vaccines included in the EPI (for example, measles and pertussis), discussed earlier. However, the accuracy of such estimates is limited because establishing a diagnosis of lower respiratory tract infection or pneumonia is difficult, particularly in settings where chest radiography is not available; many children die outside of hospitals; and other illnesses, such as malaria, make verbal autopsies (that is, post-mortem interviews of next-of-kin to determine the most likely cause of death) an unreliable means of establishing a definitive diagnosis. While pneumonia and other lower respiratory tract infections also cause substantial morbidity and mortality in older children and adults, this section will focus on these infections in infants and young children. Pneumonia in adults is discussed briefly later, in the section on AIDS.

### Etiologic Agent, Clinical Features, and Vaccine Characteristics

Lower respiratory tract infections can be caused by a variety of viral and bacterial agents, either singly or in combination. Numerous studies conducted in various countries around the world show similar results concerning the etiologic agents responsible for these infections in infants and young children. Excluding respiratory tract infections caused by agents included among the EPI vaccines, the most important viral causes of lower respiratory tract infections include influenza, parainfluenza, respiratory syncytial virus, and adenovirus (Avila et al., 1990). The most important bacterial causes of

pneumonia, as determined by lung aspirate studies (in which a needle is passed through the chest wall into affected lung parenchyma, thus avoiding contamination of samples by flora in the upper airway), include *Streptococcus pneumoniae*, *Haemophilus influenzae*, and *Staphylococcus aureus* (Shann, 1986). However, many infants and young children have evidence of dual infections (for example, a virus and a bacterium), and in as many as one-third of the cases, no etiologic agent can be found using state-of-the-art laboratory techniques.

### Descriptive Epidemiologic Features and Risk Factors

Infants and young children living in low- and middle-income environments consistently have been found to experience high incidence rates of pneumonia (Selwyn, 1990). For example, in the Highlands of Papua New Guinea, cumulative incidence rates in the range of 250 to 300 per 1,000 infants per year have been observed, compared with a rate in the range of 10 per 1,000 infants per year among upper-middle-income children in the United States. At the same time, elevated incidence rates mirroring those in Papua New Guinea have been observed among Native American children living in poverty in the United States. Verbal autopsy studies suggest that 25–50% of deaths in children under five in low- and middle-income countries are due to pneumonia and other forms of lower respiratory tract infection (Sutrisna, Reingold, Kresno, Harrison, & Utomo, 1993).

The single most important predictor of a child's risk of developing pneumonia or other lower respiratory tract infection is age. The cumulative incidence of lower respiratory tract infections is highest among young infants and drops rapidly with increasing age, reaching markedly lower levels by 2 or 3 years of age (Selwyn, 1990). Another important predictor of an increased risk of morbidity and mortality from lower respiratory tract infections is low birthweight. Other risk factors for either morbidity or mortality include exposure to indoor air pollution (from cooking, heating, and cigarette smoke); not breastfeeding; and malnutrition, including vitamin A deficiency, although these factors are closely intertwined with poverty and with each other, and their independent effects can be difficult to disentangle (Berman, 1991). HIV infection is almost certainly another important risk factor, although its role in infants and young children has not been well-studied.

Rheumatic fever following group A streptococcal pharyngitis occurs in a setting of poverty and household crowding. School-age children are primarily affected acutely, but the damage done to heart valves is usually permanent, producing life-threatening disability. Population-based data concerning the incidence of acute rheumatic fever and the prevalence of rheumatic heart disease in low- and middle-income countries are infrequently available.

### *Current Approaches to Prevention and Control*

In the 1980s WHO, together with various partners, began a multifaceted research program intended to develop an approach to reducing the substantial morbidity and mortality due to lower respiratory tract infections in infants and young children ("Clinical Management of Acute Respiratory Infections," 1981). This research program and the ARI control program that was subsequently developed were premised on the following observations:

- Upper respiratory tract infections, although frequent, are almost always benign and require only supportive care at home.
- Many lower respiratory tract infections in infants and young children are not preventable with existing vaccines.
- The major known risk factors for morbidity and mortality from lower respiratory tract infections (for example, age, low birthweight, malnutrition, and indoor air pollution) are impossible or difficult to change.

- Most morbidity and mortality from lower respiratory tract infections occur in locales where access to medical care is limited and where there are few, if any, diagnostic facilities (that is, the ability to perform chest X-rays, microbiologic cultures, and other tests).

Given the above circumstances, it was decided that an ARI control program based on a triage performed by minimally trained village health workers according to readily observable clinical signs might be feasible, inexpensive, and effective at reducing at least mortality. As a result, a large body of multidisciplinary research relating to the various aspects of such a control program was commissioned and completed. Particularly important was research relating to which readily observable clinical manifestations (for example, cough, fever, respiratory rate, and chest indrawing), singly or in combination, best distinguished infants or young children with various levels of severity of respiratory tract infection (initially classified as mild, moderate, and severe, but later as no pneumonia, pneumonia, and severe pneumonia).

Based on this research, intervention programs were developed. These were intended to train village health workers or their equivalents in how to assess and classify into one of these categories an infant or young child with signs of a respiratory tract infection. Based on their assessment, the village health workers were to recommend supportive care at home in cases of mild ARI (no pneumonia), provide an oral antimicrobial drug (either ampicillin or cotrimoxazole) and education about home care and follow-up in cases of moderate ARI (pneumonia), or refer the child immediately to the nearest hospital for assessment and inpatient care in cases of severe ARI (severe pneumonia). Well-designed intervention trials were carried out in a variety of countries to assess the efficacy of this approach in reducing mortality due to lower respiratory tract infections. As shown in a meta-analysis of these trials, they were almost all successful, reducing mortality due to lower respiratory tract infections and all cause mortality in infants and in children 1 to 4 years of age (Sazawal & Black, 1992). It is important to note, however, that virtually all these trials assessed an intervention that included regular household visits by the village health workers in search of infants and children with signs of a respiratory tract infection.

Based on these favorable results, WHO promoted and supported the implementation of ARI control programs largely based on having village health workers (or their equivalent) assess infants and young children with suspected ARI, classify them by severity of illness, and treat or refer them. The impact of such programs on mortality, as distinct from the impact seen in the intervention trials, has not been adequately assessed. However, ARI control programs that do not include a proactive, outreach component that ensures early case detection (that is, regular household visits) as was present in the intervention trials, and instead rely solely on maternal recognition of illness and appropriate, timely care-seeking are not likely to have as large an impact. On the other hand, programs that include some form of regular household visits are likely to be difficult to sustain.

For a variety of reasons, the emphasis given to ARI control programs (and "vertical" disease-specific programs in general) by WHO and others has diminished in recent years, and attention has shifted to ensuring that any sick infant or child, regardless of his or her other signs and symptoms, receives appropriate evaluation and care. This approach, referred to as the Integrated Management of Childhood Illness, is described in Exhibit 4–4 (Gove, 1997; Lambrechts, Bryce, & Orinda, 1999; Perkins, Zucker et al., 1997; Weber et al., 1997). See also Table 4–2 (Gove, 1997).

Prevention of rheumatic fever depends upon the recognition of streptococcal pharyngitis and treatment with an appropriate antimicrobial agent (for example, penicillin or erythromycin). In populations with high rates of acute rheumatic fever, school-based and other programs to detect and treat streptococcal pharyngitis have been suggested (Bach et al., 1996).

### Obstacles to Prevention and Control and Directions for Future Research

Primary prevention of lower respiratory tract infections remains a long-term goal, awaiting improvements in living conditions and socioeconomic status, as well as the availability of affordable vaccines against the major etiologic agents that are effective when given in infancy. A safe, highly effective conjugate vaccine against *H. influenzae* type b has led to the virtual disappearance of invasive infections caused by this organism in the United States and other industrialized and middle-income countries, including a number of countries in Latin America. Once problems relating to the cost of adding this vaccine to the EPI have been dealt with, this vaccine will undoubtedly have a similar effect in other low- and middle-income countries. However, it is uncertain what proportion of lower respiratory tract infection-related morbidity and mortality in such countries will be prevented by this vaccine, because serotype b accounts for only a fraction of *H. influenzae* infections.

Conjugate pneumococcal vaccines including the most important serotypes of *S. pneumoniae* have been tested and have shown excellent efficacy and safety. A conjugate pneumococcal vaccine including those serotypes that collectively account for approximately 80% of invasive infections in infants in the United States has recently been approved for use in that country, but the current cost of the vaccine makes its use in low- and middle-income countries unaffordable. Also, certain pneumococcal serotypes that are more important causes of infection in low- and middle-income countries than in the United States are not included in the recently licensed vaccine. When pneumococcal vaccines that are specifically formulated for use in low- and middle-income countries are licensed, issues relating to how to finance their inclusion in the EPI will need to be addressed. When (indeed, if) vaccines against the various viruses that cause lower

**Exhibit 4–4** Integrated Management of Childhood Illness

Throughout the 1970s and 1980s, concerted efforts were made to develop case management strategies for each of the infectious diseases that collectively accounted for the majority of morbidity and mortality among infants and young children in low- and middle-income countries— measles, malaria, diarrheal disease, and acute respiratory infections. While each of these disease-specific case management strategies has been shown to be effective at reducing severe morbidity and mortality when properly implemented, it has been recognized that having multiple distinct disease-specific programs that all target the same health care providers can lead to overlap, inefficiency, and competition for the attention of an overworked health care worker. As a result, various programs within WHO and UNICEF have collaborated in the development of the Integrated Management of Childhood Illness (IMCI), which attempts to pull together into a single more efficient program the approaches of the various disease-specific control programs (Gove, 1997). The IMCI program includes both preventive strategies and case management approaches for the illnesses that collectively account for the majority of severe morbidity, mortality, and health care provider visits among infants and young children (see Table 4–2). The results of early field assessments of the IMCI algorithm in selected countries suggest that it can be an effective tool, although some modifications may be needed to maximize its usefulness. (Lambrechts et al., 1999; Perkins, Zucker et al., 1997; Weber et al., 1997)

respiratory tract infections in infants and small children will become available is uncertain.

There are several barriers to reducing morbidity and mortality due to lower respiratory tract infections through means other than vaccination and improving living conditions. The first set of barriers relates to how to ensure that the parents or guardians of a sick child will seek and have access to appropriate care in a timely fashion. A detailed discussion of care-seeking practices and obstacles to obtaining medical care is beyond the scope of this chapter, but the obstacles are multifaceted and difficult to overcome. There are also many challenges relating to ensuring that those ill infants and children who are brought to medical care facilities receive timely and appropriate care, including adequate assessment, treatment, and follow-up. Finally, there are concerns about the likelihood that increased use of currently effective and inexpensive antimicrobial agents, particularly use of inappropriate or inadequate regimens, may lead to the development of resistant strains of bacteria (particularly *S. pneumoniae*) that may then not respond to these inexpensive, oral treatment regimens.

## BACTERIAL MENINGITIS

### Overview

*Meningitis* is a nonspecific term that encompasses inflammation of the meninges (the membranous lining that covers the brain and spinal cord), which can be caused by a wide variety of infectious and noninfectious agents. Such inflammation, regardless of its cause, tends to produce a similar clinical picture: headache, stiff neck, fever, and variable other features. There is substantial overlap between the manifestations of meningitis, which is sometimes referred to as spinal meningitis or cerebrospinal meningitis, and those of many other infectious diseases. Although meningitis can be caused by a wide variety of viruses and other infectious agents (for example, mycobacteria and parasites), meningitis caused by certain bacteria poses a substantial public health threat. Therefore, this section will be confined to a discussion of bacterial meningitis, excluding tuberculous meningitis, which is discussed briefly in the section on tuberculosis.

**Table 4–2** Child Health Interventions Included in Integrated Management of Childhood Illness

| Case Management Interventions | Preventive Interventions |
| --- | --- |
| • Pneumonia<br>• Diarrhea<br>  –Dehydration<br>  –Persistent diarrhea<br>  –Dysentery<br>• Meningitis, sepsis<br>• Malaria<br>• Measles<br>• Malnutrition<br>• Anemia<br>• Ear infection | • Immunization during sick child visits (to reduce missed opportunities)<br>• Nutrition counseling<br>• Breastfeeding support (including the assessment and correction of breastfeeding technique) |

From a public health perspective, it is important to subdivide bacterial meningitis into its endemic and epidemic forms. Endemic bacterial meningitis, while differing in a number of subtle ways between low- and middle-income and industrialized countries with regard to its descriptive epidemiologic features and the distribution of etiologic agents, poses a similar set of challenges in these two different settings. The vastly different resources available in high- and low-income countries for prevention and control of endemic bacterial meningitis, while relatively less important only a few years ago, are now assuming greater importance as a result of the development and licensure of effective but expensive conjugate vaccines against the major etiologic agents causing endemic disease. Epidemic bacterial meningitis, for reasons that remain unexplained, has virtually ceased to be a public health problem in industrialized countries since World War II, although small clusters of cases or hyperendemic disease can still be a vexing problem. In a number of low- and middle-income countries, however, particularly those in the "meningitis belt" of sub-Saharan Africa, periodic epidemics of bacterial meningitis occur on a scale never documented in industrialized countries (see below). These epidemics can be of such a magnitude and geographic scope as to be properly called public health disasters.

In industrialized countries, suspected bacterial meningitis is considered a medical emergency, requiring that appropriate clinical specimens for diagnostic testing be obtained and parenteral antimicrobial therapy in a hospital be initiated immediately. Even under these ideal conditions, case-fatality ratios for bacterial meningitis range from 3–25%, depending primarily on the specific etiologic agent and the age of the patient. Further, many patients who survive the acute episode will be left with one or more serious sequelae, including deafness, blindness, mental retardation, and seizure disorders. Although the clinical outcomes of hospitalized cases of bacterial meningitis do not, in general, differ between low- and middle-income and industrialized countries, the resources available for treating such patients are obviously much more limited in low- and middle-income countries. Furthermore, it is evident that epidemics involving tens of thousands of such cases cannot be dealt with easily by countries with extremely constrained health budgets and facilities.

## Endemic Meningitis

### Etiologic Agents

Studies of the etiology of endemic bacterial meningitis in low- and middle-income countries have been hampered by the need for a reasonably well-equipped and staffed microbiology laboratory to conduct such studies. However, a number of hospital-based studies have been conducted in areas where or in time periods when epidemic meningitis has not been present. These studies are in general agreement that the leading causes of endemic bacterial meningitis in these settings are *S. pneumoniae, H. influenzae,* and *Neisseria meningitidis,* which also are responsible for most cases of bacterial meningitis in industrialized countries, although the introduction and use of conjugate vaccines against *H. influenzae* type b has led to the virtual disappearance of cases due to this organism in such countries. Other organisms that account for a reasonable proportion of cases in industrialized countries, such as group B streptococcus and *Listeria monocytogenes,* appear to be infrequent causes in low- and middle-income countries, although this apparent difference may be artifactual. At the same time, meningitis due to salmonella appears to be more common in low- and middle-income countries than in industrialized ones.

### Descriptive Epidemiologic Features and Risk Factors

The overall cumulative incidence of endemic bacterial meningitis in low- and middle-income countries appears to be four or five times that in industrialized countries, although the available data are limited. It has been estimated that somewhere between 1 in 60 and 1 in 300 children die of bacterial meningitis before the age of five in nonepidemic areas (Greenwood, 1987). Endemic bacterial meningitis is primarily a problem in infants and young children, although age-specific incidence rates vary with the etiologic agent. Meningitis caused by *H. influenzae* occurs almost exclusively during the first 12–24 months of life. While the highest rates of meningitis due to *S. pneumoniae* and endemic meningitis due to *N. meningitidis* occur in the first 12–24 months of life, cases also occur in older children and adults. Endemic bacterial meningitis probably occurs at approximately equal rates among males and females.

Because the three leading causes of endemic bacterial meningitis are all spread via respiratory droplets, poverty and the resulting crowding increase the risk of disease. Failure to breastfeed has been shown to be a risk factor in industrialized countries and probably increases the risk in low- and middle-income countries as well. Host factors also play an important role in determining the risk of endemic bacterial meningitis, most notably sickle cell disease and HIV infection. Sickle cell disease is associated with a markedly increased risk of infection with *S. pneumoniae.* Meningitis due to *S. pneumoniae,* like that caused by salmonella, appears to occur at a substantially increased rate among HIV-infected children and adults. Malnutrition and anemia also have been suspected to be risk factors for bacterial meningitis.

### Current Approaches to Prevention and Control

In most low- and middle-income countries, little or nothing is done to prevent endemic bacterial meningitis. Bacterial meningitis due to *H. influenzae* type b is now preventable with vaccines produced by conjugating the bacterial polysaccharide to one of several protein molecules. The widespread use of these vaccines has led to its virtual eradication in industrialized countries. However, because of their substantial cost, only a few "middle-income" countries (for example, Chile) have incorporated conjugate *H. influenzae* type b vaccine into their routine childhood immunization programs thus far. Other countries in Latin America, however, are planning to add it to the vaccines routinely given to infants in the near future. While a portion of endemic meningitis caused by *N. meningitidis* could be prevented with existing purified polysaccharide vaccine against serogroup C and more recently developed vaccines against serogroup B, these vaccines are not in widespread use outside selected countries (for example, Brazil and Cuba are routinely using a vaccine against serogroup B *N. meningitidis*). Endemic meningitis due to *S. pneumoniae* has not, until recently, been vaccine preventable in infants and young children, the highest risk age groups, but a conjugate *S. pneumoniae* vaccine formulated for use in the United States has recently been approved for use in infants there. A similar vaccine formulated for use in low- and middle-income countries is not yet available but is under development.

Chemoprophylaxis, the giving of a short course of an antimicrobial agent to individuals in close contact with someone with bacterial meningitis due to *N. meningitidis* or *H. influenzae* type b. But it has been used with some success in industrialized countries, has not been widely advocated, and is virtually never used in low- and middle-income countries. The reasons for this are the small percentage of endemic cases that occur in close contacts of a known case, the cost and availability of the antimicrobial agents, the limited duration of the protection achieved, concerns about promoting the development of antimicrobial resistance, and logistical problems related to implementation.

### Obstacles to Prevention and Control and Directions for Future Research

The primary obstacle to preventing endemic meningitis due to *H. influenzae* type b in low- and middle-income countries is the cost of the highly effective and safe conjugate vaccines now used in industrialized countries. If means of dramatically reducing the cost per dose of these vaccines and paying for them can be found, and high vaccine coverage can be achieved, endemic meningitis due to this organism can be virtually eliminated. If, as expected, the conjugate *S. pneumoniae* vaccines currently being developed for use in low- and middle-income countries prove successful in preventing pneumococcal meningitis (and other invasive infections caused by this organism), similar issues of how to make the vaccines affordable for use in such countries will arise. Prevention of endemic meningococcal meningitis must await the availability of serogroup B and C conjugate vaccines that are effective in infants, provide protection

against multiple serotypes of serogroup B, and are affordable.

### Epidemic Meningitis

#### *Etiologic Agents*

Epidemic bacterial meningitis is always caused by *N. meningitidis*. More specifically, serogroup A *N. meningitidis* causes most such epidemics, although epidemics due to serogroup C also have been well documented. Serogroup B *N. meningitidis*, one of the most important causes of endemic bacterial meningitis, has caused "epidemics" in a variety of industrialized and low- and middle-income countries, but these "epidemics" are never of the scope and intensity of those caused by serogroup A, differing in overall attack rates by as much as two orders of magnitude (see below).

#### *Descriptive Epidemiologic Features and Risk Factors*

Epidemic bacterial meningitis, generally caused by serogroup A *N. meningitidis*, is one of the most interesting but least understood infectious disease problems in the world. Epidemics involving hundreds of thousands of cases and cumulative incidence rates of almost 2,000 per 100,000 total population have been observed in the "meningitis belt" of Africa (see Figure 4–3) for more than 100 years (Moore, 1992). The most recent epidemic there in the 1990s was one of the largest ever recorded and extended into parts of Africa not previously considered to be in the meningitis belt. In this region of Africa, epidemics in a given area last for 2 or 3 years and recur every 5 to 15 years. They occur only during the hot, dry season (January–April) and dissipate when the rains and cooler weather arrive, only to return the next dry season. The interepidemic period can vary from a few years to a decade or more, probably reflecting a combination of the time it takes to reaccumulate enough susceptible individuals to sustain an epidemic, the introduction of a new virulent strain of *N.*

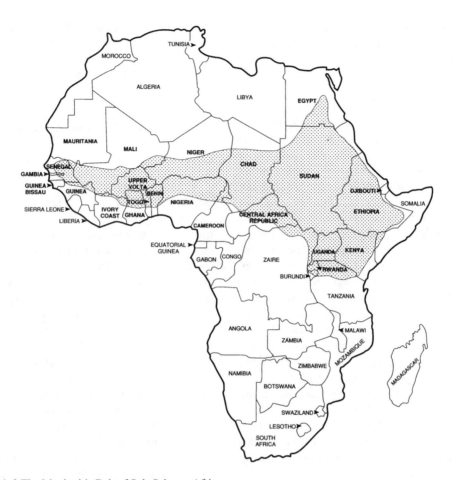

**Figure 4–3** The Meningitis Belt of Sub-Saharan Africa

*meningitidis,* prior use of polysaccharide meningococcal vaccine in the population, and other poorly defined factors (Moore, 1992).

Epidemics of meningococcal meningitis also occur in Asia and Latin America. In western China and Nepal, the epidemics follow a pattern similar to that seen in Africa, except that they occur during a cold, dry season rather than a hot, dry season. In Latin America, Brazil has borne the brunt of such epidemics, due to both serogroups A and C. Epidemics have also affected countries in the Middle East (for example, Saudi Arabia) and the Pacific (for example, New Zealand).

### Current Approaches to Prevention and Control

Historically, efforts to reduce morbidity and mortality from epidemic meningococcal meningitis have been reactive in nature. Once an epidemic is detected, a vaccination campaign is implemented as rapidly as possible, along with making more available the antimicrobial agents and other materials needed to treat cases appropriately. This approach has been rightly criticized on the grounds that there are seemingly unavoidable delays in mounting such campaigns, during which time many cases (and resulting morbidity and mortality) occur. Such reactive vaccination campaigns are almost inevitably disruptive of other health programs, and the extent to which they actually reduce the size of the epidemic is often debated.

One approach to improving the control of such epidemics that has been suggested is to improve surveillance for bacterial meningitis in areas susceptible to epidemics (for example, the meningitis belt of Africa), use a predetermined threshold rate of cases to declare an epidemic and mount a vaccination campaign, and have stockpiles of vaccine and other supplies and equipment in the immediate area ("Control of Epidemic Meningococcal Disease," 1995). However, projections suggest that even these steps would result in the prevention of no more than 40–50% of the cases that would otherwise occur, and initial attempts to establish such early detection and response capabilities have demonstrated the limitations of this approach. Others have proposed routinely vaccinating all infants, children, and young adults in areas at risk of such epidemics with currently available meningococcal A polysaccharide vaccine (Robbins, Towne, Gotschlich, & Schneerson, 1997). However, the need to give three or more doses of this vaccine, and at least one of these at age three or four years in order possibly to achieve long-term protection, has raised concerns about the costs and feasibility of such an approach (Perkins, Broome, Rosenstein, Schuchat, & Reingold, 1997).

### Obstacles to Prevention and Control and Directions for Future Research

Pilot demonstration projects that attempt to incorporate the current meningococcal A purified polysaccharide vaccine into routine vaccination programs in countries in the meningitis belt of Africa are currently being discussed. However, the ultimate prevention of such epidemics may well have to await the availability of a conjugate serogroup A and C vaccine that is immunogenic in infants, provides long-term protection when several doses are given within the first year of life, and is affordable. Such vaccines that appear promising are currently undergoing field trials in Africa, but it is unknown when they will become available or what they will cost.

## MYCOBACTERIAL INFECTIONS

### Overview

Although many species of mycobacteria can infect people, only two of them cause sufficient human illness in low- and middle-income countries to warrant discussion here—*Mycobacteria tuberculosis*, the cause of tuberculosis, and *Mycobacteria leprae*, the cause of leprosy. While *Mycobacteria bovis* (which is closely related to *M. tuberculosis*) can cause tuberculosis in humans, it accounts for a small percentage of cases, and these cases are generally not distinguishable from or in need of different treatment than cases caused by *M. tuberculosis*. Other than *M. leprae*, the various nontuberculous mycobacteria are opportunistic infections that occur almost exclusively in immunocompromised individuals. Whereas these nontuberculous mycobacteria, particularly *Mycobacteria avium* complex, have caused substantial morbidity and mortality among AIDS patients in industrialized countries, they appear to be uncommon in AIDS patients in low- and middle-income countries (see below).

Tuberculosis and infection with *M. tuberculosis* are, by every indicator available, among the most important public health problems in the world. It has been estimated that approximately one-third of the world's population (1.7 billion persons) is infected with *M. tuberculosis*, and that worldwide there were almost 8 million new cases of tuberculosis and almost 2 million deaths from tuberculosis in the year 1997 (Dye, Scheele, Dolin, Pathania, & Raviglione, 1999). Among adults, tuberculosis is responsible for more deaths than any other single infectious agent. Because suppression of the body's immune system is the most important determinant of which individuals infected with *M. tuberculosis* will subsequently develop tuberculosis, the AIDS epidemic has had disastrous consequences for the control of tuberculosis, which was underfunded and inadequate in most low- and middle-income countries even before the arrival of AIDS. In recognition of the gravity of the problems posed by it, WHO declared tuberculosis to be a global emergency in 1993.

A disease that many believe to have been leprosy was described in the Old Testament of the Bible. Leprosy occupies a unique position among human diseases, in large part because of the disfigurement that it can produce and the belief in many cultures that it represents some form of divine punishment. Although leprosy was endemic to Europe during the eleventh through thirteenth centuries, it had virtually disappeared from there by the eighteenth century, long before modern medicine arrived. There is speculation that it was the rise of tuberculosis and infection with *M. tuberculosis* that produced cross-immunity to *M. leprae* and led to the disappearance of leprosy from Europe. Some support for this theory comes from the observation that BCG, the vaccine intended to prevent tuberculosis, appears to be as or more effective in preventing leprosy. Whatever the cause of its virtual (but not complete) absence from industrialized countries, leprosy today is largely confined to a shrinking number of low- and middle-income countries.

## Tuberculosis

### *Etiologic Agent, Clinical Features, and Vaccine Characteristics*

Compared with other bacteria, mycobacteria are slow growing and have special nutritional needs. *M. tuberculosis* can be recovered from clinical specimens, particularly those from the respiratory tract, when appropriate artificial media and techniques are used, but the process takes many weeks and requires a laboratory with a modest level of sophistication and resources.

Further, it can be difficult to obtain a specimen of respiratory tract secretions, particularly from a child. As a result, most cases of tuberculosis are diagnosed and treated based on examination of respiratory tract secretions under a microscope, radiologic findings on chest X-ray, or clinical grounds.

### *Descriptive Epidemiologic Features and Risk Factors*

*M. tuberculosis* is spread via respiratory droplets produced when an individual with active pulmonary tuberculosis, particularly smear-positive tuberculosis (in which more organisms are present in the sputum), coughs or sneezes. Individuals in close contact with an untreated case, particularly household contacts, are at highest risk of becoming infected. In low- and middle-income countries, the highest incidence rates of pulmonary tuberculosis are in men and women of reproductive age, meaning that there are often infants and young children in the same household and in close daily contact with individuals with active pulmonary tuberculosis. As a result, a high proportion of individuals will be exposed to and infected with *M. tuberculosis* before they reach adulthood. Although a small proportion of infected infants and children will develop pulmonary or extrapulmonary tuberculosis soon after becoming infected, in most instances the immune system successfully walls off, but does not kill, all the *M. tuberculosis* organisms. As these infected children grow up, various factors, particularly HIV infection and malnutrition, can reduce the ability of the immune system to keep the organisms in check, and reactivation tuberculosis can occur. Before the AIDS epidemic, it was estimated that 5% of those infected as children developed tuberculosis soon after infection and another 5% developed tuberculosis at some point later in life. However, HIV infection is such a potent inhibitor of cell-mediated immunity (the part of the immune system that holds *M. tuberculosis* infection in check) that a high proportion of untreated dually infected (that is, infected with HIV and with *M. tubercu-*

*losis*) individuals can be expected to develop tuberculosis, unless they die of something else first or receive preventive therapy (see below).

It is currently estimated that 1.5 million persons die from tuberculosis each year and that 8 million persons are newly infected, with the vast majority of these deaths and infections occurring in low-income countries (WHO, 1999). While tuberculosis is a major public health problem in virtually every low-income country, the burden of disease attributable to tuberculosis varies by region and country, in part because of long-standing historical differences in the incidence of tuberculosis and the prevalence of infection with *M. tuberculosis*, in part because of local differences in the adequacy of the tuberculosis control program, and in part because of differences in the extent of the HIV/AIDS epidemic. Based on admittedly incomplete passive surveillance for reported cases of tuberculosis and on tuberculin skin test surveys, it appears that sub-Saharan Africa has the highest average annual risk of infection with *M. tuberculosis* and the highest crude incidence rate of cases of tuberculosis. However, the largest numbers of cases of tuberculosis are seen in the countries comprising the Southeast Asia and the Western Pacific regions of WHO, which collectively account for almost two-thirds of the world's cases (see Figure 4–4) (Dolin, Raviglione, & Kochi, 1994). Because of the HIV/AIDS epidemic and unrelated demographic changes (for example, population growth and increases in the numbers of individuals surviving to their thirties and forties), it has been projected that the number of new cases of tuberculosis will increase in coming years in low- and middle-income countries in all the regions of the world.

Although tuberculosis occurs in individuals in all socioeconomic strata, it is quintessentially a disease of poverty. Through its effect on crowding, poverty increases the risk of airborne transmission of *M. tuberculosis*. At the same time, through its negative effect on nutritional status, poverty increases the likelihood that someone infected with *M. tuberculosis* will develop tuberculosis. To the extent that HIV infection is more prevalent among the poor, it too increases the likelihood that an infected individual will develop tuberculosis. In addition, through its effect on access to curative medical care, poverty increases the likelihood that a patient with symptomatic pulmonary tuberculosis will remain untreated and hence infectious for a longer period of time.

### Current Approaches to Prevention and Control

Tuberculosis control programs exist in virtually all low- and middle-income countries, although there is enormous variability in the resources at their disposal and their effectiveness. The current approach to controlling tuberculosis in low- and middle-income countries is based on a strategy of rapid detection of and provision of effective multidrug therapy to all infectious cases (that is, patients with pulmonary tuberculosis, particularly smear-positive patients). Key components of a successful tuberculosis control program include a strong government commitment to the program; use of sputum smear microscopy to assess symptomatic patients who present at health care facilities; use of a standardized multidrug "short course" regimen, with direct observation of drug ingestion for at least the first 2 months of treatment (directly observed treatment, short course [DOTS]); assurance of an uninterrupted supply of all essential antituberculosis drugs; and a standardized system of recording and reporting cases, treatment, and outcome. According to a survey conducted in 1996, only 75 of the 180 countries that responded had implemented such a program, and in only 39 of these countries was there nationwide implementation (Raviglione, Dye, Schmidt, & Kochi, 1997).

In the face of the limited resources available to ensure prompt diagnosis and treatment of infectious cases of tuberculosis among those who present spontaneously to health facilities, there has been an understandable reluctance to devote scarce resources to active searching for other cases in the households of affected individuals or in the community. Similarly, prevention of

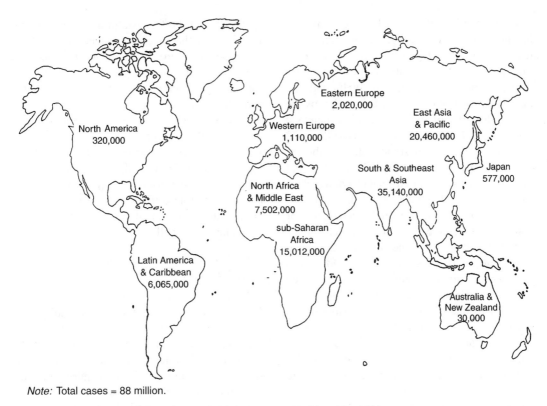

*Note:* Total cases = 88 million.

**Figure 4–4** Estimated Cumulative Tuberculosis Cases Worldwide, 1990–1999

tuberculosis in those infected either recently or longer ago in the past has not been considered a high priority or an effective use of limited resources. In addition, the use of a single drug, such as isoniazid to reduce the likelihood of tuberculosis in infected individuals (as practiced in a number of industrialized countries) has raised the specter of inadvertent single drug therapy of patients with unrecognized tuberculosis and an increased prevalence of drug-resistant strains of *M. tuberculosis*. However, recent clinical trials showing that preventive therapy is highly effective in preventing tuberculosis among HIV-infected individuals in low- and middle-income countries have focused renewed attention on the role of preventive therapy (Whalen et al., 1997).

Immunization at birth with BCG is a standard part of the EPI in every low- and middle-income country, and BCG coverage rates are high in virtually every such country. Infant immunization with BCG appears to be quite effective at reducing the risk of disseminated tuberculosis (for example, tuberculous meningitis) in infants and children, but its efficacy against pulmonary tuberculosis in this age group is probably no better than 50–60%. Infant immunization with BCG probably has, at best, only a modest effect on the risk of developing pulmonary tuberculosis as an adult and consequently has little or no impact on the spread of *M. tuberculosis* in the community.

### Obstacles to Prevention and Control and Directions for Future Research

As noted above, demographic changes and the HIV/AIDS epidemic virtually ensure that the global burden of cases of tuberculosis will rise over the coming years. At present, the principal obstacles to reducing tuberculosis-related morbidity and mortality in low- and middle-income countries are economic and operational in nature. As of 1997–1998, the most recent time period for which data are available, only 9 of 189 countries reporting to WHO had met objectives set by the WHA in 1991—that by the year 2000, 70% of incident cases be detected and 85% of detected cases be cured. Of the 22 countries with the highest incidence of tuberculosis, only two—Vietnam and Peru—had met these objectives. Increased financial and technical assistance will be needed in many countries to ensure that currently available strategies for controlling tuberculosis are fully implemented.

At the same time, further research is needed in multiple areas if control of tuberculosis is to be achieved and sustained. There is evidence that the prevalence of strains of *M. tuberculosis* resistant to one or more of the antimicrobial agents routinely used to treat tuberculosis is substantial and growing. This is occurring not only in those countries historically classified as resource poor, but also in Russia and some of the newly independent states of the former Soviet Union, where inadequate treatment of cases of tuberculosis has led to a rapid rise in drug-resistant strains. Development of new drugs that are effective against *M. tuberculosis*, are affordable and safe, and can eradicate infection with a shorter duration of treatment is a high priority, but such drugs are unlikely to be available soon. Similarly, development of a vaccine against *M. tuberculosis* that can prevent pulmonary tuberculosis is a high priority, but is not currently within view. In the meantime, operational research into how to enhance case detection and ensure dispensing of and compliance with proper treatment, as well as how to prevent tuberculosis in high-risk individuals (for example, those dually infected with *M. tuberculosis* and HIV) is urgently needed.

## Leprosy

### *Etiologic Agent, Clinical Features, and Vaccine Characteristics*

*M. leprae* cannot be grown on artificial media. In research laboratories, it can be isolated and propagated in the foot pad of a mouse or in armadillos, but these techniques have no relevance to diagnosing leprosy. The diagnosis of leprosy is made on clinical grounds, together with histopathologic examination of tissue biopsy material. *M. leprae* grows even more slowly than *M. tuberculosis*. The slow growth of both organisms is highly relevant to the control and prevention of tuberculosis and leprosy because of the consequent need to treat those who are infected for prolonged periods of time (months to years) and the resulting difficulty of ensuring compliance with antimicrobial therapy long after the individual feels well.

### *Descriptive Epidemiologic Features and Risk Factors*

While it is clear that prolonged, close contact (for example, living in the same household) with someone with untreated leprosy, particularly someone with a high burden of organisms (that is, multibacillary leprosy), is associated with a substantially increased risk of acquiring the disease, the routes of transmission are ill-defined. It is assumed that transmission occurs primarily through skin-to-skin contact or exposure to respiratory tract (for example, nasal) secretions. Environmental or animal reservoirs of *M. leprae* are thought to have little or no role in human infections. The exceedingly long incubation period for leprosy, which is believed to be years to decades, makes any study of transmission very difficult. Leprosy is primarily a disease of poverty, and even within a single relatively homogeneous community is disproportionately seen among the lowest income members. Leprosy has often been described as being more common in rural than in urban populations and as having an association with proximity to water (for example, lakes) or humidity, but clear differences in the prevalence of leprosy between neighboring communities are not well explained.

In the mid-1980s it was estimated that there were between 10 and 12 million persons with leprosy worldwide in endemic areas; the incidence of leprosy was 4 to 6 per 1,000, and the prevalence in affected countries often exceeded 10 per 1,000. However, control efforts (see below) had reduced the number of prevalent cases by more than 90% to an estimated 829,000 cases in 1998 ("Action Programme for the Elimination of Leprosy," 1998). Although leprosy previously existed throughout the world, and a handful of individuals living in industrialized countries like the United States develop leprosy each year (a few of whom have never traveled outside the United States), leprosy is now largely confined to a shrinking number of countries. In 1998, for example, more than 90% of the known cases in the world were in 16 countries, with two of those countries—India and Brazil—accounting for approximately 65% and 15%, respectively, of the cases. Other countries that continue to have substantial numbers of cases include Nigeria, Madagascar, Vietnam, Burma, Indonesia, Bangladesh, and Nepal, but other countries in Latin America, Africa, Asia, and the Middle East also have modest numbers (see Figure 4–5; WHO Expert Committee on Leprosy, 1998).

### Current Approaches to Prevention and Control

Early attempts to control leprosy were based on case-finding and prolonged (that is, multiyear) or lifetime treatment with dapsone, which had the advantages of being inexpensive and having few side effects. However, this approach failed to control leprosy, at least in part because *M. leprae* developed resistance to dapsone and it was difficult to ensure ongoing patient compliance with treatment over many years. In the early 1980s multidrug treatment with two or three (depending on the stage of leprosy) effective antimicrobial agents was introduced and has produced the greater than 90% reduction in leprosy cases referred to above. WHO has set a goal of eliminating leprosy as a public health problem (that is, a prevalence ≤ 1 case per 10,000) by the year 2000, which appears to be within reach in many, but probably not all, currently affected countries.

### Obstacles to Prevention and Control and Directions for Future Research

Because of its extremely long incubation period and the fact that infected individuals may transmit *M. leprae* for substantial periods of time prior to becoming symptomatic and being placed on multidrug therapy, it is likely that incident cases of leprosy will continue to occur in substantial numbers for years to come. The greatest threat to reducing further the prevalence and incidence of leprosy is complacency and consequent reduced funding for case detection and multidrug therapy, which is much more expensive than single-drug therapy with dapsone. The priority given to leprosy control and to leprosy-related research is likely to be reduced substantially as the prevalence of cases decreases. The role, if any, for a vaccine in the immunotherapy or the prevention of leprosy remains uncertain. Numerous studies have suggested that BCG vaccine, given primarily to prevent various forms of disseminated tuberculosis in children, offers some protection. In fact, BCG may be more effective in preventing leprosy than in preventing tuberculosis, although the estimates of its efficacy in preventing leprosy span a very large range. Whether other candidate mycobacterial vaccines will offer even greater protection than BCG remains uncertain, as does their role, if any, in leprosy control.

## SEXUALLY TRANSMITTED INFECTIONS AND AIDS

### Overview

Sexually transmitted infections (STIs) have historically been one of the most neglected areas of medicine and public health in low- and middle-income countries. Until the advent of the HIV/AIDS epidemic in the 1980s, remarkably little attention was being paid to STIs in such countries, despite the fact that they collectively cause enormous morbidity, loss of productivity, and infertility, and result in substantial health care expenditures. The fact that HIV, the cause of AIDS and all its attendant morbidity and mortality, is transmitted sexually, together with the fact that the sexual transmission of HIV is facilitated by the presence of other STIs, has focused attention on and brought an infusion of resources into this long-neglected area. However,

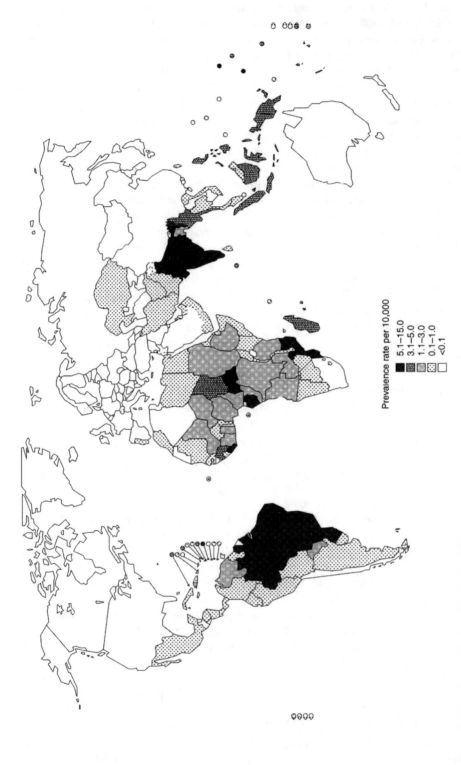

**Figure 4-5** Prevalence of Leprosy Worldwide, 1997

the myriad challenges confronting the treatment and control of STIs in low- and middle-income countries are multifaceted and complex. Among the most daunting are the difficulty of changing human sexual behavior; the frequency with which STIs are asymptomatic, particularly among women; the lack of simple, inexpensive diagnostic tests; and the lack of readily accessible, inexpensive, easy to administer, single-dose treatment regimens for most STIs.

**Etiologic Agents**

A variety of viruses and bacteria can be transmitted sexually (see Table 4–3), including some (for example, HBV) that are not traditionally grouped with other STIs. In this chapter, HBV is discussed with the other viruses that cause hepatitis. Many infectious agents that are transmitted sexually can also be transmitted via contaminated blood or injection equipment, and vertically from mother to her newborn infant.

Of the infectious agents transmitted sexually, some initially cause ulcerative lesions, primarily on or near the genitalia (for example, *Herpes simplex*, *Treponema pallidum*, and *Haemophilus ducreyii*); others initially cause urethral or vaginal discharge (for example, *Neisseria gonorrhoea*, *Chlamydia trachomatis*, and *Trichomonas vaginalis*); and others cause only systemic manifestations (for example, HIV). HPV, selected subtypes of which cause genital warts, plays an important role in the pathogenesis of cervical dysplasia and carcinoma, as well as in carcinoma of the penis, but most HPV infections are initially silent. Asymptomatic or minimally symptomatic infection with many of the sexually transmitted agents is common, greatly exacerbating the problem of interrupting transmission and reducing the prevalence and incidence of infection.

Many of the agents transmitted sexually not only produce acute symptoms referable to the lower genital tract, but also can produce other, often more serious manifestations. For example, untreated infections with *N. gonorrhoea* and *C. trachomatis* can ascend and produce pelvic inflammatory disease, tubal infertility, and ectopic pregnancy. Untreated primary syphilis in young adults can lead to life-threatening cardiac and neurologic complications due to tertiary syphilis years later, whereas congenital syphilis, the result of infection of a baby at the time of birth, produces profound systemic manifestations. As noted above, infection with HPV of selected subtypes is strongly associated with subsequent cervical dysplasia and cervical cancer. Finally, HIV causes profound damage to the host immune system and a virtually 100% case-fatality ratio in the absence of treatment with extremely expensive, antiretroviral drug regimens.

**Descriptive Epidemiologic Features and Risk Factors**

Data concerning the incidence of STIs in low- and middle-income countries are considered highly unreliable due to substantial underdiagnosis and underreporting. One recent estimate suggests that in 1995 there were 333 million new adult cases of curable STIs (for example, gonorrhea, chlamydia, syphilis, and trichomoniasis) worldwide, the vast majority of which were in low- and middle-income countries (see Figure 4–6) (Gerbase, Rowley, & Mertens, 1998). The number of noncurable STIs, including genital herpes, HPV, and HIV, is difficult to estimate. Passive surveillance for AIDS in place in most low- and middle-income countries is also not very sensitive or specific, making it necessary to estimate the number or incidence of AIDS cases. The most recent estimate is that in 1998 there were more than 33 million persons in the world living with AIDS and an additional almost 14 million who had died of AIDS since the epidemic began. The vast majority of these cases were in low-income countries, particularly sub-Saharan Africa (see Figure 4–7) ("Adults and Children," 1998). Current projections suggest that as of 2000 there are more than 40 million HIV-infected persons in the world.[*]

The prevalence of various STIs, particularly HIV, has been investigated in many low- and

---

[*]Visit the UNAIDS Website (http://UNAIDS.org/epidemic_update/index.html) for the most current information on the HIV/AIDS epidemic.

**Table 4–3** Sexually Transmitted Infections of Importance in Low- and Middle-Income Countries

| Agent | Disease | Vertical Transmission to Newborn Babies | Transmission via Blood Products |
|---|---|---|---|
| **Bacteria** | | | |
| T. pallidum | Syphilis | yes | yes |
| N. gonorrhoea | Gonorrhea, pelvic inflammatory disease | yes | no |
| C. trachomatis | Cervicitis, urethritis, lymphogranuloma vererenum, pelvic inflammatory disease | yes | no |
| H. ducreyii | Chancroid | no | no |
| **Viruses** | | | |
| Human immunodeficiency virus (HIV) | AIDS | yes | yes |
| H. simplex | Genital herpes | yes | no |
| Human papilloma virus (HPV) | Genital warts, cervical dysplasia and cervical carcinoma | ? | no |
| Hepatitis B virus* | Acute and chronic hepatitis, cirrhosis, and hepatocellular carcinoma | yes | yes |
| **Other** | | | |
| T. vaginalis | Vaginitis | no | no |

*Discussed in the section on viral hepatitis.

middle-income countries. The groups typically examined are those that can be studied easily and inexpensively—commercial sex workers, patients being treated for STIs or for tuberculosis, injection drug users, pregnant women or women giving birth, and blood donors. Prevalences of HIV infection as high as 70–80% have been seen among commercial sex workers, and in the range of 15–30% have been documented among pregnant women delivering at large urban hospitals in the worst affected urban areas of sub-Saharan Africa ("Recent HIV Seroprevalence Levels," 1999). Because an estimated 15–30% of HIV-infected pregnant women will pass the virus to their newborn babies at or soon after delivery, large numbers of HIV-infected infants are also found wherever many women of reproductive age are infected. The result of widespread HIV infection among men and women of reproductive age and among infants in the most severely affected countries has been a reversal of prior gains in life expectancy and prior reductions in infant and child mortality rates, an enormous increase in the numbers of orphaned children, and projected future declines in population size.

Given that the infectious agents under discussion are transmitted through sexual contact, it is not surprising that the highest incidences and prevalences of these infections are seen among men and women who are most sexually active, typically those 15 to 49 years of age, and that the most important risk factors for STIs—the number of sexual partners, the type of sexual partners,

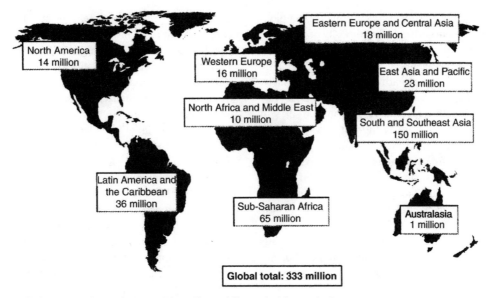

*Note:* Estimates are for gonorrhea, chlamydia, syphilis, and trichomoniasis.

**Figure 4–6** Estimates of New Adult Cases of Curable Sexually Transmitted Infections, 1995

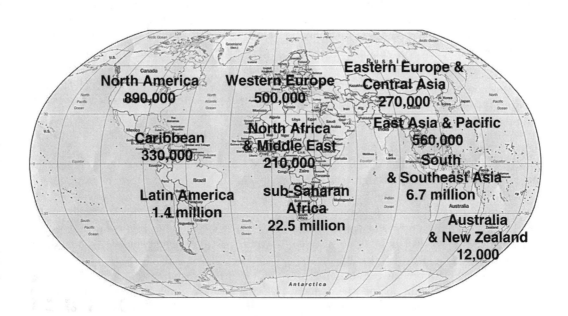

**Total: 33.4 million**

**Figure 4–7** Adults and Children Estimated To Be Living with HIV/AIDS, December 1998

and whether barrier protection (for example, a male condom) is used—are directly or indirectly related to the likelihood of exposure to one of the infectious agents. Thus individuals with large numbers of sexual partners (for example, commercial sex workers) who do not use barrier protection and those who have unprotected sex with such individuals are at highest risk. However, in societies in which it is considered acceptable for men to frequent commercial sex workers or have multiple sexual partners while women are expected to have a single partner, many monogamous women acquire STIs from their husbands. Other risk factors for STIs have been reported, such as lack of male circumcision, but are substantially less important than the number and type of sexual partners and the use or nonuse of barrier protection.

It is important to note the complex interplay between HIV infection and other STIs. There is strong evidence that infection with both ulcerative and nonulcerative STIs increases the likelihood of HIV being transmitted sexually between partners, either through the presence of disrupted mucosa or the presence in the genital tract of increased numbers of inflammatory cells and lymphocytes that can bind HIV.

## Current Approaches to Prevention and Control

The current approach to the prevention and control of STIs, including HIV, focuses on changing sexual practices through education and health promotion, increasing the availability and use of barrier methods that reduce transmission (for example, male and female condoms), improving the availability of and access to high-quality diagnostic and treatment services, shortening the time between the onset of symptoms and seeking appropriate care, reducing the stigma attached to STIs, and improving surveillance. Not surprisingly, given the enormous cultural diversity that exists, approaches to delivery of risk reduction messages (for example, school-based programs, billboards, and radio), what groups to target (for example, the entire population; individuals of reproductive age; school-age children; high-risk groups such as commercial sex workers, migrant workers, truck drivers); and what messages to deliver (for example, abstinence before marriage, monogamy, condom use) have varied greatly.

Because the laboratory facilities and trained staff needed to identify a specific etiologic agent in a given patient with a suspected STI are often lacking in many low- and middle-income countries, WHO has developed and promoted a syndromic approach to the management of STIs. This approach relies on classifying patients with a suspected STI into various groups depending on their symptoms and findings on physical examination (for example, women with a vaginal discharge, men with urethral discharge and dysuria, and patients with genital ulcer) and then treating them with a regimen designed to cover the treatable etiologic agents that are likely to be responsible (for example, *N. gonorrhoea* and *C. trachomatis* when a cervical or urethral discharge is present). Exhibit 4–5 presents a case study of the syndromic management of genital ulcer in the African country of Lesotho (Htun et al., 1998; "Management of Patients," 1991).

In general, the syndromic approach has many advantages—it removes the need for and expense of having a laboratory and a trained technician; it permits immediate treatment of the patient, without requiring the patient to return (and be abstinent in the meantime); it treats individuals who have the infection but who would have a false negative laboratory test; and it is less expensive. However, this approach can also lead to overtreatment, particularly in women with a vaginal discharge, many of whom do not have an STI.

Recently, two interesting approaches to reducing the sexual transmission of HIV through the treatment of other STIs have been tested in Africa. In the Rakai district of Uganda, a program of treating for STIs all consenting individuals of reproductive age, regardless of whether they had symptoms of an STI (that is, mass treat-

**Exhibit 4–5** Case Study of the Syndromic Management of Genital Ulcer

WHO reports that genital ulcers are commonly detected in low- and middle-income countries and may have serious consequences, including symptomatic syphilis, mutilating lesions, and enhanced transmission of HIV ("Management of patients with sexually transmitted diseases," 1991). Laboratory tests to determine the etiology of genital ulcers (for example, H. simplexvirus, *H. ducreyii, T. pallidum*, or *C. trachomatis*) are expensive and technically sophisticated, and thus generally unavailable in many health care settings in the developing world, while presumptive diagnosis based on clinical manifestations is largely unsatisfactory. WHO therefore advocates a syndromic approach to the management of genital ulcer in low- and middle-income countries.

A recent study in Lesotho illustrates the promise and drawbacks of this approach (Htun et al., 1998). In an attempt to validate STI flowcharts for the management of genital ulcer, researchers found that syndromic protocols would have provided adequate treatment for at least 90% of their patient population, while the traditional, clinically directed protocol would have provided adequate treatment for only 62% of those same patients. On the other hand, syndromic protocols also would have led to the overtreatment of primary syphilis in about 60% of patients, while the clinically directed protocols would not have resulted in any such overtreatment.

A plurality of similar studies have shown that syndromic case management of STIs using flowcharts often leads to improved treatment in many patients as well as overtreatment in some patients. In general, to determine the appropriateness of implementing the syndromic approach in a given region, the costs of overtreatment (including the cost of the drugs themselves), the risk of promoting drug resistance, and the stigma of an STI diagnosis (which can lead to domestic violence against women), must be weighed against the benefits of improved treatment, including reductions in STI and HIV transmission, decreases in sequelae from untreated infections, and increased patient satisfaction. In view of the high prevalence of STIs in many low- and middle-income countries, this trade-off is often acceptable.

ment of the community), was tried. This approach did not reduce the transmission of HIV in the community. In the Mwanza Region of Tanzania, however, an earlier, randomized, community-based study of improving the diagnosis and treatment of STIs showed an approximately 40% reduction in the incidence of HIV infection, but no change in the incidence of other STIs (Grosskurth et al., 1995).

The finding that an intensive (and expensive) regimen of AZT (zidovudine) given to HIV-infected pregnant women in the United States substantially reduced vertical transmission of HIV to their newborn babies led to trials of simpler and cheaper AZT regimens in Thailand and Ivory Coast. These trials have shown that even these simpler regimens, which are given entirely by mouth and for a shorter period of time, are partially effective in reducing vertical transmission of HIV, and plans are being made to make this regimen more widely available in low- and middle-income countries (Shaffer et al., 1999; Wiktor et al., 1999). Similar trials using an even simpler dosing regimen and a less expensive drug, nevirapine, also have shown promising results (Marseille et al., 1999). However, unless HIV testing of pregnant women can be made widely available in such settings, the availability of this regimen may not translate into marked reductions in the incidence of vertical transmission of HIV. Similarly, safe, effective, and inexpensive approaches to preventing vertical transmission during the postpartum interval will also need to be developed, given the evidence that a substantial fraction of vertical transmission of HIV may occur via breastfeeding.

## Obstacles to Prevention and Control and Directions for Future Research

There are enormous obstacles to changing the sexual behaviors of people, although there have been promising reductions in the frequency of high risk sexual behaviors and the incidence of HIV infection in Thailand (see Exhibit 4–6) (Celentano et al., 1996; Nelson et al., 1996; Rojanapithayakorn & Hanenberg, 1996) and Uganda in response to the AIDS epidemic (Kilian et al., 1999). In many societies it is considered socially acceptable, even desirable, for men to visit commercial sex workers and have multiple sex partners. Many men do not want to use condoms, and a woman may risk physical abuse, rejection, or loss of financial support if she tries to insist that a condom be used by her husband, boyfriend, or customer. Women who learn they are HIV-infected also risk abandonment or abuse if they share this information. Thus changing sexual behaviors requires the education of men as well as women, and reducing the incidence of STIs, including HIV, requires raising the status and improving the power of women in society. Similarly, economic and other practices that contribute to or promote risky sexual behaviors (for example, forcing men to live apart from their wives in order to earn a living wage) need to be rethought.

Vaccines against STIs, particularly HIV, are desperately needed, but have been difficult to develop. A vaccine against HPV is in early stages of testing and appears promising, but it is likely to be a number of years until we know whether or not it is effective in preventing cervical dysplasia and cancer. The development of vaccines against HIV has been beset by many problems, and there is disagreement about what type of vaccine (inactivated whole virus, subunit, genetically engineered, live, attenuated, and so on) is likely to be safe and effective. However, phase three trials of subunit HIV vaccines began in the United States and Thailand in 1998–1999, and trials of other vaccines are expected to begin in Uganda and elsewhere. Even under ideal circumstances, however, it is unlikely that an HIV vaccine can be available for widespread use for at least 5 to 10 years, and questions remain about who will pay the cost of making it widely available in low- and middle-income countries once it has been developed.

In the absence of vaccines against HIV and other STIs, other approaches to reducing morbidity and mortality beyond primary prevention of infection through behavior change are needed. For example, while women in industrialized countries generally have access to regular screening for cervical dysplasia, which has been shown to be a highly effective tool for the secondary prevention of invasive cervical cancer, most women in low- and middle-income countries have not had access to such screening because of the cost and need for moderately sophisticated laboratory support. Recent studies suggest that screening for cervical dysplasia using much simpler and less expensive technology may be possible in low- and middle-income countries (University of Zimbabwe/JHPIEGO Cervical Cancer Project, 1999). Similarly, even if complex and expensive combinations of antiretroviral drugs are not yet available to HIV-infected persons in most low- and middle-income countries, other treatment and prevention modalities that are far less expensive may lengthen and improve the quality of survival of such persons. Possible treatment modalities include chemoprophylaxis to prevent tuberculosis and common bacterial infections (for example, salmonella, S. pneumoniae, and others), nutritional support, and improved oral and dental hygiene, among others.

## VIRAL HEPATITIS

### Overview

Hepatitis, which means inflammation of the liver, does not represent a single disease process, and can be caused on occasion by many viruses (as well as bacteria, protozoa, chemical agents, and some noninfectious diseases). However, there are at least five viruses that specifically infect the liver—hepatitis viruses A, B, C, D, and E. Each belongs to a different family and

**Exhibit 4–6** Case Study of a Successful Public Health Program: The Declining Spread of HIV among Thai Military Conscripts

In the late 1980s heterosexual commercial sex was found to contribute significantly to the rapid spread of HIV in Thailand. Thai authorities responded swiftly to this observation and implemented public health programs that substantially increased the number of commercial sex acts protected by condoms, which in turn led to significant reductions in the rate of HIV infection among young men in Thailand. This case study tells the story of this public health success.

The first national serosurvey for HIV conducted in Thailand found that HIV was exceedingly prevalent among commercial sex workers. In June 1989, 44% of sex workers in the northern province of Chiang Mai were positive for HIV, a figure that would climb to 67% by June 1993 (Celetano et al., 1996). Commercial sex in Thailand is relatively common; for example, in 1991–1993, more than 70% of Thai military conscripts were found to have engaged in at least one commercial sex act during their period of service. Because military conscripts are selected by a national lottery, these findings are applicable to the general population of young men in Thailand, and thus commercial sex was believed to be a common source of HIV infection.

To address this situation, Thai authorities implemented an HIV/AIDS prevention and control program that included the 100% Condom Campaign to promote condom use in commercial sex establishments. Under this campaign, free condoms were distributed to all sex establishments and the use of condoms was actively enforced by Thai authorities. The campaign was accompanied by mass advertising to promote condom use during commercial sex.

In the years following the initiation of the condom campaign, the use of condoms in sex establishments increased dramatically. National behavioral surveillance data revealed that the percentage of commercial sex acts in which condoms were used rose from approximately 14% in the years prior to 1989 to more than 90% by 1993 (Rojanapithayakorn & Harenberg, 1996). Although the prevalence of HIV among sex workers has remained high, the prevalence among newly inducted military conscripts declined from 10–12% in 1991 and 1993 to approximately 7% in 1995 (Nelson et al., 1996). Further, this decline occurred in the absence of a visible AIDS epidemic (Rojanapithayakorn & Harenberg, 1996). Experts attribute these heartening findings, at least in part, to the swift implementation of the Thai HIV/AIDS prevention and control program, and especially to the success of the 100% Condom Campaign.

has unique clinical and epidemiologic features, necessitating diverse approaches to control and prevention.

Viral hepatitis is a major global public health problem. All five primary hepatitis viruses can cause acute disease. HBV, HCV, and HDV can also produce chronic infections. In many low- and middle-income countries, such persistent infections are the primary cause of serious liver disease, including chronic hepatitis, cirrhosis, and hepatocellular carcinoma, a common cancer that is almost always fatal. It is estimated that there are more than 350 million chronic carriers of HBV (WHO, 1999) and 170 million chronic carriers of HCV worldwide ("Hepatitis C: Global Prevalence," 1997).

Hepatitis A virus (HAV) and hepatitis E virus (HEV) cause acute self-limited disease; they do not cause chronic infection. Transmitted by the fecal-oral route, these viruses are endemic in many low- and middle-income countries with suboptimal environmental sanitation. HAV infections are typically asymptomatic when they occur in infants. In older children and adults, they generally produce a self-limited illness with few deaths. HEV infection results in more substantial morbidity and mortality, particularly when it occurs in pregnant women.

## Etiologic Agents

The five primary hepatitis viruses (A, B, C, D, and E) account for almost all cases of viral hepatitis. Although other viruses (for example, Epstein-Barr virus and cytomegalovirus) occasionally cause hepatitis, infections with these viruses do not principally involve the liver. Conversely, hepatitis virus G (also known as GB virus C) specifically targets liver cells, but whether this virus causes disease is not yet established (Kew & Kassianides, 1997). The following discussion is limited to the five primary hepatitis viruses.

## Descriptive Epidemiologic Features and Risk Factors

The prevalence of chronic HBV infection is high throughout low- and middle-income countries (see Figure 4–8) (Margolis, Alter, & Hadler, 1997). For example, in sub-Saharan Africa, the Amazon Basin, and a number of countries in Asia, the prevalence of chronic HBV infection exceeds 8%, and 60–85% of the population have antibody to hepatitis B surface antigen, which indicate previous HBV infection (London & Evans, 1996). In these areas, most people who acquire HBV do so at the time of birth (through vertical transmission from an infected mother) or in infancy or childhood. Most such infections produce no acute symptoms. Unfortunately, the likelihood of chronic infection and risk of progression to chronic liver disease increases significantly as the age of acquisition decreases. The most common routes of transmission of HBV in low- and middle-income settings are perinatally, from mother to child, and horizontally, from one child to another. Transmission through the use of unsterilized needles for medical injections also occurs. Less frequent modes of transmission include sexual intercourse and needle sharing among injection drug users (the two principal modes of transmission in industrialized countries). Additionally, traditional practices such as tattooing, scarification, circumcision, and body piercing with unsterile instruments can spread HBV.

HDV is a defective virus such that HDV infection can only be acquired in the presence of HBV infection. The distribution of HDV varies markedly by region but generally corresponds to the distribution of HBV, although there are some interesting exceptions to this pattern. For example, HDV infections are relatively rare in East and Southeast Asia, even though the prevalence of HBV is high in this area (Margolis et al., 1997). The primary mode of transmission of HDV is through percutaneous exposure to blood, as may occur through unsterile medical injections and the transfusion of unscreened blood. Perinatal and sexual transmission of HDV occur, but are less efficient than for HBV.

HCV virus is widespread throughout the world. Although HCV is not as infectious as HBV, HCV infection is much more likely to become chronic (as many as 80% of HCV-infected persons become chronically infected) ("Hepatitis C," 1997). In low- and middle-income countries, HCV prevalences in the general population in the range of 0–18% (see Figure 4–9) have been reported ("Hepatitis C: Global Prevalence," 1997). The principal modes of transmission of HCV in low- and middle-income countries are believed to be the reuse of needles for medical injections and the transfusion of unscreened blood. Other percutaneous exposures to blood (needle sharing among drug users and traditional practices that involve piercing the skin) are important in some settings. There is evidence that HCV also can be spread perinatally and sexually, but this is probably uncommon.

HAV infection is endemic in most low- and middle-income countries. The primary mode of transmission of HAV is fecal-oral through person-to-person contact or the ingestion of contaminated food or water. In areas with poor environmental sanitation, HAV infection is virtually universal during the first few years of life. Infection in infancy and early childhood tends to be asymptomatic or mild and produces lifelong immunity. As sanitation improves, however, individuals are more likely to escape exposure to HAV in childhood. If they then are infected as teenagers or adults, the clinical manifesta-

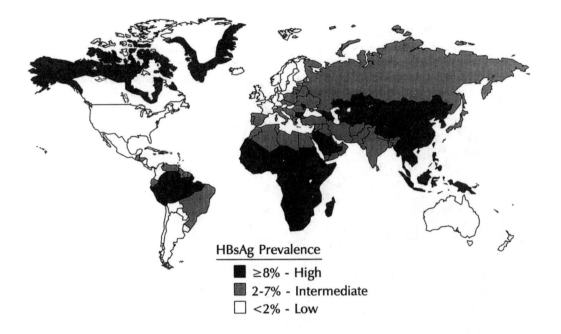

**HBsAg Prevalence**

■ ≥8% - High
▨ 2-7% - Intermediate
□ <2% - Low

**Figure 4–8** Prevalence of Chronic Hepatitis B Worldwide

tions tend to be more severe, albeit self-limited. Fatalities are uncommon.

HEV is also endemic in many low- and middle-income countries and causes substantial morbidity and mortality. HEV infection can be particularly deadly among pregnant women. For example, one study found that 28% of pregnant women who were infected with HEV during the last trimester developed fulminant, fatal hepatitis (Khuroo, Teli, Skidmore, Sofi, & Khuroo, 1981). In endemic areas, HEV can produce cyclic outbreaks, as well as sporadic cases of hepatitis. HEV is acquired through the fecal-oral route, principally through ingestion of contaminated water. Person-to-person transmission of HEV can also occur.

### Current Approaches to Prevention and Control

A safe and effective vaccine for HBV has been available since 1982. In the early 1990s the global advisory group of EPI and WHO rec-ommended integrating the vaccine into the national immunization programs of all countries by 1997. One hundred countries had achieved this goal as of 1998. However, many low- and middle-income countries have not added HBV vaccine to their childhood immunization programs because of the associated costs, even though the vaccine is available at a cost of approximately 50 cents to one U.S. dollar per dose (WHO, 1999).

Vaccination against HBV infection is also effective against HDV coinfection. (As noted above, HDV infection requires the presence of HBV.) However, additional strategies are needed to prevent HDV superinfections among chronic carriers of HBV. Because there is no vaccine against HDV *per se*, the prevention of such superinfections depends on reducing percutaneous exposures to blood in medical and nonmedical settings among those who are chronically infected with HBV.

There is also no vaccine against HCV at this time. Treatment of those who are chronically

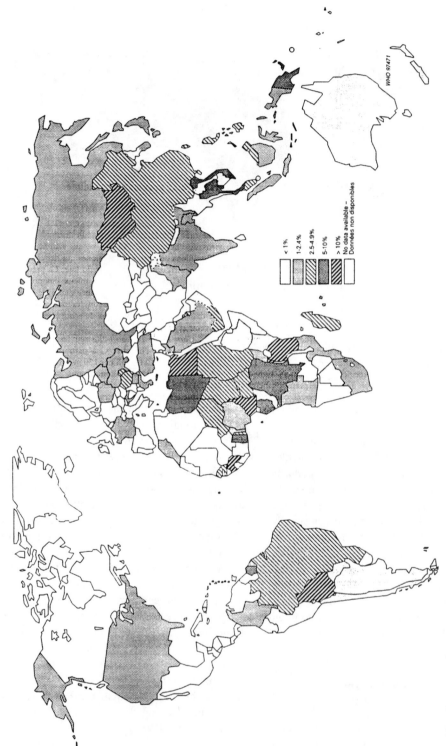

*Note:* Dotted lines on maps represent approximate border lines for which there may not yet be full agreement.

**Figure 4–9** Prevalence of Hepatitis C Worldwide

infected with HCV with interferon is effective in approximately 20% of cases, but such treatment is prohibitively expensive and thus not an option in low- and middle-income countries ("Hepatitis C," 1997). Interrupting the transmission of HCV is currently the only feasible intervention. WHO cites the following measures to prevent HCV infections: (a) screening blood and blood products worldwide, (b) effectively using universal precautions and barrier techniques, (c) destroying disposable needles and adequately sterilizing reusable injection materials, and (d) promoting public education about the risks of using unsterilized instruments to pierce the skin ("Hepatitis C," 1997).

The epidemiologic features of HAV infection vary by region and degree of sanitation, necessitating diverse approaches to control. An effective vaccine against HAV is available and may prove useful in controlling the periodic outbreaks among older children and adults that occur in areas of low endemicity. However, the current vaccine is licensed for use only in older children, not in infants. In most low- and middle-income countries, HAV infection is highly endemic and routinely acquired during infancy and early childhood, when it produces little morbidity or mortality. Consequently, the prevention of HAV infection in low- and middle-income countries is not a priority at this time, and the available vaccine is not licensed for use in the affected age group.

There is no vaccine against HEV. Improved environmental sanitation, especially the provision of clean drinking water, is the best strategy for prevention of HEV infections.

### Obstacles to Prevention and Control and Directions for Future Research

Preventing HBV and HCV infections remains a major global public health goal. Universal coverage with the HBV vaccine reduces the incidence of HBV infection and serious liver disease and represents the best hope for reducing the acute and delayed morbidity and mortality caused by this virus. Unfortunately, the cost of supplying and distributing this relatively inexpensive vaccine remains a significant barrier to achieving universal immunization. Additionally, in areas where perinatal transmission of HBV is important, the vaccine should be given within 12 hours of birth (Margolis et al., 1997)—a difficult goal to achieve in most low- and middle-income settings. The costs and logistical problems associated with achieving high levels of coverage with routinely administered childhood vaccines are exacerbated as more and more vaccines (for example, the *H. influenzae* type b vaccine) are added to the EPI. Depending upon their cost, combined vaccines may help alleviate this difficulty in the future, and research to develop and evaluate such combined vaccines is underway.

There are many obstacles to preventing HBV and HCV through means other than vaccination. The difficulty of ensuring safe medical injections and safe blood transfusions is a major barrier to reducing the bloodborne transmission of HBV and HCV. The prevention of HEV in the absence of a vaccine is no more tractable, as the problems of securing and sustaining a clean water supply are not easily overcome in low- and middle-income countries.

## MALARIA AND OTHER ARTHROPOD-BORNE DISEASES

### Overview

Blood-sucking arthropods (including mosquitoes, flies, bugs, fleas, mites, and ticks) are efficient vectors for a host of pathogenic protozoa, bacteria, viruses, and worms, which cause tremendous suffering and death around the world. Transmitted by mosquitoes, malaria is undoubtedly the most important parasitic disease in tropical regions of low- and middle-income countries (see Figure 4–10; WHO, 1993). WHO estimates that 2.3 billion people, about 41% of the world's population, live in areas at risk for malaria, resulting in 300–500 million new cases and more than 1.5 million deaths every year ("World Malaria Situation," 1997). The majority of these deaths occur in children under the age of five. Mosquitoes also transmit dengue fever (50–100 million cases per year) (Rigau-Pérez et al., 1998), yellow fever, filariasis, and Japanese encephalitis, while various other arthropods spread trypanosomiasis, leishmaniaisis, onchocerciasis (river blindness), and plague, to name but a few diseases. The public health importance of arthropod-borne diseases can scarcely be overstated—they contribute substantially to morbidity and mortality in affected countries and significantly encumber social, economic, and developmental progress.

### Etiologic Agents and Clinical Features

As noted above, arthropod-borne diseases are caused by a wide variety of pathogens. However, this section is limited to a discussion of malaria, dengue fever, yellow fever, American trypanosomiasis, and African trypanosomiasis, although many of the prevention and control issues discussed in the context of these diseases are applicable to other arthropod-borne diseases. Onchocerciasis is discussed in the section on infectious causes of blindness.

Malaria is a febrile disease caused by four species of the parasitic *Plasmodium* protozoa: *P. falciparum*, *P. vivax*, *P. malariae*, and *P. ovale*. Dengue is caused by the dengue group viruses and occurs in two forms: dengue fever, which is self-limiting and rarely fatal; and dengue hemorrhagic fever, a more severe form of the disease that is associated with bleeding and, occasionally, shock leading to death. Yellow fever is caused by a virus of the same name and is characterized by fever and, in severe cases, hemorrhage, jaundice, and liver and kidney involvement. American trypanosomiasis is caused by the protozoan parasite *Trypanosoma cruzi*. Acute infections are usually mild, but about one-third of infected individuals develop more severe chronic manifestations after several years of asymptomatic infection, including cardiac damage (most common) leading to heart failure, digestive tract damage, and neurologic involvement. African trypanosomiasis is caused by two subspecies of the protozoan parasite *Try-*

*panosoma brucei*: *T.b. rhodesiense* and *T.b. gambiense*. Individuals infected with *T.b. rhodesiense* develop symptoms within weeks to months, whereas those infected with *T.b. gambiense* develop symptoms over a period of months to years. In both cases, the disease follows a course of central nervous system derangement, coma, and certain death if left untreated.

### Descriptive Epidemiologic Features and Risk Factors

Although malaria is found in 100 countries around the world, more than 90% of cases occur in tropical Africa ("World Malaria Situation," 1997). The parasite is transmitted between humans (who serve as the reservoir) by the female *Anopheles* mosquito. In endemic areas, where transmission is constant, individuals gradually develop immunity to severe disease. As a consequence, young children (who have not yet developed immunity) and pregnant women (who have depressed immune function) experience the highest rates of malaria morbidity and mortality. Susceptible individuals who enter endemic areas (for example, migrant laborers, displaced persons, and travelers) are also at risk.

More than half the world lives in areas at risk for dengue virus infection, resulting in 50–100 million cases of dengue fever each year and 250,000–500,000 cases of dengue hemorrhagic fever, the more severe form of the disease (see Figure 4–11) (Rigau-Pérez et al., 1998). Major epidemics of dengue hemorrhagic fever to date have been largely limited to Southeast Asia and Latin America, whereas epidemics of dengue fever are more widespread. There are four dengue virus serotypes. Infection with one serotype produces long-term immunity to that serotype, but limited cross protection against the others. Evidence suggests that individuals who have preexisting antibody (for example, from a previous infection) to a given dengue virus serotype have a higher risk of developing more severe disease upon reinfection with a different

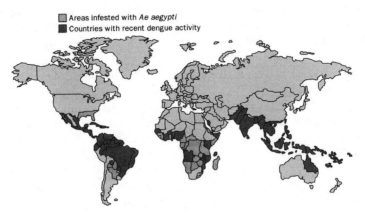

**Figure 4–11** Distribution of Dengue Worldwide

Malaria resurged in the following decades, and the goal of global malaria eradication was declared a failure and abandoned. To address the resurgence of malaria, WHO formulated a new global strategy for malaria control in 1993. The four basic technical elements of the new strategy are

1. *disease management* through the use of antimalarial drugs
2. *disease prevention* through the use of personal protection measures such as the use of repellents and insecticide-impregnated bed-nets, and vector control measures such as indoor residual spraying, larviciding, and environmental management (for example, breeding site reduction)
3. *epidemic control* through basic preparedness measures (for example, maintaining reserves of antimalarial drugs and insecticides) and disease surveillance
4. *research* to ensure that program activities are effective and responsive to changing conditions (for example, climate shifts or land-use changes) that may promote the transmission of malaria (WHO, 1993)

No antimalarial vaccines are currently available or likely to become available in the near future, although malaria vaccine development is an active area of research. Wide-scale chemoprophylaxis is not recommended because of drug resistance, cost, and feasibility.

The new strategy centers on disease control rather than vector eradication. While eradication era programs were characterized as highly prescriptive and centralized, the new approach strongly emphasizes decentralization and flexibility (Trigg & Kondrachine, 1998). It calls on countries with malaria to develop specific programs that refer to the technical elements of the global strategy, but are informed by local considerations, while the international community provides technical and financial support.

There is no specific treatment for dengue fever or dengue hemorrhagic fever beyond attentive clinical management, and there are no vaccines currently available against dengue group viruses, although a number of groups are working to develop them. Because of concerns that vaccine-induced antibody against fewer than all four serotypes could promote the development of dengue hemorrhagic fever, it is generally believed that only a vaccine that protects against all four serotypes can be safely developed, tested, and given to populations at risk. Thus the control and prevention of dengue fever currently depends on mosquito control, disease surveillance, and epidemic preparedness. Vector control measures targeting the mosquito vector of dengue (and yellow fever) use the same tools (for example, residual pesticides) as control measures targeting the mosquito vector of malaria and may provide cross-protection in areas at risk for multiple mosquito-borne diseases.

Immunization is the most important prevention measure against yellow fever. The current formulation of the yellow fever vaccine, designated 17D, is safe, effective, and relatively inexpensive at 12–25 U.S. cents per dose (Vainio & Cutts, 1998). To prevent and control yellow fever in endemic areas, WHO recommends routine infant immunization against yellow fever (within the EPI), mass immunization campaigns (for example, preventive catch-up campaigns), vigilant case and vector surveillance, reactive immunization to contain outbreaks, and careful management of the vaccine supply ("Yellow Fever Technical Consensus Meeting," 1998).

No drugs are available for the treatment of chronic American trypanosomiasis, while drugs used in the treatment of acute manifestations (benznidazole and nifurtimox) are expensive and toxic. Thus the prevention and control of American trypanosomiasis is currently focused on interrupting vectorial transmission in addition to preventing transmission via the transfusion of units of infected blood. Vector control efforts are centered on eradicating strictly domestic triatomine bugs and controlling domestic infestations of other (sylvatic) triatomine bugs predominantly through indoor residual insecticide spraying in areas at high risk for American trypanosomiasis. The prevention of transfusion-related transmission is accomplished by screening all blood donors for *T. cruzi* antibodies and rejecting infected blood. The results of these efforts have been encouraging thus far—the prevalence of *T. cruzi* infection in children and young adults has been reduced by 75–96% in countries that have implemented these control strategies (Argentina, Brazil, Chile, and Uruguay) (UNDP, 1997). Similar results can be expected elsewhere once these strategies have been more widely deployed.

The current strategy for the control and prevention of African trypanosomiasis associated with *T.b. gambiense* involves active case-finding and early treatment, which reduces the human reservoir by curing the infection. Passive surveillance for *T.b. gambiense* is unsatisfactory because infected individuals are often infectious for months to years before developing symptoms that lead to (passive) detection. However, passive surveillance and epidemic preparedness are often adequate to control the transmission of *T.b. rhodesiense*, which quickly leads to symptoms of infection.

## Obstacles to Prevention and Control and Directions for Future Research

Insecticide resistance presents a major challenge to prevention strategies based on vector control. Vectors for malaria, dengue, and yellow fever have all developed resistance to multiple insecticides including the classic insecticides (for example, DDT) and their replacements (for example, organophosphates). Alternative insecticides have been developed, but are often more costly and more toxic than the first-line agents. The dynamic ecology of vector-borne pathogens is an additional barrier to effective vector control. For example, changing land-use patterns, shifting weather patterns, urbanization, and population movements may result in new foci for disease transmission. Finally, national and international travel and commerce represent continuing opportunities for reinfestation, necessitating continuous surveillance even in areas with good vector control.

Drug resistance is a serious problem for control strategies that rely on chemotherapy to treat disease and reduce the human reservoir. Nowhere is this problem more evident than in the management of malaria. Drugs that once provided cheap and effective means of antimalarial prophylaxis and therapy are now severely compromised in many parts of the world, necessitating the use of more expensive alternative drugs. The situation is most serious in parts of Southeast Asia where multidrug resistance has been observed (Krogstad, 1996). Factors that promote drug resistance include mass chemoprophylaxis and treatment with suboptimal doses of drug.

Additional barriers to the prevention and control of arthropod-borne diseases include the intermittent disruption of public health services as a consequence of civil disturbance or war and the ever-present problem of limited resources. Other problems include the difficulty of sustaining support for successful control measures (for example, indoor insecticide spraying to control the vectorial spread of American trypanosomiasis) once the disease has been brought under control (and thus is no longer a public health priority).

Future prospects for the improved prevention of arthropod-borne disease rest primarily on vaccine development. Current research is focused on developing candidate quadrivalent dengue fever vaccines and antimalarial vaccines. Molecular technology offers additional possibilities for vector control based on genetic manipulation of the vector populations (for example, introducing Plasmodium-inhibiting genes into the *Anopheles* mosquito population) (Collins & Paskewitz, 1995).

## HELMINTHIASES

### Overview

It is estimated that more than one-third of the world's population is infected with parasitic helminths (Warren et al., 1993). The vast majority of infected individuals live in low- and middle-income countries where environmental sanitation is poor. Each parasite produces different manifestations according to the site, intensity, and length of infection. Host response also influences the clinical course of infection. In general, children experience the heaviest worm burden, and persistent infection throughout childhood is common in low- and middle-income settings. Heavy, prolonged infection produces adverse effects on growth and development, and sig-

nificantly increases childhood morbidity. In adults, helminthiases can produce acute and chronic morbidity leading to impaired productivity, chronic disability, and reduced quality of life.

In terms of global prevalence, morbidity, and mortality, the most important helminthic infections are schistosomiasis (200 million cases) ("Control of Schistosomiasis," 1993), ascariasis (1,273 million cases), trichuriasis (902 million cases), hookworm (1,277 million cases) (Chan, 1997), onchocerciasis, and lymphatic filariasis. Although many of these infections are minimally symptomatic, the number of clinically significant cases is substantial. This section focuses on schistosomiasis and the most common intestinal helminthiases (ascariasis, trichuriasis, and hookworm). Dracunculiasis, a disease of considerable historical importance, is also considered.

### Etiologic Agents and Clinical Features

Human schistosomiasis (also known as bilharziasis) is caused by a group of blood trematodes (flukes) known as schistosomes. The three main species that infect humans are *Schistosoma mansoni*, *S. japonicum*, and *S. haematobium*. Two other species, *S. mekongi* and *S. intercalatum*, also parasitize humans, but such infections are uncommon and will not be discussed further. Acute schistosomiasis (Katayama fever) is characterized by fever and chills, abdominal pain, diarrhea, and enlargement of the spleen or other organs. *S. japonicum* is most commonly associated with acute disease, although any type of schistosomiasis can cause these symptoms. Chronic disease is initiated by the deposition of schistosome eggs in the body, which induces inflammation and scarring. Chronic infection with *S. mansoni* or *S. japonicum* can lead to hepatosplenic and intestinal involvement, although most infected individuals are asymptomatic. Chronic infection with *S. haematobium* is associated with urinary tract disease and a much higher proportion (50–70%) of infected individuals are symptomatic ("Control of Schistosomiasis," 1993). *S. haematobium* infection is also associated with an increased risk for bladder cancer.

The most common intestinal helminthiases of humans are caused by *Ascaris lumbricoides*, *Trichuris trichiura* (whipworm), and two species of hookworm, *Ancylostoma duodenale* and *Necator americanus*. These parasites produce a diverse range of clinical symptoms, although light infections are generally asymptomatic. When worm burdens are heavy, *A. lumbricoides* infection is associated with malnutrition and stunted growth. *A. lumbricoides* is also the largest of the intestinal helminths, measuring 15 to 35 centimeters in length; thus single worms can cause obstruction and inflammation of the appendix, bile duct, or pancreatic duct, while a bolus of worms can cause intestinal obstruction leading to death. Trichuriasis is associated with abdominal pain, diarrhea, and general malaise when moderate worm loads are present, while nutritional deficiencies, anemia, and stunted growth can result from heavier worm loads. Hookworms attach to the intestinal mucosa where they ingest 0.03–0.26 milliliters of blood per worm per day (Warren et al., 1993). Thus the major clinical manifestations of hookworm infection are iron deficiency anemia and hypoalbuminemia resulting from chronic blood loss.

Dracunculiasis is caused by *Dracunculus medinensis* (Guinea worm), a long (60–90 centimeters), thin nematode. Symptoms of the disease are caused by the migration of the worm to the subcutaneous tissues and its eruption through the skin. Symptoms can include the formation of a blister or bleb at the site where the worm will emerge (usually the ankle or foot), hives, nausea, vomiting, diarrhea, and asthma. The blister ulcerates as the worm emerges, and local pain typically persists until the worm is expelled or extracted, which can take several weeks. Secondary infection of the worm tract is common. Severe disability generally lasting one to three months occurs in most of those infected, and permanent disability occurs in 0.5% of infected

individuals (Hunter, 1996). Even the short-term disability can have a substantial economic impact, because the worm typically emerges during the months when important agricultural work is performed (Hopkins, 1984).

## Descriptive Epidemiologic Features and Risk Factors

Schistosomiasis is the single most important helminthic disease and the second most important parasitic disease (after malaria) worldwide. At present, an estimated 200 million persons in 74 countries and territories harbor this infection, yielding 20 million cases of severe disease and approximately 100 million symptomatic infections ("Control of Schistosomiasis," 1993). *S. mansoni*, the most widespread of the schistosomes, is found in parts of Africa, the Middle East, the Caribbean, and South America; *S. haematobium* is restricted to Africa and the Middle East; and *S. japonicum* is currently found only in the Western Pacific countries. Overall, the vast majority of schistosome infections occur in sub-Saharan Africa.

The life cycle of the schistosome is quite complex, and a complete description is beyond the scope of this chapter, but a brief treatment is necessary. Adult worms live, mate, and deposit their eggs in the blood vessels lining the human intestines (*S. mansoni* and *S. japonicum*) or bladder (*S. haematobium*). These eggs migrate into the intestine or bladder and are passed out in the excreta. When deposited in fresh water, the eggs develop into immature parasites (miracidia) that infect fresh-water snails. The immature parasites then develop into infective larvae (cercariae). When released into the surrounding water, the larvae swim about, and those coming in contact with humans during this time penetrate through the skin and eventually reach the vascular system, completing the cycle. Thus the maintenance of schistosomes in a given area requires the presence of the intermediate host, the contamination of water with egg-laden excreta, and the exposure of humans to contaminated water. Because schistosomes do not multiply in the human host, the intensity of infection is largely determined by the rate at which new worms are acquired. Studies have shown that the infection rate for schistosomes typically peaks during childhood and then declines with advancing age (Butterworth, Dunne, Fulford, Ouma, & Sturrock, 1996; Hagan, 1996). This finding is thought to reflect age-dependent changes in both water exposure and immunity to infection.

The public health impact of intestinal helminthiases on low- and middle-income countries is substantial. As noted above, *A. lumbricoides*, *T. trichiura*, and hookworm each infects about 1 billion individuals globally (Chan, 1997). Although the morbidity and mortality associated with intestinal helminthiases is relatively low, the burden of illness and, to a lesser extent, death is considerable due to the extremely high prevalence of these infections (Bundy, 1990).

*A. lumbricoides*, *T. trichiura*, and hookworm share a relatively simple life cycle. The parasites mature and mate in the human intestines and produce eggs that are passed out in the feces. When deposited on moist soil, the eggs develop into the infective form of the parasite. (Because this part of the life cycle is spent in soil, these worms are collectively referred to as geohelminths.) Humans acquire the parasite when contaminated soil is ingested or, in the case of hookworm, when the infective larvae in the soil penetrate exposed skin. Thus the maintenance of these helminths requires the deposition of feces in soil and the exposure of humans to that soil. For *A. lumbricoides* and *T. trichiura* the peak intensity of infection typically occurs among young children, whereas for hookworm the peak occurs among adults (Bundy, Hall, Medley, & Savioli, 1992).

Dracunculiasis is contracted by drinking contaminated water. Parasitic larvae then migrate to the abdominal cavity where they mature into adult worms over the course of a year. After copulation, the gravid female worm migrates through the body to the subcutaneous tissue and then secretes irritants that ulcerate the skin and expose the worm. When the affected body site is immersed in water, the worm expels clouds of larvae. The larvae are consumed by copepods (minute fresh-water crustaceans, also known as water fleas), which are in turn ingested by humans who drink contaminated water. Dracunculiasis occurs in individuals of all ages, but is less common in very young children, possibly because breastfeeding reduces water consumption (Hunter, 1996).

The global campaign to eradicate dracunculiasis was launched in the 1980s as a part of the United Nations International Drinking Water Supply and Sanitation Decade (1981–1990). Since then the incidence of dracunculiasis has declined from 4 million cases per year in 1981 (Hopkins, Ruiz-Tiben, & Ruebush, 1997) to fewer than 80,000 reported cases in 1997 ("Dracunculiasis," 1998), and local eradication has occurred in many previously endemic countries. Following the eradication of the parasite in Yemen, endemic disease will be limited to Africa ("Dracunculiasis," 1998). Global eradication is considered an achievable and worthwhile goal.

In general, the degree of morbidity and mortality produced by helminthic infection is related to the intensity of infection, which varies considerably from person to person within endemic areas. Typically, a few individuals have heavy infections and experience serious clinical consequences, whereas most individuals have lighter infections and experience fewer symptoms. For example, it is estimated that 15–30% of the people carry 70% of the worm burden (Bundy et al., 1992). In addition to the clinical consequences, these individuals are usually the principal source of infection to the community (Bundy et al., 1992).

## Current Approaches to Prevention and Control

The major strategies for the control of helminthic infections are environmental sanitation and health education, chemotherapy, and control of the intermediate host. No antihelminthic vaccines are currently available.

Most helminthiases are diseases of poor sanitation. Providing for the sanitary disposal of excreta prevents the contamination of soil and water, and thus breaks the chain of transmission. However, environmental improvements must be made at the community level in order to be effective (Warren et al., 1993). Improvements in environmental sanitation are also achieved and sustained by health education to promote healthy behaviors; for example, WHO has determined that schistosomiasis could be largely prevented by eliminating indiscriminate urination and defecation and increasing compliance with medical interventions ("Control of Schistosomiasis," 1993).

Safe, effective, and relatively inexpensive oral treatments are available for many helminthiases. For schistosomiasis, praziquantel is the drug of choice. A single oral dose is well-tolerated, relatively inexpensive (30–40 U.S. cents), has an initial cure rate of 60–90%, and is effective against all species of *Schistosoma* ("Control of Schistosomiasis," 1993). Chemotherapeutic agents that act against common intestinal helminthiases are also available. For example, both albendazole and mebendazole have moderate to very good activity against five of the most common species of intestinal helminth (*A. lumbricoides*, *T. trichiura*, hookworms, *Strongyloides stercoralis*, and *Enterobius vermicularis*) ("Prevention and Control of Intestinal Parasitic Infections," 1987). These drugs are administered orally, well-tolerated, and inexpensive (for example, 10 U.S. cents per dose of mebendazole).

Selectively treating the most heavily infected individuals (often school-aged children) is usually advantageous ("Prevention and Control of Intestinal Parasitic Infections," 1987), although mass chemotherapy or a combination of strategies may be more appropriate under some circumstances. WHO recommends that strategies for the deployment of chemotherapeutic interventions be decided on a case-by-case basis according to the prevalence, intensity, and distribution of local helminthic infections, the availability of laboratory facilities, and the level of community cooperation. In addition, because the geographical distributions of the common helminthiases have considerable areas of overlap, strategies that target multiple species are desirable.

Control of the intermediate host species for certain helminths (for example, snail control for schistosomiasis) can play an important role in preventing transmission. The primary strategies for snail control include application of molluscicidal agents and environmental management. Biological control strategies, such as the introduction of competitor-snails, have not been successful and are not currently recommended ("Control of Schistosomiasis," 1993). Control of the intermediate host also plays a crucial role in preventing the transmission of dracunculiasis. Much of the success of the eradication campaign has been achieved by teaching people to pour drinking water through a finely woven cloth to filter out the tiny crustaceans that carry the *Dracunculus* parasite. Chemical eradicants have also played a role.

### Obstacles to Prevention and Control and Directions for Future Research

Major obstacles to the effective implementation of chemotherapy-based interventions are related to the logistical and financial difficulties of treating the large number of individuals in need. In addition, chemotherapy is not adequate to redress the conditions that led to the primary infection, thus posttreatment reinfection is likely to occur, necessitating repeated treatments and further cost. Resistance to the antihelminthic agents has not yet been observed in human infection; however, resistance to benzimidazoles occurs in veterinary practice, which suggests that chemotherapy-based control strategies should include provisions for detecting and, if necessary, managing emergent drug resistance.

Adequate environmental sanitation is generally viewed as the only long-term solution to the control of intestinal helminthiases and schistosomiasis. However, the provision of safe drinking water and adequate disposal facilities in low- and middle-income areas has proved to be an extremely difficult, costly, and lengthy process. At this time, control strategies must include chemotherapeutic interventions and/or vector control to relieve the immediate burden of disease while preserving universal sanitation as the long-term goal.

## ZOONOSES

### Overview

Zoonoses are defined as diseases and infections naturally transmitted between vertebrate animals and humans. Zoonotic agents include a wide variety of bacteria, viruses, protozoa, and helminths, while their nonhuman hosts include wild animals, food and draft animals, and domestic pets.

More than 200 different zoonoses are currently recognized (Hart, Trees, & Duerden, 1997). Zoonotic infections have a worldwide distribution and collectively produce significant morbidity and mortality. For example, indigenous rabies, which has a global distribution, causes an estimated 35,000–50,000 deaths per year ("World Survey of Rabies 32," 1997). *Yersinia pestis*, the bacterium that causes plague, remains enzoonotic in many parts of Africa, Asia, and South America, and in the southwestern United States. Although only 3,017 cases of human plague were reported to WHO in 1996 ("Human Plague," 1998), the control of human plague remains a public health priority because of its epidemic potential and relatively high case-fatality ratio. In low- and middle-income settings, important zoonoses include rabies, plague, anthrax, leptospirosis, leishmaniasis, African trypanosomiasis, and a number of hemorrhagic fever viruses. Food-borne zoonoses, such as salmonellosis, campylobacteriosis, and certain *E. coli* infections, also contribute to the global burden of disease, while occupational zoonoses such as brucellosis, echinococcosis, and Q fever have regional significance.

Although zoonoses have a worldwide distribution, low- and middle-income countries bear a greater burden of disease than industrialized countries. This divergence reflects, in part, differences in opportunities for exposure to zoonotic pathogens. Residents of low- and middle-income countries typically experience more frequent and more intimate contact with animals, and often live in situations of suboptimal environmental sanitation (which promotes exposure to infective material such as contaminated animal excreta). In addition, many control measures that are readily available in industrialized countries (for example, mass veterinary vaccination of domesticated animals) may not be available or affordable in low- and middle-income countries.

There are five major routes by which zoonotic pathogens are transmitted to humans:

1. *inhalation:* transmission that occurs when infective materials are aerosolized and inhaled
2. *ingestion:* transmission that occurs when humans consume contaminated meat, milk, or blood from infected animals or when foodstuffs (for example, fruits and vegetables), drinking water, or hands are contaminated with infective materials, which are then ingested
3. *nontraumatic contact:* transmission that typically occurs when pathogens enter through the skin (or mucosal surfaces or conjunctivae) as a result of direct or indirect contact with animal hides, hair, excreta, blood, or carcasses
4. *traumatic contact:* transmission via animal bites or scratches
5. *arthropod:* transmission by biting arthropods that feed on animals and humans

For some zoonoses, humans are an incidental, "dead-end" host. Human-to-human transmission of rabies or anthrax, for example, is extremely rare. For others zoonoses, humans may serve as a reservoir for infection, transmitting pathogens to other humans or even back to animals.

Zoonoses produce a wide variety of diseases with distinct clinical and epidemiologic characteristics, and are associated with many different animals occupying a number of ecologic niches, both urban and rural. Approaches to the control and prevention of zoonoses must necessarily reflect these differences. General principles, however, often include good animal husbandry (including vaccination when appropriate), environmental sanitation, vector control, and the control or elimination of animal reservoirs (for example, rats or other wild animals).

Rather than attempting to survey the entire range of zoonoses, this section is limited to a detailed discussion of rabies and leptospirosis, which are important zoonoses in many low- and middle-income countries.

### Etiologic Agents and Clinical Features

Rabies is caused by the rabies virus, which is a Lyssavirus belonging to the Rhabidoviridae family. Typically transmitted by the bite of a rabid animal, human rabies is an acute, uniformly fatal encephalitic disease. Following inoculation, there is an asymptomatic incubation period typically lasting 1–3 months, although periods as short as a few days and as long as several years have been reported (Fishbein, 1991). (Postexposure prophylaxis must be initiated during this period in order to have an effect.) The prodromal period begins with the early signs of disease, which include nonspecific symptoms (for example, fever and malaise) and abnormal sensations near the site of inoculation. This stage is followed by a 2- to 10-day period of acute neurologic dysfunction that manifests as furious rabies in about 80% of cases and paralytic (dumb) rabies in the remainder (Fishbein, 1991). Furious rabies is characterized by periods of extreme agitation and hyperactivity interspersed with periods of normalcy. Hydrophobia, aerophobia, combativeness, and hallucination may also occur. Features of paralytic rabies include paresthesia, weakness, and paralysis. The inevitable final stage of rabies (furious and paralytic) is coma followed by death.

Leptospirosis is an acute, febrile disease caused by pathogenic bacteria of the genus *Lep-*

*tospira*. The clinical course of the disease is variable, ranging from subclinical infection to severe disease involving the kidneys and liver (Weil's disease). At present, 23 *Leptospira* serogroups containing more than 212 serovars are recognized (Ellis, 1998). The case-fatality ratio among those infected with serovars that cause severe disease ranges from 5–40%, whereas infections with serovars that cause mild disease are rarely fatal (Ellis, 1998).

### Descriptive Epidemiologic Features and Risk Factors

Rabies is a disease of animals; humans are incidentally infected and only rarely transmit the virus. Animal reservoirs include dogs, cats, and wild animals (notably foxes, skunks, wolves, raccoons, mongooses, and bats). More than 99% of all human rabies cases are acquired from dogs (WHO Expert Committee on Rabies, 1992), which are the major source of human infection in low- and middle-income countries. In industrialized countries, where immunization of domestic animals is common, wild animals constitute the principal reservoir of infection and human rabies is extremely rare. Rabies virus is present in the saliva of infected animals and is typically transmitted to humans by the bite of a rabid animal. It may also be transmitted when intact mucous membranes are exposed to infective saliva. Not every exposure results in infection, but, if infection occurs, it is fatal in the absence of postexposure prophylaxis.

Leptospirosis has a worldwide distribution, but its global incidence is difficult to assess. In general, the incidence and prevalence of infection are low in industrialized countries and higher in low- and middle-income countries (for example, prevalences of infection ranging from 18% to 48% have been reported in some low- and middle-income communities) (Ellis, 1998). As with rabies, human infection with *Leptospira* is incidental, and humans do not contribute to the transmission of the bacteria. The main animal reservoirs for *Leptospira* serovars that cause human disease are rats, dogs, pigs, and cattle. Transmission of leptospires to humans typically occurs through contact with water contaminated with the urine of infected animals or through direct contact with infective animal urine. The bacteria infect humans by entering through broken skin, water-softened intact skin, mucosal surfaces, or conjunctivae. Human leptospirosis is traditionally considered an occupational disease among those whose professions involve contact with host animals (for example, dairy farmers) or water (for example, rice farmers). However, home and recreational exposures appear to be increasingly important, particularly in low- and middle-income settings. In addition, periodic flooding due to heavy rains can produce large epidemics of leptospirosis.

## Current Approaches to Prevention and Control

The control of human rabies is achieved by the prevention of human exposure to the virus and the prevention of disease through postexposure prophylaxis when exposure does occur. At present, there are no rabies vaccines suitable (that is, sufficiently inexpensive, safe, and effective) for mass pre-exposure immunization of humans.

The prevention of human exposure to rabies in low- and middle-income countries primarily depends on the control of dog rabies, which can be achieved through the widespread use of the parenteral dog rabies vaccine. The mass vaccination of owned dogs and the elimination of stray or feral dogs has proved successful in many countries. For example, in the United States, the incidence of human rabies cases was reduced from 0.03 per 100,000 per year in 1945 to less than 0.001 per 100,000 per year in the 1980s following the widespread control of dog rabies (Fishbein, 1991).

The prevention of human disease when exposure to rabies virus has occurred depends on good local wound care (for example, flushing with soap and water) and postexposure prophy-laxis, which entails passive immunization with immunoglobulin and active immunization with rabies vaccine. The complete postexposure regimen almost always prevents disease; however, the regimen must be delivered during the incubation period because neither immunization nor other treatments alter the fatal course of disease once symptoms develop.

The prevention of human leptospirosis depends on interrupting the transmission of leptospires to humans. Preventative measures include the vaccination of certain host animals (for example, cattle) or the elimination of others (for example, rats). Environmental control strategies aimed at reducing hazards such as stagnant bodies of water or the periodic flooding of residential areas, as well as educational campaigns aimed at decreasing unnecessary water exposures, may contribute to prevention efforts. Occupational improvements that curtail contact with host animals or contaminated water are also desirable. Morbidity and mortality can be lessened by the prompt administration of appropriate antibiotic therapy, which has been shown to shorten the duration and severity of human leptospirosis.

## Obstacles to Prevention and Control and Directions for Future Research

The major obstacle to the improved control of rabies is the difficulty of achieving adequate vaccine coverage of dog populations in low- and middle-income countries. WHO estimates that 75% coverage is necessary for effective control (WHO Expert Committee on Rabies, 1992). Ensuring the delivery of the parenteral vaccine to stray and feral dogs (or eliminating these dogs altogether) is especially problematic. With sustained effort, WHO considers the global elimination of urban (dog) rabies to be an attainable goal.

The future control of leptospirosis is less promising. Animal vaccination may not be economically feasible for many farmers, and vaccines are not available or appropriate for every host species. The elimination of wildlife hosts (for example, rats) is usually not feasible. Improvements in working and living conditions to reduce contact with animals and their excreta are desirable (for many reasons) but difficult to achieve in low- and middle-income settings. Until these difficulties are overcome, the control of leptospirosis must rely on health education to reduce risky behavior, veterinary education to promote good animal husbandry, and medical education to ensure the prompt diagnosis and treatment of leptospirosis.

## VIRAL HEMORRHAGIC FEVERS

### Overview

The viruses that cause hemorrhagic fever (HF) belong to four different families (see Table 4–3), and the illnesses they produce have distinct epidemiologic features. Despite their differences, these viruses produce a common clinical picture that is characterized by fever and hemorrhage, as the name suggests. Hemorrhagic manifestations can include petechiae, ecchymoses, bleeding gums, nosebleeds, vaginal bleeding, and bleeding from other mucosal surfaces, producing bloody urine, stool, and vomit. Complications can include cardiovascular and neurologic disturbances, shock, and death.

The spectrum of disease typically associated with each type of virus varies substantially. For example, Lassa virus infections result in inapparent or mild clinical symptoms in many people but cause severe life-threatening disease in others. Infections with Ebola virus and Marburg virus, on the other hand, appear to cause severe disease in virtually all those infected. The severity of the clinical illness that results from infection also varies according to differences in host response, viral virulence factors, and dose.

Infection with the HF viruses is, in general, relatively rare (Lassa virus is a notable exception). Although outbreaks are dramatic and lead to major responses on the part of public health

and other officials, HF virus infections do not have the same public health impact in terms of morbidity and mortality as the infectious diseases that more commonly afflict the peoples of most low- and middle-income countries ("Viral Haemorrhagic Fevers," 1985). However, because most HF viruses are extremely virulent and capable of epidemic spread, developing strategies to control these viruses is a public health priority. In addition, some of the viruses, such as the South American HF viruses, pose regional public health hazards within their areas of endemicity.

All HF viruses are thought to be zoonotic. These viruses are proven or suspected to be transmitted from animals to humans by an arthropod vector (for example, ticks or mosquitoes) or by direct or indirect contact with the animal reservoir (for example, rodents) of the virus (see Table 4–3). In endemic areas, the temporal distribution of many viral HFs follows seasonal changes in the activity and density of the vector or animal reservoir, or seasonal changes in human activity. The age and sex distributions of infection and disease caused by some HF viruses reflect differences in exposure to the vector or reservoir, while other viruses affect persons of all ages and both sexes.

Several of the HFs have only recently been recognized and had their agents characterized. For example, the South American HFs, Ebola HF, and Marburg HF appear to have emerged in just the past 50 years, presumably as a result of increased human activity or settlement in areas where viruses circulate among their known or presumed zoonotic hosts. In some instances, such as with Argentine HF, the geographic range of the virus has expanded beyond its initial focus (and continues to spread) (Vainrub & Salas, 1994). The development of control and prevention strategies for newly emerging infections can pose special difficulties as investigators have not had time to conduct the research needed to formulate treatment modalities, vaccines, vector-control strategies, and other preventative measures.

**Table 4–3** Distribution and Modes of Transmission of Viral Hemorrhagic Fevers

| Family Genus Virus | Disease | Principal Means of Transmission | Principal Locations |
|---|---|---|---|
| **Flaviviridae** | | | |
| *Flavivirus* | | | |
| Dengue | Dengue HF | Mosquito | Asia, Latin America |
| Yellow fever | Yellow fever | Mosquito | Sub-Saharan Africa, South America |
| Kyasanur Forest disease | Kyasanur Forest disease | Tick | India |
| Omsk HF | Omsk HF | Tick, Muskrat | Russia |
| **Arenaviridae** | | | |
| *Arenavirus* | | | |
| Lassa | Lassa fever | Rodent, Person-to-Person | West Africa |
| Junin | Argentine HF | Rodent | Argentina |
| Machupo | Bolivian HF | Rodent | Bolivia |
| Guanarito | Venezuelan HF | Rodent | Venezuela |
| Sabio | Brazilian HF | Unknown | Brazil |
| **Bunyaviridae** | | | |
| *Phlebovirus* | | | |
| Rift valley fever | Rift valley fever | Mosquito | Africa |
| *Nairovirus* | | | |
| Crimean-Congo HF | Crimean-Congo HF | Tick, Person-to-Person | Africa, Asia, eastern Europe, Middle East |
| *Hantavirus* | | | |
| Hantaan, Seoul, *Filoviridae* and others | HF with renal syndrome | Rodent | Asia, Europe |
| *Filovirus* | | | |
| Marburg | Marburg HF | Person-to-Person | Africa |
| Ebola | Ebola HF | Person-to-Person | Africa |

*Note:* HF = hemorrhagic fever.

## Etiologic Agents and Clinical Features

There are at least 14 different HF viruses (see Table 4–3). However, the public health significance of each virus differs substantially. The most prominent (in terms of annual incidence of disease) are Lassa virus, yellow fever virus, and dengue group viruses. The latter two viruses are discussed in the section on arthropod-borne diseases. Ebola virus and Marburg virus are notable for their epidemic potential and extraordinarily high case-fatality ratios, whereas the South American HFs caused by Junin, Machupo, and Guanarito viruses have regional public health importance. Detailed discussion of the remaining HF viruses is beyond the scope of this work.

## Descriptive Epidemiologic Features and Risk Factors

Ebola HF emerged in 1976 when concurrent epidemics occurred in the Democratic Republic of Congo (formerly Zaire) and Sudan. These outbreaks were caused by distinct subtypes of the virus and were characterized by high case-fatality ratios (88% in the Democratic Republic of Congo and 53% in Sudan). In total, 602 persons were infected and 431 died in the two outbreaks. Sudan experienced a second, smaller outbreak in 1979, and Gabon experienced three small outbreaks (each involving 60 or fewer cases) in the 1990s. A large outbreak occurred in Kikwit, the Democratic Republic of Congo, in 1995 and resulted in 315 cases and 244 deaths, for a case-fatality ratio of 77%. The first recognized outbreak of Marburg HF occurred in Marburg, Germany, among laboratory workers (and their contacts) who acquired the infection from monkeys imported from Uganda. Since then, three cases have been reported in South Africa (although the index case was probably exposed in Zimbabwe), and three additional cases have been reported in Kenya. The case-fatality ratio for all cases of Marburg HF reported to date is 26% (38 cases, 10 deaths).

Epidemics of Ebola HF have been sustained by person-to-person transmission through direct physical contact with infected persons or corpses (or with their bodily fluids or tissues) and the use of unsterile needles for medical injections. Person-to-person transmission is not very efficient, with secondary attack rates of 16% in household contacts (Dowell et al., 1999). Marburg virus is also transmitted by person-to-person contact. Fortunately, airborne transmission does not appear to be important for either virus. The ecologic niches of these viruses remain unknown and zoonotic vectors and reservoirs have not been identified.

Lassa virus is widely distributed across West Africa, where it causes substantial morbidity and mortality. Although its precise incidence is unknown, it is estimated that as many as 100,000 to 300,000 new infections occur each year, with an overall case-fatality ratio of about 1–2% (McCormick, Webb, Krebs, Johnson, & Smith, 1987). Fetal death and permanent deafness are common complications (Cummins et al., 1990; Monson et al., 1987). Lassa virus is

maintained in a rodent reservoir that is commonly found in the home. Virus is shed in rodent urine and droppings, and rodent-to-human transmission is believed to occur by aerosolization or ingestion of rodent excreta or by inoculation through broken skin. Rodent-to-human transmission may also occur when infected rodents are consumed as food (Ter Meulen et al., 1996). Person-to-person transmission occurs in community and hospital settings, and contributes substantially to epidemics of Lassa fever. This mode of transmission requires direct contact with infected persons. Person-to-person airborne transmission occurs rarely, if ever.

Argentine HF, which is caused by Junin virus, was first described in 1955 in agricultural workers in the Argentine pampas. Several hundred cases of Argentine HF occur each year in large, primarily agricultural regions of the pampas. The region of endemicity is expanding, and is now nearly 10 times larger than its initial compass (Vainrub & Salas, 1994). Bolivian HF, which is caused by Machupo virus, was subsequently described in northeastern Bolivia, which is the only known endemic area. Outbreaks of Bolivian HF occurred in the 1960s and early 1970s, including large epidemics that affected hundreds of individuals. Although no cases were reported from 1976 to 1992, a small outbreak in 1994 and recent sporadic cases have marked its reemergence ("Re-emergence of Bolivian Hemorrhagic Fever," 1994). Venezuelan HF, which is caused by Guanarito virus, was first recognized in 1989. During the period September 1989 to January 1997, 165 cases were reported within the small region of central Venezuela where Guanarito virus is endemic (De Manzione et al., 1998). For infections caused by all three of these viruses, the case-fatality ratio is in the range of 15–33% (De Manzione et al., 1998; Doyle, Bryan, & Peters, 1998).

Each of the three South American HF viruses is associated with a rodent reservoir that maintains the virus in the wild. As with Lassa fever, rodent-to-human transmission occurs by the aerosolization or ingestion of virus-laden rodent excreta or by inoculation through broken skin.

The rodent that carries Junin virus typically dwells in agricultural fields, whereas the rodent that carries Machupo virus readily enters the home. Rodent-control strategies must take such differences into account. Person-to-person transmission of Junin, Machupo, and Guanarito viruses is considered rare and nosocomial outbreaks are uncommon.

## Current Approaches to Prevention and Control

Recent field trials have demonstrated that a live, attenuated Junin virus vaccine is safe and provides effective protection against Argentine HF (Maiztegui et al., 1998), and may provide cross-protection against Bolivian HF as well. Vaccines are not available for Lassa fever, Ebola HF, or Marburg HF. In the absence of vaccines, reducing the morbidity and mortality caused by HF viruses depends upon preventing primary transmission by limiting exposures to virus reservoirs and vectors and controlling secondary transmission (for example, person-to-person transmission in the hospital, household, or community setting) through patient isolation and barrier nursing. In addition, the use of antiviral drugs or convalescent serum is effective in some instances.

Strategies to limit viral exposures are determined by the unique characteristics of the associated animal reservoir or vector and the distinct ways in which each of the viruses is transmitted. For example, the rodent that carries Machupo virus is frequently found in and around the home, and aggressive rodent eradication measures through trapping and poisoning appear to have been quite successful in controlling Bolivian HF (Kilgore et al., 1995). Conversely, the rodent reservoir of Junin virus lives in crop fields, where trapping and poisoning are difficult, necessitating the development of alternative rodent abatement strategies. Eradication (or even control) of the rodent reservoir of Lassa virus in West Africa is not considered feasible due to the density and wide distribution of the rodent that carries the virus. Preventing the primary transmission of Lassa virus has instead relied upon educating at-risk communities about ways to reduce opportunities for exposure, such as never leaving food items uncovered and never consuming rodents as food. The development of control strategies for Ebola virus and Marburg virus awaits identification of the reservoir(s) and vector(s).

Historically, nosocomial and person-to-person transmission of Lassa fever, Ebola HF, and Marburg HF has contributed significantly to devastating outbreaks of these diseases. (The South American HF viruses are rarely transmitted by these routes.) Field experience indicates that epidemic control is readily achieved through simple barrier nursing techniques (for example, wearing gloves, gowns, and masks; sterilizing equipment; and isolating patients), and epidemiologic studies support this conclusion. For example, serologic studies in Sierra Leone found that hospital personnel who used barrier techniques when caring for Lassa fever patients had no greater risk of infection than the local population (Helmick, Webb, Scribner, Krebs, & McCormick, 1986).

At present, few specific treatments are available for the viral HFs. Ribavirin (an antiviral drug) is effective in the treatment of Lassa fever (McCormick et al., 1986). Laboratory data suggest that ribavirin may also prove effective in treating South American HFs, although supporting clinical data are incomplete (Doyle et al., 1998). Ribavirin is unlikely to be beneficial in treating Ebola HF or Marburg HF. Convalescent serum is useful in the treatment of Argentine HF ("Viral Haemorrhagic Fevers," 1985), but donors are not plentiful. Unfortunately, most people in low- and middle-income countries are not able to afford these therapies.

## Obstacles to Prevention and Control and Directions for Future Research

The major obstacle to containing outbreaks of viral HFs (especially Ebola HF, Marburg HF, and Lassa fever) is inadequate disease surveillance, which results in delayed response and increased opportunity for epidemic spread. In many low- and middle-income countries, disease surveillance is impeded by the difficulty of making an early differential diagnosis in areas where illnesses with similar initial manifestations (for example, malaria, influenza, typhoid fever, leptospirosis, meningococcemia, and hepatitis) are prevalent. The lack of ready access to diagnostic laboratories exacerbates this difficulty. In addition, because epidemics are unpredictable in time and place, surveillance efforts are difficult to maintain. Other obstacles to the control and prevention of viral HFs include the costliness of sustaining readiness for infection-control measures (for example, maintaining supplies for barrier nursing), lack of information about the vector(s) and reservoir(s) of Ebola and Marburg viruses, the difficulties of developing and maintaining vector- and rodent-control programs, and the limited availability of ribavirin (especially for the treatment of Lassa fever).

## INFECTIOUS CAUSES OF BLINDNESS

### Overview

Severely decreased visual acuity or complete blindness is profoundly disabling in any setting, but perhaps even more so in low- and middle-income countries. Among the known causes of blindness, two infectious agents play important etiologic roles in selected regions of the world: *C. trachomatis*, the cause of trachoma, and *Onchocerca volvulus*, the cause of onchocerciasis, also known as river blindness.

### Trachoma

#### Etiologic Agents

*C. trachomatis* is a small bacterium that lives within selected types of human cells and is difficult to grow in the laboratory. Whereas *C. trachomatis* is also the cause of STIs (see above), different immunotypes of the bacterium cause trachoma and genital tract infections. Those that cause trachoma are spread person-to-person, most probably through eye and possibly nasal secretions on the hands. *C. trachomatis* is also spread mechanically by flies and probably by fomites such as washrags and handkerchiefs. Repeated episodes of infection in young (preschool) children lead to scarring of the eyelids, which in turn causes in-turned eyelashes that abrade the corneal surface, leading to subsequent corneal opacification and reduced visual acuity or blindness in adults.

#### Descriptive Epidemiologic Features and Risk Factors

Trachoma is the leading cause of preventable blindness in the world, accounting for an estimated 6 million or one-sixth of all cases (Thylefors, Négrel, Pararajasegaram, & Dadzie, 1995). In addition, roughly 150 million persons are infected with *C. trachomatis* and at risk of becoming blind. Trachoma is a disease of poverty that was described by the ancient Egyptians and previously was found throughout the world. Trachoma disappeared from Europe and virtually all of the United States long before antimicrobial agents became available in the 1930s and 1940s; improved standards of living and personal hygiene are credited with its disappearance. Trachoma is not a reportable condition, and what is known of its descriptive epidemiologic features comes from numerous surveys. Trachoma persists in hot, low- and middle-income countries, particularly in North Africa, the Middle East, sub-Saharan Africa, and drier regions of India and Southeast Asia. In hyperendemic areas, infection of the eye is virtually universal in children by their fifth birthday, but active disease is seen largely in older children. Repeated reinfection in children leads to the permanent damage to the eyes that results in subsequent blindness or visual impairment in adults. Although infection in childhood appears to be equally common in boys and girls, the blinding complications appear to be more common in women, perhaps because of repeated exposure to infected children.

Risk factors for trachoma in children largely relate to facial cleanliness, the presence of flies, and cultural practices that lead to an increased likelihood of person-to-person transmission of the etiologic agent, such as sharing washcloths and ways in which eye makeup is applied. One author has collectively referred to the various ways in which *C. trachomatis* is spread from person to person as "ocular promiscuity."

### Current Approaches to Prevention and Control

Intervention studies have demonstrated that mass treatment with a variety of topical or oral antimicrobial agents and health educational programs that lead to improved facial cleanliness can substantially reduce the prevalence of trachoma in a community as can fly control (Dawson, 1999; Emerson et al., 1999). Reductions in trachoma in low- and middle-income countries in the absence of a specific control program have also been documented as access to water, access to health care, and hygiene have improved. The current approach to reducing trachoma-associated blindness in endemic areas is summarized in the acronym SAFE, which stands for: (1) surgery to correct eyelid deformity, (2) antibiotics to treat acute eye infection and reduce sources of infection in the community, (3) facial cleanliness, and (4) environmental change that enhances availability of water and reduces the prevalence of flies. In 1997 WHO launched a new trachoma control program—Global Elimination of Trachoma by 2020 (GET2020) based on the SAFE approach.

### Obstacles to Prevention and Directions for Future Research

Trachoma is likely to remain a persistent problem in endemic areas until rising socioeconomic conditions result in better access to water, improved personal hygiene and sanitation, reductions in the numbers of flies, and improved access to health care services. While mass, communitywide treatment with antimicrobial agents can lead to reduced trachoma in such areas, these reductions have proven difficult to sustain unless such treatment is made a routine part of regularly available health services and is accompa-

nied by improvements in hygiene. Although a vaccine against trachoma has been discussed for many years, it remains unclear whether an effective vaccine can or will ever be developed.

## Onchocerciasis

*O. volvulus* is a filarial parasite that is spread through the bite of one of several species of Simulium black flies. During the bite of an infected female fly, larvae enter the body and ultimately develop into adult worms that form nodules, usually over bony prominences. Adult worms can survive inside these nodules for up to 15 years. The female adult worm produces microfilariae that migrate to the skin and the eye, and that are ingested by female flies when they bite an infected person, thus completing the cycle. In the skin, an inflammatory response to dead and dying microfilariae can lead to incapacitating itching and various types of degenerative, often unsightly, skin changes. In the eye, heavy and prolonged infection of the cornea with the microfilariae leads to opacification and reduced visual acuity or total blindness. The microfilariae can be detected by taking small snips of skin, immersing them in saline, and examining the saline microscopically.

### Descriptive Epidemiologic Features and Risk Factors

Onchocerciasis is found only in a band of sub-Saharan African countries, parts of Central America, the northern part of South America, and the Arabian peninsula. It is estimated that almost 18 million persons worldwide are currently infected with the parasite and that more than 750,000 infected individuals are either blind or have severe visual impairment as a result, with the vast majority of these individuals living in Africa (especially Nigeria, Cameroon, Uganda, the Congo, and Ethiopia) (Greene, 1992). Within these affected regions, onchocerciasis occurs in foci, largely determined by distance from the black fly breeding sites. The intensity of infection (and hence the risk of visual impairment) increases with age, as the burden of adult female worms producing microfilariae increases, and tends to be greater in men than in women, perhaps reflecting work-related exposures to the flies.

### Current Approaches to Prevention and Control

Approaches to the control of onchocerciasis and prevention of the blindness it causes have included vector control, mass treatment of infected individuals, and nodulectomy (removal of nodules to reduce the source and number of microfilariae that migrate to the eyes). Early attempts to control onchocerciasis targeted the Simulium flies that serve as vectors, the immature stages of which require running water (for example, rivers and streams) for their development. Initially, DDT was the pesticide added to rivers that served as the breeding ground for the vector, but beginning in the 1970s other agents that target the larval stages of the fly (for example, temephos) were used with great success, particularly in West Africa. These programs permitted resettlement of fertile areas that had been abandoned because of onchocerciasis, but the development of resistance of the flies to temephos required switching to other larvacidal agents in some areas.

The control of onchocerciasis was revolutionized in the late 1980s with the introduction of ivermectin, a single dose of which eliminates microfilariae for a number of months. However, because ivermectin does not kill the adult worms, repeated treatment (for example, every 6 to 12 months) of infected individuals over many years is needed to provide continued suppression of the number of microfilariae and to prevent visual damage. Fortunately, in a noteworthy humanitarian gesture, the manufacturer of ivermectin has made a commitment to provide the drug free "for as long as necessary to as many as necessary." Given the availability of ivermectin, countries affected by onchocerciasis have developed control programs in which endemic areas are identified (typically by conducting nodule surveys) and then making the drug available in those areas (Pacqué, Muñoz, Greene, & Taylor,

1991). Various approaches to making the drug available have been used (for example, passive health center-based programs and active community-based programs), and each has advantages and disadvantages.

### Obstacles to Prevention and Directions for Future Research

Although it may be possible in some endemic areas to eradicate onchocerciasis through vector control or mass ivermectin treatment programs, in the most heavily affected parts of Africa complete eradication is not likely in the foreseeable future.

## CONCLUSION

The current status of infectious diseases in low- and middle-income countries reflects both the dramatic progress that has been made in controlling some diseases and the disappointing results to date in controlling others. The eradication of smallpox, the expected imminent eradication of polio, and impressive gains made against measles and neonatal tetanus all demonstrate what can be accomplished even in the lowest-income countries with an effective vaccine when concerted efforts are made to ensure that the vaccine reaches those in need. Similar progress in reducing morbidity from dracunculiasis and onchocerciasis demonstrates that, under the right conditions and with available resources, infectious diseases can be controlled through a combination of vector control and avoidance and treatment. At the same time, the reductions in the morbidity and mortality from diarrheal diseases and acute respiratory infections that have been achieved are clear evidence that a combination of improved knowledge and access to reasonably inexpensive treatment modalities can also be highly effective.

Far less encouraging has been the progress made against malaria, dengue, tuberculosis, and AIDS, all of which continue to take a substantial toll. For diseases such as tuberculosis, much can be accomplished simply by improving diagnosis and treatment of cases using tried-and-true methods that have been available for many years. For diseases such as AIDS, behavior change and improved access to treatment of other STIs can reduce the risk of acquiring HIV infection and expanded use of antiretroviral drugs can reduce vertical transmission of the virus, but development and widespread use of an effective vaccine is the only realistic long-term solution. For vector-borne diseases such as dengue and malaria, either new approaches to vector control or effective vaccines are urgently needed.

Progress to date in controlling the morbidity and mortality from infectious diseases in low- and middle-income countries demonstrates that much can be accomplished even in the absence of marked improvements in socioeconomic conditions. Ultimately, however, widespread improvements in education and socioeconomic conditions will be needed if such progress is to be maintained.

---

## DISCUSSION QUESTIONS

1. What are the major different types of approaches that have been used to prevent morbidity and mortality from infectious diseases in low- and middle-income countries?
2. What are the major obstacles that have had and will have to be overcome in implementing various approaches to preventing morbidity and mortality from infectious diseases in low- and middle-income countries?
3. In the year 2000, what infectious diseases account for the most mortality in low-income countries? The most morbidity?
4. If you were working in the Ministry of Health of a low-income country and needed to set priorities concerning resource allocation, how could you go about determining the relative importance of various infectious diseases as causes of mortality in your country? The causes of morbidity/disability?

---

## REFERENCES

Aaby, P., Samb, B., Simondon, F., Knudsen, K., Seck, A.M., Bennett, J., Markowitz, L., Rhodes, P., & Whittle, H. (1994). Sex-specific differences in mortality after high-titre measles immunization in rural Senegal. *Bulletin of the World Health Organization, 72,* 761–770.

Action programme for the elimination of leprosy: Status report 1998. (1998). Document WHO/LEP/98.2. Geneva, Switzerland: World Health Organization.

Adults and children estimated to be living with HIV/AIDS as of end 1998. (1998). World Health Organization UNAIDS website. (www.unaids.org/highband/document/epidemio/index.html).

Avila, M., Salomón, H., Carballal, G., Ebekian, B., Woyskovsky, N., Cerqueiro, M.C., & Weissenbacher, M. (1990). Role of viral pathogens in acute respiratory tract infections. *Reviews of Infectious Diseases, 12,* S974–S981.

Bach, J.F., Chalons, S., Forier, E., Elana, G., Jouanelle, J., Kayemba, S., Delbois, D., Mosser, A., Saint-Aime, C., & Berchel, C. (1996). 10-year educational programme

aimed at rheumatic fever in two French Caribbean islands. *Lancet, 347,* 644–648.

Berman, S. (1991). Epidemiology of acute respiratory infections in children of developing countries. *Reviews of
Infectious Diseases, 13,* S454–S462.

Bern, C., Martines, J., de Zoysa, I., & Glass, R.I. (1992).
The magnitude of the global problem of diarrhoeal dis-
ease: A ten-year update. *Bulletin of the World Health
Organization, 70,* 705–714.

Black, R.E. (1993). Persistent diarrhea in children of developing countries. *Pediatric Infectious Disease Journal,
12,* 751–761.

Black, R.E., Merson, M.H., Rahman, A.S., Yunus, M., Alim,
A.R., Huq, I., Yolken, R.H., & Curlin, G.T. (1980). A
two-year study of bacterial, viral, and parasitic agents
associated with diarrhea in rural Bangladesh. *Journal of
Infectious Diseases, 142,* 660–664.

Bundy, D.A. (1990). New initiatives in the control of helminths. *Transactions of the Royal Society of Tropical
Medicine and Hygiene, 84,* 467–468.

Bundy, D.A., Hall, A., Medley, G.F., & Savioli, L. (1992).
Evaluating measures to control intestinal parasitic infections. *World Health Statistics Quarterly, 45,* 168–179.

Butterworth, A.E., Dunne, D.W., Fulford, A.J., Ouma, J.H.,
& Sturrock, R.F. (1996). Immunity and morbidity in
*Schistosoma mansoni* infection: Quantitative aspects.
*American Journal of Tropical Medicine and Hygiene,
55,* 109–115.

Celentano, D.D., Nelson, K.E., Suprasert, S., Eiumtrakul,
S., Tulvatana, S., Kuntolbutra, S., Akarasewi, P., Mata-
nasarawoot, A., Wright, N.H., Sirisopana, N., & Theet-
ranont, C. (1996). Risk factors for HIV-1 seroconversion
among young men in northern Thailand. *Journal of the
American Medical Association, 275,* 122–127.

Chan, M.-S. (1997). The global burden of intestinal nematode infections: Fifty years on. *Parasitology Today, 13,*
438–443.

Cholera Working Group, International Centre for Diarrhoeal Diseases Research, Bangladesh. (1993). Large
epidemic of cholera-like disease in Bangladesh caused
by *Vibrio cholerae* O139 synonym Bengal. *Lancet, 342,*
387–390.

Clinical management of acute respiratory infections in children: A WHO memorandum. (1981). *Bulletin of the
World Health Organization, 59,* 707–716.

Collins, F.H., & Paskewitz, S.M. (1995). Malaria: Current
and future prospects for control. *Annual Review of En-
tomology, 40,* 195–219.

*Control of epidemic meningococcal disease: WHO practical
guidelines.* (1995). Lyon, France: World Health Organization and Fondation Marcel Mérieux.

Control of schistosomiasis: The second report of the WHO
Expert Committee. (1993). WHO technical report series
830. Geneva, Switzerland: World Health Organization.

Cummins, D., McCormick, J.B., Bennett, D., Samba, J.A.,
Farrar, B., Machin, S.J., & Fisher-Hoch, S. P. (1990).
Acute sensorineural deafness in Lassa fever. *Journal of
the American Medical Association, 264,* 2093–2096.

Cutts, F.T., & Vynnycky, E. (1999). Modelling the incidence
of congenital rubella syndrome in developing countries.
*International Journal of Epidemiology, 28,* 1176–1184.

Dawson, C. (1999). Flies and the elimination of blinding
trachoma. *Lancet, 353,* 1376–1377.

De Manzione, N., Salas, R.A., Paredes, H., Godoy, O.,
Rojas, L., Araoz, F., Fulhorst, C.F., Ksiazek, T.G., Mills,
J.N., Ellis, B.A., Peters, C.J., & Tesh, R.B. (1998). Venezuelan hemorrhagic fever: Clinical and epidemiological studies of 165 cases. *Clinical Infectious Diseases,
26,* 308–313.

Dolin, P.J., Raviglione, M.C., & Kochi, A. (1994).
Global tuberculosis incidence and mortality during
1990–2000. *Bulletin of the World Health Organization,
72,* 213–220.

Dove, A.W., & Racaniello, V.R. (1997). The polio eradication effort: Should vaccine eradication be next? *Science,
277,* 779–780.

Dowdle, W.R., & Hopkins, D.R. (1998). *The eradication of
infectious diseases: Report of the Dahlem Workshop on
the Eradication of Infectious Diseases, Berlin, March
16–22, 1997.* Chichester, England: John Wiley & Sons.

Dowell, S.F., Mukunu, R., Ksiazek, T.G., Khan, A.S., Rollin,
P.E., & Peters, C.J. (1999). Transmission of Ebola hem-
orrhagic fever: A study of risk factors in family mem-
bers, Kikwit, Democratic Republic of the Congo, 1995.
Commission de Lutte contre les Epidémies à Kikwit.
*Journal of Infectious Diseases, 179,* S87–S91.

Doyle, T.J., Bryan, R.T., & Peters, C.J. (1998). Viral hemorrhagic fevers and hantavirus infections in the Americas. *Infectious Disease Clinics of North America, 12,*
95–110.

Dracunculiasis: Global surveillance summary, 1997. (1998).
*Weekly Epidemiological Record, 73,* 129–135.

Dye, C., Scheele, S., Dolin, P., Pathania, V., & Raviglione,
M. (1999). Global burden of tuberculosis: estimated
incidence, prevalence, and mortality by country. *Journal
of the American Medical Association, 282,* 677–686.

Ekwanzala, M., Pépin, J., Khonde, N., Molisho, S., Bruneel,
H., & De Wals, P. (1996). In the heart of darkness:
Sleeping sickness in Zaire. *Lancet, 348,* 1427–1430.

El Samani, E.F., Willett, W.C., & Ware, J.H. (1998). Association of malnutrition and diarrhea in children aged under
five years: A prospective follow-up study in a rural
Sudanese community. *American Journal of Epidemiology, 128,* 93–105.

Ellis, W.A. (1998). Leptospirosis. In S.R. Palmer, E.J.L.
Soulsby, & D.I.H. Simpson (Eds.), *Zoonoses: Biology,
clinical practice, and public health control* (pp.
115–126). New York: Oxford University Press.

El-Rafie, M., Hassouna, W.A., Hirschhorn, N., Loza, S., Miller, P., Nagaty, A., Nasser, S., & Riyad, S. (1990). Effect of diarrhoeal disease control on infant and childhood mortality in Egypt: Report from the National Control of Diarrheal Diseases Project. *Lancet, 335,* 334–338.

Emerson, P.M., Lindsay, S.W., Walraven, G.E., Faal, H., Bøgh, C., Lowe, K., & Bailey, R.L. (1999). Effect of fly control on trachoma and diarrhoea. *Lancet, 353,* 1401–1403.

EPI information system: Global summary, September 1998. (1998). Document WHO/EPI/GEN/98.10. Geneva, Switzerland: World Health Organization.

Expanded programme on immunization, Global Advisory Group. (1994). Part II. Achieving the major disease control goals. *Weekly Epidemiological Record, 69,* 29–31, 34–35.

Fishbein, D.B. (1991). Rabies in humans. In G.M. Baer (Ed.), *The natural history of rabies* (2nd ed., pp. 519–549). Boca Raton, FL: CRC Press.

Gerbase, A.C., Rowley, J.T., & Mertens, T.E. (1998). Global epidemiology of sexually transmitted diseases. *Lancet, 351,* 2–4.

Glass, R.I., Libel, M., & Brandling-Bennett, A.D. (1992). Epidemic cholera in the Americas. *Science, 256,* 1524–1525.

Goodgame, R.W., & Greenough, W.B. (1975). Cholera in Africa: A message for the West. *Annals of Internal Medicine, 82,* 101–106.

Gove, S. (1997). Integrated management of childhood illness by outpatient health workers: Technical basis and overview. The WHO Working Group on Guidelines for Integrated Management of the Sick Child. *Bulletin of the World Health Organization, 75,* 7–24.

Graham, N.M. (1990). The epidemiology of acute respiratory infections in children and adults: A global perspective. *Epidemiologic Reviews, 12,* 149–178.

Greene, B.M. (1992). Modern medicine versus an ancient scourge: Progress toward control of onchocerciasis. *Journal of Infectious Diseases, 166,* 15–21.

Greenwood, B.M. (1987). The epidemiology of acute bacterial meningitis in tropical Africa. In J.D. Williams & J. Burnie (Eds.), *Bacterial meningitis* (pp. 61–91). London: Academic Press.

Grosskurth, H., Mosha, F., Todd, J., Mwijarubi, E., Klokke, A., Senkoro, K., Mayaud, P., Changalucha, J., Nicoll, A., ka-Gina, G., Newell, J., Mugeye, K., Mabey, D., & Hayes, R. (1995). Impact of improved treatment of sexually transmitted diseases on HIV infection in rural Tanzania: Randomised controlled trial. *Lancet, 346,* 530–536.

Gubler, D.J. (1998). Dengue and dengue hemorrhagic fever. *Clinical Microbiology Reviews, 11,* 480–496.

Guerrant, R.L., Hughes, J.M., Lima, N.L., & Crane, J. (1990). Diarrhea in developed and developing countries: Magnitude, special settings, and etiologies. *Reviews of Infectious Diseases, 12,* S41–S50.

Hagan, P. (1996). Immunity and morbidity in infection due to *Schistosoma haematobium. American Journal of Tropical Medicine and Hygiene, 55,* 116–120.

Hart, C.A., Trees, A.J., & Duerden, B.I. (1997). Zoonoses. *Journal of Medical Microbiology, 46,* 4–6.

Helmick, C.G., Webb, P.A., Scribner, C.L., Krebs, J.W., & McCormick, J.B. (1986). No evidence for increased risk of Lassa fever infection in hospital staff. *Lancet, 2,* 1202–1205.

Hepatitis C. (1997). *Weekly Epidemiological Record, 72,* 65–69.

Hepatitis C: Global prevalence. (1997). *Weekly Epidemiological Record, 72,* 341–344.

Hopkins, D.R. (1984). Eradication of dracunculiasis. In P.G. Bourne (Ed.), *Water and sanitation: Economic and sociological perspectives* (pp. 93–114). Orlando, FL: Academic Press.

Hopkins, D.R., Ruiz-Tiben, E., & Ruebush, T.K. (1997). Dracunculiasis eradication: Almost a reality. *American Journal of Tropical Medicine and Hygiene, 57,* 252–259.

Htun, Y., Morse, S.A., Dangor, Y., Fehler, G., Radebe, F., Trees, D.L., Beck-Sague, C.M., & Ballard, R.C. (1998). Comparison of clinically directed, disease specific, and syndromic protocols for the management of genital ulcer disease in Lesotho. *Sexually Transmitted Infections, 74,* S23–S28.

Hull, H.F., Ward, N.A., Hull, B.P., Milstien, J.B., & de Quadros, C. (1994). Paralytic poliomyelitis: Seasoned strategies, disappearing disease. *Lancet, 343,* 1331–1337.

Human plague in 1996. (1998). *Weekly Epidemiological Record, 73,* 366–369.

Hunter, J.M. (1996). An introduction to guinea worm on the eve of its departure: Dracunculiasis transmission, health effects, ecology and control. *Social Science and Medicine, 43,* 1399–1425.

Hussey, G.D., & Klein, M. (1990). A randomized, controlled trial of vitamin A in children with severe measles. *New England Journal of Medicine, 323,* 160–164.

Huttly, S.R., Morris, S.S., & Pisani, V. (1997). Prevention of diarrhoea in young children in developing countries. *Bulletin of the World Health Organization, 75,* 163–174.

Keusch, G.T., & Cash, R.A. (1997). A vaccine against rotavirus: When is too much too much? [Editorial]. *New England Journal of Medicine, 337,* 1228–1229.

Kew, M.C., & Kassianides, C. (1997). HGV: Hepatitis G virus or harmless G virus? *Lancet, 348,* SII10.

Khuroo, M.S., Teli, M.R., Skidmore, S., Sofi, M.A., & Khuroo, M.I. (1981). Incidence and severity of viral hepatitis in pregnancy. *American Journal of Medicine, 70,* 252–255.

Kilgore, P.E., Peters, C.J., Mills, J.N., Rollin, P.E., Armstrong, L., Khan, A.S., & Ksiazek, T.G. (1995). Prospects for the control of Bolivian hemorrhagic fever [Editorial]. *Emerging Infectious Diseases, 1,* 97–100.

Kilian, A.H., Gregson, S., Ndyanabangi, B., Walusaga, K., Kipp, W., Sahlmüller, G., Garnett, G.P., Asiimwe-Okiror, G., Kabagambe, G., Weis, P., & von Sonnenburg, F. (1999). Reductions in risk behaviour provide the most consistent explanation for declining HIV-1 prevalence in Uganda. *AIDS, 13,* 391–398.

Krogstad, D.J. (1996). Malaria as a reemerging disease. *Epidemiologic Reviews, 18,* 77–89.

LaForce, F.M., Lichnevski, M.S., Keja, J., & Henderson, R.H. (1980). Clinical survey techniques to estimate prevalence and annual incidence of poliomyelitis in developing countries. *Bulletin of the World Health Organization, 58,* 609–620.

Lambrechts, T., Bryce, J., & Orinda V. (1999). Integrated management of childhood illness: A summary of first experiences. *Bulletin of the World Health Organization, 77,* 582–594.

London, W.T., & Evans, A.A. (1996). The epidemiology of hepatitis viruses B, C, and D. *Clinics in Laboratory Medicine, 16,* 251–271.

Maiztegui, J.I., McKee, K.T., Jr., Barrera Oro, J.G, Harrison, L.H., Gibbs, P.H., Feuillade, M.R., Enria, D.A., Briggiler, A.M., Levis, S.C., Ambrosio, A.M., Halsey, N.A., & Peters, C.J. (1998). Protective efficacy of a live attenuated vaccine against Argentine hemorrhagic fever. AHF Study Group. *Journal of Infectious Diseases, 177,* 277–283.

Management of patients with sexually transmitted diseases: Report of a WHO Study Group. (1991). WHO technical report series 810. Geneva, Switzerland: World Health Organization.

Margolis, H.S., Alter, M.J., & Hadler, S.C. (1997). Viral hepatitis. In A.S. Evans & R.A. Kaslow (Eds.), *Viral infections of humans: Epidemiology and control* (4th ed., pp. 363–418). New York: Plenum Medical Books.

Markowitz, L.E., Nzilambi, N., Driskell, W.J., Sension, M.G., Rovira, E.Z., Nieburg, P., & Ryder, R.W. (1989). Vitamin A levels and mortality among hospitalized measles patients, Kinshasa, Zaire. *Journal of Tropical Pediatrics, 35,* 109–112.

Marseille, E., Kahn, J.G., Mmiro, F., Guay, L., Musoke, P., Fowler, M.G., & Jackson, J.B. (1999). Cost effectiveness of single-dose nevirapine regimen for mothers and babies to decrease vertical HIV-1 transmission in sub-Saharan Africa. *Lancet, 354,* 803–809.

McCormick, J.B., King, I.J., Webb, P.A., Scribner, C.L., Craven, R.B., Johnson, K.M., Elliott, L.H., & Belmont-Williams, R. (1986). Lassa fever: Effective therapy

with ribavirin. *New England Journal of Medicine, 314,* 20–26.

McCormick, J.B., Webb, P.A., Krebs, J.W., Johnson, K.M., & Smith, E.S. (1987). A prospective study of the epidemiology and ecology of Lassa fever. *Journal of Infectious Diseases, 155,* 437–444.

Medina, E., & Yrarrazaval, M. (1983). Typhoid fever in Chile: Epidemiological considerations. *Revista Medica de Chile, 111,* 609–615.

Mølbak, K., Wested, N., Højlyng, N., Scheutz, F., Gottschau, A., Aaby, P., & da Silva, A.P. (1994). The etiology of early childhood diarrhea: A community study from Guinea-Bissau. *Journal of Infectious Diseases, 169,* 581–587.

Monson, M.H., Cole, A.K., Frame, J.D., Serwint, J.R., Alexander, S., & Jahrling, P.B. (1987). Pediatric Lassa fever: A review of 33 Liberian cases. *American Journal of Tropical Medicine and Hygiene, 36,* 408–415.

Moore, P.S. (1992). Meningococcal meningitis in sub-Saharan Africa: A model for the epidemic process. *Clinical Infectious Diseases, 14,* 515–525.

Murray, C.J.L., & Lopez, A.D. (1994). Global comparative assessments in the health sector: Disease burden, expenditures, and intervention packages: Collected reprints from the Bulletin of the World Health Organization. Geneva, Switzerland: World Health Organization.

Nair, G.B., Ramamurthy, T., Bhattacharya, S.K., Mukhopadhyay, A.K., Garg, S., Bhattacharya, M.K., Takeda, T., Shimada, T., Takeda, Y., & Deb, B.C. (1994). Spread of *Vibrio cholerae* O139 Bengal in India. *Journal of Infectious Diseases, 169,* 1029–1034.

Nelson, K.E., Celentano, D.D., Eiumtrakol, S., Hoover, D.R., Beyrer, C., Suprasert, S., Kuntolbutra, S., & Khamboonruang, C. (1996). Changes in sexual behavior and a decline in HIV infection among young men in Thailand. *New England Journal of Medicine, 335,* 297–303.

Otten, M.W., Jr., Deming, M.S., Jaiteh, K.O., Flagg, E.W., Forgie, I., Sanyang, Y., Sillah, B., Brogan, D., & Gowers, P. (1992). Epidemic poliomyelitis in the Gambia following the control of poliomyelitis as an endemic disease. I. Descriptive findings. *American Journal of Epidemiology, 135,* 381–392.

Pacqué, M., Muñoz, B., Greene, B.M., & Taylor, H.R. (1991). Community-based treatment of onchocerciasis with ivermectin: Safety, efficacy, and acceptability of yearly treatment. *Journal of Infectious Diseases, 163,* 381–385.

Pan America Health Organization. (1994, October). Measles elimination by the year 2000. *EPI Newsletter, 16,* 1–2.

Patriarca, P.A., Wright, P.F., & John, T.J. (1991). Factors affecting the immunogenicity of oral poliovirus vaccine in developing countries: Review. *Reviews of Infectious Diseases, 13,* 926–939.

Perkins, B.A., Broome, C.V., Rosenstein, N.E., Schuchat, A., & Reingold, A.L. (1997). Meningococcal vaccine in sub-Saharan Africa [Letter]. *Lancet, 350,* 1708.

Perkins, B.A., Zucker, J.R., Otieno, J., Jafari, H.S., Paxton, L., Redd, S.C., Nahlen, B.L., Schwartz, B., Oloo, A.J., Olango, C., Gove, S., & Campbell, C.C. (1997). Evaluation of an algorithm for integrated management of childhood illness in an area of Kenya with high malaria transmission. *Bulletin of the World Health Organization, 75,* 33–42.

Prevention and control of intestinal parasitic infections: Report of a WHO Expert Committee. (1987). WHO technical report series 749. Geneva, Switzerland: World Health Organization.

Progress toward elimination of neonatal tetanus: Egypt, 1988–1994. (1996). *Morbidity and Mortality Weekly Report, 45,* 89–92.

Progress toward poliomyelitis eradication: West Africa, 1997–September 1998. (1998). *Morbidity and Mortality Weekly Report, 47,* 882–886.

Raviglione, M.C., Dye, C., Schmidt, S., & Kochi, A. (1997). Assessment of worldwide tuberculosis control. WHO Global Surveillance and Monitoring Project. *Lancet, 350,* 624–629.

Recent HIV seroprevalence levels by country: February 1999. (1999). (Research Note No. 26). Washington, DC: Health Studies Branch, International Program Center, Population Division, U.S. Bureau of the Census.

Re-emergence of Bolivian hemorrhagic fever. (1994). *Epidemiological Bulletin, 15,* 4–5.

Rigau-Pérez, J.G., Clark, G.G., Gubler, D.J., Reiter, P., Sanders, E.J., & Vorndam, A.V. (1998). Dengue and dengue haemorrhagic fever. *Lancet, 352,* 971–977.

Robbins, J.B., Towne, D.W., Gotschlich, E.C., & Schneerson, R. (1997). "Love's labours lost": Failure to implement mass vaccination against group A meningococcal meningitis in sub-Saharan Africa. *Lancet, 350,* 880–882.

Rojanapithayakorn, W., & Hanenberg, R. (1996). The 100% condom program in Thailand. *AIDS, 10,* 1–7.

Sazawal, S., & Black, R.E. (1992). Meta-analysis of intervention trials on case-management of pneumonia in community settings. *Lancet, 340,* 528–533.

Schofield, F. (1986). Selective primary health care: Strategies for control of disease in the developing world. XXII. Tetanus: A preventable problem. *Reviews of Infectious Diseases, 8,* 144–156.

Selwyn, B.J. (1990). The epidemiology of acute respiratory tract infection in young children: Comparison of findings from several developing countries. Coordinated Data Group of BOSTID Researchers. *Reviews of Infectious Diseases, 12,* S870–S888.

Shaffer, N., Chuachoowong, R., Mock, P.A., Bhadrakom, C., Siriwasin, W., Young, N.L., Chotpitayasunondh, T., Chearskul, S., Roongpisuthipong, A., Chinayon,

P., Karon, J., Mastro, T.D., & Simonds, R.J. (1999). Short-course zidovudine for perinatal HIV-1 transmission in Bangkok, Thailand: A randomised controlled trial. *Lancet, 353,* 773–780.

Shann, F. (1986). Etiology of severe pneumonia in children in developing countries. *Pediatric Infectious Disease, 5,* 247–252.

Sinha, A., Sazawal, S., Kumar, R., Sood, S., Reddaiah, V.P., Singh, B., Rao, M., Naficy, A., Clemens, J.D., & Bhan, M.K. (1999). Typhoid fever in children aged less than 5 years. *Lancet, 354,* 734–737.

Stanfield, J.P., & Galazka, A. (1984). Neonatal tetanus in the world today. *Bulletin of the World Health Organization, 62,* 647–669.

Sutrisna, B., Reingold, A., Kresno, S., Harrison, G., & Utomo, B. (1993). Care-seeking for fatal illnesses in young children in Indramayu, West Java, Indonesia. *Lancet, 342,* 787–789.

Sutter, R.W., Patriarca, P.A., Brogan, S., Malankar, P.G., Pallansch, M.A., Kew, O.M., Bass, A.G., Cochi, S.L., Alexander, J.P., Hall, D.B., Suleiman, A.J.M., Al-Ghassany, A.A.K., & El-Bualy, M.S. (1991). Outbreak of paralytic poliomyelitis in Oman: Evidence for widespread transmission among fully vaccinated children. *Lancet, 338,* 715–720.

Ter Meulen, J., Lukashevich, I., Sidibe, K., Inapogui, A., Marx, M., Dorlemann, A., Yansane, M.L., Koulemou, K., Chang-Claude, J., & Schmitz, H. (1996). Hunting of peridomestic rodents and consumption of their meat as possible risk factors for rodent-to-human transmission of Lassa virus in the Republic of Guinea. *American Journal of Tropical Medicine and Hygiene, 55,* 661–666.

Thylefors, B., Négrel, A.D., Pararajasegaram, R., & Dadzie, K.Y. (1995). Global data on blindness. *Bulletin of the World Health Organization, 73,* 115–121.

Trigg, P.I., & Kondrachine, A.V. (1998). Commentary: Malaria control in the 1990s. *Bulletin of the World Health Organization, 76,* 11–16.

United Nations Development Programme (UNDP), World Bank, WHO Special Programme for Research and Training in Tropical Diseases (TDR). (1997). Tropical disease research: Progress 1995–96: Thirteenth programme report. Geneva, Switzerland: World Health Organization.

University of Zimbabwe/JHPIEGO Cervical Cancer Project. (1999). Visual inspection with acetic acid for cervical-cancer screening: Test qualities in a primary-care setting. *Lancet, 353,* 869–873.

Vainio, J., & Cutts, F. (1998). Yellow fever. Document WHO/EPI/GEN/98.11. Geneva, Switzerland: World Health Organization.

Vainrub, B., & Salas, R. (1994). Latin American hemorrhagic fever. *Infectious Disease Clinics of North America, 8,* 47–59.

Viral haemorrhagic fevers: Report of a WHO Expert Committee. (1985). WHO technical report series 721. Geneva, Switzerland: World Health Organization.

Walsh, J.A. (1983). Selective primary health care: Strategies for control of disease in the developing world. IV. Measles. *Reviews of Infectious Diseases, 5,* 330–340.

Warren, K.S., Bundy, D.A., Anderson, R.M., Davis, A.R., Henderson, D.A., Jamison, D.T., Prescott, N., & Senft, A. (1993). Helminth infection. In D.T. Jamison, W.H. Mosley, A.R. Measham, & J.L. Bobadilla (Eds.), *Disease control priorities in developing countries* (pp. 131–160). New York: Oxford University Press.

Weber, M.W., Mulholland, E.K., Jaffar, S., Troedsson, H., Gove, S., & Greenwood, B.M. (1997). Evaluation of an algorithm for the integrated management of childhood illness in an area with seasonal malaria in the Gambia. *Bulletin of the World Health Organization, 75,* 25–32.

Whalen, C.C., Johnson, J.L., Okwera, A., Hom, D.L., Huebner, R., Mugyenyi, P., Mugerwa, R.D., & Ellner, J.J. (1997). A trial of three regimens to prevent tuberculosis in Ugandan adults infected with the human immunodeficiency virus. Uganda–Case Western Reserve University Research Collaboration. *New England Journal of Medicine, 337,* 801–808.

WHO Expert Committee on Leprosy. (1998). Seventh report (pp. 1–43). WHO technical report series 874. Geneva, Switzerland: World Health Organization.

WHO Expert Committee on Rabies. (1992). Eighth report. WHO technical report series 824. Geneva, Switzerland: World Health Organization.

Wiktor, S.Z., Ekpini, E., Karon, J.M., Nkengasong, J., Maurice, C., Severin, S.T., Roels, T.H., Kouassi, M.K., Lackritz, E.M., Coulibaly, I., & Greenberg, A.E. (1999). Short-course oral zidovudine for prevention of mother-to-child transmission of HIV-1 in Abidjan, Côte d'Ivoire: A randomised trial. *Lancet, 353,* 781–785.

World Health Organization. (1993). A global strategy for malaria control. Geneva, Switzerland: Author.

World Health Organization. (1999). World Health Organization report on infectious diseases: Removing obstacles to healthy development. Document WHO/CDS/99.1. Geneva, Switzerland: Author.

World malaria situation in 1994. (1997). Part I. Population at risk. *Weekly Epidemiological Record, 72,* 269–274.

World survey of rabies 32 for the year 1996. (1997). Document WHO/EMC/ZDI/98.4. Geneva, Switzerland: World Health Organization.

Yellow fever technical consensus meeting. (1998). Document WHO/EPI/GEN/98.08. Geneva, Switzerland: World Health Organization.

Yellow fever, 1996–1997. (1998). Part II. *Weekly Epidemiological Record, 73,* 370–372.

# CHAPTER 5

# Nutrition

*Keith P. West, Jr., Benjamin Caballero, and Robert E. Black*

Nutritional concerns in low-income countries remain largely ones of deprivation and hunger, conditions that lead to deficiencies and ensuing health consequences, and their alleviation. Undernutrition, due to chronic dietary deficiency of protein, energy, and micronutrients, is viewed both as a consequence and cause of poor human health, development, and achievement (World Bank, 1993). While severe forms of undernutrition, evident by classical, clinical manifestations, often have profound and clearly recognized consequences with respect to morbidity, disability, and mortality, they tend to be rare events in populations. More prevalent are clinically inapparent, less severe, "hidden" forms of undernutrition, to which are linked a constellation of health consequences that adversely affect child growth and development, general health and well-being, productivity, and economic progress (Administration Committee on Coordination/Sub-Committee on Nutrition [ACC/SCN], 2000). Groups at highest risk of being undernourished are the impoverished, who lack food security and the necessary resources to adequately feed and care for themselves. Within a population, those at highest risk of undernutrition are individuals who, at certain stages in their lives, are often exposed to its causes and most vulnerable to its consequences: the fetus, infant, young child, and woman of reproductive age. Implicit in this membership is a generally held need to preserve the future. The nutritional plight of older persons,

the most rapidly growing demographic group in the world, is beginning to receive attention (Roubenoff, 1999), although little evidence on nutritional health yet exists for this group on which to base nutrition policy in low-income countries (Chilima & Ismail, 1998).

At the other end of the nutritional spectrum is the rapidly evolving "nutrition transition," a process marked by a shift in the paradigm from one of undernutrition to overnutrition in previous low- and middle-income countries, or economically advancing segments of society within these countries (ACC/SCN, 2000). It is marked by changes in diet toward increased energy (calorie) consumption, resulting from increased intakes of fat and refined sugars and decreased intakes of dietary fiber and roughage as highly refined, processed foods replace traditional diets (Popkin, 1998). The nutrition transition parallels, and contributes to, rapid economic, demographic, and epidemiologic transitions underway in many previously underdeveloped societies. Thus the rise from dietary deficit to adequacy has likely contributed to improved health and longevity across the globe (World Bank, 1993), but these changes also bring excessive shifts in dietary patterns and obesity that, along with reduced activity and other exposures of industrialization, increase risk of degenerative, cardiovascular, and neoplastic (that is, noncommunicable) diseases that are rapidly becoming leading causes of adult morbidity and mortality throughout middle-income countries (World Bank, 1993).

The diversity and breadth of nutritional need in practically all countries, and the urgency to act to correct malnutrition, were formally brought to the global political stage in the form of the International Conference on Nutrition in Rome in 1992. From this conference emerged a World Declaration and Plan of Action, which continue to guide the development of national nutrition plans for many countries into the new millennium (see Exhibit 5–1).

It is possible to address only a limited number of public health nutrition problems in a treatise about known and emerging nutrition priorities in low-income countries. Still, several spheres of malnutrition that are motivating concern, research, and national and international response at the start of the twenty-first century are addressed. These include undernutrition and its components of protein-energy malnutrition and micronutrient deficiencies (specifically, of vitamin A, iron, iodine, and zinc) and their in-

teractions with infection and effects on health, human capacity, and survival; the roles of adequate breast- and complementary feeding in shaping healthy children and productive lives; and the diverse nutritional concerns among the adults, from undernutrition in older persons to the transition from under- to overnutrition in more affluent segments of rapidly developing societies. Throughout the chapter attention is drawn to approaches for prevention.

## THE NUTRITIONAL SPECTRUM

It should be kept in mind that the general definition of the term *malnutrition* does not differentiate undernutrition from overnutrition; thus, except when discussing "protein-energy malnutrition," the term *undernutrition* is used here predominantly to capture deficiencies in protein, energy, and micronutrients. It is recognized that there may be three separate groups of individuals in a population who are normal in nutriture, undernourished, and overnourished, as depicted

---

**Exhibit 5–1** Nutrition: A National Priority and Human Right

The International Conference on Nutrition (ICN) was organized by the Food and Agricultural Organization and World Health Organization and held in Rome in December 1992, attended by representatives of 159 countries from around the world to commit their states to the principles of a World Declaration and Plan of Action for Nutrition (Food and Agriculture Organization, 1992). Broad goals to which governments pledged were, before the year 2000, to eliminate (1) famine and famine-related deaths, (2) starvation and nutritional deficiency diseases in communities affected by natural and man-made disasters, and (3) iodine and vitamin A deficiencies. Countries were called upon to develop and implement national nutrition plans based on situational analyses within each country, using the ICN Plan of Action as a guide.

In retrospect, the ICN and the follow-up that has occurred have galvanized world opinion about the importance of nutrition in development, ag-

riculture, trade, health, security, and quality of life. It stimulated both government and private sectors to address formally issues such as food security; micronutrient malnutrition; nutritional vulnerability; dietary needs of pregnant women, their fetuses, and children; and older persons as they relate to human and national development. Through the ICN, national commitments were made to act on behalf of the malnourished. By 1996 national nutrition plans were being prepared or had been completed in 39 countries. Many had been adopted at the highest levels of state, reflecting a national commitment to ICN goals.

While the world fell short in meeting the literal goals of the ICN as the century turned, the momentum continues as governments refine plans and, increasingly, initiate programs. The ICN set the stage for a global movement in the 1990s to recognize adequate nutrition as a human right, which will be "tested" many times in the decades ahead.

in Figure 5–1, and that indicators of nutritional status are imperfect in identifying who and how many individuals are malnourished in a population. In the figure, the heavy line represents all individuals in a population. The more bell-shaped (dashed) curve represents the normative distribution of healthy individuals, some of whom would appear under- or overnourished by usual indicators of status, but are not. Malnutrition is represented by the other two distributions of individuals (that is, those who are deficient in energy, protein, essential fatty acids, or micronutrients, for example, and those who are overnourished, due to excessive intakes of energy and nutrients leading to obesity, toxicity, and so on), in relation to their requirements. In those two subgroups, the severity of malnutrition and associated morbidity presumably increases with distance from the norm (with intensity of shading). Drawing a cutoff through either tail of the overall distribution to estimate the extent of malnutrition (prevalence) or screen those at risk reveals the challenges facing nutritional assessment for purposes of estimating prevalence, screening, surveillance, and program evaluation.

## UNDERNUTRITION

Undernutrition combined with hunger, which is defined here as a chronic lack of adequate food to meet normal need, remains the most pervasive human malady in the world. Undernutrition is the result of a complex interaction between a diet that is chronically inadequate in protein, energy, and essential micronutrients and infection, modified by needs at certain stages of life (for example, periods of rapid growth during fetal life or early childhood, or periods of high nutritional demand, such as during pregnancy and lactation in women).

### Extent of Undernutrition

The magnitude of undernutrition can be gauged, globally and by region, by estimating the daily per capita availability of energy in the food supply, from national food balance sheets maintained by the Food and Agricultural Organization of the United Nations (Table 5–1) (United Nations Development Programme [UNDP], 1999); the prevalence and number of underweight, stunted, and wasted children (with abnormally low weight for age, height for age, and weight for height, respectively) (Table 5–2); and the prevalence and severity of micronutrient deficiencies (discussed later), based on national survey databases maintained by the World Health Organization (WHO) (ACC/SCN, 1996; De Onis, Monteiro, Akres, & Clugston, 1993; WHO, 1993, 1995a) and numerous other sources.

Unfortunately, regions are not always summarized along the same boundaries, making direct comparisons sometimes difficult. Nonetheless, Table 5–1 amply reflects the increased availability of food within most regions over a 26-year period (1970–1996), as well as the profound lack of increase in dietary energy in sub-Saharan Africa and "least developed countries," a group of 43 countries (23 in Africa) with lowest calculated values for the Human Development Index (HDI) and the Human Poverty Index (HPI) (UNDP, 1999).[*] Comparison of 1996 per capita daily energy supply data across regions suggests a high degree of food insecurity among sub-Saharan (2,205 kcal), South Asian (2,402 kcal) populations, and the group of least industrialized countries (2,095 kcal) compared to other advancing or industrialized regions of the world. Differences in protein availability parallel those of energy. The situation is even more bleak than suggested by balance sheet data, however, because average food (energy) availability is always greater than average intake, neither of which recognizes enormous disparities in food consumption across socioeconomic, cultural,

---

[*]The HDI is a score assigned by the United Nations Development Programme to each country based on life expectancy at birth, adult literacy, school enrollment, and gross domestic product; the HPI reflects quality of life issues such as longevity, knowledge/ literacy, economic well-being, and social inclusion (UNDP, 1999).

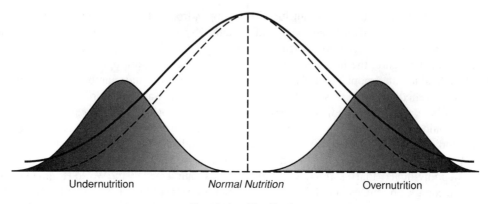

Undernutrition          *Normal Nutrition*          Overnutrition

**Population Distribution**

**Figure 5–1**  Spectrum of Nutritional Status in a Hypothetical Population

age, and gender strata within a country. Nor does food energy availability reflect adequacy of intakes of food sources of micronutrients that do not necessarily "track" dietary energy (Bouis & Novenario-Reese, 1997).

Food balance data point toward a dire and deteriorating food security situation, first and foremost in sub-Saharan Africa. The level of human stress is further accented by setbacks in life expectancy in countries such as Zimbabwe, Zambia, Botswana, and Uganda, largely due to the human immunodeficiency virus (HIV)/ acquired immune deficiency syndrome (AIDS)

epidemic (UNDP, 1999). Yet, a different impression of geographic need with respect to nutrition emerges when the prevalence of early childhood undernutrition, based on surveys of weight for age, height for age (stunting), and weight for height (wasting), are examined; these indicators are widely considered to be informative indexes of food adequacy and development (see below). These data show that the largest percentages and numbers of malnourished children reside in South Asia, where approximately 60% of pre-schoolers are estimated to be underweight and stunted, more than 15% wasted (Table 5–2).

**Table 5–1**  Energy and Protein Supply on a Per Capita Per Day Basis, by Region of the World

| Region | Energy Supply (kcal) | | Protein Supply (g) |
|---|---|---|---|
| | *1970* | *1996* | *1996* |
| Southern Asia | 2,094 | 2,402 | 58 |
| Southeast Asia | 1,957 | 2,659 | 62 |
| Sub-Saharan Africa | 2,226 | 2,205 | 53 |
| Arab States | 2,206 | 2,907 | 77 |
| East Asia | 2,033 | 2,862 | 76 |
| Latin America and Caribbean | 2,491 | 2,812 | 72 |
| Least developed countries* | 2,090 | 2,095 | 51 |
| Industrialized countries | 2,986 | 3,377 | 105 |
| World | 2,336 | 2,751 | 74 |

*Includes 43 countries based on UNDP indexes

**Table 5–2** Regional Estimates for the Prevalence and Numbers of Underweight, Stunted, and Wasted Children in Developing Countries, Ranked in Descending Order of Prevalence for Each Indicator

| | Underweight | | | Stunted | | | Wasted | |
|---|---|---|---|---|---|---|---|---|
| | % | No. (×10⁶) | | % | No. (×10⁶) | | % | No. (×10⁶) |
| South Asia | 61 | 101.2 | South Asia | 60 | 100.9 | South Asia | 17 | 28.9 |
| Southeast Asia | 33 | 21.8 | East Africa | 47 | 17.5 | West Africa | 10 | 3.5 |
| West Africa | 33 | 12.2 | Southeast Asia | 43 | 24.9 | Southeast Asia | 8 | 4.4 |
| East Africa | 31 | 11.5 | Melanesia | 42 | 0.3 | East Africa | 6 | 2.2 |
| Melanesia | 30 | 0.2 | West Africa | 38 | 14.1 | North Africa | 6 | 1.2 |
| East Asia | 21 | 26.0 | East Asia | 32 | 39.2 | Melanesia | 6 | 0 |
| Caribbean | 19 | 0.6 | Central America | 30 | 4.8 | Central America | 5 | 0.7 |
| Central America | 18 | 2.8 | Caribbean | 26 | 0.9 | East Asia | 4 | 4.4 |
| North Africa | 11 | 2.4 | North Africa | 25 | 5.5 | Caribbean | 2 | 0.1 |
| South America | 8 | 2.9 | South America | 18 | 6.4 | South America | 2 | 0.7 |

*Note:* Prevalence is the percentage below −2 standard normal deviates from the WHO/NCHS reference (median) value of weight for age (underweight), height for age (stunted), and weight for height (wasted), based on data from national surveys of children <6 years of age carried out from 1980–1992 in 79 countries.

In contrast, half these proportions of children are underweight and wasted, and two-thirds the proportion are stunted, in rural Africa. While the prevalence of childhood malnutrition is projected to continue to slowly decrease over the next 20 years, from approximately 180 million in the mid-1980s (ACC/SCN, 1992; De Onis et al., 1993) to approximately 135–150 million (Pinstrup-Andersen, Pandya-Lorch, & Rosegrant, 1997), the relative positions of sub-Saharan Africa and South Asia are to remain unchanged (James, 1998; Pinstrup-Andersen et al., 1997). From the Asian perspective, the paradox has been explained as the "Asian Enigma," whereby the relatively worse nutritional status of South Asian children, compared to African children, in the presence of seemingly more food, may be due to many factors unique to South Asia. These include a characteristically lower birthweight, in the region where approximately 75% of all births with intrauterine growth retardation (slow fetal growth manifested by a small size for gestational age) in the world occur (De Onis, Blossner, & Villar, 1998). Typically, South Asian infants are exposed to inadequate "exclusive" breastfeeding and late timing of complementary foods, occurring against a background of chronic undernutrition and profound neglect of the status of females throughout much of rural South Asia (Ramalingaswami, Jonsson, & Rohde, 1996). This inference is reinforced by differences in the rates of wasting among women, estimated to affect 30–50% versus 10–15% of women of reproductive age in South Asia and sub-Saharan Africa, respectively (ACC/SCN, 2000). From the African perspective, the paradox of exceedingly low food availability without apparent deterioration in nutritional status remains unexplained, perhaps reflecting, in part, widespread dependence on indigenous food crops not accounted for in the formal agricultural sector, and mortality of vulnerable groups due to the HIV/AIDS epidemic, festering civil wars, and periodic famines that grip the continent, which lowers the prevalence (proportion of the population affected) of undernutrition.

The nature of undernutrition varies in Latin America and the Caribbean, where young children tend to be mildly underweight and moderately stunted but not wasted (Table 5–2). Similarly, except for Haiti, where nearly 20% of women are wasted, national survey data suggest that only approximately 5% of women of reproductive age in this region have a low body mass index (<18.5), a ratio measure of body weight adequacy for a given height (that is, weight in kg ÷ height$^2$ in m). This percentage is comparable to that found among women in the United States (ACC/SCN, 2000). Rather, a tendency toward being overweight for height (with approximately 10% having a body mass index >30, versus >20% in the United States) is an emerging adult concern, providing evidence of a nutrition transition in this region (ACC/SCN, 2000; Popkin, 1998).

Under relatively intransigent conditions of food insecurity and poverty, undernutrition at the population level appears to persist within a given region, over time and across most vulnerable groups. Such persistence has been observed in United Nations' reports, for example, as a strong ecological correlation between the prevalence of low birthweight (% <2,500 g) and percent of preschool children with low weight for age (% <–2 Z-scores). Similar linear associations exist across regions in terms of the percent of low-weight women (<45 kg) and both the percent of low birthweight infants and underweight preschool children (ACC/SCN, 1992). The relative position for each region remains approximately the same for each comparison, with South Asia uniformly exhibiting the highest joint prevalences. The associations reflect "robust" differences between regions in the burden of undernutrition as well as a degree of "inertia" between generations within regions that must be overcome to improve nutritional status permanently in undernourished populations. The inertia is further reflected by familial correlations between preschool child and maternal size (height or weight) in low-income countries, r~0.3 (Hautvast et al., 2000; Lindtjorn & Alemu,

1997), that are similar to estimates obtained in industrialized countries (Mueller, 1986), despite the marked left displacement of the former on the nutritional spectrum. Although these relationships are expressed anthropometrically, micronutrient deficiencies, at least in terms of their severity, can also be expected to cluster by region and over time. The health consequences associated with undernutrition are considered next.

## Undernutrition as a Risk Factor for Infection and Related Mortality

Undernutrition must be considered as a possible risk factor for infectious morbidity and associated case-fatality among children in low-income countries. As gestational age and size for gestation age are possibly correlated with nutritional status during early childhood, it is appropriate to consider these as part of a continuum of possible risk. Nevertheless, studies have generally examined separately the risk related to status at birth in the neonatal or infant period and the risk related to nutritional status throughout childhood, at least up to age 5 years.

### Low\ Birthweight

Low birthweight is usually defined as weight at birth less than 2,500 grams (approximately 5 lb. 14 oz.). The incidence of low weight births varies inversely with level of economic development (ACC/SCN, 1992), as does the proportion of these births that is due to fetal malnutrition (that is, intrauterine growth retardation) versus preterm delivery of less than 37 weeks gestation (De Onis et al., 1998). Intrauterine growth retardation is usually defined as a birth that is more than 2 standard deviations (SDs) below the median weight expected for that gestational age (or, alternatively but not equivalently, <10th percentile). The rate of low birthweight deliveries in low- and middle-income countries ranges from approximately 10% in most countries in Latin American to 30–50% in South Asian coun-

tries (De Onis et al., 1998). In settings with a high incidence of low birthweight, two-thirds or more of these low weight births are due to intrauterine growth retardation. In settings with a low incidence of low birthweight, most are due to preterm delivery.

To examine the role of nutritional risk factors for morbidity and mortality, it is important to evaluate births that have intrauterine growth retardation. Unfortunately, many of the studies provide information only on low birthweight births rather than distinguish these by the cause of the low weight. Low birthweight babies have the largest increase in risk during the neonatal period, and they continue to have additional risk in the postneonatal period of infancy. In high-income countries, birthweights of 3,500–4,500 grams (7 lb. 11 oz.–9 lb. 14 oz.) are associated with the lowest risk of neonatal mortality. The relative risk of neonatal mortality increases with birthweights below 2,500 grams and increases even more for very low birthweight babies of less than 1,500 grams (3 lb. 3 oz.) (Ashworth, 1998). In low-income countries, the data are more limited due to the difficulty of obtaining accurate birthweight measurements for deliveries that are predominantly in the home. In most low-income country populations, at least 20–40% of births are classified as low birthweight, which appears to be predominantly due to intrauterine growth retardation. In these settings the neonatal mortality rates range to 50 deaths per 1,000 live births and increase with decreasing birthweight. In two studies that were able to cross-classify births by nutritional status for gestational age (to determine if the birth had intrauterine growth retardation) and gestational age, the results varied substantially. In Brazil babies with intrauterine growth retardation had a five-fold increase in the risk of death (Barros, Victora, Vaughan, Teixeira, & Ashworth, 1987), while in Bangladesh the increased risk was only slightly increased (El-Arifeen, 1997). During the postneonatal period, low weight births continued to have higher mortality than babies born with a higher weight. Again the data are limited, but in Brazil babies born with intrauterine growth retardation had a fourfold increase in postneonatal mortality, and such births in Bangladesh had about a 50% increase in postneonatal deaths (Barros et al., 1987; El-Arifeen, 1997).

Because of the importance of diarrhea and pneumonia as causes of death in children in low-income countries, a few studies have evaluated whether low birthweight confers additional risk for deaths from these two causes. In three studies in low-income countries, the increased risk of diarrheal deaths during infancy was 2.5–2.8-fold for low birthweight babies (Ashworth & Feachem, 1985). Likewise, the risks of death from acute lower respiratory infections were increased, but with more variability with a relative risk ranging from 1.6 to 8.0 (Victora et al., 1999).

As might be expected from these studies of infant mortality, low birthweight has also been shown to be a risk factor for diarrheal and respiratory morbidity (Ashworth & Feachem, 1985; Victora et al., 1999). Studies in Papua New Guinea (Bukenya, Barnes, & Nwokolo, 1991), Thailand (Ittiravivongs, Songchitratna, Ratthapalo, & Pattara-Arechachai, 1991), and Brazil (Victora, Barros, Kirkwood, & Vaughan, 1990) found a relative risk adjusted for other possible determinants of illness ranging from 1.6 to 3.9 for acute diarrhea. Studies in China (Chen, Yu, & Li, 1988), Argentina (Cerquerio, Murtagh, Halac, Avila, & Weissenbacher, 1990), and Brazil (Victora et al., 1990; Victora, Smith, Barros, Vaughan, & Fuchs, 1989) found a relative risk ranging from 1.4 to 2.2 for acute lower respiratory infection or pneumonia hospitalization.

The consequences of low birthweight, however, may extend into adulthood. In recent years, it has been hypothesized that nutritional insult during fetal life, reflected by intrauterine growth retardation, may lead to increased risk of coronary heart disease (Barker, Osmond, Winter, Margetts, & Simmonds, 1989), hypertension (Barker, Bull, Osmond, & Simmonds, 1990), and diabetes (Hales et al., 1991). While studies

to date have been unable to explain such associations by confounding socioeconomic and dietary influences (Leon, 1998), the hypothesis remains controversial (Joseph & Kramer, 1996). In the Gambia, however, the risk of all-cause mortality in a cohort of individuals more than 14.5 years of age, followed from birth, was fourfold greater among individuals born during the preharvest "hungry" than in the postharvest season. Death beyond 25 years of age was 10 times more likely among individuals born during the hungry season (Moore et al., 1999). Most known causes of death were reportedly infectious-related causes. The etiological importance of maternal undernutrition in hungry season low birthweight incidence has been confirmed by low maternal weight gain and birthweight (Prentice, Whitehead, Watkinson, Lamb, & Cole, 1983), and the responsiveness of birthweight and neonatal survival to maternal supplementation with food (providing approximately 1,000 kcal per day) in this season (Ceesay et al., 1997). Both seasonal birth cohorts were comparable in nutritional status in their second year of life, however, suggesting a latent effect of gestational insult on subsequent health and survival. It has been hypothesized that intrauterine or early postnatal undernutrition may leave an "imprint" on an individual, for example through defects of thymic and other lymphoid tissues at critical developmental periods that could impair host resistance to infection (Moore et al., 1999; Prentice, 1998) or otherwise predispose individuals to disease (Barker et al., 1989; Leon, 1998) later in life.

### Childhood Undernutrition

This section focuses on the risk of infectious disease and related mortality in early childhood as a function of anthropometric status, as risk from micronutrient deficiency is considered separately in the chapter. It is clear that severe malnutrition carries a risk of death, but it is the potentially causal interaction of undernutrition with common infectious diseases in low-income countries that is of far greater importance. It has long been postulated that there is a "synergy" between undernutrition and infectious diseases in which the combination of these conditions results in much greater mortality than either independently (Scrimshaw, Taylor, & Gordon, 1967). This appears to be because infectious diseases are more severe in undernourished children and carry a higher case fatality rate, although an increased incidence of infectious diseases may also play some role.

A review of the observational studies of anthropometric status as a risk factor for child mortality in low-income countries demonstrated that each level of worsening weight for age below the international median is associated with increased mortality (Figure 5–2) (Pelletier, Frongillo, & Habicht, 1993). Similar increases in mortality risk have been observed with decrements in mid-upper arm circumference (MUAC), adjusted (Sommer & Loewenstein, 1975) or unadjusted (Briend, Wojtyniak, & Rowland, 1987; Briend & Zimicki, 1986; West et al., 1991) for height, across all preschool ages, including early infancy once arm size is adjusted for age (De Vaquera, Townsend, Arroyo, & Lechtig, 1983; West et al., 1991). Stunting early in life (<3 years), adjusted for wasting, carries a disproportionate risk of mortality (Katz, West, Tarwotjo, & Sommer, 1989; Smedman, Sterky, Mellander, & Wall, 1987).

It is important to note that even mild undernutrition puts a child at increased risk of mortality. Since the greatest number of undernourished children have mild to moderate rather than severe malnutrition, most of the excess risk of death is attributable to the less severe forms of undernutrition. Also important is the observation that with worsening levels of weight for age the mortality rate increases logarithmically (Figure 5–2). Across studies, children were estimated to experience an approximately 7% compound increase in risk of dying for every percent decrease in weight for age below the referent median (Pelletier et al., 1993), suggesting the absence of an often posited "threshold" phenomenon (Pelletier, 1994). The effect is consistent, however, with the postulated synergistic interaction between nutrition and infection, as nearly all the deaths are due to infectious diseases. It was suggested that 56% of all childhood deaths could be explained by the potentiating effects of undernutrition on infectious morbidity, 83% of which could be expected among children with mild-to-moderate malnutrition (Pelletier et al., 1993). The implication of this estimate is illustrated in Figure 5–3. Thus reductions in mortality may be achieved either through improving nutritional status or by reducing the incidence or case fatality from infectious diseases; however, improvements in both at the same time would be expected to have a synergetic benefit. In addition, improving nutritional well-being to reduce these excess deaths will require approaches that correct underlying inequities in impoverished communities through broad-based programs that improve food security and diets (or nutrient intakes through fortification) since poor screening specificity (that correctly excludes large numbers of children unlikely to die) in a mildly to moderately malnourished population could overwhelm targeted nutrition programs.

Diarrheal diseases and pneumonia are the two most important causes of death in children under five years of age in low-income countries. These two conditions have a higher case fatality rate in undernourished children compared to those who are well nourished. For example, malnourished children who were discharged from a hospital after treatment for diarrheal illness in Bangladesh had a 14-fold greater risk of dying comparing with better nourished controls (Roy, Chowdhury, & Rahaman, 1983). In a community-based study in rural India, severely malnourished children had a 24-fold higher diarrheal case fatality rate compared with better nourished children (Bhandari, Bhan, & Sazawal, 1992) and, in Mexico, undernourished children had an 8-fold greater risk of death with severe diarrhea (Tome, Reyes, Rodriguez, Guiscafre, & Gutierrez, 1996). Studies in the Philippines (Tupasi et al., 1990), Papua New Guinea (Shann, Barker, & Poore, 1989), Bangladesh (Rahman et al., 1990), and Argentina (Weissenbacher et al., 1990) ) of acute lower respiratory infection and pneumonia found a 2- to 3-fold increase in case fatality

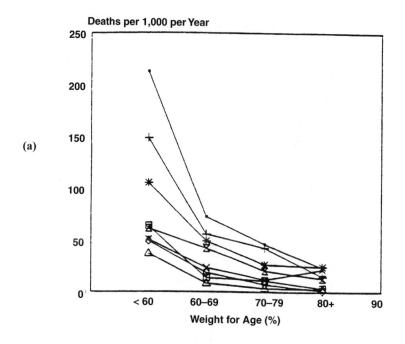

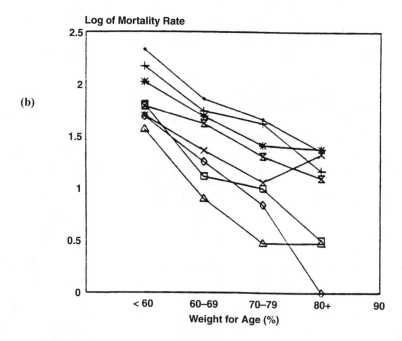

**Figure 5–2** Association between Weight for Age and Risk of Mortality among Children 6 to 59 Months of Age at Baseline, Followed for Periods of 6 to 24 Months, in 8 Longitudinal Population Studies in Six Countries, Ordered from Highest to Lowest at <60% Weight for Age: Tanzania, Papua New Guinea, Malawi, Bangladesh, India, and Indonesia. Panel (a): mortality rate by study; panel (b): log mortality rate per 1,000 children per year by study.

Country

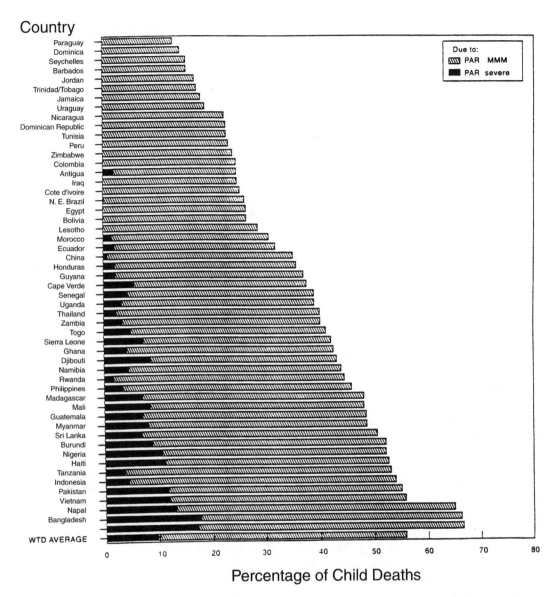

**Percentage of Child Deaths**

**Figure 5–3** Population-Attributable Risk (PAR) of Preschool Child Death Due to the Potentiating Effects of Mild to Moderate Malnutrition (MMM) and Severe Malnutrition on Infectious Disease in 53 Countries

rate in undernourished versus better nourished children.

Prospective studies to evaluate the role of undernutrition, assessed by anthropometry, in predisposing children to cause-specific mortality have found a progressively increased risk with worsening nutritional status. For example, in the Philippines the risk of mortality for diarrhea and acute lower respiratory infections nearly doubled with each one unit decrease in weight for age Z-score (Yoon, Black, Moulton, & Becker, 1997). Likewise, in Brazil pneumonia mortality was found to increase by a factor of 4 to 5, even in children who were below the median but above –2 Z-score weight for age (explained below), whereas children who were below –2 Z-score had a 21-fold increase in pneumonia mortality (Victora et al., 1989).

It has long been observed that measles has been associated with undernutrition in children in low-income countries. This association and the apparent higher case fatality rate for measles in malnourished children led many to conclude that there was again a synergistic relationship. More recently some investigators have questioned this interpretation. Studies, particularly from West Africa, have not found an increased risk of illness, greater severity of illness, or risk of death from measles in malnourished children (Aaby, 1988). These investigators found that a determining factor in measles severity is the intensity of the exposure to the measles virus; for example, secondary cases exposed in the home have more intense exposure than sporadic cases that are presumably infected in the community. Frequent association between malnutrition and crowding in the home, poor health services utilization (that is, measles immunization) and thus longer sibling exposure to the virus, may partly explain a measles-malnutrition relationship, where observed (Aaby, 1988). While the role of undernutrition, as assessed by anthropometry, in measles mortality is in question, the observation in several African settings that vitamin A supplementation during acute measles can substantially reduce the severity and case fatality of measles (Barclay, Foster, & Sommer, 1987; Coutsoudis, Kiepiela, Coovadia, & Broughton, 1992; Hussey & Klein, 1990) still speaks for the importance of nutritional risk factors in affecting survival from measles.

The role of undernutrition in predisposing children to malaria is also controversial. Early observations from the nineteenth century reported that malaria was more frequent in those with inadequate diets or with undernutrition (Garnham, 1954). However, studies in the latter part of the twentieth century appeared to show that malnutrition could be actually protective for malaria. This was based on observational studies (Hendrickse, Hasan, Olumide, & Akinkunmi,

1971) or on interventions such as the refeeding of famine victims (Murray, Murray, Murray, & Murray, 1975) in which an exacerbation of malaria appeared to occur. Animal studies seemed to support the suppressive effects of a poor diet on malaria leading to the belief that undernourished children are less susceptible to the infection and consequences of malaria. More recent studies, however, indicate strongly that the relationship between nutritional status and malaria is complex and that undernutrition serves as a risk factor for increased malaria mortality and morbidity (Shankar et al., 1997). Additional studies indicate that specific micronutrients, such as vitamin A, zinc, iron, and others, affect the risk of infection and severity of illness with malaria as well (discussed below). While it is now believed that undernutrition is a risk factor for malaria, it is also a consistent observation that refeeding a malaria-infected, starved host can reactivate the low-grade infection that could make it more severe. One implication is that antimalarial measures should be included during nutritional rehabilitation of famine victims who are likely to have malaria infection.

Nutritional status has been assessed widely as a risk factor for the severity and incidence of diarrheal diseases. As might be expected with the reported higher case fatality rate in undernourished children, there is an association with disease severity. One measure of this is the duration of the illness. In studies in several countries, the duration of diarrhea in mild to moderately malnourished children was shown to be up to 3-fold longer than for better nourished (Black, Brown, & Becker, 1984b). Undernutrition is also an important risk factor for the occurrence of persistent diarrhea (Baqui et al., 1993). This relationship has also been demonstrated for specific types of diarrhea such as episodes due to *Shigella species* and enterotoxigenic *Escherichia coli* where the illness duration in Bangladeshi children was 2.5-fold longer in undernourished children (Black, Brown, & Becker, 1984b). Poorer nutritional status has also been documented to be associated with increased rate of stool output in children, leading to an increased risk of dehydration (Black et al., 1984). These mechanisms likely explain the increased risk for hospitalization and length of hospital stay due to diarrhea in undernourished children (Man et al., 1998; Victora et al., 1990). The effect of undernutrition on diarrheal incidence has been more variable in different settings. Some studies show no increased risk of overall incidence while others have found a 30–70% increased risk of incident diarrhea in undernourished children (Black et al., 1984; El Samani, Willett, & Ware, 1986; Guerrant, Schorling, McAuliffe, & de Souza, 1992). Some enteropathogens causing diarrhea, such as *Cryptosporidium parvum*, may be particularly selected as a cause of infection in undernourished children (Checkley et al., 1998).

The role of undernutrition as a risk factor for severity or incidence of acute lower respiratory infections or pneumonia has also received extensive study. Evidence would support an association between undernutrition and severity of respiratory infection, with such associations being found in both hospital-based and community-based studies. Undernutrition has been found to increase the likelihood that a child will have bacteremia, pleural effusion, and other complications (Johnson, Aderele, & Gbadero, 1992). Studies in the Philippines, Costa Rica (James, 1972), or Brazil (Fonseca et al., 1996; Victora et al., 1989) found a modestly increased incidence of acute lower respiratory infections in undernourished children, but studies in Papua New Guinea (Smith, Lehman, Coakley, Spooner, & Alpers, 1991), Uruguay (Selwyn, 1990), and Guatemala (Cruz et al., 1990) did not find any relationship. One study in the Gambia found that the development of pneumococcal infection was associated with a history of poor weight gain prior to the illness compared with other children in the community (O'Dempsey et al., 1996). At this point, it appears that undernutrition is consistently associated with increased severity and complications of illness, as well as case fatality, and in some settings may also be associated with a modestly increased incidence of these infections.

## Contributions of Infection to Undernutrition

Infections in childhood have long been recognized to influence physical growth and rates of malnutrition among children in low- and middle-income countries. After initial observation of the relationship, more recent work has assessed the size of this effect and moderating influences. This has been done largely in prospective community-based studies, which use intensive surveillance to assess episodes of illness and growth performance. These studies examined the most frequent childhood infectious diseases, especially diarrhea and respiratory diseases. Some have assessed the effects of measles, malaria, and other infections, such as those of the skin. It is clear from the studies to date that infectious morbidity, particularly diarrheal disease, has an important effect on weight gain (Table 5–3). A similar effect on linear growth was generally observed in these studies.

The negative effect of diarrhea on weight and often height gain of children during and after an episode of acute diarrhea has been documented in diverse low-income country settings. Nevertheless, the magnitude of the effect on growth faltering has varied widely in these studies (Black, Brown, & Becker, 1983). Some studies, such as those in Guatemala (Martorell, Yarbrough, Lechtig, Habicht, & Klein, 1975), Mexico (Condon-Paoloni, Joaquin, Johnston, deLicardi, & Scholl, 1977), and Bangladesh (Black et al., 1984a) have reported that 10% to 24% of the growth faltering could be explained statistically by the prevalence of diarrhea, whereas studies in other countries such as Uganda (Cole & Parkin, 1977), the Gambia (Rowland, Cole, & Whitehead, 1977), and Sudan (Zumrawi, Dimond, & Waterlow, 1987) have reported that diarrhea could explain as much as 40–80% of observed faltering. In nearly all instances, these percentages of growth faltering explained by diarrhea were higher than those explained by other infectious diseases, again demonstrating the quantitative importance of the diarrhea-growth faltering relationship. Infec-

**Table 5–3** Reported Effects of Pediatric Infectious Diseases on Weight Gain from Prospective Studies in Selected Developing Countries

| Country | Diarrhea | Respiratory | Malaria | Measles | Other |
|---|---|---|---|---|---|
| Bangladesh | yes | no | — | — | no |
| Bangladesh | yes | — | — | — | — |
| Brazil | yes | no | — | — | — |
| Colombia | yes | — | — | — | — |
| The Gambia | yes | no | yes | — | no |
| The Gambia | yes | yes | no | — | no |
| Guatemala | yes | no | — | — | — |
| Guatemala | yes | — | — | — | — |
| Mexico | yes | no | — | — | — |
| The Philippines | yes | yes | — | — | — |
| Sudan | yes | yes | — | — | — |
| Taiwan | no | no | — | — | — |
| Tanzania | — | — | yes | — | — |
| Uganda | yes | no | no | yes | no |
| Zimbabwe | no | — | — | — | — |

tious diseases generally result in poorer weight gain or weight loss, which may be due to loss of appetite (Brown, Black, Robertson, & Becker, 1985) or increased metabolism. With diarrhea there may also be intentional withholding of food, as well as malabsorption of ingested food in the damaged intestine (Behrens, Lunn, Northrop, Hanlon, & Neale, 1987; Lunn, Northrop-Clewes, & Downes, 1991). Variation in these factors may explain some of the differences in the magnitude of effect in various low-income country settings, but it is necessary also to consider factors such as the etiology of diarrhea, the age pattern of infection, feeding pattern and dietary intake, treatment practices, and the length of the convalescent period.

Few studies have examined the differential effect of diarrhea due to specific etiologic agents on growth. In Bangladesh, enterotoxigenic *Escherichia coli* and *Shigella species* had the strongest effects on growth, while rotavirus and other enteropathogens, in part due to their lower prevalence, did not have a significant effect (Black et al., 1984a). The seasonal pattern of particular enteropathogens causing diarrhea may explain part of the seasonality in growth seen in some low-income country settings. In regard to clini-

cal syndromes, it has been noted that dysentery (that is, bloody diarrhea) or persistent diarrhea (that is, defined by the World Health Organization as an episode lasting >14 days) have particularly important adverse effects on the growth of children (Black, 1993). As one might expect, the magnitude of the weight deficit is inversely related to the duration of the diarrheal episode. Persistent diarrheal episodes usually occur in children who also have, in general, a higher burden of diarrhea, so that both the persistent episodes and the high prevalence of diarrhea adversely affect growth.

Asymptomatic as well as symptomatic infections can have an adverse effect on growth. Infection with *C. parvum,* with or without illness, in Peruvian children was associated with a reduction in weight gain, controlling for other variables (Checkley et al., 1998). Even though the effect size was lower with asymptomatic infections than with symptomatic ones, because of their higher prevalence asymptomatic infections had a greater overall impact on growth than symptomatic infections. Children after illness have the potential to grow more rapidly than they were growing previously; this is known as "catch-up growth." Children with a *C. parvum* infection in the first six months of life did not have catch-up growth, showing that there was a long-lasting adverse effect on linear growth, whereas children with infections at an older age did have some catch-up growth.

The feeding practices of a child at the time of illness can modify the effect of diarrhea on growth. Infants who are exclusively or predominantly breastfeeding experience less adverse effects of diarrhea (Launer, Habicht, & Kardjati, 1990). This may be because breastfeeding ameliorates the severity of the illness or because breastfeeding generally seems to be continued without reduction in most circumstances during illness (Brown et al., 1985; Hoyle, Yunus, & Hen, 1980), whereas other foods may be reduced due to medical or cultural practices or anorexia because of the illness. Aside from studies mentioned previously showing that infection with certain pathogens early in life may adversely affect growth (Checkley et al., 1998), the effect of diarrheal disease in the first 6 months of life is generally less than the effects observed at older ages. Thus children in the first 6 months of life who are exclusively or predominantly breastfed may have less severe consequences of diarrhea or other infectious diseases (Khin-Maung-U et al., 1985; Launer et al., 1990; Rowland, Rowland, & Cole, 1988).

There is also a modifying effect of diet on the relationship between diarrhea and growth (Brown et al., 1988). Diarrhea has a lesser effect among children whose usual dietary intake is greater or of better quality, or among children who receive food supplements, compared to children with poorer diets or those not receiving food supplements in the same setting (Lutter et al., 1989).

Appropriate treatment of diarrheal illnesses may reduce the adverse effects of diarrhea on growth. The replacement of fluid and electrolytes with oral rehydration therapy may restore appetite and improve bowel function. Also, continued feeding during the illness has been demonstrated in clinical trials to result in improved weight gain in comparison to partial withholding of food during the acute phase (Brown et al., 1988). While antibiotics are not necessary for most cases of acute diarrhea, appropriate antibiotic treatment of dysentery would be expected to shorten the illness and, therefore, the period of adverse effects on growth.

Catch-up growth seems possible without specific supplementary feeding programs, due to the child's increased consumption of available food; however, some diarrheal disease control programs recommend additional feeding in the convalescent period after illness. Unfortunately, the opportunity for catch-up growth may be limited by the duration of the healthy period between illnesses. Studies in Bangladesh (Black et al., 1983) and Zimbabwe (Moy, Marshall, Choto, McNeish, & Booth, 1994) have shown that it requires about 2 weeks following diarrhea for children to recover to their pre-illness weight and about 4 weeks to grow to the weight expected if these children had continued the rate of growth that they had prior to the illness. Another illness occurring during this month-long convalescent period may result in insufficient time for catch-up growth to occur and could add additional nutritional insult. The net effect in the long term is a reduction in both ponderal and linear growth.

Acute respiratory infections, predominantly upper respiratory infections, have a high prevalence worldwide. Children in low-income countries, while having a similar prevalence of upper respiratory infections as children in more industrialized countries, have a substantially higher rate of acute lower respiratory infections or pneumonia (Graham, 1990). Most of the studies of the effect of acute respiratory infections on growth have included both upper and lower respiratory infections and have generally not found an effect of the illnesses on growth. In a Gambian study, children under two years of age with acute lower respiratory infections diagnosed by a pediatrician had a loss of 14.7 grams of weight per day of illness, slightly but not significantly greater than the reduction observed with diarrheal diseases (Rowland et al., 1988). However, the prevalence of diarrhea was much higher than that of acute lower respiratory infections, so that diarrheal diseases explained one-half and respiratory infections only one-quarter of the observed weight deficit. Other studies in the Philippines (Adair et al., 1993), Papua New Guinea (Smith et al., 1991), Guatemala (Cruz et al., 1990), and Brazil (Victora et al., 1990) have also indicated that acute lower respiratory infections adversely affected growth.

Acute respiratory illnesses have been shown to be associated with a 10% to 20% reduction in food intake, possibly due to a reduction in the child's appetite (Brown et al., 1985; Mata, Cromal, Urrutia, & Garcia, 1977). As with other illnesses, catabolism may also play a role. Further studies are required to assess the magnitude of the adverse effects of acute lower respiratory infections on growth and to document if there are modifying factors, as there appear to be with diarrheal diseases.

A few studies have attempted to document whether malaria has an adverse effect on growth in children in low-income countries. In the Gambia malaria prevalence adversely affected weight gain but not linear growth (Rowland et al., 1977). Subsequent studies in Uganda (Cole & Parkin, 1977) and the Gambia (Rowland et al., 1988) were not able to demonstrate an effect of malaria on the growth of children.

Although it has been believed for many years that measles causes a reduction in growth, this has been difficult to document on a population basis. This is in part because of the low incidence of measles found in prospective studies, which in some cases was due to the administration of measles vaccine in the study cohort. Older studies suggest that children with measles lose weight or have reduced growth velocity (Reddy, 1991), but measles has been best recognized as an illness that precipitates severe clinical forms of malnutrition. In children with previous undernutrition, measles can precipitate kwashiorkor or marasmus (DeMaeyer & Adiels-Tegman, 1985), as well as xerophthalmia (Sommer, 1982). Measles can also predispose to subsequent diarrhea and pneumonia, which will have additional adverse effects on nutritional status.

Intestinal helminthic infections, especially with *Acaris lumbricoides*, in children in low- and middle-income countries have been associated with poor growth (Rousham & Mascie-Taylor, 1994). In such populations, periodic deworming of children using a mass treatment approach has been demonstrated to improve growth (Adams, Stephenson, Latham, & Kinoti, 1994; Stoltzfus et al., 1998; Willett, Kilama, & Kihamia, 1979). Because children are reinfected rapidly after treatment, such approaches should be routine and combined with environmental sanitation and hygiene education.

## Conceptual Models Related to Undernutrition

From the foregoing, it is clear that poor growth and undernutrition adversely affect child health and survival. In recent years two conceptual models have been proposed to help visualize the continuum of undernutrition, its complex causation and consequences. The first proposes a sequence of life events during which undernutrition may interact with infection, care, and other factors, throughout life and across generations (Figure 5–4). In this model, surviving infants who may be growth-retarded and developmentally delayed due to undernutrition face increased nutritional, health, and developmental risks throughout childhood, adolescence, the reproductive years (for women, with implications for offspring), and older years of life (ACC/SCN, 2000). It identifies various times in the life cycle where malnutrition may occur and what outcomes may be altered by effective and timely intervention.

The second conceptual design is a slight modification of a well-known UNICEF model (Figure 5–5) that attempts to hierarchically link effects of diverse basic (or root), underlying, and immediate causes of malnutrition into a unified causal framework (UNICEF, 1997). Implied in this organization is the fact that there is no single cause of malnutrition. Rather, malnutrition results from a set of interacting causes that vary in intensity, duration, specificity, and proximity to the individual. These may be viewed as "component causes" (Rothman & Greenland,

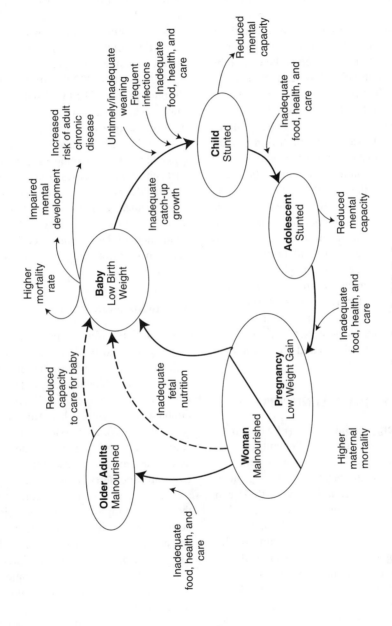

**Figure 5–4** Conceptual Model of the Effects of Undernutrition throughout the Life Cycle

1998). Which are operating, and how they interact, determine the type and severity of malnutrition, the health or functional consequences, and offer insight into prevention. The level of risk associated with any one cause depends on the presence and strength of other factors acting in the causal path. For example, corneal xerophthalmia, a manifestation of severe vitamin A deficiency (Sommer, 1995), could be caused by the joint impact of a diet chronically inadequate in vitamin A (Tarwotjo, Sommer, Soegiharto, Susanto, & Muhilal, 1982), multiple previous episodes of infection that drain nutrient stores (Sommer, 1982), wasting malnutrition reflecting protein-energy depletion that may restrict mobilization of vitamin A (Sommer, 1982; Gopalan, Venkatachalam, & Bhavani, 1960), and a precipitating episode of measles (Foster & Sommer, 1987). These immediate causes could result from entitlement failure in a household (Sen, 1992), leading to nonavailability of nutritious complementary foods, neglect to be immunized against measles, and inaccessibility to a health center for treatment or earlier prophylaxis (underlying causes), and so on. Correction of any one of these factors could interrupt a particular causal path and prevent corneal destruction.

## PROTEIN-ENERGY MALNUTRITION

Protein-energy malnutrition (PEM) constitutes a spectrum of pathological conditions arising from chronic deficiencies in protein and energy to meet requirements for tissue growth, function, maintenance, and activity. PEM can range from clinically inapparent, chronic undernutrition, usually only discerned by anthropometric criteria but carrying measurable public health risk (Figure 5–2), to an acute clinical syndrome, manifest by extreme muscle wasting and fat loss that characterizes marasmus to edema, skin, hair, liver, and other classic changes associated with kwashiorkor (DeMaeyer, 1976). The condition results from an insufficient protein and energy-dense diet (primary PEM); impaired

absorption, digestion, or use of dietary constituents due to other disease (secondary PEM); or a combination of the two. Although micronutrient deficiencies contribute to suboptimal growth (Allen, 1994; Brown, Peerson, & Allen, 1998), primary PEM is considered to be the dominant cause of depressed child growth leading to high proportions of underweight, stunted, and wasted children in the low-income countries (Table 5–2) (ACC/SCN, 2000; Waterlow, 1972, 1973). Chronic, primary PEM is also the likely cause of low-weight prevalence observed among women of reproductive age in low-income countries (ACC/SCN, 1992). Secondary PEM, on the other hand, may develop as a complication of gastrointestinal diseases (for example, diarrhea or dysentery), severe trauma or surgery, and other medical conditions. Commonly found in hospital settings, secondary PEM is a frequent component of the "vicious cycle," or interaction, between nutrition and infection (Scrimshaw et al., 1967).

### Mild to Moderate PEM

It is difficult, if not impossible, to distinguish primary, mild-to-moderate PEM from general, mild-to-moderate undernutrition, with its numerous dietary, biochemical, and socioeconomic correlates (Ahmed et al., 1991, 1992, 1993; Graham & Cordano, 1969; Hussain, Lindtjorn, & Kvale, 1996). At this level of PEM, clinical signs are few, mild, and unreliable, causing its assessment to rely almost entirely on comparative anthropometry, most frequently based on measurements of weight, stature, and arm size that usually employ age and, occasionally, gender-specific and locally derived, normative, reference criteria (Frisancho, 1981; WHO, 1995). The aspect of malnutrition of interest and the purpose of assessment (for example, to estimate prevalence, screen for intervention, monitor a situation) will guide the most appropriate choice of indicator(s) with which to assess protein-energy status (Habicht, Meyers, & Brownie, 1982; Habicht & Pelletier, 1990). Anthropometric pro-

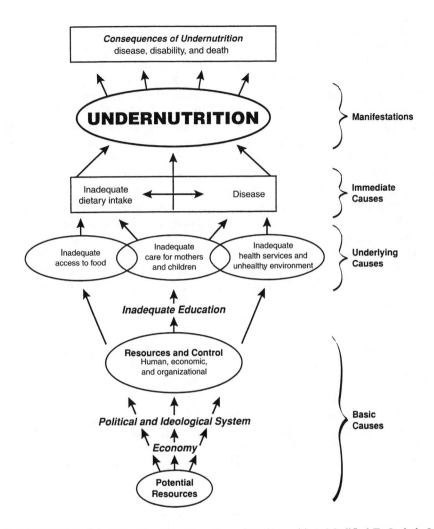

**Figure 5–5** UNICEF Conceptual Model of the Causation of Undernutrition, Modified To Include Its Consequences

cedures are well-standardized for obtaining reliable measures of weight, length, height, MUAC, and skinfolds (Cameron, 1978; Gibson, 1990; Lohman, Roche, & Martorell, 1988).

Measurement of child length (<2 yr.) or height (>2 yr.), compared against a referent value for age, reveals the adequacy of linear growth (Hamill et al., 1979; WHO, 1995). "Stunting," discerned by a child's stature being, say, two standard normal deviates (Z-scores) below the

median of a referent distribution, is taken to represent the effects of chronic PEM (Waterlow et al., 1977). Wasting, which is revealed by a child's weight being <1 or 2 Z-scores below the reference median weight for height, identifies acute PEM (Waterlow et al., 1977). Because growth deceleration is a gradual process, stunting is often associated with other indicators of poverty and neglect (Martorell, Mendoza, & Castillo, 1988). MUAC, which detects a thin arm, is an alternative indicator of wasting (Jelliffe, 1966; WHO, 1995) that, when used with tricipital skinfold measurement to calculate upper arm muscle and fat areas, provides a relative measure of body composition (Frisancho, 1981; Heymsfield, McManus, Stevens, & Smith, 1982; Trowbridge, Hiner, & Robertson, 1981; West, 1986). Although interpreted as an acute condition, wasting can also persist for long periods of time. Ponderal or weight change, on the other hand, is the sum effect of bone growth and soft tissue accretion (or loss). This means that a low weight for age, alone, cannot reliably distinguish between stunting and wasting. Consideration of both of these aspects of PEM provides useful information about the long-standing and current nutritional status of individuals and communities. Still, growth monitoring that requires only weight to be routinely plotted on a growth chart (Morley, 1976), as widely practiced throughout the low-income countries (Ruel, Rivera, & Habicht, 1995), can permit detection of early growth deviance and malnutrition in primary care settings (Ruel et al., 1990; Tulchinsky, Acker, El Malki, Socolar, & Reshef, 1985), although for many reasons related to implementation, this has not been effectively done (George, Latham, Abel, Ethirajan, & Frongillo, 1993; Hendrata & Rohde, 1988; Martorell & Shekar, 1994).

Typically, estimates of the prevalence of malnutrition are derived by calculating the percentage of children below indicator cutoffs (Table 5–4). This was originally proposed by Gomez for classifying children according to categories in weight for age, expressed as a percent of a reference median (Gomez et al., 1956). This indicator, however, fails to place a child's weight in the context of a distribution of normal weight values. The use of standard normal deviates, or Z-scores, has become the convention for comparing the nutritional status of children against a referent population distribution (Waterlow et al., 1977). In addition to the use of cutoffs, which provide empirical estimates of prevalence, estimates of the percentage of children whose status lies outside the referent distribution ("standard-

ized prevalence") can also be calculated (Figure 5–6) (Mora, 1989; WHO, 1995). Under reasonable assumptions of normality of referent and test population anthropometric values, the standardized prevalence provides a valid estimate of the total burden of malnutrition as it adjusts for proportions of false negatives and false positives not accounted for in a cutoff-based estimate. However, it cannot be used to screen individuals or estimate the prevalence at degrees of severity (Mora, 1989). Discrepancies between estimators lessen with greater separation of the malnourished from the referent population (Yip & Scanlon, 1994). The "standardized" approach was first proposed for assessing the prevalence of anemia (Cook et al., 1971; Meyers, Habicht, Johnson, & Brownie, 1973; Yip, 1994).

Regions of the world differ markedly by their levels of wasting and stunting PEM (Table 5–2) and by the degree to which these indicators covary within populations. For example, the prevalences of both (based on cutoffs) are highly correlated across populations of South Asia but lack any ecological relationship throughout Africa or Latin America, where far less wasting is found (Victora, 1992). Perhaps not unexpectedly, prevalences of stunting and wasting PEM vary in their ability to predict preschool child mortality rates by region, with ecological correlations for both being high in South Asia (0.87 and 0.73, respectively) but much lower to nonexistent in Africa (0.10 and 0.28) and Latin America (0.43 and 0.02) (Victora, 1992).

## Severe PEM

Typical clinical manifestations of severe PEM (skin lesions, hair discoloration, and edema) were first described in 1865 by F. Hinojosa in weaned children of the village of La Magdalena, Mexico (Hinojosa, 1864). Decades later, Cicely Williams introduced into the literature the term *kwashiorkor*, by which the Ge tribe of what is now Ghana described a similar syndrome, associated with "displacing the older child from the breast" (Williams, 1933). The term has since remained in dominant usage,

**Table 5–4** Common Anthropometric Indicators with Cross-sectional Cutoffs for Classifying Preschool Children by Severity of Undernutrition

| Indicator | Interpretation | Classification System | Degree of Severity | | | References |
|---|---|---|---|---|---|---|
| | | | Moderate or Severe | Worse | Mild or Worse | |
| Weight-for-age | underweight | % median | <60% | <75% | <90% | (Gomez et al., 1956; Jelliffe, 1966) |
| | | standardized | –3 Z | –2 Z | –1 Z | (Hamill et al., 1995; Waterlow et al., 1977; WHO, 1995) |
| Height-for-age or Length-for-age | stunting | % median | <85% | <90% | <95% | (Jelliffe, 1966) |
| | | standardized | –3 Z | –2 Z | –1 Z | (Hamill et al., 1995; Waterlow et al., 1977; WHO, 1995) |
| Weight-for-height | wasting | % median | <70% | <80% | <90% | (Jelliffe, 1966) |
| | | standardized | –3 Z | –2 Z | –1 Z | (Hamill et al., 1995; Waterlow et al., 1977; WHO, 1995) |
| MUAC | wasting | absolute | <11.5 cm | <12.5 cm | <13.5 cm | (West et al., 1991) |

*Notes*: Cutoffs between classification system are only approximately equal. Comparisons are most suitable for children 12–59 months of age; below 12 months care should be taken in interpreting populations against current WHO reference (WHO, 1995; Victora et al., 1998). MUAC = mid-upper arm circumference.

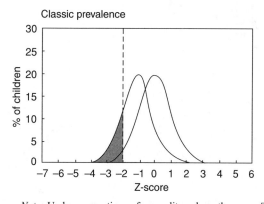
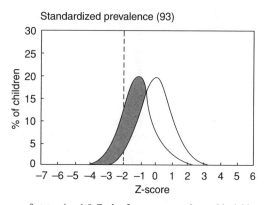

*Note:* Under assumptions of normality, where the mean Z-score of status is –1.0 Z, the former approach would yield a prevalence of 16% below the conventional cutoff of –2.0 Z, the latter would indicate 38% of the population being malnourished (WHO, 1995; Mora, 1989).

**Figure 5–6**  Classic and Standardized Approaches to Estimating Prevalence of Undernutrition

replacing other descriptors such as "Mehl-nahrschaden," "sugar baby," "bwaki," and "en-fants rouges" (DeMaeyer, 1976). An equally severe, but distinct, clinical expression of PEM is *marasmus*, represented by marked wasting of muscle and fat and near cessation of linear growth, considered to represent a form of "bal-anced starvation" (Figure 5–7, right child). Often, both clinical syndromes coexist as ma-rasmic-kwashiorkor (Brown et al., 1981; Reddy, 1991). Excellent treatises on both aspects of severe PEM exist (DeMaeyer, 1976; Reddy, 1991; Torun & Chew, 1999). The major clinical and laboratory characteristics that distinguish marasmus and kwashiorkor are listed in Table 5–5 (Torun & Chew, 1999).

A reduction in protein and energy intake ini-tially triggers a series of adaptive responses. Protein and tissue turnover are reduced, and use of indispensable amino acids is maximized (Golden, Waterlow, & Picou, 1977). As the di-etary deficit persists, the process of adaptation leads to *accommodation*, which implies that the metabolic equilibrium can be maintained only at the expense of alterations in structure and func-tion of tissues and systems (Waterlow, 1985). One of the first such alterations is a reduction or cessation of growth. Energy expenditure is

also reduced, and protein-energy malnourished children usually appear quiet and even lethargic in more severe cases. As the deficit progresses, high-turnover tissues are not adequately re-placed, leading to clinical manifestations in the skin, hair, and the gastrointestinal tract. Typical high exposure to environmental contamination and communicable disease, coupled with im-paired immune competence and lowered host re-sistance (Bhaskaram & Sivakumar, 1986; Chan-dra, 1977; Keusch et al., 1987; Keusch, 1993; Smyth, Hetherton, Smith, Radcliff, & O'Herlihy, 1997), makes infection an almost universal com-plication of severe PEM (Brown et al., 1981). The clinical picture may thus be altered by the development of skin infections, bacterial or viral diarrhea, pneumonia, and urinary tract infec-tions. Symptoms may be aggravated by concur-rent micronutrient deficiencies (Golden, Golden, Harland, & Jackson, 1978). Infection further impairs appetite and food intake (Martorell, Yar-brough, Yarbrough, & Klein, 1980), and in-creases nutrient deficit by increasing require-ments and losses (Caballero, 1997). Thus even moderate infectious diseases carry a very high case fatality for the presenting, acute malnour-ished child, ranging from approximately 3–4% to 20% or more for younger cases (Brown et

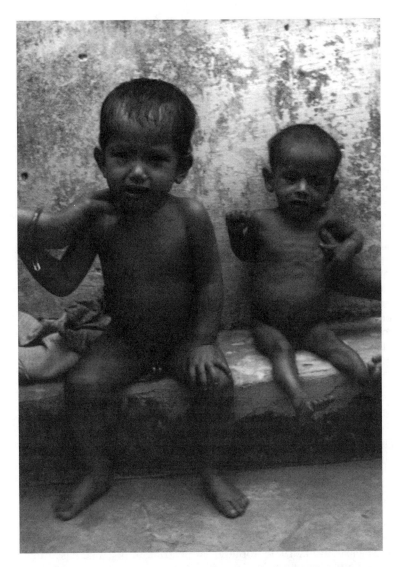

**Figure 5–7** Mild PEM (clinically normal appearance) and Marasmus (evident by extreme wasting of limbs and torso) 1-Year-Old Bangladeshi Children; child on left is a boy, child on right is a girl.

al., 1981; Galvan & Canderon, 1965; McLaren, Shirajiane, Tchalian, & Khoury, 1965; Sommer, 1982).

The management of acute PEM can be divided in two phases: stabilization and refeeding. In the first, the aim is to correct hydration and acid-base alterations, and institute antimicrobial therapy as appropriate. Antibiotics should be included only when there is documented or clear clinical evidence of infection (Torun & Chew, 1999).

Refeeding can be initiated as soon as the child is stable and rehydration is almost complete. The initial regime will depend on the assessment of the gastrointestinal tract. In kwashiorkor and marasmic-kwashiorkor, severe damage of the intestinal mucosa must be assumed, and initiation of refeeding must be done with caution. Feeding

**Table 5–5** Major Characteristics of Marasmus and Kwashiorkor

|  | Marasmus | Kwashiorkor |
| --- | --- | --- |
| Usual age | infancy | second and third years |
| Clinical signs |  |  |
| Odema | absent | present |
| Dermatosis | rare, mild | common |
| Hair changes | common | very common |
| Hepatomegaly | rare | very common |
| Psychomotor change | alert, hungry | miserable |
| Wasting of fat and muscle | severe | mild |
| Anemia | common | very common |
| Laboratory tests |  |  |
| Total body water | high | high |
| Extracellular water | some increase | more increase |
| Body potassium | some depletion | much depletion |
| Renal function | impaired | impaired |
| Glucose tolerance | normal | impaired |
| Albumin, transferrin, etc. | slightly low | very low |
| Nonessential/essential amino acids | normal | high |
| Non-esterified fatty acids | normal | high |
| 3-Methylhistidine | very high | high |

is gradually increased from around 0.7 g/kg of good quality protein and 60 kcal/kg of energy to several times these levels (Graham, 1977, 1979; Graham, Morales, Placko, & MacLean, 1979; Graham, Placko, Acevedo, Morales, & Cordano, 1969; Lopez de Romana, Graham, Mellits, & MacLean, 1980; MacLean & Graham, 1979; Maclean, Klein, Lopez de Romana, Massa, & Graham, 1978; Maclean et al., 1979; Torun et al., 1983). In severe PEM regular milk can be well tolerated by severely malnourished children if gradually administered (Torun et al., 1983). The full recovery of weight and body composition may require as much as three months of optimal feeding. Few centers can afford to keep the child for such a long period of time, and patients are usually discharged from the recovery center before they reach their target recovery weight.

After apparent recovery from acute malnutrition, young children returning to poor living conditions remain at high risk of subsequent infectious disease, poor growth (Baertl, Adrian-zen, & Graham, 1976), and mortality for a year or longer after discharge (Khanum, Ashworth, & Huttly, 1998; Reddy, 1991; West, Goetghebuer, Milligan, Mulholland, & Weber, 1999). Uncomplicated cases of severe PEM have been successfully and less expensively rehabilitated (achieving >80% of weight for height) by supervised, extended home-care programs compared to hospitalization or clinic-based treatment regimens (Khanum, Ashworth, & Huttly, 1994).

## MICRONUTRIENT DEFICIENCIES

Essential micronutrients comprise vitamins and minerals that are required by the body in minute amounts from the diet to support tissue growth, development, function, maintenance, and repair. Micronutrient deficiency, frequently accompanied by degrees of PEM, progressively impairs normal physiologic processes with increasing severity, duration, and mix of dietary deficits, depending on concurrent health conditions and timing with respect to stage of life. Historically, the severity of micronutrient deficiency has been interpreted to parallel its progression in clinical signs (for example, mild eye signs of xerophthalmia = mild vitamin A deficiency), with little attention given to subacute deficiency, similar to historic neglect of the extent and consequences of mild weight deficit in children (Pelletier et al., 1993). However, improved methods to assess biochemical and functional aspects of deficiency in populations, greater cognizance that clinical signs reflect moderate-to-severe nutrient depletion ("tip of the iceberg"), and revelations about the morbidity and mortality risks associated with more prevalent subclinical stages of deficiency, have prompted global efforts to address the full spectrum of micronutrient deficiencies and their impact on health and survival (Humphrey, West, & Sommer, 1992; Stoltzfus, 1997). Estimates of the extent of micronutrient undernutrition vary widely, from 20% of the world's population—or more than 1 billion persons—being deficient in one or more essential micronutrients (Trowbridge et al., 1993) to more than 2 billion being iron deficient alone (UNICEF, 1997). Despite imprecision of global estimates, dietary deficit or imbalance in essential micronutrients represents an enormous problem of "hidden hunger" (Ramalingaswami, 1995), with global health consequence, especially in the low-income countries (Howson, Kennedy, & Horwitz, 1998; McGuire & Galloway, 1994; Trowbridge et al., 1993). Among the multiple micronutrient deficiencies affecting health, four have gained widespread attention for their relevance to child and maternal health, development, and survival: vitamin A, iron, iodine, and zinc. These are each discussed in the following sections.

## Vitamin A Deficiency

Vitamin A deficiency is the leading cause of preventable pediatric blindness and a major determinant of childhood morbidity and mortality in low-income countries (Sommer & West, 1996). Based on population-based biochemical and clinical status surveys, 200–250 million children in more than 70 low- and middle-income countries are vitamin A deficient, of whom at least 3 million, or >1% of all deficient children globally (Figure 5–8), are estimated to present its ocular manifestations, xerophthalmia (WHO, 1993). Projecting earlier incidence rates from Southeast Asia (Sommer, Tarwotjo, Hussaini, Susanto, & Soegiharto, 1981), some 500,000 or more children develop corneal xerophthalmia worldwide, of whom half can be expected to go blind (Sommer et al., 1981). Importantly, estimates are emerging to reveal the extent of vitamin A deficiency among women of reproductive age. Surveys in South Asia typically find 10–20% of women experiencing night blindness during pregnancy (Christian et al., 1998a; Kamal, Ahsan, & Salam, 1998; Katz et al., 1995; Pradhan, Aryal, Regmi, Ban, & Govindasamy, 1997), a condition attributed largely to vitamin A deficiency (Christian et al., 1998b; Dixit, 1966; Mandal, Nanda, & Bose, 1969). Similar preliminary prevalence estimates have been reported from Africa and Central America (Shankar, 2000). Based on the numbers of women of childbearing age, their total fertility (Parikh & Shane, 1998) and likely regional prevalence of maternal night blindness, at least 4 million pregnant women develop night blindness each year (West, 2000). The number of pregnant women with subclinical vitamin A deficiency (for example, based on serum retinol <30 μg/dl or poor dark adaptation) can be expected to be two to three times the prevalence of night blindness (Christian et al., 1998b).

### Function and Assessment

Vitamin A is an essential nutrient that participates in the visual cycle and, at the genomic level, in regulating cell proliferation and differentiation (Blomhoff, 1994). Normally, rod (and cone) photoreceptor cells in the retina of the eye produce photosensitive pigments that respond to light, triggering neural impulses along the optic nerve to the brain that results in vision. Rhodopsin ("visual purple") is the vitamin A-dependent photosensitive pigment that accumulates in rod

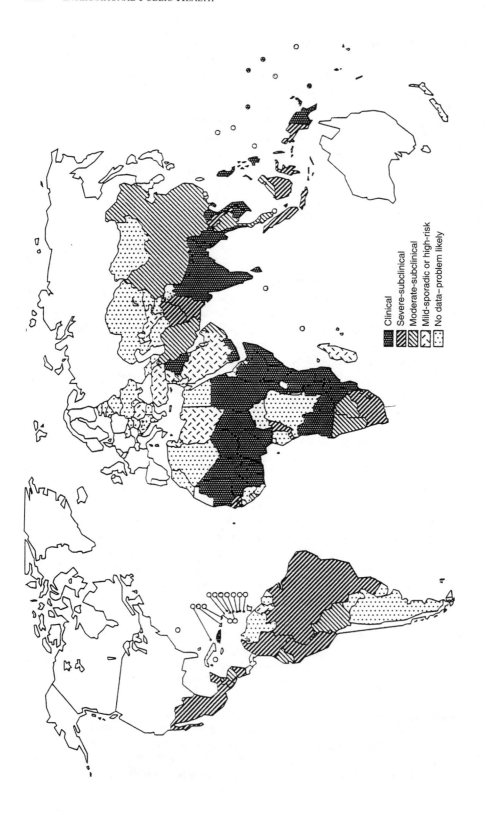

**Figure 5–8**  Countries Categorized by Degree of Public Health Importance of Vitamin A Deficiency

cells, enabling vision under conditions of low illumination (scotopic vision) (Wald, 1955). Vitamin A deficiency leads to decreased availability of retinaldeyhde (retinal) and decreased production of rhodopsin, raising the minimum threshold of light required to see in the dark. This impairment of rod function leads to "night blindness," a condition that is readily recognized by affected individuals (Sommer & West, 1996). Other, more pervasive functions of vitamin A draw on its role in gene regulation, especially evident in rapidly dividing, bipotential cells. Within the nucleus, vitamin A metabolic intermediates (retinoic acids) interact with receptor proteins that, in turn, influence transcription by activating or inhibiting nearby target genes (Kastner, Chambon, & Leid, 1994), thereby directing protein synthesis and cell differentiation and proliferation. Adequate vitamin A nutriture, therefore, helps to maintain, for example, the function and integrity of mucus-secreting, epithelial, immunologic, and osteogenic cells in the body. Deficiency of vitamin A can change the types of cells produced, causing keratinizing metaplasia of epithelial surfaces, evident by xerotic changes (drying) on ocular surfaces (leading to xerophthalmia) (Sommer, 1995). These cellular changes may disrupt the "barrier function" of epithelial surfaces. Further, vitamin A deficiency can alter the expression and function of immune effect or cells and their ability to clear pathogens (Ross, 1996). These pathophysiologic processes can lead to impaired host resistance to infection (Semba, 1994).

Vitamin A status is commonly assessed by clinical, biochemical, and function indicators. Assessment and staging of xerophthalmic eye signs, following a widely accepted WHO classification system (Table 5–6) (Sommer, 1995), provide standardized criteria for evaluating the extent of moderate to severe deficiency, screening individuals for treatment and, because xerophthalmia clusters (Katz, Zeger, & Tielsch, 1988; Katz, Zeger, West, Tielsch, & Sommer, 1993), identifying communities at risk. Biochemical and functional indicators, in the absence of clinical signs, are best applied toward estimating levels of deficiency in groups of individuals. Serum (plasma) retinol is the most commonly measured biochemical indicator of vitamin A status. Although homeostatically controlled within a broad range of nutritional adequacy, plasma retinol concentration falls progressively with liver and total body vitamin A depletion (Olson, 1992; Underwood, 1990). Serum retinol eluted from a filter paper blood spot has shown promise as a practical and inexpensive field approach to population assessment (Craft et al., 2000). Serum retinol response tests following receipt of a standard, small oral dose of vitamin A are based on retinol kinetics (relative dose response [RDR] and modified RDR) that allow relative liver adequacy of vitamin A to be estimated (Loerch, Underwood, & Lewis, 1979; Flores, Campos, Araujo, & Underwood, 1984; Tanumihardjo et al., 1990). Other functional, preclinical measures for evaluating community vitamin A status include breast milk retinol concentration (Stoltzfus & Underwood, 1995), conjunctival impression cytology (Wittpenn, Tseng, & Sommer, 1986; Natadisastra et al., 1988; Stoltzfus, Miller, Hakimi, & Rasmussen, 1993), and dark adaptometry (Congdon et al., 1995). Cutoffs for evaluating community risk by these various means are in Table 5–6 (WHO, 1996a).

### Health Consequences

Consequences of vitamin A deficiency that are of public health importance in low-income countries relate to increased risks of xerophthalmia and its blinding sequelae, infectious morbidity and mortality, and, to some extent, poor growth.

***Xerophthalmia.*** Active stages of xerophthalmia, due to vitamin A deficiency, include night blindness, conjunctival xerosis (dryness), usually with Bitot's spots, corneal xerosis, ulceration, and necrosis ("keratomalacia" or softening of the cornea). Corneal lesions may heal to form a scar (leukoma), become phthisic (shrunken globe), or form a staphyloma (bulging eye) (Sommer, 1995). Noncorneal xerophthalmia indicates mild eye disease but moderate-to-severe

**Table 5–6** WHO Classification and Minimum Prevalence Criteria for Xerophthalmia and Vitamin A Deficiency as a Public Health Program

| Definition (Code) | Minimum Prevalence | Highest Risk Groups |
|---|---|---|
| Night blindness (XN) | 1.0% | Children 2–5 years; pregnant/lactating women |
| Conjunctival xerosis (X1A) | — | |
| Bitot's spots (X1B) | 0.5% | |
| Corneal xerosis (X2) | | |
| Corneal ulceration keratomalacia (X3) | 0.01% | children 1–3 years |
| Xerophthalmic corneal scar (XS) | 0.05% | cumulative >1 year |
| Serum retinol   <0.35 mol L | 5.0% | |
|                 <0.70 mol L | 10.0% | |
| Abnormal CIC/RDR/MRDR | 20.0%* | |

*Provisional cut-offs above which community interventions may be warranted.
*Note:* CIC = conjunctival impression cytology; RDR = relative dose response; MRDR = modified RDR.

deficiency, revealed by a low serum retinol concentration and accompanied increases in risk of morbidity and mortality (Sommer & West, 1996). Corneal involvement is a medical emergency as it is potentially blinding and associated with a case fatality rate of 5–25% (Sommer, 1982). WHO has classified stages of xerophthalmia and provided prevalence estimates as minimum criteria for defining vitamin A deficiency as a public health problem (Table 5–6). The vitamin A treatment schedule for xerophthalmia is well standardized (Table 5–7) (Sommer, 1995; WHO/UNICEF/IVACG, 1997).

*Morbidity and Mortality.* A dose-responsive, strong and consistent association has been shown to exist between clinical vitamin A deficiency, represented by mild xerophthalmic eye signs, and short-term risk of child mortality (Sommer, Hussaini, Tarwotjo, & Susanto, 1983; Sommer & West, 1996). The causality of this association has been born out by eight community intervention trials, enrolling more than 165,000 children, conducted in South and Southeast Asia and Africa over the past 20 years (Figure 5–9). Overviews indicate that the findings from these trials are compatible with reductions of 23–34% in preschool child mortality following vitamin A prophylaxis by direct supplementation or rou-

tine consumption of vitamin A-fortified food (Beaton et al., 1993; Fawzi, Chalmers, Herrera, & Mosteller, 1993; Glasziou & Mackerras, 1993; Tonascia, 1993). Embedded in this impact on all-cause death are likely to be strong effects of vitamin A supplementation in reducing the severity and case-fatality of measles, as seen in both community (Rahmathullah et al., 1990; West et al., 1991) and hospital-based clinical trials (Barclay et al., 1987; Coutsoudis et al., 1992; Ellison, 1932; Hussey & Klein, 1990), diarrhea and dysentery (Arthur et al., 1992), and possibly *Plasmodium falciparum* malaria (Shankar et al., 1999). Recent studies in Nepal have shown maternal night blindness during pregnancy to be associated with increased risks of infectious and reproductive morbidity, general malnutrition (Christian et al., 1998b), and prolonged mortality through the first two years after delivery and the episode of maternal night blindness (Christian et al., in press). Further, routine, low-dose vitamin A or ß-carotene supplementation of women was reported to reduce mortality related to pregnancy by more than 40% (West et al., 1999), although no reductions were observed in fetal or early infant death (Katz et al., in press).

*Poor Growth.* Vitamin A is required for mammalian growth. The discovery of vitamin A early

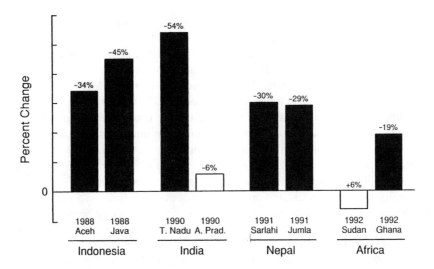

**Figure 5–9** Summary of Percent Change in Mortality of Children (~≥6 mo to 72 mo) Receiving Vitamin A versus No Vitamin A (controls) in Eight Field Intervention Trials. Black bars represent statistically significant reductions, white bars nonsignificant change. Total *N* (across trials) >165,000 children. Meta-analyses show overall 23% to 34% reductions in mortality with Vitamin A.

in the twentieth century was prompted by observations that young animals deprived of an ether-soluble fraction in egg yolk and milk ("fat-soluble factor A") failed to gain weight and eventually died (McCollum & Davis, 1915). Children, who may wax and wane in vitamin A nutriture throughout preschool years, decelerate in linear growth as they enter a mildly xerophthalmic state, only to recover height growth more slowly relative to weight as apparent vitamin A intake improves (Tarwotjo, Katz, West, Tielsch, & Sommer, 1992), possibly explaining a rather consistent association between mild xerophthalmia and stunting (Khatry et al., 1995; Mele et al., 1991; Sommer & West, 1996). However, growth responses to population-based vitamin A supplementation have been mixed, with many studies finding neither a linear nor ponderal effect (Fawzi et al., 1997; Kirkwood et al., 1996; Lie, Ying, En-Lin, Brun, & Geissler, 1993; Ramakrishnan, Latham, & Abel, 1995; Rahmathullah, Underwood, Thulasiraj, & Milton, 1991). Others have reported improvement in weight without height (Bahl, Bhandar, Taneja, & Bhan, 1997; West et al., 1988), height without weight gain (Humphrey et al., 1998; Muhilal, Permeisih, Idjradinata, Muherdiyantiningsih, & Karyadi, 1988), or acceleration in both aspects of growth in high risk subgroups (West et al., 1997; Donnen et al., 1998; Hadi et al., 2000). Presence of infection may also blunt a potential growth response (Hadi et al., 1999). Thus the ability to demonstrate effects of vitamin A on child growth may depend on the severity of other intercurrent risk factors. On balance, it appears that some aspect of growth may improve following vitamin A supplementation among children for whom, or during seasons when, vitamin A deficiency is moderate to severe and "growth limiting" compared to other nutritional and disease factors.

*Prevention*

Prevention of vitamin A deficiency should be guided by epidemiologic insight. For example, mild xerophthalmia has been observed to cluster by region (Cohen et al., 1987), community (Katz et al., 1988; Mele et al., 1991; Sommer, 1982), and household, where siblings of cases have been reported to be 7–13 times more likely also to have or develop xerophthalmia (Katz et al., 1993) and twice as likely to die (Khatry et al., 1995) than children living in homes with no history of xerophthalmia. Vitamin A deficiency often exhibits seasonality (Sinha & Bang, 1973). Both patterns of clustering can help target high-risk groups and seasons for programs.

Three broad strategies exist to prevent vitamin A deficiency: direct supplementation with high-potency vitamin A, food fortification, and a wide range of dietary approaches to increase vitamin A intake. In addition, measures taken to prevent and control infection, which depletes vitamin A stores through increased use and excretion in the body (Campos, Flores, & Underwood, 1987; Mitra, Alvarez, & Stephensen, 1998), may conserve vitamin A status and, therefore, be viewed as a complementary approach to prevent vitamin A deficiency.

High potency vitamin A supplementation is the most common, direct strategy to increase vitamin A intake and status. Typically, a large oral dose of vitamin A (Table 5–7) is delivered either as a gelatinous capsule or in oily syrup to preschool children on a periodic basis, providing a theoretically sufficient supply of the nutrient for a 4- to 6-month period (Bloem et al., 1995). Improvement in serum retinol concentration can be variable, ranging from a few weeks to a few months, although prophylactic efficacy against xerophthalmia and child mortality can last for 6 to 8 months (Sommer & West, 1996). Vitamin A can be delivered as a community-based intervention (Bloem et al., 1995), or through clinic-based treatment and prevention programs (West & Sommer, 1987). UNICEF supports national vitamin A delivery programs through distribution of more than 400 million supplements to low- and middle-income countries each year (see Exhibit 5–2) (Dalmiya, 1999). WHO recommends that a 200,000 IU oral dose of vitamin A be given to women within 6 to 8 weeks postpartum as a means to improve maternal and infant stores (Table 5–7). Although effective in improving short-term vitamin A status of women and their breastfed infants, other dietary or supplementary means are required to sustain

such improvement (Rice et al., 1999; Stoltzfus et al., 1993).

Fortification is increasingly assuming importance as a means to improve routine consumption of vitamin A. Many food "vehicles" can be technically fortified with vitamin A in that the nutrient can be added in nutritionally efficacious amounts without affecting organoleptic qualities under ambient conditions of production and consumer use. Successful commercial candidate foods should, ideally, be produced or processed centrally in a limited number of units (to maintain quality control), have wide market penetration in high-risk areas, be consumed by target groups within a relatively narrow band of intake (to set effective and safe nutrient levels), and be produced and packaged to maintain adequate shelf life at low cost, while maintaining standards set by government regulatory bodies. A few products have been fortified with vitamin A that have been shown to be effective in improving and maintaining adequate vitamin A status in high-risk populations. Most successful has been the fortification of sugar in Guatemala and elsewhere in Central and South America; this has been convincingly shown to improve vitamin A intake and status over the course of two decades (Arroyave, Mejia, & Aguilar, 1981; Dary, 1994; Krause, Delisle, & Solomons, 1998). Monosodium glutamate fortification with vitamin A was conclusively shown to improve status and reduce mortality in South East Asia (Sommer & West, 1996; Muhilal, Permeisih, et al., 1988; Solon, Fernandez, Latham, & Popkin, 1979), but organoleptic changes hindered its further use (Solon et al., 1985). Other successfully tested products include nonrefrigerated margarine (Solon et al., 1996) and centrally processed wheat flour (Solon et al., in press) in the Philippines, and a variety of long-standing food aid commodities such as dried skim milk powder, vegetable oil, and cereal grain flours.

Improved intake of vitamin A through other food-based means inevitably leads to a substantially diversified diet and increased intakes of many micronutrients (Combs, Welch, Duxbury, Uphoff, & Nesheim, 1996). Highly bioavailable,

**Table 5–7** Vitamin A Treatment and Prevention Schedules

| Age | Treatment at Diagnosis* | Prevention | |
| | | Dosage | Frequency |
| --- | --- | --- | --- |
| < 6 months | 50,000 IU | 50,000 IU | every 4–6 months |
| 6–12 months | 100,000 IU | 100,000 IU | every 4–6 months |
| ≥ 1 year | 200,000 IU | 200,000 IU | every 4–6 months |
| Women | 200,000 IU** | 200,000 IU | ≤ 8 weeks after delivery |

*Treat all cases of xerophthalmia and measles with the same age-specific dosage the next day and again 1 to 4 weeks later.
**For women of reproductive age, give 200,000 IU only for corneal xerophthalmia; for milder eye signs (night blindness or Bitot's spots), give women 5,000–10,000 IU per day or ≤ 25,000 IU per week for ≥ 4 weeks.

preformed vitamin A is found in liver, fish liver oil, cheese, milk, and other full-fat dairy products. Such foods, however, typically comprise 10–15% of all food sources of vitamin A in low-income settings. Provitamin A carotenoids (for example, ß-carotene) derived from deeply colored yellow and orange fruits and vegetables, and dark green leaves, contribute more than 85% of food-based vitamin A in the developing world (Food and Agriculture Organization of the UN, 1988). While apparently effective in preventing moderate-to-severe vitamin A deficiency (Sommer & West, 1996), the efficiency of bioconversion of plant-based carotenoids to retinol may be lower than previously calculated, particularly from dark green leaves, possibly

**Exhibit 5–2** The Vitamin A "Campaign" Trail

Field research has shown that vitamin A supplementation can reduce preschool child mortality by 25–35% and can virtually eliminate nutritional blindness in many low- and middle-income countries (Sommer & West, 1996). In recent years, high-potency vitamin A delivery has been redesigned as a semiannual national campaign, with widely advocated, highly organized distribution days set six months apart. On 2 days each year, government; communities; and local, national, and international agencies focus on distributing a US 2-cent vitamin A capsule (VAC) to the country's children. In some settings, vitamin A distribution has been integrated into WHO Expanded Programme for Immunization or National Immunization Days (WHO, 1998), or into other programs such as "Operation Timbang," a national child weighing day program in the Philippines (Klemm et al., 1997). In Bangladesh, where VACs have been distributed since 1973, the campaign approach launched in 1995 as National Vitamin A Week nearly doubled coverage, from 40–45% to 80–85%, a level that has been sustained (Helen Keller International, 1998). Similar rates of coverage have been reinstated in Indonesia, where VAC distribution also began in the mid-1970s (Soewarta & Bloem, 1999). In mountainous Nepal, a "model" national program was launched in 1993, starting in only eight districts. Supported by USAID and UNICEF, the program was organized around community mobilization from its outset. As of the year 2000, 60 of 75 districts consistently achieve semiannual coverage of approximately 90%, reaching more than 2 million children and preventing blindness through the efforts of more than 25,000 local female community health volunteers (Houston, 1999). Knowledge that vitamin A saves lives coupled with a reinvigorated campaign approach to VAC delivery has led vitamin A delivery to be considered an essential component of child survival strategies in these and other countries.

limiting the ability of a strict vegetarian diet to optimize vitamin A status (De Pee, Bloem, Gorstein et al., 1998; De Pee et al., 1999; De Pee, West, Muhilal, Karyadi, & Hautvast, 1995).

Children with xerophthalmia are breastfed less frequently, weaned from the breast at an earlier age, and given foods that are high in vitamin A content less often than clinically normal children (Mahalanabis, 1991; Mele et al., 1991; Sommer & West, 1996; Tarwotjo et al., 1982; West, Chirambo, Katz, Sommer, & Malawi Survey Group, 1986). Thus infant and child feeding approaches should encourage continued breastfeeding into the third year of life, while nutritious complementary foods such as egg, ripe mango and papaya, cooked carrot and dark green leaves are introduced at appropriate times (De Pee, Bloem, Satoto et al., 1998; Kuhnlein, 1992; Seshadri, 1996; Tarwotjo et al., 1982). With whom children eat their meals may also affect the quality of their diet (Shankar et al., 1998). Social marketing programs have been effective in increasing household purchases and intakes of vitamin A food sources such as dark green leaves (Smitasiri, Attig, & Dhanamitta, 1992) and egg (De Pee, Bloem, Satoto et al., 1998). Home gardening, where commonly practiced, provides an excellent means to increase the variety of provitamin A carotenoid-rich foods (Talukder, Islam, Klemm, & Bloem, 1993). Although effects of homestead gardening on vitamin A status remain inconclusive, other food security, nutritional, and economic benefits can accrue from such programs (Marsh, 1998).

**Iron Deficiency and Anemia**

Iron deficiency is the most common micronutrient deficiency in the world, with anemia, characterized by abnormally low blood hemoglobin concentration, being its major clinical manifestation. Although anemia is not specific to iron deficiency, the two conditions are inseparable in most malnourished populations, making anemia the most frequently reported clinical index of iron deficiency in the low-income countries (Yip, 1994).

An estimated 1.3 to more than 2 billion women, children, and men in the world are anemic (DeMaeyer & Adiels-Tegman, 1985; WHO, 1992a). Approximately half of the global burden of anemia is due solely to iron deficiency. On the other hand, depletion of body iron stores with or without impaired red cell production, is likely to be twice as prevalent as anemia (Cook, Finch, & Smith, 1976; Yip, 1994), leading to roughly similar global estimates of the prevalence of anemia (from all causes) and iron deficiency. The term *nutritional anemia* includes the anemic burden due to deficiency in iron plus other vitamins, particularly folate, vitamin B12 (Fishman, Christian, & West, in press), and vitamin A (Sommer & West, 1996), and trace elements that participate in erythropoiesis (WHO, 1992a). Major "nonnutritional" causes of red cell mass loss or destruction and consequent anemia are hookworm (Albonico et al., 1998; Brooker et al., 1999; Hopkins et al., 1997; Stoltzfus et al., 1997; Stoltzfus et al., 1998) and malarial (Beales, 1997) infections, respectively, both of which occur in large areas of the low-income countries. HIV/AIDS has emerged as an important cause of anemia in sub-Saharan Africa (Vetter et al., 1996).

Pregnant women, infants, and young children are at highest risk of iron deficiency anemia. Based on population surveys conducted between 1970 through the late 1980s, more than half of all pregnant women in the world are anemic, and 95%—or approximately 56 million women (at that time)—of them reside in the low-income countries (Table 5–8) (WHO, 1992a). As with wasting and stunting malnutrition (ACC/SCN, 1992a), South Asia shoulders the greatest burden of iron deficiency, where 75% of pregnant women and nearly 60% of nonpregnant women are anemic. High rates of anemia are also observed in Southeast Asia, most of Africa, Oceania, and the Caribbean. Recent data from Central Asia suggest 40–60% of women of reproductive ages are anemic (Sharmanov, 1998). Moderate-to-severe maternal anemia, defined at hemoglobin cutoffs ranging from <90 or <100 g/L, affects far fewer women, but its use may

**Table 5–8** Estimated Prevalence of Anemia in Women (circa 1988)

| Region | Pregnant Women Hb below 110 g/L | | Nonpregnant Women Hb below 120 g/L | |
|---|---|---|---|---|
| | % | (in thousands) | % | (in thousands) |
| World | 51 | 58,270 | 35 | 399,250 |
| Developed countries* | 18 | 2,520 | 12 | 35,460 |
| Developing countries | 56 | 55,750 | 43 | 363,800 |
| Africa | 52 | 11,450 | 42 | 47,940 |
| eastern | 47 | 3,380 | 41 | 13,540 |
| middle | 54 | 1,290 | 43 | 5,330 |
| northern | 53 | 2,240 | 43 | 11,450 |
| southern | 35 | 380 | 30 | 2,500 |
| western | 56 | 4,170 | 47 | 15,120 |
| Asia* | 60 | 40,140 | 44 | 294,960 |
| eastern* | 37 | 7,290 | 33 | 105,760 |
| southeastern | 63 | 6,300 | 49 | 47,230 |
| southern | 75 | 24,760 | 58 | 133,180 |
| western | 50 | 1,790 | 36 | 8,790 |
| Latin-America | 39 | 4,030 | 30 | 28,640 |
| Caribbean | 52 | 340 | 36 | 2,790 |
| Central | 42 | 1,210 | 39 | 9,550 |
| South | 37 | 2,480 | 25 | 16,310 |
| Northern America | 17 | 570 | 10 | 7,050 |
| Europe | 17 | 920 | 10 | 12,100 |
| Oceania* | 71 | 130 | 66 | 780 |
| Former USSR** | 15 | 640 | 12 | 7,770 |

* Japan, Australia and New Zealand have been excluded from the regional estimates but are included in the total for developed countries. *Note:* Figures may not add to totals due to rounding.
 ** Data collected prior to recent political changes.

differentiate, with greater clarity, populations lying along an anemia-health risk continuum (Stoltzfus, 1997). Severe anemia (Hb cutoffs ranging from <50 to < 70 g/L) generally occurs in less than 5% of women in high-risk populations (Stoltzfus, 1997; Sharmanov, 1998).

Nationally representative prevalence rates of anemia for young children are less available, but existing data suggest that nearly half of preschoolers in the low-income countries are anemic (DeMaeyer & Adiels-Tegman, 1985) compared, for example, to rates of less than 10% among toddlers in the United States, of which only about one-third is due to iron deficiency (Looker, Dallman, Carroll, Gunter, & Johnson, 1977).

### Function and Assessment

In the body, iron is found in metabolically active "functional" and "storage" pools, accounting for approximately 75% and approximately 25% of total body iron, respectively (Lynch, 1999). Approximately 80% of functional iron complexes with hemoglobin during erythropoiesis, where it plays a central role in oxygen transport to cells. Approximately 10% of this metabolic iron pool is incorporated into intracellular myoglobin, where oxygen is stored for use during muscle contraction. In addition, iron serves as a cofactor in 200 or more heme and nonheme enzymes involved in cellular respiration, division, and growth (Dallman, 1986; Ryan, 1997; Viteri, 1998). Thus iron is required for normal cellular energy production, muscle contraction, hormonal regulation, intestinal function, neural tissue growth, function, and repair among other physiologic processes that confer vital roles for iron to perform physical work, achieve a normal pregnancy outcome, and achieve full motor and cognitive potential (Ryan, 1997; Viteri, 1998).

Total body iron balance is largely regulated at the point of absorption. Dietary heme iron (for example, from red meat) is readily taken up by the small intestinal mucosa, with 12–25% typically being absorbed (Bothwell & Charlton, 1981), versus a much smaller fraction of dietary nonheme iron, typically less than 5% from cereal-based diets. Absorption depends on the iron status and requirements of the host, food matrix, and the presence of dietary factors that inhibit or enhance absorption (Bothwell et al., 1982). Plasma transferrin transports newly absorbed iron as well as endogenous iron released from normal macrophage degradation of senescent red blood cells in the marrow, liver, and spleen. Although virtually all cells require iron, approximately 80% of transferrin-bound iron is delivered to erythroid precursors in bone marrow for red cell production. Tissue uptake of the transferrin-iron complex is mediated by a specific transferrin receptor, the cell surface density of which is directly related to tissue iron need (Skikne, Flowers, & Cook, 1990). Normally, up to approximately 30% of body iron is stored in association with the intracellular protein, ferritin, from which iron can be released into circulation to maintain homeostasis, or as hemosiderin, which is a less available, longer term intracellular storage form of tissue iron (Dallman, 1986).

During prolonged dietary deficit, iron is released from intracellular ferritin into circulation for transferrin-mediated delivery to the erythron to support hematopoiesis, resulting in decreased iron stores. As iron depletion progresses, transferrin carries less iron, diminishing the supply of iron to the marrow and other tissues. This stage of iron deficiency without anemia is reflected by increased transferrin receptor expression on cell surfaces, a low level of transferrin saturation with iron, and increased amounts of circulating erythrocyte protoporphyrin, an iron-free heme precursor (Skikne et al., 1990). Finally, iron deficiency anemia develops as hemoglobin concentration falls, red cells become microcytic and hypochromic, and mean corpuscular volume decreases (Ryan, 1997).

A sizable number of iron status indicators that track the above changes in iron status leading to anemia exist; however, only a few commonly used ones are discussed here. Assessment of hemoglobin or hematocrit concentrations, evaluating their distributions against conventional cutoffs by age, life stage, and gender (Table 5–9), is the standard approach for diagnosing and estimating the prevalence of anemia. Field assessment of hemoglobin has been advanced greatly through development of the HemoCue, a battery operated portable photometer (Anglholm, Sweden) (Yip, 1994). In populations where iron deficiency is known to be the single, major cause of anemia, comparing the distribution of Hb values against a referent Hb distribution of individuals known to be free of iron deficiency, can reveal the total burden of anemia that should be amenable to iron intervention (Yip, 1994; Yip, Johnson, & Dallman, 1984). Estimating the prevalence of moderate-to-severe anemia that likely carries greater health risk (Dallman, 1986), and would be more responsive to intervention, may improve the interpretation of population anemia burden over currently accepted cutoffs for mild anemia or worse (Stoltzfus, 1997). Assessing hemoglobin response to supplementation provides another, more accurate but complex, approach to estimating the extent of iron deficiency anemia (Yip, 1994).

Ferritin occurs in circulation, giving rise to its use as an indicator of tissue iron stores (Cook, Lipschitz, Miles, & Finch, 1974), with each 1

**Table 5–9** Hemoglobin and Hematocrit Cutoffs Used To Define Anemia

| Target Group | Hemoglobin Cutoff (g/L) | | Hematocrit Cutoff (%) |
| | Any | Moderate to Severe* | Any |
| --- | --- | --- | --- |
| Children 6 months–5 years | <11 | <9 | <33 |
| Children 6–11 years | <11 | <9 | <34 |
| Children 12–13 years | <12 | <10 | <36 |
| Nonpregnant women | <12 | <10 | <36 |
| Pregnant women | <11 | <9 | <33 |
| Men | <13 | <11 | <39 |

*Suggested cutoffs motivated by discussions of Stoltzfus (1997) and Yip (1994), indicating a cutoff for moderate anemia at ~20 g/L below that for mild anemia, and findings of Garn et al., from the US National Collaborative Perinatal Project (1981).

µg/L concentration of plasma ferritin reflecting approximately 8–10 mg of tissue iron. Concentrations below 12 µg/L are conventionally taken to represent a state of body iron depletion (Bothwell & Charlton, 1981), although plasma ferritin may be elevated in response to acute infection or chronic inflammation (Walter, Olivares, Pizarro, & Munoz, 1997). Measurement of soluble transferrin receptor in plasma has been shown to provide a dependable estimate of tissue iron need (Cook, Baynes, & Skikne, 1994) under conditions of chronic disease or inflammation (Ferguson, Skikne, Simpson, Baynes, & Cook, 1992), undernutrition (Kuvibidila, Warrier, Ode, & Yu, 1996), and pregnancy (Akesson, Bjellerup, Berglund, Bremme, & Vahter, 1998) but remains to be widely used in low-income countries. Another common measure of iron status is percent transferrin saturation, which reflects the adequacy of iron delivery to tissues (Bothwell & Charlton, 1981). The conceptual spectrum of deficiency with illustrated cutoffs for serological indicators commonly used in low-income countries is depicted in Figure 5–10 (Bothwell & Charlton, 1981).

Simple diagnostic tools available to assess anemia in primary care settings include the clinical diagnosis of pallor (palmar, tarsal conjunctival, and nail bed), which can diagnose severe anemia (Hb <50 to <70 g/L or Hct <15%) with approximately 10–50% sensitivity and 90–100% specificity (Kalter et al., 1997; Stoltzfus et al.,

1999; Luby et al., 1995; Zucker et al., 1997). A simple "color scale" has shown promise as a tool for field use in diagnosing low hemoglobin from a fresh blood spot (Stott & Lewis, 1995; Lewis, Stott, & Wynn, 1998). Inexpensive instruments for detecting anemia in primary care settings have recently been compiled (Robinett, Taylor, & Stephens, 1996).

### Health Consequences

Highest risk groups in terms of both probability of becoming anemic from iron deficiency and suffering its consequences are women of reproductive age, especially during pregnancy; infants older than 6 months of age; and young children.

*Maternal Morbidity.* Women are at high risk of anemia due to periodic menstrual blood loss and increased requirements during pregnancy associated with expanded red blood cell mass and accretion of iron in fetal tissue and placenta. Thus gestational iron deficiency anemia is likely to be harmful to the mother, fetus, and infant, but evidence remains controversial and potentially confounded by other factors influencing health (Allen, 1997). A severalfold higher risk of maternal mortality has been observed among pregnant women with moderate-to-severe anemia (Hb <40 to <90 g/L) (Harrison, 1989; Llewellyn-Jones, 1965; Sarin, 1995), possibly related to greater risk of puer-

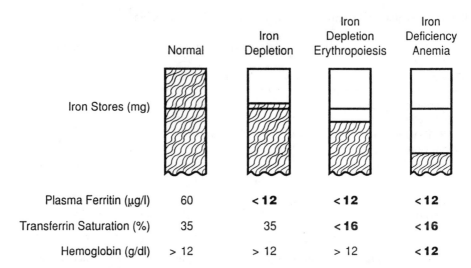

**Figure 5–10** Relationship between Depletion in Body Iron Stores and Change in Selected Indicators of Iron and Anemia Status. Bold values represent deficient status.

peral cardiac failure or hemorrhage (Allen, 1997). Severe anemia has been estimated to account for 10–20% of all maternal deaths in low-income countries (UNICEF, 1997), but data revealing the incidence and severity of maternal morbidity relative to hematologic status are lacking (Allen, 1997). Risks of preterm delivery, low birthweight, fetal malformations, and fetal deaths have been found to follow a U-shaped curve with respect to maternal hemoglobin (hematocrit) measured early in pregnancy, with an elevation in hemoglobin (for example, >130 g/L) posing as much or more risk of an adverse outcome as a lower (<90 g/L) hemoglobin concentration (Dreyfuss, 1998; Scholl, Hediger, Fischer, & Shearer, 1992; Steer, Alam, Wadsworth, & Welch, 1995; Yip et al., 1984; Zhou et al., 1998). Causal mechanisms that may underlie these risks are not well understood. Maternal iron deficiency anemia may also place newborns at risk of low iron stores during infancy (Hokama et al., 1996; Kilbride et al., 1999; Preziosi et al., 1997). Recently, iron supplementation during pregnancy was found to improve newborn length, Apgar score, and survival (Christian, 1998; Preziosi et al., 1997) and lead to larger plasma ferritin concentrations at three months of age, but more

trials are needed to clarify the benefit of maternal iron supplementation to infants.

***Poor Growth.*** Late infancy and early childhood is a high-risk period for becoming iron deficient and anemic because of high iron requirements to support rapid growth coupled with poor dietary intake of bioavailable iron (Gibson, Ferguson, & Lehrfeld, 1998; Ryan, 1997). Iron deficiency anemia has been associated with stunted growth (Chwang, Soemantri, & Pollitt, 1988) and in some trials iron supplementation (for example, at approximately 2–3 mg/kg/body weight/day) has improved both ponderal and linear growth of initially anemic and iron-deficient children (Angeles, Schultink, Matulessi, Gross, & Sastroamidjojo, 1993; Aukett, Parks, Scott, & Wharton, 1986; Chwang, Soemantri, & Pollitt, 1988; Lawless, Latham, Stephenson, Kinoti, & Pertet, 1994). Yet in other trials, including studies done in populations where iron deficiency anemia prevails, daily iron had no effect on child growth (Rahman, Akramuzzaman, Mitra, Fuchs, & Mahalanabis, 1999; Rosado, Lopez, Munoz, Martinez, & Allen, 1997), and in one study supplemental iron mildly suppressed weight gain (Idjradinata, Watkins, & Pollitt, 1994). Positive effects on growth of school-aged children in Kenya (Lawless et al., 1994), qualitatively different growth responses within similar populations (Chwang et al., 1988; Idjradinata et al., 1994) and the lack of effect observed in wasted (Rahman et al., 1999) as well as nonwasted (Rasado et al., 1997) populations suggests that a growth effect from increased iron intake can not be expected.

***Developmental Deficits.*** Persistent deficits in learning, psychomotor, behavioral interactions, and educational achievement have been observed more often in anemic infants and young children than in children with normal hematologic status (Aukett et al., 1986; Lozoff et al., 1998; Pollitt, Gorman, Engle, Rivera, & Matorell, 1995), but such abnormalities may also result from malnutrition, other health problems (Heywood, Oppenheimer, Heywood, & Jolley, 1989), and inadequate stimulation at home (Lozoff et al., 1998). Perhaps not surprisingly, some trials have reported improved behavioral (Oski, Honig, Helu, & Howanitz, 1983), developmental (Aukett et al., 1986), and learning-achievement scores with daily iron supplementation of children (Bruner, Joffe, Duggan, Casella, & Brandt, 1996; Soemantri, Pollitt, & Kim, 1985), while other trials have failed to reverse early psychomotor deficits with iron (Lozoff, Wolf, & Jimenez, 1996; Walter, 1989). Still, the potential for infantile and early childhood iron deficiency to compromise child development provides strong impetus to advance both iron deficiency prevention program and research agendas.

### Prevention

Programs should seek first to prevent iron deficiency anemia among pregnant and postpartum women and infants 6–24 months of age (Stoltzfus & Dreyfuss, 1998). Ideally, women entering their reproductive years (Viteri, 1998) and preschool children provide additional groups to target, especially in areas of high anemia prevalence (Stoltzfus & Dreyfuss, 1998). Effective planning should establish proportions of the anemic burden attributable to iron deficiency, malaria, hookworm, or other causes (Yip, 1997).

Anthelminthic programs may prove highly effective where hookworm and *trichuris* are endemic (Albonico et al., 1998; Brooker et al., 1999; Hopkins et al., 1997; Stoltzfus et al., 1998). Malarial prophylaxis programs may reduce risk of anemia (Beales, 1997; Huddle, Gibson, & Cullinan, 1999). Iron deficiency is the underlying cause of anemia, however, in most populations, which can be directly addressed through iron supplementation, food fortification, or other dietary measures.

***Iron Supplementation.*** Guidelines have been developed for the effective use of iron and folic acid supplements to prevent and treat iron deficiency anemia (Table 5–10) (Stoltzfus & Dreyfuss, 1998). Daily iron supplementation can be highly effective in raising blood hemoglobin and plasma ferritin levels among pregnant women. Inclusion of folic acid can guard against megaloblastic anemia, neural tube abnormalities among women supplemented periconceptionally (MRC Vitamin Study Research Group, 1991), and other consequences of folate deficiency that may affect malnourished populations (Fishman et al., in press). A long-standing debate over whether prophylactic iron may be contraindicated where malaria is endemic appears to be finding some resolution (Murray et al., 1975; Oppenheimer, 1998). Recent findings of a randomized trial in Tanzania show that iron supplementation can effectively prevent severe anemia in infants without increasing the risk of malaria (Menendez et al., 1997). In addition, a recent meta-analysis of field trials carried out to date suggests that, in malaria-infected persons, an approximately 5% increase in circulating parasite density may be expected to occur with iron supplementation, but this risk increment is associated with little, if any, increase in clinical malaria (INACG Secretariat, 1999). To date, though, low-cost systems for routine and high-compliance delivery of oral iron to infants and young children in typical low-income country settings remain to be implemented (Nestle & Alnwick, 1997).

***Fortification.*** Iron fortification of foodstuffs such as fish sauces, curry powder, sugar, salt,

**Table 5–10** Guidelines for Supplementing Pregnant Women and Infants with Iron

| Prevalence of Anemia | Daily Dosage | | Condition | Duration |
| | Iron (mg) | Folic Acid (µg) | | |
| --- | --- | --- | --- | --- |
| Pregnant Women | | | | |
| <40% | 60 | 400 | in pregnancy | 6 months* |
| ≥40% | 60 | 400 | in pregnancy | 6 months* |
| | | | postpartum | 3 months |
| Infants | | | | |
| <40%** | 12.5*** | 50 | birth weight ≥2,500 g | 6–12 months |
| | | | birth weight <2,500 g | 2–24 months |
| ≥40%** | 12.5*** | 50 | birth weight ≥2,500 g | 6–24 months |
| | | | birth weight <2,500 g | 2–24 months |

* If 6-month duration cannot be achieved in pregnancy, continue supplement to 6 months postpartum or increase dose to 120 mg iron/day.
** If prevalence in infants is not known, assume same prevalence as observed in pregnant women in same population.
*** Iron dosage based on 2 mg iron/kg body weight/day.

dairy products, and infant formulas, has been successfully carried out in a number of settings (Stoltzfus & Dreyfuss, 1998), though few iron fortification programs exist in low- and middle-income countries at present (Yip, 1997). Several food-grade forms of iron are available for use, depending on the type of food vehicle, methods of preparation, storage, and other factors. For example, ferrous sulfate can be used in liquids but may discolor dry foods or make fatty foods rancid (INACG, 1997). Iron EDTA (ethylenediaminetetraacetic acid) has been shown to be an effective fortificant that permits efficient absorption of nonheme iron in the presence of dietary inhibitors of absorption (Lynch, Hurrell, Bothwell, & MacPhail, 1993). As with supplementation, two target groups exist for fortification—infants and young children and women—for whom different food vehicles may need to be considered. Powdered milk, frequently given to children in low-income, aid-recipient families, was fortified with both iron and vitamin C to improve iron status of young children in Chile (Yip, 1997). The use of coated "sprinkles" containing iron sulfate has been proposed to fortify meals at home (Nestle & Alnwick, 1997). Some Caribbean, South American, and South Asian countries have begun to fortify wheat flour with iron, although rigorous evaluation of the impact on iron status and anemia is generally lacking (Yip, 1997).

*Dietary Approach.* Typically, the iron density of diets in low-income regions ranges from 4.5 to 7.5 mg per 1,000 kilocalories (ACC/SCN, 1992), largely consisting of nonheme iron from grains, nuts, vegetables, and fruits from which iron is poorly absorbed (Bothwell et al., 1982; Lynch, 1997). Phytates in foods, tannins and polyphenols in tea, calcium in dairy products and green leaves, and animal protein from whole milk, cheeses, and egg whites further inhibit the absorption of nonheme iron (Hallberg, Brune, Erlandsson, Sandberg, & Rossander-Hulten, 1991; Lynch, 1997; Ryan, 1997). Concurrent intakes of ascorbic acid (for example, from citrus) or meat, poultry, and fish (Bothwell et al., 1982; Monsen et al., 1978) can enhance nonheme absorption in a dose-response manner. However, dietary programs to prevent anemia in low-income countries have been few and have achieved little success (Yip, 1997).

### Iodine Deficiency

Iodine is an essential component of thyroid hormones that control cellular metabolism and neuromuscular tissue growth and development. Deficiency in iodine and consequent thyroid hormone production during critical periods of organogenesis can thus damage the brain and nervous tissue, causing irreversible mental retardation and other developmental abnormalities. The spectrum of mild through severe health consequences causally linked to iodine deficiency at different stages of life (Exhibit 5–3) are collectively known as iodine deficiency disorders, or IDD (Hetzel, 1987). While these effects vary in their specificity with respect to deficiency of iodine, the term has propelled greater understanding of the multiple health and societal consequences of this nutrient deficiency. Informative treatises exist on the histories of goiter and cretinism, the two most notable clinical syndromes of iodine deficiency (Hetzel, 1989).

As an element in the Earth's crust, iodine can be either sufficient or in varying stages of depletion in areas of the world. Thus iodine adequacy of all flora and fauna, and therefore food, in a general locale is dependent on the adequacy of the nutrient in soil (Houston, 1999). Major mountainous regions of the world, such as the Himalayas, Andes, and Alps, are severely de-pleted in soil iodine, resulting from erosion due to glacier activity, rain, and deforestation (Dunn & van der Haar, 1990). However, plains regions of central Africa, Asia, and Europe, as well as major riverine and deltaic areas affected by frequent flooding, such as Gangetic South Asia and valleys of the Yellow, Rhine, and the Amazon, also lack iodine (Dunn & van der Haar, 1990) (Figure 5–11). In some areas of Central Africa, such as Zaire, where environmental iodine and intake are marginal-to-low, iodine deficiency is augmented by routine consumption of goitrogenic substances, such as linamarin, a cyanide-containing compound found in the root of cassava (Delange et al., 1982). Thiocyanates, which result from detoxification of linamarin in the liver, decrease iodine uptake by the thyroid gland and suppress circulating thyroid hormone, leading to secondary iodine deficiency.

As of the early 1990s an estimated 1.6 billion persons, or nearly 30% of the world's population, were thought to be at risk of iodine deficiency (WHO, 1993), based on documented occurrence of goiter (prevalence >5%) and the sizes of populations living in iodine-depleted regions of the world (Houston, 1999). Data from

---

**Exhibit 5–3** Spectrum of Iodine Deficiency Disorders

**Fetus**
- abortions
- stillbirths
- congenital anomalies
- increased perinatal mortality
- increased infant mortality
- neurological cretinism: mental deficiency, deaf mutism, spastic diplegia, squint
- myxedematous cretinism: dwarfism, mental deficiency
- psychomotor defects

**Neonate**
- neonatal goiter
- neonatal hypothyroidism
- increased susceptibility to nuclear radiation*

**Child and Adolescent**
- goiter
- juvenile hypothyroidism
- impaired mental function
- retarded physical development
- increased susceptibility to nuclear radiation*

**Adult**
- goiter with its complications
- hypothyroidism
- impaired mental function
- iodine-induced hyperthyroidism
- increased susceptibility to nuclear radiation*

*Due to increased uptake of radioactive iodine.

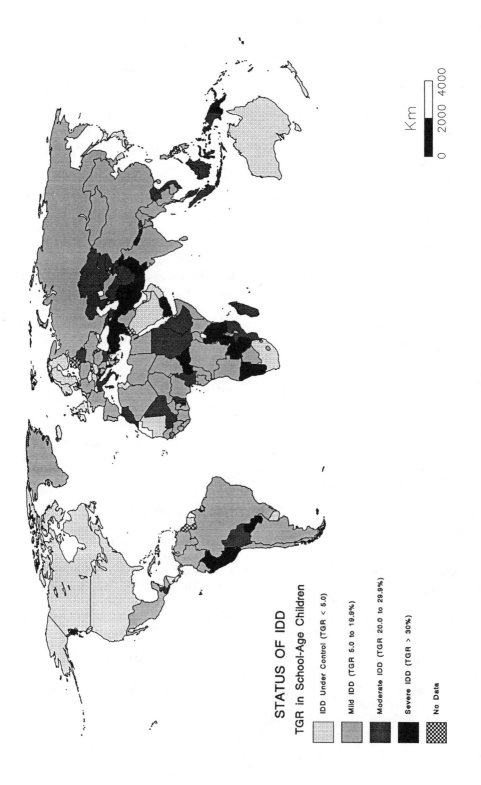

**Figure 5–11** Prevalence of Worldwide of Iodine Deficiency Disorders (IDD) Based on Assessment of the Total Goiter Rate (TGR) in School-Aged Children

existing population-based surveys, compiled as part of a global micronutrient deficiency surveillance system (WHO, 1993), suggest there are approximately 655 million or more persons affected by goiter, more than 11 million cretins (Table 5–11), and, perhaps of greatest concern, more than 43 million persons in 118 affected countries throughout the world with some degree of mental impairment resulting from iodine deficiency (WHO, 1994).

*Function*

Iodine, ingested as iodide or iodate, is an essential constituent of thyroid hormones. Once in circulation, nearly all body iodide is actively trapped by follicle cells of the thyroid gland where it is oxidized to iodine and bound to tyrosine amino acids, catalyzed by an iron-containing peroxidase, to form the thyroid hormones, T3 (tri-iodothyronine) and T4 (tetra-iodothyronine, or thyroxine) (Houston, 1999; Tortora & Grabowski, 1996). T3 and T4 are stored in the thyroid gland in association with the glycoprotein thyroglobulin.

Following stimulation from the hypothalamus, thyroid-stimulating hormone (TSH) is released from the anterior pituitary gland that induces thyroid hormone release into circulation bound to circulatory carrier proteins (Houston, 1999). As T3 and T4 levels rise, the hypothalamic-anterior pituitary-thyroid axis maintains homeostasis by reducing thyroid hormone re-

lease. Within target cells, thyroid hormones regulate oxygen use, basic metabolic rate, protein synthesis, and thermogenesis; this is accomplished largely by influencing gene transcription (Stein, 1994). During gestation, both maternal as well as fetally derived T3 and T4 contribute to the regulatory thyroxine pool that, acting in concert with other hormones (for example, growth hormone, insulin), directs fetal tissue function, growth, and development. In particular, thyroid hormones influence the development of the brain and other neural tissue, giving rise to their, and iodine's, key role in regulating fetal and infant growth, and physical and mental function, and development (Tortora & Grabowski, 1996). Paradoxically, excess build-up of iodine in the thyroid gland can suppress the release of T3 and T4, leading to concern about risks of toxicity associated with rapid correction of iodine deficiency in some endemic areas (Corvilain, Van Sande, Dumont, Bourdoux, & Ermans, 1998; Dunn, Semigran, & Delange, 1998; Stanbury et al., 1998), similar to risks observed in areas of chronically high iodine intake (Konno, Makita, Yuri, Iizuka, & Kawasaki, 1994).

*Health Consequences*

Among the disorders caused by lack of iodine, fetal and neonatal hypothyroidism due to maternal iodine depletion is by far the most serious, with widespread consequence. This disorder permanently alters the structure and function

**Table 5–11** Number (%) of Persons at Risk of Iodine Deficiency Disorders by WHO Region

| WHO Region | Population (Millions) | At Risk of IDD Millions (%) | Population Goitrous Millions (%) | Population Cretinous Millions (%) |
|---|---|---|---|---|
| Africa | 550 | 181 (33) | 86 (16) | 1.1 (0.2) |
| Americas | 727 | 168 (23) | 63 (9) | 0.6 (0.9) |
| Eastern Mediterranean | 406 | 173 (43) | 93 (23) | 0.9 (2.3) |
| Europe | 847 | 141 (17) | 97 (11) | 0.9 (1.1) |
| Southeast Asia | 1,355 | 486 (36) | 176 (13) | 3.2 (1.3) |
| Western Pacific | 1,553 | 423 (27) | 141 (9) | 4.5 (2.9) |
| **Total** | 5,438 | 1,572 (29) | 656 (12) | 11.2 (2.0) |

of the brain and other nervous tissue during critical stages of development, giving rise to permanent neurological and developmental abnormalities (Stein, 1994; Hetzel, 1994). Postnatal iodine deficiency perpetuates thyroid failure that, depending on its duration and severity, can lead to continued hypothyroidism, growth retardation, sexual immaturity, and impaired cognition and motor development (Halpern, 1994).

Severe iodine deficiency can result in spontaneous abortion, stillbirth, and congenital abnormalities among surviving offspring (Pharoah, Buttfield, & Hetzel, 1971). Cretinism (Figure 5–12), representing the most severe clinical spectrum of the IDD, is usually manifest by severe mental and growth retardation, paraplegia, rigidity, deaf-mutism, and facial disturbances (Hetzel, 1994). The type and severity of brain and other neurological and musculoskeletal deficits appear to arise from the timing, duration, and severity of insult. For example, the central nervous system defects associated with cretinism can be linked to severe gestational iodine deficiency in the second trimester of pregnancy (DeLong et al., 1994; Halpern, 1994), a period when the cerebral cortex, basal ganglia, and cochlea undergo rapid growth and development. Severe fetal hypothyroidism thus gives rise to the *neurologic* cretin. Severe growth retardation, sexual delay, and musculoskeletal deformity, with continued neurological damage, can be attributed largely to severe postnatal iodine deficiency, giving rise to the *myxedemetous* cretin (Boyages, 1994).

Mild, biochemical, or noncretinous hypothyroidism due to iodine deficiency is a major public health concern due to its frequency in infancy and early childhood. Decreased infant survival may be a little-suspected consequence of mild neonatal hypothyroidism (Cobra et al., 1997). More fully appreciated is the observation that children living in iodine-deficient communities, usually exhibiting one or more indications of iodine deficiency, exhibit a lower intelligence quotient and perform more poorly in cognition, motor function, and school achievement tests than peers with normal status growing up

under iodine-sufficient surroundings (Bleichrodt & Born, 1994; Huda, Grantham-McGregor, Rahman, & Tomkins, 1999). Historically, the strength of evidence for a unique contribution of mild iodine deficiency to impaired cognition, however, has been tempered by lack of control in studies for community differences in nutritional, health, education, and socioeconomic factors that can also influence child stimulation and achievement. Some of these concerns for confounders, however, are being addressed. A recent observational study of young, mildly hypothyroid, and euthyroid Bangladeshi school children, matched on school, grade, and local area and controlled for numerous potential confounders related to child health and household status, still observed deficient performance of hypothyroid children in terms of abilities to spell and read (Huda et al., 1999). Recognition and quantification of this subclinical "base of the IDD iceberg" have been key motivating factors for invigorated efforts to prevent iodine deficiency (Hetzel, 1989).

Goiter is an enlarged thyroid gland and is the most commonly observed clinical manifestation of iodine deficiency. Chronic deficiency of iodine lowers thyroid hormone output that, in turn, leads to increased TSH release from the anterior pituitary to stimulate increased T3 and thyroxine production. Failure results in compensatory growth of the thyroid gland (Kavishe, 1999). Goiter size can range from barely palpable with the neck extended to grotesquely visible from a distance. An enlarged thyroid due to iodine deficiency poses little known health risk. However, hyperthyroidism reflecting a state of thyrotoxicosis may serve as an indicator of cardiac risk in some elderly groups who respond abnormally to iodine prophylaxis (Corvilain et al., 1998; Dunn et al., 1998; Stanbury et al., 1998).

### Assessment

Iodine status can be assessed through clinical and biochemical means. Indicators with suggested cutoffs, target populations for assessment, and criteria related to severity of iodine

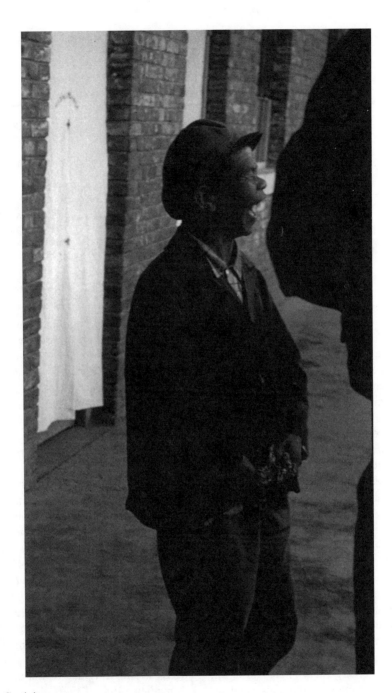

**Figure 5–12** Cretinism

deficiency as a public health problem have been published by WHO and the ICCIDD (WHO, 1994) (Table 5–12).

Virtually all goiter occurring in iodine-deficient areas can be attributed to iodine deficiency, and, thus, goiter prevalence can serve as a useful

**Table 5–12** WHO Minimum Criteria for Iodine Deficiency as a Public Health Problem

| Indicator | Cutoff | Target Population | Severity of IDD | |
|---|---|---|---|---|
| | | | Mild | Severe |
| | | | Percent Affected | |
| Goiter | grade >0 | schoolchildren | 5–19 | ≥30 |
| Thyroid volume* | >97th percentile | schoolchildren | 5–19 | ≥30 |
| TSH** | >5 mu/L | neonates | 3–19 | ≥40 |
| | Unit | | Median Concentration | |
| Urinary iodine | ug/L | schoolchildren | 50–99 | <20 |
| Thyroglobulin | ng/ml | children and adults | 10–19 | ≥40 |

*Assessed by ultrasonography.
**Whole blood thyroid stimulating hormone.

population indicator of risk. Reliable thyroid examination by palpation requires well-trained observers (Peterson et al., 2000). In 1960 the WHO established a five-stage goiter classification system (Perez, Scrimshaw, & Munoz, 1960) that served as the basis for evaluating the public health significance of iodine deficiency over the subsequent three decades (WHO, 1993). The minimum clinical cutoff for estimating the total goiter rate (TGR) was a palpable glandular mass with each lobe being at least as large as the distal phalanx of the subject's thumb. A TGR of >10% was set as the minimum for iodine deficiency public health criterion (Perez et al., 1960). In 1994 the WHO simplified the scheme to two clinical grades, defining goiter as a palpable mass of any size with the neck in a normal position, and lowered the minimum TGR of public health significance to >5% (WHO, 1994). Although motivated to improve diagnostic reliability, the reverse may have occurred by changing the minimum cutoff to a milder, less discernible stage of thyroid enlargement (Peterson et al., 2000). Thyroid volume is more reliably and accurately assessed by ultrasonography than by palpation, providing a clear method of choice where resources permit (Pardede et al., 1998; Tajtakova et al., 1990). In recent years, normative standards have been developed for evaluating

ultrasound-derived thyroid volume distributions (Delange et al., 1997). Still, responsiveness, in terms of goiter reduction, to even long-term (for example, >6 month to 4 year duration) iodine intervention is variable (Elnagar et al., 1995; Hintze et al., 1988), suggesting the need to depend on other indicators of iodine status for program evaluation.

Urinary iodine (UI) concentration serves as the conventional, biochemical measure of current iodine intake and status of a population. Fasting morning samples of urine can be used to assess iodine status of a community (Thomson et al., 1997; WHO, 1994), although high day-to-day variability requires 24-hour urine collection on more than one day for reliable individual assessment (Rasmussen, Ovesen, & Christiansen, 1999; Thomson et al., 1997). UI is preferably reported as µg/L (WHO, 1994) although creatinine-adjusted concentrations are frequently used and, at least in otherwise normally nourished populations, the two measures can be equated (1 µg/L ~= 1 µg/g) (Dunn & van der Haar, 1990). A median value of more than 100 µg/L urine is considered to be reflective of a normal (average) iodine intake (that is, >150 µg per day) and adequate status in the community (Dunn & van der Haar, 1990). Notably, median urinary iodine concentrations correlate negatively with the prevalence of goiter across communities (Bar-Andziak, Lazecki, Radwanowska, & Nauman, 1993; Caron et al., 1997; Delange et al., 1997; Kimiagar, Azizi, Navai, Yassai, & Nafarabadi, 1990; Pardede et al., 1998; Rasmussen et al., 1999), and correlate positively with iodine intake (for example, r = 0.3 to 0.6) (Bar-Andziak et al., 1993; Brussard, Brants, Hulshof, Kistemaker, & Lowik, 1997; Kim, Moon, Kim, Sohn, & Oh, 1998), serving to affirm population-based assessments of risk based on this measure.

Additional iodine status indicators include serum, whole blood or whole blood spot TSH and serum thyroglobulin concentration. TSH measurement is recommended for screening neonates for hypothyroidism, which also can indicate population iodine status (Delange, 1998; Dunn, 1996; Lixin et al., 1995). Neonatal TSH tends to be negatively correlated (for example, r = –0.5) with maternal urinary iodine, thus reflecting the status of the materno-fetal dyad (Lixin et al., 1995). Thyroglobulin concentration reflects increased turnover of thyroid cells due to hypertrophy and hyperplasia. Both indicators rise with increasingly severe iodine deficiency (decreasing median iodine intakes and UI excretion levels) (WHO, 1994).

### Prevention

Unlike other micronutrient deficiencies that might be corrected by diversifying the local diet, iodine deficiency correction in an endemic area is largely dependent on consuming foods grown in iodine sufficient soil or fortified with iodine (iodization). Pilot projects in China have successfully demonstrated the beneficial impact of iodinating irrigation water used for crop production on iodine status of humans and animal herds.

An average dietary iodine intake of approximately 150 μg/d is recommended for adults to maintain adequate iodine status (Delange, 1993; National Research Council, 1989). A usual intake of 50 μg/d is considered a minimum requirement, below which thyroid enlargement can be expected (Delange, 1993). U.S. Recommended Dietary Allowances (RDAs) during in-

fancy through age three years, which range from 40 μg/d to 70 μg/d, are premised on an adequate maternal iodine intake and breast milk iodine concentration. The questionable applicability of these assumptions in iodine deficient regions of the world has motivated some experts to suggest raising the recommendation to 90 μg/d for these young ages (Delange, 1993).

Universal salt iodization (USI) remains the longest standing, most adapted, and most cost-effective approach to preventing iodine deficiency and its disorders throughout the world. Begun in the United States and selected European countries in the 1920s, USI programs are now underway in at least 82 of the 118 countries where risk of IDD is a public health concern (Underwood, 1994). Salt iodization technology is straightforward, typically involving the dry-mixing or spraying potassium iodate or iodide with food grade salt (Mannar & Dunn, 1995). Levels of iodization vary across and within countries, after considering salt consumption patterns, iodine gap in the diet, ambient exposures, packaging, transport, and other conditions. Often the iodine concentration will range from 10 ppm to 80 ppm of elemental iodine (Mannar & Dunn, 1995). In addition to the expected efficacy of the intended dosage, the success of salt iodization rests on numerous other political, legislative, management, and marketing and salt use factors that must be synchronous to be effective (see Exhibit 5–4). Failure in these other program elements has led to disappointingly small changes in iodine status in many settings, even after decades of salt iodization (Langer, Tajtakova, Podoba, Kostalova, & Gutekunst, 1994; Lindberg, Andersson, & Lamberg, 1989; Metges et al., 1996; Syrenicz et al., 1993). Still, USI remains a viable goal in most countries in need of iodine deficiency control.

Where salt iodization is not practical, other means must be found to deliver adequate iodine to high-risk groups (Solomons, 1998). Annual or biannual supplementation with iodized oil improves iodine status (Peterson et al., 2000) and has been shown to markedly lower risk of maternal hypothyroidism, cretinism, and fetal/infant

**Exhibit 5–4** Salt Iodization: Ensuring Quality, Maintaining Impact

---

Salt remains a common dietary item for people of all ages, cultures, and geographic and socio-economic bounds. Industrialized countries have had iodized salt to prevent iodine deficiency for several decades; yet the full impact of salt iodization has yet to be achieved in, especially, most low- and middle-income countries. Iodizing salt is straightforward, but many factors impede progress. Key steps for cost-effective salt iodization were laid out in a 1996 quality assurance workshop for producers, policy makers, scientists, and programmers (Quality Assurance Workshop, 1997). These include:

- **Producers:** Upgrade raw salt production through quality control and training; batch process salt and iodate by a mechanized, noncorrosive blender or mixer, with manual backup for power outage; or for continuous processing, use screw/auger mixer during or after adding iodate dosing pumps and spray methods for uniform iodization; package bulk salt in lined or laminated bags ≤50 kg, using semiautomated filling, sealing, and stitching procedures; label bulk bags with "Use No Hooks," "Iodized Salt," producer's name/address, and bag weight; retail salt in smaller (<1 kg), heat sealed bags; support government efforts to monitor and achieve iodized salt standards; monitor with salt test kits; self-police through producer associations.

- **Governments:** Pass and review as needed enabling salt iodization legislation (setting ranges versus absolute concentrations for iodine content) that includes packaging, labeling, transport, and marketing policies; hold "stakeholder" meetings to provide updates on IDD control and discuss new technology; develop methods for small producers to meet standards; create national database of producers to ensure training; strictly monitor and provide incentives for compliance, focusing on low coverage areas; modernize test laboratories; accelerate consumer demand for small (<1 kg) retail packages; enforce policies related to national standards; monitor IDD impact.

- **Agencies:** Develop and distribute information for producers; help improve government-industry-international exchange; monitor and inform on potassium iodate market; help increase consumer demand for small packages of salt; assist in capacity building and quality assurance agenda.

---

mortality (Pharoah et al., 1971). An annual dose of 200 mg of iodine has been shown to optimize iodine status while minimizing risk of toxicity in adults (Peterson et al., 2000). Under consideration is the possibility of delivering a single, oral dose of iodized oil to young infants at the time of oral polio vaccine, possibly through the WHO Expanded Programme for Immunization. In one randomized trial, neutralizing antibody responses to oral polio vaccine were unaffected by iodized oil intake (Taffs et al., 1999) while infant mortality was reduced (Cobra et al., 1997).

Irrespective of the choice of iodine intervention, sound programming principles must be followed, which include involving key stakeholders (from government to private sector) in planning, educating the targeted public (especially important with voluntary salt iodization), proper moni-

toring, and taking adequate steps to solve problems and ensure sustainability (Dunn, 1996).

## Zinc Deficiency

Zinc is essential for mammalian cell life, function, growth, differentiation, and replication (Hambidge & Krebs, 1999; Keen & Gershwin, 1990; Solomons, 1999). Such ubiquitous need can be expected to confer on zinc a central role in protecting the health of individuals.

Zinc deficiency remains one of the least "visible" micronutrient deficiencies. Global estimates of its extent, severity, and health impact in populations are lacking due to absence of adequate, nationally representative data on zinc status (ACC/SCN, 2000). This uncertainty, attributed to a lack of reliable indicators or lack of consensus with respect to their use, interpretation, and target groups to assess (Caulfield, Zavaleta, Shankar, & Merialdi, 1998), coupled with limited experience to date in prevention programs (Gibson & Ferguson, 1998), may have been factors that led to the near exclusion of zinc on the global micronutrient agenda a decade ago ("Ending Hidden Hunger," 1992; McGuire & Galloway, 1994; Trowbridge et al., 1993). Limited survey data, however, suggest that 25% or more of prepubescent children in grain-dependent areas of the low-income world have low zinc status, expressed by serum zinc (<70 µg/dl) or hair zinc (<1.68 µmol/g) concentrations (Ferguson et al., 1993; Smith, Makdani, Hegar, Rao, & Douglass, 1999; Udomkesmalee et al., 1992). Similar prevalences have been observed in women of reproductive age (Gross et al., 1998).

Dietary data estimating intakes of zinc as well as, often, phytate (naturally occurring inhibitor of zinc absorption in food), suggest a larger, though more variable, percentage of the world's undernourished are at risk of zinc inadequacy (Caulfield et al., 1998; Ferguson et al., 1993; Gibson & Huddle, 1998; Murphy, Beaton, & Calloway, 1992). Suspicion of high prevalence, coupled with marked health risks being attributed to zinc deficiency (Black, 1998; Prasad, 1985), lend an urgency to the need to measure and establish the public health significance of zinc deficiency (Black, 1997; Sandstead et al., 1998).

### Function and Assessment

Zinc is found in all cells, serving as a constituent of more than 200 enzymes and numerous transcription proteins (as a "zinc finger") that regulate nucleic acid synthesis, metabolism of protein, lipid, carbohydrate, and cell differentiation (Cousins & Hempe, 1990; Stipanuk, 2000). These functions confer on zinc important roles in organogenesis, tissue growth, functional development, and immunity (Shankar & Prasad, 1998; Stipanuk, 2000). Such broad involvement in metabolism virtually assures zinc an important role in maintaining health. Zinc is absorbed by both passive diffusion across a concentration gradient and by energy-dependent processes when intake is low (Stipanuk, 2000). In mixed diets, the efficiency of zinc absorption can vary widely, from practically nil to 40%, with the lowest absorption associated with high grain and plant consumption and the highest with breast milk and meat. Absorption tends to be higher in zinc deficiency (Solomons, 1999). Zinc is primarily transported to the liver bound to albumin from which it is released in association with a carrier protein, $\alpha_2$-macroglobulin. Uptake into tissues appears to be regulated, although mechanisms are poorly understood. About 90% of total body zinc resides in skeletal muscle, calcified bone, and marrow, mostly bound to the storage protein, metallothionein. This leaves only a small exchangeable body pool that can respond to short-term variation in zinc intake. Less than 1% of body zinc is in circulation (Cousins & Hempe, 1990).

Zinc status may be assessed by a combination of clinical, biochemical, test-response, and dietary methods (Gibson, 1990; Gibson & Huddle, 1998). Clinical signs of moderate to severe zinc deficiency, including marked growth retardation, dermatitis and other skin changes, poor appetite, and mental lethargy, are either rare or lack sufficient specificity to be useful for population assessment. Diagnosis of more prevalent mild zinc deficiency usually rests on determining serum or plasma zinc concentration (Gibson, 1990). Although unreliable for individual assessment, the distribution of plasma zinc concentrations or responsiveness of the lower end of the distribution to intervention can identify groups at risk. A (morning, fasting) plasma cutoff of <60 µg/dl (<9.2 µmol/L) has been suggested for classifying individuals as zinc deficient (Gibson, 1990), although cutoffs ranging from <50 µg/dl (<7.7 µmol/L) to <80 µg/dl (<12.3 µmol/L) have been used. Hair zinc concentration may be used as a static indicator to identify groups of individuals likely to be zinc deficient, with 1.68 µmol/g suggested as a cutoff (Gibson & Huddle, 1998). Stable isotope dilution methods may be used to assess total body zinc stores, though the cost and complexity of this approach limits its use to evaluating small numbers of individuals and validating other indicators (Hambidge & Krebs, 1995; Hambidge, Krebs, & Miller, 1998). Dietary assessment can provide valuable insight with respect to the distribution and probable bioavailability of dietary zinc from local food resulting from concurrent estimation of phytate content, but alone cannot reflect status of an individual or population (Gibson & Ferguson, 1998).

### Health Consequences

As predicted by Prasad (1991), the past decade has witnessed an "explosion" of research to elucidate zinc's role in health. Preschool children who exhibit low serum zinc level are more likely to develop diarrhea and experience more severe episodes of diarrhea or acute respiratory infection than children with adequate zinc status (Bahl, Bhandari, Hambidge, & Bhan, 1998). The causality of this association has been examined by quantifying the impact of zinc supplementation on the incidence, duration, and severity of acute and persistent diarrhea or dysentery (Faruque, Mahalanabis, Haque, Fuchs, & Habte, 1999; Penny et al., 1999; Rosado, 1997; Roy et al., 1999; Ruel, Rivera, Santizo, Lonnerdal, & Brown, 1997; Sazawal et al., 1995, 1996; Sazawal, Black, et al., 1997; Sazawal, Jalla, et al., 1997; Sazawal et al., 1998; Zinc Investigators' Collaborative Group, 1999), acute respiratory infections (Roy et al., 1999; Ruel et al., 1997; Sazawal et al., 1998), malaria (Shankar & Prasad, 1998), immune competence (Sazawal, Jalla, et al., 1997; Shankar & Prasad, 1998) and growth (Brown, Peerson, & Allen, 1998; Rosado et al., 1997) in young children. The number, specificity, and timeliness of the trials, coupled with an urgent need to grasp health implications of adequate zinc nutriture for policy and program purposes, have stimulated overview analyses to better discern the health benefits of improved zinc nutriture, especially for high-risk populations.

**Diarrhea.** Evidence for a role of zinc in reducing the incidence, severity, and duration of diarrhea is remarkably consistent. Data from seven clinical trials evaluating the efficacy of continuous, daily zinc supplementation of preschool children were recently pooled for analysis (Zinc Investigators' Collaborative Group, 1999). Eligible trials provided 1–2 RDAs of zinc (that is, 5–20 mg as sulfate, gluconate, or methionate), with or without other micronutrients, for periods of 12 to 54 weeks to preschoolers who had recovered, or were recovering, from a recent episode of diarrhea or who were initially malnourished by anthropometric indicators (weight for height or height for age). The benefit of zinc supplementation was consistent with average reductions of 18% in the incidence (odds ratio = 0.82; 95% confidence interval [CI]: 0.72–0.93) (Figure 5–13, Panel A) and 25% (OR = 0.75; 95% CI: 0.63–0.88) in the prevalence (days ill/100 person-days) (Figure 5–13, Panel B) of diarrhea. The apparent, greater impact on prevalence can be expected because prevalence includes episodic duration, which was also reduced by zinc supplementation (Faruque et al., 1999; Hambidge et al., 1998; Roy et al., 1997; Ruel et al., 1997). Zinc therapy also reduced the frequency of persistent diarrhea (R.E. Black, 1998).

**Respiratory Infection.** Fewer studies have evaluated the effects of zinc on acute lower respiratory infection. Four continuous-supplementation trials examined this question (Ninh et al., 1996; Penny et al., 1999; Sazawal et al., 1998; Zinc Investigators' Collaborative Group, 1999). These studies revealed an average reduction of 41% in the incidence of pneumonia among zinc-supplemented versus control children (OR = 0.59; 95% CI: 0.41–0.83). A 25–40% reduction in risk of acute lower respiratory infection with zinc compares favorably with an approximately 33% reduction in pneumonia that has been projected if low weight for age (below –2 Z-scores) were to be eliminated (Victora et al., 1999).

**Malaria.** Experimental zinc deficiency impairs host defenses against malarial infection (Shankar & Prasad, 1998). *Plasmodium falciparum (pf)* parasitemia has also been negatively

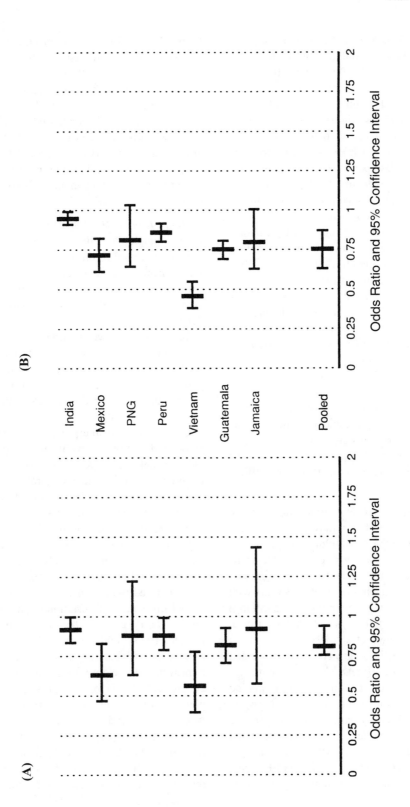

**Figure 5–13** Individual and Pooled Effects (Odds Ratio and 95% Confidence Interval) of Daily Zinc Supplementation on Incidence (Panel A) and Prevalence (Panel B) of Early Childhood Diarrhea in Seven Randomized, Double-Masked, Continuous Supplementation Trials

associated with measures of zinc status or intake in Africa (Gibson & Huddle, 1998) and Southeast Asia (Gibson et al., 1991). The public health impact of this association has been tested in three randomized, double-masked field trials. The largest and most rigorous was conducted among 274 children aged 6 to 60 months in Papua New Guinea. Children who received 10 mg of zinc, six days per week for 10 months, experienced a 38% reduction (95% CI: 3 to 60%) in *pf* malaria episodes (fever plus parasitemia >9200 per µL), and a 69% reduction in episodes with heavy parasitemia (>100,000 µL) (Shankar et al., 2000). Similar reductions in malarial illness have been reported from the Gambia (30%, not statistically significant) (Bates et al., 1993) and another trial among nursery school children in Uganda where zinc supplementation throughout the school year was associated with a 25% reduction in weekly illness event rates (p<0.05), >80% of which were classified as malaria attacks (Kikafunda, Walker, Allan, & Tumwine, 1998).

With mounting evidence that adequate zinc nutriture can reduce the incidence and intensity of infections, it is plausible that child mortality could be reduced by preventing even "mild" zinc deficiency through supplementation or fortification of food.

***Poor Growth.*** A recent overview has clarified the extent and type of growth response that may occur when prepubescent children are given zinc on a daily basis. Twenty-five controlled trials were included in a meta-analysis that examined the effect of dosing children under 13 years with approximately 14 mg zinc (range of 1.5–50 mg) daily for periods of 10 days to 16 months (mean ~7 months) (Brown et al., 1998). Differences in ponderal and linear growth were expressed as an "effect size" ([mean change in treatment group – mean change in control group] / pooled standard deviation of the difference between groups), weighted by sample size, expressed as a standard deviation. The analysis revealed modest but statistically significant increases in weight (0.26 SD, p<0.001) and height (0.22 SD, p<0.0001) (Figure 5–14), with larger effects

seen for weight (0.38 SD) in zinc-undernourished children (where baseline mean serum zinc concentration was <80 µg/dl) and for height/length (0.49 SD) in more stunted study children (Brown et al., 1998). Zinc supplementation has, in some settings, also increased tricipital skinfold size (Kikafunda et al., 1998), mid-upper arm circumference (Cavan et al., 1993; Kikafunda et al., 1998), and lean body mass, supporting a role for zinc in maintaining body composition.

***Reproductive Health.*** Zinc is required for normal maternal health, fetal growth, and development and parturition (Caulfield et al., 1998). Experimental zinc deficiency leads to poor pregnancy outcomes (Apgar, 1985; Bunce, Lytton, Gunesekera, Vessal, & Kim, 1994), but evidence linking human maternal zinc deficiency to intrauterine growth retardation, prematurity, low birthweight, and complications at delivery is conflicting (Caulfield et al., 1998; Tamura, Goldenberg, Johnston, & Dubard, 2000). Maternal plasma zinc concentration decreases throughout gestation (Tamura et al., 2000), possibly reflecting deficiency, an interpretation supported by associated complications at labor and delivery (McMichael et al., 1982). However, decreasing maternal plasma zinc may also reflect increased feto-placental uptake, hormonal influences, or effects of plasma volume expansion (Lonnerdal, 1998; Tamura et al., 2000), which may partly explain a lack of association between zinc status and fetal growth in relatively well-nourished populations (Tamura et al., 2000). Several trials have reported modest increases (approximately 0.5 wk) in length of gestation (Caulfield et al., 1998; Cherry et al., 1989; Garg, Singhla, & Arshad, 1993; Goldenberg et al., 1995; Kynast & Saling, 1986; Ross, Nel, & Naeye, 1985) and improved birthweight (Garg et al., 1993; Goldenberg et al., 1995) following maternal zinc supplementation, while others carried out in low-income countries have failed to find any effect on newborn size (Caulfield, Zavaleta, Figueroa, & Leon, 1999; Osendarp et al., 2000; Ross et al., 1985), possibly due, in part, to mothers having a relatively normal zinc status at the outset. Gross

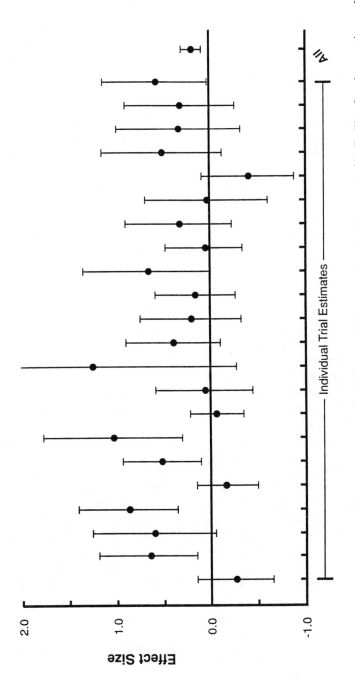

**Figure 5–14** Individual and Overview ("All") Effect Size Estimates (Expressed as a Standardized Distance) of Daily Zinc Supplementation on Height Growth Based on 22 Individual Trials among Preschool Aged Children

benefit to reproductive health from increased maternal zinc intake appears to require an initial maternal zinc deficiency to correct. However, more subtle benefit may often escape detection, such as improved fetal neurobehavioral development following maternal zinc supplementation (Merialdi, Caulfield, Zavaleta, Figueroa, & DiPietro, 1998). Zinc also plays a known role in mammalian cell differentiation and turnover, ontogeny of mammalian systems, and thymic and other lymphoid tissue development and function (Cousins & Hempe, 1990), which, for example, could predispose individuals deprived of essential zinc in utero to permanent impairment in immunity and host resistance (Beach, Gershwin, & Hurley, 1982). Chronic, postnatal, and even intergenerational effects of deviations in maternal zinc nutriture fit well with emerging theories of fetal malnutrition and lifelong disease risk (Leon, 1998).

### Prevention

The ubiquitous role of zinc in nature and its potential to affect many facets of health make zinc deficiency one of the most compelling of all micronutrient deficiencies to address. Yet little has been done to prevent zinc deficiency to date. Prevention strategies could employ dietary, fortification, supplementary, and agricultural approaches. Excellent sources of bioavailable zinc include red meat, liver and other organ meats, poultry, shellfish, eggs, and milk. These foods often contribute <10% of dietary zinc among low-income populations (Gibson & Ferguson, 1998). Also, the adequacy of dietary zinc depends on both its quantity and bioavailability, the latter being a function of the presence of compounds in foods that inhibit absorption of zinc. These compounds include phytates, found abundantly in whole grain cereals and legumes; dietary fiber; oxalates; polyphenols; and other binding compounds (Oberleas & Harland, 1981; Solomons, 1999). A dietary phytate-to-zinc molar ratio of >15 (Gibson, 1990), common in many traditional diets in low- and middle-income countries (Ferguson et al., 1993), has been associated with low zinc status (WHO, 1996b). Phytates may be reduced in some whole

grains (for example, wheat, rice, and sorghum) by milling that can remove the phytate-rich aleurone layer, or by methods that induce enzymatic (phytase) hydrolysis of phytic acid, thereby disabling its ability to complex with zinc in the gut (Lonnerdal, Sandberg, Sandstrom, & Kunz, 1989). These latter methods include soaking of cereals or legumes, germination and fermentation of cereals and related products (Gibson, Yeudall, Drost, Mtitimuni, & Cullinan, 1998), methods that are easily applied in rural areas. Plant breeding strategies may provide new generations of staple crops in the future that increase zinc and decrease phytic acid content, while enhancing yield (Gibson & Ferguson, 1998; Graham, Ascher, & Hynes, 1992; Ruel & Bouis, 1998).

Fortification, either with zinc alone, but more likely along with other micronutrients, offers promise as processed staple grains and other food commodities increasingly penetrate the low-income markets. Micronutrient premixes containing zinc have been proposed for complementary and special transitional foods for children in refugee settings (Gibson & Ferguson, 1998) based on estimated needs of infants and young (Brown, Dewey, & Allen, 1998). Direct supplementation offers the most immediate approach for improving zinc status of mothers and children, most probably in combination with other micronutrients. However, zinc interactions with other nutrients such as nonheme iron (Solomons, 1986), copper (Yadrick, Kenney, & Winterfeldt, 1989), and calcium (Wood & Zheng, 1997), which are only beginning to be understood, may influence bioavailability and efficacy, and, therefore, choice of the form and dosage of zinc in supplements (Gibson, Yeudall, et al., 1998). Recommended daily intakes of zinc for infants, young children, and women are 5, 10, and 12 mg, respectively (National Research Council, 1989).

### DIET AND UNDERNUTRITION

From the foregoing sections, it should be apparent that young children, in particular, are vulnerable to protein, energy, and micronutrient deficiencies. Diet in childhood should be adequate to meet all normal energy and nutrient requirements to support tissue growth, maintenance and function, and physical activity. Health and developmental consequences can occur when diet continually fails to meet these nutritional demands. Family and mealtime conditions under which food is eaten often reflect broader issues of child care and nurturing in the home that can influence child development. Most childhood undernutrition results directly from a diet that is chronically inadequate in quantity, conventionally taken to mean low in energy and protein; and quality, more broadly reflecting poor biological value of protein (for example, low amino acid score), low or imbalanced micronutrient density, or bioavailability due to high "antinutrient" content (for example, phytate, fiber, oxalates, and so on). Poor quality may also refer to nonhygienic aspects of food consumed, which could lead to food contamination and increased disease risk. Often the diet of the undernourished encompasses most of these features to varying degrees. Nutrient supplements are generally not viewed as part of the diet. Fortified food, though still rare in the diets of most low-income people, is increasingly being viewed as contributing to dietary quality. Dietary needs and the major ways these are met in infancy and early childhood are the focus of this section.

## Breastfeeding to Complementary Feeding Continuum

Ideally, the infant-to-child feeding continuum should be viewed as a process, involving first breast and then transitional feeding, that results in adequate nourishment of children to support normal growth, health, and development from birth through the early childhood years. The process of establishing exclusive breastfeeding, followed by phasing in complementary feeding and eventual further transition to family foods, is illustrated in Figure 5–15. The concept is advanced by clear definitions of feeding states that have emerged in recent years. Thus exclusive and almost exclusive (or predominant) breastfeeding are differentiated due to potential pathogen exposure and risk of infection that accompanies the latter (Labbok & Karsovec, 1990). Partial breastfed infants are usefully subdivided according to their consumption of nonhuman milk, solid foods, and frequency of breastfeeding or percent of total daily energy consumed from breast milk (Piwoz, Creed de Kanashiro, Lopez de Romana, Black, & Brown, 1996). Complementary feeding begins with the onset of partial breastfeeding. Complementary foods, or "special transitional foods," are "any nutrient-containing foods or liquids other than breast milk given to young children during the period of complementary feeding" (Brown et al., 1998). Their purpose is to adequately nourish an infant who is gradually weaning from the breast, while trying to minimize breast milk displacement. It has been suggested that the term *weaning food* be avoided as it may convey the wrong goal of displacing breast milk with another, even if nutritious, food (Brown et al., 1998). Finally, the complementary feeding period passes when an infant is fully weaned from the breast, although infrequent, "token" breastfeeding may persist prior to complete cessation, with likely little nutritional or growth benefit (Labbok & Karsovec, 1990; Piwoz et al., 1996). By that age, often 3 to 4 years, a child has passed through the period of highest risk for growth faltering, serious infectious illness, and mortality. Dietary progression to a full household diet is likely to follow patterns established during complementary feeding.

An empirical example of the breast-to-complementary feeding continuum can be derived from data on breastfeeding prevalence among nearly 21,000 children participating in the Botswana Nutritional Surveillance System (Figure 5–16) (Michaelson, 1988). The pattern is typical of many rural areas of Africa and other low-income regions, whereby initial, (almost) exclusive breastfeeding rapidly gives way to partial breastfeeding by 6 months of age, and gradual weaning by 3 years of age. The "slopes" of the transition curves depend on cultural and socioeconomic norms, and especially maternal, caregiver, and family preferences related to breastfeeding initiation; frequency and duration; the

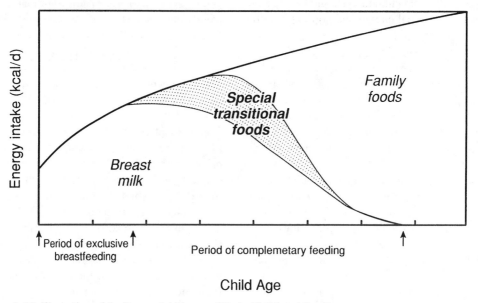

**Figure 5–15**  Illustration of the Sequential Phases of Early Childhood Feeding

availability of hygienic (Rowland, Barrell, & Whitehead, 1978), affordable, and nutritious complementary foods; emerging changes in women's roles in communities; and other lifestyle, socioeconomic, and food security factors (Begin, Frongillo, & Delisle, 1999; Galler, Ramsey, Harrison, Brooks, & Weiskopf-Bock, 1998; Underwood & Hofvander, 1982). Reflecting regional variation in these determinants, breastfeeding tends to extend for a longer duration in South and Southeast Asia, indicated by prevalences of, often, 50–80% at age 2 years (Brown, Black, & Becker, 1982; Grummer-Strawn, 1996; Huffman, Chowdhury, Chakraborty, & Simpson, 1980; Khatry et al., 1995), and lower in Latin America (Grummer-Strawn, 1996) and China (Taren & Chen, 1993).

**Breastfeeding**

Exclusive breastfeeding is generally believed to provide adequate energy and nutrients to an infant through the first 4 to 6 months of life,

during which average intakes have been observed to range between 700 and 800 ml per day in both low-income and industrialized countries (Brown et al., 1998). Feeding early nutrient and energy-dense colostrum is important in this process. Exclusively breastfed infants reared in industrialized countries (Dewey, Heinig, & Nommsen-Rivers, 1995) and in families of high socioeconomic standing in low-income countries (Pathak, Shah, & Tataria, 1993) tend to follow or exceed the WHO/NCHS median weight for age curve through the first 3 months of life (Victora et al., 1998; WHO Working Group on Infant Growth, 1994). Lower milk production (for example, 400 to 600 ml/d), as has been observed in some malnourished populations of women (Jelliffe & Jelliffe, 1978), might suggest the age of complementary food introduction to be closer to 4 than 6 months, but this remains a matter of debate (Brown et al., 1998). It is inadequately known the degree to which frequent exposure to infection, as often occurs among young infants in poor societies, changes energy and nutrient requirements and the consequent ability

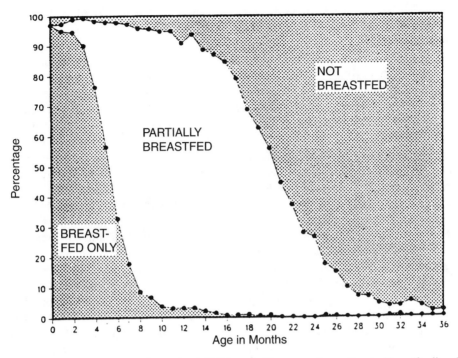

**Figure 5–16** Actual Distributions of Preschool Children in Botswana According to Breastfeeding Status. "Partially breastfed" implies period of complementary feeding and "not breastfed" can be interpreted to denote transition to family foods.

of exclusive breastfeeding to meet these needs (Brown et al., 1998; Butte, 1996). In some studies, infection has been noted to have relatively little effect on breast milk intake during early infancy (Brown et al., 1985; Brown, Stallings, Creed de Kanashiro, Lopez de Romana, & Black, 1990). Interaction with infection, however, could partly explain the frequent occurrence of growth failure among almost exclusively breastfed infants during the first 3 to 6 months of life in poorly nourished groups (Rivera & Ruel, 1997).

Beyond energy and nutrients, breast milk contains a repertoire of antimicrobial and anti-inflammatory factors, hormones, digestive enzymes, transport molecules, and growth modulators that appear to confer substantial protection from infection and other harmful agents (Prentice, 1996). These factors, along with the nutritional qualities of human milk, provide bio-

logical plausibility for observed reductions in persistent or severe diarrheal morbidity (Victora, Fuchs, Kirkwood, Lombardi, & Barros, 1992), including episodes of cholera and shigellosis (Clemens et al., 1986, 1990) among breastfed versus nonbreastfed infants and young children. Lower risk of sick child visits and reported episodes of diarrhea, ear infection, and respiratory infection have also been associated with early breastfeeding in industrialized countries (Raisler, Alexander, & O'Campo, 1999). Breastfeeding appears to markedly improve an infant's chances of surviving the first 2–3 months of life, an age at which a pooled analysis of studies in three countries revealed a 75–80% lower risk of death among breastfed infants relative to nonbreastfed infants. A stronger, protective effect was observed against diarrhea-related (85% reduction) than acute respiratory infection-related (58% reduction) fatality at that age (WHO Collaborative Study Team, 2000). Continued breast-feeding in mid-infancy (4 to 8 months) through the second year of life was associated with approximately 50% and approximately 33% reductions in risk of death, respectively. The "survival effect" of breastfeeding appears to disproportionately benefit those at highest risk: severely malnourished children (Briend, Wojtyniak, & Rowland, 1988), among whom breastfeeding has been associated with a strong protective effect into the third year of life (Briend & Bari, 1989), and children from low-income households, evident, for example, by high maternal illiteracy and poor sanitation. The likely benefits to survival among low-income children are fully consistent with observations linking extended, partial breastfeeding to protection against consequences of moderate-to-severe micronutrient deficiencies, such as xerophthalmia (Mahalanabis, 1991; West et al., 1986). Better educated women, on the other hand, while less likely to breastfeed, are also more likely to use promotive and curative health services (Becker, Peters, Gray, Gultiano, & Black, 1993) and ensure a more nutritious diet that can lead to improved child survival (Bairagi, 1980; Bouis & Novenario-Reese, 1997).

One paradoxical, largely cross-sectional observation in recent years has been that breastfed children in late infancy through the third year of life are generally, though not always (Taren & Chen, 1993), lower in weight and shorter in height than their weaned peers of the same age (Brakohiapa et al., 1988; Castillo, Atalah, Riumallo, & Castro, 1996; Caulfield, Bentley, & Ahmed, 1996; Grummer-Strawn, 1996; Victora, Vaughan, Martines, & Barcelos, 1984). The finding has persisted despite repeated attempts to adjust for multiple possible confounding factors. It has been difficult, however, to develop plausible explanations for how breastfeeding could depress physical growth, while improving survival and reducing risks of micronutrient deficiencies, lacking evidence that breastfeeding specifically increases the risk of infection or reduces appetite and, thus, nutrient delivery to the infant. The association is more likely to be ex-

plained by factors related to (1) cross-sectional study designs that cannot reveal the temporal dimension of the breastfeeding-nutritional status relationship; (2) residual confounding, despite adjustment for multiple factors as measured that may influence both the mother's decision to breastfeed and the nutritional health of children; and (3) reverse causality, which could lead mothers to continue breastfeeding their children because they are malnourished (Caulfield et al., 1996). Relevant to understanding this phenomenon, a recent prospective study in Kenya assessed the growth of 264 partially breastfed children between approximately 14 to 20 months of age, by their longitudinal breastfeeding and weaning habits over a 6-month period. Children who continued to breastfeed for the entire follow-up period gained more in height (+0.6 cm) and weight (+230 g) than children who breastfed for a medium duration (50–99% of the 6-month follow-up) and 3.4 cm and 370 g more in weight and height, respectively, than children whose breastfeeding duration was shortest (<50% of the follow-up period) (Onyango, Esrey, & Kramer, 1999). These findings agree with two other recent longitudinal studies of breastfeeding and growth (Adair et al., 1993; Marquis, Habicht, Lanata, Black, & Rasmussen, 1997), indicating that prospective studies that collect sufficient data on breastfeeding, diet, morbidity, care, and other factors are required to clarify this issue, short of an (unlikely) randomized trial.

Among few negative effects of breastfeeding, that of greatest public health importance is the potential for breast milk to carry HIV and thus serve as a vehicle for vertical transmission of the virus from mother to infant (Dunn, Newell, Ades, & Peckham, 1992; Kreiss, 1997). It is estimated that breastfeeding may account for 5–15% of all postnatal HIV infection among infants (Leroy et al., 1998). HIV infection is associated with marked changes in maternal wasting and micronutrient status, which could affect the pathogenesis and transmission of disease (Mostad et al., 1997; Semba & Tang, 1999) and infant survival (Fawzi et al., 1998). Viral load and mastitis may interact to increase risk of vertical transmission to breastfed infants (Semba et al., 1999). Because of the lack of suitable feeding alternatives and the known, protective effects of breastfeeding in reducing risk of infant mortality due to infection (WHO Collaborative Study Team, 2000), presently mothers living in impoverished areas, where risk of infant mortality due to infection is high, are recommended to breastfeed, irrespective of maternal HIV status. Where infection plays a lesser role in infant mortality, HIV-positive mothers are encouraged to feed other appropriate complementary foods to their infants ("Current consensus on HIV transmission," 1995; WHO, 1992).

Interventions to promote breastfeeding have in recent years targeted the medical and health care establishment in low-income countries to formally change policies and programs to promote exclusive breastfeeding early in life and, in recent years, to offer sound advice to mothers in HIV-endemic areas. The most widely adapted and cost-effective program to date has been the global "Baby Friendly Hospital Initiative" developed and promoted by WHO and UNICEF (see Exhibit 5–5) (Sanghvi & Murray, 1997). Promotion and adoption by women of appropriate breastfeeding practices is considered one of the most cost-effective interventions within the low-income world for increasing disability-adjusted life years (DALYs, a quantitative index of burden of disease) (Horton et al., 1996; Murray & Lopez, 1997; Sanghvi & Murray, 1997; World Bank, 1993) (Figure 5–17).

## Complementary (and Supplementary) Feeding

While considerable agreement exists about the basic sequences of early childhood feeding, opinions vary widely around the world about the exact month of age at which complementary feeding should begin, the specific types of foods infants can tolerate, their order of introduction, frequency and mode of feeding, preparation, and the degree to which variation in these "delivery-related" facets of child feeding affect the short- and long-term health, growth, and development of children (Dewey, in press). Among these questions, most available evidence relates to the effects of diverse feeding interventions on growth and developmental indexes of children. In this section, findings are grouped together from both complementary and supplementary feeding trials where types of intervention, age groups, and study designs permit some degree of assimilation.

### Impact on Growth

The effects of infant and child feeding, beyond breastfeeding alone, on growth vary with age and with other study-specific factors. Randomized complementary feeding trials were carried out among Honduran infants between 4 and 6 months of age who had been normal (Cohen, Brown, Canahuati, Rivera, & Dewey, 1994) and small (Dewey, Cohen, Brown, & Rivera, 1999) for gestational age at birth. No concurrent, or extended, growth differences through 12 months of age could be attributed to infant receipt of a nutritious menu of complementary foods during the 3-month period compared to control infants who remained exclusively breastfed. In both studies, early complementary feeding appeared mildly to displace breast milk intake, despite maintaining a normal frequency of breastfeeds, by 6 months of age. In only one of four randomized feeding trials conducted in Senegal, the Congo, Bolivia, and New Caledonia did intake of a standardized, fortified instant gruel, providing approximately 200 kcal daily to 4- to 7-month old infants, have any impact on growth. In Senegal, where malnutrition was highest, linear growth improved by approximately 0.5 cm among supplemented over nonsupplemented infants (Simondon et al., 1996). These results generally agree with observational studies indicating that the growth of exclusively breastfed infants either parallels or exceeds that of partially or fully weaned infants through the first 6 months of life (Brown et al., 1998). An exception lies in a well-described trial in Colombia during which mothers were randomized in the third trimester of pregnancy to receive a family food package each week, including a skim-milk

**Exhibit 5–5** Breastfeeding Promotion: The Baby Friendly Hospital Initiative

---

The Baby Friendly Hospital Initiative (BFHI) is a global campaign, initiated by WHO and UNICEF and supported by international and national agencies to ensure that hospital practices promote establishing and continuing exclusive breastfeeding immediately after delivery. The campaign seeks to have hospitals develop and implement a coherent policy to:

- inform pregnant women about the benefits of breastfeeding
- help mothers initiate breastfeeding within 30 minutes after birth
- give newborns no food or drink other than breast milk (except medicines)
- practice "rooming-in" with no planned separations of mother and infant
- encourage breastfeeding on demand
- give no pacifiers or artificial teats to breastfeeding infants
- prohibit distribution of gifts or samples of formula

- promote formation of and refer mothers to breastfeeding support groups

Delivery of these and other BFHI services requires hospitals to develop and strictly enforce policies to achieve breastfeeding goals, to provide staff with training, to develop and distribute only reviewed and approved brochures, and to evaluate outcomes such as compliance, maternal intention to breastfeed, in-hospital and home lactational performance, among other measures, with follow-up action to address problems (WHO, 1989). Evaluations of the BFHI in several countries between 1992 to 1995 showed high hospital compliance in establishing policies and adhering to rules related to rooming-in, separations, prohibition of prelacteals and other fluids, and distribution of gift samples, but poor achievement with respect to educating mothers prenatally about breastfeeding, assisting mothers to establish breastfeeding, developing informational brochures, providing reliable home follow-up, and counseling of mothers (Sanghvi, 1995).

---

and vegetable protein mixture for their infants beginning at 3 months of age (sufficient to provide 670 kcal and 23 g of protein daily). Supplemented infants exhibited a 0.6 cm and 162 g increase in length and weight, respectively, over controls from 3 to 6 months of age (Lutter et al., 1990; Mora, Herrera, Suescun, de Navarro, & Wagner, 1981), although breastfeeding patterns were not reported and the effect may been partly influenced by maternal supplementation.

In the latter half of infancy and early childhood, purposeful supplementary feeding appears to increase growth over that observed in non-supplemented children. The results of a study from 1969 to 1977 by the Instituto Nutricional de Central America y Panama (INCAP) showed that supplementation of infants daily for 3 years with *atole*, a high-protein, multinutrient supplement (providing 90 to 170 kcal/d), led to a 2.5 cm height advantage over children given *fresca*, a low-calorie supplement, with most of the effect attributed to supplementation in the latter half of the first year (Habicht, Martorell, & Rivera, 1995). Notable growth effects in older preschool

years were not observed, but the early height difference persisted into adolescence (Ruel, Rivera, Habicht, & Martorell, 1995). In Ghana the efficacy of "Weanimix," a cereal-legume transitional food (containing maize, soybean, and groundnut) developed by UNICEF, was tested without and fortified with added vitamins and minerals, as well as with other local ingredients (fish powder and koko, a fermented maize porridge). At 6 months of age, infants were randomized to one of these four mixtures for daily consumption. Compared to a cross-sectional, local referent group, all four supplemented groups appeared to have accelerated in weight and length for age, but no differences in growth or morbidity were noted among infants receiving the various feeding mixtures. Vitamin and mineral-fortified Weanimix intake appeared to increase plasma ferritin and retinol concentrations over other mixtures (Lartey, Manu, Brown, Peerson, & Dewey, 1999). In the Colombian infants, continued supplementation with the protein-calorie gruel stimulated additional increments in weight (+110 g) and length (+0.45 cm) between 9 and

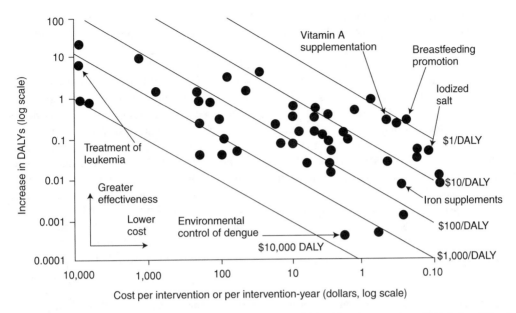

**Figure 5–17** Comparison of the Cost-Effectiveness of Several Nutrition Interventions (Labeled as Vitamin A Supplementation, Breastfeeding Promotion, and Iodized Salt) in Relation to Other Public Health and Treatment Programs in Terms of Disability-Adjusted Life Years (DALYs) Gained (Horton et al., 1996), a Summary Measure of "Life Years Lost Due to Premature Mortality and Years Lived with Disability Adjusted for Severity" (Murray & Lopez, 1997). *Note:* Calculated DALYs gained due to vitamin A did not consider impact on child mortality (World Bank, 1993), leading to an underestimate of effectiveness.

12 months of age, and smaller increments thereafter, through 36 months of age (Lutter et al., 1990). In Jamaica children 9 to 24 months of age given a weekly take-home milk formula supplement (providing a home intake-adjusted approximately 100 kcal/day) showed improved weight, length, and head circumferential growth over controls during an initial 6-month period, but not thereafter (Walker, Powell, Grantham-McGregor, Himes, & Chang, 1991). In Indonesia, providing a 400 kcal/d dietary supplement for 3 months to children 6 to 20 months of age accelerated gain in weight but not height, suggesting the intervention may have been too short to induce change in linear growth (Husaini et al., 1991). These outcomes, coupled with the varied effects noted with different micronutrient supplements, suggest that the growth impact of feeding depends on many local dietary, disease, and seasonal factors that may limit to different

degrees ponderal and linear growth and changes in body composition of children.

### Development Effects

Complementary or supplementary feeding early in life may improve childhood developmental indexes. In the INCAP study, the sustained increment in growth observed in *atole* recipients was accompanied by subsequent gains over *fresca* recipients on aptitude and cognitive tests (Pollitt et al., 1995). Four years after completion of the Jamaican trial, previously supplemented children showed a modest increase in perceptual-motor scores over those not supplemented. However, children who had been stunted and had smaller head circumferences at the trial's outset had significantly lower intelligence scores, irrespective of supplement receipt (Grantham-McGregor, Walker, Chang, & Powell, 1997), a possible indication of early cognitive impairment that has been observed in children born with IUGR (Villar, Smeriglio, Martorell, Brown, & Klein, 1984). Mental and psychomotor test scores also improved over the 3-month period Indonesian infants had been given the energy and protein-dense supplement (Husaini et al., 1991). Observed effects of zinc (Bentley et al., 1997; M.M. Black, 1998), iron (Aukett et al.,1986;  Bruner et al., 1996; Oski et al., 1983; Soemantri et al., 1985), and iodine (Bleichrodt & Born, 1994; Huda et al., 1999) supplementation on early childhood cognition and development suggest that a usual dietary intake of foods rich in such micronutrients could exert similar, or perhaps greater, benefit.

## UNDERNUTRITION AMONG OLDER PERSONS

Until recently, a largely unrecognized group at high risk of undernutrition was the rapidly growing segment of older persons (>60 years), particularly those living in impoverished settings where deteriorating health, strength, and capability are further stressed by the need to continue working to support themselves. Aging in such populations is often accompanied by decreased access to resources that are essential to maintain a minimum standard of quality of life, including adequate food, health and dental care, social and welfare services, family support, and so forth. As life expectancy continues to rise (Roubenoff, 1999; World Bank, 1993), so too will the number of older persons, expected to exceed 1.2 billion by the year 2025, two-thirds of whom will live in the low- and middle-income countries (ACC/SCN, 2000).

Undernutrition, due to coexisting primary deficiency and malnutrition secondary to disease, is likely to be widely prevalent among older urban and rural people in low- and middle-income countries. For example, limited survey data obtained from periurban slums of Mumbai, India[*] and rural villages of Malawi (Chilima &

---

[*]Based on unpublished survey data from the London School for Hygiene and Tropical Medicine, as reported in reference (ACC/SCN, 2000).

Ismail, 1998) suggest that 25–35% of free-living older persons in low-income populations may be in a chronic state of acute undernourishment, reflected by a low body mass index (<18.5 kg of weight per $m^2$ of height). An undernutrition-chronic disease interaction likely exists among older persons in many low- and middle-income countries, both sharing underlying and basic causes in poverty and its determinants (Figures 5–4 and 5–5). Specific age-related disorders that may be exacerbated by intercurrent malnutrition and disease, and are likely to be of considerable public health importance in the low-income countries but for which little to no data exist, include sarcopenia with consequent muscle weakness, impaired mobility, and body function (Kehayias, Fiatarone, Zhuang, & Roubenoff, 1997; Roubenoff, 1999); osteoporosis with resultant bone fractures (Wark, 1999); and various dementias of potential nutritional origin (Riggs, Spiro, Tucker, & Rush, 1996; Rosenberg & Miller, 1992; Tucker, 2000). Evidence that exists suggests that undernutrition among older persons is an immense and growing problem in low- and middle-income countries, providing impetus to define accurately the extent and severity of nutritional deficiencies in this age group, understand their likely causes, and identify resources that could better enable healthy aging in undernourished populations of the world, for whom programs are virtually nonexistent at present.

## THE NUTRITION TRANSITION

In contrast to emerging concerns about undernutrition among older persons, the changes in demographic, social, and economic conditions of many low- and middle-income countries are modifying rapidly the patterns of diet-related diseases, particularly in those countries with emerging market economies (Murray & Lopez, 1997). Health problems traditionally associated with abundance, such as obesity, diabetes, and cardiovascular diseases, are increasing at an alarming rate such that noncommunicable diseases count among the top 10 causes of death and disability in many low- and middle-income countries (see Chapter 6). The shift in disease and death from communicable and undernutrition-related to noncommunicable causes has been termed the *health or epidemiologic transition*. The changes in food availability, dietary intake, and diet-related disease patterns underlying this process are known as the *nutrition transition* (Popkin, 1994).

Although the association between diet and noncommunicable chronic diseases is clearly multifactorial, two elements are at the center of the nutrition transition as it relates to health status: changes in dietary patterns and in lifestyle, specifically physical activity. A change in dietary pattern toward higher total fat and saturated fat intake, and consumption of more refined carbohydrates and less fiber, are all linked to increased risk of chronic diseases such as cardiovascular disease, diabetes, obesity, and cancer. A sedentary lifestyle, by favoring a positive energy balance, promotes the development of excess weight and poor cardiovascular health.

Changes in dietary patterns are driven primarily by the globalization of food production and marketing, which is changing rapidly the type and amount of foods available to consumers in many low- and middle-income countries. Policies regarding local production, import regulations, and subsidies can also greatly alter the kind of foods that appear in the market and lower their cost relative to income. It has been suggested that the dietary shift toward higher fats and refined sugars observed in many low- and middle-income countries has more to do with these policies than with the cultural adoption of Western style diets (Popkin, 1999). On the other hand, "westernization" may indeed be the predominant factor driving those same changes in industrialized nations, such as Japan. In either case, the end result is a diet with increasing energy content as fat and more consumption of refined sugars.

Social and economic advancement tends to change patterns of dietary intake of populations by increasing the percent of animal protein sources and total fat. Even low-quality foods consumed by the urban poor tend to have higher energy density and fat content than rural foods. The perception that fat-rich foods are status symbols of socioeconomic advancement is likely to influence change in food preferences associated with migration to urban areas (Caballero & Rubinstein, 1997). It has been pointed out that the number of different foods in the usual diet, an index of diversity, also increases with urbanization (Drewnowski et al., 1996).

Reliable data on dietary intake in transitional countries are still too scarce to allow a global assessment of trends in macronutrient intake. Data on food production suggest that the main contribution to the increase in fat intake in low- and middle-income regions may come from vegetable oils. The global production of soy, palm, and rapeseed oils rose substantially over the past 15 years (71 million metric tons by 1996), while animal fat remained unchanged at around 12 metric tons (Drewnowski & Popkin, 1997). The increased availability of vegetable oils in low- and middle-income countries is probably related to its increased use in industrialized countries, resulting in low-cost production. In addition, subsidies and marketing strategies of international corporations may further facilitate product penetration in low- and middle-income markets.

Sedentary lifestyle may be facilitated by two phenomena resulting from certain economic development trends: urbanization and switch to a service economy. Urbanization is usually associated with increasing use of automobiles and mechanized transportation, at the expense of walking and bicycling; reduction in availability of open areas for recreational activities; increased percentage of women entering the workforce; and increased consumption of meals outside the home. The trend toward a service economy leads toward a predominance of less energy-demanding jobs, compared to manufacturing or agriculture jobs. Combined with the reduction in physical activity related to urbanization, these trends facilitate the positive energy balance and the development of excess body weight. A typical example of these factors is South Korea, where agriculture, forestry, and fisheries jobs declined from 40% of all occupations in 1964 to less than 10% in 1993. In the same period, service jobs increased from 44% to 64% (Kim, Moon, & Popkin, 2000). A similar trend has been shown throughout the low- and middle-income countries (Popkin, 1999).

Urbanization, another component of the transition, also affects dietary patterns in low- and middle-income countries. The few surveys comparing rural and urban diets report slight improvements in the micronutrient content of urban diets (Alarcon & Adrino, 1991), which tend to have higher content of saturated fats and of artificial and natural sweeteners (Popkin, 1994).

Migration to an urban environment is usually associated with a decrease in the energy demands of daily living. Mechanization of transportation and a reduced energy output of labor are major factors. Trends in employment in low- and middle-income countries indicate that service-type jobs are increasing at the expense of agriculture and other more physically demanding activities (Popkin & Doak, 1998). Thus energy requirements for urban work are likely to be less compared to rural areas. Energy spent in survival activities such as carrying water or gathering wood, which are routine in rural areas, are also likely to be less in the urban setting.

In summary, diet-related chronic diseases are increasing in many low- and middle-income areas, fueled by three major factors: (1) population and health trends leading to more individuals reaching adulthood and living longer; (2) changes in dietary patterns leading to increased consumption of energy from fat and refined sugars; and (3) increase in sedentary time with the consequent reduction in energy expenditure and positive energy balance. Several other factors, including the impact of dietary changes on genetic polymorphism and of other, yet unidentified environmental factors, may also play a role in the increasing trend in chronic noncommunicable diseases in low- and middle-income regions.

## CONCLUSION

Malnutrition will remain a complex and evolving challenge in the twenty-first century, with large numbers of individuals in low-income countries undernourished with respect to quality and quantity of diet for the stage in their lives. In many low-income countries, the burdens of disease and death are unquestionably linked to protein-energy and micronutrient deficiencies, exacerbated by infectious diseases (Gwatkin, Guillot, & Heuveline, 1999). The vicious cycle of undernutrition and infection is revealed at the community level by higher rates of mortality attributed to diarrhea and acute respiratory infection among underweight children and by the poor nutritional recovery of children exposed to repeated bouts of infection. Micronutrient deficiencies, highlighting especially the poor quality of diet, also interact with infection. Children who are vitamin A deficient are less able to resist infection; this then leads to more severe disease and risk of fatality. In addition, severe infection, especially evident with measles and diarrhea, depletes vitamin A stores and raises the odds of a child developing xerophthalmia. Zinc deficiency predisposes children to both increased incidence and duration of diarrhea, respiratory infection, and other infections. Deficiencies are partly amended by controlling infection, and the incidence or severity of infection can be modulated by supplementing children with these micronutrients. The health and chances of survival of women of reproductive age, exposed to the nutritional stresses of pregnancy and lactation, appear similarly compromised by chronic undernutrition. Newborns of protein-energy and micronutrient-deficient women appear to face unfavorable risks with respect to health and survival.

The importance of normal nutrition extends beyond the spiral of infection and death. Iodine- and iron-deficient children are slower to learn and develop intellectually, which curbs their capacity to achieve their full human potential and contribute fully to society. Supplementing children with these micronutrients may partially reverse these sequelae, if caught in time. A normal, nutritious diet given from birth through early childhood would appear to be the most attractive and efficacious approach to accrue these individual nutrient benefits simultaneously, though science lags in clearly demonstrating such dietary effects. Breastfeeding through early infancy, followed by a nutrient and energy-dense, hygienic diet thereafter that allows breastfeeding to extend into early childhood, appears to offer the best chances for children to grow, develop, and defend themselves against an often hostile environment.

The consequences of undernutrition, and the responses of the malnourished to intervention, have led to compelling estimates of the benefits to individuals and societies of preventing such forms of malnutrition in low-income countries (Figure 5–17). Measured in terms of DALYs (see Chapter 1), interventions such as promoting breastfeeding, supplementing children (and probably women) with vitamin A, delivering iron (and probably folate) supplements to women and children, and assuring availability of iodized salt in a population are widely viewed to be among the most cost-effective approaches for extending and improving the quality of life (ACC/SCN, 2000; Gwatkin et al., 1999; Horton et al., 1996; Murray & Lopez, 1997). Such efforts can be grouped into feasible, minimum packages that can facilitate policy development and affordable integrated approaches to prevent undernutrition (see Exhibit 5–6). Doubtless, there are other approaches that can be taken to both define and measure the benefits of additional nutrition interventions that can prevent undernutrition (Hyder, Rotllant, & Morrow, 1998). As the risks along the nutritional spectrum shift, for increasing numbers of societies, from undernutrition to overnutrition, the need to assure a healthful diet will continue to challenge public health researchers and practitioners in the decades ahead.

**Exhibit 5–6** The Minimum Nutrition Package

As the importance of dietary deficiencies as underlying causes of child and maternal morbidity and mortality have become better appreciated, nutritional approaches that are affordable, effective, and complementary have been packaged together for primary care and other community outreach programs, collectively called the Nutrition Minimum Package. The concept of packaging simple interventions to achieve major public health benefit building on the growth monitoring, oral rehydration, breastfeeding and immunization effort originated by UNICEF 2 decades ago, complementing the WHO/UNICEF Integrated Management of Childhood Illness Programme. Ideally, the "doctrine" of good nutrition should be a national policy derived from the International Conference on Nutrition in Rome in 1992 (see Exhibit 5–1). A reasonable, evidence-based minimum nutrition package could include

- exclusive breastfeeding for 4–6 months
- appropriate complementary feeding between 4 to 24 months
- adequate vitamin A intake for infants, children, and women
- appropriate dietary "case management" during and after illness
- iron-folate supplementation of pregnant women
- regular use of iodized salt by all families

These are best carried out by (1) prioritizing each according to local needs and resources, (2) choosing nutrient/message delivery systems that make local sense, and (3) monitoring, evaluating, and acting in a timely manner on new findings, seeking always to improve coverage, achieve greater impact, and reduce costs.

## DISCUSSION QUESTIONS

1. The same population may be affected by multiple micronutrient deficiencies, although different life stages and socioeconomic or geographic groups may be more vulnerable to certain individual nutrient deficiencies. Discuss ways in which single micronutrient deficiency prevention strategies might be combined, integrated, or coordinated to achieve cost-effective control.
2. A developing country may be afflicted with high rates of undernutrition while undergoing a nutrition transition among economically advanced segments of its population. Discuss the challenges this situation poses for the government in developing food and nutrition policies as well as national guidelines for healthy eating.
3. The Ministry of Health of a country has decided to institute a national, community-based, daily supplementary feeding scheme aimed at improving preschool child growth and development in high-risk populations. Discuss approaches the government may take in identifying target groups, initiating the feeding program, and evaluating its effects.

## REFERENCES

Aaby, P. (1988). Malnutrition and overcrowding/intensive exposure in severe measles infection: Review of community studies. *Review of Infectious Diseases, 10,* 478–491.

Adair, L., Popkin, B.M., Van Derslice, J., Akin, J., Guilkey, D., Black, R., Briscoe, J., & Flieger, W. (1993). Growth dynamics during the first two years of life: A prospective study in the Philippines. *European Journal of Clinical Nutrition, 47,* 42–51.

Adams, E.J., Stephenson, L.S., Latham, M.C., & Kinoti, S.N. (1994). Physical activity and growth of Kenyan school children with hookworm: *Trichuris trichiura* and *Ascaris lumbricoides* infections are improved after treatment with albendazole. *Journal of Nutrition, 124,* 1199–1206.

Administrative Committee on Coordination/Subcommittee on Nutrition (ACC/SCN). (1992, October). *Second report on the world nutrition situation: Volume I—Global and regional results.* Geneva, Switzerland: World Health Organization.

Administrative Committee on Coordination/Subcommittee on Nutrition (ACC/SCN). (1996, November). *Update on the nutrition situation.* Geneva, Switzerland: World Health Organization.

Administrative Committee on Coordination/Subcommittee on Nutrition (ACC/SCN). (2000). *Fourth report on the world nutrition situation: Nutrition throughout the life cycle.* Washington, DC: International Food Policy Research Institute.

Ahmed, F., Barua, S., Mohiduzzaman, M., Shaheen, N., Bhuyan, M.A.H., Margetts, B.M., & Jackson, A.A. (1993). Interactions between growth and nutrient status in school-age children of urban Bangladesh. *American Journal of Clinical Nutrition, 58,* 334–338.

Ahmed, F., Bhuyan, A.H., Shaheen, N., Barua, S., Margetts, B.M., & Jackson, A.A. (1991). Effect of socio-demographic conditions on growth of urban school children of Bangladesh. *European Journal of Clinical Nutrition, 45,* 327–330.

Ahmed, F., Mohiduzzaman, M., Barua, S., Shaheen, N., Margetts, B.M., & Jackson, A.A. (1992). Effect of family size and income on the biochemical indices of urban school children of Bangladesh. *European Journal of Clinical Nutrition, 46,* 465–473.

Akesson, A., Bjellerup, P., Berglund, M., Bremme, K., & Vahter, M. (1998). Serum transferrin receptor: A specific marker of iron deficiency in pregnancy. *American Journal of Clinical Nutrition, 68,* 1241–1246.

Alarcon, J.A., & Adrino, F.J. (1991). Diferencias urbano-rurales en la ingesta de alimentos de familias pobres de Guatemala. *Archivos Latinamericanos de Nutrición, 51,* 327–335.

Albonico, M., Stoltzfus, R.J., Savioli, L., Tielsch, J.M., Chwaya, H.M., Ercole, E., & Cancrini, G. (1998). Epidemiological evidence for a differential effect of hookworm species, *Ancylostoma duodenale* or *Necator americanus*, on iron status of children. *International Journal of Epidemiology, 27,* 530–537.

Allen, L.H. (1994). Nutritional influences on linear growth: A general review. *European Journal of Clinical Nutrition, 48,* S75–S89.

Allen, L.H. (1997). Pregnancy and iron deficiency: Unresolved issues. *Nutrition Reviews, 55,* 91–101.

Angeles, I.T., Schultink, W.J., Matulessi, P., Gross, R., & Sastroamidjojo, S. (1993). Decreased rate of stunting among anemic Indonesian preschool children through iron supplementation. *American Journal of Clinical Nutrition, 58,* 339–342.

Apgar, J. (1985). Zinc and reproduction. *Annual Review of Nutrition, 5,* 43–68.

Arroyave, G., Mejia, L.A., & Aguilar, J.R. (1981). The effect of vitamin A fortification of sugar on the serum vitamin A levels of preschool Guatemalan children: A longitudinal evaluation. *American Journal of Clinical Nutrition, 34,* 41–49.

Arthur, P., Kirkwood, B., Ross, D., Morris, S., Gyapong, J., Tomkins, A., & Addy, H. (1992). Impact of vitamin A supplementation on childhood morbidity in northern Ghana. *Lancet, 339,* 361–362.

Ashworth, A. (1998). Effects of intrauterine growth retardation on mortality and morbidity in infants and young children. *European Journal of Clinical Nutrition, 52,* S34–S42.

Ashworth, A., & Feachem, R.G. (1985). Interventions for the control of diarrhoeal diseases among young children: Prevention of low birthweight. *Bulletin of the World Health Organization, 63,* 165–184.

Aukett, M.A., Parks, Y.A., Scott, P.H., & Wharton, B.A. (1986). Treatment with iron increases weight gain and psychomotor development. *Archives of Diseases in Childhood, 61,* 849–857.

Baertl, J.M., Adrianzen, B., & Graham, G.G. (1976). Growth of previously well-nourished infants in poor homes. *American Journal of Diseases in Children, 130,* 33–35.

Bahl, R., Bhandari, N., Hambidge, K.M., & Bhan, M.K. (1998). Plasma zinc as a predictor of diarrheal and respiratory morbidity in children in an urban slum setting. *American Journal of Clinical Nutrition, 68,* 414S–417S.

Bahl, R., Bhandari, N., Taneja, S., & Bhan, M.K. (1997). The impact of vitamin A supplementation on physical growth of children is dependent on season. *European Journal of Clinical Nutrition, 51,* 26–29.

Bairagi, R. (1980). Is income the only constraint on child nutrition in rural Bangladesh? *Bulletin of the World Health Organization, 58,* 767–772.

Baqui, A.H., Sack, R.B., Black, R.E., Chowdhury, H.R., Yunus, M., & Siddique, A.K. (1993). Cell-mediated immune deficiency and malnutrition are independent risk factors for persistent diarrhea in Bangladeshi children. *American Journal of Clinical Nutrition, 58,* 543–548.

Bar-Andziak, E., Lazecki, D., Radwanowska, N., & Nauman, J. (1993). Iodine intake and goiter incidence among schoolchildren living in Warsaw region (Warsaw and Ciechanow Voivodships—Warsaw Coordinating Center). *Edokrynologia Polska, 44,* 288–295.

Barclay, A.J.G., Foster, A., & Sommer, A. (1987). Vitamin A supplements and mortality related to measles: A randomised clinical trial. *British Medical Journal, 294,* 294–296.

Barker, D.J.P., Bull, A.R., Osmond, C., & Simmonds, S.J. (1990). Fetal and placental size and risk of hypertension in adult life. *British Medical Journal, 301,* 259–262.

Barker, D.J.P., Osmond, C., Winter, P.D., Margetts, B., & Simmonds, S.J. (1989). Weight in infancy and death from ischaemic heart disease. *Lancet, 2,* 577–580.

Barros, F.C., Victora, C.G., Vaughan, J.P., Teixeira, A.M.B., & Ashworth, A. (1987). Infant mortality in southern Brazil: A population based study of causes of death. *Archives of Diseases in Childhood, 62,* 487–490.

Bates, C.J., Evans, P.H., Dardenne, M., Prentice, A., Lunn, P.G., Northrop-Clewes, C.A., Hoares, S., Cole, T.J., Horan, S.J., Longman, S.C., Stirling, D., & Aggett, P.J. (1993). A trial of zinc supplementation in young rural Gambian children. *Journal of Nutrition, 69,* 243–255.

Beach, R.S., Gershwin, M.E., & Hurley, L.S. (1982). Gestational zinc deprivation in mice: Persistence of immunodeficiency for three generations. *Science, 218,* 469–471.

Beales, P.F. (1997). Anaemia in malaria control: A practical approach. *Annals of Tropical Medicine and Parasitology, 91,* 713–718.

Beaton, G.H., Martorell, R., Aronson, K.J., Edmonston, B., McCabe, G., Ross, A.C., & Harvey, B. (1993). Effectiveness of vitamin A supplementation in the control of young child morbidity and mortality in developing countries. ACC/SCN State of the Art Series Nutrition Policy Discussion Paper, No. 13. Geneva, Switzerland: Administrative Committee on Coordination/Subcommittee on Nutrition (ACC/SCN).

Becker, S., Peters, D.H., Gray, R.H., Gultiano, C., & Black, R.E. (1993). The determinants of use of maternal and child health services in Metro Cebu, the Philippines. *Health Transition Reviews, 3,* 77–89.

Begin, F., Frongillo, E.A., & Delisle, H. (1999). Caregiver behaviors and resources influence child height-for-age in rural Chad. *Journal of Nutrition, 129,* 680–686.

Behrens, R.H., Lunn, P.G., Northrop, C.A., Hanlon, P.W., & Neale, G. (1987). Factors affecting the integrity of the intestinal mucosa of Gambian children. *American Journal of Clinical Nutrition, 45,* 1433–1441.

Bentley, M.E., Caulfield, L.E., Ram, M., Santizo, M.C., Hurtado, E., Rivera, J.A., Ruel, M.T., & Brown, K.H. (1997). Zinc supplementation affects the activity patterns of rural Guatemalan infants. *Journal of Nutrition, 127*, 1333–1338.

Bhandari, N., Bhan, M.K., & Sazawal, S. (1992). Mortality associated with acute watery diarrhea, dysentery, and persistent diarrhea in rural north India. *Acta Paediatrica Supplement, 381*, 3–6.

Bhaskaram, P., & Sivakumar, B. (1986). Interleukin-1 in malnutrition. *Archives of Diseases in Childhood, 61*, 182–185.

Black, M.M. (1998). Zinc deficiency and child development. *American Journal of Clinical Nutrition, 68*, 464S–469S.

Black, R.E. (1993). Persistent diarrhea in children of developing countries. *Pediatric Infectious Diseases Journal, 12*, 751–761.

Black, R.E. (1997). Zinc for child health: Child Health Research Project special report. Johns Hopkins University, Baltimore, MD.

Black, R.E. (1998). Therapeutic and preventive effects of zinc on serious childhood infectious diseases in developing countries. *American Journal of Clinical Nutrition, 68*, 476S–479S.

Black, R.E., Brown, K.H., & Becker, S. (1983). Influence of acute diarrhea on the growth parameters of children. In J.A. Bellanti (Ed.), *Acute diarrhea: Its nutritional consequences* (pp. 75–84). New York: Vevey-Raven Press.

Black, R.E., Brown, K.H., & Becker, S. (1984a). Effects of diarrhea associated with specific enteropathogens on the growth of children in rural Bangladesh. *Pediatrics, 73*, 799–805.

Black, R.E., Brown, K.H., & Becker, S. (1984b). Malnutrition is a determining factor in diarrheal duration, but not incidence, among young children in a longitudinal study in rural Bangladesh. *American Journal of Clinical Nutrition, 39*, 87–94.

Black, R.E., Merson, M.H., Eusof, A., Huq, I., & Pollard, R. (1984). Nutritional status, body size, and severity of diarrhoea associated with rotavirus or enterotoxigenic *Escherichia coli. Journal of Tropical Medical Hygiene, 87*, 83–89.

Bleichrodt, N., & Born, M.P. (1994). A metaanalysis of research on iodine and its relationship to cognitive development. In J.B. Stanbury (Ed.), *The damaged brain of iodine deficiency* (pp. 195–200). New York: Cognizant Communication Corporation.

Bloem, M.W., Hye, A., Wijnroks, M., Ralte, A., West, K.P., Jr., & Sommer, A. (1995). The role of universal distribution of vitamin A capsules in combating vitamin A deficiency in Bangladesh. *American Journal of Epidemiology, 142*, 843–855.

Blomhoff, R. (1994). Introduction: Overview of vitamin A metabolism and function. In R. Blomhoff (Ed.), *Vitamin A in health and disease* (pp. 1–35). New York: Marcel Dekker.

Bothwell, T.H., & Charlton, R.W. (1981). *Iron deficiency in women*. Report for the International Nutritional Anemia Consultative Group (INACG). Washington, DC: Nutrition Foundation.

Bothwell, T.H., Hallberg, L., Clydesdale, F.M., Van Campen, D., Cook, J.D., Wolf, W.J., & Dallman, T.R. (1982, June). The effects of cereals and legumes on iron bioavailability. Report for the International Nutritional Anemia Consultative Group (INACG). Washington, DC: Nutrition Foundation.

Bouis, H.E., & Novenario-Reese, M.J.G. (1997). The determinants of demand for micronutrients: An analysis of rural households in Bangladesh. FCND Discussion Paper No. 32. Washington, DC: International Food Policy Research Institute.

Boyages, S.C. (1994). The damaged brain of iodine deficiency: Evidence for a continuum of effect on the population at risk. In J.B. Stanbury (Ed.), *The damaged brain of iodine deficiency* (pp. 251–257). New York: Cognizant Communication Corporation.

Brakohiapa, L.A., Bille, A., Wuansah, E., Kishi, K., Yartey, J., Harrison, E., Armar, M.A., & Yamamoto, S. (1988). Does prolonged breastfeeding adversely affect a child's nutritional status? *Lancet, 2*, 416.

Briend, A., & Bari, A. (1989). Breastfeeding improves survival, but not nutritional status, of 12–35-months-old children in rural Bangladesh. *European Journal of Clinical Nutrition, 43*, 603–608.

Briend, A., & Zimicki, S. (1986). Validation of arm circumference as an indicator of risk of death in one- to four-year-old children. *Nutrition Research, 6*, 249–261.

Briend, A., Wojtyniak, B., & Rowland, M.G.M. (1987). Arm circumference and other factors in children at high risk of death in rural Bangladesh. *Lancet, 2*, 725.

Briend, A., Wojtyniak, B., & Rowland, M.G.M. (1988). Breast feeding, nutritional state, and child survival in rural Bangladesh. *British Medical Journal, 296*, 879.

Brooker, S., Peshu, N., Warn, P.A., Mosobo, M., Guyatt, H.L., Marsh, K., & Snow, R.W. (1999). The epidemiology of hookworm infection and its contribution to anaemia among pre-school children on the Kenyan Coast. *Transactions of the Royal Society for Tropical Medical Hygiene, 93*, 240–246.

Brown, K.H., Black, R.E., & Becker, S. (1982). Seasonal changes in nutritional status and the prevalence of malnutrition in a longitudinal study of young children in rural Bangladesh. *American Journal of Clinical Nutrition, 36*, 303–313.

Brown, K.H., Black, R.E., Robertson, A.D., & Becker, S. (1985). Effects of season and illness on the dietary intake of weanlings during longitudinal studies in rural

Bangladesh. *American Journal of Clinical Nutrition, 41,* 343–355.

Brown, K.H., Dewey, K., & Allen, L. (1998). Complementary feeding of young children in developing countries: A review of current scientific knowledge. WHO/NUT/98. Geneva, Switzerland: World Health Organization.

Brown, K.H., Gastanaduy, A.S., Saavedra, J.M., Lembcke, J., Rivas, D., Robertson, A.D., Yolken, R., & Sack, R.B. (1988). Effect of continued oral feeding on clinical and nutritional outcomes of acute diarrhea in children. *Journal of Pediatrics, 112,* 191–200.

Brown, K.H., Gilman, R.H., Gaffar, A., Alamgir, S.M., Strife, J.L., Kapikian, A.Z., & Sack, R.B. (1981). Infections associated with severe protein-calorie malnutrition in hospitalized infants and children. *Nutrition Research, 1,* 33–46.

Brown, K.H., Peerson, J.M., & Allen, L.H. (1998). Effect of zinc supplementation on children's growth: A meta-analysis of intervention trials. *Bibliotheca Nutritio et Dieta Dieta, 54,* 76–83.

Brown, K.H., Stallings, R.Y., Creed de Kanashiro, H., Lopez de Romana, G., & Black, R.E. (1990). Effects of common illnesses on infants' energy intakes from breastmilk and other foods during longitudinal community-based studies in Huascar (Lima), Peru. *American Journal of Clinical Nutrition, 52,* 1005–1013.

Bruner, A.B., Joffe, A., Duggan, A.K., Casella, J.F., & Brandt, J. (1996). Randomised study of cognitive effects of iron supplementation in non-anaemic iron-deficient adolescent girls. *Lancet, 348,* 992–996.

Brussard, J.H., Brants, H.A.M., Hulshof, K.F.A.M., Kistemaker, C., & Lowik, M.R.H. (1997). Iodine intake and urinary excretion among adults in the Netherlands. *European Journal of Clinical Nutrition, 51,* S59–S62.

Bukenya, G.B., Barnes, T., & Nwokolo, N. (1991). Low birthweight and acute childhood diarrhoea: Evidence of their association in an urban settlement of Papua New Guinea. *Annals of Tropical Paediatrics, 11,* 357–362.

Bunce, G.E., Lytton, F., Gunesekera, B., Vessal, M., & Kim, C. (1994). Molecular basis for abnormal parturition in zinc deficiency in rats. In L. Allen, J. King, & B. Lonnerdal (Eds.), *Nutrient regulation during pregnancy, lactation, and infant growth.* New York: Plenum Press.

Butte, N.F. (1996). Energy requirements of infants. *European Journal of Clinical Nutrition, 50,* S24–S36.

Caballero, B. (1997). Nutritional requirements of the sick child. In A. O'Donnell, J.M. Bengoa, B. Torun, B. Caballero, E. Lara Pantin, & M. Pena (Eds.), *Nutricion y alimentacion del nino en los primeros anos de vida* (pp. 335–364). Washington, DC: Pan American Health Organization.

Cameron, N. (1978). The methods of auxological anthropometry. In F. Falkner & J.M. Tanner (Eds.), *Human growth: A comprehensive treatise.* Vol. 3: *Methodology, ecological, genetic, and nutritional effects on growth* (2nd ed.) (pp. 3–46). New York: Plenum Press.

Campos, F.A.C.S., Flores, H., & Underwood, B.A. (1987). Effect of an infection on vitamin A status of children as measured by the relative dose response (RDR). *American Journal of Clinical Nutrition, 46,* 91–94.

Caron, P., Hoff, M., Bazzi, S., Dufor, A., Faure, G., Ghandour, I., Lauzu, P., Lucas, Y., Maraval, D., Mignot, F., Ressigeac, P., Vertongen, F., & Grange, V. (1997). Urinary iodine excretion during normal pregnancy in healthy women living in the southwest of France: Correlation with maternal thyroid parameters. *Thyroid, 7,* 749–754.

Castillo, C., Atalah, E., Riumallo, J., & Castro, R. (1996). Breast-feeding and the nutritional status of nursing children in Chile. *Bulletin of the Pan American Health Organization, 30,* 125–132.

Caulfield, L.E., Bentley, M.E., & Ahmed, S. (1996). Is prolonged breastfeeding associated with malnutrition? Evidence from nineteen demographic and health surveys. *International Journal of Epidemiology, 25,* 693–703.

Caulfield, L.E., Zavaleta, N., Figueroa, A., & Leon, Z. (1999). Maternal zinc supplementation does not affect size at birth or pregnancy duration in Peru. *Journal of Nutrition, 129,* 1563–1568.

Caulfield, L.E., Zavaleta, N., Shankar, A.H., & Merialdi, M. (1998). Potential contribution of maternal zinc supplementation during pregnancy to maternal and child survival. *American Journal of Clinical Nutrition, 68,* 499S–508S.

Cavan, K.R., Gibson, R.S., Grazioso, C.F., Isalgue, A.M., Ruz, M., & Solomons, N.W. (1993). Growth and body composition of periurban Guatemalan children in relation to zinc status: a longitudinal zinc intervention trial. *American Journal of Clinical Nutrition, 57,* 344–352.

Ceesay, S.M., Prentice, A.M., Cole, T.J., Ford, F., Weaver, L.T., Poskitt, E.M.E., & Whitehead, R.G. (1997). Effects on birthweight and perinatal mortality of maternal dietary supplements in rural Gambia: 5-year randomised controlled trial. *British Medical Journal, 315,* 786–790.

Cerqueiro, M.C., Murtagh, P., Halac, A., Avila, M., & Weissenbacher, M. (1990). Epidemiologic risk factors for children with acute lower respiratory tract infection in Buenos Aires, Argentina: A matched case-control study. *Reviews of Infectious Diseases, 12,* S1021–1028.

Chandra, R.K. (1977). Lymphocyte subpopulations in human malnutrition: Cytotoxic and suppressor cells. *Pediatrics, 59,* 423–427.

Checkley, W., Epstein, L.D., Gilman, R.H., Black, R.E., Cabrera, L., & Sterling, C.R. (1998). Effects of *Cryptospo-*

*ridium parvum* infection in Peruvian children: Growth faltering and subsequent catch-up growth. *American Journal of Epidemiology, 148,* 497–506.

Chen, Y., Yu, S., & Li, W. (1988). Artificial feeding and hospitalization in the first 18 months of life. *Pediatrics, 81,* 58–62.

Cherry, F.F., Sandstead, H.H., Rojas, P., Johnson, L.K., Batson, H.K., & Wang, X.B. (1989). Adolescent pregnancy: Associations among body weight, zinc nutriture, and pregnancy outcome. *American Journal of Clinical Nutrition, 50,* 945–954.

Chilima, D.M., & Ismail, S.J. (1998). Anthropometric characteristics of older people in rural Malawi. *European Journal of Clinical Nutrition, 52,* 643–649.

Christian, P. (1998). Antenatal iron supplementation as a child survival strategy. Letter to the editor. *American Journal of Clinical Nutrition, 68,* 403–404.

Christian, P., West, K.P., Jr., Khatry, S.K., Katz, J., LeClerq, S., Pradhan, E.K., & Shrestha, S.R. (1998a). Vitamin A or B-carotene supplementation reduces but does not eliminate maternal night blindness in Nepal. *Journal of Nutrition, 128,* 1458–1463.

Christian, P., West, K.P., Jr., Khatry, S.K., Katz, J., Shrestha, S.R., Pradhan, E.K., LeClerq, S.C., & Pokhrel, R.P. (1998b). Night blindness of pregnancy in rural Nepal: Nutritional and health risks. *International Journal of Epidemiology, 27,* 231–237.

Christian, P., West, K.P., Jr., Khatry, S.K., Kimbrough-Pradhan, E., LeClerq, S.C., Katz, J., Shrestha, S.R., Dali, S.M., & Sommer, A. (in press). Night blindness during pregnancy and subsequent mortality among women in Nepal: Effects of vitamin A and B-carotene supplementation. *American Journal of Epidemiology.*

Chwang, L., Soemantri, A.G., & Pollitt, E. (1988). Iron supplementation and physical growth of rural Indonesian children. *American Journal of Clinical Nutrition, 47,* 496–501.

Clemens, J.D., Sack, D.A., Harris, J.R., Khan, M.R., Chakraborty, J., Chowdhury, S., Rao, M.R., van Loon, F.P., Stanton, B.F., & Yunus, M. (1990). Breastfeeding and the risk of severe cholera in rural Bangladeshi children. *American Journal of Epidemiology, 131,* 400–411.

Clemens, J.D., Stanton, B., Stoll, B., Shadid, N.S., Banu, H., & Chowdhury, A.K. (1986). Breastfeeding as a determinant of severity in shigellosis: Evidence for protection throughout the first three years of life in Bangladeshi children. *American Journal of Epidemiology, 123,* 710–720.

Cobra, C., Muhilal, Rusmil, K., Rustama, D., Djatnika, Suwardi, S.S., Permaesih, D., Muherdiyantiningsih, Martuti, S., & Semba, R.D. (1997). Infant survival is improved by oral iodine supplementation. *Journal of Nutrition, 127,* 574–578.

Cohen, N., Rahman, H., Mitra, M., Sprague, J., Islam, S., Leemhuis de Regt, E., & Jalil, M.A. (1987). Impact of massive doses of vitamin A on nutritional blindness in Bangladesh. *American Journal of Clinical Nutrition, 45,* 970–976.

Cohen, R.J., Brown, K.H., Canahuati, J., Rivera, L.L., & Dewey, K.G. (1994). Effects of age of introduction of complementary foods on infant breast milk intake, total energy intake, and growth: A randomised intervention study in Honduras. *Lancet, 344,* 288–293.

Cole, T.J., & Parkin, J.M. (1977). Infection and its effect on the growth of young children: A comparison of The Gambia and Uganda. *Transactions of the Royal Society for Tropical Medicine and Hygiene, 71,* 196–198.

Combs, G.F., Jr., Welch, R.M., Duxbury, J.M., Uphoff, N.T., & Nesheim, M.C. (1996). *Food-based approaches to preventing micronutrient malnutrition: An international research agenda.* Ithaca, NY: Cornell International Institute for Food, Agriculture, and Development.

Condon-Paoloni, D., Joaquin, C., Johnston, F.E., deLicardi, E.R., & Scholl, T.O. (1977). Morbidity and growth of infants and young children in a rural Mexican village. *American Journal of Public Health, 67,* 651–656.

Congdon, N., Sommer, A., Severns, M., Humphrey, J., Friedman, D., Clement, L., Wu, L.S., & Natadisastra, G. (1995). Pupillary and visual thresholds in young children as an index of population vitamin A status. *American Journal of Clinical Nutrition, 61,* 1076–1082.

Cook, J.D., Alvarado, J., Gutnisky, A., Labardini, J., Lavrisse, M., Linares, J., Loria, A., Maspes, V., Restrepo, A., Reynafarje, C., Sanchez-Medal, L., Velez, H., & Viteri, F. (1971). Nutritional deficiency and anemias in Latin America: A collaborative study. *Blood, 38,* 591–603.

Cook, J.D., Baynes, R.D., & Skikne, B.S. (1994). The physiological significance of circulating transferrin receptors. In L. Allen, J. King, & B. Lonnerdal (Eds.), *Nutrient regulation during pregnancy, lactation, and infant growth.* New York: Plenum Press.

Cook, J.D., Finch, C.A., & Smith, N.J. (1976). Evaluation of the iron status of a population. *Blood, 48,* 449–455.

Cook, J.D., Lipschitz, D.A., Miles, L.E.M., & Finch, C.A. (1974). Serum ferritin as a measure of iron stores in normal subjects. *American Journal of Clinical Nutrition, 27,* 681.

Corvilain, B., Van Sande, J., Dumont, J.E., Bourdoux, P., & Ermans, A.M. (1998). Autonomy in endemic goiter. *Thyroid, 8,* 107–113.

Cousins, R.J., & Hempe, J.M. (1990). Zinc. In M.L. Brown (Ed.), *Present knowledge in nutrition* (6th ed.) (pp. 251–260). Washington, DC: ILSI Press, 28.

Coutsoudis, A., Kiepiela, P., Coovadia, H.M., & Broughton, M. (1992). Vitamin A supplementation enhances specific IgG antibody levels and total lymphocyte numbers while improving morbidity in measles. *Pediatric Infectious Diseases Journal, 11,* 203–209.

Craft, N.E., Haitema, T., Brindle, L.K., Yamini, S., Humphrey, J.H., & West, K.P., Jr. (2000). Retinol analysis in dried blood spots by HPLC. *Journal of Nutrition, 130,* 882–885.

Cruz, J.R., Pareja, G., de Fernandez, A., Peralta, F., Caceres, P., & Cano, F. (1990). Epidemiology of acute respiratory tract infections among Guatemalan ambulatory preschool children. *Reviews of Infectious Diseases, 12,* S1029–S1034.

Current consensus on HIV transmission and breastfeeding. (1995). *PVO Child Survival Technical Report, 4,* 3–5.

Dallman, P.R. (1986). Biochemical basis for the manifestation of iron deficiency. *Annual Review of Nutrition, 6,* 13–40.

Dalmiya, N. (1999). Personal communication.

Dary, O. (1994). Avances en el proceso de fortificacion de azucar con vitamina A en Centro America. *Boletin de la Oficina Sanitaria Pan Americana, 117,* 529–536.

Delange, F. (1993). Requirements of iodine in humans. In F. Delange (Ed.), *Iodine deficiency in Europe.* New York: Plenum Press.

Delange, F. (1998). Screening for congenital hypothyroidism used as an indicator of the degree of iodine deficiency and of its control. *Thyroid, 8,* 1185–1192.

Delange, F., Benker, G., Caron, P., Eber, O., Ott, W., Peter, F., Podoba, J., Simescu, M., Szybinsky, Z., Vertongen, F., Vitti, P., Wiersinga, W., & Zamrazil, V. (1997). Thyroid volume and urinary iodine in European schoolchildren: Standardization of values for assessment of iodine deficiency. *European Journal of Endocrinology, 136,* 180–187.

Delange, F., Thilly, C., Bourdoux, P., Hennart, P., Courtois, P., & Ermans, A.M. (1982). Influence of dietary goitrogens during pregnancy in humans on thyroid function of the newborn. In F. Delange, F.B. Iteke, & A.M. Ermans (Eds.), *Nutritional factors involved in goitrogenic action of cassava* (pp. 40–50). Ottawa: International Developmental Research Centre Publications.

DeLong, R., Tai, M., Xue-Yi, C., Xin-Min, J., Zhi-Hong, D., Rakeman, M.A., Ming-Li, Z., & Heinz, R. (1994). The neuromotor deficit in endemic cretinism. In J.B. Stanbury (Ed.), *The damaged brain of iodine deficiency* (pp. 9–13). New York: Cognizant Communication Corporation.

DeMaeyer, E.M. (1976). Protein-energy malnutrition. In G.H. Beaton & J.M. Bengoa (Eds.), *Nutrition in preventive medicine: The major deficiency syndromes, epidemiology, and approaches to control* (pp. 23–54). Geneva, Switzerland: World Health Organization.

DeMaeyer, E.M., & Adiels-Tegman, M. (1985). The prevalence of anemia in the world. *World Health Statistics Quarterly, 38,* 302–316.

De Onis, M., Blossner, M, & Villar, J. (1998). Levels and patterns of intrauterine growth retardation in developing countries. *European Journal of Clinical Nutrition, 52,* S5–S15.

De Onis, M., Monteiro, C., Akres, J., & Clugston, G. (1993). The worldwide magnitude of protein-energy malnutrition: An overview from the WHO Global Database on Child Growth. *Bulletin of the World Health Organization, 71,* 703–712.

De Pee, S., Bloem, M.W., Gorstein, J., Sari, M., Satoto, Yip, R., Shrimpton, R., & Muhilal. (1998). Reappraisal of the role of vegetables in the vitamin A status of mothers in Central Java, Indonesia. *American Journal of Clinical Nutrition, 68,* 1068–1074.

De Pee, S., Bloem, M.W., Satoto, Yip, R., Sukaton, A., Tjiong, R., Shrimpton, R., Muhilal, & Kodyat, B. (1998). Impact of a social marketing campaign promoting dark-green leafy vegetables and eggs in Central Java, Indonesia. *International Journal of Vitamin and Nutrition Research, 68,* 389–398.

De Pee, S., Bloem, M.W., Tjiong, R., Martini, E., Satoto, Gorstein, J., Shrimpton, R., & Muhilal. (1999). Who has a high vitamin A intake from plant foods, but a low serum retinol concentration? Data from women in Indonesia. *European Journal of Clinical Nutrition, 53,* 288–297.

De Pee, S., West, C.E., Muhilal, Karyadi, D., & Hautvast, J.G.A.J. (1995). Lack of improvement in vitamin A status with increased consumption of dark-green leafy vegetables. *Lancet, 346,* 75–81.

De Vaquera, M.V., Townsend, J.W., Arroyo, J.J., & Lechtig, A. (1983). The relationship between arm circumference at birth and early mortality. *Journal of Tropical Pediatrics, 29,* 167–174.

Dewey, K.G. (in press). Approaches for improving complementary feeding of infants and young children. Background paper for WHO/UNICEF technical consultation on infant and young child feeding. Geneva, Switzerland: World Health Organization.

Dewey, K.G., Cohen, R.J., Brown, K.H., & Rivera, L.L. (1999). Age of introduction of complementary foods and growth of term, low-birth-weight, breast-fed infants: A randomized intervention study in Honduras. *American Journal of Clinical Nutrition, 69,* 679–686.

Dewey, K.G., Heinig, M.J., & Nommsen-Rivers, L.A. (1995). Differences in morbidity between breast-fed and formula-fed infants. *Journal of Pediatrics, 126,* 696–702.

Dixit, D.T. (1966). Night blindness in third trimester of pregnancy. *Indian Journal of Medical Research, 54,* 791–795.

Donnen, P., Brasseur, D., Dramaix, M., Vertongen, F., Zihindula, M., Muhamiriza, M., & Hennart, P. (1998). Vitamin A supplementation but not deworming improves growth of malnourished preschool children in eastern Zaire. *Journal of Nutrition, 128,* 1320–1327.

Drewnowski, A., Henderson, S.A., Shore, A.B., Fischler, C., Preziosi, P., & Hercberg, S. (1996). Diet quality and dietary diversity in France: Implications for the French paradox. *Journal of the American Dietary Association, 96,* 663–669.

Drewnowski, A., & Popkin, B.M. (1997). The nutrition transition: New trends in the global diet. *Nutrition Reviews, 55,* 31–43.

Dreyfuss, M.L. (1998). *Anemia and iron deficiency during pregnancy: Etiologies and effects on birth outcomes in Nepal.* Thesis, Johns Hopkins University, Baltimore, MD.

Dunn, J.T. (1996). Seven deadly sins in confronting endemic iodine deficiency, and how to avoid them. *Journal of Clinical Endocrinological Metabolism, 81,* 1332–1335.

Dunn, D.T., Newell, M.L., Ades, A.E., & Peckham, C.S. (1992). Risk of human immuno-deficiency virus type 1 transmission through breastfeeding. *Lancet, 340,* 585–588.

Dunn, J.T., Semigran, M.J., & Delange, F. (1998). The prevention and management of iodine-induced hyperthyroidism and its cardiac features. *Thyroid, 8,* 101–106.

Dunn, J.T., & van der Haar, F. (1990). *A practical guide to the correction of iodine deficiency.* The Netherlands: International Council for Control of Iodine Deficiency Disorders (ICCIDD).

El Samani, F.Z., Willett, W.C., & Ware, J.H. (1986). Predictors of simple diarrhoea disease surveillance in a rural Ghanaian pre-school child population. *Transactions of the Royal Society for Tropical Medicine and Hygiene, 80,* 208–213.

El-Arifeen, S. (1997). Birthweight, intrauterine growth retardation and prematurity: A prospective study of infant growth and survival in the slums of Dhaka, Bangladesh. Doctoral thesis, Johns Hopkins School of Public Health, Baltimore, MD.

Ellison, J.B. (1932). Intensive vitamin therapy in measles. *British Medical Journal, 2,* 708–711.

Elnagar, B., Eltom, M., Karlsson, F.A., Ermans, A.M., Gebre-Medhin, M., & Bourdoux, P.P. (1995). The effects of different doses of oral iodized oil on goiter size, urinary iodine, and thyroid-related hormones. *Journal of Clinical Endocrinological Metabolism, 80,* 891–897.

Ending hidden hunger. (1992). Montreal: Policy Conference on Micronutrient Malnutrition.

Faruque, A.S.G., Mahalanabis, D., Haque, S.S., Fuchs, G.J., & Habte, D. (1999). Double-blind, randomized, controlled trial of zinc or vitamin A supplementation in young children with acute diarrhoea. *Acta Paediatrica, 88,* 154–160.

Fawzi, W.W., Chalmers, T.C., Herrera, G., & Mosteller, F. (1993). Vitamin A supplementation and child mortality: A meta-analysis. *Journal of the American Medical Association, 269,* 898–903.

Fawzi, W.W., Herrera, G., Willett, W.C., Nestle, P., El Amin, A., & Mohamed, K.A. (1997). The effect of vitamin A supplementation on the growth of preschool children in the Sudan. *American Journal of Public Health, 87,* 1359–1362.

Fawzi, W.W., Msamanga, G.I., Spiegelman, D., Urassa, E.J.N., McGrath, N., Mwakagile, D., Antelman, G., Mbise, R., Herrera, G., Kapiga, S., Willett, W.C., & Hunter, D.J., for the Tanzania Vitamin and HIV Infection Trial Team. (1998). Randomised trial of effects of vitamin supplements on pregnancy outcomes and T cell counts in HIV-1-infected women in Tanzania. *Lancet, 351,* 1477–1482.

Ferguson, B.J., Skikne, B.S., Simpson, K.M., Baynes, R.D., & Cook, J.D. (1992). Serum transferrin receptor distinguishes the anemia of chronic disease from iron deficiency anemia. *Journal of Laboratory Clinical Medicine, 19,* 385–390.

Ferguson, E.L., Gibson, R.S., Opare-Obisaw, C., Ounpuu, S., Thompson, L.U., & Lehrfeld, J. (1993). The zinc nutriture of preschool children living in two African countries. *Journal of Nutrition, 123,* 1487–1496.

Fishman, S.M., Christian, P., & West, K.P., Jr. (in press). The role of vitamins in the prevention and control of anaemia: A review of current knowledge, controlled trials, and research priorities. *Public Health and Nutrition.*

Flores, H., Campos, F., Araujo, C.R.C., & Underwood, B.A. (1984). Assessment of marginal vitamin A deficiency in Brazilian children using the relative dose response procedure. *American Journal of Clinical Nutrition, 40,* 1281–1289.

Fonseca, W., Kirkwood, B.R., Victora, C.G., Fuchs, S.R., Flores, J.A., & Misago, C. (1996). Risk factors for childhood pneumonia among the urban poor in Fortaleza, Brazil: A case-control study. *Bulletin of the World Health Organization, 74,* 199–208.

Food and Agriculture Organization of the United Nations and World Health Organization (1992). World declaration and plan of action for nutrition. Rome: International Conference on Nutrition.

Food and Agriculture Organization of the United Nations. (1988). Requirements of vitamin A, iron, folate, and vitamin B12: Report of a joint FAO/WHO expert consultation. Rome: Food and Agriculture Organization.

Foster, A., & Sommer, A. (1987). Corneal ulceration, measles, and childhood blindness in Tanzania. *British Journal of Ophthalmology, 71,* 331–343.

Frisancho, A.R. (1981). The norms of upper limb fat and muscle areas for assessment of nutritional status. *American Journal of Clinical Nutrition, 34,* 2540–2545.

Galler, J.R., Ramsey, F.C., Harrison, R.H., Brooks, R., & Weiskopf-Bock, S. (1998). Infant feeding practices in Barbados predict later growth. *Journal of Nutrition, 128,* 1328–1335.

Galvan, R.R., & Canderon, J.M. (1965). Deaths among children with third-degree malnutrition. *American Journal of Clinical Nutrition, 16,* 351–355.

Garg, H.K., Singhla, K.C., & Arshad, Z. (1993). A study of the effect of oral zinc supplementation during pregnancy on pregnancy outcome. *Indian Journal of Physiology and Pharmacology, 37,* 276–284.

Garn, S.M., Ridella, S.A., Petzold, A.S., & Falkner, F. (1981). Maternal hematologic levels and pregnancy outcomes. *Seminars in Perinatology, 5,* 155–162.

Garnham, P.C.C. (1954). Malaria in the African child. *East African Medical Journal, 31,* 155–159.

George, S.M., Latham, M.C., Abel, R., Ethirajan, N., & Frongillo, E.A., Jr. (1993). Evaluation of effectiveness of good growth monitoring in south Indian villages. *Lancet, 342,* 348–352.

Gibson, R.S. (1990). *Principles of nutritional assessment.* New York: Oxford University Press.

Gibson, R.S., & Ferguson, E.L. (1998a). Assessment of dietary zinc in a population. *American Journal of Clinical Nutrition, 68,* 430S–434S.

Gibson, R.S., & Ferguson, E.L. (1998b). Nutrition intervention strategies to combat zinc deficiency in developing countries. *Nutrition Research Reviews, 11,* 115–131.

Gibson, R.S., Ferguson, E.L., & Lehrfeld, J. (1998). Complementary foods for infant feeding in developing countries: Their nutrient adequacy and improvement. *European Journal of Clinical Nutrition, 52,* 764–770.

Gibson, R.S., Heywood, A., Yaman, C., Sohlstrom, A., Thompson, L.U., & Heywood, P. (1991). Growth in children from the Wosera subdistrict, Papua New Guinea, in relation to energy and protein intakes and zinc status. *American Journal of Clinical Nutrition, 53,* 782–789.

Gibson, R.S., & Huddle, J.M. (1998). Suboptimal zinc status in pregnant Malawian women: Its association with low intakes of poorly available zinc, frequent reproductive cycling, and malaria. *American Journal of Clinical Nutrition, 67,* 702–709.

Gibson, R.S., Yeudall, F., Drost, N., Mtitimuni, B., & Cullinan, T. (1998). Dietary interventions to prevent zinc deficiency. *American Journal of Clinical Nutrition, 68,* 484S–487S.

Glasziou, P.P., & Mackerras, D.E.M. (1993). Vitamin A supplementation in infectious diseases: A meta-analysis. *British Medical Journal, 306,* 366–370.

Golden, M.H.N., Golden, B.E., Harland, P.S.E.G., & Jackson, A.A. (1978). Zinc and immunocompetence in protein-energy malnutrition. *Lancet, 1,* 1226.

Golden, M.H.N., Waterlow, J.C., & Picou, D. (1977). Protein turnover, synthesis, and breakdown before and after recovery from protein-energy malnutrition. *Clinical Science and Molecular Medicine, 53,* 473–477.

Goldenberg, R.L., Tamura, T., Neggers, Y., Copper, R.L., Johnston, K.E., DuBard, M.B., & Hauth, J.C. (1995). The effect of zinc supplementation on pregnancy outcome. *Journal of the American Medical Association, 274,* 463–468.

Gomez, F., Ramos-Galvan, R., Frenk, R., Cravioto, J.M., Chavez, R., & Vasquez, J. (1956). Mortality in second and third degree malnutrition. *Journal of Tropical Pediatrics, 2,* 77–85.

Gopalan, C., Venkatachalam, P.S., & Bhavani, B. (1960). Studies of vitamin A deficiency in children. *American Journal of Clinical Nutrition, 8,* 833–840.

Graham, G.G. (1977). *Nutritional evaluation of cereal mutants.* Vienna: International Atomic Energy Agency.

Graham, G.G. (1979). Resolving nutrition deficiency in developing countries: The importance of animal protein in the diets of infants and children. In *Animal disease prevention in developing countries: Its relationship to health, nutrition, and development* (Scientific Publication No. 380). Washington, DC: Pan American Health Organization/World Health Organization.

Graham, G.G., & Cordano, A. (1969). Copper depletion and deficiency in the malnourished infant. *Johns Hopkins Medical Journal, 124,* 139–150.

Graham, G.G., Morales, E., Placko, R.P., & MacLean, W.C., Jr. (1979). Nutritive value of brown and black beans for infants and small children. *American Journal of Clinical Nutrition, 32,* 2362–2366.

Graham, G.G., Placko, R.P., Acevedo, G., Morales, E., & Cordano, A. (1969). Lysine enrichment of wheat flour: Evaluation in infants. *American Journal of Clinical Nutrition, 22,* 1459–1468.

Graham, N.M.H. (1990). The epidemiology of acute respiratory infections in children and adults: A global perspective. *Epidemiologic Reviews, 12,* 149–178.

Graham, R.D., Ascher, J.S., & Hynes, S.C. (1992). Selecting zinc-efficient cereal genotypes for soils of low zinc status. *Plant and Soil, 146,* 241–250.

Grantham-McGregor, S.M., Walker, S.P., Chang, S.M., & Powell, C.A. (1997). Effects of early childhood supplementation with and without stimulation on later development in stunted Jamaican children. *American Journal of Clinical Nutrition, 66,* 247–253.

Gross, R., Hansel, H., Schultink, W., Shrimpton, R., Matulessi, P., Gross, G., Tagliaferri, E., & Sastroamdijojo,

S. (1998). Moderate zinc and vitamin A deficiency in breast milk of mothers from East-Jakarta. *European Journal of Clinical Nutrition, 52,* 884–890.

Grummer-Strawn, L.M. (1996). The effect of changes in population characteristics on breastfeeding trends in fifteen developing countries. *International Journal of Epidemiology, 25,* 94–102.

Guerrant, R.I., Schorling, J.B., McAuliffe, J.F., & de Souza, M.A. (1992). Diarrhea as a cause and an effect of malnutrition: Diarrhea prevents catch-up growth and malnutrition increases diarrhea frequency and duration. *American Journal of Tropical Medicine and Hygiene, 47,* 28–35.

Gwatkin, D.R., Guillot, M., & Heuveline, P. (1999). The burden of disease among the global poor. *Lancet, 354,* 586–589.

Habicht, J.P., Martorell, R., & Rivera, J.A. (1995). Nutritional impact of supplementation in the INCAP longitudinal study: Analytic strategies and inferences. *Journal of Nutrition, 125,* 1042S–1050S.

Habicht, J.P., Meyers, L.D., & Brownie, C. (1982). Indicators for identifying and counting the improperly nourished. *American Journal of Clinical Nutrition, 35,* 1241–1254.

Habicht, J.P., & Pelletier, D.L. (1990). The importance of context in choosing nutritional indicators. *Journal of Nutrition, 120,* 1519–1524.

Hadi, H., Stoltzfus, R.J., Dibley, M.J., Moulton, L.H., West, K.P., Jr., Kjolhede, C.L., & Sadjimin, T. (2000). Vitamin A supplementation selectively improves the linear growth of Indonesian preschool children: Results from a randomized controlled trial. *American Journal of Clinical Nutrition, 71,* 507–513.

Hadi, H., Stoltzfus, R.J., Moulton, L.H., Dibley, M.J., & West, K.P., Jr. (1999). Respiratory infections reduce the growth response to vitamin A supplementation in a randomized controlled trial. *International Journal of Epidemiology, 28,* 874–881.

Hales, C.N., Barker, D.J.P., Clark, P.M.S., Cox, L.J., Fall, C., Osmond, C., & Winter, P.D. (1991). Fetal and infant growth and impaired glucose tolerance at age 64. *British Medical Journal, 303,* 1019–1022.

Hallberg, L., Brune, M., Erlandsson, M., Sandberg, A.S., & Rossander-Hulten, L. (1991). Calcium: Effects of different amounts on nonheme-and heme-iron absorption in humans. *American Journal of Clinical Nutrition, 53,* 112–119.

Halpern, J.P. (1994). The neuromotor deficit in endemic cretinism and its implications for the pathogenesis of the disorder. In J.B. Stanbury (Ed.), *The damaged brain of iodine deficiency* (pp. 15–24). New York: Cognizant Communication Corporation.

Hambidge, K.M., & Krebs, N.F. (1995). Assessment of zinc status in man. *Indian Journal of Pediatrics, 62,* 169–180.

Hambidge, K.M., & Krebs, N.F. (1999). Zinc, diarrhea, and pneumonia. *Journal of Pediatrics, 135,* 661–664.

Hambidge, K.M., Krebs, N.F., & Miller, L. (1998). Evaluation of zinc metabolism with use of stable-isotope techniques: Implications for the assessment of zinc status. *American Journal of Clinical Nutrition, 68,* 410S–413S.

Hamill, P.V.V., Drizid, T.A., Johnson, C.L., Reed, R.B., Roche, A.F., & Moore, W.M. (1979). Physical growth: National Center for Health statistics percentiles. *American Journal of Clinical Nutrition, 32,* 607–629.

Harrison, K.A. (1989). Tropical obstetrics and gynecology: Maternal mortality. *Transactions of the Royal Society for Tropical Medicine and Hygiene, 83,* 449–453.

Hautvast, J.L.A., Tolboom, J.J.M., Kafwembe, E.M., Musonda, R.M., Mwanakasale, V., van Staveren, W.A., van't Hof, M.A., Sauerwein, R.W., Willems, J.L., & Monnens, L.A.H. (2000). Severe linear growth retardation in rural Zambian children: The influence of biological variables. *American Journal of Clinical Nutrition, 71,* 550–559.

Helen Keller International. (1998). *Current status of preschool vitamin A capsule supplementation program in rural Bangladesh.* Bangladesh: Helen Keller International.

Hendrata, L., & Rohde, J.E. (1988). Ten pitfalls of growth monitoring and promotion. *Indian Journal of Pediatrics, 55,* S9–S15.

Hendrickse, R.G., Hasan, A.H., Olumide, L.O., & Akinkunmi, A. (1971). Malaria in early childhood: An investigation of five hundred seriously ill children in whom a "clinical" diagnosis of malaria was made on admission to the children's emergency room at University College Hospital, Ibadan. *Annals of Tropical Medicine and Parasitology, 65,* 1–20.

Hetzel, B.S. (1987). An overview of the prevention and control of iodine deficiency disorders. In B.S. Hetzel, J.T. Dunn, & J.B. Stanbury (Eds.), *The prevention and control of iodine deficiency disorders* (pp. 7–31). Netherlands: Elsevier Science Publishers.

Hetzel, B.S. (1989). *The story of iodine deficiency: An international challenge in nutrition.* Oxford and Delhi: Oxford University Press.

Hetzel, B.S. (1994). Historical development of the concepts of the brain-thyroid relationships. In J.B. Stanbury (Ed.), *The damaged brain of iodine deficiency* (pp. 1–7). New York: Cognizant Communication Corporation.

Heymsfield, S.B., McManus, C., Stevens, V., & Smith, J. (1982). Muscle mass: Reliable indicator of protein-energy malnutrition severity and outcome. *American Journal of Clinical Nutrition, 35,* 1192–1199.

Heywood, A., Oppenheimer, S., Heywood, P., & Jolley, D. (1989). Behavioral effects of iron supplementation in infants in Madang, Papua New Guinea. *American Journal of Clinical Nutrition, 50,* 630–640.

Hinojosa, F. (1864). Apuntes sobre una enfermedad del pueblo de La Magdalena. *Gaceta Médica Mexicana, 1,* 137–139.

Hintze, G., Emrich, D., Richter, K., Thal, H., Wasielewski, T., & Kobberling, J. (1988). Effect of voluntary intake of iodinated salt on prevalence of goitre in children. *Acta Endocrinologica* (Copenhagen), *117,* 333–338.

Hokama, T., Takenaka, S., Hirayama, K., Yara, A., Yoshida, K., Itokazu, K., Kinjho, R., & Yabu, E. (1996). Iron status of newborns born to iron deficiency anaemic mothers. *Journal of Tropical Pediatrics, 42,* 75–77.

Hopkins, R.M., Gracey, M.S., Hobbs, R.P., Spargo, R.M., Yates, M., & Thompson, R.C.A. (1997). The prevalence of hookworm infection, iron deficiency, and anaemia in an Aboriginal community in north-west Australia. *Medical Journal of Australia, 166,* 241–244.

Horton, S., Sanghvi, T., Phillips, M., Fieldler, J., Perez-Escamilla, R., Lutter, C., Rivera, A., & Segall-Correa, A.M. (1996). Breastfeeding promotion and priority setting. *Health Policy and Planning, 11,* 156–168.

Houston, R. (1999). Iodine: Physiology, dietary sources, and requirements. In M.J. Sadler, J.J. Strain, & B. Caballero (Eds.), *Encyclopedia of human nutrition* (pp. 1138–1146). San Diego: Academic Press.

Houston, R. (1999). The Napal national vitamin A program. Elements of success. Nepali Technical Assistance Group and John Snow Inc, for the Ministry of Health, U.S. Agency for International Development, and UNICEF Nepal, Kathmandu.

Howson, C.P., Kennedy, E.T., & Horwitz, A. (1998). *Prevention of micronutrient deficiencies: Tools for policymakers and public health workers.* Washington, DC: National Academy Press.

Hoyle, B., Yunus, M., & Hen, L.C. (1980). Breast-feeding and food intake among children with acute diarrheal disease. *American Journal of Clinical Nutrition, 33,* 2365–2371.

Huda, S.N., Grantham-McGregor, S.M., Rahman, K.M., & Tomkins, A. (1999). Biochemical hypothyroidism secondary to iodine deficiency is associated with poor school achievement and cognition in Bangladeshi children. *Journal of Nutrition, 129,* 980–987.

Huddle, J.M., Gibson, R.S., & Cullinan, T.R. (1999). The impact of malarial infection and diet on the anaemia status of rural pregnant Malawian women. *European Journal of Clinical Nutrition, 53,* 792–801.

Huffman, S.L., Chowdhury, A.K.M., Chakraborty, J., & Simpson, N.K. (1980). Breast-feeding patterns in rural Bangladesh. *American Journal of Clinical Nutrition, 33,* 144–154.

Humphrey, J.H., Agoestina, T., Juliana, A., Septiana, S., Widjaja, H., Cerreto, M.C., Wu, L.S.F., Ichord, R.N., Katz, J., & West, K.P., Jr. (1998). Neonatal vitamin A supplementation: Effect on development and growth at 3 years of age. *American Journal of Clinical Nutrition, 68,* 109–117.

Humphrey, J.H., West, K.P., Jr., & Sommer, A. (1992). Vitamin A deficiency and attributable mortality among under-5-year-olds. *Bulletin of the World Health Organization, 70,* 225–232.

Husaini, M.A., Karyadi, L., Husaini, Y.K., Sandjaja, B., Karyadi, D., & Pollitt, E. (1991). Developmental effects of short-term supplementary feeding in nutritionally-at-risk Indonesian infants. *American Journal of Clinical Nutrition, 54,* 799–804.

Hussain, A., Lindtjorn, B., & Kvale, G. (1996). Protein energy malnutrition, vitamin A deficiency, and night blindness in Bangladeshi children. *Annals of Tropical Paediatrics, 16,* 319–325.

Hussey, G.D., & Klein, M. (1990). A randomized, controlled trial of vitamin A in children with severe measles. *New England Journal of Medicine, 323,* 160–164.

Hyder, A.A., Rotllant, G., & Morrow, R.H. (1998). Measuring the burden of disease: Healthy life-years. *American Journal of Public Health, 88,* 196–202.

Idjradinata, P., Watkins, W.E., & Pollitt, E. (1994). Adverse effect of iron supplementation on weight gain of iron-replete young children. *Lancet, 343,* 1252–1254.

International Nutritional Anemia Consultative Group (INACG). (1997). *Iron EDTA for food fortification.* Washington, DC: Nutrition Foundation.

International Nutritional Anemia Consultative Group (INACG) Secretariat. (1999). Safety of iron supplementation programs in malaria-endemic regions. INACG consensus statement. Washington, DC: International Life Sciences Institute.

Ittiravivongs, A., Songchitratna, K.S., Ratthapalo, S., & Pattara-Arechachai, J. (1991). Effect of low birthweight on severe childhood diarrhea. *Southeast Asian Journal of Tropical Medicine and Public Health, 22,* 557–562.

James, J.W. (1972). Longitudinal study of the morbidity of diarrheal and respiratory infections in malnourished children. *American Journal of Clinical Nutrition, 25,* 690–694.

James, P. (1998). The global nutrition challenge in the millennium. In *Challenges for the 21st century: A gender perspective on nutrition through the life cycle,* ACC/SCN symposium report, Nutrition Policy Paper #17. Geneva, Switzerland: World Health Organization.

Jelliffe, D.B. (1966). *The assessment of the nutritional status of the community.* WHO Monograph Series No. 53. Geneva, Switzerland: World Health Organization.

Jelliffe, D.B., & Jelliffe, E.F.P. (1978). The volume and composition of human milk in poorly nourished communities: A review. *American Journal of Clinical Nutrition, 31,* 492–515.

Johnson, W.B., Aderele, W.I., & Gbadero, D.A. (1992). Host factors and acute lower respiratory infections in pre-school children. *Journal of Tropical Pediatrics, 38,* 132–136.

Joseph, K.S., & Kramer, M.S. (1996). Review of the evidence on fetal and early childhood antecedents of adult chronic disease. *Epidemiology Reviews, 18,* 158–174.

Kalter, H.D., Burnham, G., Kolstad, P.R., Hossain, M., Schillinger, J.A., Khan, N.Z., Saha, S., de Wit, V., Kenya-Mugisha, N., Schwartz, B., & Black, R.E. (1997). Evaluation of clinical signs to diagnose anaemia in Uganda and Bangladesh, in areas with and without malaria. *Bulletin of the World Health Organization, 75*(S), 103–111.

Kamal, M.K., Ahsan, R.I., & Salam, A.K.M.A. (1998). *Achieving the goals for children in Bangladesh.* Bangladesh Bureau of Statistics/Ministry of Planning/Government of the People's Republic of Bangladesh/Dhaka: UNICEF.

Kastner, P., Chambon, P., & Leid, M. (1994). Role of nuclear retinoic acid receptors in the regulation of gene expression. In R. Blomhoff (Ed.), *Vitamin A in health and disease* (pp. 189–238). New York: Marcel Dekker.

Katz, J., Khatry, S.K., West, K.P., Jr., Humphrey, J.H., LeClerq, S.C., Pradhan, E.K., Pokhrel, R.P., & Sommer, A. (1995). Night blindness is prevalent during pregnancy and lactation in rural Nepal. *Journal of Nutrition, 125,* 2122–2127.

Katz, J., West, K.P., Jr., Khatry, S.K., Pradhan, E.K., LeClerq, S.C., Christian, P., Wu, L.S.F., Adhikari, R.K., Shrestha, S.R., & Sommer, A., & the NNIPS-2 Study Group. (in press). Maternal low-dose vitamin A or B-carotene supplementation has no effect on fetal loss and early infant mortality: A cluster randomized trial in Nepal. *American Journal of Clinical Nutrition.*

Katz, J., West, K.P., Jr., Tarwotjo, I., & Sommer, A. (1989). The importance of age in evaluating anthropometric indices for predicting mortality. *American Journal of Epidemiology, 130,* 1219–1226.

Katz, J., Zeger, S.L., & Tielsch, J.M. (1988). Village and household clustering of xerophthalmia and trachoma. *International Journal of Epidemiology, 17,* 865–869.

Katz, J., Zeger, S.L., West, K.P., Jr., Tielsch, J.M., & Sommer, A. (1993). Clustering of xerophthalmia within households and villages. *International Journal of Epidemiology, 22,* 709–715.

Kavishe, F.P. (1999). Iodine: Iodine deficiency disorders. In M.J. Sadler, J.J. Strain, & B. Caballero (Eds.), *Encyclopedia of human nutrition* (pp. 1146–1153). San Diego: Academic Press.

Keen, C.L., & Gershwin, M.E. (1990). Zinc deficiency and immune function. *Annual Review of Nutrition, 10,* 415–431.

Kehayias, J.J., Fiatarone, M.F., Zhuang, H., & Roubenoff, R. (1997). Total body potassium and body fat: Relevance to aging. *American Journal of Clinical Nutrition, 66,* 904–910.

Keusch, G.T. (1993). Malnutrition and the thymus gland. In S. Cunningham-Rundles (Ed.), *Nutrient modulation of the immune response* (pp. 283–299). New York: Marcel Dekker.

Keusch, G.T., Cruz, J.R., Torun, B., Urrutia, J.J., Smith, H., Jr., & Goldstein, A. (1987). Immature circulating lymphocytes in severely malnourished Guatemalan children. *Journal of Pediatric Gastroenterology and Nutrition, 6,* 265–270.

Khanum, S., Ashworth, A., & Huttly, S.R.A. (1994). Controlled trial of three approaches to the treatment of severe malnutrition. *Lancet, 344,* 1728–1732.

Khanum, S., Ashworth, A., & Huttly, S.R.A. (1998). Growth, morbidity, and mortality of children in Dhaka after treatment for severe malnutrition: A prospective study. *American Journal of Clinical Nutrition, 67,* 940–945.

Khatry, S.K., West, K.P., Jr., Katz, J., LeClerq, S.C., Pradhan, E.K., Wu, L.S., Thapa, M.D., & Pokhrel, R.P. (1995). Epidemiology of xerophthalmia in Nepal: A pattern of household poverty, childhood illness, and mortality. *Archives of Ophthalmology, 113,* 425–429.

Khin-Maung-U, Nyunt-Nyunt-Wai, Myo-Khin, Mu-Mu-Khin, Tin-U, & Thane-Toe. (1985). Effect on clinical outcome of breast feeding during acute diarrhoea. *British Medical Journal, 290,* 587–589.

Kikafunda, J.K., Walker, A.F., Allan, E.F., & Tumwine, J.K. (1998). Effect of zinc supplementation on growth and body composition of Ugandan preschool children: A randomized, controlled intervention trial. *American Journal of Clinical Nutrition, 68,* 1261–1266.

Kilbride, J., Baker, T.G., Parapia, L.A., Khoury, S.A., Shuqaidef, S.W., & Jerwood, D. (1999). Anaemia during pregnancy as a risk factor for iron-deficiency anaemia in infancy: A case-control study in Jordan. *International Journal of Epidemiology, 28,* 461–468.

Kim, J.Y., Moon, S.J., Kim, K.R., Sohn, C.Y., & Oh, J.J. (1998). Dietary iodine intake and urinary iodine excretion in normal Korean adults. *Yonsei Medical Journal, 39,* 355–362.

Kim, S., Moon, S., & Popkin, B.M. (2000). The nutrition transition in South Korea. *American Journal of Clinical Nutrition, 71,* 44–53.

Kimiagar, M., Azizi, F., Navai, L., Yassai, M., & Nafarabadi, T. (1990). Survey of iodine deficiency in a rural area near Tehran: Association of food intake and endemic goitre. *European Journal of Clinical Nutrition, 44,* 17–22.

Kirkwood, B.R., Ross, D.A., Arthur, P., Morris, S.S., Dollimore, N., Binka, F.N., Shier, R.P., Gyapong, J.O., Addy, H.A., & Smith, P.G. (1996). Effect of vitamin A supplementation on the growth of young children in northern Ghana. *American Journal of Clinical Nutrition, 63,* 773–781.

Klemm, R.D.W., Villate, E.E., Tuason-Lopez, C., Puertollano, E.P., Triunfante, J., del Rosario, A., & Dimaano, M.V. (1997). Integrating vitamin A capsule supplementation into child weighing: a monitoring study on Philippine OPT Plus. Philippines: Helen Keller International.

Konno, N., Makita, H., Yuri, K., Iizuka, N., & Kawasaki, K. (1994). Association between dietary iodine intake and prevalence of subclinical hypothyroidism in the coastal regions of Japan. *Journal of Clinical Endocrinology and Metabolism, 78,* 393–397.

Krause, V.M., Delisle, H., & Solomons, N.W. (1998). Fortified foods contribute one half of recommended vitamin A intake in poor urban Guatemalan toddlers. *Journal of Nutrition, 128,* 860–864.

Kreiss, J. (1997). Breastfeeding and vertical transmission of HIV-1. *Acta Paediatrica, 421,* 113–117.

Kuhnlein, H.V. (1992). Food sources of vitamin A and provitamin A. *Food and Nutrition Bulletin, 14,* 3–5.

Kuvibidila, S., Warrier, R.P., Ode, D., & Yu, L. (1996). Serum transferrin receptor concentrations in women with mild malnutrition. *American Journal of Clinical Nutrition, 63,* 596–601.

Kynast, G., & Saling, E. (1986). Effect of oral zinc application during pregnancy. *Gynecology and Obstetrics Investigations, 21,* 117–123.

Labbok, M., & Karsovec, K. (1990). Toward consistency in breastfeeding definitions. *Studies in Family Planning, 21,* 226–230.

Langer, P., Tajtakova, M., Podoba, J., Jr., Kostalova, L., & Gutekunst, R. (1994). Thyroid volume and urinary iodine in school children and adolescents in Slovakia after 40 years of iodine prophylaxis. *Experimental Clinical Endocrinology, 102,* 394–398.

Lartey, A., Manu, A., Brown, K.H., Peerson, J.M., & Dewey, K.G. (1999). A randomized, community-based trial of the effects of improved, centrally processed complementary foods on growth and micronutrient status of Ghanaian infants from 6 to 12 months of age. *American Journal of Clinical Nutrition, 70,* 391–404.

Launer, L.J., Habicht, J.P., & Kardjati, S. (1990). Breast feeding protects infants in Indonesia against illness and weight loss due to illness. *American Journal of Epidemiology, 131,* 322–331.

Lawless, J.W., Latham, M.C., Stephenson, L.S., Kinoti, S.N., & Pertet, A.M. (1994). Iron supplementation improves appetite and growth in anemic Kenyan primary school children. *Journal of Nutrition, 124,* 645–654.

Leon, D.A. (1998). Fetal growth and adult disease. *European Journal of Clinical Nutrition, 52,* S72–S82.

Leroy, V., Newell, M.L., Dabis F., Peckham, C., Van de Perre, P., Buterys, M., Kind, C., Simmonds, R.J., Wiktor, S., & Msellati, P. (1998). International multicentre pooled analysis of late postnatal mother-to-child transmission of HIV-1. Ghent International Working Group on Mother-to-Child Transmission of HIV. *Lancet, 352,* 597–600.

Lewis, S.M., Stott, G.J., & Wynn, K.J. (1998). An inexpensive and reliable new haemoglobin colour scale for assessing anaemia. *Journal of Clinical Pathology, 51,* 21–24.

Lie, C., Ying, C., En-Lin, W., Brun, T., & Geissler, C. (1993). Impact of large-dose vitamin A supplementation on childhood diarrhoea, respiratory disease, and growth. *European Journal of Clinical Nutrition, 47,* 88–96.

Lindberg, O., Andersson, L.C., & Lamberg, B-A. (1989). The impact of 25 years of iodine prophylaxis on the adult thyroid weight in Finland. *Journal of Endocrinology Investigations, 12,* 789–793.

Lindtjorn, B., & Alemu, T. (1997). Intra-household correlations of nutritional status in rural Ethiopia. *International Journal of Epidemiology, 26,* 160–165.

Lixin, S., Zhongfu, S., Jiaxiu, Z., Qilin, M., Deming, K., Lifu, Y., & Ying, T. (1995). The measurement and application of Tsh-Irma levels among different age groups in areas with iodine deficiency disorders. *Chinese Medical Science Journal, 10,* 30–33.

Llewellyn-Jones, D. (1965). Severe anaemia in pregnancy (as seen in Kuala Lumpur, Malaysia). *Australia and New Zealand Journal of Obstetrics and Gynaecology, 5,* 191–197.

Loerch, J.D., Underwood, B.A., & Lewis, K.C. (1979). Response of plasma levels of vitamin A to a dose of vitamin A as an indicator of hepatic vitamin A reserves in rats. *Journal of Nutrition, 109,* 778–786.

Lohman, T.G., Roche, A.F., & Martorell, R. (1988*). Anthropometric standardization reference manual.* Champaign, IL: Human Kinetics Publishers.

Lonnerdal, B. (1998). Zinc metabolism during pregnancy: Interactions with vitamin A. *Bibliotheca Nutritio et Dieta Dieta, 54,* 93–102.

Lonnerdal, B., Sandberg, A.S., Sandstrom, B., & Kunz, C. (1989). Inhibitory effects of phytic acid and other inositol phosphates on zinc and calcium absorption in suckling rats. *Journal of Nutrition, 119,* 211–214.

Looker, A.C., Dallman, P.R., Carroll, M.D., Gunter, E.W., & Johnson, C.L. (1977). Prevalence of iron deficiency in the United States. *Journal of the American Medical Association, 277,* 973–976.

Lopez de Romana, G., Graham, G.G., Mellits, E.D., & MacLean, W.C., Jr. (1980). Utilization of the protein and energy of the white potato by human infants. *Journal of Nutrition, 110,* 1849–1857.

Lozoff, B., Klein, N.K., Nelson, E.C., McClish, D.K., Manuel, M., & Chacon, M.E. (1998). Behavior of infants with iron-deficiency anemia. *Child Development, 69,* 24–36.

Lozoff, B., Wolf, A.W., & Jimenez, E. (1996). Iron-deficiency anemia and infant development: Effects of extended oral iron therapy. *Journal of Pediatrics, 129,* 382–399.

Luby, S.P., Kazembe, P.N., Redd, S.C., Ziba, C., Nwanyanwu, O.C., Hightower, A.W., Franco, C., Chitsulo, L., Wirima, J.J., & Olivar, M.A. (1995). Using clinical signs to diagnose anaemia in African children. *Bulletin of the World Health Organization, 73,* 477–482.

Lunn, P.G., Northrop-Clewes, C.A., & Downes, R.M. (1991). Intestinal permeability, mucosal injury, and growth faltering in Gambian infants. *Lancet, 338,* 907–910.

Lutter, C.K., Mora, J.O., Habicht, J.P., Rasmussen, K.M., Robson, D.S., & Herrera, M.G. (1990). Age-specific responsiveness of weight and length to nutritional supplementation. *American Journal of Clinical Nutrition, 51,* 359–364.

Lutter, C.K., Mora, J.O., Habicht, J.P., Rasmussen, K.M., Robson, D.S., Sellers, S.G., Super, C.M., & Herrera, M.G. (1989). Nutritional supplementation: Effects on child stunting because of diarrhea. *American Journal of Clinical Nutrition, 50,* 1–8.

Lynch, S.R. (1997). Interaction of iron with other nutrients. *Nutrition Reviews, 55,* 102–110.

Lynch, S.R. (1999). Iron: Physiology, dietary sources, and requirement. In M.J. Sadler, J.J. Strain, & B. Caballero (Eds.), *Encyclopedia of human nutrition* (pp. 1153–1159). San Diego: Academic Press.

Lynch, S.R., Hurrell, R.F., Bothwell, T.H., & MacPhail, A.P. (1993). *Iron EDTA for food fortification.* A report of the International Nutritional Anemia Consultative Group (INACG). Washington, DC: Nutrition Foundation.

MacLean, W.C., Jr., & Graham, G.G. (1979). The effect of level of protein intake in isoenergetic diets on energy utilization. *American Journal of Clinical Nutrition, 32,* 1381–1387.

MacLean, W.C., Jr., Klein, G.L., Lopez de Romana, G., Massa, E., & Graham, G.G. (1978). Protein quality of conventional and high protein rice and digestibility of glutinous and non-glutinous rice by preschool children. *Journal of Nutrition, 108,* 1740–1747.

MacLean, W.C., Jr., Lopez de Romana, G., Klein, G.L., Massa, E., Mellits, E.D., & Graham, G.G. (1979). Digestibility and utilization of the energy and protein of wheat by infants. *Journal of Nutrition, 109,* 1290–1298.

Mahalanabis, D. (1991). Breast feeding and vitamin A deficiency among children attending a diarrhoea treatment centre in Bangladesh: A case-control study. *British Medical Journal, 303,* 493–496.

Man, W.D., Weber, M., Palmer, A., Schneider, G., Wadda, R., Jaffar, S., Mulholland, E.D., & Greenwood, B.M. (1998). Nutritional status of children admitted to hospital with different diseases and its relationship to outcome in The Gambia, West Africa. *Tropical Medicine and International Health, 3,* 678–686.

Mandal, G.S., Nanda, K.N., & Bose, J. (1969). Night blindness in pregnancy. *Journal of Obstetrics and Gynecology of India, 19,* 453–458.

Mannar, M.G.V., & Dunn, J.T. (1995). *Salt iodization for the elimination of iodine deficiency.* Netherlands: International Council for Control of Iodine Deficiency Disorders (ICCIDD).

Marquis, G.S., Habicht, J.P., Lanata, C.F., Black, R.E., & Rasmussen, K.M. (1997). Breast milk or animal-product foods improve growth of Peruvian toddlers consuming marginal diets. *American Journal of Clinical Nutrition, 66,* 1102–1109.

Marsh, R. (1998). Building on traditional gardening to improve household food security. *Food, Nutrition, and Agriculture, 22,* 4–14.

Martorell, R., Mendoza, F., & Castillo, R. (1988). Poverty and stature in children. In J.C. Waterlow (Ed.), *Linear growth retardation in less developed countries* (pp. 57–73). Nestle Nutrition Workshop Series, vol. 14. New York: Vevey-Raven Press.

Martorell, R., & Shekar, M. (1994). Growth-faltering rates in California, Guatemala, and Tamil Nadu: Implications for growth-monitoring programmes. *Food and Nutrition Bulletin, 15,* 185–191.

Martorell, R., Yarbrough, C., Lechtig, A., Habicht, J.P., & Klein, R.E. (1975). Diarrheal diseases and growth retardation in preschool Guatemalan children. *American Journal of Physical Anthropology, 43,* 341–346.

Martorell, R., Yarbrough, C., Yarbrough, S., & Klein, R. E. (1980). The impact of ordinary illnesses on the dietary intakes of malnourished children. *American Journal of Clinical Nutrition, 30,* 345–350.

Mata, L.J., Cromal, R.A., Urrutia, J.J., & Garcia, B. (1977). Effect of infection of food intake and the nutritional state: Perspectives as viewed from the village. *American Journal of Clinical Nutrition, 30,* 1215–1227.

McCollum, E.V., & Davis, M. (1915). The essential factors in the diet during growth. *Journal of Biological Chemistry, 23,* 231–254.

McGuire, J., & Galloway, R. (1994). *Enriching lives: Overcoming vitamin and mineral malnutrition in developing countries.* Washington, DC: World Bank.

McLaren, D.S., Shirajiane, E., Tchalian, M., & Khoury, G. (1965). Xerophthalmia in Jordan. *American Journal of Clinical Nutrition, 17,* 117–130.

McMichael, A.J., Dreosti, I.E., Gibson, G.T., Hartshorne, J.M., Buckley, R.A., & Colley, D.P. (1982). A prospective study of serial maternal serum zinc levels and pregnancy outcome. *Early Human Development, 7,* 59–69.

Mele, L., West, K.P., Jr., Kusdiono, Pandji, A., Nendrawati, H., Tilden, R.L., Tarwotjo, I., & ACEH Study Group. (1991). Nutritional and household risk factors for xerophthalmia in Aceh, Indonesia: A case-control study. *American Journal of Clinical Nutrition, 53,* 1460–1465.

Menendez, C., Kahigwa, E., Hirt, R., Vounatsou, P., Aponte, J.J., Font, F., Acosta, C.J., Schellenberg, D.M., Galindo, C.M., Kimario, J., Urassa, H., Brabin, B., Smith, T.A., Kitua, A.Y., Tanner, M., & Alonso, P.L. (1997). Randomised placebo-controlled trial of iron supplementation and malaria chemoprophylaxis for prevention of severe anaemia and malaria in Tanzanian infants. *Lancet, 350,* 844–850.

Merialdi, M., Caulfield, L.E., Zavaleta, N., Figueroa, A., & DiPietro, J.A. (1998). Adding zinc to prenatal iron and folate tablets improves fetal neurobehavioral development. *American Journal of Obstetrics and Gynecology, 180,* 483–490.

Metges, C.C., Greil, W., Gartner, R., Rafferzeder, M., Linseisen, J., Woerl, A., & Wolfram, G. (1996). Influence of knowledge on iodine content in foodstuffs and prophylactic usage of iodized salt on urinary iodine excretion and thyroid volume of adults in southern Germany. *Zeitschrift Ernahrungswiss, 35,* 6–12.

Meyers, L.D., Habicht, J.P., Johnson, C.L., & Brownie, C. (1973). Prevalences of anemia in black and white women in the United States estimated by two methods. *American Journal of Public Health, 73,* 1042–1049.

Michaelsen, K.F. (1988). Value of prolonged breastfeeding. Letter to the editor. *Lancet, 2,* 788–789.

Mitra, A.K., Alvarez, J.O., & Stephensen, C.B. (1998). Increased urinary retinol loss in children with severe infections. *Lancet, 351,* 1033–1034.

Monsen, E.R., Hallberg, L., Layrisse, M., Hegsted, D.M., Cook, J.D., Mertz, W., & Finch, C.A. (1978). Estimation of available dietary iron. *American Journal of Clinical Nutrition, 31,* 134.

Moore, S.E., Cole, T.J., Collinson, A.C., Poskitt, E.M.E., McGregor, I.A., & Prentice, A.M. (1999). Prenatal or early postnatal events predict infectious deaths in young adulthood in rural Africa. *International Journal of Epidemiology, 28,* 1088–1095.

Mora, J.O. (1989). A new method for estimating a standardized prevalence of child malnutrition from anthropometric indicators. *Bulletin of the World Health Organization, 67,* 133–142.

Mora, J.O., Herrera, M.G., Suescun, J., de Navarro, L., & Wagner, M. (1981). The effects of nutritional supplementation on physical growth of children at risk of malnutrition. *American Journal of Clinical Nutrition, 34,* 1885–1892.

Morley, D. (1976). *Paediatric priorities in the developing world.* London: Butterworths.

Mostad, S.B., Overbaugh, J., DeVange, D.M., Welch, M.J., Chohan, B., Mandaliya, K., Nyange, P., Martin, J.L., Jr., Ndinya-Achola, J., Bwayo, J.J., & Kreiss, J.K. (1997). Hormonal contraception, vitamin A deficiency, and other risk factors for shedding of HIV-1 infected cells from the cervix and vagina. *Lancet, 350,* 922–927.

Moy, R.J.D., Marshall, T.F.de C., Choto, R.G.A.B., McNeish, A.S., & Booth, I.W. (1994). Diarrhoea and growth faltering in rural Zimbabwe. *European Journal of Clinical Nutrition, 48,* 810–821.

MRC Vitamin Study Research Group. (1991). Prevention of neural tube defects: Results of the Medical Research Council vitamin study. *Lancet, 338,* 131–137.

Mueller, W.H. (1986). The genetics of size and shape in children and adults. In F. Falkner & J.M. Tanner (Eds.), *Human growth: A comprehensive treatise.* Vol. 3: *Methodology, ecological, genetic, and nutritional effects on growth* (2nd ed.) (pp. 145–168). New York: Plenum Press.

Muhilal, Permeisih, D., Idjradinata, Y.R., Muherdiyantiningsih, & Karyadi, D. (1988). Vitamin A-fortified monosodium glutamate and health, growth, and survival of children: A controlled field trial. *American Journal of Clinical Nutrition, 48,* 1271–1276.

Murphy, S.P., Beaton, G.H., & Calloway, D.H. (1992). Estimated mineral intakes of toddlers: Predicted prevalence of inadequacy in village populations in Egypt, Kenya, and Mexico. *American Journal of Clinical Nutrition, 56,* 565–572.

Murray, C.J.L., & Lopez, A.D. (1997). Global mortality, disability, and the contribution of risk factors: Global burden of disease study. *Lancet, 349,* 1436–1442.

Murray, M.J., Murray, N.J., Murray, A.B., & Murray, M.B. (1975). Refeeding-malaria and hyperferraemia. *Lancet, 1,* 653–654.

Natadisastra, G., Wittpenn, J.R., Muhilal, West, K.P., Jr., Mele, L., & Sommer, A. (1988). Impression cytology: A practical index of vitamin A status. *American Journal of Clinical Nutrition, 48,* 695–701.

National Research Council. (1989). *Recommended dietary allowances* (10th ed.). Washington, DC: National Academy Press.

Nestle, P., & Alnwick, D. (1997). Iron/Multi-micronutrient supplements for young children. Summary and conclusions of a consultation held at UNICEF, Copenhagen, Denmark, August 19–20, 1996. Washington, DC: INACG Secretariat.

Ninh, N.X., Thissen, J.P., Collette, L., Gerard, G.G., Khoi, H.H., & Ketelslegers, J.M. (1996). Zinc supplementation increases growth and circulating insulin-like growth factor I (IGF-I) in growth-retarded Vietnamese children. *American Journal of Clinical Nutrition, 63,* 514–519.

Oberleas, D., & Harland, B.F. (1981). Phytate content of foods: Effect on dietary zinc bioavailability. *Journal of the American Dietetic Association, 79,* 433–436.

O'Dempsey, T.J., McArdle, R.F., Lloyd-Evans, N., Baldeh, I., Lawrence, B.E., Secka, O., & Greenwood, B. (1996).

Pneumococcal disease among children in a rural area of west Africa. *Pediatric Infectious Disease Journal, 15,* 431–437.

Olson, J.A. (1992). Measurement of vitamin A status. *Netherlands Journal of Nutrition, 53,* 163–167.

Onyango, A.W., Esrey, S.A., & Kramer, M.S. (1999). Continued breastfeeding and child growth in the second year of life: A prospective cohort study in western Kenya. *Lancet, 354,* 2041–2045.

Oppenheimer, S.J. (1998). Iron and infection in the tropics: Paediatric clinical correlates. *Annals of Tropical Paediatrics, 18,* S81–S87.

Osendarp, S.J.M., van Raaij, J.M.A., Arifeen, S.E., Wahed, M.A., Baqui, A.H., & Fuchs, G.J. (2000). A randomized, placebo-controlled trial of the effect of zinc supplementation during pregnancy on pregnancy outcome in Bangladeshi urban poor. *American Journal of Clinical Nutrition, 71,* 114–119.

Oski, F.A., Honig, A.S., Helu, B., & Howanitz, P. (1983). Effect of iron therapy on behavior performance in non-anemic, iron-deficient infants. *Pediatrics, 71,* 877–880.

Pardede, L.V.H., Hardjowasito, W., Gross, R., Dillion, D.H.S., Totoprajogo, O.S., Yosoprawoto, M., Waskito, L., & Untoro, J. (1998). Urinary iodine excretion is the most appropriate outcome indicator for iodine deficiency at field conditions at district level. *Journal of Nutrition, 128,* 1122–1126.

Parikh, L., & Shane, B. (1998). *Women of our world.* Washington, DC: Population Reference Bureau.

Pathak, A., Shah, N., & Tataria, A. (1993). Growth of exclusively breastfed infants. *Indian Pediatrics, 30,* 1291–1300.

Pelletier, D.L. (1994). The potentiating effects of malnutrition on child mortality: Epidemiologic evidence and policy implications. *Nutrition Reviews, 52,* 409–415.

Pelletier, D.L., Frongillo, E.D., & Habicht, J.P. (1993). Epidemiologic evidence for a potentiating effect of malnutrition on child mortality. *American Journal of Public Health, 83,* 1130–1133.

Penny, M.E., Peerson, J.M., Marin, M., Duran, A., Lanata, C.F., Lonnerdal, B., Black, R.E., & Brown, K.H. (1999). Randomized, community-based trial of the effect of zinc supplementation, with and without other micronutrients, in the duration of persistent childhood diarrhea in Lima, Peru. *Journal of Pediatrics, 135,* 208–217.

Perez, C., Scrimshaw, S., & Munoz, A. (1960). Technique of endemic goitre surveys. In *Endemic goitre* (pp. 360–383). Geneva, Switzerland: World Health Organization.

Peterson, S., Sanga, A., Eklof, H., Bunga, B., Taube, A., Gebre-Medhin, M., & Rosling, H. (2000). Classification of thyroid size by palpation and ultrasonography in field surveys. *Lancet, 355,* 106–110.

Pharoah, P.O.D., Buttfield, I.H., & Hetzel, B.S. (1971). Neurological damage to the fetus resulting from severe iodine deficiency during pregnancy. *Lancet, 1,* 308–310.

Pinstrup-Andersen, P., Pandya-Lorch, R., & Rosegrant, M.W. (1997). The world food situation: Recent developments, emerging issues, and long-term prospects. 2020 Vision Food Policy Report. Washington, DC: IFPRI.

Piwoz, E.G., Creed de Kanashiro, H., Lopez de Romana, G., Black, R.E., & Brown, K.H. (1996). Feeding practices and growth among low-income Peruvian infants: A comparison of internationally recommended definitions. *International Journal of Epidemiology, 25,* 103–114.

Pollitt, E., Gorman, K.S., Engle, P.L., Rivera, J.A., & Martorell, R. (1995). Nutrition in early life and the fulfillment of intellectual potential. *Journal of Nutrition, 125,* 1111S–1118S.

Popkin, B.M. (1994). The nutrition transition in low-income countries: An emerging crisis. *Nutrition Reviews, 52,* 285–298.

Popkin, B.M. (1998). The nutrition transition and its health implications in lower-income countries. *Public Health and Nutrition, 1,* 5–21.

Popkin, B.M. (1999). Urbanization, lifestyle changes, and the nutrition transition. *World Development, 27,* 1905–1915.

Popkin, B.M., & Doak, C.M. (1998). The obesity epidemic is a worldwide phenomenon. *Nutrition Reviews, 56,* 106–114.

Pradhan, A., Aryal, R.H., Regmi, G., Ban, B., & Govindasamy, P. (1997). *Nepal Family Health Survey 1996.* Kathmandu, Nepal, and Calverton, MD: Ministry of Health (Nepal), New ERA, and Macro International.

Prasad, A.S. (1985). Clinical manifestations of zinc deficiency. *Annual Review of Nutrition, 5,* 341–363.

Prasad, A.S. (1991). Discovery of human zinc deficiency and studies in an experimental human model. *American Journal of Clinical Nutrition, 53,* 403–412.

Prentice, A.M. (1996). Constituents of human milk. *Food and Nutrition Bulletin, 17,* 305–312.

Prentice, A.M. (1998). Early nutritional programming of human immunity. In *Annual Report, 1998* (pp. 53–64). Laussanne: Nestle Foundation for the Study of Problems of Nutrition in the World.

Prentice, A.M., Whitehead, R.G., Watkinson, M., Lamb, W.H., & Cole, T.J. (1983). Prenatal dietary supplementation of African women and birth-weight. *Lancet, 1,* 489–492.

Preziosi, P., Prual, A., Galan, P., Daouda, H., Boureima, H., & Hereberg, S. (1997). Effect of iron supplementation on the iron status of pregnant women: Consequences for newborns. *American Journal of Clinical Nutrition, 66,* 1178–1182.

Quality Assurance Workshop for Salt Iodized Programs. (1997). Program Against Micronutrient Malnutrition, Opportunities for Micronutrient Interventions, and John Snow, Inc.

Rahman, M.M., Huq, F., Sack, D.A., Butler, T., Azad, A.K., Alam, A., Nahar, N., & Islam, M. (1990). Acute lower respiratory infections in hospitalized patients with diarrhea in Dhaka, Bangladesh. *Reviews of Infectious Diseases, 12,* S899–S906.

Rahman, M.M., Akramuzzaman, S.M., Mitra, A.K., Fuchs, G.J., & Mahalanabis, D. (1999). Long-term supplementation with iron does not enhance growth in malnourished Bangladeshi children. *Journal of Nutrition, 129,* 1319–1322.

Rahmathullah L., Underwood, B.A., Thulasiraj, R.D., & Milton, R.C. (1991). Diarrhea, respiratory infections, and growth are not affected by a weekly low-dose vitamin A supplement: A masked, controlled field trial in children in southern India. *American Journal of Clinical Nutrition, 54,* 568–577.

Rahmathullah, L., Underwood, B.A., Thulasiraj, R.D., Milton, R.C., Ramaswamy, K., Rahmathullah, R., & Babu, G. (1990). Reducing mortality among children in Southern India receiving a small weekly dose of vitamin A. *New England Journal of Medicine, 323,* 929–935.

Raisler, J., Alexander, C., & O'Campo, P. (1999). Breastfeeding and infant illness: A dose-response relationship. *American Journal of Public Health, 89,* 25–30.

Ramakrishnan, U., Latham, M.C., & Abel, R. (1995). Vitamin A supplementation does not improve growth of preschool children: A randomized, double-blind field trial in South India. *Journal of Nutrition, 125,* 202–211.

Ramalingaswami, V. (1995). New global perspectives on overcoming malnutrition. *American Journal of Clinical Nutrition, 61,* 259–263.

Ramalingaswami, V., Jonsson, U., & Rohde, J. (1996). The Asian enigma. In Peter Abramson (Ed.), *The progress of nations* (pp. 11–17). New York: UNICEF.

Rasmussen, L.B., Ovesen, L., & Christiansen, E. (1999). Day-to-day and within-day variation in urinary iodine excretion. *European Journal of Clinical Nutrition, 53,* 401–407.

Reddy, V. (1991). Protein-energy malnutrition. In P. Stanfield, M. Brueton, M. Chan, M. Parkin, & T. Waterston, *Diseases of children in the subtropics and tropics* (4th ed.) (pp. 335–357). London: Hodder & Stoughton.

Rice, A.L., Stoltzfus, R.J., de Francisco, A., Chakraborty, J., Kjolhede, C.L., & Wahed, M.A. (1999). Maternal vitamin A or b-carotene supplementation in lactating Bangladeshi women benefits mothers and infants but does not prevent subclinical deficiency. *Journal of Nutrition, 129,* 356–365.

Riggs, K.M., Spiro, A.L.I., Tucker, K., & Rush, D. (1996). Relations of vitamin B12, vitamin B6, folate, and homocysteine to cognitive performance in the Normative Aging Study. *American Journal of Clinical Nutrition, 63,* 306–314.

Rivera, J., & Ruel, M.T. (1997). Growth retardation starts in the first three months of life among rural Guatemalan children. *European Journal of Clinical Nutrition, 1,* 92–96.

Robinett, D., Taylor, H., & Stephens, C. (1996). *Anemia detection in health services: Guidelines for program managers* (2nd ed.). Seattle: Program for Appropriate Technology in Health (PATH).

Rosado, J.L., Lopez, P., Munoz, E., Martinez, H., & Allen, L.H. (1997). Zinc supplementation reduced morbidity, but neither zinc nor iron supplementation affected growth or body composition of Mexican preschoolers. *American Journal of Clinical Nutrition, 65,* 13–19.

Rosenberg, I.H., & Miller, J.W. (1992). Nutritional factors in physical and cognitive functions of elderly people. *American Journal of Clinical Nutrition, 55,* 1237S–1243S.

Ross, A.C. (1996). The relationship between immunocompetence and vitamin A status. In A. Sommer & K.P. West, Jr. (Eds.), *Vitamin A deficiency: Health, survival, and vision* (pp. 251–273). New York: Oxford University Press.

Ross, S.M., Nel, E., & Naeye, R. (1985). Differing effects of low- and high-bulk maternal dietary supplements during pregnancy. *Early Human Development, 10,* 295–302.

Rothman, K.J., & Greenland, S. (1998). Causation and causal inference. In K.J. Rothman & S. Greenland (Eds.), *Modern epidemiology* (2nd ed.) (pp. 7–28). Philadelphia: Lippincott-Raven.

Roubenoff, R. (1999). Sarcopenia: Inevitable, but treatable. *SCN News, 19,* 27–29.

Rousham, E.K., & Mascie-Taylor, C.G. (1994). An 18-month study of the effect of periodic anthelminthic treatment on the growth and nutritional status of pre-school children in Bangladesh. *Annals of Human Biology, 21,* 315.

Rowland, M.G.M., Barrell, R.A.E., & Whitehead, R.G. (1978). Bacterial contamination in traditional Gambian weaning foods. *Lancet, 1,* 136–138.

Rowland, M.G.M., Cole, T.J., & Whitehead, R.G. (1977). A quantitative study into the role of infection in determining nutritional status in Gambian village children. *British Journal of Nutrition, 37,* 441–450.

Rowland, M.G.M., Rowland, S.G.J.G., & Cole, T.J. (1988). Impact of infection on the growth of children from 0 to 2 years in an urban West African community. *American Journal of Clinical Nutrition, 47,* 134–138.

Roy, S.K., Chowdhury, A.K., & Rahaman, M.M. (1983). Excess mortality among children discharged from hospital after treatment for diarrhoea in rural Bangladesh. *British Medical Journal, 287,* 1097–1099.

Roy, S.K., Tomkins, A.M., Akramuzzaman, S.M., Behrens, R.H., Haider, R., Mahalanabis, D., & Fuchs, G. (1997) Randomised controlled trial of zinc supplementation in malnourished Bangladeshi children with acute diarrhoea. *Archives of Diseases in Childhood, 77,* 196–200.

Roy, S.K., Tomkins, A.M., Haider, R., Behrens, R.H., Akramuzzaman, S.M., Mahalanabis, D., & Fuchs, G.J. (1999). Impact of zinc supplementation on subsequent growth and morbidity in Bangladeshi children with acute diarrhoea. *European Journal of Clinical Nutrition, 53,* 529–534.

Ruel, M.T., & Bouis, H.E. (1998). Plant breeding: A long-term strategy for the control of zinc deficiency in vulnerable populations. *American Journal of Clinical Nutrition, 68,* 488S–494S.

Ruel, M.T., Pelletier, D.L., Habicht, J.P., Mason, J.B., Chobokoane, C.S., & Maruping, A.P. (1990). Comparison of mothers' understanding of two child growth charts in Lesotho. *Bulletin of the World Health Organization, 68,* 483–491.

Ruel, M.T., Rivera, J., & Habicht, J.P. (1995). Length screens better than weight in stunted populations. *Journal of Nutrition, 125,* 1222–1228.

Ruel, M.T., Rivera, J., Habicht, J.P., & Martorell, R. (1995). Differential response to early nutrition supplementation: Long-term effects on height at adolescence. *International Journal of Epidemiology, 24,* 404–412.

Ruel, M.T., Rivera, J.A., Santizo, M.-C., Lonnerdal, B., & Brown, K.H. (1997). Impact of zinc supplementation on morbidity from diarrhea and respiratory infections among rural Guatemalan children. *Pediatrics, 99,* 808–813.

Ryan, A.S. (1997). Iron-deficiency anemia in infant development: Implications for growth, cognitive development, resistance to infection, and iron supplementation. *Yearbook of Physical Anthropology, 40,* 25–62.

Sandstead, H.H., Penland, J.G., Alcock, N.W., Dayal, H.H., Chen, X.C., Li, J.S., Zhao, F., & Yang, J.J. (1998). Effects of repletion with zinc and other micronutrients on neuropsychologic performance and growth of Chinese children. *American Journal of Clinical Nutrition, 68,* 470S–475S.

Sanghvi, T.G. (1995). *Improving the cost-effectiveness of breastfeeding promotion in maternity services.* Summary of the USAID/LAC HNS Study in Latin America (1992–1995). Arlington, VA: U.S. Agency for International Development.

Sanghvi, T., & Murray, J. (1997). *Improving child health through nutrition: The Nutrition Minimum Package.* Arlington, VA: Basic Support for Institutionalizing Child Survival (BASICS) Project, for the US Agency for International Development, Washington, DC.

Sarin, A.R. (1995). Severe anemia of pregnancy, recent experience. *International Journal of Gynaecology and Obstetrics, 2,* S43–S49.

Sazawal, S., Black, R.E., Bhan, M.K., Bhandari, N., Sinha, A., & Jalla, S. (1995). Zinc supplementation in young children with acute diarrhea in India. *New England Journal of Medicine, 333,* 839–844.

Sazawal, S., Black, R.E., Bhan, M.K., Jalla, S., Bhandari, N., Sinha, A., & Majumdar, S. (1996). Zinc supplementation reduces the incidence of persistent diarrhea and dysentery among low socioeconomic children in India. *Journal of Nutrition, 126,* 443–450.

Sazawal, S., Black, R.E., Bhan, M.K., Jalla, S., Sinha, A., & Bhandari, N. (1997). Efficacy of zinc supplementation in reducing the incidence and prevalence of acute diarrhea: A community-based, double-blind, controlled trial. *American Journal of Clinical Nutrition, 66,* 413–418.

Sazawal, S., Black, R.E., Jalla, S., Mazumdar, S., Sinha, A., & Bhan, M.K. (1998). Zinc supplementation reduces the incidence of acute lower respiratory infections in infants and preschool children: A double-blind controlled trial. *Pediatrics, 102,* 1–5.

Sazawal, S., Jalla, S., Mazumder, S., Sinha, A., Black, R.E., & Bhan, M.K. (1997). Effect of zinc supplementation on cell-mediated immunity and lymphocyte subsets in preschool children. *Indian Pediatrics, 34,* 589.

Scholl, T.O., Hediger, M.L., Fischer, R.L., & Shearer, J.W. (1992). Anemia vs iron deficiency: Increased risk of preterm delivery in a prospective study. *American Journal of Clinical Nutrition, 55,* 985–988.

Scrimshaw, N.S., Taylor, C.E., & Gordon, J.E. (1967). *Interactions of nutrition and infection.* WHO Monograph Series. Geneva, Switzerland: World Health Organization.

Selwyn, B.J. (1990). The epidemiology of acute respiratory tract infection in young children: Comparison of findings from several developing countries. *Reviews of Infectious Diseases, 12,* S870–888.

Semba, R.D. (1994). Vitamin A, immunity, and infection. *Clinical Infectious Disease, 19,* 489–499.

Semba, R.D., Kumwenda, N., Hoover, D.R., Taha, T.E., Quinn, T.C., Mtimavalye, L., Biggar, R.J., Broadhead, R., Miotti, P.G., Sokoll, L.J., van der Hoeven, L., & Chiphangwi, J.D. (1999). Human immunodeficiency virus load in breast milk, mastitis, and mother-to-child transmission of human immunodeficiency virus type 1. *Journal of Infectious Diseases, 180,* 93–98.

Semba, R.D., & Tang, A.M. (1999). Micronutrients and the pathogenesis of human immunodeficiency virus infection. *British Journal of Nutrition, 81,* 181–189.

Sen, A. (1992). Food entitlements and economic chains. In L.F. Newman, W. Crossgrove, R.W. Kates, R. Matthews, & S. Millman, *Hunger in history: Food short-*

*age, poverty, and deprivation* (pp. 374–386). Oxford: Blackwell.

Seshadri, S. (Ed.). (1996). *Use of carotene-rich foods to combat vitamin A deficiency in India: A multicentric study*. Scientific report 12. New Delhi: Nutrition Foundation of India.

Shankar, A. (2000). Personal communication.

Shankar, A.H., Genton, B., Semba, R.D., Baisor, M., Paino, J., Tamja, S., Adiguma, T., Wu, L., Rare, L., Tielsch, J.M., Alpers, M.P., & West, K.P., Jr. (1999). Effect of vitamin A supplementation on morbidity due to Plasmodium falciparum in young children in Papua New Guinea: A randomised trial. *Lancet, 354,* 203–209.

Shankar, A.H., Genton, B., Tamja, S., Arnold, S., Wu, L., Baisor, M., Paino, J., Tielsch, J.M., West, K.P., Jr., & Alpers, M.A. (1997). Zinc supplementation can reduce malaria-related morbidity in preschool children. *American Journal of Tropical Medicine and Hygiene, 57,* A434.

Shankar, A.V., Gittelsohn, J., West, K.P., Jr., Stallings, R., Gnywali, T., & Faruque, F. (1998). Eating from a shared plate affects food consumption in vitamin A-deficient Nepali children. *Journal of Nutrition, 128,* 1127–1133.

Shankar, A.H., & Prasad, A.S. (1998). Zinc and immune function: The biological basis of altered resistance to infection. *American Journal of Clinical Nutrition, 68,* 447S–463S.

Shann, F., Barker, J., & Poore, P. (1989). Clinical signs that predict death in children with severe pneumonia. *Pediatric Infectious Disease Journal, 8,* 852–855.

Sharmanov, A. (1998). Anaemia in Central Asia: Demographic and health survey experience. *Food and Nutrition Bulletin, 19,* 307–317.

Simondon, K.B., Gartner, A., Berger, J., Cornu, A., Massamba, J.P., San Miguel, J.L., Ly, C., Missotte, I., Simondon, F., Traissac, P., Delpeuch, F., & Maire, B. (1996). Effect of early, short-term supplementation on weight and linear growth of 4–7-month-old infants in developing countries: A four-country randomized trial. *American Journal of Clinical Nutrition, 64,* 537–545.

Sinha, D.P., & Bang, F.B. (1973). Seasonal variation in signs of vitamin-A deficiency in rural West Bengal children. *Lancet, 2,* 228–231.

Skikne, B.S., Flowers, C.H., & Cook, J.D. (1990). Serum transferrin receptor: A quantitative measure of tissue iron deficiency. *Blood, 75,* 1870–1876.

Smedman, L., Sterky, G., Mellander, L., & Wall, S. (1987). Anthropometry and subsequent mortality in groups of children aged 6–59 months in Guinea-Bissau. *American Journal of Clinical Nutrition, 46,* 369–373.

Smitasiri, S., Attig, G.A., & Dhanamitta, S. (1992). Participatory action for nutrition education: Social marketing vitamin A-rich foods in Thailand. *Ecology of Food and Nutrition, 28,* 199–210.

Smith, J.C., Makdani, D., Hegar, A., Rao, D., & Douglass, L.W. (1999). Vitamin A and zinc supplementation of preschool children. *Journal of the American College of Nutrition, 18,* 213–222.

Smith, T.A., Lehman, D., Coakley, C., Spooner, V., & Alpers, M.P. (1991). Relationships between growth and acute lower-respiratory infections in children <5 years in a highland population of Papua New Guinea. *American Journal of Clinical Nutrition, 53,* 963–970.

Smyth, P.P.A., Hetherton, A.M.T., Smith, D.F., Radcliff, M., & O'Herlihy, C. (1997). Maternal iodine status and thyroid volume during pregnancy: Correlation with neonatal iodine intake. *Journal of Clinical Endocrinology and Metabolism, 82,* 2840–2843.

Soemantri, A.G., Pollitt, E., & Kim, I. (1985). Iron deficiency anemia and educational achievement. *American Journal of Clinical Nutrition, 42,* 1221–1228.

Soewarta, K., & Bloem, M.W. (1999). The role of high-dose vitamin A capsules in preventing a relapse of Vitamin A deficiency due to Indonesia's current crisis. *Helen Keller International Indonesia Crisis Bulletin* 1999;1:1–4

Solomons, N.W. (1986). Competitive interaction of iron and zinc in the diet: Consequences for human nutrition. *Journal of Nutrition, 116,* 927–935.

Solomons, N.W. (1998). There needs to be more than one way to skin the iodine deficiency disorders cat: Novel insights from the field in Zimbabwe. *American Journal of Clinical Nutrition, 67,* 1104–1105.

Solomons, N.W. (1999). Malnutrition: Secondary malnutrition. In M.J. Sadler, J.J. Strain, & B. Caballero (Eds.), *Encyclopedia of human nutrition* (pp. 1254–1259). San Diego, CA: Academic Press.

Solon, F.S., Fernandez, T.L., Latham, M.C., & Popkin, B.M. (1979). An evaluation of strategies to control vitamin A deficiency in the Philippines. *American Journal of Clinical Nutrition, 32,* 1445–1453.

Solon, F.S., Klemm, R.D.W., Sanchez, L., Darnton-Hill, I., Craft, N.E., Christian, P., & West, K.P., Jr. (in press). Evaluation of the efficacy of vitamin A-fortified wheat-flour bun on the vitamin A status of Filipino school children. *American Journal of Clinical Nutrition.*

Solon, F.S., Latham, M.C., Guirriee, R., Florentino, R., Williamson, D.F., & Aguilar, J. (1985). Fortification of MSG with vitamin A: The Philippines experience. *Food Technology, 39,* 71–79.

Solon, F.S., Solon, M.S., Mehansho, H., West, K.P., Jr., Sarol, J., Perfecto, C., Nano, T., Sanchez, L., Isleta, M., Wasantwisut, E., & Sommer, A. (1996). Evaluation of the effect of vitamin A-fortified margarine on the vitamin A status of preschool Filipino children. *European Journal of Clinical Nutrition, 50,* 720–723.

Sommer, A. (1982). *Nutritional blindness, xerophthalmia, and keratomalacia.* New York: Oxford University Press.

Sommer, A. (1995). *Vitamin A deficiency and its consequences: A field guide to their detection and control* (3rd ed.). Geneva, Switzerland: World Health Organization.

Sommer, A., Hussaini, G., Tarwotjo, I., & Susanto, D. (1983). Increased mortality in children with mild vitamin A deficiency. *Lancet, 2,* 585–588.

Sommer, A., & Loewenstein, M.S. (1975). Nutritional status and mortality: A prospective validation of the QUAC stick. *American Journal of Clinical Nutrition, 28,* 287–292.

Sommer, A., Tarwotjo, I., Hussaini, G., Susanto, D., & Soegiharto, T. (1981). Incidence, prevalence, and scale of blinding malnutrition. *Lancet, 1,* 1407–1408.

Sommer, A., & West, K.P., Jr. (1996). *Vitamin A deficiency: Health, survival, and vision.* New York: Oxford University Press.

Stanbury, J.B., Ermans, A.E., Bourdoux, P., Todd, C., Oken, E., Tonglet, R., Vidor, G., Braverman, L.E., & Medeiros-Neto, G. (1998). Iodine-induced hyperthyroidism: Occurrence and epidemiology. *Thyroid, 8,* 83–100.

Steer, P., Alam, M.A., Wadsworth, J., & Welch, A. (1995). Relation between maternal haemoglobin concentration and birthweight in different ethnic groups. *British Medical Journal, 310,* 489–491.

Stein, S.A. (1994). Molecular and neuroanatomical substrates of motor and cerebral cortex abnormalities in fetal thyroid hormone disorders. In J.B. Stanbury (Ed.), *The damaged brain of iodine deficiency* (pp. 67–102). New York: Cognizant Communication Corporation.

Stipanuk, M.H. (2000). *Biochemical and physiological aspects of human nutrition.* Philadelphia: W.B. Saunders.

Stoltzfus, R.J. (1997). Rethinking anaemia surveillance. *Lancet, 349,* 1764–1766.

Stoltzfus, R.J., Albonico, M., Chwaya, H.M., Tielsch, J.M., Schulze, K.J., & Savioli, L. (1998). Effects of the Zanzibar school-based deworming program on iron status of children. *American Journal of Clinical Nutrition, 68,* 179–186.

Stoltzfus, R.J., Chwaya, H.M., Tielsch, J.M., Schulze, K.J., Albonico, M., & Savioli, L. (1997). Epidemiology of iron deficiency anemia in Zanzibari school children. *American Journal of Clinical Nutrition, 65,* 153–159.

Stoltzfus, R.J., & Dreyfuss, M.L. (1998). *Guidelines for the use of iron supplements to prevent and treat iron deficiency anemia.* International Nutrition Anemia Consultative Group/World Health Organization/United Nations Children's Fund. Washington, DC: ILSI Press.

Stoltzfus, R.J., Edward-Raj, A., Dreyfuss, M.L., Albonico, M., Montresor, A., Thapa, M.D., West, K.P., Jr., Chwaya,

H.M., Savioli, L., & Tielsch, J. (1999). Clinical pallor is useful to detect severe anemia in populations where anemia is prevalent and severe. *Journal of Nutrition, 129,* 1675–1681.

Stoltzfus, R.J., Hakimi, M., Miller, K.W., Rasmussen, K.M., Dawiesah, S., Habicht, J.P., & Dibley, M.J. (1993). High-dose vitamin A supplementation of breast feeding Indonesian mothers: Effects on the vitamin A status of mother and infant. *Journal of Nutrition, 123,* 666–675.

Stoltzfus, R.J., Miller, K.W., Hakimi, M., & Rasmussen, K.M. (1993). Conjunctival impression cytology as an indicator of vitamin A status in lactating Indonesian women. *American Journal of Clinical Nutrition, 58,* 167–173.

Stoltzfus, R.J., & Underwood, B.A. (1995). Breast-milk vitamin A as an indicator of the vitamin A status of women and infants. *Bulletin of the World Health Organization, 73,* 703–711.

Stott, G.J., & Lewis, S.M. (1995). A simple and reliable method for estimating haemoglobin. *Bulletin of the World Health Organization, 73,* 369–373.

Syrenicz, A., Napierala, K., Celibala, R., Majewska, U., Krzyzanowska, B., Gulinska, M., Gozdzik, J., Widecka, K., & Czekalski, S. (1993). Iodized salt consumption, urinary iodine concentration, and prevalence of goiter in children from four districts of north-western Poland (Szczecin Coordinating Center). *Endokrynologia Polska, 44,* 343–350.

Taffs, R.E., Enterline, J.C., Rusmil, K., Muhilal, Suwardi, S.S., Rustama, D., Djatnika, Cobra, C., Semba, R.D., Cohen, N., & Asher, D.M. (1999). Oral iodine supplementation does not reduce neutralizing antibody responses to oral poliovirus vaccine. *Bulletin of the World Health Organization, 77,* 484–491.

Tajtakova, M., Hancinova, D., Langer, P., Tajtak, J., Foldes, O., Malinovsky, E., & Varga, J. (1990). Thyroid volume by ultrasound in boys and girls 6–16 years of age under marginal iodine deficiency as related to the age of puberty. *Klinisce Wochenschrift, 68,* 503–506.

Talukder, A., Islam, N., Klemm, R., & Bloem, M. (1993). *Home gardening in South Asia: The complete handbook.* Dhaka, Bangladesh: Helen Keller International.

Tamura, T., Goldenberg, R.L., Johnston, K.E., & Dubard, M. (2000). Maternal plasma zinc concentrations and pregnancy outcome. *American Journal of Clinical Nutrition, 71,* 109–113.

Tanumihardjo, S.A., Muhilal, Yuniar, Y., Permaeshi, D., Sulaiman, Z., Karyadi, D., & Olson, J.A. (1990). Vitamin A status in preschool-age Indonesian children as assessed by the modified relative-dose-response assay. *American Journal of Clinical Nutrition, 52,* 1068–1072.

Taren, D., & Chen, J. (1993). A positive association between extended breast-feeding and nutritional status in rural Hubei Province, People's Republic of China. *American Journal of Clinical Nutrition, 58,* 862–867.

Tarwotjo, I., Katz, J., West, K.P., Jr., Tielsch, J.M., & Sommer, A. (1992). Xerophthalmia and growth in pre-school Indonesian children. *American Journal of Clinical Nutrition, 55,* 1142–1146.

Tarwotjo, I., Sommer, A., Soegiharto, T., Susanto, D., & Muhilal. (1982). Dietary practices and xerophthalmia among Indonesian children. *American Journal of Clinical Nutrition, 35,* 574–581.

Thomson, C.D., Colls, A.J., Conaglen, J.V., Macormack, M., Stiles, M., & Mann, J. (1997). Iodine status of New Zealand residents as assessed by urinary iodide excretion and thyroid hormones. *British Journal of Nutrition, 78,* 891–912.

Tome, P., Reyes, H., Rodriguez, L., Guiscafre, H., & Gutierrez, G. (1996). Death caused by acute diarrhea in children: A study of prognostic factors. *Salud Publica de Mexico, 38,* 227–235.

Tonascia, J.A. (1993). Meta-analysis of published community trials: Impact of vitamin A on mortality. In Helen Keller International (Ed.), *Bellagio Meeting on Vitamin A Deficiency and Childhood Mortality* (pp. 49–51). Proceedings of Public Health Significance of Vitamin A Deficiency and Its Control. New York: Helen Keller International.

Tortora, G.J., & Grabowski, S.R. (1996). The endocrine system. In G.J. Tortora & S.R. Grabowski (Eds.), *Principles of anatomy and physiology* (8th ed.) (pp. 501–550). New York: HarperCollins.

Torun, B., & Chew, F. (1999). Protein-energy malnutrition. In M.E. Shils, J.A. Olson, M. Shike, & A.C. Ross (Eds.), *Modern nutrition in health and disease* (pp. 963–988). Baltimore: Williams & Wilkins.

Torun, B., Solomons, N.W., Caballero, B., Flores-Huerta, S., Orozco, G., & Batres, R. (1983). Intact and lactose-hydrolyzed milk to treat malnutrition in Guatemala. In J. Delmont (Ed.), *Milk intolerances and rejection* (pp. 109–115). Basel, Switzerland: Karger.

Trowbridge, F.L., Harris, S.S., Cook, J., Dunn, J.T., Florentino, R.F., Kodyat, B.A., Mannar, M.G.V., Reddy, V., Tontisirin, K., Underwood, B.A., & Yip, R. (1993). Coordinated strategies for controlling micronutrient malnutrition: a technical workshop. *Journal of Nutrition, 123,* 775–787.

Trowbridge, F.L., Hiner, C.D., & Robertson, A.D. (1981). Arm muscle indicators and creatinine excretion in children. *American Journal of Clinical Nutrition, 36,* 691–696.

Tucker, K. (2000). B vitamins, homocysteine, heart disease, and cognitive function. *SCN News, 19,* 30–33.

Tulchinsky, T.H., Acker, C., El Malki, K., Socolar, R.S., & Reshef, A. (1985). Use of growth charts as a simple epidemiological monitoring system of nutritional status of children. *Bulletin of the World Health Organization, 63,* 1137–1140.

Tupasi, T.E., Mangubat, N.V., Sunico, M.E., Magdangal, D.M., Navarro, E.E., Leonor, Z.A., Lupisan, S., Medalla, F., & Lucero, M.G. (1990). Malnutrition and acute respiratory tract infections in Filipino children. *Review of Infectious Diseases, 12,* S1047–S1054.

Udomkesmalee, E., Dhanamitta, S., Sirisinha, S., Charoenkiatkul, S., Tuntipopipat, S., Banjong, O., Rojroongwasinkul, N., Kramer, T.R., & Smith, J.C., Jr. (1992). Effect of vitamin A and zinc supplementation on the nutriture of children in Northeast Thailand. *American Journal of Clinical Nutrition, 56,* 50–57.

Underwood, B.A. (1990). Methods for assessment of vitamin A status. *Journal of Nutrition, 120,* 1459–1463.

Underwood, B.A. (1994). Current status of iodine deficiency disorders: A global perspective. *NU News on Health Care in Developing Countries, 8,* 4.

Underwood, B.A., & Hofvander, Y. (1982). Appropriate timing for complementary feeding of the breast-fed infant: A review. *Acta Paediatrica Scandinavica, 294*(S), 1–32.

UNICEF. (1997). *The state of the world's children 1998.* New York: Oxford University Press.

United Nations Development Programme (UNDP). (1999). *Human development report 1999* (pp. 127–258). New York: Oxford University Press.

Vetter, K.M., Djomand, G., Zadi, F., Diaby, L., Brattegaard, K., Timite, M., Andoh, J., Adou, J.A., & DeCock, K.M. (1996). Clinical spectrum of human immunodeficiency virus disease in children in a west Africa city. Project RETRO-CI. *Pediatric Infectious Disease Journal, 15,* 438–442.

Victora, C.G. (1992). The association between wasting and stunting: An international perspective. *Journal of Nutrition, 122,* 1105–1110.

Victora, C.G., Barros, F.C., Kirkwood, B.R., & Vaughan, J.P. (1990). Pneumonia, diarrhea, and growth in the first 4 year of life: A longitudinal study of 5914 urban Brazilian children. *American Journal of Clinical Nutrition, 52,* 391–396.

Victora, C.G., Fuchs, S.C., Kirkwood, B.R., Lombardi, C., & Barros, F.C. (1992). Breast-feeding, nutritional status, and other prognostic factors for dehydration among young children with diarrhoea in Brazil. *Bulletin of the World Health Organization, 70,* 467–475.

Victora, C.G., Kirkwood, B.R., Ashworth, A., Black, R.E., Rogers, S., Sazawal, S., Campbell, H., & Gove, S. (1999). Potential interventions for the prevention of childhood pneumonia in developing countries: improving nutrition. *American Journal of Clinical Nutrition, 70,* 309–320.

Victora, C.G., Morris, S.S., Barros, F.C., de Onis, M., & Yip, R. (1998). The NCHS reference and the growth of breast- and bottle-fed infants. *Journal of Nutrition, 128,* 1134–1138.

Victora, C.G., Smith, P.G., Barros, F.C., Vaughan, J.P., & Fuchs, S.C. (1989). Risk factors for deaths due to respiratory infections among Brazilian infants. *International Journal of Epidemiology, 18,* 918–925.

Victora, C.G., Vaughan, J.P., Martines, J.C., & Barcelos, L.B. (1984). Is prolonged breast-feeding associated with malnutrition? *American Journal of Clinical Nutrition, 39,* 307–314.

Villar, J., Smeriglio, V., Martorell, R., Brown, C.H., & Klein, R.E. (1984). Heterogeneous growth and mental development of intrauterine growth-retarded infants during the first 3 years of life. *Pediatrics, 74,* 783–791.

Viteri, F.E. (1998). A new concept in the control of iron deficiency: Community-based preventive supplementation of at-risk groups by the weekly intake of iron supplements. *Biomedical and Environmental Sciences, 11,* 46–60.

Wald, G. (1955). The photoreceptor process in vision. *American Journal of Ophthalmology, 40,* 18–41.

Walker, S.P., Powell, C.A., Grantham-McGregor, S.M., Himes, J.H., & Chang, S.M. (1991). Nutritional supplementation, psychosocial stimulation, and growth of stunted children: The Jamaican study. *American Journal of Clinical Nutrition, 54,* 642–648.

Walter, T. (1989). Infancy: Mental and motor development. *American Journal of Clinical Nutrition, 50,* 655–666.

Walter, T., Olivares, M., Pizarro, F., & Munoz, C. (1997). Iron, anemia, and infection. *Nutrition Reviews, 55,* 111–124.

Wark, J.D. (1999). Osteoporosis: A global perspective. *Bulletin of the World Health Organization, 77,* 424–426.

Waterlow, J.C. (1972). Classification and definition of protein-calorie malnutrition. *British Medical Journal, 3,* 566–569.

Waterlow, J.C. (1973). Note on the assessment and classification of protein-energy malnutrition in children. *Lancet, 2,* 87–89.

Waterlow, J.C. (1985). What do we mean by adaptation? In K. Blaxter & J.C. Waterlow (Eds.), *Nutritional adaptation in man* (pp. 1–10). London: John Libbey.

Waterlow, J.C., Buzina, R., Keller, W., Lane, J.M., Nichaman, M.Z., & Tanner, J. (1977). The presentation and use of height and weight data for comparing the nutritional status of groups of children under the age of 10 years. *Bulletin of the World Health Organization, 55,* 489–498.

Weissenbacher, M., Carballal, G., Avila, M, Salomon, H., Harisiadi, J., Catalano, M., Cerqueizo, M.C., & Murtagh, P. (1990). Hospital-based studies on acute respiratory tract infection in young children. *Review of Infectious Diseases, 12,* S889–S898.

West, K.P., Jr. (1986). Peri-urban malnutrition in Bangladesh: Differential energy, protein, and growth status of children. *Ecology of Food and Nutrition, 19,* 99–112.

West, K.P., Jr. (2000). Unpublished calculations.

West, K.P., Jr., Chirambo, M., Katz, J., Sommer, A., & Malawi Survey Group. (1986). Breast-feeding, weaning patterns, and the risk of xerophthalmia in southern Malawi. *American Journal of Clinical Nutrition, 44,* 690–697.

West, K.P., Jr., Djunaedi, E., Pandji, A., Kusdiono, Tarwotjo, I., Sommer, A., & ACEH Study Group. (1988). Vitamin A supplementation and growth: A randomized community trial. *American Journal of Clinical Nutrition, 48,* 1257–1264.

West, K.P., Jr., Katz, J., Khatry, S.K., LeClerq, S.C., Pradhan, E.K., Shrestha, S.R., Connor, P.B., Dali, S.M., Christian, P., Pokhrel, R.P., Sommer, A., & the NNIPS-2 Study Group. (1999). Double blind, cluster randomised trial of low-dose supplementation with vitamin A or B-carotene on mortality related to pregnancy in Nepal. *British Medical Journal, 318,* 570–575.

West, K.P., Jr., LeClerq, S.C., Shrestha, S.R., Wu, L.S.-F., Pradhan, E.K., Khatry, S.K., Katz, J., Adhikari, R., & Sommer, A. (1997). Effects of vitamin A on growth of vitamin A-deficient children: Field studies in Nepal. *Journal of Nutrition, 127,* 1957–1965.

West, K.P., Jr., Pokhrel, R.P., Katz, J., LeClerq, S.C., Khatry, S.K., Shrestha, S.R., Pradhan, E.K., Tielsch, J.M., Pandey, M.R., & Sommer, A. (1991). Efficacy of vitamin A in reducing preschool child mortality in Nepal. *Lancet, 338,* 67–71.

West, K.P., Jr., & Sommer, A. (1987). *Delivery of oral doses of vitamin A to prevent vitamin A deficiency and nutritional blindness.* ACC/SCN State-of-the-Art Series. Nutrition Policy Discussion Paper No. 2. Rome: United Nations Administrative Committee on Coordination, Subcommittee on Nutrition.

West, T.E., Goetghebuer, T., Milligan, P., Mulholland, E.K., & Weber, M.W. (1999). Long-term morbidity and mortality following hypoxaemic lower respiratory tract infection in Gambian children. *Bulletin of the World Health Organization, 77,* 144–148.

WHO Collaborative Study Team on the Role of Breastfeeding on the Prevention of Infant Mortality. (2000). Effect of breastfeeding on infant and child mortality due to infectious diseases in less developed countries: A pooled analysis. *Lancet, 355,* 451–455.

WHO Working Group on Infant Growth. (1994). *An evaluation of infant growth.* Geneva, Switzerland: World Health Organization, Nutrition Unit.

Willett, W.C., Kilama, W.L., & Kihamia, C.M. (1979). Ascaris and growth rates: A randomized trial of treatment. *American Journal of Public Health, 69,* 987–991.

Williams, C.D. (1933). A nutritional disease of childhood associated with a maize diet. *Archives of Diseases in Childhood, 8,* 423–433.

Wittpenn, J.R, Tseng, S.C.G., & Sommer, A. (1986). Detection of early xerophthalmia by impression cytology. *Archives of Ophthalmology, 104,* 237–239.

Wood, R.J., & Zheng, J.J. (1997). High dietary calcium intakes reduce zinc absorption and balance in humans. *American Journal of Clinical Nutrition, 65,* 1803–1809.

World Bank. (1993). *World development report 1993: Investing in health.* New York: Oxford University Press.

World Health Organization. (1989). *Protecting, promoting, and supporting breast-feeding—the special role of maternity services.* A Joint WHO/UNICEF Statement. Geneva, Switzerland: World Health Organization.

World Health Organization. (1992a). *Maternal health and safe motherhood programme. The prevalence of anaemia in women: A tabulation of available information* (2nd ed.). WHO/MCH/MSM/92.2. Geneva, Switzerland: World Health Organization.

World Health Organization. (1992b). Office of Information consensus statement: HIV and breast-feeding. Press Release WHO/30. Geneva, Switzerland: World Health Organization.

World Health Organization. (1993). Global prevalence of iodine deficiency disorders. MDIS Working Paper No. 1. Geneva, Switzerland: Micronutrient Deficiency Information System/World Health Organization.

World Health Organization. (1994). Indicators for assessing iodine deficiency disorders and their control through salt iodization. WHO/NUT/94.6. Geneva, Switzerland: World Health Organization.

World Health Organization. (1995a). The global prevalence of vitamin A deficiency. MDIS Working Paper No. 2. WHO/NUT/95.3. Geneva, Switzerland: World Health Organization.

World Health Organization. (1995b). Physical status: The use and interpretation of anthropometry. WHO Technical Report Series 854. Geneva, Switzerland: World Health Organization.

World Health Organization. (1996a). Indicators for assessing vitamin A deficiency and their application in monitoring and evaluating intervention programs. WHO/NUT/96.10. Geneva, Switzerland: World Health Organization.

World Health Organization. (1996b). *Trace elements in human health and nutrition.* Geneva, Switzerland: World Health Organization.

World Health Organization/UNICEF/IVACG. (1997). *Vitamin A supplements: a guide to their use in the treatment and prevention of vitamin A deficiency and xerophthalmia* (2nd ed.). Geneva, Switzerland: World Health Organization.

World Health Organization. (1998). *Integration of vitamin A supplementation with immunization: Policy and programme implications.* Report of a meeting 12–13 January, 1998, UNICEF: New York. Global Program for Vaccines and Immunization Expanded Program on Immunization. Geneva, Switzerland: World Health Organization.

Yadrick, M.K., Kenney, M.A., & Winterfeldt, E.A. (1989). Iron, copper, and zinc status: Response to supplementation with zinc or zinc and iron in adult females. *American Journal of Clinical Nutrition, 49,* 145–150.

Yip, R. (1994). Iron deficiency: Contemporary scientific issues and international programmatic approaches. *Journal of Nutrition, 124,* 1479S–1490S.

Yip, R. (1997). The challenge of improving iron nutrition: Limitations and potentials of major intervention approaches. *European Journal of Clinical Nutrition, 51,* S16–S24.

Yip, R., Johnson, C., & Dallman, P.R. (1984). Age-related changes in laboratory values used in the diagnosis of anemia and iron deficiency. *American Journal of Clinical Nutrition, 39,* 427–436.

Yip, R., & Scanlon, K. (1994). The burden of malnutrition: A population perspective. *Journal of Nutrition, 124,* 2043S–2046S.

Yoon, P.W., Black, R.E., Moulton, L.H., & Becker, S. (1997). The effect of malnutrition on the risk of diarrheal and respiratory mortality in children <2 years of age in Cebu, Philippines. *American Journal of Clinical Nutrition, 65,* 1070–1077.

Zhou, L.-M., Yang, W.-W., Hua, J.-Z., Deng, C.-Q., Tao, X., & Stoltzfus, R.J. (1998). Relation of hemoglobin measured at different times in pregnancy to preterm birth and low birthweight in Shanghai, China. *American Journal of Epidemiology, 148,* 998–1006.

Zinc Investigators' Collaborative Group: Bhutta, Z.A., Black, R.E., Brown, K.H., Meeks Gardner, J., Gore, S., Hidayat, A., Khatun, F., Martorell, R., Ninh, N.X., Penny, M.E., Rosado, J.L., Roy, S.K., Ruel, M., Sazawal, S., & Shankar, S. (1999). Prevention of diarrhea and pneumonia by zinc supplementation in children in developing countries: Pooled analysis of randomized controlled trials. *Journal of Pediatrics, 135,* 689–697.

Zucker, J.R., Perkins, B.A., Jafari, H., Otieno, J., Obonyo, C., & Campbell, C.C. (1997). Clinical signs for the recognition of children with moderate or severe anaemia in western Kenya. *Bulletin of the World Health Organization, 78*(S), 97–102.

Zumrawi, F.Y., Dimond, H., & Waterlow, J.C. (1987). Effects of infection on growth in Sudanese children. *Human Nutrition: Clinical Nutrition, 41,* 453–461.

# CHAPTER 6

# Chronic Diseases and Injury

*David V. McQueen, Matthew T. McKenna, and David A. Sleet*

This chapter provides an overview of chronic diseases and injury. The emphasis is on low- and middle-income countries, but information is often included on industrialized countries for comparison and to provide a more complete depiction of the global situation. Chronic diseases, often called *noncommunicable* or *degenerative diseases* in international health literature, are generally characterized by uncertain risk factors, a long latency period, prolonged course of illness, noncontagious origin, functional impairment or disability, and incurability. Many important diseases, as well as the consequences of serious injuries, have chronic characteristics. In recent years the attention to chronic diseases and injury has revealed the great potential cost of these conditions, both in financial and human suffering terms. More recently this financial cost and suffering have come to be expressed as the burden of chronic diseases and injury. Despite this growing recognition of burden, the available data worldwide are limited. In the industrialized world there is an abundance of data, albeit they are often analyzed only superficially. In the low- and middle-income countries, data are generally lacking or suspect. The student of international public health should bear this in mind when reading this chapter and the references cited.

This chapter first discusses the rise of interest in chronic diseases and injury as a public health problem and the emerging terminology. Attention is then given to the general context for the growth of chronic diseases as a global problem. Key risk factors are discussed, such as aging and personal behavior. The chapter then devotes attention to the current epidemiology of specific chronic diseases and injury in low- and middle-income countries. Special attention is given to those diseases and risk factors where there is reasonably good information, namely cardiovascular disease (CVD), stroke, cancer, diabetes, injury, tobacco use, eating behaviors, physical activity, and alcohol consumption. Relatively little attention is given to global efforts to prevent these diseases or to promote healthier behaviors. This stems more from a lack of available information than of interest among the authors.

## RECENT VIEWS ON THE BURDEN OF CHRONIC DISEASES AND INJURY

Although viewed historically as a burden to industrialized nations, chronic diseases are expected to alter the health of the globe over the next decade dramatically. In 1990 chronic diseases superseded communicable diseases as the cause of death in all areas of the world except sub-Saharan Africa and the Middle East. Epidemiologists estimate that by the year 2020 chronic diseases will account for "seven of ten deaths in low-income regions of the world compared with less than half today" (Murray & Lopez, 1997). These projections suggest that morbidity and mortality associated with chronic diseases will soon reach global proportions and demonstrate the need to prepare accordingly.

Recently, the World Bank, the World Health Organization (WHO), and the Harvard School of Public Health produced a systematic and comprehensive estimate of the relative impact of the major diseases affecting populations around the world (Murray & Lopez, 1996a, 1996b). In this joint study, the *Global Burden of Disease* (GBD), Murray and Lopez presented estimates of mortality, incidence, and morbidity for major regions of the world and introduced an index called the disability-adjusted life year (DALY), which combines the number of years of life lost from premature death with the loss of health from disease and disability. Thus the DALY provides an approach that calculates the contribution of mortality and morbidity health outcomes to the burden of disease and injury. Although some controversy exists around the ethical and value choices incorporated into the DALY, the measure has provided a valuable reference point for documenting current global health problems. In fact, a major finding of the GBD study was that chronic diseases and injury are already sources of substantial disability and premature mortality in low- and high-income countries. The GBD study also provides a tool for assessing future health problems, asserting that within the next 2 decades conditions such as ischemic heart disease, diabetes, depression, and injuries from road traffic accidents will become the predominant global health problems.

Although a detailed presentation of the methodology and results from the GBD study is provided in Chapter 1, four major findings of the study are highlighted here. First, the relative importance of major causes of death and disability are dominated by conditions in low- and middle-income countries because approximately 80% of the world's population live in these countries. The mortality and incidence rates of infectious diseases and maladies of childhood, such as diarrhea and pneumonia, are high. However, the absolute rates of disability and death from chronic diseases and injury are also frequently higher in low- and middle-income countries than in industrialized countries.

Second, life expectancy has on average increased in most countries with an attendant increase in the importance of chronic health problems associated with old age (Figure 6–1). This improvement in life span has resulted from two main factors. First, socioeconomic conditions have generally improved throughout the world during the past century, and these trends are expected to continue. Second, public health programs, such as water sanitation and immunizations, have been increasingly successful at controlling the impact of infectious diseases. This shift from diseases associated with poverty, such as maternal and childhood illnesses and infectious conditions, to diseases of affluence, such as ischemic heart disease and diabetes, is frequently referred to as the *epidemiologic transition* (Orman, 1971). Statistical models designed to project major health burdens in the future were developed as part of the GBD analysis. These projections suggest that this transformation from acute to chronic conditions will accelerate in the next 20 to 30 years, so that in the year 2020 the changes in the major sources of mortality will reflect a truly global epidemiologic transition (see Chapter 1).

A third finding of the GBD study is that injuries, particularly road traffic accidents, are also a major source of disability and premature death in low- and middle-income countries. Many of these nations, especially in Latin America, have rudimentary road systems and automobile manufacturing practices that do not incorporate many of the safety features considered standard in the industrialized world. Persons living in the densely populated urban centers of many low- and middle-income countries also frequently experience an excessive number of injuries associated with natural events such as earthquakes and hurricanes. Finally, the ravages of war-related injuries have a much greater impact on the military personnel and civilian populations in low- and middle-income countries than among those in industrialized countries (Murray & Lopez, 1996a, 1997).

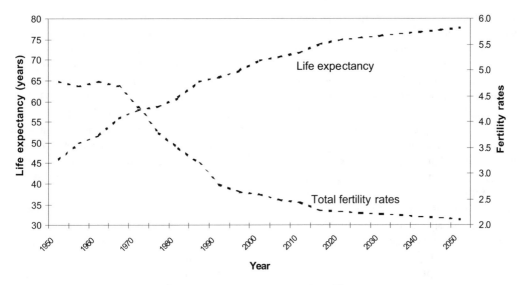

**Figure 6–1** Known and Projected Worldwide Life Expectancy and Fertility Rates

The final factor that has led to an increased relative burden of chronic conditions is the dramatic decline in birth and fertility rates in most countries (Figure 6–1). The lower birth rates imply that there will be fewer children and pregnant women and thus fewer problems associated with childhood and childbirth. For low- and middle-income countries, lower birth rates, an increase in life expectancy, and the already elevated rates of chronic diseases portend dramatic increases in the *relative* and *absolute* importance of chronic conditions, including ischemic heart disease, stroke, diabetes, and depression.

## DEFINITIONS OF TERMS

Many terms are used to describe chronic diseases, and they are used interchangeably (McKenna, Taylor, Marks, & Koplan, 1998). "Chronic diseases have been referred to as chronic illnesses, noncommunicable diseases, and degenerative diseases" (Breslow, 1997). WHO and many other health organizations use the acronym NCD for noncommunicable diseases. Whatever terminology is used, chronic

diseases are generally characterized by a long latency (chronic) period, a prolonged course of illness with the unlikelihood of cure, noncontagious origin, functional impairment or disability, and complex causality. Because many communicable or infectious diseases have chronic sequelae, it is sometimes difficult and problematic to provide an exact dichotomous separation of chronic from acute diseases.

What distinguishes most chronic diseases is that they are the result of a combination of socioenvironmental and behavioral risks. Thus, in contrast to infectious diseases, the causal agents are complex and multifactorial (Diez-Roux, 1998; Krieger, 1994). Many of the sociocultural factors influencing the development, increased incidence, and persistence of chronic diseases are tied to macro-level factors such as poverty, race, social status, education, and income. These factors make chronic diseases especially pertinent globally because of their wide variation throughout the world.

Injury comes from the Latin *in-juris*, which literally means "not right." Injury, or trauma, is defined as physical damage to the body caused by rapid transfer of mechanical, electrical, chemical, thermal, or radiation energy, or as a lack of essentials, such as oxygen in the case of drowning and heat in the case of frostbite (Sleet & Rosenberg, 1997). Chronic exposures to energy over long periods of time can also cause many disabilities and some diseases (for example, skin cancer and repetitive stress syndrome), but the acute nature of rapid transfer of energy beyond human tissue threshold is what distinguishes injury from other maladies. Injury prevention is the study, identification, and implementation of strategies to prevent, reduce, or eliminate the transfer of energy to the human body or to ensure the supply of such essentials as heat or oxygen to the body to maintain normal functioning (Forjuoh, 1996).

Injuries are typically classified according to whether they are intentional or unintentional. *Intentional* injuries, or violence, include those that result from homicide, interpersonal violence, war, collective violence, suicide, attempted suicide, and self-harm. *Unintentional* injuries are those previously considered "accidents" and include poisonings, fires, burns and scalds, drowning, suffocation, falls, sports injuries, and motor-vehicle and transportation-related injuries.

## MAJOR SOCIAL, ECONOMIC, AND DEMOGRAPHIC TRENDS

During the past century, in general, urban areas grew and rural areas declined. However, in the past half century, urbanization leveled off in the industrialized countries at around 75% urban; the less industrialized countries are becoming more urban, but in the lowest-income countries less than 50% of the population still resides in urban areas. The long-term effects of this rural-to-urban settlement pattern on chronic diseases and injury are mixed, though one can speculate that chronic diseases are likely to become a greater burden for urban areas.

As the incidence and prevalence of infectious diseases in low- and middle-income countries declines, the effects of other health problems, such as trauma, increase. Globally, injuries take

an enormous toll on children, adolescents, and young adults. Ranking fifth among the leading causes of death, unintentional injuries account for 5.2% of the total mortality and are responsible for 10–30% of all hospital admissions (Jacobs & Cutting, 1986; Mackay, 1993; Taket, 1986). In low- and middle-income countries, injuries are often viewed as the inevitable consequences of technology and economic development (Stansfield, Smith, & McGreevey, 1993). Nevertheless, the reverse is also true. Without advanced technology and economic growth, injury risks continue to pose significant hazards to the population. WHO has recognized this problem and adopted a "Manifesto for Safe Communities" that emphasizes the rights and responsibilities to provide safety and equity for all (WHO, 1993).

Although relevant information on all the social, economic, and demographic trends in all the low- and middle-income countries could not be covered systematically here, many current resources provide details on specific countries. WHO's Internet site provides relatively up-to-date information on trends in socioeconomic development and health status, health and environment, health resources, and health services (WHO, 1999). It also provides links to other sources, including WHO regional offices, the World Bank, the United Nations, and the United Nations Educational, Scientific and Cultural Organization (UNESCO). The World Bank website is useful for making economic comparisons and for pursuing the changing role of poverty in the world (www.worldbank.org), and the U.S. Census Bureau maintains a website (www.census.com) that monitors global population trends and provides summary data on the world's 227 countries. The accuracy and consistency of these websites are highly varied, but they provide comparative data of relevance to chronic diseases.

At the close of the twentieth century there were 10 countries with populations greater than 100 million: China, India, Indonesia, the United States, Brazil, Japan, Pakistan, Bangladesh, the Russian Federation, and Nigeria. This number will undoubtedly increase in the twenty-first century. Mexico is nearing the 100 million mark. It is notable that most of these are low- or middle-income countries, and this will continue to be the case. China, India, and the United States are predicted to remain the three most populated countries on the globe through 2050, the three constituting a cumulative population of around 3.5 billion. It is notable that the least industrialized of these countries, India, will have the largest population at around 1.7 billion, followed by China with 1.3 billion, and the United States with around 400 million. Of the 18 countries estimated to have more than 100 million persons in 1050, only Japan and the United States will have highly developed economies, and it is notable that the United States and Canada are among the few highly industrialized economies predicted to have an increase in population during the next 50 years. Economically, few countries are getting rich before they are getting older. This forecast suggests profound consequences for health care costs and other resources required for managing chronic diseases in aging populations.

## Aging

In the year 2000 more than half the population of older adults—that is, persons aged 65 years or older—lived in low- and middle-income countries; by 2025 this will increase to nearly 70%. The proportion of the world population over 65 years of age will continue to grow throughout the next decades. In all level-income nations the traditional population "pyramid" familiar to demographers in the past will be replaced by a population "rectangle." The U.S. Census Bureau website (www.census.gov) displays traditional population pyramids to demonstrate the dramatic changes in population aging for different countries and to show projected or future changes in population. These displays illustrate clearly the disappearance of the pyramidal population structure of most countries and the emergence of a rectangular population structure with older populations.

If present trends continue, the proportion of the oldest old—that is, those 80 years or older—will also increase dramatically.

This drastic population transition will have many notable effects. Its economic impact will be pronounced and exacerbated by declining labor force participation rates in most low- and middle-income countries. In seemingly direct contradiction to the increase in life span has been a lowering of the retirement age. These factors have placed heavy burdens on old-age economic security programs, and the effect on health care expenditures will also be great. The World Bank estimates that by 2050 in most industrialized countries pension and health care costs will consume one-quarter of public funding. Many low- and middle-income countries will soon have a similar age structure and thus face the impact of increased incidence of chronic diseases. The challenge for political leaders will be to develop and implement appropriate health care programs for older adults in these nations.

One significant consequence of this changing demographic pattern is the concurrent rise of illnesses with long-term morbidity, particularly among populations in low-income countries. Historically, epidemiologists and health demographers were concerned with mortality rates because death was the chief outcome of the diseases afflicting the population and often occurred rapidly. With chronic diseases, the disease process and all its ramifications becomes much more relevant. Most of the chronic diseases with high mortality, such as CVD, cancer, and chronic obstructive pulmonary disease (COPD), are accompanied by long periods of decline; many chronic diseases and injuries also have long periods of disability. One may expect that in many low-income countries persons with these conditions may simply receive little or no medical attention.

## Chronic Diseases as a Consequence of Personal Behaviors

Considerable research in the second half of the twentieth century has shown that personal behaviors, or lifestyles, are highly associated with chronic disease morbidity and mortality (Belloc, 1973; Berkman & Breslow, 1983). Much of this research has emphasized four principal lifestyle behaviors: tobacco use, eating behaviors, physical activity, and alcohol consumption. More recently, sexual behavior has been added to the lifestyle list. The relationship of these lifestyle behaviors and aging is significant because the behaviors that tend to be associated with many chronic diseases occur over a long period of time before the chronic condition becomes evident. Although the literature on lifestyle and health is extensive, most is based on research carried out in North America and Europe. Many of the observed relationships between behavior and illness, however, may also be found among populations in low- and middle-income countries. This assertion can already be observed in these countries with regard to sexual behavior and the spread of human immunodeficiency virus (HIV).

Although lifestyle has been a central concept in the behavioral risk factor approach to health and illness, many regard the concept as only one component among the sociocultural or sociostructural factors related to health and illness. Additional variables are now considered to be critical in defining the etiology of chronic diseases. These include social class, culture, social networks, education, occupation, income, race, and gender. The literature supporting the causal relationships between these variables and chronic diseases is vast and beyond the scope of this chapter. It is also largely the product of research institutions in industrialized countries.

## EPIDEMIOLOGY OF CHRONIC DISEASES AND INJURY

### Cardiovascular Disease

Cardiovascular disease refers to a number of diverse heart and blood vessel diseases. In the industrialized world CVD has long been the leading cause of death and disability. At the end of the millennium, CVDs accounted for about 20% percent of all deaths globally. They are emerging causes of death and disability among persons in the low-income countries and are already the leading causes of death in many middle-income countries. It is expected that the most populated countries will eventually cite CVD as the major cause of death and disability.

The pattern of CVD mortality is diverse; even within individual countries CVD mortality and morbidity vary considerably by age, race, and gender. For example, in the United States the age-adjusted mortality rate in 1995 was 55% higher for men than women and was considerably less for White men and women than for Black men and women. Ethnic variation is also considerable, with Asian and Hispanic Americans displaying considerable variation from the European-derived White population. The reason for this observed variability within a single country is undoubtedly a complex combination of risk factors, genetics, and cultural and socioenvironmental differences. It is notable that the United States is in the middle of the industrialized nations, ranking 16th among 35 countries in CVD mortality rates, although the country has experienced a fairly steady decline in mortality during the last 2 decades of the past century. The U.S. experience illustrates the complex issues involved in making any simple generalizations about country comparisons at the global level; that is, there is often as much variation within a large country as one observes between countries. A recent report by the Institute of Medicine summarized the burden of CVD globally:

> Although is it not surprising that cardiovascular disease (CVD) is the leading cause of death worldwide because of its predominance in developed countries, it is surprising that CVD ranked second as a cause of death in all developing countries in 1990, with its burden almost equal to that of the leading cause–lower respiratory infections. . . . In fact, given the falling rates of infectious and

parasitic diseases and the increasing rates of CVD in developing countries, CVD was most likely the developing world's leading cause of death by the mid-1990s. If ignored, this epidemic will increase drastically in the coming years. Not only is CVD the largest cause of mortality in older age groups and in men, it is also a very significant contributor to mortality in persons of economically productive ages (i.e., 30–69 years) and in women. ... Evidence shows that in 1990, CVD contributed to three times as many deaths worldwide in 30- to 69-year-old men and women as did infectious and parasitic diseases. This is true for all regions of the world except Sub-Saharan Africa. In this region, the numbers of deaths from CVD and infectious or parasitic diseases were about equal in 1990, and it is possible that CVD will soon dominate mortality in this region as well. This burden of disease and death in the economically most productive age stratum has important consequences for health care resources and for the economy in general. . . . (Howson, Reddy, Ryan, & Bale, 1998, p. 77)

### Coronary Heart Disease

Of the many CVD conditions, coronary heart disease (CHD) has been the most widely studied. Essentially, CHD refers to atherosclerosis of the arteries that supply blood to the muscles of the heart. A coronary event or heart attack refers to the occlusion of the blood supply to the heart muscles resulting in an abrupt inadequacy of blood supply (ischemia). CHD is the leading cause of CVD-related mortality and morbidity in the industrialized countries. It is also likely to become the leading cause of death in low- and middle-income economies. CHD mortality varied greatly over the past century. This variation is particularly notable in the United States,

where the mortality rate began at about 200 deaths per 100,000 persons at the beginning of the century, peaked in the 1950s at about 300 deaths per 100,000, and then declined toward the end of the century to about the same level as at the beginning of the century. The explanations for this "epidemic" are diverse and beyond the scope of this chapter, except to note the phenomenon in an advanced, industrialized country as it passed through a long period from early industrialization to postindustrialism. Exhibit 6–1 emphasizes some of the chief concerns for low- and middle-income countries.

The largest, ongoing study of CHD is the WHO MONICA project (Tunstall-Pedoe, Kuulasmaa, Mahonen, Tolonen, & Ruokokoski, 1999). This project was designed to examine the epidemiologic characteristics of CHD in 21 countries over the last 2 decades of the twentieth century. Most of the studied countries were in Europe, but Australia, China, New Zealand, and the United States were also included. The data collected from this project represent the most comprehensive international profile of CHD to date. What has emerged is a diverse relationship between economic levels of countries and CHD mortality and variations of CHD mortality among countries with similar levels of economic development.

The global implications of the CHD data raise more questions than answers. The principal question is whether the low- and middle-income countries and regions of the world are destined to follow the same epidemic pattern that characterized Europe and North America. The difficulty in making any firm prediction or giving a firm answer to this question is that relatively little is understood about the reasons for the decline in CHD mortality. Nonetheless, that component of CHD morbidity and mortality that is attributable to known risk factors, particularly behavioral risk factors, is better understood. However, without systematic surveillance of such factors in low- and middle-income countries, there may not be sufficient information to understand fully the epidemic when and if it develops.

**Exhibit 6–1** Special Case: Controlling Cardiovascular Disease in Low- and Middle-Income Countries

The United States Institute of Medicine (IOM) recently issued a definitive report on the control of CVD in developing countries (Howson et al., 1998). In general, this report was fairly optimistic. IOM supported the view that with proper attention to risk factor reduction and relatively low cost management of known diseases that the developing countries could reduce CVD-related morbidity and mortality. Unfortunately, the dominant view among many developing countries is that all available health resources should be used to control communicable disease and that until these diseases are eliminated efforts in public health should not be diluted by attention to the major chronic diseases.

The IOM laid out major criteria for investing in CVD research in low- and middle-income countries. First, it recognized a need for improved vital statistics for CVD and pointed out the dearth of in-formation in several large countries. For example, India, which contributes 17% of global deaths for CVD, has no comprehensive registration of deaths. Serious deficits in vital registration exist for most of Africa and the Middle East. Second, the IOM report asserted a need for systematic surveys of behavioral risk factors for CVD. Third, it pointed out that little information exists on the therapeutic effects of different drugs and inter-ventions among different ethnic communities in low-income countries. Finally, the IOM stated that implementing tobacco-control programs and tobacco policies is clearly needed to develop a coherent plan of research and prevention devel-opment in low- and middle-income countries. Clearly, a need exists to begin building a com-prehensive public health infrastructure that will respond to the obviously rising problem of CVD in low- and middle-income countries.

### Stroke

The second predominant form of vascular dis-ease is stroke. Stroke is a syndrome character-ized by the loss of either cognitive or physical functioning caused by damage to blood vessels that supply nutrients and oxygen to the brain. Usually the loss of function is focused, such as the paralysis of a portion of the body; coma and death may result if large sections of the brain are involved. Damage to the brain can result either from leakage of blood directly into brain tissue (hemorrhagic) or from occlusion of a vessel (ischemic). Hemorrhage usually results from a combination of elevated blood pressure and blood vessel disease. Ischemic strokes are usually the result of dislodged fragments from friable plaques of atherosclerosis that line large vessels such as the carotid artery. These frag-ments, called emboli, can also originate from clots in the chambers of the heart. Emboli course through the bloodstream and can become lodged in smaller vessels supplying the brain. Occasion-ally they are large enough to serve as loci of enlarging clots that occlude vessels.

If a person survives the initial effects of a stroke, much functional capacity can often be restored with intensive rehabilitation efforts, particularly in younger patients. In industrial-ized countries stroke is the third most common cause of death and the leading cause of dis-ability among people living in their own homes (Poungvarin, 1998). Because of this large burden, epidemiologists in Europe and the United States have studied stroke extensively. There is little variability in the incidence of stroke across Western countries (including Europe and the United States) except for France, where rates of all vascular-related diseases are unexpect-edly low (Sudlow & Warlow, 1997). Rates of stroke, particularly hemorrhagic events, are high in Japan. Major risk factors for stroke have been identified, with increasing age and hypertension playing a major role (Exhibit 6–2). Large cam-paigns to identify and treat high blood pressure, such as the National High Blood Pressure Edu-cation Program in the United States, have been credited with contributing a large part to the 60% reduction in the death rate from this disease since the 1960s. A similar trend of decreasing

**Exhibit 6–2** Well-Documented Risk Factors for Stroke

**Modifiable**
- Hypertension
- Heart disease
  - atrial fibrillation
  - infective endocarditis
  - mitral stenosis
  - recent large myocardial infarction
- Cigarette smoking
- Sickle-cell disease
- Previous transient ischemic attacks (ministrokes)
- Asymptomatic carotid disease
- Excessive alcohol consumption (mostly hemorrhagic)

**Potentially Modifiable**
- Diabetes mellitus
- Left-ventricular hypertrophy

**Nonmodifiable**
- Age
- Sex
- Hereditary/familial factors

rates has been observed in most industrialized countries (NIH, 1997).

Because populations in low- and middle-income countries have traditionally been younger and because stroke tends to be a condition affecting older adults, epidemiologists have not studied this disease so intensely in these countries. Therefore, information on the incidence, prevalence, and mortality of stroke in these countries is limited. However, as life expectancies in these countries increase, it is anticipated that stroke will become a larger contributor to morbidity and mortality. The few studies that exist in low- and middle-income countries reveal that the risk factors for stroke are similar to those in industrialized countries (Poungvarin, 1998). The available data suggest that the rates of stroke are higher in Asian countries such as Taiwan and Korea (Poungvarin, 1998). Because hypertension is less likely to be treated in low- and middle-income countries, researchers have found

that the type of vascular disease in these countries is slightly different from that observed in industrialized countries. Also, the mechanism of brain damage is more likely to involve the spontaneous rupture and bleeding of small vessels deep in the brain rather than occlusion of large- and medium-sized arteries.

Besides the slightly greater preponderance of hemorrhagic versus ischemic stroke in low- and middle-income countries, infectious causes of vascular disease, such as tuberculosis, syphilis, and parasitic diseases (for example, schistosomiasis), are more common causes of stroke. Other than the prevention and treatment of these infectious causes of stroke, the principles for preventing stroke in low- and middle-income countries are similar to those in industrialized countries. Mild elevations in blood pressure can be ameliorated by reducing salt intake, limiting alcohol consumption, and engaging in physical activity; higher elevations generally require medical therapy.

Information about the diagnosis and treatment as well as the natural history of stroke in low- and middle-income countries is sparse. Optimal care includes the use of expensive diagnostic technologies such as computerized tomography scanning of the brain as well as complex medications that inhibit blood clots for patients with ischemic strokes. Rehabilitation is best coordinated by specialized teams. Other than rudimentary neurosurgical techniques designed to remove large blood clots within and around the brain that can result from hemorrhagic strokes, resources for stroke care are generally unavailable to the largely rural populations living in low- and middle-income countries.

## Cancer

Any overview of the public health dimensions of cancer must emphasize two major issues. First, cancers are usually classified according to the organ where the abnormal cellular growth begins and by the specific type of tissue that becomes malignant within the organ. Thus, cancer cannot be considered a single disease; rather, it is a collection of more than 100 separate conditions. What these conditions have in common is the proliferation of disorganized cells that invade adjacent structures of the body and spread through the blood and lymphatic system to distant organs. These afflictions frequently have different causes, clinical manifestations, natural histories, and treatments. Given this complex nosology, any presentation must consider at least a few of the major types of cancer.

The second issue that must be considered when describing the global burden of cancer is that the diagnosing and the recording, reporting, and collating of data necessary to maintain a reliable cancer registration system are technically complex and enormously expensive. Thus the information on the incidence of cancer in low- and middle-income countries is sparse. Where information is available, the data must be interpreted with great caution because rates frequently vary due to incomplete registration, a paucity of trained medical providers, or inadequate reporting and registration procedures.

The agency within WHO responsible for coordinating international public health efforts in cancer research, surveillance, prevention, and treatment is the International Agency for Research on Cancer (IARC), located in Lyons, France. This agency produces numerous publications on cancer, including a detailed compilation of cancer incidence data from high-quality registries (Parkin, Whelan, Ferlay, Raymond, & Young, 1992). The data compiled by this agency served as the basis for global estimates of cancer provided in the GBD study. Although most of the data presented in this chapter are derived from the GBD estimates, the authors suggest that the reader refer to the IARC publications for primary data and information on the details of international cancer epidemiology.

Major differences in the relative importance of specific cancers currently exist between industrialized and low- and middle-income countries (Figure 6–2). In the industrialized world, cancers of the lung, breast, colon, and prostate are the most frequent types. In low- and middle-income countries, malignancies are most common in the mouth and oropharynx, stomach, and liver. Although lung cancer is relatively less common in low- and middle-income countries, it is a growing source of morbidity and mortality as tobacco use becomes more prevalent (Peto, 1997; Peto et al., 1992). Gross comparisons such as the relative frequency of cancers by anatomical site can mask immense variation in cancer rates. For example, there is an almost 50-fold difference in the incidence of liver cancer between Thailand and the state of Iowa in the United States. For many cancers with such profoundly large variations in rates, the causes and interventions are well understood. However, interventions are frequently difficult to implement because of their cost or because of social and economic factors. For example, the major causes of liver cancer in the world are infections with viruses and parasites that invoke a chronic inflammatory process. This inflammation leads to malignant transformation of liver cells in a certain proportion of infected individuals. Because these infections are much more prevalent in low- and middle-income countries, such as those in Southeast Asia, liver cancer is more frequent there. An effective vaccination is available to prevent mother-to-child transmission of the virus—hepatitis B—that is recognized as a major cause of this disease. These immunizations, however, are relatively expensive for low- and middle-income countries to distribute and administer (see Chapter 4).

Tobacco use—the major cause of lung cancer—is the most important example of a carcinogen that is difficult to control because of social and economic factors. Tobacco products are a great source of revenue for businesses at the level of their production (farmers and producers) and distribution (retail stores). They are also a major source of tax revenue for many governments (Taylor, 1984). In a country like Thailand, where the production of tobacco has been a government-owned monopoly, there are obvious disincentives for the government to control the spread of this lethal habit.

Although researchers have elucidated the chain of causality for some relatively common

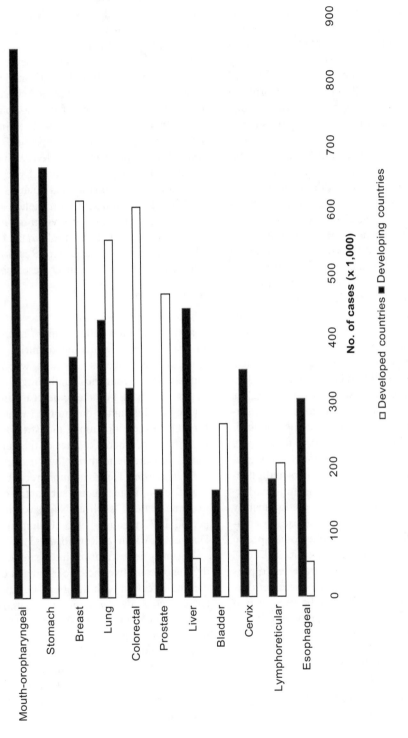

**Figure 6–2** Ten Most Common Cancers in Developed and Developing Countries (in thousands)

cancers, others with wide geographic variations in incidence, such as breast cancer, are frequently attributed to general, but incompletely characterized lifestyle factors such as diet. The major risk factors and preventive measures available for each of the major cancers will be briefly reviewed here. A common theme for all malignancies associated with significant morbidity in low- and middle-income countries is that state-of-the-art medical treatments with surgery or chemotherapeutic medicines are not widely available. Therefore, the concentration is on prevention rather than treatment. Even in an industrialized country such as the United States, where enormous resources are devoted to treating cancer, prevention efforts have proven the most successful means of decreasing mortality from this disease over the course of the twentieth century (Bailar & Gornick, 1997). A recent publication produced by IARC compared the survival patterns in high- and low-income countries for some of the most common and preventable cancers, such as those of the mouth, stomach, liver, and lung. The report demonstrated uniformly poor outcomes in all registries studied, including those in high-income countries (Sankaranarayanan, Black, Swaminathan, & Parkin, 1998). Differences in the average length of survival between high- and low-income countries were greatest for those sites where multimodal therapy (that is, radiation, surgery, and chemotherapy) is most effective. Such malignancies include subtypes of testicular tumors, leukemia, and lymphoma that occur predominantly among younger persons. Using these observations, WHO has classified chemotherapeutic agents for these cancers as "essential drugs." WHO has also recommended strategies to provide these treatments in low-resource settings (WHO, 1994). However, it must be remembered that for the most part treatable subtypes of these tumors are relatively rare.

### Mouth and Oropharyngeal Cancer

This category denotes a heterogeneous group of tumors, including cancer of the lip, tongue, oral cavity, nose, and pharynx. Heavy use of alcohol and tobacco (smoked and chewed) are the major risk factors for these tumors. Thus these cancers tend to be much more common among men than women. An exception to this gender inequality exists in India where a nut called betel quid is commonly chewed by men and women and is strongly associated with oral cancer. In China and a few other Asian countries the incidence of cancer of the nasopharynx is high. Dietary practices, such as eating salted fish, and infection with the Epstein-Barr virus (etiologic agent of mononucleosis) have been implicated as major risk factors. Synergistic interactions of noxious agents such as alcohol, betel quid, and tobacco with dietary deficiencies of trace elements and vitamins have also been proposed as playing a role in the causation of these tumors (World Cancer Research Fund/American Institute for Cancer Research, 1997).

### Stomach Cancer

Cancer of the stomach is one of the most common and most lethal tumors in the world. In low- and middle-income countries, the incidence of this cancer is very high, whereas most industrialized countries, including the United States, observed a dramatic decrease in the frequency of this tumor during the twentieth century. One exception among industrialized countries is Japan, where the rates of this tumor tend to be comparable to many low- and middle-income countries. However, more recent trends in incidence in Japan indicate substantial decreases in some regions, such as Nagasaki during the period 1973 through 1985 (Coleman, Esteve, Damiecki, Arslan, & Renard, 1993).

Recently investigators have suggested that the major causative factor of stomach cancer is chronic infection with the gram–negative spiral bacteria *Helicobacter pylori*. This pathogen also causes peptic ulcer disease and atrophic inflammation in the stomach. Infection is more common among persons from lower socioeconomic strata and among children in low- and middle-income countries where infection appears to be endemic (Vaira et al., 1998). The routes of transmission of *Helicobacter pylori* have not been clearly elucidated. Because most persons who become infected do not develop cancer, investigators believe that certain cofactors, such as genetic susceptibility and dietary intake of fruits, vegetables, and trace elements such as selenium, may modify the influence of the oncogenic effects of this bacterial infection.

### Breast Cancer

In industrialized countries early detection with screening mammograms and the use of pharmaceutical agents such as tamoxifen that modify the proliferative influence of estrogen on breast tissue are interventions frequently promoted to prevent breast cancer mortality. These complex and expensive technologies are used because the established risk factors of family history, early menarche, late menopause, late age at first pregnancy, and nulliparity are essentially nonmodifiable. There is a fivefold difference in the risk of breast cancer between the high rates observed in North America and western Europe as compared to Asia. Although Japan is a highly industrialized country, breast cancer rates among Japanese women are very low (Coleman et al., 1993).

Epidemiologists have found that the incidence of breast cancer among White European, Asian, and Latin American immigrant women residing in the United States increases to the risk observed among U.S.-born White women as long as they reside in the United States. Among non-Whites, particularly Asians, the rates increase modestly with increasing duration of residence, but the incidence remains much lower than that of native-born inhabitants (Thomas & Karagas, 1996). These findings, coupled with the vast international differences in the rates of this disease, suggest a strong environmental influence on the risk of breast cancer. These observations have prompted many investigators to invoke diet, especially consumption of saturated fats, and obesity as risk factors for breast cancer (Rose, Boyar, & Wynder, 1986). Though plausible in light of the international comparisons, analytic investigations such as case-control and cohort studies within industrialized and low-income countries have not provided a clear link between dietary factors and breast cancer incidence (Willett, 1998). Some investigations support a protective effect for vigorous physical activity, but, just as with the connection to dietary factors, the findings from various studies are inconsistent (Latikka, Pukkala, & Vihko, 1998).

### Lung Cancer

Lung cancer is a rare disease in populations where there is an absence of tobacco use. An increase in smoking tobacco, particularly in the form of cigarettes, is inevitably accompanied by an epidemic of lung cancer (Peto, Chen, & Boreham, 1999). The consistent and strong link between the population prevalence of smoking and lung cancer death rates has enabled epidemiologists to estimate accurately the population-level exposure to this risk factor using lung cancer mortality as a surrogate measure (Peto et al., 1992). There are few other risk factors in chronic disease epidemiology that have been so consistently and strongly linked to a specific disease.

Scientists have documented other environmental exposures as strong risk factors for lung cancer, including inhaled arsenic, asbestos, chloromethyl ethers, polycyclic hydrocarbons, chromium, nickel, and radiation (Blot & Fraumeni, 1996). Exposures to these are important, primarily in the occupational setting (see Chapter 8). The potential contribution of radon, a radioactive but chemically inert gas that arises from natural subterranean deposits, has recently been highlighted in the United States (Centers for Disease Control and Prevention, 1989). The risk of lung cancer associated with radon was first documented in uranium miners (Samet, Kutvirt, Waxweiler, & Key, 1984). Subsequently, the discovery that household levels are elevated in focal areas of the United States has raised concerns about radon as a potentially significant public health problem. Because the accumulation of radon in any home requires high-quality, energy-efficient building practices that "seal in" the household air, it is unlikely that this is a widespread contributor to lung cancer risk in low- and middle-income countries where energy-efficient construction is not common.

In specific regions of China the domiciliary use of inadequately ventilated open coal pits to heat homes has been convincingly associated with an increased risk of lung cancer (Lan, Chen, Chen, & He, 1993; see Chapter 8). In recent studies in China, however, investigators found that tobacco is the preeminent cause of lung cancer mortality in that country (Liu et al., 1998).

### Colorectal Cancer

Cancers of the colon and rectum have similar epidemiologic characteristics and are primarily diseases of industrialized countries. These cancers generally affect both sexes equally. Screening techniques using chemical tests to detect occult blood in the stool and endoscopic inspection have been found to be highly effective in preventing mortality from these diseases (Frame & Atkins, 1996). However, the expense of these technologies would not appear to make them cost-effective interventions in low- and middle-income countries with low-incidence rates. Studies on immigrant populations and analytic epidemiologic investigations strongly suggest that diets rich in fruits and vegetables and increased physical activity are protective mediators of risk (Haenszel & Kurihara, 1968). The precise constituents of plant food that protect against colorectal malignancies have not been definitively determined. One of the most popular theories is that indigestible vegetable fiber promotes retention of water within the lumen of the colon and decreases the transit time of stool through the alimentary canal. This decrease in transit time could theoretically dilute carcinogens and decrease the exposure of the colonic mucosa to cancer-causing agents (Howe et al., 1992), but this theory is still disputed. Despite international comparisons and case-control studies supporting this theory, prospective cohort studies have not shown a consistent link between dietary fiber and the risk of colorectal cancer (Fuchs et al., 1999).

### Prostate Cancer

Prostate cancer is a disease that occurs predominantly in men aged 70 years and older in affluent countries. The etiology of this disease is poorly understood, and family history is the only consistently identified risk factor. Screening techniques to prevent mortality using digital rectal exams and a blood test called prostate specific antigen (PSA) have not been shown to be effective or cost-effective. Other than in the United States, these technologies are rarely used. The incidence and prevalence of prostate cancer will inevitably increase as the populations of low- and middle-income countries age, but effective interventions to prevent this cancer will require further basic science and epidemiologic research.

### Liver Cancer

The importance of infectious agents as causative agents for liver cancer is undeniable. In a recent comprehensive review, IARC concluded that 81% of the worldwide incidence of liver cancer is attributable to hepatitis B and C viruses and to parasites such as schistosomes and liver flukes (Pisani, Parkin, Munoz, & Ferlay, 1997). Hepatitis B is particularly important, and the prevalence of this infection in any population is a strong predictor of mortality from liver cancer (Beasley & Hwang, 1991). Worldwide, hepatitis B is generally transmitted through sexual intercourse or from mother to newborn during the perinatal period. Hepatitis C is also transmitted parenterally, but sexual intercourse and the birth process appear to be less common modes of transmission for this virus. People in low-income countries may become infected with schistosomes and liver flukes by bathing in and drinking water infested with these parasites.

A vaccination against hepatitis B has been effective in curtailing the incidence of liver cancer. In 1984 in Taiwan a mass vaccination against hepatitis B was launched. The average annual incidence of hepatocellular carcinoma (the major form of liver cancer) among children aged 6 to 14 years decreased by 37% between 1981 and 1986 and between 1986 and 1990. During this same period rates among younger children declined by more than 50% (Chang, Chen, & Lai, 1997). WHO has launched a similar vaccination program in Gambia, Africa, with plans to follow the long-term rates of liver cancer in this country among the vaccinated population (Fortuin, Chotard, & Jack, 1993).

In low-incidence countries, such as the United States, cirrhosis induced by heavy alcohol consumption plays a more prominent role in the genesis of liver cancer. In low- and middle-income countries, naturally occurring environmental chemicals probably also mediate the carcinogenic effects of chronic infections as well as promote the development of liver cancer in their own right. One such group of substances that have been studied extensively are the aflatoxins. These compounds are produced by fungi that grow on foods such as peanuts, corn, and cassava. Though well documented as hepatic carcinogens in animal studies, epidemiologic data in humans are less consistent. The variability in these studies arises from difficulties in measuring the long-term exposure to these chemicals over a lifetime as well as genetic variability in the ability of individuals to metabolize aflatoxins. However, strong laboratory evidence suggests that these compounds, as well as other naturally occurring carcinogens, play some role as a cause of liver cancer (Stuver, 1998).

Besides naturally occurring carcinogens, environmental epidemiologists have also identified a variety of industrially produced chemicals, such as vinyl chloride, as hepatic carcinogens. Exposure to many of these chemicals occurs in occupational settings. In the industrialized world occupational regulations have reduced worker's exposure to many of the known hepatic carcinogens and lowered their cancer risk. In low- and middle-income countries, however, occupational regulations are less frequently legislated or enforced. Thus work-related liver cancer will become more important in emerging market economies unless occupational health protections are promoted and implemented (see Chapter 8).

## Bladder Cancer

Bladder cancer is much more common in men than women in most countries. No single etiologic agent has been identified that explains the occurrence of a majority of cases. However, infection with urinary schistosomes appears to be the most important preventable cause in low-income countries where the parasite exists, whereas occupational exposure to arylamine chemicals and cigarette smoking have been most strongly associated with this disease in industrialized countries (Pisani et al., 1997; Ross, Jones, & Yu, 1996). Though not as strongly associated with bladder cancer as are occupational carcinogens, tobacco-related tumors are more common because there is much more exposure to tobacco smoke in industrialized as well as low- and middle-income countries.

## Uterine Cervix Cancer

Uterine cervical cancer is one of the 10 most common cancers in the world (Figure 6–2), and second only to breast cancer in incidence among women. In many low- and middle-income countries, especially in Latin America, this is the most frequent malignancy diagnosed in women. In industrialized countries, cervical cancer incidence and mortality have declined because of the widespread use of cytologic sampling of the cervix using a laboratory evaluation procedure known as the Pap smear (Coleman et al., 1993; Koss, 1989). Through the detection and ablative treatment of precancerous lesions, frank malignancy can be prevented. However, this screening technique is technically difficult and too expensive to implement in most low-and middle-income countries. WHO has tentatively promoted the use of direct visual inspection of the cervix with ablative treatment of suspicious lesions (WHO, 1994). Unfortunately, systematic studies of this approach suggest that it is not very specific and results in unnecessary medical expenditures and discomfort due to overtreatment of nonneoplastic lesions (Kitchener & Symonds, 1999).

Promising laboratory and public health re-search now focuses on developing an effective vaccine against the human papilloma virus (HPV) (Murakami, Gurski, & Steller, 1999). This pathogen has more than 100 separate, anti-genically distinct strains. Transmission occurs through direct person-to-person contact and usu-ally results in transient warts on the hands, feet, or genitalia. Each of the strains is specific for anatomical sites where the warts proliferate, and the most common types associated with genital warts are types 8 and 11. Researchers have definitively identified several other types, most importantly 16 and 18, as major causative agents for cervical cancer (Franco, Rohan, & Villa, 1999). Initially, infection with the onco-genic forms of HPV usually produce flat warts on the cervix that frequently remain unnoticed by the affected women. Most studies suggest that type 16 is responsible for approximately half of the cervical cancer occurring worldwide. If a vaccine is developed against the major can-cer-related strains of HPV, mass vaccination programs to prevent cervical cancer may be im-plemented and thus replicate the programs de-veloped to prevent liver cancer.

### Lymphoreticular Cancers

This group of malignancies includes leuke-mia, lymphomas, and multiple myeloma. There are few public health measures currently avail-able to prevent these cancers, as the etiology for most have not been identified. Two prominent exceptions are Burkitt's lymphoma and adult T cell leukemia/lymphoma. Burkitt's lymphoma is a non-Hodgkin's type of malignancy of the lymph gland that is histologically distinct. It is the most common form of childhood lymphoma in much of Africa. This lymphoma has been epidemiologically linked to Epstein-Barr virus infection at a young age. Because this cancer is most common in countries where malaria is holoendemic, it is thought to arise from the in-teraction between this protozoan infection and proliferating lymphocytes induced by early in-fection with the Epstein-Barr virus (Mueller,

Evans, & London, 1996). Treatment with the chemotherapeutic agent methotrexate of the form of this tumor found in low-income coun-tries is highly effective.

### Esophageal Cancer

In the industrialized world most cases of esophageal cancer are attributable to heavy use of alcohol and tobacco, and the incidence of this cancer is two to three times higher among men than women. However, the highest rates are ob-served in specific regions of eastern China and central Asia, an observation made even before the widespread dissemination of tobacco prod-ucts. It is estimated that half the incident cases of esophageal cancer in the world occur in China. In this country the ratio of rates between men and women is closer to one as compared to that observed in industrialized countries. Numerous hypotheses have been proposed to explain these geographic variations in the incidence of this disease, but no definitive explanation has been found. Esophageal cancer is a disabling and uni-formly lethal disease even in countries where advanced medical therapy is available. The aver-age estimated survival time after diagnosis is generally less than 2 years worldwide (Murray & Lopez, 1996b).

### Cancer Prevention

Using information developed in the GBD, WHO has developed a "Cancer Priority Ladder" (Exhibit 6–3) to guide individual countries toward implementing the most feasible and po-tentially effective cancer prevention programs given their economic resources, epidemiologic situation, and technical capacity. Prevention strategies, including discouraging tobacco use and controlling infectious diseases associated with specific cancers, are the cornerstones for preventing cancer even in the lowest-income countries. Ironically, just as infectious diseases seem to be receding, tobacco use is on the rise, and the cancers and chronic diseases associated with its use are increasing (Peto et al., 1999). It is also of note that infection control measures

**Exhibit 6–3** World Health Organization Ladder of Cancer Control Priorities, from Highest to Lowest

- Tobacco control
- Infection control, for example, hepatitis B, *H. pylori*, schistosomiasis
- Cancer treatment
- Effective pain control
- Sample cancer registries
- Healthy eating programs (low-fat, emphasize fruits and vegetables)
- Treatment and referral guideline development
- Nurse education programs
- National cancer networks
- Specialized clinical evaluation units and cancer centers
- Clinical research
- Basic research
- International aid program

that will prevent mortality directly attributable to infection may also indirectly mitigate the future burden of cancer.

## Other Leading Chronic Diseases of International Importance

Although the chronic diseases that cause the greatest mortality and morbidity are maladies of the cardiovascular and cerebrovascular systems and cancer, there are other chronic diseases of importance. Diabetes, while an enormously prevalent and strong risk factor for cardiovascular diseases, is a major direct source of disability throughout the world. Other chronic conditions that are also growing sources of morbidity and mortality in low- and middle-income countries include COPD, musculoskeletal conditions, and neuropsychiatric conditions such as blindness, depression, and dementia.

### Diabetes

Diabetes is a metabolic disorder. The hallmark finding is an elevated glucose level in the blood, and the disease is commonly attributed to a deficiency in the amount of insulin secreted by the pancreas. Diabetes has two distinct types of pathogenesis. The first, usually called type 1, is also known as insulin-dependent diabetes mellitus (IDDM) or juvenile-onset diabetes mellitus; it is characterized by immune destruction of the cells of the pancreas that secrete insulin. Type 2 diabetes, noninsulin-dependent diabetes mellitus (NIDDM) or adult-onset diabetes mellitus, is characterized by a high level of serum glucose and elevated levels of insulin. This paradoxical situation exists because of cellular resistance to the actions of insulin.

Diabetes can result in weight loss, metabolic acidosis, and, if left untreated, death. With insulin therapy, persons with type 1 diabetes can avoid the major metabolic complications of their disease but must learn to manage the chronically elevated glucose levels (called hyperglycemia) that often cause damage to microscopic blood vessels in the eyes and kidneys as well as decrements in the function of peripheral nerves. These sequelae lead to the major complications of diabetes, including blindness, renal failure, and injuries and chronic infections of the extremities, which frequently require amputation. A patient who escapes the direct complications of microvascular and neurologic damage often succumbs to disorders associated with large vessel disease, such as ischemic heart disease.

IDDM usually occurs in youth and appears to have a strong genetic component (Dorman, 1997). Research findings also indicate that unknown environmental conditions, such as dietary factors and infectious agents, may influence the incidence of the disease. A current theory suggests that a virus, such as Coxsackie or mumps, may evoke an autoimmune reaction that destroys the islet cells of the pancreas. However, researchers have not yet identified a specific viral infection that can explain most cases.

In many countries, health officials and WHO have established IDDM registries (Karvonen, Tuomilehto, Libman, & LaPorte, 1993). These registries demonstrate substantial variation in IDDM rates by racial group and country (Figure 6–3). IDDM rates are usually highest among

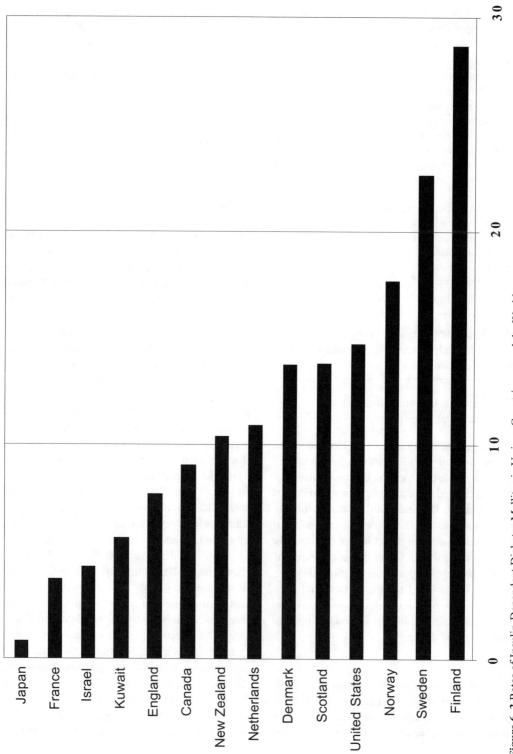

**Figure 6–3** Rates of Insulin-Dependent Diabetes Mellitus in Various Countries around the World

White populations in northern climates; Finland and Sweden have the highest rates. The lowest rates are seen in Asian countries, Mexico, Chile, and Peru, and among Native Americans in the United States. In regions with moderate IDDM incidence rates, such as North and South America, central Europe, Africa, and Australia, Whites generally experience higher rates of the disease than do people of African descent or Hispanic ethnicity.

People with IDDM are usually treated with parenteral insulin. In many low- and middle-income countries, this type of insulin is difficult to obtain or is too expensive to administer to many patients. Training for health professionals is also limited, which sometimes leads to iatrogenic deaths from hypoglycemia due to insulin overdoses (Savage, 1993).

NIDDM is the result of insulin resistance rather than insulin deprivation, so glucose is able to enter cells. Persons with NIDDM do not usually experience severe metabolic disorders. However, because of chronic hyperglycemia, they often have many of the same complications as persons with IDDM.

NIDDM has a genetic component, as well as two major environmental factors that contribute to its occurrence: obesity and inactivity. In societies where obesity is rare and people have a high level of ambient activity due to physical labor and manual transportation, this form of diabetes is rare. A recent comprehensive analysis of surveys from around the world of blood glucose levels after an oral glucose load indicate that the prevalence of NIDDM among persons older than 20 years of age is increasing (King, Aubert, & Merman, 1998). This analysis found that 135 million persons had type 2 diabetes in 1995 and that more than 60% of them lived in the low- and middle-income countries. Using United Nations estimates of the age-specific growth in populations, the analysis concluded that by the year 2025 the total number of adults with diabetes will increase by 120% and that more than 75% of these adults will be living in these countries. The investigators assumed that this increase would be attributable to the

aging of the global population. However, studies conducted by WHO suggest that NIDDM is increasing in prevalence among populations experiencing modernization with decreases in physical activity and increases in average body mass. Particularly high rates of NIDDM have been observed among Pacific Islanders in Micronesia, Polynesia, and Melanesia; Australian aborigines; Asian Indians; and certain subsets of Native Americans (Taylor, 1993). Therefore, the United Nations estimates probably represent conservative prognostications unless prevention and control programs for diabetes are widely disseminated. Such programs must encourage weight maintenance, and loss where necessary, as well as increased physical activity. The impending problems associated with this increase have prompted WHO to promote diabetes as a major priority in noncommunicable disease control.

Malnutrition-related diabetes mellitus (MRDM) is another distinct type of diabetes observed in low- and middle-income countries located in the tropics and subtropics. It is the result of childhood malnutrition that appears to induce calcification of the pancreas. Persons with MRDM require insulin to ameliorate their hypoglycemia, but they are not prone to the major metabolic problems observed with IDDM (Tripathy & Samal, 1997). Few studies on the long-term follow-up of these patients have been conducted, and the pathophysiologic link between early nutritional deprivation and pancreatic calcifications has not been elucidated.

### Chronic Obstructive Pulmonary Disease

This category of chronic lung diseases includes chronic bronchitis and emphysema. Although these diseases have different pathologic attributes, both are characterized by increasing breathlessness and a chronic cough that worsens over time. Using projections from the GBD, it is estimated that COPD will rise from the sixth to the third leading cause of death in the world by the year 2020 (Murray & Lopez, 1996a, 1996b). The major risk factor for this disease is cigarette smoking. It is most prevalent in industrialized countries where cigarette smoking has been prevalent for an extended period of time. Although COPD is growing in importance in low- and middle-income countries with the global spread of tobacco use, COPD is also highly prevalent in such areas as Papua New Guinea and Nepal, where tobacco use has not been widespread, but there is substantial air pollution as a result of the use of indoor fires for heating and cooking (see Chapter 8) (Taylor, 1993).

### Musculoskeletal Conditions

Musculoskeletal conditions such as osteoporosis, osteoarthritis, and rheumatoid arthritis are major sources of disability and suffering, though they are frequently underappreciated as major health problems because they do not usually directly result in fatalities. In surveys from industrialized countries, one-third to one-half of adults claim to experience some level of joint pain and decreased functional capacity that are reported to be caused by "arthritis" (Centers for Disease Control and Prevention, 1999). Data from low- and middle-income countries suggest that their impact is the same or perhaps even higher.

Medical treatment for the inflammatory joint diseases of osteoarthritis and rheumatoid arthritis aims to reduce pain and maintain optimal function. However, pharmacologic treatment with older medications, such as aspirin, can cause gastrointestinal bleeding; the newer anti-inflammatory agents that help to suppress the immune system are very expensive. Physical activity regimens that are nontraumatic to joints and avoidance of excessive weight gain are the mainstays of preventing osteoarthritis, which is sometimes called degenerative joint disease (National Arthritis Foundation, 1990). Osteoporosis is characterized by demineralization of the bone matrix with increased fragility of the skeleton. Persons with this condition are at increased risk of debilitating fractures of the hip and spine. This condition is much more prevalent among White women. Taking adequate amounts of dietary calcium, getting sufficient physical activity, and avoiding tobacco products are the main

lifestyle activities that help prevent this condition.

### Neuropsychiatric Conditions

One of the major conclusions of the GBD was that mental illnesses were among the leading causes of disability in the world (Murray & Lopez, 1996a, 1996b). An estimated 45 million persons are affected by schizophrenia, and 340 million persons experience depression at any given time. Effective pharmacologic treatments exist for these conditions but are not fully distributed to those most in need, even in industrialized countries (WHO, 1998a; see Chapter 7).

Dementia will inevitably become more prevalent as the global population ages. The major causes of this condition are Alzheimer's disease and cerebrovascular disease. The latter can be prevented by eating a low-fat diet, engaging in physical activity, identifying and controlling hypertension, and avoiding cigarette smoking. Two other highly prevalent and debilitating neurologic diseases are blindness and epilepsy, which affect 25 million and 40 million persons, respectively, worldwide. Infectious causes of these conditions, such as bacterial meningitis, onchocerciasis, and trachoma, are much more common in low- and middle-income countries. Their prevention and treatment present major opportunities to improve the health of persons in these countries (see Chapter 4). As the population in low- and middle-income countries ages, researchers expect diabetes and cataracts to grow in importance as causes of blindness. Some investigators anticipate a doubling of blindness cases by the year 2020 (WHO, 1998a).

## Chronic Diseases Related to Malnutrition

An energy-rich diet consisting of few unrefined plants and dominated by processed foods that are high in saturated fats from animal sources has repeatedly been implicated as a major risk factor for numerous chronic diseases, such as atherosclerosis, cancer, and diabetes (Kushi & Foerster, 1998). The prevalence of obesity increases along with the associated problems of hypertension, NIDDM, and musculoskeletal disorders when such a diet is combined with the sedentary lifestyle frequently cultivated within industrialized countries. Another hypothesis that has ascended in the public health community suggests countries in the midst of rapid economic development may be particularly vulnerable to the ravages of such a "Western" diet. This proposition, frequently called the Barker hypothesis because it has been vigorously promoted in the medical literature by a British researcher named D.J.P. Barker, posits that nutritional deprivation during the prenatal period and low weights at birth and at one year of age cause children to have greater susceptibility to a variety of diseases in later life (Barker, 1990).

A number of correlative studies by Barker and others have supported this theory. However, a contemporary exhaustive review of the subject suggests that many of the findings were based on ecologic studies that drew their conclusions from correlations between historic periods of nutritional deficiency in a particular country or region and subsequent rates of chronic diseases (Joseph & Kramer, 1996). Unmeasured intermediaries between group-level exposures and population rates of disease make such studies of questionable use when trying to evaluate a biologic mechanism operating at the level of individuals. More recent studies making use of individual-level data on nutritional status during the perinatal period and subsequent health events have not supported the Barker hypothesis as a mechanism for chronic disease etiology beyond the accepted deleterious effects of a sedentary lifestyle and energy-rich diet (Kannisto, Christensen, & Vaupel, 1996; Susser & Levin, 1999).

In reality, whether current or previously high levels of malnutrition in the low- and middle-income world portend a global epidemic of chronic diseases does not alter the basic public health dimensions of an aging world population with increasing access to a diet high in fat. Such a diet can result in increased rates of diabetes, cardiovascular disease, and hypertension regardless of whether there were antecedent periods

of perinatal starvation (Taylor, 1993). Mounting the interventions necessary to forestall adoption of such a diet in low- and middle-income countries is a profound challenge to public health practice. Data recently published by WHO from 79 low- and middle-income countries and a number of industrialized countries suggest that about 22 million children less than 5 years old are already currently considered overweight (>2 standard deviations above reference for height and weight) (WHO, 1998a).

## Aging, Disability, Frailty, and Health-Related Quality of Life

A recurrent theme in this chapter is that the aging of the global population will inevitably lead to an increase in the incidence, morbidity, and mortality from chronic diseases. An underlying assumption is that advanced age is invariably associated with failing health and the increased likelihood of illness. The biologic mechanisms controlling the progressive loss of cells in most organs of the body and decreases in function, capacity, and resiliency are not well understood. The ultimate goal of future research should be to elucidate the determinants of the aging process and thereby design efforts to ameliorate the disability, general frailty, and illnesses associated with this process.

Currently, two perspectives dominate the thinking about the process of aging. The first posits that aging is essentially a surrogate for the sum total of time-dependent "insults" inflicted on the human organism that result in cellular destruction and in many cases discrete illnesses. This perspective holds that health can be maintained, aging forestalled, and death delayed by studying and resolving the mechanisms behind the individual diseases (Peto et al., 1997). Within this theoretical framework the primary explanation for the greater number of untoward health events associated with older age is that time must pass for a critical number of stresses and insults to accumulate. Even apparently age-related events, such as menopause, are not viewed as inherently dependent on age per se within this construct. Proponents believe that if the discrete biologic mechanisms leading to menopause could be elucidated, then this event could also be altered by medicine.

Another perspective suggests that the aging process of cellular degradation is inevitable and programmed. Hence, disease prevention and treatment can prolong life by preventing overwhelming stress on a gradually less resilient system, but the mechanisms of aging inherently facilitate disease (Fossel, 1998). Investigators with this view generally support the notion that mechanistic research at the molecular and cellular level should concentrate on the common processes involved in time-related cellular death. Understanding these processes may provide insight into the genesis of many different diseases. The recognition that these "programmed" components of cellular dysfunction have a large genetic contribution is one rationale for the human genome project being conducted in the United States. This effort is resulting in the DNA sequencing of all the genes constituting the human genome. The expectation is that this information will greatly facilitate understanding of basic biologic mechanisms in human chemistry and cellular function, and as a result lead to many preventive and curative treatments (Collins, 1999).

Aside from the biologic conceptions of age, there is growing evidence from industrialized countries that reducing exposure to major chronic disease risk factors, such as lack of physical inactivity, tobacco use, and obesity, prolongs life, reduces disability, and improves health-related quality of life (Vita, Terry, Hubert, & Fries, 1998). A theory called the *compression of morbidity* attempts to accommodate these observations with the more reductionistic views of the aging process described above. This theory was posited by James Fries 20 years ago and propounds that there is a programmed limit to the human life span (estimated at between 90 and 100 years). Prevention and effective treatment not only extend the length of life toward this programmed limit, but also decrease the relative and absolute period of time lived in poor health (Fries, 1980). The results from the

GBD support this theory in that countries with high premature mortality rates also exhibited an elevated prevalence of disabilities (Murray & Lopez, 1997). In industrialized countries where life expectancies improved in previous decades, growing evidence suggests that disability rates among older adults are rapidly diminishing (Manciaux & Romer, 1991). Data from the United States illustrate this point (Figure 6–4). A study of older Americans demonstrated that the prevalence rate of chronic disability and institutionalization declined by almost 15% from 1982 to 1994. This suggests that even though the number of persons over 65 years of age is increasing in the United States, the absolute number of dependent persons with disabilities in this age group has remained relatively stable (Manton, Corder, & Stallard, 1997).

Regardless of the precise intricacies of the aging process, it is clear that as mortality rates decline and the number of older adults increases, promotion of health-related quality of life (HRQOL) will become an important public health goal. Defining, measuring, and facilitating HRQOL has generated an enormous and frequently contentious literature (Murray & Lopez, 1996a, 1996b). Most indexes of HRQOL attempt to ascertain the impact of illness or disability on several health-related domains of life that include physical (pain, mobility), psychological (cognition), and social (the ability to maintain social interactions) dimensions. The methods and procedures for conducting these measures are highly varied. Because of the complexity of measuring health, no firm international consensus has been established on the best approach to quantifying HRQOL (WHO, 1998a). The DALY has been adopted provisionally by WHO as a means to introduce nonfatal health outcomes into the analysis of health data. Many industrialized countries, such as Canada, the Netherlands, and the United States, are exploring numerous measures similar to the DALY to accommodate the increasing importance of HRQOL into health policy considerations.

The immense increases in the older population in low-and middle-income countries ex-

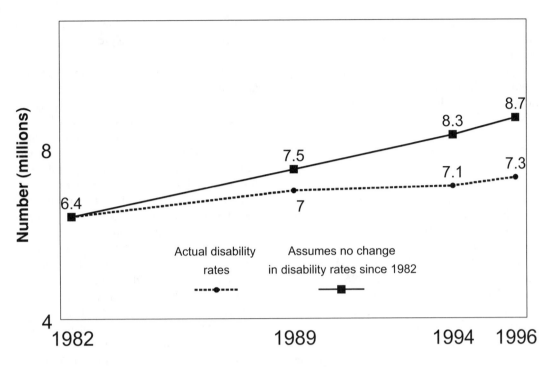

**Figure 6–4** Chronically Disabled Americans, Age 65 Years and Above

pected over the next 30 years present enormous challenges to international public health efforts. This challenge is greater than a simple increase in the total volume of discrete diseases associated with older age. The average productivity of the entire population is compromised if efforts are not adopted to support, or better yet prevent, the potential dependency needs of large numbers of older adults. For example, it is estimated that by the year 2020 there will be 274 million persons over age 60 in China alone—more than the current population of the entire United States (WHO, 1998b). The WHO has highlighted aging as a major health issue in recent reports and meetings (WHO, 1998a, 1998b). The central theme of the WHO strategy is to promote the adoption of healthy lifestyles and ready access to effective preventive and curative care throughout the life course. This comprehensive strategy is currently the best approach for promoting a healthy and productive older population (Krug, 1999).

**Injury**

Injuries are among the 10 leading causes of death worldwide. Every day almost 16,000 persons die from injuries (Krug, 1999). In 1998 unintentional and intentional injuries accounted for an estimated 5.8 million deaths, which corresponded to a death rate of 97.9/100,000 population, of which 3.8 million (128.6/100,000 population) were men and 2.0 million (66.7/100,000 population) were women (Krug, 1999).

Injury incidence and severity are affected by age, sex, race, and occupation, as well as by economic and geographic factors. Worldwide, children, young adults, and older adults are at increased risk of death, and their associated death rates are higher for males than for females throughout the life cycle. Injuries are also higher among populations of lower socioeconomic status and among those living in substandard physical environments. About half of all deaths to those age 10–24 years are the result of injuries and violence. Nonfatal injuries greatly affect those over age 60. Advanced technology and increased availability of motor vehicles and weapons will likely lead to higher rates of traffic injuries and violence, as well as injuries related to poisonings and burns (Zwi, Msika, & Smetannikov, 1993).

Types of injuries differ in urban and rural settings. This is often related to exposures to different hazards (violence in large urban centers, exposure to pesticides in rural and farming areas). Whereas a greater concentration of automobiles increases the number of vehicle crashes in urban areas, in rural areas vehicle speed tends to be higher, road conditions generally poorer, and medical care to individuals sustaining injuries less available (Mathai, 1996). Each of these factors may lead to higher injury rates and poorer outcomes from vehicle accidents in rural areas.

Injuries can also be viewed from a regional perspective. They appear to cause the greatest mortality in low- and middle-income countries and in areas where war and civil violence are prevalent. By interpreting the data of Murray and Lopez it can be seen that sub-Saharan Africa manifests the highest injury death rate among the major world regions. Its rate is more than twice that of India's and is mainly due to violence. More industrialized regions of the world, such as Europe, Australia, Scandinavia, North America, and Japan, have some of the lowest injury death rates.

The burden of injury is particularly evident in countries where communicable, infectious diseases have been substantially controlled. Where these diseases used to account for the greatest number of lives lost, medical treatments and prevention efforts have brought them under greater control such that injury has replaced them as a major cause of mortality. As infectious diseases continue to diminish, unintentional injuries and violence will occupy an even more dominant place as a major health threat throughout the life span.

Injuries account for one in seven years of life lost worldwide. By the year 2020 they will ac-

count for one in five, with low- and middle-income countries bearing the greatest percentage of this increase. Worldwide, violence (suicide, homicide, war) in 1990 accounted for almost the same number of DALYs lost as either human immunodeficiency virus (HIV) or tuberculosis. Unintentional injuries cause as many DALYs lost as diarrhea and more than cardiovascular disease or cancers. In low- and middle-income regions in 1990, injuries were responsible for more than one-third of all DALYs lost from all causes among males aged 15–44 years old.

Despite the immense burden of injury worldwide, the disparity in the burden between industrialized and low- and middle-income countries continues to widen. A vast majority of unintentional injuries in the world occur in low-income countries. Specifically, low-income nations are responsible for more than 70% of the world's motor-vehicle injuries. Of the violence-related injuries, 1,183,000 of the 1,423,000 occurred in low-income countries (World Bank, 1993). Lopez and his colleagues in 1990 estimated that violence-related mortality ranked nineteenth as a cause of death worldwide. If current trends continue, violence will increase to twelfth place by the year 2020 (Branche, 1998).

The burden of injuries was highest in the formerly socialist countries of Europe, where almost 19% of all disease burden was attributable to injuries in 1990. China had the second highest injury burden, Latin America and the Caribbean the third, and sub-Saharan Africa the fourth. In almost all regions, unintentional injuries were a much bigger health burden than violence (Murray & Lopez, 1996a, 1996b).

The lead cause of injury deaths globally is motor-vehicle accidents, followed by other unintentional injuries, suicide, homicide, drowning, war-related injuries, falls, burns, and poisonings (Figure 6–5). Whereas motor-vehicle injury rates have decreased dramatically in most industrialized countries, many low- and middle-income nations continue to show a worsening situation. Estimates from WHO indicate that of the 865,000 traffic deaths occurring worldwide annually, 74% are in low-income coun-

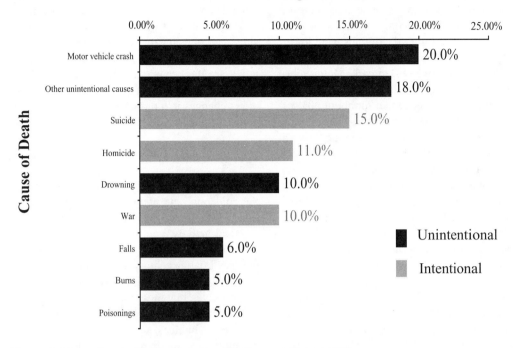

**Figure 6–5** Injury Deaths Worldwide by Leading Cause and Intent, 1990

tries (WHO, 1984; Soderlund & Zwi, 1995). The number of temporary and permanent disabilities resulting from traffic injuries is many times greater than the number of deaths. Motor-vehicle crashes were ranked ninth in worldwide disease burden in 1990. If present trends continue, by the year 2020 they will be ranked third. One reason motor-vehicle injuries in low- and middle-income countries and indeed around the world have not seen the major declines that have been realized by infectious diseases is that many people still consider injuries as mere "accidents," unpredictable and unpreventable. Also, investigators have cited a number of factors that specifically contribute to the continuing motor-vehicle injury problem in low- and middle-income countries, including rapid population growth, increasing motorization, little access to emergency care, lack of safety features in cars, crowded roads, poor road maintenance, and lack of police enforcement.

Intentional injuries (suicide and homicide) are ranked third and fourth, respectively (Figure 6–5). Suicide represents 15% of injury deaths, whereas criminal homicide represents 11% of injury deaths worldwide. Factors often responsible for intentional injuries such as homicide and suicide include poverty, racism, social injustice, isolation, drug trafficking, and drug and alcohol use (Rosenberg et al., 1987).

Among adults aged 15–44, traffic accidents were the leading cause of death for men and the fifth leading cause of death for women worldwide in 1990. For women aged 15–44, suicide was the second leading cause of death. For young adults, traffic accidents, suicide, war-related injuries, fire and burns, and violence all were included in the 10 leading causes of death. In China alone more than 180,000 women committed suicide in 1990. In India, more than 87,000 Indian women died in fires (Murray & Lopez, 1996b).

In an international comparative analysis, a number of differences were found in injury mortality among 11 high-income countries. For example, the annual injury death rates were lower in England, Wales, Israel, and the Netherlands, and higher in France and Denmark. Motor-vehicle accidents, firearms, poisoning, falls, suffocation, and drowning accounted for about 60% of all injury deaths in the 11 countries. The rates of death from motor-vehicle injuries ranged from a low of 6 per 100,000 population in England and Wales to a high of 21 per 100,000 in New Zealand, which also had the highest rate of deaths in motorcycle crashes. Motor-vehicle–related injuries were the leading cause of death among children age 1–14 in all 11 countries. In four of the comparison countries—the United States, Norway, Israel, and France—firearms were the second leading cause of injury deaths at ages 15–24 years. In the United States, the majority of the firearm-related deaths were homicides (62%), whereas in all other countries they were primarily suicides (51–93%). The homicide rate in the United States is four to nine times the rates in comparison countries (Fingerhut, Cox, & Warner, 1998).

## EPIDEMIOLOGY OF PRINCIPAL BEHAVIORAL RISK FACTORS FOR CHRONIC DISEASES

Nearly all chronic diseases are seen as complex products of genetic, sociodemographic, sociocultural, and behavioral factors. Many of these are viewed as immutable, such as gender, age, and race; others are seen as moderately modifiable, such as education, income, and social support; still others are seen as highly modifiable, such as eating behaviors, physical activity, tobacco use, and substance use. Modifiability is largely viewed in terms of what individuals are able to change, rather than what can be achieved at the group or organization level. Indeed, modifiability of the factors causing disease is highly dependent on other capabilities. For instance, it may be possible in the future to modify genetic factors and predispositions

for chronic disease that were once seen as immutable. With powerful political will and group consensus it may be possible to affect social support, cohesion, or social capital. What remains clear is that the most modifiable factors today are the behavioral ones, and most of the research and practical intervention efforts to affect changes in long-term chronic disease outcomes have addressed these personal risks.

### Four Risk Factors

Four behavioral risk factors predominate in the epidemiologic literature of chronic disease: tobacco use (mainly smoking), eating behaviors, physical activity, and alcohol consumption. As noted earlier, since the HIV/AIDS epidemic of the past quarter century, sexual behaviors have been increasingly studied. It is worth emphasizing, however, that these four behavioral risk factors cannot easily be disentangled from their societal influences. Cigarette use and alcohol consumption can hardly be seen outside the social factors leading to their wide adoption and popularization in films, media, and sporting events. Similarly, eating behaviors and dietary patterns cannot be easily separated from the growth of the fast-food industry and an emphasis on high-fat, high-sugar content foods. Also, the observed decrease in physical activity in some countries can be linked to an excessive reliance on automobiles and a growing number of sedentary hours in front of a television or video screen. It is the complexity of these interrelationships that makes it difficult to understand the meaning of risk for chronic diseases. Most of the behavioral risk factors are complex because they culminate in other risk factors. For example, while obesity is considered a risk factor for cancer, CVD, diabetes, injuries, and other chronic diseases and conditions, it must be viewed as a product of many forces operating at genetic, sociocultural, and behavioral levels.

This complex risk-factor approach was explored and researched extensively in the latter half of the twentieth century in North America, Europe, and Australia. Most of the vast literature from the fields of epidemiology, health promotion, the social and behavioral sciences, and other relevant fields and disciplines has been based on the experience of populations living in the economically advanced, industrial countries. Although it may be assumed that the same constellation of factors operate universally in the causation of chronic diseases, given the complicated interaction of the biologic, social, cultural, and behavioral factors, one cannot guarantee that the components will interact in the same way in low- and middle-income countries. Thus it is difficult to know whether the CHD "epidemic" experienced in the industrialized countries will be mirrored in low- and middle-income countries. While it has been asserted (McGinnis & Foege, 1993) that behavioral factors may account for most of the variance in chronic disease etiology in industrialized countries, this pattern may be different in low- and middle-income countries. Indeed, it is possible that the influence of sociocultural and behavioral factors may be more pronounced in low- and middle-income countries.

The difficulties in assessing the nature of risk factors at the global level are not simply methodological. They arise from the lack of an appropriate public health infrastructure in much of the world. Probably the best data are on tobacco use. However, the comparative data on other behavioral risk factors remain often sketchy and problematic to interpret.

## Tobacco Use

Tobacco use is often simply translated into cigarette smoking. Cigarettes are the predominant delivery form of addictive nicotine in North America and Europe, but not the only use of tobacco. Other forms include chewing and snorting tobacco, pipe and cigar use, and various mixtures of tobacco with other substances, for example tobacco mixed with betel nuts. The focus on cigarette smoking has been based on several reasons: (1) it is relatively easy to measure and verify its use; (2) it is a product supported by a powerful international business community; (3) it is viewed as the major modifiable behavioral risk factor in cancer and heart disease; and (4) it is a behavior that has few redeeming values associated with its use, in marked contrast to eating and drinking behaviors.

The reported prevalence of cigarette smoking varies considerably across the globe. Although the national picture in the United States is complex when one considers state-by-state data and age-specific rates and race differences, the overall trend is encouraging. In the past 30 years, there has been a steady decline to just below 30% in cigarette smoking among both men and women (Giovino, Henningfield, Tomar, Escobedo, & Slade, 1995). In many ways, the U.S. experience is hopeful because the decline has been sustained over a long period. However, there are some disturbing aspects as well. One is whether there is a bottoming out of the trend, indicating that there is a hard-core addicted group whose behavior will be exceedingly difficult to change. The second is the disturbing trend at the end of the past century of a slight increase in smoking among young people, notably in young women. From an international perspective, many Western countries may follow these same trends.

In the low- and middle-income countries, the observed and measured patterns of cigarette smoking are mixed. Nonetheless, some broad generalizations seem apparent at the beginning of the twenty-first century. First, adult male smoking prevalence is very high in many countries, more than 50% in Bangladesh, China, Japan, Korea, Russia, Indonesia, and Vietnam. Second, with the exception of Russia, the smoking rates for females in these countries are low. However, the possibility of a sharp rise in smoking rates among women represents a major public health concern. Third, given the economic importance of the tobacco industry, cigarette use will probably remain a major behavioral risk factor globally. Finally, were there to be a major global decline in smoking rates, given the lag time between behavior change and health outcomes, the effect on chronic diseases would not be seen for several decades, especially for lung cancer. Thus there is every reason to predict that smoking-related diseases will continue to be of major significance globally (see Exhibit 6–4).

### Alcohol Consumption

Alcohol abuse is a major contributor to chronic diseases and injuries. Documenting morbidity and mortality of alcohol use is complicated by the daily or regular consumption of alcohol in many countries. At the same time, many countries prohibit or restrict alcohol use. There is more certainty in assessing the alcohol-attributable deaths from injuries. For motor vehicle injuries, there appears to be a dose-response effect, with high blood alcohol levels leading to more severe injuries. Alcohol also contributes to other injuries, such as drowning, fires, falls, and pedestrian and occupational injuries. The contribution of alcohol to injuries is extremely high in Latin America and the Caribbean, where it accounts for almost 10% of the total disease and injury burden. Alcohol consumption in low- and middle-income countries has increased by 146% since the early 1960s (Stansfield et al., 1993).

Unlike cigarette smoking, for which individuals can fit nicely into a categorization scheme (for example, never smoked, former smoker, current smoker), alcohol use and abuse is not so easily defined. Many investigations have attempted to define alcohol use on the basis of quantity, frequency, and variability, but an accurate classification of use versus abuse remains dependent upon many social and cultural factors. Drinking patterns vary greatly by country and within countries. Some of the factors that define these patterns are religion, ethnicity, race, gender, and socioeconomic status. Drinking patterns in the United States are more moderate than those in Europe. The pattern for most of the latter half of the last century has been one where the majority of the female population are nondrinkers and nearly half of males are abstainers or former drinkers. Less than 15% of the U.S. population is considered to be "heavy drinkers," which is classified as more than 14 drinks per week. Serious alcohol abuse and its effects, such as injuries, liver cirrhosis, and alcohol-related syndromes, appear to be minor problems in many of the low- and middle-income countries, but of critical importance in Russia and the former Soviet states.

### Eating Behaviors and Physical Activity

Although eating behaviors and physical activity are considered important behavioral risk factors in the etiology of chronic diseases, the data available on their influence are problematic. Eating behaviors per se have been relatively little studied except by anthropologists. Generally, the public health literature has focused on nutrition and diet content, which are the products of eating behavior. This has made meaningful interpretation of any global data difficult, primarily because of the idiosyncratic nature of foodstuffs consumed within any given cultural group. Much of the relevant literature on eating behaviors concentrates on definable, recognizable outcomes, such as malnutrition or obesity, which can be more credibly measured and compared.

Few reliable sources of global data on obesity exist. The most comprehensive data are from the WHO MONICA study (Tunstall-Pedoe et al., 1999). Although these data stem from population-based surveys within countries and are therefore not generalizable to the entire country population, they do provide comparable data collected from many countries across the globe. What is remarkable is the wide geographic range of those considered obese (that is, bodymass index [BMI] $\geq 30$). Malta and France have high proportions of obese men aged 35–64, while Sweden and China have the lowest proportions. Among women aged 35–64, the former Soviet Union and Malta have the highest proportions, with New Zealand and China having the lowest proportions. However, in nearly all MONICA countries the majority of men in this age group

**Exhibit 6–4** A Chronic Disease Behavioral Risk Factor Example: Tobacco Use and Control in China

Smoking and the use of tobacco is a widely recognized risk factor in disease. It is a critical risk factor in several severe chronic diseases, including CVD, cancer, and respiratory diseases. Moreover, it is totally a self-induced behavior. Smoking remains the single most dangerous and wholly modifiable human behavior associated with chronic disease.

In 1996 investigators carried out a national survey to study smoking patterns in China (Yang et al., 1997). They conducted interviews with approximately 65,000 men and 57,000 women, using a three-stage sampling of households chosen from 145 disease surveillance points. The survey results mirror the 1990 census data from China in terms of the distributions of age, sex, place of residence (urban/rural), education, occupation, and geographic distribution. In brief, the survey provides a national overview of smoking patterns in a large, complex nation.

Some key findings of this survey are noteworthy. Smoking rates in China are very high; nearly 70% of adult men reported being current smokers. Despite this high rate, there is some variation by social status. Higher educated and professional males have a lower smoking rate, though the effect seems to be largely related to education with only university education having a notable effect. However, even for the college educated males, the rate was greater than 50%. In marked distinction, the smoking rate among women was highly influenced by educational level with a very low prevalence of around 1% reported for college-educated women.

It is clear that with a high prevalence rate passive smoking would be commonplace. More than half the nonsmokers in the survey reported exposure to the smoke of others for a period of more than 15 minutes per day and more than 1 day per week. The home and workplace were the common sites for passive smoking. Clearly, exposure to passive smoking in China is a significant added risk for chronic disease for both smokers and nonsmokers.

The survey also contained questions on knowledge and attitudes toward smoking. This type of information provides the basic background for designing public health initiatives for the control of smoking. In industrialized countries the knowledge of the harm caused by smoking is high in both smokers and nonsmokers, but in China the knowledge base was very weak. More than half of smokers and nonsmokers believed there was little harm in smoking. Although respondents had relatively accurate knowledge about the relationship between smoking and chronic bronchitis, only 4% reported awareness of the dangers of smoking and heart disease.

This survey illustrates the type of in-depth epidemiologic knowledge needed for all countries if a concerted public health effort is to be undertaken to reduce smoking behavior. The survey also found interest in policies to prevent young people from smoking.

This survey also provides background to illustrate the immensity of the tobacco problem in emerging economies. It provides a view of what many of the global issues will be in the next century. Tobacco control will have to overcome some powerful obstacles. First, the prevalence of smoking is very high and will probably not decline precipitously. Second, more women, especially in urban areas, are smoking. Third, knowledge of risks remains low in the population, indicating the need for considerable health education. Finally, the total impact of smoking on chronic disease, as the populations exposed to this high level of smoking age, will result in an enormous health care burden.

were overweight (BMI of 25 or more). Globally the observed pattern is of a symmetrical increase in the proportion of a population with high BMI as the proportion of the population with low BMI increases (WHO Study Group, 1990). This relationship holds with countries as diverse as India, Ethiopia, China, Mexico, Brazil, and Peru, to name just a few. The implications of this finding are puzzling in that obesity does not relate simply to economic development; it appears compounded by other factors. Much basic research remains to be done.

Obesity is highly affected by levels of physical activity in a population. Unfortunately, physical activity has been difficult to measure and conceptualize universally. Like eating behavior, it is tied to many cofactors, such as income, work, transportation, leisure time, and drinking behavior. Most measurements of physical activity routinely used in industrialized countries are based on physical activity related to exercise and leisure time activities. The issue of physical movement within the context of total daily routines remains complex. Although the calculated global burden of disease attributable to physical inactivity remains lower than that of smoking, it has been estimated at nearly 4% of total deaths (Murray & Lopez, 1996c).

## Some Observations

In 1985 Doll and Peto estimated that nearly 70% of the cancers occurring in industrialized countries were attributable to tobacco (30%), alcohol (3%), and a high-fat diet low in plant constituents (35%). In their study, these investigators estimated that about 10% of cancers were the result of infections, but they speculated that the actual fraction attributable to microbes could be much higher (Doll & Peto, 1985). It may be asserted that in the future the attributable causes of cancer may well have a similar distribution globally as that of the United States more than 15 years ago. Currently infection seems to play a larger role in low- and middle-income countries. The IARC recently estimated that in 1990 21% of cancer cases in low- and middle-income countries were attributable to identified microbial pathogens; only 9% of cancer cases in the industrialized world could be attributed to such infections (Pisani et al., 1997).

## SPECIAL PROBLEMS AND ISSUES FOR CHRONIC DISEASES AND INJURY IN THE GLOBAL CONTEXT

In the latter half of the twentieth century chronic disease and injury became the predominant global source of morbidity and mortality. After millennia of deaths in childbirth and infancy, and relatively short life spans, populations around the globe are now faced with the fruits of medical success and the practice of public health. Nonetheless, these benefits were not evenly distributed in the past and those living in highly industrialized economies had a significant advantage over individuals living in low- and middle-income countries in life expectancy and ultimate development of chronic diseases. This "burden of wealth" has now been transformed to a "burden of aging," and the experience of chronic disease is becoming endemic.

Most of the issues regarding chronic diseases that prevail in industrialized countries pertain also to low- and middle-income countries. Nevertheless, two issues are particularly pertinent. First, the science of public health is often underdeveloped in low- and middle-income countries. Chronic disease surveillance systems are spotty, behavioral risk surveillance is uncommon, and disease registries are incomplete. Where there is measurement of chronic diseases and injury, multiple methodological problems make it difficult to replicate public health research undertaken in the West. For example, much public health research has relied on survey methodology. Survey methodology is not simple to carry out, even in a country such as the United States, which has massive resources to allocate to this practice.

Second, the etiologic research that has informed Western epidemiology for decades may or may not be applicable to low- and middle-income countries. For example, the concept of "disparities" in Sweden or the United States may be different in its dimensions in India or Bangladesh. Similarly, many other hybrid notions such as "social capital" may be unique to the Western world. With the possible exception of smoking, the major behavioral risks associated with physical activity and eating behaviors show great variation globally. Measurement of these behaviors in any ongoing surveillance system would be challenging.

## Health Care and Public Health Leadership

Data on the availability of health care professionals in countries from around the world are regularly collected by WHO. These data have identified three major forms of imbalance between health workers and the medical care needs of populations. First, great variability exists in the numbers of health care providers (Figure 6–6). Globally, industrialized countries have more than 250 physicians per 100,000 persons, but the ratio is only 14 per 100,000 persons in the low- and middle-income countries (WHO, 1998a). This variability reflects enormous disparities in the relationship between the numbers of health care professionals available and the number needed in many countries. Second, few international standards have been developed to train professionals in the health sciences. Thus a substantial gap exists between the skills of the provider and the complexity of the tasks to be performed. Most low- and middle-income countries do not have the resources to train adequate numbers of physicians, nurses, or medi-

cal technicians to meet the growing medical care needs of an aging population. In line with the traditional public health focus of many donor agencies and governments, training and staffing have tended to concentrate on maternal and child health issues. Therefore, the largest group of health care providers is nurses and midwives. As chronic diseases increase in importance and as the major health care priorities of the low- and middle-income countries change, more health care professionals will be needed to identify chronic conditions and provide home-based care (WHO, 1998a). Reassigning emphasis away from issues primarily concerned with maternal and child health and toward the health needs of older women and men presents a major challenge to the traditional international public health community (Birn, 1999).

The third problem is a tendency for providers to cluster in urban centers. The major cities of low- and and middle-income and industrialized countries tend to have an overabundance of highly specialized, tertiary-care services, while the rural regions of countries do not receive

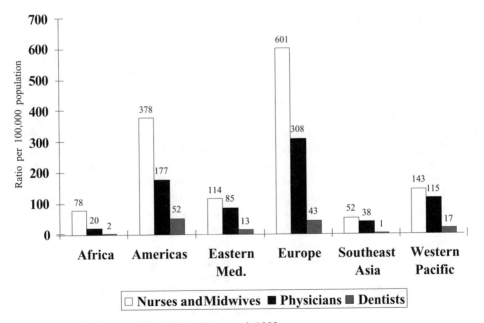

**Figure 6–6** Regional Estimates of Health Care Personnel, 1993

basic health needs. Besides these clear mismatches in the numbers of direct health care providers, such as doctors, nurses, and dentists, the availability and training of other important personnel such as laboratory technicians and pharmacists are also highly variable across the world. By monitoring these disparities, WHO has attempted to influence training and resource allocation policies in individual countries. However, comprehensive and coordinated efforts to redirect skilled health care workers have not been launched and are not likely to be carried out in the near future.

Leadership for injury prevention is normally found within the government, at the federal, state, or local level. Nongovernmental organizations and local coalitions can also play key roles in advancing injury control and in advocating for changes in education, social policy, engineering and product technology, and for police enforcement to prevent injuries. The private sector, too, can take an active role in promoting community safety and security. The development of effective pubic health strategies in middle-income countries (such as the former Soviet Union) and in low-income nations is a continuing challenge because of the numerous political and economic hardships they face (European Centre on Health of Societies in Transition, 1998).

The scale of the injury problem has not yet been recognized or addressed in low- and middle-income nations, and international assistance to combat injuries pales in comparison to assistance to fight other health problems. In 1990 global assistance for leprosy and onchocerciasis was about $50 per DALY lost, $7 for blindness, $4 for HIV and sexually transmitted infections, but only $0.01 for injuries (Michaud & Murray, 1994). This failure to appreciate the magnitude of the injury problem together with an absence of leadership in injury prevention has meant that many countries have no injury prevention programs or the available efforts are uncoordinated (see Exhibit 6–5).

To be effective, injury control interventions need to target behaviors, products, and environments—the main determinants of injury. The three strategies used to prevent and control injuries include education and behavior-change strategies (to modify behaviors), legislation and enforcement strategies (to modify environments), and technology and engineering strategies (to modify products). However, overlap in using strategies for more than one target often occurs, as in the use of education and behavior change to modify regulations and to increase police enforcement (Sleet & Gielen, 1998). Used together, these strategies can complement one another in efforts to prevent and control injuries.

Despite these obstacles, many low- and middle-income countries have made progress in strengthening injury prevention. In a 1989 survey 11 of 32 developing countries had established a coordinating body for injury prevention, and many had established strategies for planning and financing research activities. The WHO has an injury prevention program that assists member countries in building capacity and locating support for injury-control activities (Stansfield et al., 1993).

## CONCLUSION

It is difficult to summarize such a broad area of public health as chronic diseases and injury in the global context. There are enormous methodological difficulties in using available data to assess the scope and size of the problems associated with chronic diseases and injuries. Although many countries have reasonably well-developed systems of vital statistics for communicable diseases, they have not developed or implemented systems to track chronic diseases. In fact, comprehensive data on chronic diseases and injury are lacking worldwide. Also, few countries have sophisticated methods of obtaining surveillance data on behavioral risk factors; thus, there is a lack of basic action on the leading behavioral associations with the major chronic diseases. A parallel situation exists with disease registries. Where information is available, researchers are often skeptical of the data-collection systems used. This is not a criticism of the

**Exhibit 6–5** Bicycle Injuries as an Example of a Global Injury Issue

Bicycle injuries are a relatively understudied and unrecognized transportation safety problem in many developing countries (Barss, Smith, Baker, & Mohan, 1998; Manciaux & Romer, 1991). The little information that exists points to a major transportation injury problem. China is one of the few developing countries where public policy has encouraged bicycling as a form of commuting. Data on bicycle trips as a percentage of all daily passenger trips range from 77% in Tianjin, China, to 1% in Sydney, Australia. There are estimated to be more than 300 million bicycles in China. More than 1 in 4 Chinese own a bicycle, while only 1 in 74,000 own an automobile (Barss et al., 1998). As bicycling increases, so will bicycle-related injuries. In Beijing, about one-third of all traffic deaths occur among bicyclists. In Wuhan, bicycle helmet use is nonexistent, despite the fact that bicyclists comprise 45% of all traffic fatalities.

To reduce these injuries in China and elsewhere, several levels of intervention can be effective. Personal behavioral changes include use of a bicycle helmet, safe bicycling practices, and courtesy in sharing the road among vehicle drivers. Legislative and regulatory changes include laws that require helmet use, strict legal limits on alcohol use while bicycling, speed restrictions, and enforcement of traffic laws. Environmental changes may include separating bicyclists from other traffic, bicycle lanes, bicycling-oriented traffic signals and signs, painted edge lines on the road, removal of pathway and street obstacles and obstructions, clear visual lines of sight, and repair of road surfaces to remove potholes and dangerous curbs. Simultaneous use of these approaches can dramatically reduce bicycle-related injuries in all countries.

public health practitioners in these countries; rather, it is the recognition of the poor state of surveillance infrastructure in most countries. Indeed, even the more industrialized countries often lack in-depth comprehensive surveillance systems for chronic diseases and their associated risks.

There is an even greater dearth of information on the social determinants of health and illness in low- and middle-income countries. Recent efforts to assess the global burden of disease have helped to broaden our understanding of social determinants, but there is much information yet to be obtained. Years of careful work in the United States, Britain, Australia, and several European countries have shown that there are powerful relationships between poverty, racism, and many sociocultural disparities and chronic disease morbidity and mortality. It can logically be assumed that these same factors operate in low- and middle-income countries. The influence of these factors is yet to be determined. Any one of these factors or variables could act quite differently in some contexts from what has been witnessed in the industrialized world. Part

of the problem is that any social variable, for example industrialization, may be experienced in a different context from that of, say, the United States or Germany. These are countries that are long past their building of an industrial base, having experienced this buildup in another century. At the end of the twentieth century the new industrialization occurring in low- and middle-income countries was of another type entirely. So the epidemiologic question remains as to whether the same chronic disease patterns will be observed.

There is reason for concern with the global chronic disease and injury picture in the twenty-first century. The experience of the industrialized countries in the twentieth century may well be repeated, but more rapidly. This will most likely be the case with the continued heavy use of tobacco, less physical activity, higher-fat diets, and increasing use of the automobile. Furthermore, the pervasiveness of mass media, advertising, and the Internet means that the risk factors and social determinants related to chronic diseases and injury may spread virulently. The rise of chronic diseases will unduly burden the poor infrastructure for their care and treatment, and the aging of the population will add to this burden. In addition, it is unclear whether there is a political will to address chronic diseases in low- and middle-income countries, given the continued mortality caused by infectious diseases.

All these factors are critical concerns for the building of a new public health infrastructure. One notable change is the recognition by the traditional public health agencies of the need to develop complicated partnerships to address chronic diseases and to aid the public health infrastructure. Thus global agencies, such as WHO and national agencies such as the Centers for Disease Control and Prevention in the United States, embrace the idea of significant cooperation at various levels of government as well as with nongovernment agencies and the private sector. The future of chronic disease amelioration and injury prevention in low- and middle-income countries will probably rest on their ability to establish an adequate public health infrastructure.

## DISCUSSION QUESTIONS

1. In planning a global health strategy for public health, what should be the balance of concern between communicable and noncommunicable diseases?
2. Given that cardiovascular disease is the leading cause of mortality in most of the world, what actions are needed to reduce this burden?
3. There is overwhelming evidence that the single most important behavioral risk factor contributing to chronic diseases in low- and middle-income countries is tobacco use. Discuss possible solutions and impediments to eliminating this risk factor in the future.
4. Lack of good global statistical information about chronic diseases and injury is apparent. How can this situation be improved? Who should improve it?
5. What steps can be taken to reduce the burden of injury in low- and middle-income countries?

## REFERENCES

Bailar, J.C., & Gornick, H.L. (1997). Cancer undefeated. *New England Journal of Medicine, 336,* 1569–1574.

Barker, D.J.P. (1990). Fetal and infant origins of adult disease. *British Medical Journal, 301,* 1111.

Barss, P., Smith, G., Baker, S., & Mohan, D. (1998). *Injury prevention: An international perspective.* New York: Oxford University Press.

Beasley, R.P., & Hwang, L.-Y. (1991). Overview of the epidemiology of hepatocellular carcinoma. In F.B. Hollinger, S.M. Lemon, & H.S. Margolis (Eds.), *Viral hepatitis and liver disease* (pp. 532–535). Baltimore: Williams & Wilkins.

Belloc, N.B. (1973). Relationship of health practices and mortality. *Preventive Medicine, 2*(1), 67–81.

Berkman, L.F., & Breslow, L. (1983). Health and ways of living: The Alameda County study. New York: Oxford University Press.

Biemer, P.P., et al. (Eds.). (1991). *Measurement errors in surveys.* New York: John Wiley & Sons.

Birn, A.E. (1999). Skirting the issue: Women and international health in historical perspective. *American Journal of Public Health, 89,* 399–407.

Blot, W.J., & Fraumeni, J.F. (1996). Cancers of the lung and pleura. In D. Schottenfeld & J.F. Fraumeni (Eds.),

*Cancer epidemiology and prevention* (pp. 637–665). New York: Oxford University Press.

Branche, C. (1998, February). Burden of disease: Injuries and violence worldwide. Paper presented at the 15th annual meeting of INCLEN, Queretaro, Mexico.

Breslow, L. (1997). Social origins of cardiopulmonary disease: The need for population-focused prevention studies. *Annals of Epidemiology, 7,* 57, 54–57.

Centers for Disease Control and Prevention. (1989). Lung cancer and exposure to radon in women: New Jersey. *Morbidity and Mortality Weekly Report, 38,* 715–718.

Centers for Disease Control and Prevention. (1999). Impact of arthritis and other rheumatic conditions on the healthcare system: United States, 1997. *Morbidity and Mortality Weekly Report, 48,* 349–353.

Chang, M.H., Chen, C.J., & Lai, M.S. (1997). Universal hepatitis B vaccination in Taiwan and the incidence of hepatocellular carcinoma in children. *New England Journal of Medicine, 336,* 1855–1859.

Coleman, M.P., Esteve, J., Damiecki, P., Arslan, A., & Renard, H. (Eds.). (1993). Trends in cancer incidence and mortality. (IARC Scientific Publication No. 121). Lyon, France: International Agency for Research on Cancer.

Collins, F.S. (1999). Shattuck lecture: Medical and societal consequences of the Human Genome Project. *New England Journal of Medicine, 341,* 28–37.

Diez-Roux, A.V. (1998). Bringing context back into epidemiology: Variables and fallacies in multilevel analysis. *American Journal of Public Health, 88,* 216–221.

Doll, R., & Peto, R. (1985). The causes of cancer. New York: Oxford University Press.

Dorman, J.S. (1997). Molecular epidemiology of insulin-dependent diabetes mellitus. *Epidemiologic Reviews, 19,* 91–98.

Epstein, F.H. (1989). The relationship of lifestyle to international trends in C.H.D. *International Journal of Epidemiology, 18*(3 Suppl. 1), S203–S209.

European Centre on Health of Societies in Transition. (1998, September). *Childhood injuries: A priority area for the transition countries of Central and Eastern Europe and the newly independent states.* Final Report. London: London School of Hygiene and Tropical Medicine.

Fingerhut, L.A., Cox, C.S., & Warner, M. (1998, October 7). Advance data from vital and health statistics. *International comparative analysis of injury mortality: Findings from the ICE on injury statistics,* No. 303. Hyattsville, MD: National Center for Health Statistics, Centers for Disease Control and Prevention.

Forjuoh, S.N. (1996). Injury control in developing nations: What can we learn from industrialized countries? *Injury Prevention, 2*(2), 90–92.

Fortuin, M., Chotard, J., & Jack, A.D. (1993). Efficacy of hepatitis B vaccine in the Gambian Expanded Programme on Immunisation. *Lancet, 341,* 1129–1131.

Fossel, M. (1998). Telomerase and the aging cell: Implications for human health. *Journal of the American Medical Association, 279,* 1732–1735.

Frame, P., & Atkins, D. (1996). Screening for colorectal cancer. In Report of the U.S. Preventive Services Task Force, *Guide to Clinical Preventive Services* (2nd ed.) (pp. 105–118). Baltimore, MD: Williams & Wilkins.

Franco, E.L., Rohan, T.E., & Villa, L.L. (1999). Epidemiologic evidence and human papillomavirus infection as a necessary cause of cervical cancer. *Journal of the National Cancer Institute, 91,* 506–511.

Fries, J.F. (1980). Aging, natural death, and the compression of morbidity. *New England Journal of Medicine, 303,* 130–135.

Fuchs, C.S., Giovannucci, E.L., Colditz, G.A., Hunter, D.J., Stampfer, M.J., Rosner, B., Speizer, F.E., & Willett, W.C. (1999). Dietary fiber and the risk of colorectal cancer and adenoma in women. *New England Journal of Medicine, 340,* 169–176.

Giovino, G.A., Henningfield, J.E., Tomar, S.L., Escobedo, L.G., & Slade, J. (1995). Epidemiology of tobacco use and dependence. *Epidemiology Reviews, 17,* 48–65.

Goldman, L. (1984). The decline in ischemic heart disease mortality rates. *Annals of International Medicine, 101,* 825–836.

Haenszel, W., & Kurihara, M. (1968). Studies of Japanese migrants: Mortality from cancer and other diseases among Japanese in the United States. *Journal of the National Cancer Institute, 40,* 43–68.

Howe, G.R., Benito, E., Castelleto, R., Cornee, J., Esteve, J., Gallagher, R.P., Iscovich, J.M., Deng-ao, J., Kaaks, R., Kune, G.A., et al. (1992). Dietary intake of fiber and decreased risk of cancers of the colon and rectum: Evidence from the combined analysis of 13 case-control studies. *Journal of the National Cancer Institute, 84,* 1887–1896.

Howson, C.P., Reddy, K.S., Ryan, T.J., & Bale, J.R. (Eds.). (1998). *Control of cardiovascular diseases in developing countries: Research, development, and institutional strengthening.* Washington, DC: National Academy Press.

Jacobs, G.D., & Cutting, C.A. (1986, April). Further research on accident rates in developing countries. *Accident Analysis and Prevention, 18*(2), 119–127.

Joseph, K.S., & Kramer, M.S. (1996). Review of the evidence on fetal and early childhood antecedents of adult chronic disease. *Epidemiologic Reviews, 18,* 158–174.

Kannisto, V., Christensen, K., & Vaupel, J.W. (1996). No increased mortality in later life for cohorts born during famine. *American Journal of Epidemiology, 145,* 987–995.

Karvonen, M., Tuomilehto, J., Libman, I., & LaPorte, R. (1993). A review of the recent epidemiological data on the worldwide incidence of type I (insulin-dependent) diabetes mellitus. World Health Organization Diamond Project Group. *Diabetologia, 36,* 883–892.

King, H., Aubert, R., & Merman, W.H. (1998). Global burden of diabetes, 1995–2025: Prevalence, numerical estimates, and projections. *Diabetes Care, 21,* 1414–1431.

Kitchener, H.C., & Symonds, P. (1999). Detection of cervical intraepithelial neoplasia in developing countries. *Lancet, 353,* 856–857.

Koss, L.G. (1989). The Papanicolaou test for cervical cancer detection: A triumph and a tragedy. *Journal of the American Medical Association, 261,* 737–743.

Krieger, N. (1994). Epidemiology and the web of causation: Has anyone seen the spider? *Social Science and Medicine, 39,* 887–903.

Krug, E. (Ed.). (1999). Injury: A leading cause of the global burden of disease. Document # WHO/HSC/PVI/99.11. Geneva, Switzerland: World Health Organization.

Kushi, L.H., & Foerster, S.B. (1998). Diet and nutrition. In R.C. Brownson, P.L. Remington, & J.R. David (Eds.), *Chronic disease epidemiology and control* (pp. 216–260). Washington, DC: American Public Health Association.

Lan, Q., Chen, W., Chen, H., & He, X.Z. (1993). Risk factors for lung cancer in non-smokers in Xuanwei County of China. *Biomedical and Environmental Sciences, 6,* 112–118.

Latikka, P., Pukkala, E., & Vihko, V. (1998). Relationship between the risk of breast cancer and physical activity: An epidemiological perspective. *Sports Medicine, 26,* 133–143.

Liu, B.Q., Peto, R., Chen, Z.M., Boreham, J., Wu, Y.P., Li, J.Y., Campbell, T.C., & Chen, J.S. (1998). Emerging tobacco hazards in China: 1. Retrospective proportional mortality study of one million deaths. *British Medical Journal, 317,* 1411–1422.

Mackay, J. (1993). *The state of health atlas.* New York: Simon & Schuster.

Manciaux, M., & Romer, C.J. (Eds.). (1991). *Accidents in childhood and adolescence: The role of research.* Geneva, Switzerland: World Health Organization/INSERM.

Manton, K.G., Corder, L., & Stallard, E. (1997). Chronic disability trends in elderly United States populations: 1982–1994. *Proceedings of the National Academy of Science, 94,* 2593–2598.

Mathai, W. (1996, April). *The epidemiology and risk factors associated with motor vehicle injuries in developing countries.* Master's thesis, Rollins School of Public Health, Emory University, Atlanta, Georgia.

McGinnis, J.M., & Foege, W.H. (1993). Actual causes of death in the United States. *Journal of the American Medical Association, 270,* 2207–2212.

McKenna, M.T., Taylor, W.R., Marks, J.S., & Koplan, J.P. (1998). Current issues and challenges in chronic disease control. In R.C. Brown, P.L. Remington, & J.R. Davis (Eds.), *Chronic disease epidemiology and control* (pp. 1–26). Washington, DC: American Public Health Association.

Michaud, C., & Murray, C.J.L. (1994). External assistance to the health sector in developing countries: A detailed analysis, 1972–1990. In C.J.L. Murray & A.D. Lopez (Eds.), *Global comparative assessments in the health sector: Disease burden, expenditures, and intervention packages* (pp. 157–169). Geneva, Switzerland: World Health Organization.

Mueller, N.E., Evans, A.S., & London, W.T. (1996). Viruses. In D. Schottenfeld & J.F. Fraumeni (Eds.), *Cancer epidemiology and prevention* (pp. 502–531). New York: Oxford University Press.

Murakami, M., Gurski, K.J., & Steller, M.A. (1999). Human papillomavirus vaccines for cervical cancer. *Journal of Immunotherapy, 22,* 212–218.

Murray, C.J.L., & Lopez, A.D. (1996a). *The global burden of disease 1990.* Geneva, Switzerland: World Health Organization.

Murray, C.J.L., & Lopez, A.D. (1996b). *Global health statistics 1990.* Geneva, Switzerland: World Health Organization.

Murray, C.J.L., & Lopez, A.D. (Eds.). (1996c). *The global burden of disease: Summary.* Cambridge, MA: Harvard University Press.

Murray, C.J.L., & Lopez, A.D. (1997). Regional patterns of disability-free life expectancy and disability-adjusted life expectancy: Global Burden of Disease Study. *Lancet, 349,* 1347–1352.

National Arthritis Foundation. (1990). *National arthritis action plan: A public health strategy* (pp. 10–12). Atlanta, GA: National Arthritis Foundation, CDC, ASTHO.

National Institutes of Health. (1997) The sixth report of the joint national committee on prevention, detection, evaluation, and treatment of high blood pressure. NIH publication no. 98–4080. Washington, DC: 1997.

Orman, A.R. (1971). The epidemiologic transition: A theory of the epidemiology of population change. *Milbank Memorial Fund Quarterly, 49,* 509–538.

Over, M., Ellis, R.P., Huber, J.H., & Solon, O. (1994). The consequences of adult ill-health. In *The health of adults in the developing world* (pp. 161–199). New York: Oxford University Press.

Papers from a workshop on trends and determinants of coronary heart disease mortality: International comparisons.

(1989). *International Journal of Epidemiology, 18*(3 Suppl. 1), S1–S230.

Parkin, D.M., Whelan, S.J., Ferlay, J., Raymond, L., & Young, J. (Eds.). (1992). *Cancer incidence in five continents.* (Vol. 7.) IARC science publication no. 143. Lyon, France: International Agency for Research on Cancer.

Pearson, T.A., Jamison, D.T., & Trejo-Gutierrez, J. (1993). Cardiovascular disease. In D.T. Jamison et al. (Eds.), *Disease control priorities in developing countries* (pp. 577–594). New York: Oxford University Press.

Peto, R. (1997, August 24). *Global tobacco mortality: Monitoring the growing epidemic.* Presentation at the Tenth World Conference on Tobacco and Health, Beijing.

Peto, R., Chen, Z.M., & Boreham, J. (1999). Tobacco: The growing epidemic. *Nature Medicine, 5*(1), 15–17.

Peto, R., Lopez, A.D., Boreham, J., Thun, M., & Heath, C., Jr. (1992). Mortality from tobacco in developed countries: Indirect estimation from national vital statistics. *Lancet, 339,* 1268–1278.

Peto, R., et al. (1997, October 25). There is no such thing as aging. *British Medical Journal, 315,* 1030–1032.

Pisani, P., Parkin, D.M., Munoz, N., & Ferlay, J. (1997). Cancer and infection: Estimates of the attributable fraction in 1990. *Cancer Epidemiology, Biomarkers and Prevention, 6,* 387–400.

Popkin, B.M. (1994). The nutrition transition in low-income countries: An emerging crisis. *Nutrition Reviews, 52,* 285–298.

Poungvarin, N. (1998). Stroke in the developing world. *Lancet, 352*(Suppl. 3), 19–22.

Powell, K.E., & Blair, S.N. (1994). The public health burdens of sedentary living habits: Theoretical but realistic estimates. *Medicine and Science in Sports and Exercise, 26,* 851–856.

Rose, D.P., Boyar, A.P., & Wynder, E.L. (1986). International comparisons of mortality rates for cancer of the breast, ovary, prostate, and colon, and per capita food consumption. *Cancer, 58,* 2363–2371.

Rose, G. (1989). Causes of the trends and variations in C.H.D. mortality in different countries. *International Journal of Epidemiology, 18*(3, Suppl. 1), S174–S179.

Rosenberg, M.L., Gelles, R.J., Hollinger, P.C., Zahn, M.A., Stark, E., Conn, J.M., Fajman, N.M., & Karlson, T.A. (1987). Violence: Homicide, assault, and suicide. *American Journal of Preventive Medicine, 3*(Suppl. 5), 164–178.

Ross, R.K., Jones, P.A., & Yu, M.C. (1996). Bladder cancer epidemiology and pathogenesis. *Seminars in Oncology, 23,* 536–545.

Sackett, D.L., Richardson, W.S., Rosenberg, W., & Haynes, R.B. (1997). *Evidence-based medicine.* London: Churchill Livingstone.

Sackett, D.L., & Rosenberg, W.M.L. (1995). On the need for evidence-based medicine. *Health Economics, 4,* 249–254.

Samet, J.M., Kutvirt, D.M., Waxweiler, R.J., & Key, C.R. (1984). Uranium mining and lung cancer in Navajo men. *New England Journal of Medicine, 310,* 1481–1484.

Sankaranarayanan, R., Black, R.J., Swaminathan, R., & Parkin, D.M. (1998). An overview of cancer survival in developing countries. In R. Sankaranarayanan, R.J. Black, & D.M. Parkin (Eds.), *Cancer survival in developing countries.* IARC science publication no. 145. Lyon, France: International Agency for Research on Cancer.

Savage, A. (1993). Diabetes in the developing world. *Lancet, 341,* 900.

Skinner, C.J., Holt, D., & Smith, T.M. (Eds.). (1989). *Analysis of complex surveys.* London: John Wiley & Sons.

Slattery, M.L., & Randle, D.E. (1988). Trends in coronary heart disease mortality and food consumption in the United States between 1909 and 1980. *American Journal of Clinical Nutrition, 47,* 1600–1067.

Sleet, D.A., & Gielen, A. (1998). Injury prevention. In J. Arnold & S. Gorin (Eds.), *Health promotion handbook* (pp. 247–275). St. Louis, MO: Mosby.

Sleet, D.A., & Rosenberg, M.L. (1997). Injury control. In D. Scutchfield & C.W. Keck (Eds.), *Principles of public health practice* (pp. 337–349). Albany, NY: Delmar Publishers.

Smith, G.S., & Barss, P. (1991). Unintentional injuries in developing countries: The epidemiology of a neglected problem. *Epidemiology Reviews, 13,* 228–266.

Smith, J.P., & Kington, R. (1997). Demographic and economic correlates of health in old age. *Demography, 34*(1), 159–170.

Soderlund, R.N., & Zwi, A.B. (1995). Traffic-related mortality in industrialized and less developed countries. *Bulletin of the World Health Organization, 73*(2), 175–182.

Stansfield, S.K., Smith, G.S., & McGreevey, W.P. (1993). Injury. In D.T. Jamison, W.H. Mosley, A.R. Measham, & J.L. Bobadilla (Eds.), *Disease control priorities in developing countries* (pp. 609–633). New York: Oxford University Press.

Stuver, S.O. (1998). Towards global control of liver cancer? *Seminars in Cancer Biology, 8,* 299–306.

Sudlow, C.L.M., & Warlow, C.P. (1997). Comparable studies of the incidence of stroke and its pathological types: Results from an international collaboration. *Stroke, 28,* 491–499.

Susser, M., & Levin, B. (1999). Ordeals for the fetal programming hypothesis. *British Medical Journal, 318,* 885–886.

Taket, A. (1986). Accidents in children, adolescents, and young adults: A major public health problem. *World Health Statistics Quarterly, 39,* 232–256.

Taylor, P. (1984). *Smoke ring: The politics of tobacco.* London: Bodley Head.

Taylor, R. (1993). Non-communicable diseases in the tropics. *Medical Journal of Australia, 159,* 266–270.

Thomas, D.B., & Karagas, M.R. (1996). Migrant studies. In D. Schottenfeld & J.F. Fraumeni (Eds.), *Cancer epidemiology and prevention* (pp. 236–254). New York: Oxford University Press.

Tripathy, B.B., & Samal, K.C. (1997). Overview and consensus statement on diabetes in tropical areas. *Diabetes/ Metabolism Review, 13,* 63–76.

Tunstall-Pedoe, H., Kuulasmaa, K., Mahonen, M., Tolonen, H., & Ruokokoski, E. (1999). Contribution of trends in survival and coronary-event rates to changes in coronary heart disease mortality: 10 year results from 37 WHO MONICA project populations. *Lancet, 353,* 1547–1557.

Vaira, D., Holten, J., Menegatti, M., Gatta, L., Ricci, C., Ali, A., Landi, F., Moretti, C., & Miglioni, M. (1998). Routes of transmission of *Helicobacter pylori* infection. *Italian Journal of Gastroenterology and Hepatology* (Suppl. 3), S279–S285.

Vita, A.J., Terry, R.B., Hubert, H.B., & Fries, J.F. (1998). Aging, health risks, and cumulative disability. *New England Journal of Medicine, 338,* 1035–1041.

Willett, W.C. (1998). Dietary fat intake and cancer risk: A controversial and instructive story. *Seminars in Cancer Biology, 8,* 245–253.

World Bank. (1993). *World development report 1993: Investing in health.* New York: Oxford University Press.

World Cancer Research Fund/American Institute for Cancer Research. (1997). *Food, nutrition, and the prevention of cancer: A global perspective.* Washington, DC: American Institute for Cancer Research.

World Health Organization. (1984). Road traffic accidents in developing countries: A report of a WHO meeting. WHO technical report series 703. Geneva, Switzerland: Author.

World Health Organization. (1993). *Manifesto for safe communities: Safety—A universal concern and responsibility for all.* Resolution adopted at the First World Conference on Accident and Injury Prevention, Stockholm, Sweden, September 1989.

World Health Organization. (1994). Essential drugs for cancer chemotherapy. *Bulletin of the World Health Organization, 72,* 693–698.

World Health Organization. (1998a). *The world health report 1997: Conquering suffering, enriching humanity.* Geneva, Switzerland: Author.

World Health Organization. (1998b). *The world health report: Life in the 21st century—A vision for all.* Geneva, Switzerland: Author.

World Health Organization. (1999). *WHO Programme on cancer control: Developing a global strategy for cancer.* Geneva, Switzerland: Author. http://who-pcc.iarc.fr/ Publications/Publications.html.

World Health Organization Study Group. (1990). Diet, nutrition, and the prevention of chronic diseases. WHO Technical Report Series 797, 161a. Geneva, Switzerland: World Health Organization.

Yang, G., et al. (1997). *Smoking and health in China: 1996 national prevalence survey of smoking patterns.* Beijing: China Science and Technology Press.

Zwi, A.B., Msika, B., & Smetannikov, E. (1993, January/ February). Causes and remedies. *World Health, 1,* 18–20.

# CHAPTER 7

# Mental Health

*Mitchell G. Weiss, Alex Cohen, and Leon Eisenberg*

Although mental health has now just begun to receive appropriate attention commensurate with the enormous impact of mental illness in low- and middle-income countries, until recently it has been little more than a footnote to the broader discussion of international health priorities. This chapter reviews key concepts and issues in psychiatry, psychiatric epidemiology, and mental health as they apply to international health. Conditions in low- and middle-income tropical countries are analyzed, identifying issues with particular impact on indigenous peoples and special populations, such as women, children, older adults, and minorities. After discussing mental health-related mortality from suicide, the chapter reviews key categories of mental disorders (schizophrenia, mood and anxiety disorders, substance abuse, and disorders in childhood and adolescence) and their contribution to the global burden of disease in low- and middle-income countries.

Because questions about diagnosis, classification, and assessment have been predominant influences in the fields of psychiatry and psychiatric epidemiology since the 1960s, the framework and orientations of the diagnostic systems of the American Psychiatric Association (APA) and the World Health Organization (WHO) for the classification of mental disorders are discussed. Attention to international and cross-cultural differences has also focused on the importance of local meanings of mental disorders as a complementary consideration to diagnostic assessment. The chapter therefore examines the impact and promise of cultural formulation in clinical practice and development of a cultural epidemiology concerned with the experience of illness, its meaning, and related risk and health-seeking behaviors, which complement the standard approach to psychiatric epidemiology.

Recognizing distinctive historical influences and ecological settings that affect life and health in many low- and middle-income tropical countries, the chapter considers the impact of colonial history and various ways that tropical diseases affect mental health. The impact on mental health of major social changes, such as urbanization and migration, and the impact of war and violence, which are all accompanied by a set of intense experiences with important effects on mental health, are discussed. The chapter concludes with a review of approaches used by international and local agencies to prevent and treat mental illness and to promote mental health, citing examples of specific policies and programs.

## BURDEN OF MENTAL DISORDERS

Recent developments in the assessment of global disease burden have underscored the im-

Support of the Swiss National Science Foundation (grant # 32-51068.97) to the first author, and secretarial assistance of Cornelia Naumann are gratefully acknowledged.

portance of mental disorders and stimulated re-examination of international health priorities. Notably neglected in the past because of their limited mortality, recent accounts indicate more clearly than ever the relatively high burden of mental disorders and related conditions. A recent assessment of disability-adjusted life years (DALYs) lost in different regions for various diseases, conditions, and injuries has upwardly revised the burden of disease in low- and middle-income countries attributable to neuropsychiatric conditions to 10.5%, with an additional 1.5% attributed to intentional self-injuries, including suicide (Figure 7–1). Corresponding figures in high-income countries are 23.5% for neuropsychiatric conditions and 2.2% for intentional self-inflicted injuries (WHO, 1999a). Age-specific figures illustrate the relative scope of the problem even more dramatically. Five of the 10 leading causes of disability in low- and middle-income countries among persons 15–44 years old are mental health and behavioral problems (Murray & Lopez, 1996). Unipolar major depression is the leading cause of disability, accounting for 9.9% of all DALYs in this age group. All together, these five conditions account for almost 22% of all DALYs in the most productive years of life (Table 7–1). Projections from analysis of the global burden of disease suggest that mental disorders will increase as the epidemiologic health transition continues; they will account for 15% of the disease burden worldwide by the year 2020, with unipolar major depression becoming the second-ranked cause of lost DALYs.

Although the burden of mental illness is enormous, attention to mental health policy in international health planning often falls far short of needs, an especially tragic state of affairs because many mental disorders are now treatable. The full extent of the shortfall is difficult to assess because international databases do not show the percentage of national health budgets devoted to mental health services. Neither WHO nor the World Bank keeps track of these data. Low- and middle-income countries in Asia, Africa, South America, and the Western Pacific do not have the resources—neither the facilities nor trained personnel—to provide even basic psychiatric services (Desjarlais, Eisenberg, Good, & Kleinman, 1995). In the face of competing priorities, effective advocacy has more successfully focused the attention of policy makers on infectious and chronic diseases. Other factors, such as stigma, disinterest of international donors, and the failure to appreciate the value and potential impact of effective mental health policy and programs on health promotion and illness prevention, continue to play a role in maintaining the relative inattention to mental health on the global health agenda.

The impact on international mental health priorities that has resulted from innovations in assessing the global disease burden with DALYs highlights the significance and potential impact of better data on mental health morbidity. It is important to note, however, that the recent attention is not the result of new data or any particular epidemiologic study, but rather interpretation of existing data viewed through a new lens, constructed with indicators that account for disability as well as mortality (see Chapter 1). Various landmark studies in psychiatric epidemiology had previously demonstrated the scope of mental illness, but it had been difficult to present the findings from such research in a convincing enough manner to draw the attention of international public health policy makers. WHO's International Pilot Study of Schizophrenia, launched in 1967, was conceived with that aim, as a component of a long-term program in psychiatric epidemiology to provide morbidity data to guide planning and evaluation of mental health services. It developed the Present State Examination and used it for the 12-site collaborative study (WHO, 1979).

Motivated initially by the need for data to fill gaps identified in the report of a 1978 President's Commission on Mental Health, the NIMH (National Institutes of Mental Health) Epidemiological Catchment Area (ECA) Program in the United States studied a broader set of mental disorders among nearly 20,000 persons at five sites. Using the Diagnostic Interview Schedule,

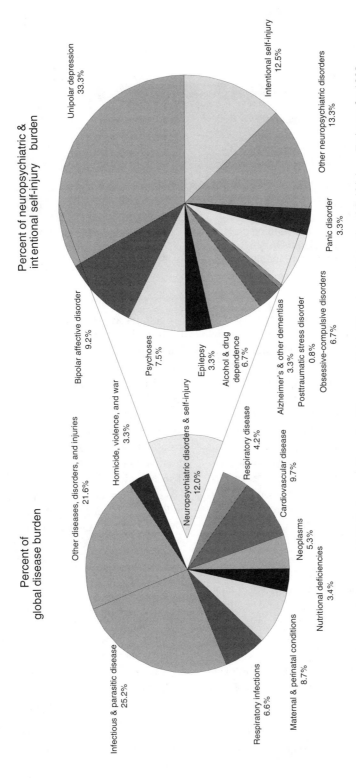

**Figure 7–1** Burden of Disease in Low- and Middle-Income Countries: Neuropsychiatric Disorder and Intentional Self-injury, Estimate for 1998

**Table 7–1** Ten Leading Causes of DALYs Lost at Ages 15–44 Years in Developing Regions, 1990

| Rank | Disease or injury | Number (in thousands) | Total DALYs |
|---|---|---|---|
| | All causes | 357,437 | 100.0% |
| 1 | Unipolar major depression | 35,398 | 9.9% |
| 2 | Tuberculosis | 19,451 | 5.4% |
| 3 | Road traffic accidents | 14,321 | 4.0% |
| 4 | War | 12,382 | 3.5% |
| 5 | Iron-deficiency anemia | 12,033 | 3.4% |
| 6 | Self-inflicted injuries | 12,004 | 3.4% |
| 7 | Violence | 11,448 | 3.2% |
| 8 | Bipolar disorder | 10,948 | 3.1% |
| 9 | Schizophrenia | 9,514 | 2.7% |
| 10 | Alcohol use | 9,371 | 2.6% |
| | Total DALYs from 10 leading causes | 146,870 | 41.1% |
| | Mental health-related DALYs (shaded) among 10 leading causes | 77,235 | 21.7% |

Note: DALY = disability-adjusted life year.

it examined the prevalence, incidence, and use of health services for specific mental disorders in the general population. Regier and Burke (1995) review the methods employed in the ECA study and other major population studies of mental disorders in Europe and North America.

Among the landmark studies in Africa and Asia, a collaboration between the Aro Hospital for Nervous Diseases near Abeokuta, Nigeria, and Cornell University studied psychiatric disorders among the Yoruba people. It set out to compare the occurrence of mental disorders affecting people in African and Euro-American cultures, integrating sociocultural and epidemiologic aims and methods. Predating the development of criteria-based diagnoses and structured interviews in psychiatric epidemiology, it based diagnoses on the descriptive accounts in what then was the current American diagnostic manual, DSM–II *(Diagnostic and Statistical Manual of the American Psychiatric Association*, 2nd edition). Psychiatrist interviewers were encouraged to use their clinical judgment and pursue interesting leads or unclear statements. The research methods were adapted from experience in previous research conducted by the investigators in a Canadian community, the Stirling County Study (Leighton et al., 1963).

Carstairs and Kapur (1976) studied mental disorders in a coastal community of Karnataka State, India. Rather than taking the more common path of adapting an existing instrument from Europe or North America, they developed and pilot-tested a new instrument, the Indian Psychiatric Schedule. Like Leighton and Lambo, Carstairs and Kapur were interested in cross-cultural comparisons and were especially attentive to questions about the cultural validity of such epidemiologic comparisons.

WHO is currently initiating a new series of studies through an International Consortium in Psychiatric Epidemiology, under the banner of the World Mental Health 2000 Survey. This population-based survey is examining the epidemiology of mental disorders in the context of general health problems in more than 10 countries throughout the world. With 5,000 interviews planned for each country, it will produce the most comprehensive psychiatric epidemiologic database of its kind, assessing mental and chronic physical disorders, health status and disabilities, risk factors, treatment, and adverse consequences of mental disorders. Improved estimates of the global burden of mental disorders, an expected result, should provide a useful baseline for regional comparisons, changes over time, and assessing the impact of mental health programs (Üstün, 1999). Research examining the effectiveness and cost of particular interventions and control approaches is also needed, given the often precarious balance of needs and available financing. Cowley and Wyatt (1993) suggest an approach to calculating the cost and benefits of psychiatric treatment with reference to DALYs lost to schizophrenia or bipolar disorder and gained from treatment.

Although the epidemiology of mental disorders and computation of DALYs provide important indicators of the magnitude of suffering arising from impaired mental health and useful data for evaluating the effectiveness and economics of program strategies, they do not tell the whole story. In addition to the defined burden specified by DALYs, which account for age of disease-related death or disability (keeping in mind that disease refers here also to mental disorders, other conditions that are not strictly diseases, and injuries), other aspects of the burden are especially important in assessing the suffering arising from mental illness. WHO strategy for improving the mental health of underserved populations also recognizes an *undefined burden* and a *hidden burden*. While the defined burden refers to effects on the person identified with a mental disorder, the undefined burden acknowledges the emotional and socioeconomic impact on the family, community, and all those affected by the impaired social role imposed by the disorder. The hidden burden arises from the humiliation, isolation, and social consequences, such as unemployment, that may result from stigma and human rights violations. The distinctive social contexts of many indigenous populations and effects on their mental health are indicated in Exhibit 7–1.

## MAJOR MENTAL DISORDERS AND ASSOCIATED PROBLEMS

This section reviews the major mental disorders and associated problems of relevance to low- and middle-income countries.

## Suicide

Suicide, the taking of one's own life intentionally, is a major public health problem. The *World Development Report* (World Bank, 1993) estimated that 818,000 persons committed suicide in 1990, accounting for about 1.6% of total world mortality. WHO projections for the year 2000 estimate there will be approximately 1 million suicides and 10–20 times that number of attempts. More people die from suicides than in all the world's armed conflicts, and the number is about the same or a little more than fatalities in road traffic accidents. Suicide is among the three leading causes of death in the 15–35-year-old age group in all countries reporting to WHO. Although it predominated in the past among older adults, suicide now occurs more among younger people in one-third of countries (WHO, 1999b).

Reported rates vary by age and sex. Thus, U.S. data for 1996 cite an overall rate of 10.8 (per 100,000)—4.0 for women and 18.0 for men. The rate for white males was 19.1, for black males 11.8, and for Native American males 20.0. Male death rates for suicide were 22.0 between ages 15 and 24; 25.0 between ages 25 and 44; 22.6 between 45 and 64; and they rose steadily after age 65 to 28.0 from 65 to 74, 45.0 from 75 to 84, and to 63.0 for those 85 and older. Rates for females varied relatively little over the life span, so that with increasing age, female rates are an ever smaller fraction of the total (National Center for Health Statistics, 1998).

U.S. data are cited here because they are among the most accurate population-based statistics. Even so, official data almost certainly significantly underestimate actual rates because suicide is so stigmatized that family members often enlist the cooperation of their physicians to conceal its occurrence in a relative. The fact that suicide is illegal in some countries and requires medico-legal documentation and processing provides incentives to police and government health workers to classify suicides as accidents. As expected, active surveillance typically shows higher rates than passive reporting in the same region. Attempts at suicide are esti-

**Exhibit 7–1** Mental Health of the World's Indigenous Peoples

Indigenous populations, numbering 5,000 to 6,000 distinct groups with 250 million persons, are found throughout the world. These diverse peoples include Amerindians of the Western Hemisphere, Pygmies of central Africa, the Maori of New Zealand, scheduled tribes of India, and the Saami of northern Europe. Relatively little research has focused on their mental health, but what is known points to high rates of various neuropsychiatric and behavioral problems. Throughout the Western Hemisphere indigenous peoples suffer from high rates of alcoholism and suicide. By no means a local problem, the same can be said of the peoples of the Pacific Islands, northern Russia, and the aboriginal population of Taiwan. Disturbingly similar processes of dislocation, epidemics, depopulation, and subjugation put indigenous peoples throughout the world at high risk of depression and anxiety. Poor health status and lack of access to public health programs and medical care are likely contributors to high rates of epilepsy and mental retardation among indigenous peoples. Despite common problems, because their cultures, histories, social organizations, political contexts, and lifestyles differ markedly, generalizations about the mental health problems of indigenous peoples are often misleading.

Case studies are particularly informative, especially when the findings apply to a large group. Australian aborigines are a particularly good example; their plight illustrates the mix of unique features and common problems that also apply for other indigenous peoples. The census of 1991 estimated that the aboriginal population (including the people of Torres Strait) totaled 265,458, about 1.6% of the Australian population. On all socioeconomic indicators, they were clearly disadvantaged. Their unemployment rate (more than

30%) was 2.6 times higher than in the general population; their household income levels were lower; they were less well educated; and nearly one-third lived in overcrowded housing conditions. Aborigines were markedly overrepresented in the criminal justice system, as indicated by statistics for arrest and imprisonment. Measures of health status reflected similar disparities. Infant mortality rates among aborigines were 3 times and age-specific mortality rates were between 2 and 7 times higher than those of the general population; life expectancies were much shorter (17 and 15 years less for men and women, respectively) (Swan & Raphael, 1995). In addition, aborigines suffered from significantly higher rates of such diseases as diabetes, respiratory disorders, hepatitis B, and sexually transmitted infections.

These conditions—in addition to a history of colonization and loss of land, high levels of domestic violence, sexual and physical abuse, child abuse, and forced family separations—have made grief and trauma central experiences of aboriginal life (Hunter, 1997; McKendrick, Cutter, Mackenzie, & Chiu, 1992). High levels of substance use, especially alcoholism, contribute to social malaise (Cawte, 1991; McLaren, 1995), and suicide rates are high among male aboriginal youth (Clayer & Czechowicz, 1991; Hunter 1991a, 1991b). Not surprisingly, a 1995 report concluded that mental health was a major problem in most aboriginal communities: although available data were limited, rates of depression, suicide, nonfatal deliberate self-harm, trauma and grief, substance abuse, domestic violence, and child abuse rates appeared to be quite high generally. A shortage of services amplifies the impact of these problems (Swan & Raphael, 1995).

mated to be 3–10 times higher than completed suicides; because there is no official requirement for reporting attempts, estimates are extrapolations from local studies.

In the United States and other industrial countries, completed suicides are 3 to 4 times more common among men than women, although at-

tempts are far more common among women; men employ more lethal methods. In contrast, suicide rates are higher in women in Southeast Asia, compared with other regions, with pesticide ingestion a major mode in rural areas.

The case of the People's Republic of China (PRC) is particularly instructive. Data on suicide were not reported to WHO during the 1970s and 1980s. Suspected suicides were investigated by the police rather than the health department; to the extent that any data existed, they were in police files. It was dangerous to inquire too closely about suicide data, because suicide was "politically incorrect." Suicide was believed to reflect social pathology, and because such pathology had been abolished by the socialist revolution, it was regarded as a criticism of the political order. Some U.S. health workers, sympathetic to the goals of the PRC, issued reports on the abolition of suicide, an absurd contention.

In 1989 the Chinese government began to release figures on suicide. It is now acknowledged to be a major public health problem. Because China does not have an integrated national death registration system, calculation of deaths by cause are extrapolations from population-based samples. Among the 39 countries that provide suicide rates to WHO, China has the second highest rate for 15- to 24-year-olds and the third highest for those age 65–74 years. There are more female suicides; rural rates are three times urban rates. Although China is the only country reporting higher female than male rates, other countries in the region report male/female ratios approximating unity, in contrast to the threefold higher rates for males in industrialized countries. The *Global Burden of Disease* study by Murray and Lopez (1996) estimates that 56% of all female suicides in the world in 1990 occurred in China. Phillips, Liu, and Zhang (1999) estimate that suicide rates for women under 45 are 40% higher than those for men, particularly in rural areas, whereas the male/female ratio is about equal for those over 45. Suicide rates among older adults are very high.

Although some believe that there is a "cultural proclivity toward suicide" among Chinese, much lower rates in Taiwan, Hong Kong, and among the Chinese in Singapore make it clear that whatever the "cultural proclivity," psychosocial and socioeconomic factors must be significant modifiers. Western psychiatrists believe that suicide most often results from mental ill-

ness, because it is known that suicide rates are elevated among patients with affective disorders, schizophrenia, and substance abuse. In contrast, mental health professionals in Southeast Asia regard suicide primarily as a social problem. In the absence of data for the years before 1987, it is difficult to ascribe the high rates to recent social changes in the PRC.

Articles in the Chinese popular press associate suicide with major economic losses for individual families, with increasing rates of infidelity and alcohol abuse, rapidly increasing cost of health care, migration from the countryside to the city, and the increasing gap between high- and low-income people. Phillips et al. (1999) suggest that five interacting factors are at work: (1) the cultural acceptability of suicide as a solution for certain problems, (2) social circumstances that increasingly place individuals in morally ambiguous and socially constrained positions, (3) a high prevalence of mental disorders that limit individuals' ability to adapt to stress, (4) access to convenient and effective methods of suicide, and (5) the lack of suicide prevention services.

In Micronesia, Polynesia, and Melanesia, suicide has reached almost epidemic proportions in adolescent males, among whom suicide has become the leading cause of death (Rubinstein, 1995). In Truk, Micronesia, rates in the 1980s among 15- to 24-year-old males reached more than 200 per 100,000. (The comparable U.S. rate was 23.) These suicides appear to represent a response to untenable social conflict under conditions where there are few traditional modes of resolution. The younger generation has become alienated at a time when the development of a wage economy has eliminated traditional men's organizations that provided an outlet for diffusing intrafamilial authority conflicts. The explanation within the culture is that the adolescent who is socially withdrawn commits an ambivalent suicide reflecting both his despair and his wish to correct strained social relations.

In Sri Lanka, national rates of suicide are high, in contrast to previously low rates in the

1950s; the profound violent social upheaval in that country is a likely explanation. Terrorist groups glorify suicidal self-destruction in pursuit of political goals; many of the young people recruited into terrorism routinely carry cyanide amulets to commit suicide, should they be captured. In a study of suicides among a population in a resettlement program, analysis of individual suicides identified personal reasons, such as infidelity, shattered romance, and poverty as common causes.

In the past, culturally sanctioned forms of suicide in India included the self-immolation of Hindu widows and religious suicides at the end of life. The ancient practice of a virtuous widow, cremating herself on her husband's funeral pyre, came to be known as *sati*; it was believed to confer merit on the widow, her deceased husband, and family. Many accounts indicate, however, that this practice was not always voluntary. The burden of the widow to the family, the benefits of pilgrimage to the site of a sati, and a desire to control the deceased husband's property offered incentives that explain accounts of various degrees of coercion, including murder, of the burdensome widow. Although the practice is now illegal and widely condemned, in the late 1980s after a widely reported instance, some conservative politicians condoned the practice. More recently, in November 1999 another possible case in Uttar Pradesh sparked similar controversy. Even when the act was "voluntary," the motivation to become a sati undoubtedly reflected the misery a woman could expect from life as a widow, a socially stigmatized identity for many of the diverse peoples of India.

To the extent that suicide is explainable as stemming from psychopathology, it highlights the needs for mental health professionals to intervene early. It is essential for effective community programs that health workers be trained to identify relevant local risk factors, typical themes, and stresses associated with suicidal behavior. Insofar as depression is the key intervening mechanism, treatment can be decisive. One outcome of a program in Gotland, Sweden, that

educated general practitioners in the recognition and treatment of depression was a lowering of suicide rates (Rutz, von Knorring, & Walinder, 1992). There is also a need for effective health education measures disseminated through the mass media to advise the population of the transient nature of many self-destructive impulses and the benefit from available services.

Because the social contexts of suicide differ dramatically from one community to another, regional centers for suicide research should be established to study the factors associated with variation in rates. Interdisciplinary field studies are essential to identify relationships among suicidal behaviors, cultural beliefs, and sociopolitical environments. Programs to increase the equality and autonomy of women can be expected to reduce suicide rates in China. Restricting access to handguns could substantially reduce homicide as well as suicide. In agricultural societies, where lethal insecticides are the most common method for suicide, research to develop less toxic alternatives must be undertaken. Health education for clinicians and workers should ensure that expertise and antidotes are available to respond to ingestions as promptly and effectively as possible. One reason for the high lethality of insecticide ingestion in rural communities is the lack of access to emergency poison treatment centers.

## Schizophrenia

The schizophrenias are a group of severe mental disorders that first appear in late adolescence or early adulthood. In every society, it is highly stigmatized whatever theories people hold about its causes. In some societies, madness is thought to be contagious or inherited. Patient and family may be shunned; chances for marriage, not only for the patient but also for siblings, are limited. Stigma leads to isolation and neglect. Patients are often hidden, to avoid shaming the family; others are institutionalized under deplorable conditions—sometimes caged in groups, without clothing, on starvation rations.

According to Kramer (1989), there were about 23 million persons with schizophrenia in the world in 1985, 75% in the low- and middle-income countries. By the year 2000 projected demographic profiles suggest that the absolute number in these countries will have risen by 45% as a consequence of the increase in the number of persons living into the age of risk (between 15 and 45).

In an acute presentation of schizophrenia, the manifest clinical signs and symptoms include delusions (false beliefs), hallucinations (disembodied voices or visions), jumbled and incoherent thoughts, a mood out of keeping with thoughts, and lack of insight about being ill. The patient's strange and excited behavior is often disruptive and disturbing to the community. In chronic schizophrenia, the "positive" symptoms of the acute syndrome (delusions and hallucinations) are replaced by "negative" symptoms (underactivity, apathy, lack of drive, and social withdrawal).

Brief reactive psychosis, which can mimic an early presentation of schizophrenia, is a transient disorder with good prognosis, sometimes difficult to distinguish from an organic mental disorder in patients with an acute medical condition. Because of the importance—and difficulty—of distinguishing schizophrenia from acute and transient psychotic disorders, the ICD–10 of WHO requires that delusions, hallucinations, and other symptoms be present for a minimum of one month to make a diagnosis of schizophrenia. In DSM–IV of the American Psychiatric Association (1994), continuous signs of disturbance must be present for at least 6 months. Thus, patients whose symptoms remit before the end of the 6-month period would be classified as schizophrenic by ICD–10 but not by DSM–IV. Evidence suggests that the ratio of brief reactive psychoses to schizophrenia is greater in some low- and middle-income societies than in Europe and North America.

Prevalence estimates of schizophrenia in low- and middle-income countries vary from study to study. Epidemiologic research in Europe shows a more restricted range of prevalence from 2.5 to 5.3 per thousand. The most comprehensive study undertaken in China reported a point prevalence of 6.06 per thousand in urban and 3.42 per thousand in rural areas. With a population of 1.1 billion and a rural to urban ratio of 3:1, the reported prevalence leads to an estimate of 4.5 million people with schizophrenia at any given time. Less than 2% are hospitalized in China's 414 psychiatric hospitals; about 3.4% live on their own; less than 4% can be found in prisons, in nursing homes, or on the streets. More than 90% live with their families, more than double the percentage who do so in the United States (Phillips, Pearson, & Wang, 1994). However, social changes in China over the past several decades (smaller families, reduced availability of free health care, greater competition for jobs, and the greater value given to personal autonomy) are making it increasingly difficult for families to cope with patients with schizophrenia at home.

In Europe and North America, schizophrenia is more prevalent in lower socioeconomic classes. Most investigators have concluded that this disparity among the low-income people, in cities, and among some immigrant populations results from "drift" down the social ladder because of psychopathology rather than "stress" as a cause of the illness (Dohrenwend et al., 1992). However, research provides strong support for the hypothesis that social and cultural factors affect the course and prognosis (rather than the cause) of schizophrenia. A chronic course of schizophrenia is less common with schizophrenia in low- and middle-income countries (Figure 7–2). A WHO (1979) team carried out a 2-year follow-up study of patients with schizophrenia in nine countries. Outcome varied enormously. Two years after the first treated episode, 58% of patients were reported to be recovered in Nigeria and 50% in India, compared to only 8% in Denmark. These findings were surprising because schizophrenia has been regarded as a chronic illness with severe, persisting symptoms that decline over time. Comparability of samples was immediately suspect.

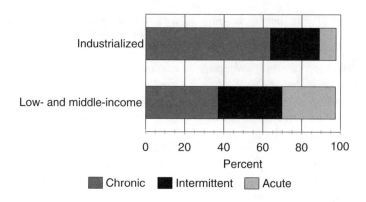

*Note:* Chronic—one or more episodes with incomplete remission in between; intermittent—partial remissions with no further episodes. acute—full remission, no further episode. Both total less than 100% because some patients could not be classified chronic, acute, or intermittent.
Low-income sites: Agra, India; Cali, Colombia; and Ibadan, Nigeria
Industrialized regions: Aarhus, Denmark; London, England; Moscow, Russia; Prague, Czechoslovakia; and Washington, DC, United States.

**Figure 7–2** Course of Schizophrenia in Low- and Middle-Income and Industrialized Countries, 1993

To investigate possible sources of variation in outcome, WHO launched a second international study that used more rigorous diagnostic criteria and obtained a more complete sample of first admission cases at all sites. Results were similar (Jablensky et al., 1992).

How might social and cultural factors influence the course of mental illness? First, beliefs about the cause and course of schizophrenia held by members of a society or group within that society, including mental health professionals, strongly influence their response to people who are ill and influence the way patients view their illness (Waxler, 1979). Where such illness is considered an essential part of the self that cannot be expected to change (for example, "*the* schizophrenic" as opposed to "the person *with* schizophrenia"), it is more likely to be chronic. In contrast, beliefs that the ill person is possessed by spirits that can be exorcised presume that recovery is possible and will occur.

Second, extended families in many countries can provide a supportive environment to lessen the severity of mental illness (El-Islam, 1982). The impact of the extended family, however, is far from uniform across societies, and all families are not necessarily supportive of a mentally ill member.

Third, a difference may exist in how improvement is evaluated in different environments. Families living under the conditions of extreme poverty and lacking access to health services may readily decide that an ill member is not in need of care. Similarly, strained health services likely exhibit a tendency to have a relatively low threshold of "no problem," when there are overwhelming numbers of patients waiting to see a mental health worker.

Fourth, severity of illness seems to be linked to work environments and level of involvement in the wage economy. Greater opportunity for patients to engage in meaningful labor in some nonindustrial countries can contribute to better outcomes (Warner, 1985).

Finally, characteristics of treatment settings, as well as specific treatments, can influence outcomes both negatively and positively. Prolonged hospitalization in understaffed large institutions interacts with the schizophrenic disease process to produce a *social breakdown syndrome* that is no less devastating than the disease itself (Gruenberg, 1967). Mental health systems may have a financial stake in maintaining a population of patients (for example, the old state hospital) rather than promoting empowerment and independence. A large census means more jobs in the hospital. Psychosocial interventions may also inadvertently produce dependency. Basic research on treatment settings and mental health policy is essential if we are to socially design more effective systems for promoting recovery.

Despite the evidence supporting the belief that the outcome for schizophrenia is better in low- and middle-income countries, methods employed in these research projects have been questioned (Cohen, 1992; Edgerton & Cohen, 1994; Hopper, 1991). The International Pilot Study of Schizophrenia (IPSS) was hospital-based and subject to sample bias. A number of sites in the determinants of outcome in severe mental disorders (DOSMD) study experienced difficulties in identifying all first-incident cases of schizophrenia in the designated catchment areas, which also suggests the possibility of sample bias. Subsequent statistical analysis suggested that center groupings not strictly defined by "developed" vs. "developing" interact with other variables, raising questions about the predictive validity of this variable (Craig, Siegel, Hopper, Lin, & Sartorius, 1997). The reliability of informants' abilities to reconstruct and accurately report the course of illness has also been questioned (Pulver & Carpenter, 1983; Raphael, Cloitre, & Dohrenwend, 1991).

More fundamentally, direct observation of the relevant sociocultural environments was not undertaken in either IPSS or DOSMD. Thus neither study provides systematic evidence regarding the cultural factors that putatively impel persons with schizophrenia toward better outcomes. One study by El-Islam (1982) demonstrated a better outcome for persons with schizophrenia if they were members of an extended family. The data suggested, however, that these better outcomes resulted more from extended families effectively monitoring medication regimens than providing psychosocial supports.

## Mood (Affective) Disorders

*Bipolar affective disorder* (manic-depressive disorder) is characterized by recurrent episodes in which the patient's mood, energy, and activity are markedly disturbed, at times toward elation and overactivity (mania) and at others toward lowered mood and decreased energy (depression). Mood states are usually alternating or mixed, but bipolar disorder must be differentiated from mania without a previous depressive episode. Manic episodes are characterized by elevated mood, varying from carefree joviality to uncontrollable excitement, accompanied by incessant talking, decreased sleep, and loss of normal social inhibitions. It may be accompanied by delusions and hallucinations. Acute manic episodes can be halted by neuroleptic drugs; the likelihood of recurrence is diminished by maintenance lithium treatment. The lifetime prevalence of bipolar disorder is estimated at 1.3%, affecting men and women equally and with age of onset at the end of the second decade.

Unipolar major depression is mood disorder that can occur as a single episode in a lifetime (uncommon) or as one of many episodes (most common). Depressive symptoms are an unavoidable aspect of everyone's life at various times. A major depressive episode—more intense, distressing, and characterized by a constellation of symptoms well beyond the normal range of emotional experience—is another matter. Major depression is characterized by sadness or diminished pleasure in daily life and involves a number of additional symptoms, such as weight change, disturbed sleep patterns, fatigue, feelings of worthlessness and self-blame, diminished ability to concentrate, indecisiveness, and changes in motor patterns (retardation or agitation). Patients with major depressive disorder or bipolar disorder suffer intense emotional and physical anguish; the illness disrupts their ability to function in family, job, and social life. The worst consequence of depression is suicide. It is estimated that between 40–70% of all suicide victims in the United States suffer from major depression. The onset of unipolar major depression is in the mid-20s, and lifetime incidence is estimated at 16.1%; it affects about twice as many women as men. A less intense chronic depression (dysthymia) is characterized by the persistence of symptoms over several years. More than twice as many women are affected, and it continues to increase up to age 65.

Whereas schizophrenia is a "low-prevalence, high-severity" disorder, depression is more typically characterized by high prevalence and moderate severity (Eisenberg, 1992). For example, the 1-year prevalence of depression was 10 times higher than that for schizophrenia in one large U.S. population study. Surveys of patients attending primary health care clinics in sub-Saharan Africa and in Latin America indicate that depression is the principal or a contributing reason for seeking care in as many as one-fifth to one-third of cases (Üstün & Sartorius, 1995); these findings are similar to those from North America and Europe (Goldberg & Huxley, 1992). In the aggregate, depression produces far more morbidity than schizophrenia. Because suicide is a far greater risk in depression, depression has a greater impact on premature mortality. Although we lack comparable mental health economic estimates in low- and middle-income countries, in the United States depression resulted in a cost to the nation in 1990 of about $44 billion, about the same as that resulting from heart disease; it accounted for about 30% of the total cost of all mental illness in that year (Rice, Kelman, & Miller, 1991).

It is widely believed that rates for depression have been increasing in the United States, western Europe, Puerto Rico, Lebanon, and Taiwan in recent decades; depression is now seen at younger ages and in greater frequency. How social experiences are transformed into psychopathology is unknown, although urbanization, changes in family structure, and poverty have been postulated to have a role (Cross-National Collaborative Group, 1992). Some researchers maintain, however, that the apparent increases in rates of depression are artifacts of methodological problems, primarily the reliance on cross-sectional studies to reconstruct lifetime prevalence of depression in different cohorts (Simon et al., 1995).

## Anxiety Disorders

Anxiety disorders are subclassified into panic disorder, phobias, obsessive-compulsive disorder, generalized anxiety disorder, and posttraumatic stress disorder. Epidemiologic studies in Latin America have identified a high prevalence of anxiety disorders, with an excess of cases in lower socioeconomic strata. A census of the mental health status of villagers in the area of Sao Francisco, Bahia, Brazil, reported a 14% prevalence for anxiety disorders; rates in women were twice as high as those in men (Almeido-Filho, 1993). Highly prevalent idioms of distress—"nerves" (*nervios*) or "attacks" (*ataques*), for example, in Hispanic cultures, or elaborate somatic idioms ("heart distress" in Iran, the "fatigue and dizziness" characteristic of "neurasthenia" [*shenjing shuairuo*] in China)— make direct translation of categories across cultures difficult (Kleinman & Good, 1985).

*Panic disorder* is marked by episodes of intense fear and discomfort, which occur unpredictably and for no apparent reason, and which last for minutes to hours; it includes additional symptoms, such as shortness of breath, dizziness, palpitations, tremor, sweating, and often a fear of dying or "going crazy." *Agoraphobia* is present if the patient is fearful of being in situations where escape would be difficult in the event of panic; as a result, the person is unable to leave home or is able to leave only if accompanied. *Social phobia* is a persistent fear of particular social situations (such as speaking in public, eating, or writing when someone is looking) because of the anticipation of embarrassment and humiliation. So persistent is the fear that the need to avoid such exposure interferes with work and social activity. *Specific phobias* (formerly known as simple phobias or isolated phobias) are uncontrollable fears of particular stimuli, such as dogs, snakes, insects, blood, or heights.

*Obsessive-compulsive disorder* is characterized by intrusive, distressing, and senseless thoughts (obsessions) and by behaviors (such as hand washing) that are repetitive, illogical efforts to ward off misfortune through ritualized performance (compulsions). The obsessions and compulsions are distressing to the affected persons, who recognize at some point that they are excessive and unreasonable, and who may also try to suppress or neutralize such thoughts and impulses. The disorder is moderately responsive to cognitive behavioral therapy and psychotropic drugs.

*Generalized anxiety disorder* is manifested by motor tension and overactivity of the autonomic nervous system (shortness of breath, palpitations, dry mouth, dizziness). Symptoms include constant fears and worries about impending misfortune in the absence of a visible threat. Lifetime prevalence rates for generalized anxiety disorder vary from 5–12% in urban and rural communities in Taiwan and from 5–10% in regions of the United States (Compton et al., 1991).

Anxiety disorders can have serious effects on social function, work, personal well-being, and use of health services. Agoraphobia can make someone housebound. If panic disorder is missed by the doctor, fruitless medical test procedures, risky and ineffective treatments, and frustration can result. With proper diagnosis and treatment, psychopharmacologic agents and psychotherapy have been shown to be effective in treating anxiety disorders. Many of these problems are less likely to come to the attention of psychiatrists or other clinicians in resource-poor settings, where the existence of services to treat these disorders, if available, may not be widely known. For example, in Nepal most people first seek the help of *jhankris*, or traditional healers, for anxiety disorders.

*Posttraumatic stress disorder* (PTSD) is a persistent response (often after a delay) to a catastrophic experience. Distress is common among all victims subjected to overwhelming experiences (for example, earthquake, flood, war, or torture) but in PTSD persists long after the event and interferes with function in some of those who have been exposed. Typical symptoms include flashbacks and bad dreams, numbness and blunting of emotional responsiveness, detachment from other people, and avoidance of activities and situations that reawaken memories. There is usually a state of autonomic hyperarousal, hypervigilance, an enhanced startle reaction, and insomnia. PTSD is commonly described among victims of natural or manmade disasters. PTSD is recognized as a disorder with characteristic features arising in response to trauma. It is not the only response to overwhelming trauma, however; depression or other mental disorders may also result.

### Substance Abuse

Substance abuse is a serious source of morbidity and mortality the world over. The 1993 World Development Report estimates that alcohol-related diseases affect 5–10% of the world's population each year and account for about 2% of the global burden of disease. Firm data on heroin and cocaine abuse are not available, but their effects are devastating. The most lethal of the addicting substances is tobacco, which exacts an enormous and growing toll by inducing cancer, progressive respiratory impairment, cardiovascular disease, and stroke (see Chapter 6).

The profits to be made from the sale of licit drugs (alcohol and tobacco) and the criminal industry providing illicit drugs (heroin, cocaine, and the like) rival oil and automotive industries, while expenditures on education to prevent use and treatment for addicted persons are trivial by comparison. Beyond its effects on morbidity and mortality, substance abuse tears at the social fabric of communities. Government functionaries and police officials can be regularly corrupted by criminal bribes. At a national level, the use and sale of both illicit and licit substances have produced substantial and alarming levels of violence in many Latin American countries, such as Colombia and Mexico.

Substance use occurs in a social context in which it is legitimized and, for most users, effectively governed by cultural norms. Use becomes abuse when the user is unable to fulfill social and work roles, suffers medical consequences, experiences drastic physical and psychological symptoms on withdrawal, and is unable to stop seeking the drug despite knowing its harmful effects. Because the term *abuser* stigmatizes the victim, WHO emphasizes dependence and its health consequences to highlight the relevant medical issues. The APA's DSM–IV considers dependence to be a more severe condition than abuse, classifying both as disorders of substance use.

Drug abuse increases during rapid social destabilization, particularly in the case of adolescents and young men moving from traditional village settings to urban environments. Culture shock, conflict, value loss, and marginality frequently result as family ties weaken. Drugs are available and offer a temporary "escape" from the despair of daily life.

### Alcohol Abuse

The countries of Africa, Asia, and Latin America constitute the fastest growing import region for both hard liquor and beer, representing one-fifth to one-quarter of global import totals. The effects of alcohol on the user range from disinhibition and relaxation to a sequence of maladaptive behavioral changes, including aggression and violence in some, and depression, slurred speech, stupor, and incoherence in others. Prolonged and excessive drinking gives rise to delirium tremens, hallucinations, and psychotic states. Persons with alcohol dependence or alcohol-related problems suffer from a range of physical and mental problems. For example, a study in primary care settings in Nigeria found that such persons had relatively high rates of mental disorders, used health care facilities more often, and were more likely to be separated, divorced, or widowed (Abiodun, 1996).

Culture can be important to control overuse. Traditional Chinese culture emphasized social drinking and discouraged solitary drinking.

Drinking occurred almost exclusively with meals; ritual toasting at dinner tables promoted bonds of friendship. In the past it was believed that alcoholism was nonexistent among Chinese, but new data indicate a steadily increasing prevalence in urban areas with much lower rates in the countryside. A Beijing Medical University study found alcohol abuse rates of 6.61% in urban and 0.83% in rural areas (Shen, 1987). In Africa the breakdown of traditional village life has been accompanied by the commercialization of beer production. It is different from social drinking in the past, which typically occurred in small groups with the host fermenting a home brew. Loss of social controls increases rates of alcoholism.

Alcohol abuse not only has medical consequences for the user but serious repercussions on others in the community. It also contributes to traffic accidents, violence, suicide, and homicide (for example, Hunter, 1991a, 1991b). Alcohol is responsible for more violent behavior, most notably wife battering, than any other drug. Research among the Inuit of Baffin Island, for example, shows that problems of assault and sexual abuse of women were often associated with alcohol use (Abbey, Hood, Young, & Malcolmson, 1993).

### Cocaine, Heroin, and Other Abused Substances

The use of cocaine and heroin has serious health and social consequences. Because drug abuse occurs covertly and is illegal, treatment is usually delayed. Users run a risk of death from overdose, infection, violence, sexually transmitted infection, and circulatory and respiratory diseases as a direct consequence of use. Intravenous drug use carries a high risk of infection, both bacterial and viral, and is second only to sexual activity as the route of transmission of HIV infection. The cardiotoxic effects of cocaine are a leading cause of sudden death. Heroin users are vulnerable to sudden death from intravenous use, sometimes because of miscalculating the dose, but also from deliberate poisoning by the supplier (who increases purity covertly) to punish an addict thought to be revealing information to the police.

The abuse of licit drugs, notably psychoactive drugs, through inappropriate prescription practices and the street sale of illegally obtained prescription medication, has been a problem since the introduction of such drugs. In earlier years it was principally connected with the use of barbiturates and opioids, but it has since spread to include benzodiazepines and other psychoactive drugs. Most recently, the overprescription and the overuse of serotonin uptake inhibitors (such as fluoxetine) has been a topic of much contention, given the readiness of some physicians to prescribe antidepressants for inappropriate indications. In more affluent societies, anabolic steroids are also abused by young people who take them to enhance muscle development and athletic performance. Inhalant use (gasoline, paint thinner, industrial glue) is an important problem in many low- and middle-income communities in South America among adolescents and young adults. Habitual inhalation causes severe damage to the central nervous system, liver, bone marrow, and kidneys.

In the debate on controlling substance abuse, opinions are polarized between those who emphasize reducing supply and those who advocate efforts to reduce demand. Control of supply has proven to be remarkably ineffective as well as very costly. In addition to the necessity of maintaining armies of law enforcement agencies, attempts at control often lead to corruption of local governments, because producers bribe officials. Criminalization of drug use leads to the incarceration of anyone caught in possession of drugs, both sellers and users alike. The result is an ever-growing prison population in the United States (more than 2 million at last count). Because the drug trade is one of the few lucrative options available to many low-income populations, subsistence farmers may often turn to growing illegal crops.

The United Nations estimates that about 8 million people use heroin each year. Of the illegal drugs, it leads to the highest known mortality and the most emergency room episodes (United Nations International Drug Control Program, 1997). The goal of treatment is to overcome dependence and enable users to be reintegrated into society. While direct detoxification is possible, this is rarely successful. Methadone maintenance markedly damps the response to heroin, greatly reduces illicit drug use, and improves health and social behavior. The experience with daily oral administration of methadone in countries that can support such programs has made it the treatment of first choice for stabilization (Bammer, Dobler-Mikola, Fleming, Strang, & Uchtenhagen, 1999).

Legalization of substances of abuse, such as heroin and cocaine, has been proposed as a way to reduce criminal sanctions and thus social cost. Such proposals arouse strong political, legal, and social concerns. For example, would legal availability result in increased use? There is no clear answer to that question. In countries where relatively adequate treatment services and social supports exist, such as the Netherlands, legalization of access to drugs at regulated sites has not been accompanied by an epidemic of use. In England heroin prescription in an overall context of prohibition has been legal for decades, although controversial. Overprescribing by some practitioners contributed to the rise of a black market, which ultimately led to restrictions in 1968, whereby specialized clinics were established and prescribing rights were limited to selected doctors. Experience with heroin distribution programs in Switzerland, as reported from a series of studies comprising the Swiss National Cohort Study of more than 1,000 heroin-dependent individuals in 17 clinics and a prison, has also been positive (Uchtenhagen, 1998). Other experience in Geneva, however, was not fully consistent with these optimistic findings; it was unclear whether substantiated benefits resulted from methadone itself or from the intensive medical and psychosocial services that were also made available to the study group. Improvements in work, housing, physical health, and lessened use of other drugs, as reported in the National Cohort Study, were not found in the Geneva study (Rusche, 1999).

However controversial and complex the situation reflected by European experience may be, the questions become even more difficult when policy makers try to generalize from such experience in small, wealthy European nations to large, heterogeneous low- and middle-income countries in other parts of the world. Historically, colonial administrations focused on regulating supply, an especially controversial policy in a setting where the motives of the regulators and their regard for the population were questionable (Saldanha, 1995). The effect of industrialization, urbanization, and environmental changes on the increasing rates of substance abuse, especially as it affects particularly vulnerable populations, such as child laborers (Saldanha, 1995), reflects distinctive social issues that receive too little attention (Bansal & Banerjee, 1993). Health policy and substance abuse in India has focused on "de-addiction" and the physiology of drug dependence; more attention is needed to the social contexts and behavioral dimensions of demand.

In industrialized countries as well, emphasis on demand reduction by the treatment and rehabilitation of drug users is honored more in rhetoric than practice. For example, in the United States, despite widespread governmental condemnation of drug abuse, no administration has ever provided sufficient funds to treat more than a fraction of the users willing to enter treatment. The relatively small allocation of resources to services for treatment and prevention is remarkable, a sharp contrast to the huge investment in attempts at controlling supply, even though such attempts have been clearly ineffective.

Interventions to reduce substance abuse and dependence that focus only on treating individuals are unlikely to be effective (Currie, 1993), especially in low- and middle-income countries where the cost of treating individuals is difficult to bear. Policy formulations and empirical research must be directed at the complex economic and social forces that support the initiation and maintenance of substance abuse. Little progress can be foreseen without confronting of the underlying social and economic factors and pertinent processes of development and social change, human rights, and local cultural values.

## Disorders in Childhood and Adolescence

As already indicated, neuropsychiatric disorders secondary to central nervous system malfunction (such as epilepsy) are more common in low- and middle-income countries because of the increased prevalence of complications of pregnancy and parturition, bacterial and parasitic infections of the brain, and malnutrition sufficient to hamper brain development. They also have a worse prognosis than in industrialized countries because of limited access to treatment. On similar grounds, one would expect higher rates of learning disabilities, but they become evident only where schooling is available and sufficient numbers of students are enrolled to detect them. Consequently, in many low- and middle-income countries, meaningful data on the prevalence of learning disorders are not available because of limited access to education. The same is true for other child psychiatric disorders; few cases are registered officially because of the paucity of services. Obtaining sound data on the prevalence of child psychiatric and adolescent disorders in the community remains a challenge in middle- and high-income countries, as well.

Roberts, Attkisson, and Rosenblatt (1998) have reviewed more than 50 epidemiologic studies carried out over the past 4 decades to estimate the overall prevalence of child and adolescent psychiatric disorders. Most studies have been undertaken in the United States and the United Kingdom, some in Europe and Asia, and only a handful in low- and middle-income countries. The most prominent finding is that methodologic difficulties continue to plague child psychiatric epidemiology.

The robustness of prevalence estimates has been sharply limited by problems with inadequate sampling methods and limited sample sizes, with inconsistencies in case ascertainment and in case definition from one study to another, and with lack of uniformity in data presentation and analysis. Reported figures range from less than 5% to almost 50% (with a mean of 16%). From the studies they included in their survey, Roberts et al. (1998) computed the following median rates: 8% for preschoolers, 12% for preadolescents, and 15% for adolescents.

The few studies in low- and middle-income countries report highly variable rates: 29.0% for the Sudan (Rahim & Cederblad, 1984); 6.1% for Malaysia (Kasmini et al., 1993); and 8.3% (Wang, Shen, Gu, Jia, & Zhang, 1989), 7.0% (Matsuura et al., 1993), and 17.3% (Ekblad, 1990) in several studies in the PRC. Given the wide range of uncertainty surrounding all these estimates, meaningful cross-country comparisons are not possible.

## CLASSIFICATION AND ASSESSMENT OF MENTAL DISORDERS

Diagnostic categories used by mental health professionals indicate how they and society think about mental illness. The way mental disorders are defined and classified is a matter of fundamental importance for psychiatric epidemiology and public health. Efforts to advance the mental health of populations rely heavily on data from diagnostic assessment and the power of epidemiology to interpret those data. The utility of the diagnostic process on which epidemiologic studies are based requires confidence in the validity of the categories of disorder that are being counted and analyzed. The classification and assessment of mental disorders have in recent years become predominant concerns for the field.

Various challenges, both from outside and within psychiatry, motivated mental health professionals to focus on the development of new systems of classification for psychiatric disorders and to consider questions about the validity and the reliability of assessment. Leaders in the field regarded this as an essential task, required

for progress and to maintain psychiatry as a medical specialty. Although the discipline had become fragmented in the 1960s by competing theoretical orientations—biological, psychodynamic, behavioral, and social—a degree of rapprochement to guide practice and research was achieved by George Engel's (1977) biopsychosocial model. Speaking as a psychiatrist, he convinced medical colleagues that psychiatry had something to offer them and facilitated reintegration of psychiatry and medicine. Contributing to the development of psychiatric epidemiology, comparable advances resulted from addressing fundamental questions about the classification of mental disorders, the validity of diagnostic categories, and efforts to achieve reproducible assessment. Criteria-based diagnosis as a standard facilitated development of large population studies of the epidemiology, determinants, and related features of mental disorders. The new framework also brought fundamental changes to the practice of clinical psychiatry, substantial enough that many characterized them as a paradigm shift (Rogler, 1997).

### Development of DSM–III and ICD–10

Efforts to construct a more scientific foundation for psychiatry made the 1970s a period of ascendancy for psychiatric epidemiology. This discipline also benefited from advancing technologies in other fields, such as educational testing, statistics, and development of high-speed computers, which made it possible to work with multivariate statistical analyses of large samples. As diagnostic reliability became imperative, the kappa statistic developed by Joseph Fleiss (Fleiss, Spitzer, Endicott, & Cohen, 1972), which compares the assessment of two raters and corrects for chance agreement, provided a better way to assess interrater reliability, which helped to further improve the diagnostic process by highlighting problems in achieving reliable assessment.

The new approach to diagnosis, developed in the 1970s and controversial at first, relied on specific diagnostic criteria. Inclusion and exclusion criteria replaced the descriptive accounts of diagnostic concepts, published in WHO and APA manuals, based on clinical impressions and ideas about diagnostic entities that clinicians constructed in the course of training and practice. This new diagnostic approach was embodied in the APA's *Diagnostic and Statistical Manual of Mental Disorders, Third Edition* (DSM–III) in 1980. With further refinement in subsequent revisions (DSM–III-R in 1989 and DSM–IV in 1994) (see APA, 1994), and subsequently incorporated in WHO's *International Classification of Diseases, Tenth Edition* (ICD–10) (see WHO, 1992), first published in 1992 (Rogler, 1997; Klerman, 1983), this approach became firmly established as a standard in the field.

Identifying the three components of this process helps to explain the nature and significance of these developments. First, it was necessary to *clarify the ideal of a valid diagnosis*. Acknowledging their limitations, guidelines conceived originally for schizophrenia were generalized to provide an approach for examining the validity of a broad range of diagnostic categories. These guidelines were considered by some to represent an ideal, unachievable in practice, but they served to stimulate further thinking and research on validity and reinvigorated psychiatric epidemiology (Robins & Barrett, 1989). Eventually the focus on schizophrenia and the presumption of its hereditary basis limited the usefulness and application of these guidelines. Even for schizophrenia itself, efforts to find biological criteria capable of informing clinical practice have consistently fallen short of expectations.

Second, *development of diagnostic criteria* became a priority, so that a clinician or researcher could determine whether someone's condition fulfilled criteria for a diagnosis. Efforts to advance this agenda also began with a focus on schizophrenia, producing the so-called St. Louis Research Criteria (also known as Feighner Criteria) (Feighner et al., 1972). An expanded set of categories, which included affective (now called mood) disorders, followed in

the Research Diagnostic Criteria (RDC) (Spitzer, Endicott, & Robins, 1978). The DSM–III included diagnostic criteria for a much expanded collection of disorders.

Third, *instruments and methods were developed for systematic assessment* of patients in the clinic and of individuals in the community, with reference to diagnostic criteria and systematic methods to ensure the reliability of diagnosis, based on interrater agreement. The Renard Diagnostic Interview was used to diagnose patients with reference to the St. Louis Criteria. The Schedule for Affective Disorders and Schizophrenia (SADS) was used for assessing patients with reference to RDC criteria, and a variation of the SADS that queried lifetime occurrence of symptoms (SADS-L) was used for community studies. Among the diagnostic instruments that were developed for DSM and ICD, a subset was intended for use by experienced clinicians to assess patients (Structured Clinical Interview for DSM, and Schedules for Clinical Assessment in Neuropsychiatry [SCAN]). Others were more highly structured diagnostic instruments for use by lay interviewers to determine the epidemiology of mental illness in the community (Diagnostic Interview Schedule, and Composite International Diagnostic Interview [CIDI]); data were based on direct responses to questions, because these interviews aimed to eliminate the need for interviewer judgments about symptoms that require clinical experience. Development of these instruments also benefited from experience in the WHO International Pilot Study of Schizophrenia with the Present State Examination (PSE). That too was a criteria-based diagnostic instrument, but the specific criteria were embedded in a complex computer program known as CATEGO, which lacked the transparency required for review, critique, and development of the criteria. Now that criteria-based diagnosis is an established standard, however, such transparency is essential, and an unspecified computer program is no longer accepted uncritically as authoritative.

It was an explicit aim of DSM–III to avoid endorsing any particular theoretical orientation, wherever possible, either biological or psychological. The manual concerned itself with mental *disorders* (based on demonstrable distress, functional impairment, or imposition of risk) instead of considering mental *diseases* (based on elusive pathology). This reorientation provided a rational basis for systematic assessment—considering the presence, severity, duration, and context of symptoms. Innovations and changes introduced as new features of DSM–III have been retained in the current version (DSM–IV) and were to a greater or lesser extent also incorporated in ICD–10. These new features included explicit inclusion and exclusion criteria for most disorders; attention to the validity of disorders; a multiaxial approach that also considers social stressors and level of functioning; and an emphasis on descriptive accounts rather than the psychodynamic theory as the framework for classification, which excluded some time-honored concepts, like *neurosis*, and reformulated others, like *hysteria*.

These new features reflected an agenda set by the chair of the DSM–III Task Force, Robert Spitzer, to rethink the psychiatric nosology and shift the orientation from its Freudian psychoanalytic focus on the structure of the mind and unconscious motives, drives, and other mental or emotional processes, collectively known as psychodynamics. In its place, following the teachings of Emil Kraepelin, the new framework regarded mental disorders as analogous to physical diseases. Careful observation of psychiatric symptoms—that is, psychopathology—and an empirical approach were advocated as the best way to learn about mental disorders. The task force gave priority to inputs from research over experience from clinical practice (Bayer & Spitzer, 1985).

The impact of the American DSM–III was dramatic in the United States and throughout the world. The manual or its abridgement was translated into more than a dozen languages. The interim revision in 1989 (DSM–III-R) and full revision in 1994 (DSM–IV) maintained the basic style and underlying conceptual framework and attempted to incorporate updates based on the promised validation studies of diagnostic disorders. DSM–IV called on the contributions of a more elaborately structured task force and 13 working groups.

The influence of DSM–III and IV on international psychiatry is also reflected in WHO's ICD–10, which incorporated criteria-based definitions of diagnostic categories. It developed an abbreviated multiaxial system, considering contextual factors that may influence the diagnosis, treatment, or course of mental disorders on Axis III (Janca, 1997). Several versions of ICD–10 have been published to serve different constituencies, one with clinical descriptions and diagnostic guidelines, another with diagnostic criteria for research, and a third for use in primary care. Field trials evaluated the categories of ICD–10 in 40 countries and the text of the published version, with acknowledgments listing contributions from 32 countries.

## Cultural Critique

Although the DSM–III was produced primarily for use in psychiatry in the United States, international experience with it has stimulated some of the most useful commentary and critique. N. N. Wig, a leading figure in Indian psychiatry with extensive experience in other low- and middle-income countries, discussed some of the contributions and shortcomings, providing a "third-world view," in *International Perspectives on DSM–III* (Wig, 1983). Although every country has its own distinctive cultural and historical traditions, he pointed out that many low- and middle-income countries in Africa, Asia, and Latin America share limitations in the mental health component of their health systems as a result of limited economic resources. He emphasized the need in such settings for a simple, unbiased, and clinically relevant system to guide mental health services, but he also recognized the need to remain within and benefit from the body of research and advances of international psychiatry. Managing the distinct, and sometimes competing, priorities of each constitutes a difficult dilemma for many psychiatrists and mental health workers in low- and middle-income countries.

Reliance on field trials to guide revisions and the introduction of a multiaxial system were both welcome innovations, but the sheer bulk of the manual and complexity of some categories seemed too cumbersome for practical application. Somatization Disorder, for example, requires a minimum of 14 symptoms for women and 12 for men among a list of 37. Some of this complexity, including criteria for that disorder, has been reduced in the revisions, but other problems remain. Paradoxically, Wig found the diagnostic criteria both a strength and a weakness. He suggested that the imposing structure of the manual may fix ideas about psychopathology prematurely without conveying the tentativeness of the categories. Despite its assertions to the contrary, the DSM has been used like a textbook, and it has clearly inspired and influenced the style of other textbooks. "One feels that whatever has been neatly put down in the form of crisp criteria is absolute truth. The criteria, however, are seldom more than a crystallization of clinical knowledge accumulated to date" (Wig, 1983, p. 82). Both the ICD and the DSM acknowledge this point, but vigilance among users is required nevertheless.

Another serious problem resulted from the failure of DSM–III to consider any role for culture, an omission the task force developing DSM–IV subsequently attempted to address. Wig pointed out:

> Many of the current criteria of DSM–III, as would be expected, are based heavily on American experience, which in many cases is not universal. Examples given in the clinical descriptions and criteria are often so culture bound that they provide only poor guidelines for use in developing countries. This is perhaps an inherent problem in modern psychiatry—wherever knowledge of a biological base for a disorder is weak, the diagnostic descriptions or criteria become highly culture-specific (Wig, 1983, p. 83).

The value of the section on childhood mental disorders was felt to be especially compromised by the culture-bound formulation of categories and examples. The section on organic mental disorders required such a specific reference to a known organic condition as the source of symptoms that it could not be readily applied for many patients presenting with a fever, and for whom one could only speculate about the contribution of a medical illness. Spitzer responded to this point by suggesting that although it may compromise the desired goal of supporting exclusive categories—inasmuch as *delimitation from other disorders* is a criterion for the validity he advocates—it may be advisable to specify when it was thought an organic condition may play some role, even though uncertain.

The category of Brief Psychotic Disorder, as it has been reconceptualized in the DSM–IV, appears to address Wig's concerns about the earlier formulation. The more recent criteria permit a time course of one day to one month, which better fits the clinical experience of Asian and African practitioners, and permit specification of stressors or postpartum onset. Because so many patients in primary care appear not to have an organic basis for their somatic symptoms, somatoform disorders are a very important category (Üstün & Sartorius, 1995). For these disorders the nature of the symptoms and the organization of symptom categories require more careful consideration. Recent research highlights the nature of this persisting problem for both DSM–IV and ICD–10 (Janca & Isaac, 1997).

Wig's discussion indicates how the choice of symptoms acknowledged and emphasized by a health or diagnostic system reflects cultural and historical values. International psychiatry represented in the DSM and ICD manuals, which to some extent is a product of European cultural history, has elevated the status of depression and anxiety. Other emotions, however, emphasized in other cultural histories may also be distressing and could as well have served as a focus of clinical attention, as they do in some traditional medical systems—emotions such as anger, greed, jealousy, hate, and eroticism. If clinical experience in India had the same impact on the international psychiatric nosology as did experience in Western Europe, then the current emphasis on depression might have been replaced by somatization. Instead of the masked depression that has figured prominently in clinical reports in nonindustrialized practice settings, perhaps the field might instead have elaborated a notion of masked somatization to characterize clinical patterns of common disorders in western European and North American psychiatry. Such a masked somatization would account for patients whose emphasis on emotional symptoms and absence of somatic pains would be at odds with expectations from clinical experience in India, Africa, and other non-industrialized settings. Research findings lend credence to such speculation (Weiss, Raguram, & Channabasavanna, 1995).

## Local Meaning of Mental Disorder

The diagnoses presented in ICD–10 and DSM–IV represent professional formulations of mental disorders. It might be asked how these compare with the way people with mental illness, their families, and others in their communities think about these problems that so profoundly affect their lives. Because the professional nosologies do not address that question, what frameworks are available to communicate and compare local views of impaired mental health? Several key concepts in medical anthropology and cultural psychiatry elaborate the distinction between local and professional concepts of sickness and health (Table 7–2). It has been especially useful to distinguish the insider and outsider perspectives and to specify the difference between illness and disease. The explanatory model framework has also stimulated considerable research and influenced clinical practice, although it is now often replaced by more specific concepts focusing on illness experience, causal explanations, and illness behavior in a broader context of illness representations.

Kenneth Pike formulated the concept and advocated the terms *etic* and *emic* to distinguish the outsider and insider points of view. An *etic* orientation specified a descriptive or analytic framework based on concepts coming from *outside* the local social system under consideration. An *emic* orientation emphasized concepts that either originated locally or were introduced from the outside and acquired substantial local meaning *within* the social system; it is the insider's orientation (Headland, Pike, & Harris, 1990). Medical anthropologists commonly use these terms to distinguish professional and local concepts of sickness and health (see Chapter 2).

Eisenberg (1977) elaborated technical meanings of the familiar terms *illness* and *disease* to specify a similar distinction, but with a medical focus from the outset. Disease represented a professional way of looking at sickness—a way of characterizing abnormal structure or function. Illness referred to the experience of sickness according to the affected person (usually a patient in the clinic) and others in the social network affected by the problem. Psychiatric illness provided relevant examples to show how clinicians had a responsibility to address illness in the absence of disease, even though medical training usually emphasizes disease with less attention to illness. The distinction between illness and disease has become a linchpin in the foundation of medical anthropology. It has also helped to clarify implications of the social construction of mental illness and the way ideas of both patients and clinicians influence the course and outcomes of illness (Eisenberg, 1988).

The illness explanatory model has been described as "notions about an episode of sickness and its treatment that are employed by all those engaged in the clinical process" (Kleinman, 1980). The term was introduced to bridge the interests of psychiatry, medicine, and medical anthropology, providing a framework to motivate culturally sensitive clinical practice

**Table 7–2** Orientations to Sickness and Health

| Local | Professional |
|---|---|
| *emic* | *-etic* |
| Illness | Disease |
| | |
| Health/help seeking | Treatment delay |
| Illness behavior | Treatment plan |
| | Compliance/adherence |
| | |
| Explanatory model | Psychopathology |
| Cultural model | Diagnosis |
| Illness experience | Etiology |
| Causal explanation | |
| Illness representation | |

and clinically sophisticated anthropological research. When Kleinman elaborated the concept, it encompassed: "(1) etiology; (2) time and mode of onset of symptoms; (3) pathophysiology; (4) course of sickness . . . and (5) treatment" (Kleinman, 1980, p. 105). Some researchers and the text of the cultural formulation for DSM–IV, however, have emphasized a narrower view of the explanatory model, focusing on causal attribution, the first of the five aspects of the broader concept. Some medical anthropologists refer to *causal explanations* to specify this aspect of the explanatory model. The term *illness experience* has come to specify more precisely the broader scope of the illness explanatory model framework, and the idea of *illness representations* has provided a useful overarching framework for health research.

**Clinical Cultural Formulation**

Despite the undeniable importance of its contribution and the considerable appeal of its innovations, DSM–III was deeply flawed as a guide for international psychiatry, especially in low- and middle-income countries. Wig's balanced critique made this point. The parochial emphasis on a middle-class, majority-culture subset of Americans of European origin provided examples too constricted for psychiatric practice in other countries, and for psychiatric practice in the multicultural environment in much of

North America as well. Recognizing this problem, when charged to produce a revision, the DSM–IV Task Force tried to correct these shortcomings by constituting a Committee on Culture and Diagnosis. The committee was asked to advise on diagnostic categories and criteria, provide accounts of cultural features of many disorders, and develop an appendix that included guidelines for a cultural formulation and a glossary of culture-bound syndromes. Psychiatrists and social scientists on the committee also contributed to a section on cultural issues for DSM–IV in the DSM–IV source book (Widiger et al., 1997, sec. VI, chs. 41–56).

The cultural formulation listed below was probably the committee's most significant contribution to DSM–IV. It provided a needed framework for dealing with questions of culture, social class, and minority status—issues that because of prior neglect had diminished the credibility of the field. The following are the key points of this cultural formulation:

- cultural identity of the individual
- cultural explanations of the individual's illness
- cultural factors related to psychosocial environment and levels of functioning
- cultural elements of the relationship between the individual and the clinician
- overall assessment for diagnosis and care*

This outline of cultural formulation, though inadequate according to leaders in cultural psychiatry (Kleinman, 1997), has had substantive impact (Rogler, 1996) and has provided a framework for training programs, case conferences, and research (Mezzich, 1995).

**Validity**

Among the three tasks that were priorities for developing psychiatric epidemiology—validating specific mental disorders, creating diagnostic

*\*Source:* Data from American Psychiatric Association, *Diagnostic and Statistical Manual of Mental Disorders, 4th Edition,* © 1994, American Psychiatric Press.

criteria, and developing instruments for assessment—the first remains the most problematic today. The dilemma of cultural validity makes it even more vexing for international and cross-cultural interests. Much of the literature in psychiatric epidemiology concerns itself with questions of minimizing diagnostic error, but this assumes confidence in the validity of the disorder accepted as a reference point. Even if one were confident of the biological basis of mental disorders, one could not assume they would be precisely revealed by symptomatology. Emil Kraepelin, who defined the concept of dementia praecox that influenced the later formulation of schizophrenia, himself made this point:

> We must seriously consider how far the phenomena on which we normally base our diagnosis really do afford insight into the basic pathological process. While it may be admitted that this procedure is generally valuable, there is a fairly extensive area in which such distinguishing criteria are lacking: either they are insufficiently well marked or they are unreliable (Kraepelin, 1920).

The current criteria-based nosology defines disorders by the coherence of symptom patterns. Insofar as the declared successes of the field trials for the DSM and the ICD refer primarily to the ability of investigators to agree on diagnostic assessment, they did not resolve questions about the validity of the mental disorders. Reliability of assessment does not ensure the validity of a disorder. Psychiatric epidemiologists and statisticians recognize that overzealous efforts to improve reliability may actually diminish the validity of a criteria-based disorder:

> Validity might actually worsen as reliability improves. One might, for example, make the criteria for a given diagnostic category so limited but so precise that interexaminer agreement on presence versus absence is excellent, but the patients one ends up with as cases of that disorder are atypical

of the population of cases (Fleiss & Shrout, 1989, p. 279).

DSM–IV, renewing the promise of the previous edition to validate categories of disorder with research, outlined indicators of the validity of diagnostic categories in the introduction under the heading "limitations of the categorical approach." People with the same diagnosis should be a homogeneous group; their diagnosis should be clearly distinguishable from other diagnoses, and their diagnoses should be mutually exclusive. Family history and laboratory verification in the Robins and Guze (1970) criteria were too closely linked to organic hypotheses and technical limitations to retain (Table 7–3). The manual acknowledges that the categories of DSM–IV disorders fell short of the ideal:

> There is no assumption that each category of mental disorder is a completely discrete entity with absolute boundaries. . . . There is also no assumption that all individuals described as having the same mental disorder are alike in all important ways. . . . Individuals sharing a diagnosis are likely to be heterogeneous even in regard to the defining features of the diagnosis (APA, 1994, p. xxii).

If the influences of history, culture, environment, medical illness, and other localizing features are also accounted for, expectations for the validity of mental disorders defined solely by their symptomatology must be even more modest. Recognition and acceptance of the need for periodic revisions of the ICD and the DSM provide a means for accommodating historical changes. These revisions should be guided not only by additional research findings, but also by acceptance that things change, and that nosology must also change. Norman Sartorius, who was director of the Division of Mental Health at WHO from 1974 to 1993, pointed out in the introduction of ICD–10 that "a classification is a way of seeing the world at a point in time." Questions about the influence of culture, environment, and other localizing features require additional consideration.

**Table 7–3** Approach to Establishing Validity of Mental Disorders

| | Indicator of Validity | Robins & Guze (1970) | Spitzer & Williams (1988) | APA (1994) |
|---|---|---|---|---|
| Clinical description | Clinical picture of the disorder with reference to its most striking features | X | X | X |
| Laboratory studies | Characteristic findings from chemical, tissue, and radiological studies | X | X | |
| Response to somatic treatment | Placebo-controlled double-blind clinical trial | | X | |
| Delimitation from other disorders | Distinctiveness of the disorder, not overlapping with other diagnostic categories | X | X | X |
| Follow-up study | Homogeneity of members of the diagnostic group, recognizing marked differences among them, raises questions about validity, but some conditions have variable course and outcome | X | X | |
| Family study | Increased prevalence among close relatives as evidence for the validity of the disorder | X | X | |

## Cultural Epidemiology

Accounting for cultural differences is not so straightforward a matter as dealing with historical changes. Periodic revisions may account for the latter, but it is less clear how to achieve the right mix of international standards and local variants. Nevertheless, that is what must be done. WHO has made considerable efforts to achieve a common language and a standard for regional comparisons (Sartorius et al., 1993). International psychiatry has a greater stake in ensuring the cultural validity of mental disorders than does any regional group; if there are questions about the coherence and validity of the categories among diverse groups to be compared across regions or in multicultural urban settings, how can confidence be placed in findings that are based on these categories, or how can these findings be used to guide mental health policy and planning? If the concepts of a mental disorder do not fit local conditions, however, how can local clinicians work with them?

Questions about the cultural validity of diagnostic concepts arose even before DSM–III appeared, based on concerns articulated by Kleinman (1977) with reference to depression and somatization. He discussed a problem he called the *category fallacy*, that is, the mistaken assumption that a clinical category that is valid or meaningful in one setting, where it may have originated, remains valid or meaningful somewhere else where it is actually understood differently or not at all. He argued that the effort to work with some professional categories of mental disorder in some settings constitutes a category fallacy. Culture-bound syndromes— that is, local patterns and concepts of illness— provide obvious examples: the dhat syndrome of South Asia (emotional and somatic symptoms attributed to semen loss) would be an unproductive focus of clinical inquiry in other places where people do not attribute such symptoms to this cause. Although the category fallacy raises questions about whether the validity of a particular concept should be accepted outside its culture of origin, questions about cultural validity apply to more subtle and more commonplace issues as well.

It is recognized that the reliability of assessment does not ensure the validity of the categories, as explained above; such caution is likely to be even more salient in international and multicultural settings where the heterogeneity of cultural differences requires more attention. How to take cultural validity into account is an open question for the field (Guarnaccia, Good, & Kleinman, 1990). Even if a concept like depression is meaningful in different cultures, there is no assurance that the symptom clusters and criteria now endorsed as diagnostic criteria apply equally well everywhere. Suppose the DSM–IV criteria for major depression is considered (namely, five of nine symptoms, including either intense sadness or loss of interest in previously pleasurable activities over a period of at least 2 weeks) as the mark of a valid disorder. *Valid,* of course, means something more than the reliability of assessment, which has been the operational standard for much research in psychiatric epidemiology. A valid category is expected to be a relevant account of the problem, meaningful in the context of psychiatric principles, or useful as a guide to clinical management and treatment—ideally, all three. Even if patients can be found in India, Tanzania, Cambodia, and Nicaragua who fulfill DSM–IV or ICD–10 criteria for major depression, it must still be asked whether some other configuration of symptom criteria for depression, which have been called "alternative criteria sets," would identify more relevant, meaningful, and clinically useful configurations locally (Spitzer & Williams, 1988).

Although depression, schizophrenia, or other disorders can be defined according to the ICD or DSM, assessing cultural validity is another matter. Local clinicians can provide valuable insights concerning the relevance, meaning, and clinical usefulness of the category specified by the international criteria. That is a first step, but systematic research is also needed to address two other sets of questions. The first set concerns whether the standard criteria are relevant, meaningful, and clinically useful in the local health system. Formulation of the outcome variables should be sensitive to local conditions, especially in low- and middle-income countries where the expense of health research without local benefit is difficult to justify. Might some other configuration of the criteria, specified with reference to the international standard, be more valid locally—perhaps fewer or more symptoms, longer or shorter duration, additional or dropped criteria? Statistical methods that examine the internal consistency of alternative configurations of symptom criteria, and the relationship between clinically significant features and outcomes with reference to the alternative configurations of categories, are appropriate. The SCAN and CIDI already provide both ICD and DSM diagnoses from the same raw data set, and identifying other alternative configurations is now technically feasible, not nearly so daunting with present-day computers as it would have been a decade ago. Such an approach, based on evaluation of the internal coherence of the concept, has been used for the development and local validation of stigma scales, recognizing that although the concept is meaningful in different settings, the indicators of self-perceived stigma and the process of stigmatization may vary across cultures (Raguram, Weiss, Channabasavanna, & Devins, 1996; Vlassoff et al., 2000).

A second set of questions concerns the local experience and meaning of specific mental disorders. The need for that is also clear; for example, in WHO collaborative studies of Somatoform Disorders, Janca and Isaac (1997) found that neither ICD–10 nor DSM–IV included culture-specific symptoms that were "important and necessary for their diagnosis in specific cultures." Perhaps more to the point, it is also evident that the local language of distress and disorder needs to be understood, so that clinicians and health workers can relate what they are taught to the problems they confront in their clinics

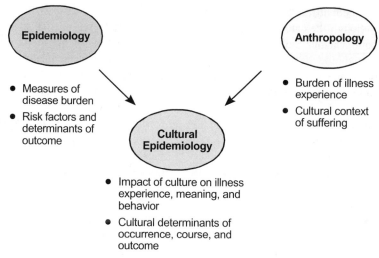

**Figure 7–3** Intregrative Framework for Cultural Epidemiology

and communities. To address these issues, knowing the best criteria set for major depression is not enough. Ethnographic research and a cultural epidemiology of illness-related experience, meaning, and behavior, ascertained with locally appropriate instruments complementing the psychiatric epidemiology of mental disorders, should also play a role (Figure 7–3).

A framework and family of interviews known as the EMIC, originally for Explanatory Model Interview Catalogue, have been developed to study illness experience (patterns of distress), its meaning (perceived causes), and associated behavior (risk related and help seeking). Variants of the EMIC have been locally adapted for research with patients, laypersons, and health care providers in India, Africa, and other parts of the world for study of mental illness and tropical medical diseases (Weiss, 1997). This research informs culturally sensitive clinical practice and mental health policy. Other approaches to cultural research are examining the interactions between biology, behavior, and culture; studies in the psychobiology of ethnicity consider how these interactions affect the choice of drugs, their side effects, safe and optimal dosing, and the diversity of psychotropic responses (Lin & Smith, 2000).

## HISTORICAL, ENVIRONMENTAL, AND SOCIAL CONTEXTS

The values and effectiveness of health systems reflect important influences of their history and structure, the impact of environmental factors (especially tropical diseases in many low- and middle-income countries), and the social processes of urbanization, migration, and war. Each plays a key role in all aspects of public health, but because the experience of mental illness and maintenance of mental health is particularly intertwined with these historical and contextual factors, they are crucial considerations for understanding the mental health of populations. Recognizing that formerly colonized countries are not wholly uniform, characteristic features of colonial history that explain how mental health services developed as they did are examined below; in addition, the ways in which environmental and social contexts continue to exert their influence are considered.

### Historical Priorities of Colonial Medicine

During the colonial period in the history of many low- and middle-income African and Asian countries, preoccupations with racial comparisons, geographical pathology, and global politics shaped professional views concerning the occurrence of tropical medical and mental disorders, and ideas about whom they affected. Medical authorities at the end of the nineteenth century speculated that indigenous populations were resistant to tropical diseases—such as malaria, typhoid, and yellow fever—that devastated Europeans in Africa and Asia, and Americans in the Philippines (Anderson, 1996; Harrison, 1996). Over the next 25 years, however, more careful observations showed malaria frequently affected Africans, and previous assertions that other tropical diseases spared the indigenous populations also proved to be incorrect or misleading when they failed to appreciate the effects of long-term exposure.

A similar transition took place in the clinical recognition and epidemiologic accounts of depression (Weiss & Kleinman, 1988). British psychiatrists who staffed the so-called lunatic asylums in India were struck by differences between "native" patients they were treating and European patients they had previously treated in England. A superintendent of such an institution in the Punjab, G. F. W. Ewens (1908, p. 2), explained, "Simple quiet suicidal melancholia, such as one sees so many of at home, are practically unknown here." Raymond Prince (1968) suggested four factors to explain the low rates of depression reported in Africa during the colonial period, compared with higher rates after independence, which were similar to those found in Europe and North America:

1. In Europe, depression had been thought to be a disease affecting only people who were sufficiently sensitive and intellectually aware. Those who became the subjects of colonial rule were not considered vulnerable, and the question of their having clinical depression seemed irrelevant.
2. Cultural differences in depressive symptoms, especially a preponderance of somatic presentations, produced a so-called masked depression, which was unrecognized.
3. People with depression were reluctant to come to the highly stigmatized mental hospitals, and thus psychiatrists, who were most likely to identify the disorder, did not see such patients.
4. Urbanization and other social changes in the postcolonial era may have played a role in actually increasing rates of depression.

For the colonial medical services in Asia and Africa, it was not the problems of the indigenous populations, but the psychiatric problems of Europeans that were their prime mental health concerns. Attention focused on the particular stressors routinely confronting the outsiders—adjustment, isolation, and climate—as well as the problems arising from some of the common coping strategies, such as alcohol abuse. The interactions between medical disease, psychological problems, and social context often presented a clinically challenging dilemma. For example, a condition known as tropical neurasthenia—characterized by tiredness, restlessness, irritability, and impaired concentration—was identified as an organic condition, or perhaps the effects of several organic conditions, combined with the effects of climate, social stressors, and the influence of an individual's psychological profile. Debate in the medical literature grappled with questions about the relative role of organic and psychological factors, a controversy resembling the current debate about the organic or psychological basis of chronic fatigue syndrome, neurasthenia, and myalgic encephalomyelitis. Malaria was also believed to play a role in tropical neurasthenia for many patients. According to the 1940 edition of *Manson's Tropical Medicine,* neurasthenia "has superseded tropical diseases" as a cause of disability among Europeans (Manson, 1940).

Clinical attention to the psychiatric problems and conditions of the indigenous population of colonized countries was often motivated mainly by a desire to maintain an orderly society, rather than efforts to relieve their suffering. In Papua New Guinea, for example, Goddard (1992) emphasized social control as the principal motivation of the Australian colonial administrations when they established limited mental health services at the end of World War II. Although some effort was also made to provide treatment, the structure and operation of the mental health system indicated the priorities. Admission was typically by magistrate's order, rather than a response to seeking treatment, and the institutions, which developed initially in the prison system, were used mainly for serious psychotic disorders with behavioral disturbances that might be considered a threat to others. As in other parts of the world, the structure and nature of mental health services fostered, and too often continued to perpetuate, stigma. Recognizing problems with these institutional policies and the public image of these services, and in an effort to address the issue, the term *lunatic asylum* was replaced by *mental hospital*, but in India, for example, this only came about in 1925.

## Impact of Tropical Disease Burden on Mental Health

The persisting burden of infectious diseases in societies at an early stage of the epidemiologic health transition compromises emotional well-being and the functioning of social institutions in various ways. Some of these effects are nonspecific and social, such as the emotional toll of preventable mortality and bereavement that development seeks to reduce. Others are more direct and disease-specific, such as organic mental disorders and characteristic psychological problems resulting from the emotional impact of symptoms of a medical illness or the neuropathophysiology of endemic parasitic diseases (Weiss, 1994). The higher frequency of acute brief psychosis in low- and middle-income tropical countries, compared with Europe and North America, is striking; evidence from the WHO study of the determinants of outcome of severe mental disorders suggests an association with nonspecific fevers (Collins et al., 1999). Direct effects on the central nervous system, reactiva-

tion of a latent virus, and activation of autoantibody responses have been considered as possible mechanisms. Effects of poor nutrition and trauma predisposing to both fever and psychosis have also been considered.

Malaria provides a good example of the various ways that a parasitic infection is known to affect mental health. In addition to weakness and debility from anemia in chronic malaria, several acute organic brain syndromes are also observed. These include (1) neurasthenic symptoms that may be associated with fever, (2) delirium and coma, and (3) psychosis that usually begins with paranoid or manic features and may subsequently lead to depression over time. Cerebral malaria is a major cause of acute encephalopathy in regions endemic for *falciparum* infections. In some cases, atypical because of the absence of a fever, a sudden personality change, or even disturbed behavior that brings a person to jail instead of the hospital, may lead to a fatality from untreated malaria (Marsden & Bruce-Chwatt, 1975). As is shown in Exhibit 7–2, other interests, not readily anticipated, also link malaria and mental health.

Neurocysticercosis may be the most common cause of epilepsy in low- and middle-income tropical countries. It is also responsible for hydrocephalus and other neurological and neuropsychiatric disorders. Ingestion of eggs of the pork tapeworm, *Taenia solium*, results in the deposition of larvae at various sites in the central nervous system, causing symptoms as a result of the mass effects of the lesions and inflammatory reactions that follow when the larvae within the cysts die. Although the neurological symptoms are usually prominent, psychoses resembling schizophrenia and depression, which may lead to suicide, have also been reported (Dixon & Lipscomb, 1961).

Other parasitic diseases associated with fatigue, weakness, lethargy, and inactivity include hookworm infections and schistosomiasis. Depression may be a feature of amebiasis and giardiasis. Sleeping sickness (human African trypanosomiasis, HAT) produces mood swings, mania, and depression. The onset of the charac-

**Exhibit 7–2** Malaria Therapy for Mental Illness

Malaria is a disease of special interest to psychiatry for a reason unrelated to its psychiatric morbidity; it played a key role in the work leading to the only Nobel Prize ever awarded to a psychiatrist, Julius Wagner-Jauregg. He received the prize in physiology of medicine in 1927 for his discovery that inducing fever in patients with neurosyphilis by infecting them with malaria provided an effective treatment for general paralysis of the insane (neurosyphilis). Despite some fatalities, "malaria therapy" remained the accepted treatment for this condition until the advent of penicillin (Raju, 1998).

teristic daytime drowsiness of HAT may come late in the course of the illness; the disease may also produce a wide variety of emotional and behavioral changes delaying diagnosis and treatment. Gambian HAT is more likely than the Rhodesian variety to produce emotional liability, confusion, hallucinations, and assaultive or other antisocial behavior.

Although rare, organic mental disorders have been reported for loaiasis, bancroftian filariasis, and onchocerciasis. The emotional distress, depression, and even suicidal thinking and behavior arising from the demoralizing effects of relentless itching and disfigurement of the skin from onchocercal skin disease are far more common than blindness and impaired vision in the villages of sub-Saharan Africa where onchocerciasis is endemic. The adverse emotional and social effects of onchocercal skin disease, including stigma, are closely related to fulfillment of social roles, cultural values, and gender (Brieger, Oshiname, & Ososanya, 1998; Vlassoff et al., 2000).

In recent years questions have also been raised about the role of Borna disease virus (BDV) in neuropsychiatric illness, especially mood disorders and depression. This zoonotic condition affects cattle, sheep, and other animals, producing variable behavioral disturbances suggestive of mood disorders in humans. People may be in-

fected with the virus, but infection is not clearly associated with specific symptoms. Studies suggest, however, that rates of infection are higher among people with mood disorders, schizophrenia, and possibly some neurological disorders, such as hippocampal sclerosis. Research is underway in the United States and Europe to clarify the epidemiology of BDV infection and its neuropsychiatric significance.

A study of the seroprevalence of BDV in Africa is noteworthy here for findings that people with malaria or schistosomiasis were more likely to be infected (9.8%) than controls (2.1%) (Bode, Riegel, Lange, & Ludwig, 1992). If it can be confirmed that people with chronic tropical diseases have higher rates of BDV infection, it would be reasonable to question the neuropsychiatric impact of infection and its implications for mental health. In many rural societies of low- and middle-income tropical countries where sanitation is poor, tropical diseases endemic, and people are in close proximity to animals, they may be at increased risk for zoonotic infections. This shows how particular organic causes of psychiatric morbidity may be more significant in such settings; research should consider the impact of social and tropical environmental conditions on BDV infection and its role in neuropsychiatric illness (Hatalski, Lewis, & Lipkin, 1997). The wide range of responses to infections among both animals and humans suggests that different subtypes have different effects and may also indicate the value of molecular epidemiologic research to address this question. Such considerations underscore the significance of interactions among environmental factors, genetic predisposition, social stressors, and the pathophysiology of specific infectious diseases that may account for unrecognized neuropsychiatric illness in low-income settings. Because the disability worldwide from mental disorders is so pervasive, even if only a small percentage were found to result from organic conditions that may ultimately be or become treatable, the number of people who would benefit could still be very large (McSweegan, 1998).

Greater sensitivity to the possibility of organic causes of psychiatric morbidity should be complemented by recognition of the social contexts that favor the proliferation of disease and clarification of the mechanisms by which these social factors operate. Human African trypanosomiasis is a good example. In the early 1900s the causal agent and role of the tsetse fly in transmission had become clear, but it was not until the 1960s that control measures addressing animal reservoirs, vector control, case finding, and treatment drastically reduced the impact and rates of the disease to a very low level (Lyons, 1992). In recent decades, however, poor surveillance, inadequate vector control, neglected national health programs, mass migrations of infected individuals who travel with their parasites, and social disruptions have all contributed to a resurgence of the disease, most notably in war-torn African countries such as Angola, Sudan, and the Democratic Republic of Congo (formerly Zaire) (Barrett, 1999; Smith, Pepin, & Stich, 1998).

**Urbanization**

Among all the social, political, economic, and cultural changes that have taken place in the second half of the twentieth century, the rapid urbanization of low- and middle-income countries has been extraordinary. Between 1950 and 1990 urban populations in Asia, Africa, Central and South America, and the Pacific region increased from 285 million (16% of the total) to 1.5 billion (27% of the total) (Harpham & Blue, 1995). Estimates for the year 2000 indicate that the urban residents of these regions will constitute 50% of their population, whereas in 1800 only 14% of people lived in cities (Marsella, 1995). In 1950 the populations of Mexico City and São Paulo were 3.1 million and 2.8 million, respectively, but the estimated population of each for the year 2000 was expected to reach 24 million (Desjarlais et al., 1995). In Asia the process is similar; Seoul, Teheran, Karachi, Manila, New Delhi, and Bangkok were all expected to have populations between 10 and 13.5 million by the year 2000, remarkable considering that

none of them had more than 1.5 million residents in 1950 (Hobsbawm, 1994).

Approximately 50% of urban populations in low- and middle-income countries live in extreme poverty, and of these some 100 million adults and another 80 million children are homeless (Desjarlais et al., 1995). More troubling is the fact that the disparities between high- and low-income people are widening, and poverty is becoming concentrated in the cities of low- and middle-income countries, where it is confined increasingly to low-income neighborhoods—a process that is likely to intensify social problems (Massey, 1996).

Concern about the oppressive conditions of life in cities is not new. More than 2,000 years ago Plato considered the effects of urban life to be negative. The view that urbanization engenders mental distress and behavioral problems has been a recurring theme among philosophers, such as Jean-Jacques Rousseau and Henry David Thoreau (Marsella, 1998). According to Harpham (1994; see also Harpham & Blue, 1995), urbanization takes its toll on mental health in low- and middle-income countries through increased stressors and adverse life events (for example, overcrowded and polluted physical environments, dependence on a cash economy, and high levels of violence) in combination with reduced social supports (for example, separation from partner, breakup of extended families, and separation from traditional social networks); together they contribute to increased levels of distress (Figure 7–4). The impact of urbanization in low- and middle-income countries is especially burdensome for children, women, and older adults (Blanc, 1994). The impact of traumatic life events and the role of grief from bereavement, fears, and insoluble problems arising from personal crises have been shown to account for high rates of depression among women in Harare, the capital city of Zimbabwe; this rate is twice as high as for women in London (Broadhead & Abas, 1998).

On the other hand, urban life is not all bad, and it is not invariably more stressful than living in rural areas. Orley and Wing (1979) reported rates of depression among women in

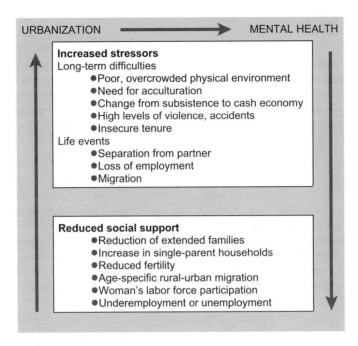

Model of social factors of urbanization in developing countries likely to affect mental health.

**Figure 7–4** Urbanization and Mental Health

rural Uganda that were higher than those in both London and Harare. In China suicide rates are higher in rural areas, especially among women (Phillips et al., 1999). Epidemiologic studies in Taiwan also indicate lower rates of depression in urban areas (Cheng, 1989; Cheng, Soong, Chong, & Lin, 1995). Cities offer more health and mental health services than rural areas. Virtually all the mental health resources in low- and middle-income countries are found in cities where there are greater economic and social opportunities for professionals.

The rural-urban comparison may itself be simplistic; each urban setting and the processes by which urbanization proceeds vary throughout the world. Factors such as environmental pollution, population density, economic opportunity, health status, health services, and social supports are distinctive in different settings (Marsella, 1998). Also, conditions that are unacceptable according to middle-class standards may be considered attractive to urban migrants from the countryside, leading to the ironic questions

raised in the newspaper article with the paradoxical headline, "Bombay needs more slums" (see Exhibit 7–3). To appreciate the problems of urbanization, attention to the specific local features of the environment, political power structures, social networks, and cultural contexts is required for useful insights to guide effective health policy. The worldwide momentum of urbanization appears to be irresistible, and the real questions concern not so much whether urbanization will continue, but how it will proceed. This is an area where government policies can make a great difference. Provision of public health services, decent housing, education, and economic opportunities can make cities habitable for all their citizens.

**Migration**

Unprecedented numbers of people are now migrating cross-nationally, and by the beginning of the 1990s approximately 100 million persons were living outside their country of

**Exhibit 7–3** We Need More Slums

According to conventional wisdom, urbanization is a process that brings with it many problems. But a more provocative, less conventional analysis suggests the slums that proliferate in urban centers, and even in smaller towns, are in fact a boon to their inhabitants and their country, however inconvenient these slums and the massive rural-urban shift may be for urban elites. An article in a Bombay newspaper, *Indian Express*, argued that slums should be looked upon not so much as problems, but rather as solutions:

For years people have been moaning and groaning about the explosion of slums in our cities. Hundreds of new rural immigrants pour every day into our big cities. They occupy public land, green spaces and pavements. They build shanty towns having no water or sanitation, which stink to the high heavens and breed bacteria in trillions. Their wretched hovels are flooded every time it rains, with refuse floating into each shanty. Their influx has brought congestion, pollution and filth on an unprecedented scale to cities . . .

All this moaning and groaning is hopelessly misguided. The urban slums of India represent a great economic and social evolution that is raising the income and social conditions of the poor on an unprecedented scale. The urban elite cannot see this evolution because it is cloaked in so much filth and excreta. But the main problem lies in the vision of the elite, not in the slums.

Who are the gainers and losers of the slum explosion? The gainers are the millions of rural poor that have flooded into cities to take advantage of higher incomes there. The immigrants also enjoy better access to medical care, education and entertainment than they would ever dream of in their villages. The caste barriers that stop the lower castes in rural areas from rising are much less evident in cities. . . .

This is not, of course, an ideal state of affairs. It would be far better if we had honest politicians, honest municipalities and honest taxpayers. In that case the elite would pay heavy taxes that would be efficiently used by politicians to create better infrastructure and amenities that would protect the urban quality of life while benefitting immigrants. But since we don't have honesty among either tax-payers, tax-collectors or politicians who dispense tax revenue, we have to look at second-best solutions. The slum explosion is one of them. . . .

We need to provide our slums with sanitation and drinking water. We need to start schools and primary health centres wherever possible. We need to create bus services for slum-dwellers. But we must not get hung up on the mere existence or proliferation of slums. Above all we must see the influx into cities as a positive sign of progress that has many more winners than losers. Let us have more slum improvement and upgradation. But above all, let us have more and more slums (Anklesaria Aiyar, 1988, p. 8).

origin. The process of migration entails considerable stress—reestablishment of social networks, reinsertion into a new socioeconomic system, and adaptation to a new culture—and the effects on mental health of so many changes and adaptations are of course complex. A suitable framework to explain and work with the effects of this process should consider several factors, such as the circumstances that brought about the migration, how the migrants are received in the host country, and the age and gender of the migrants (Beiser, Dion, Gotowiec, Hyman, & Vu, 1995; Rogler, 1994). Several examples illustrate how these factors operate.

Three migrant groups in New Zealand include Indochinese refugees, Pacific Islanders, and people from the United Kingdom. A study by Pernice and Brook (1994) found that Indochinese refugees had the highest levels of emotional distress, as measured by the Hopkins Symptom Checklist-25, a screening instrument used to detect symptoms of depression, anxiety, somatic aches and pains, and other symptoms that identify clinically significant mental health problems. Distress among the Pacific Islander immigrants was nearly as high, but although it was similar in magnitude to the refugees, it was different in character, apparently resulting from widespread racism in New Zealand. In contrast, immigrants from the United Kingdom, who had a cultural affinity for New Zealand, saw migration as an opportunity; they were not subject to discrimination, and they reported much lower levels of mental distress than either the Indochinese refugees or the Pacific Islander immigrants.

A comparison of Ethiopian and Russian Jewish immigrants to Israel provides a second example (Ponizovsky et al., 1998). If only the similarities in the cultural backgrounds of the immigrant and host country populations were considered, as indicated by the experience in New Zealand, it might be expected that Russian immigrants would have an easier time adjusting to life in Israel than Ethiopian immigrants. The Russians were well-educated Europeans with many sociocultural similarities to Israelis, whereas the Ethiopians, coming from an insular traditional African society, might reasonably be expected to find more to which they needed to adjust in a modern westernized nation. In this case, however, evidence shows this assumption to be misleading. First, although men in both groups displayed similar levels of psychological distress, Russian women were more distressed than Ethiopian women. This appeared to result from the fact that migration brought a decline in status and professional opportunities to the Russian women, whereas it brought many new opportunities for education, economic benefits, and equal rights to Ethiopian women.

Symptom profiles of distress were different in the two groups: Russian immigrants had more anxiety and hostility, and Ethiopians had more paranoid ideation. This, too, was consistent with the impact of thwarted professional aspirations and lack of opportunities for economic advancement confronting the Russians, and the marginalizing experience of the Ethiopians, as an isolated African minority living in a largely European society. Elderly persons, especially among the Russians, were more distressed than those who were younger. As time passed, distress was reduced among the Ethiopians but remained the same among the Russians. These findings indicate how the impact of migration on mental health is shaped by pre- and postmigration factors, as well as by the interaction of the cultural and socioeconomic backgrounds of the migrant groups and their host cultures.

The vast majority of people who migrate do so because of factors beyond their control (see Chapter 9). Tens of millions of people have left their native countries in search of economic opportunity only to be subjected to exploitation, inadequate living conditions, racism, and xenophobia. Between 1960 and 1992 the number of refugees from war and starvation increased almost tenfold, from less than 2 million to more than 18 million; the great majority fled from one low- or middle-income country to another. Another 20 million have been displaced within their own countries because of civil conflict or adverse effects of economic development. Given their circumstances, migrants are at increased risk of depression, anxiety, and posttraumatic stress (Desjarlais et al., 1995; Fullilove, 1996). For example, in South America economic development is forcing increasing numbers of indigenous peoples to migrate to urban areas in search of a viable livelihood. Insofar as South American societies are highly stratified and exclusionary, migration does not necessarily bring improved social well-being; more often it has resulted in displacement and uprooting of indigenous peoples, high rates of unemployment, and squalid living conditions. It has also exposed them to uncertainty and social stress in the absence of supportive social networks, which result in higher risk of acute and chronic mental disorders (Almeido-Filho, 1987; Gaviria et al., 1986).

Although stressful, migration is typically motivated by a quest for more or better opportunities, which may in fact become available. Many problems of relocation could be alleviated to some extent by appropriate supports and social services. More specialized mental health services, if they are to be effective, should require that personnel are trained to recognize and respond to the specific needs of migrant populations. Language and cultural differences may be discomforting to health professionals, whose experience in their home culture may not prepare them for the special problems of immigrants and refugees. Planning health services for immigrants requires attention to the circumstances of relocation that are quite different from the experience of the host population. Depending on the policies of the host government, immigrants may be either welcomed or admitted reluctantly with suspicion. Immigration policy may be linked closely with local and regional politics and the social and economic conditions of the host countries. Tensions between policies that emphasize hospitality and welfare, or hostility and exclusion, may reflect efforts to rationalize compassion and the strains on economic and social welfare systems already burdened by demands for limited resources. These tensions may also reflect local politics and the interplay of different ideologies.

Such tensions in host country societies and governments are likely to influence health policy. Sensitive to these conflicts, patients may be suspicious of health services, especially if they appear to function more as gatekeepers instead of health service providers. Inasmuch as mental health professionals are more likely than others in the health system to be hearing about and working with sensitive issues concerning the migration experience, they must be aware of how they and their role in the health system are perceived. The need to establish a credible, effective treatment alliance is most obviously crucial for the success of mental health services, but important for all health care providers; government policy must be sensitive to this need. Distinguishing such obligations to patients from obligations to the government and bureaucracy presents a challenge to health professionals, and quality of care often requires that they learn something about the culture of immigrant peoples, and their expectations and needs. Research

and training to upgrade professional expertise and skills are required to fulfill this obligation.

## Vulnerability and the Needs of Special Populations

Mental health and variation in the risk of mental illness reflect particular vulnerabilities and needs among various special populations. In general, as described earlier in this chapter, women throughout the world have much higher rates of depression (2 to 3 times greater) and lower risk of suicide and substance abuse than men. The higher rates of depression likely reflect socially based gender differences, rather than biologically based sex differences. Economic dependence and particular stressors at various stages of the life cycle play a role; victimization from domestic violence is a serious problem throughout the world, not just in low- and middle-income countries. Better appreciation of how emotional distress and mental illness are mediated through gender can be expected to improve the quality of health services significantly with particular benefits for mental health.

Older adults have relatively high rates of suicide and are at risk for dementia. Children in low- and middle-income countries more regularly fail to reach developmental milestones, suffer from seizure disorders (both febrile seizures and epilepsy), and manifest aggressive and antisocial behavior disorders (Desjarlais et al., 1995). Homelessness and child labor deprive many children of opportunities for education and development that leave them disadvantaged to compete in an adult world. Just as the mental health effects of migration depend on many factors, the mental health of special populations is contingent on the various social, cultural, economic, and biological environments that locally define the stressors, supports, and experience of these groups.

## War and Violence

An important book, *War and Public Health* (Levy & Sidel, 1997), recently examined the question of war from a public health perspective, considering its impact and ways the field might prevent the effects of war and war itself. In his foreword, former U.S. president Jimmy Carter summarized the impact of war:

> War and militarism have catastrophic effects on human health and well-being. These effects include casualties during war, long-lasting physical and psychological effects on noncombatant adults and children, the reduction of human and financial resources available to meet social needs, and the creation of a climate in which violence is a primary mode of dealing with conflict.

Mental health is clearly among the interests at stake. Violence remains a pervasive feature of life in the twentieth century. It is now perhaps even more disturbing that technologies and capacities, which if used constructively would be a source of pride and a measure of progress, are being used to perpetrate that violence. King Leopold's slaughter of millions of Central Africans in the pursuit of ivory and rubber, two world wars, the genocide of European Jews, the massacre of Armenians, the horrors of the Khmer Rouge in Cambodia, the "dirty wars" in Argentina and Chile, the multitude of so-called low-intensity wars in Africa and Central America, massive state repression in the former Soviet Union and China, planned genocide in Rwanda, and ethnic cleansing in the states of the former Yugoslavia provide an indication of the pervasiveness and impact of state-organized violence. Recent decades have also brought changes with them in the nature of warfare, which now more frequently targets civilian populations. Rape, murder, mutilation, and other forms of terror have increasingly become widely used instruments of political violence and social control.

Mental health concerns about violence extend beyond the global political issues of war to local murders, muggings, kidnappings, and other kinds of assault that have become pervasive in some countries and in too many neighborhoods throughout the world, where security at home is not so secure. The results of these large- and small-scale, global, local, and individual conflicts, and the terror, torture, and other forms of violence that accompany them present a host of overwhelming social, economic, and personal problems. Violence makes orphans of children, and widows and widowers of spouses, and it brings irretrievable loss to parents who lose their sons and daughters to an untimely death or disablement. The devastation of infrastructures gives way to poverty, malnutrition, and ill health. Dislocation shreds the fabric of family life and destroys social networks. The trauma of these experiences produces immense emotional suffering—fear, pain, loss, grief, guilt, anxiety, hatred, and sadness. In the case of political violence, ethnic strife, and low-intensity warfare, the psychiatric consequences are often severe and long-standing (Desjarlais et al., 1995).

Violence is the medium through which many vulnerable groups within populations are put at risk and experience subjugation. Obvious examples include the impact of domestic violence on women and the effects of war on children. Many of the world's indigenous peoples have been especially vulnerable to violence of all kinds over extended periods. During the nineteenth century many indigenous peoples of North America were killed or died in epidemics, with the survivors forced to live on reservations. Australian aborigines have a similar history in that regard. Indigenous peoples in El Salvador and Guatemala have been the targets of political violence; Amnesty International (1992) has called for inquiries into killings of tribal peoples in the Chittagong Hill Tracts of Bangladesh; human rights violations against indigenous peoples in Myanmar; political killings of tribal peoples in the Cordillera region of the Philippines; and the torture, rape, and death in caste and communal conflicts in India. During the 1994 war in Rwanda, as many as 30% of the Twa died or were killed in massacres, and another 30% were forced to flee the country. A review of headlines at the beginning of the current millenium brings attention to the ethnic cleansing, murders, and systematic rape that were an integral feature of the conflict in Kosovo; the systematic amputations in Sierra Leone, where civilians were not accidental victims, but intended targets; and many other equally horrendous accounts.

The tale and toll of violence in our age is regrettably a much longer story. Such events confront the skills of mental health professionals, who are called upon to respond and to help the victims as much as they can. The training and available guidance to prepare them to deal with such needs is often inadequate and based on models of disorder that are less than pertinent to the needs of the victims of violence. Mental health professionals need more useful frameworks and strategies to respond and help with the varieties of stress reactions that follow from violence and disaster. The nature of these stress reactions needs to be better understood, and principles of intervention need to be examined more critically and tested to improve approaches to treatment and prevention based on realistic expectations. Torture treatment centers already play a useful role as a specialized resource for treatment; their expertise should be used to train mental health professionals and provide consultative advice when needed.

As Levy and Sidel (1997) and the contributors to their book argue clearly and convincingly, war and its prevention should be prominent among the mainstream interests and curriculum of public health (see Chapter 9). Because the emotional, psychological, and social issues arising from war and other kinds of violence are so clearly pertinent to its interests, mental health policy also needs to include these issues within the scope of its concern. Mental health practitioners have special responsibilities for responding to the emotional impact of violence and treating mental disorders that may result. Analysis and discussion in the psychiatric literature of the report of the Carnegie Commission on Preventing Deadly Conflict asked how the social and behavioral sciences, as well as psychiatry itself, can assess and influence the decision-making process and leadership to minimize the risk of mortal conflicts (Hamburg, George, & Ballentine, 1999). Although preventing and stopping war and violence are not only (or primarily) mental health issues, they are a special interest for mental health professionals and are among the foremost concerns and challenges for all of us.

## MENTAL HEALTH POLICIES AND PROGRAMS FOR LOW- AND MIDDLE-INCOME COUNTRIES

Notwithstanding notable exceptions, mental health services are inadequate in many low- and middle-income countries. Historically lacking priority in the health system and receiving scant attention in the curriculum of medical training, the quality of mental health care is often poorer than that defined by international standards. Difficult to verify but frequently cited statistics suggest that more than 30% of the world's population lacks access to basic drugs for treatment of mental disorders, and in sub-Saharan Africa less than 5% of those in need receive treatment for depression. Insofar as a lack of resources may be responsible, low- and middle-income countries should not be blamed for being poor, but insofar as a commitment is lacking for use of available resources or for developing additional resources and meaningful policy for mental health, more effective advocacy is required.

Additional policy objectives include translation of mental health priorities into program activities, their integration into the health sector of all countries, and assurance of the availability of mental health services. However reasonable this may be, it is not necessarily clear how to achieve these aims, and the matter is further complicated by the fact that no single solution can be expected to work everywhere. Thoughtful consideration of the nature of local needs highlights the importance of developing local service models or carefully adapting imported service models for locally appropriate mental health care. WHO's *World Health Report 2000* has focused on the performance and impact of health systems, and the implications of the concepts and criteria developed for that analysis need to be considered with respect to specific needs for mental health services. Innovation and research are required to implement the key elements of a mental health service system for low- and middle-income countries. These include:

- crisis intervention, especially for addressing the psychological basis of deliberate self-harm
- Identification and resource-appropriate treatment of common mental disorders typically encountered in primary care
- development of specialist referral networks for backup and support
- development of community awareness and support for mental health problems

Although a medical model is appropriate and necessary to promote awareness of the need for accessible services to provide appropriate treatment, a public health model suggests that critical questions of health promotion and illness prevention cannot be ignored. Although not specific to mental health, this point is especially salient because of the web of interrelationships that link mental disorders, emotional distress, and social stressors at all levels (personal, familial, community, and so forth); because of the important role of social supports in the family and community; and because the impact of social policy is so compelling. Careful consideration of the overall relationship between health and development with a particular focus on mental health can be expected to identify valuable resources in the social structure of communities, social networks, and cultural values that may be mobilized to advance mental health policy aims—not only for recognition and treatment, but also to prevent mental illness and promote mental health.

Although low- and middle-income countries are disadvantaged by limited resources for the health sector generally, ongoing development programs, where they exist, may provide a comparative advantage if the value is recognized and means are available to incorporate mental health policy aims in the agenda for community development. Insofar as development programs often recognize the importance of an infrastructure for various degrees of community involvement and participation, such infrastructures offer opportunities for extending policy and programs beyond curative services. The nature of interacting forces of globalization and localization has been explored in the *World Bank's World Development Report 1999/2000* (World Bank 2000), suggesting distinctive advantages of global and local levels of policy making.

Over the past 2 decades WHO and the government of India have supported efforts to develop strategies for community psychiatry in low-income rural areas, such as Raipur Rani in Haryana, North India, and Sakalawara and Bellary in Karnataka, South India. Despite promising initial results, expectations have remained unfulfilled. Nevertheless, these initiatives managed for a time to capture the attention of policy makers. Publication in 1993 of the World Bank's annual report has also influenced policy makers and brought mental health to a more prominent position than ever before on the public health agenda. It is not just in psychiatry conferences or psychiatric journals that a large number of presentations and articles (including this chapter) dutifully begin with a recitation of the mental health-related DALYs. More important, by situating mental disorders in a broader context of global disease, these data have caught the attention of health professionals and bureaucrats who would otherwise pay scant attention to statistics, no matter how dramatic, from research in psychiatric epidemiology and mental health.

Following the World Bank report, publication of *The World Mental Health Report* (Desjarlais et al., 1995) sharpened the focus on the scope of mental health needs and took advantage of a process that had been set in motion. A carefully planned release of that volume through the United Nations resulted in the establishment in 1996 of a global initiative, Nations for Mental Health (1997), coordinated by WHO, to improve the mental health and psychosocial well-being of underserved populations. Activities of this program continue in the reorganized WHO Department (previously Division of Mental Health before restructuring in 1998) of Mental Health within the mandate of one of its three teams concerned with mental health promotion, development, and policy.

Another team in the department focuses on mental and behavioral disorders, and a third is concerned with basic services for neurological disorders and neuroscience. The mental and behavioral disorders group has made suicide prevention its top priority. Other priorities include reduction of the burden of mental disorders, especially depression, identifying ways to support people disabled by mental illness, and improving mental health services. The department is also examining how best to respond to mental health needs that result from natural disasters and violent conflicts. Aiming to reduce vulnerabilities and minimize the impact of such experiences, as much as possible, WHO and other agencies, including NIMH in the United States, are searching for a better understanding and ways to treat the variety of stress reactions that result from disasters, war, and the experience of other extraordinary psychological traumas.

Within the WHO Department of Mental Health, the Nations for Mental Health program has been most directly concerned with explicit interests of low- and middle-income countries. When it was established, it focused on five mental and neurological disorders affecting underserved populations: dementia, mental retardation, depression, schizophrenia, and epilepsy. Underserved populations include people in extreme poverty, abused women, abandoned older adults, indigenous peoples, and other identifiably disadvantaged groups. It operates through support to local demonstration projects that are likely to be generalizable and sustainable, applying existing knowledge and aiming to develop human capital (that is, engendering competence and developing additional skills and expertise among existing program personnel). Priority interests include reducing the stigma of mental illness and promoting human rights; it works through partners in the United Nations system, other multilateral organizations (such as the World Bank), various academic institutions, and nongovernmental organizations (NGOs).

Reducing stigma is also a priority of other international and national mental health groups, such as the World Federation of Mental Health and the Royal College of Psychiatry in the United Kingdom (Byrne, 1999), which has mounted a Changing Minds campaign against stigma. Stigma is a highly complex phenomenon

with many facets. A survey conducted at the Oxford University indicated that young people are less tolerant of the mentally ill than their elders, suggesting that knowledge may not be enough to counter the emotions that fuel stigmatizing opinions (Yamey, 1999). Some health communications may inadvertently make matters even worse.

The Nations for Mental Health program funds projects and helps governments support the development of innovative strategies and implementation of locally applicable mental health policies. In Belize, for example, it has supported mental health workshops attended by the medical staff of district health centers, established a mobile psychiatric unit that can provide services to villages lacking other access to care, arranged regular supervision for psychiatric staff at the district hospital, developed various mental health education activities, established a mental health referral and information system, and improved community-based management of severe mental disorders.

In Khayelitsha, a low-income community outside Cape Town, South Africa, this program has provided funding to implement and evaluate a program to prevent mental health problems in deprived children of depressed mothers. It aims to counteract the adverse effects of difficult social environments on children's emotional, social, cognitive, and physical development by improving mother-infant interactions. In Mongolia the Nations for Mental Health Program is fostering a shift from specialist to community-oriented services to promote mental health and prevent mental illness. The program supports postgraduate training of psychiatrists in community mental health care and trains general practitioners to recognize and treat mental disorders in primary care clinics. Other demonstration projects have been supported in Argentina to reintegrate people with mental illness back into their families, communities, and the workplace; in Bolivia to strengthen community networks; in China to improve the well-being of students; in Egypt to train primary care providers; in Ghana to reduce stigma; in the Marshall Islands to counter suicide and deliberate self-harm; in Mozambique to integrate mental health care in general health services; in Sri Lanka to support community rehabilitation of psychiatric patients; and in Yemen to create community mental health services. Exhibit 7–4 provides a case study from Mexico illustrating the nature of mental health needs, their social context, and

the available opportunities for help in the community and through the mental health system.

Although data generated initially by the World Bank have stimulated much of the recently increased attention to mental health, the bank does not have a designated mental health program. Recognizing the importance of mental health

---

**Exhibit 7–4** Mental Health Needs and Services in Mexico

Olivia is a 43-year-old woman who lives in a small village in the Mexican state of Jalisco with her seven children, ages 8 to 15. Five years ago her husband, Arturo, became desperate when he realized that his two-job income was insufficient to support his family. He left Olivia and the children to travel to the United States to find a job. Olivia has not heard from Arturo since. She explains now that she suffers from *nervios*, a culturally defined disorder among Latin American people, especially common among women. The condition is often associated with stressful social circumstances, and symptoms are wide ranging (Salgado de Snyder, Diàz-Pérez, & Ojeda, in press). Unlike most low-income Mexican women, Olivia has been to see a psychiatrist for her emotional problems. Her sister took her to see a specialist because her *nervios* prevented her from functioning adequately and meeting her responsibilities. She lost her appetite, could not sleep, and became irritable and moody. "I felt like I was going crazy," she explained.

Olivia and her family are among many Mexicans adversely affected by the rapid growth of the country. Mexico is currently undergoing an active process of demographic, economic, educational, political, and epidemiologic transition that affects the lives of its nearly 92 million persons. The majority (70%) are concentrated in cities, which are notable less for the benefits of an urban infrastructure and availability of services than they are for the crushing number of inhabitants. The rural population (30%) is dispersed in thousands of small villages throughout the country, and the 56 ethnic groups that constitute 15% of the total population have the lowest standard of living.

In most regions of Mexico, access to any formal mental health services is limited. Specialists are available only in large cities, mainly Mexico City. The Mexican Institute of Psychiatry is one of the 11 National Institutes of Health that provide outpatient treatment and inpatient care for the general public. Psychiatrists and psychologists in private practice are also available in most large urban centers, but their cost is beyond the reach of most people in Mexico, where the minimum daily wage is approximately US$4, and the cost of a consultation with a private specialist is about US$30.

What do most Mexicans do when they suffer from mental health problems? Efforts to find relief include self-care and use of home remedies, over-the-counter medication, and "self-control." They also seek emotional support from friends, family, and community. Some people may also consult a general practice physician, a priest, a pharmacist, a nurse, or a folk healer; whom they see depends on what they understand the cause of their problem to be, the cost of treatment, and the availability of a desired health care provider (Salgado de Snyder, Diàz-Pérez, Maldonado, & Bautista, 1998).

From 1995 to 2000 the Mexican Ministry of Health began implementing a reform of its national health system, aiming both to extend the coverage of health services to disadvantaged rural and urban populations and to increase the quality of services nationally. Mental health has been included among the designated priorities of the reform. Nevertheless, in view of what remains to be done and the impact of the ongoing epidemiologic health transition in Mexico, needs for mental health services of many Mexicans, like Olivia, are likely to remain unmet without substantial additional input.

for many of its development programs, however, a short-term mental health advisor, identified through a committee of the World Federation of Mental Health, has recently joined the Bank to facilitate mental health interests broadly in its various development activities.

With its focus on mental health policy and emphasizing the need to influence government programs, the Institute of Psychiatry in London, a WHO Collaborating Centre working with the Nations for Mental Health program, has begun developing a global mental health information database. It will consist of country profiles accessible on the World Wide Web, so that government policy makers may see how their country compares with others with respect to the status of a variety of mental health-related issues. As such, the database would not only provide a useful source of information, but also serve as an effective advocacy tool to foster comparisons and improvements in mental health policies and programs. The structure of these country profiles includes five sections: (1) mental health of the population, (2) factors influencing mental health, (3) health and social services for people with mental illness, (4) an account of specific policies and programs, and (5) other policies and programs that affect mental health.

In addition to the work of international agencies and external partners, a variety of national and local NGO-sponsored mental health programs and development activities are also playing a significant role in advancing international mental health. The work of the Samaritans, Befrienders, and associated agencies in suicide prevention is well known. Other agencies are involved in a host of additional health services and programs, encompassing a full range of activities from the mundane to the highly innovative. The question of how to transform a prior focus on specialty, hospital-based medical training into effective community-based activities involving paraprofessional health and general development workers—activities that are capable of mobilizing the support of local communities—remains a formidable challenge for mental health policy makers and planners.

Inasmuch as government bureaucracies responsible for health may not be able to marshal the required assets on their own—financial, technical, intellectual, or organizational—new partnerships involving governments, NGOs, research and training institutes, and international agencies may be necessary to advance these efforts. Policy makers in low- and middle-income countries, where mental illness has been widely ignored, must first acknowledge the burden and the needs and commit themselves to developing effective mental health policies. The next steps should then be both professionally informed and locally appropriate; innovation, resources, and commitment are required to make it happen.

## CONCLUSION

The importance of mental health on the international public health agenda has been seriously underestimated, resulting in considerable preventable suffering, disability, and mortality. Acceptance of the DALY as an indicator of the burden of disease and related conditions has begun to change this, because it is more sensitive to the disabilities imposed by mental disorder than other, previously more influential, indicators. Appreciation of the nature and power of the epidemiologic health transition helps explain the anticipated increase in the prominence of depression and other mental disorders, as their contribution to the total burden of disease and related conditions in low- and middle-income countries increases toward the level of high-income countries. Depression and other common mental disorders are particularly sensitive to adverse byproducts of development and social change, which adds to this effect. Consequently, the prominence of mental illness can be expected to become greater than might be accounted for solely by the shift from acute to chronic health problems in the health transition and by demographic changes that increase the proportion of people reaching an age at risk.

In the fields of psychiatry and psychiatric epidemiology major developments in the classification, diagnosis, and assessment of mental disorders have been easiest to integrate in practice and research in North America and Europe, particularly in settings where cultural diversity is minimal. However, cultural diversity may result in a mismatch between clinical experience and theory needed to guide policy and practice if the theory is based on clinical experience with patients from another cultural group. Transnational and cross-cultural comparisons, and research in multicultural settings, require complementary data from cultural epidemiology to clarify not only the distribution of disorders in designated populations, but also the local experience, meaning, and behaviors that characterize mental illness. These must be taken into account for effective mental health policy to reach the underserved in greatest need.

The history of psychiatry, especially in former colonial countries, indicates the powerful effect of social values and political process on health policy. Consideration of psychiatric epidemiology, oppressive hierarchies, the variety of social systems, ecology, and general health status in settings where tropical diseases persist suggests the complexity of the web of interactions that influence mental health and illness. It is widely recognized, at least in principle, that biological, psychological, and social factors all play a role, individually and collectively. They affect the occurrence of health problems of all kinds (not just mental illness), their clinical course, outcomes, and success in controlling them.

This biopsychosocial principle helps to explain why the challenges to mental health policy are so imposing in low- and middle-income tropical countries. In addition to all the usual factors, endemic parasitic diseases and other medical diseases of poverty, such as malnutrition, have a social and psychological impact, and some of these are also responsible for organic mental disorders. Social and demographic changes affecting people worldwide—such as urbanization, migration, and social dislocation—have

even greater effects where resources to deal with them are less available. The impact of war and violence, which low- and middle-income countries are less able to resist and cope with, also has serious effects on mental health.

Innovative models, policies, and programs are needed to build effective clinical and community mental health services in socially and culturally distinctive rural and urban settings of low- and middle-income countries. Such models are also needed to better account for the social determinants of mental illness and its epidemiology, prevention, and control. The design of mental health services requires careful coordination of clinic- and community-based activities, and it must also be sensitive to the critical balance of decentralized services and centralized backup in settings where specialists are few, and careful planning is required to make them available.

The needs for case identification, treatment, and support for patients with varying degrees of psychiatric disability provide the rationale for policy development and implementation of new mental health programs. Because the determinants of mental health and illness are so intertwined with social forces and cultural values, and because these interrelationships are so complex, broader public health objectives to prevent mental illness and promote mental health in low- and middle-income countries have been especially difficult to achieve or even to consider. Additional attention to these issues is needed.

Hopeful signs indicate positive change from notable neglect by public health authorities and international agencies. Nevertheless, the problems are long-standing, and recognition of the priority of mental health is a recent phenomenon. It is reasonable to expect that sustaining awareness of this priority will require considerable effort. Designing new and locally appropriate models, policy, and programs to meet these needs remains among the most formidable challenges on the international health agenda.

## DISCUSSION QUESTIONS

1. Psychiatric epidemiology is concerned with the occurrence and determinants of specific mental disorders, and DALYs indicate how mental disorders contribute to the global burden of diseases and related conditions. What are the particular advantages and limitations of each approach? How do other accounts of mental illness inform mental health policy and programs?

2. How can mental health programs promote the need for identifying and treating common mental disorders, such as depression and anxiety, without enhancing stigma that may lead some people to minimize or deny these conditions?

3. Mental health is particularly sensitive to the impact of social changes that may be influenced by public policy. What obligations and limits should mental health professionals consider to guide their participation in formulating public policy?

4. In what ways can mental health systems accommodate the particular needs of the communities they serve? With reference to the policies of international health organizations and an appropriate standard of care, how much consistency and variation is desirable and possible across nations, regions, districts, and communities?

5. Based on current understanding of mental health problems and their social contexts, what measures should be considered to prevent mental illness and promote mental health? What additional research would you suggest to better inform such policy and programs?

## REFERENCES

Abbey, S.E., Hood, E., Young, L.T., & Malcolmson, S.A. (1983). Psychiatric consultation in the eastern Canadian Arctic: III. Mental health issues in Inuit women in the eastern Arctic. *Canadian Journal of Psychiatry, 38,* 32–35.

Abiodun, O.A. (1996). Alcohol-related problems in primary care patients in Nigeria. *Acta Psychiatrica Scandinavica, 93,* 235–239.

Almeido-Filho, N. (1987). Social epidemiology of mental disorders: A review of Latin American studies. *Acta Psychiatrica Scandinavica, 75,* 1–10.

Almeido-Filho, N. (1993). Becoming modern after all these years: Social change and mental health in Latin America. Working paper, Project on International Mental and Behavioral Health, Department of Social Medicine, Harvard Medical School, Boston.

American Psychiatric Association. (1994). *Diagnostic and statistical manual of mental disorders* (4th ed.). Washington, DC: American Psychiatric Press.

Amnesty International. (1992). *Human rights violations against indigenous peoples.* New York: Author.

Anderson, W. (1996). Immunities of empire: Race, disease, and the new tropical medicine, 1900–1920. *Bulletin of the History of Medicine, 70,* 94–118.

Anklesaria Aiyar, S.S. (1988, August 31). We need more slums. *Indian Express* (Bombay edition).

Bammer, G., Dobler-Mikola, A., Fleming, P.M., Strang, J., & Uchtenhagen, A. (1999). The heroin prescribing debate: Integrating science and politics. *Science, 284,* 1277–1278.

Bansal, R.K., & Banerjee, S. (1993). Substance use by child laborers. *Indian Journal of Psychiatry, 35,* 159–161.

Barrett, M.P. (1999). The fall and rise of sleeping sickness. *Lancet, 353,* 1113–1114.

Bayer, R., & Spitzer, R.L. (1985). Neurosis, psychodynamics, and DSM–III. *Archives of General Psychiatry, 42,* 187–196.

Beiser, M., Dion, R., Gotowiec, A., Hyman, I., & Vu, N. (1995). Immigrant and refugee children in Canada. *Canadian Journal of Psychiatry, 40,* 67–72.

Blanc, C.S. (1994). *Urban children in distress: Global predicaments and innovative strategies.* Langhorne, PA: Gordeon and Breach.

Bode, L., Riegel, S., Lange, W., & Ludwig, H. (1992). Human infections with Borna disease virus: Seroprevalence in patients with chronic diseases and healthy individuals. *Journal of Medical Virology, 36,* 309–315.

Brieger, W.R., Oshiname, F.O., & Ososanya, O.O. (1998). Stigma associated with onchocercal skin disease among those affected near the Ofiki and Oyan Rivers in Western Nigeria. *Social Science and Medicine, 47*(7), 841–852.

Broadhead, J.C., & Abas, M.A. (1998). Life events, difficulties and depression among women in an urban setting in Zimbabwe. *Psychological Medicine, 28,* 29–38.

Byrne, P. (1999). Stigma of mental illness: Changing minds, changing behaviour. Editorial. *British Journal of Psychiatry, 174,* 1–2.

Carstairs, G.M., & Kapur, R.L. (1976). *The great universe of Kota: Stress, change and mental disorder in an Indian village.* Berkeley, CA: University of California Press.

Cawte, J. (1991). Aboriginal alcoholism. *Medical Journal of Australia, 154,* 365.

Cheng, T.A. (1989). Urbanisation and minor psychiatric morbidity: A community study in Taiwan. *Social Psychiatry and Psychiatric Epidemiology, 24,* 309–316.

Cheng, T.A., Soong, W.T., Chong, M.Y., & Lin, T.Y. (1995). Urbanization, psychosocial stress, and minor mental illness in Taiwan. In T. Harpham & I. Blue (Eds.), *Urbanization and mental health in developing countries* (pp. 61–72). Aldershot, United Kingdom: Avebury.

Clayer, J.R., & Czechowicz, A.S. (1991). Suicide by aboriginal people in South Australia: Comparison with suicide deaths in the total urban and rural populations. *Medical Journal of Australia, 154,* 683–685.

Cohen, A. (1992). Prognosis for schizophrenia in the Third World: A reevaluation of cross-cultural research. *Culture, Medicine and Psychiatry, 16,* 53–75, 101–106.

Collins, P.Y., Varma, V.K., Wig, N.N., Mojtabai, R., Day, R., & Susser, E. (1999). Fever and acute brief psychosis in urban and rural settings in north India. *British Journal of Psychiatry, 174,* 520–524.

Compton, W.M., 3rd., Helzer, J.E., Hwu, H.G., Yeh, E.K., McEvoy, L., Tipp, J.E., & Spitznagel, E.L. (1991). New methods in cross-cultural psychiatry: Psychiatric illness in Taiwan and the United States. *American Journal of Psychiatry, 148,* 1697–1704.

Cowley, P., & Wyatt, R.J. (1993). Schizophrenia and manic-depressive illness. In D.T. Jamison, W.H. Mosley, A.R. Measham, & J.L. Bobadilla (Eds.), *Disease control priorities in developing countries* (pp. 662–670). Oxford: Oxford University Press for World Bank.

Craig, T.J., Siegel, C., Hopper, K., Lin, S., & Sartorius, N. (1997). Outcome in schizophrenia and related disorders compared between developing and developed countries: A recursive partitioning re-analysis of the WHO DOSMD data. *British Journal of Psychiatry, 170,* 229–233.

Cross-National Collaborative Group. (1992). The changing rate of major depression. *Journal of the American Medical Association, 268,* 3098–3105.

Currie, E. (1993). *Reckoning: Drugs, the cities, and the American future.* New York: Hill and Wang.

Desjarlais, R., Eisenberg, L., Good, B., & Kleinman, A. (1995). *World mental health: Problems and priorities in low-income countries.* New York: Oxford University Press.

Dixon, H.B.F., & Lipscomb, F.M. (1961). *Cysticercosis: An analysis and follow-up of 450 cases.* Privy Council, Medical Research Council Special Report Series No. 299. London: Her Majesty's Stationery Office.

Dohrenwend, B., Levav, I., Shrout, P.E., Schwartz, S., Naveh, G., Link, B.G., Skodol, A.E., & Stueve, A. (1992). Socioeconomic status and psychiatric disorders: The causation-selection issue. *Science, 255,* 946–951.

Edgerton, R.B., & Cohen, A. (1994). Culture and schizophrenia: The DOSMD challenge. *British Journal of Psychiatry, 164,* 222–231.

Eisenberg, L. (1977). Disease and illness: Distinctions between professional and popular ideas of sickness. *Culture, Medicine and Psychiatry, 1*(1), 9–23.

Eisenberg, L. (1988). The social construction of mental illness. *Psychological Medicine, 18,* 1–9.

Eisenberg, L. (1992). Treating depression and anxiety in primary care. *New England Journal of Medicine, 326,* 1080–1084.

Ekblad, S. (1990). The Children's Behavior Questionnaire for completion by parents and teachers in a Chinese sample. *Journal of Child Psychology and Psychiatry, 31,* 775–791.

El-Islam, M.F. (1982). Rehabilitation of schizophrenics by the extended family. *Acta Psychiatrica Scandinavica, 65,* 112–119.

Engel, G.L. (1977). The need for a new medical model: The challenge for biomedicine. *Science, 196,* 129–136.

Ewens, G.F.W. (1908). *Insanity in India: Its symptoms and diagnosis with reference to the relation of crime and insanity.* Calcutta: Thacker, Spink.

Feighner, J.P., Robins, E., Guze, S.B., Woodruff, R.A., Winokur, G., & Munz, R. (1972). Diagnostic criteria for use in psychiatric research. *Archives of General Psychiatry, 26,* 57–63.

Fleiss, J.L., & Shrout, P.E. (1989). Reliability considerations in planning diagnostic validity studies. In L.N. Robins & J.E. Barrett (Eds.), *The validity of psychiatric diagnosis* (pp. 279–291). New York: Ravel Press.

Fleiss, J.L., Spitzer, R.L., Endicott, J., & Cohen, J. (1972). Quantification of agreement in multiple psychiatric diagnosis. *Archives of General Psychiatry, 26,* 168–171.

Fullilove, M.T. (1996). Psychiatric implications of displacement: Contributions from the psychology of place. *American Journal of Psychiatry, 153,* 1516–1523.

Gaviria, F.M., Richman, J., Flaherty, J.A., Wintrob, R.M., Martinez, H., Garcia Pacheco, C., Pathak, D.S., Mitchell, T., & Birz, S. (1986). Migration and mental health in Peruvian society: Toward a psychosocial model. *Social Psychiatry, 21,* 193–199.

Goddard, M. (1992). Bedlam in paradise: A critical history of psychiatry in Papua New Guinea. *Journal of Pacific History, 27,* 55–72.

Goldberg, D., & Huxley, P. (1992). *Common mental disorders: A bio-social model.* London: Routledge.

Gruenberg, E.M. (1967). The social breakdown syndrome: Some origins. *American Journal of Psychiatry, 123,* 1481–1489.

Guarnaccia, P.J., Good, B.J., & Kleinman, A. (1990). A critical review of epidemiological studies of Puerto Rican mental health. *American Journal of Psychiatry, 147*(11), 1449–1456.

Hamburg, D.A., George, A., & Ballentine, K. (1999). Preventing deadly conflict: The critical role of leadership. *Archives of General Psychiatry, 56,* 971–976.

Harpham, T. (1994). Urbanization and mental health in developing countries: A research role for social scientists, public health professionals and social psychiatrists. *Social Science and Medicine, 39,* 233–245.

Harpham, T., & Blue, I. (Eds.). (1995). *Urbanization and mental health in developing countries.* Aldershot, United Kingdom: Avebury.

Harrison, M. (1996). "The tender frame of man": Disease, climate, and racial difference in India and the West Indies, 1760–1860. *Bulletin of the History of Medicine, 70,* 68–93.

Hatalski, C.G., Lewis, A.J., & Lipkin, W.I. (1997). Borna disease. *Emerging Infectious Diseases, 3*(2), 129–135.

Headland, T.N., Pike, K.L., & Harris, M. (Eds.). (1990). *Emics and etics: The insider/outsider debate.* Frontiers of Anthropology Series, No. 7. Newbury Park, CA: Sage Publications.

Hobsbawm, E. (1994). *The age of extremes: A history of the world, 1914–1991.* New York: Pantheon.

Hopper, K. (1991). Some old questions for the new cross-cultural psychiatry. *Medical Anthropology Quarterly, 5,* 299–330.

Hunter, E. (1991a). Out of sight, out of mind—1. Emergent patterns of self-harm among aborigines of remote Australia. *Social Science and Medicine, 33,* 655–659.

Hunter, E. (1991b). Out of sight, out of mind—2. Social and historical contexts of self-harmful behaviour among aborigines of remote Australia. *Social Science and Medicine, 33,* 661–671.

Hunter, E. (1997). Double talk: Changing and conflicting constructions of indigenous mental health. *Australian and New Zealand Journal of Psychiatry, 31,* 820–827.

Jablensky, A., Sartorius, N., Ernberg, G., Anker, M., Korten, A., Cooper, J.E., Day, R., & Bertelsen, A. (1992). Schizophrenia: Manifestations, incidence and course in different cultures—A World Health Organization ten-country study. Monograph. *Psychological Medicine,* Supplement 20.

Janca, A. (Ed). (1997). *Multiaxial presentation of the ICD–10 for use in adult psychiatry.* Cambridge, United Kingdom: Cambridge University Press.

Janca, A., & Isaac, M. (1997). ICD–10 and DSM–IV symptoms of somatoform disorders in different cultures. *Keio Journal of Medicine, 46*(3), 128–131.

Kasmini, K., Kyaw, O., Krishnaswamy, S., Kasmini, K., Kyaw, O., Krishnaswamy, S., Ramli, H., & Hassan, S. (1993). A prevalence survey of mental disorders among children in a rural Malaysian sample. *Journal of Child Psychology and Psychiatry, 87,* 253–257.

Kleinman, A. (1977). Depression, somatization and the "new cross-cultural psychiatry." *Social Science and Medicine, 11*(1), 3–10.

Kleinman, A. (1980). *Patients and healers in the context of culture.* Berkeley, CA: University of California Press.

Kleinman, A. (1997). Triumph or pyrrhic victory? The inclusion of culture in DSM–IV. *Harvard Review of Psychiatry, 4*(6), 343–344.

Kleinman, A., & Good, B. (1985). *Culture and depression.* Berkeley, CA: University of California Press.

Klerman, G.L. (1983). The significance of DSM–III in American psychiatry. In R.L. Spitzer, J.B.W. Williams, & A.E. Skodol (Eds.), *International perspectives on DSM–III* (pp. 3–25). Washington, DC: American Psychiatric Press.

Kraepelin, E. (1920). Die Erscheinungsformen des Irreseins. *Zeitschrift für die gesamte Neurologie und Psychiatrie, 62,* 1–29. Translated by H. Marshall. Patterns of mental disorder. In S.R. Hirsch & M. Shepherd (Eds.), *Themes and variations in European psychiatry.* Charlottesville, VA: University Press of Virginia, 1974.

Kramer, M. (1989). Barriers to prevention. In B. Cooper & T. Helgason (Eds.), *Epidemiology and the prevention of mental disorders* (pp. 30–55). London: Routledge.

Leighton, A.H., Lambo, T.A., Hughes, C.C., Leighton, D.C., Murphy, J.M., & Macklin, D.B. (1963). *Psychiatric disorder among the Yoruba: A report form the Cornell-Aro Mental Health Research Project in the western region, Nigeria.* Ithaca, NY: Cornell University Press.

Levy, B.S., & Sidel, V.W. (Eds.). (1997). *War and public health.* New York and Oxford: Oxford University Press in cooperation with the American Public Health Association.

Lin, K.M., & Smith, M.W. (2000). Psychopharmacotherapy in the context of culture and ethnicity. In P. Ruiz (Ed.), *Ethnicity and psychopharmacology (Review of Psychiatry,* vol. 19). Washington, DC: American Psychiatric Press.

Lyons, M. (1992). *The colonial disease: A social history of sleeping sickness in Northern Zaire, 1900–1940.* Cambridge, United Kingdom: Cambridge University Press.

Manson, P. (1940). *Manson's tropical diseases: A manual of the diseases of warm climates* (11th ed., rev.), P. Manson-Bahr (Ed.). Baltimore: Williams & Wilkins.

Marsden, P.D., & Bruce-Chwatt, L.J. (1975). Cerebral malaria. Contemporary neurology series. *Topics on Tropical Neurology, 12,* 29–44.

Marsella, A.J. (1995). Urbanization, mental health and psychosocial well-being: Some historical perspectives and considerations. In T. Harpham & I. Blue (Eds.), *Urbanization and mental health in developing countries* (pp. 17–38). Aldershot, United Kingdom: Avebury.

Marsella, A.J. (1998). Urbanization, mental health, and social deviancy: A review of issues and research. *American Psychologist, 53,* 624–634.

Massey, D.S. (1996). The age of extremes: Concentrated affluence and poverty in the twenty-first century. *Demography, 33,* 395–412.

Matsuura, M., Okubo, Y., Kojima, T., Matsuura, M., Okubo, Y., Kojima, T., Takahashi, R., Wang, Y.F., Shen, Y.C., & Lee, C.K. (1993) A cross-national prevalence study of children with emotional and behavioral problems: A WHO Collaborative study in the Western Pacific Region. *Journal of Child Psychology and Psychiatry, 34,* 307–315.

McKendrick, J., Cutter, T., Mackenzie, A., & Chiu, E. (1992). The pattern of psychiatric morbidity in a Victorian urban aboriginal general practice population. *Australian and New Zealand Journal of Psychiatry, 26,* 40–47.

McLaren, N. (1995). Shrinking the Kimberley: Remote area psychiatry in Australia. *Australian and New Zealand Journal of Psychiatry, 29,* 199–206.

McSweegan, E. (1998). Infectious diseases and mental illness: Is there a link? *Emerging Infectious Diseases, 4*(1), 123–124.

Mezzich, J.E. (1995). Cultural formulation and comprehensive diagnosis: Clinical and research perspectives. *Psychiatric Clinics of North America, 18*(3), 649–657.

Murray, C.J.L., & Lopez, A.D. (Eds.) (1996). *The global burden of disease: A comprehensive assessment of mortality and disability from diseases, injuries, and risk factors in 1990 and projected to 2020.* Global burden of disease and injury series (Vol. I). Cambridge, MA: Harvard University Press.

National Center for Health Statistics. (1998). *Health, United States,* Hyattsville, MD: Author.

Nations for Mental Health. (1997). *An overview of a strategy to improve the mental health of underserved populations.* Geneva, Switzerland: World Health Organization.

Orley, J., & Wing, J.K. (1979). Psychiatric disorders in two African villages. *Archives of General Psychiatry, 36,* 513–520.

Pernice, R., & Brook, J. (1994). Relationship of migrant status (refugee or immigrant) to mental health. *International Journal of Social Psychiatry, 40,* 177–188.

Phillips, M.R., Liu, H., & Zhang, Y. (1999). Suicide and social change in China. *Culture, Medicine and Psychiatry, 23,* 25–50.

Phillips, M.R., Pearson, V., & Wang, R. (1994). Psychiatric rehabilitation in China: Models for change in a changing society. *British Journal of Psychiatry Supplement, 24,* 11–18.

Ponizovsky, A., Ginath, Y., Durst, R., Wondimeneh, B., Safro, S., Minuchin-Itzigson, S., & Ritsner, M. (1998). Psychological distress among Ethiopian and Russian Jewish immigrants to Israel: A cross-cultural study. *International Journal of Social Psychiatry, 44,* 35–45.

Prince, R. (1968). The changing picture of depressive syndromes in Africa. *Canadian Journal of African Studies, 1,* 177–192.

Pulver, A.E., & Carpenter, W.T. (1983). Lifetime psychotic symptoms assessed with the DIS. *Schizophrenia Bulletin, 9,* 377–382.

Raguram, R., Weiss, M.G., Channabasavanna, S.M., & Devins, G.M. (1996). Stigma, depression, and somatization: A report from South India. *American Journal of Psychiatry, 153,* 1043–1049.

Rahim, S.I., & Cederblad, M. (1984). Effects of rapid urbanization on child behavior and health in a part of Khartoum, Sudan. *Journal of Child Psychology and Psychiatry, 25,* 629–641.

Raju, T.N.K. (1998). The Nobel chronicles. *Lancet, 352,* 1714.

Raphael, K.G., Cloitre, M., & Dohrenwend, B.P. (1991). Problems of recall and misclassification with checklist methods of measuring stressful life events. *Health Psychology, 10,* 62–74.

Regier, D.A., & Burke, J.D., Jr. (1995). Epidemiology (section 5.1, Quantitative and experimental method in psychiatry). In H.I. Kaplan & B.J. Sadock (Eds.), *Comprehensive Textbook of Psychiatry* (6th ed., 2 vols., pp. 377–397). Baltimore: Williams & Wilkins.

Rice, D.P., Kelman, S., & Miller, L.S. (1991). Estimates of economic costs of alcohol and drug abuse and mental illness, 1985 and 1988. *Public Health Reports, 106,* 280–291.

Roberts, R.E., Attkisson, C.C., & Rosenblatt, A. (1998). Prevalence of psychopathology among children and adolescents. *American Journal of Psychiatry, 1555,* 715–725.

Robins, E., & Guze, S.B. (1970). Establishment of diagnostic validity in psychiatric illness: Its application to schizophrenia. *American Journal of Psychiatry, 126*(7), 107–111.

Robins, L.N., & Barrett, J.E. (Eds.). (1989). *The validity of psychiatric diagnosis.* New York: Ravel Press.

Rogler, L.H. (1994). International migrations: A framework for directing research. *American Psychologist, 49,* 701–708.

Rogler, L.H. (1996). Framing research on culture in psychiatric diagnosis: The case of DSM–IV. *Psychiatry, 59*(2), 145–155.

Rogler, L.H. (1997). Making sense of historical changes in the *Diagnostic and Statistical Manual of Mental Disorders*: Five propositions. *Journal of Health and Social Behavior, 38,* 9–20.

Rubinstein, D.H. (1995). Love and suffering: adolescent socialization and suicide in Micronesia. *Contemporary Pacific, 7*(1), 21–53.

Rusche, S. (1999). Prescribing heroin. *Science, 285,* 531.

Rutz, W., von Knorring, L., & Walinder, J. (1992). Long-term effects of an educational program for general practitioners given by the Swedish Committee for the Prevention and Treatment of Depression. *Acta Psychiatrica Scandinavica, 85,* 83–88.

Saldanha, I.M. (1995). On drinking and 'drunkenness': History of liquor in colonial India. *Economic and Political Weekly, 30,* 2323–2331.

Salgado de Snyder, V.N., Díaz-Pérez, M.J., Maldonado, M., & Bautista, E. (1998). Pathways to mental health service utilization among rural inhabitants of a Mexican village with a high migratory tradition to the United States. *Health and Social Work, 23,* 249–261.

Salgado de Snyder, V.N., Díaz-Pérez, M.J., & Ojeda, V. (in press). The prevalence of *nervios* and associated symptomatology among inhabitants of Mexican rural communities. *Culture, Medicine and Psychiatry.*

Sartorius, N., Kaelber, C.T., Cooper, J.E., Roper, M.T., Rae, D.S., Gulbinat, W., Üstün, T.B., & Regier, D.A. (1993). Progress toward achieving a common language in psychiatry. *Archives of General Psychiatry, 50,* 115–124.

Shen, Y. (1987). Recent epidemiological data on alcoholism in China. *Chinese Mental Health Journal, 1*(6), 251–252.

Simon, G.E., VonKorff, M., Üstün, T.B., Gater, R., Gureje, O., & Sartorius, N. (1995). Is the lifetime risk of depression actually increasing? *Journal of Clinical Epidemiology, 48,* 1109–1118.

Smith, D.H., Pepin, J., & Stich, A.H.R. (1998). Human African trypanosomiasis: An emerging public health crisis. *British Medical Bulletin, 54*(2), 341–355.

Spitzer, R.L., Endicott, J., & Robins, E. (1978). Research diagnostic criteria: Rationale and reliability. *Archives of General Psychiatry, 35,* 773–789.

Spitzer, R.L., & Williams, J.B.W. (1988). Having a dream: A research strategy for DSM–IV. *Archives of General Psychiatry, 45*(9), 871–874.

Swan, P., & Raphael, B. (1995). *"Ways forward": National consultancy report on aboriginal and Torres Strait Islander mental health.* Canberra, Australia: Government Publishing Service.

Uchtenhagen, A. (1998). *Narcotics prescription for heroin addicts: Main results of the Swiss National Cohort Study.* Basel, Switzerland and New York: Karger.

United Nations International Drug Control Program. (1997). *World drug report.* Oxford: Oxford University Press.

Üstün, T.B. (1999). The global burden of mental disorders. *American Journal of Public Health, 89,* 1315–1318.

Üstün, T.B., & Sartorius, N. (1995). *Mental illness in general health care: An international study.* Chichester: John Wiley & Sons.

Vlassoff, C., Weiss, M.G., Ovuga, E.B.L., Eneanya, C., Nwel, P.T., Babalola, S.S., Awedoba, A.K., Theophilus, B., Cofie, P., & Shetabi, P. (2000). Gender and the stigma of onchocercal skin disease in Africa. *Social Science and Medicine, 50,* 1353–1368.

Wang, Y.F., Shen, Y.C., Gu, B.M., Jia, M.X., & Zhang, A.L. (1989). An epidemiological study of behavior problems in school children in urban areas of Beijing. *Journal of Child Psychology and Psychiatry, 30,* 907–912.

Warner, R. (1985). *Recovery from schizophrenia: Psychiatry and political economy.* London: Routledge and Kegan Paul.

Waxler, N.E. (1979). Is outcome for schizophrenia better in non-industrial societies? The case of Sri Lanka. *Journal of Nervous and Mental Disease, 167,* 144–158.

Weiss, M.G. (1994). Parasitic diseases and psychiatric illness. *Canadian Journal of Psychiatry, 39*(10), 623–628.

Weiss, M.G. (1997). Explanatory Model Interview Catalogue: Framework for comparative study of illness experience. *Transcultural Psychiatry, 34*(2), 235–263.

Weiss, M.G., & Kleinman, A.M. (1988). Depression in cross-cultural perspective: Developing a culturally informed model. In P. Dasen, N. Sartorius, & J. Berry (Eds.), *Psychology, culture and health: Towards applications* (pp. 179–206). Beverly Hills, CA: Sage.

Weiss, M.G., Raguram, R., & Channabasavanna, S.M. (1995). Cultural dimensions of psychiatric diagnosis: Comparing DSM–III-R and illness explanatory models in South India. *British Journal of Psychiatry, 166,* 353–359.

Widiger, T.A., Frances, A.J., Pincus, H.A., Ross, R., First, M.B., & Davis, W. (Eds.). (1997). *DSM–IV Sourcebook* (Vol. 3). Washington, DC: American Psychiatric Association.

Wig, N.N. (1983). DSM–III: A perspective from the Third World. In R.L. Spitzer, J.B.W. Williams, & A.E. Skodol (Eds.), *International perspectives on DSM–III* (pp. 79–89). Washington, DC: American Psychiatric Press.

World Bank. (2000). *World development report 1999/2000: Entering the 21st century: The changing development landscape.* New York: Oxford University Press.

World Bank. (1993). *World development report 1993: Investing in health.* New York: Oxford University Press.

World Health Organization. (1979). *Schizophrenia: An international follow-up study.* New York: Wiley.

World Health Organization. (1992). *The ICD–10 classification of mental and behavioral disorders.* Geneva, Switzerland: Author.

World Health Organization. (1999a). *The world health report 1999: Making a difference.* Geneva, Switzerland: Author.

World Health Organization. (1999b). *Figures and facts about suicide.* Division of Mental Health. Geneva, Switzerland: Author.

World Health Organization. (2000). *The World health report 2000: Health systems: Improving performance.* Geneva, Switzerland: Author.

Yamey, G. (1999). Young less tolerant of mentally ill than the old. News item. *Lancet, 319,* 1092.

# CHAPTER 8

# Environmental Health

*Anthony J. McMichael, Tord Kjellström, and Kirk R. Smith*

This chapter explores the definition of *environment,* taking note of the several disciplinary perspectives, the international spectrum of environmental health issues, and the ongoing emergence of larger-scale environmental problems. Conceptual and methodological issues that characterize the area of mainstream environmental health research and public health action are discussed. Subsequently, using a five-way subdivision of environment classified by scale and setting, the profiles of environmental health hazards are discussed within the domestic setting, in the workplace and community, and on regional and global scales. Illustrative case studies are presented.

The final section considers the issues and prospects that bear on the future of environmental health research and policy. What priorities apply in an unequal world? What are the environmental hazards of globalization, in its several guises? How can the environmental influences on human population health be conceptualized so as to develop a more integrated "ecological" understanding of the interplay between human populations and the natural environment, and the consequences for human health of contaminating, depleting, or overloading that environment?

## DEFINITION AND SCOPE OF ENVIRONMENT

*Environment* is an elastic term. In this chapter *environment* refers to external physical, chemical, and microbiological exposures and processes that impinge upon individuals and groups, and are beyond the immediate control of individuals. This definition excludes exposures that occur largely because of individual choice— such as active cigarette smoking and personal dietary habits. It also excludes risk factors that arise within the social-cultural environment, such as violent crime and community stress (see Chapter 9). Further, environmental conditions associated with risk of physical injury (such as traffic, workplace, and home) will only be discussed briefly (for further details, see Chapter 6).

The environment can be categorized several ways, including in relation to environmental media (air, water, soil, and food), economic sector (transport, land use, and energy generation), physical scale (local, regional, global), setting (household, workplace, and urban environment), and disease outcomes (cancers, congenital anomalies, and others). A classification that comprises five categories is used here, defined jointly by physical scale and by setting. They are

1. household
2. occupational
3. community
4. regional
5. global

A sixth category, that of cross-scale, should also be recognized. The scale at which an environmental health impact eventually occurs may not be the scale at which the exposure was initiated.

Consider the hierarchy of environmental health consequences of energy use. The environmental impacts of energy production and use comprise a significant proportion of the total human impact on the environment at each of the six above-mentioned levels. The extraction, harvesting, processing, distribution, and use of fuels and other energy sources have major environmental impacts at all scales, from individual households to the globe itself. Combustion occurs locally, causing local air pollution—but it also contributes to regional acid rain and, globally, to the accumulation of carbon dioxide as a heat-trapping greenhouse gas in the lower atmosphere.

In defining *environment*, there are two other points to note.

First, some environmental exposures arise because of natural variation, whereas others are due to human interventions. Natural exposures arise from seasonal, latitudinal, or altitudinal gradients in solar irradiation, extremes of hot and cold weather, the occurrence of physical disasters, and local micronutrient deficiencies in soil. The usual "environmental" concern, however, is with exposure to human-made hazards. In industrialized countries attention has focused in recent years on the many chemical contaminants entering the air, water, soil, and food and on physical hazards such as ionizing radiation, urban noise, and road trauma. In low- and middle-income countries, the major environmental concerns are with the microbiological quality of drinking water and food, the physical safety of housing and work, indoor air pollution, and road hazards. Those hazards are kept under control in industrialized countries through major investments into good quality housing and community infrastructure (drinking water supply, sewerage, solid waste collection, and others).

Second, on another axis are two fundamentally different dimensions of environment. There is the familiar local physicochemical and microbiological environment as vehicle for diverse specific hazards able to cause injury, toxicity, nutritional deficiency, or infection. Less familiar are today's emerging disruptions to the biosphere's various ecologic and geophysical systems that stabilize, replenish, recycle, cleanse, and produce, thereby providing climatic stability, food yields, clean freshwater, nutrient cycling, and sustained biodiversity (see also "Environment: Encompassing Both 'Hazard' and 'Habitat'").

## SCALE AND DISTRIBUTION OF ENVIRONMENTAL RISKS TO HEALTH

The relative importance of "environmental" exposures as a cause of human disease and premature death remains contentious. The question is difficult, because knowledge about disease etiology is incomplete—and because the statistic is a moving target that reflects the latency period between environmental change and nonacute health outcomes. Many of today's chronic diseases are the result of past exposures that have either changed (such as urban air pollution) or ceased.

The complex bidirectional relationships between environmental conditions, socioeconomic circumstances, demographic change, and human health present a further difficulty in estimating the environmental contribution to disease burden (Shahi, Levy, Binger, Kjellstrom, & Lawrence, 1997). For example, the combination of population pressure and poverty among rural populations in low- and middle-income countries often leads to land degradation, deforestation, flooding, further impoverishment, and increased risks to health from infectious disease, food shortages, and nutritional deficiencies. The plight of sub-Saharan Africa, with its persistent poverty, environmental stresses, and marginalization in the global economy, illustrates well these complex relationships. Erstwhile gains in sub-Saharan Africa's health, education, and living standards have reversed in the past 2 decades: a majority of people live in absolute poverty; more than 50% still lack safe drinking water, and 70% lack proper sanitation; and the spread of desertification and deforestation is affecting some regions (Logie & Benatar, 1997). According to the World Health Organization (WHO, 1999), infant mortality rates are 55% higher than in other low- and middle-income countries, and average life expectancy is about a decade less.

In general, there is a tendency for environmental health risks to shift during the economic development process, first from household to community and then to regional and global scales, as part of the "environmental risk transition" (Smith, 1997). Environmental risks in low- and middle-income societies are dominated by poor food, water, and air quality at the household level from inadequate sanitation, contaminated water, and low-quality fuels (WHO, 1997). Some of the activities that help solve these problems act to transfer problems to the community level in the form of urban air pollution, hazardous waste, and chemical pollution. In the industrialized societies, where most community and household problems have come under considerable control, problems have been shifted to the global scale, for example, through greenhouse-gas emissions.

As discussed in Chapter 1, the shift in diseases during the epidemiologic transition—although its details vary substantially in different places and times—has been one of the most important features of economic development. Before there can be a shift in age-specific disease patterns, however, there needs to be a shift in the within-population pattern of risks that lead to disease. Another important characteristic that shifts is temporal scale. Many important infectious diseases, such as diarrhea, malaria, and measles, for example, have relatively short latency periods (hours to weeks) between exposure to risk factors and development of disease. Cancer and other chronic noninfectious diseases, however, often entail time delays of several decades. Global processes such as anthropogenic climate change may involve even longer time periods. Thus the risk transition tends to involve a shift in temporal characteristics, and this has important implications for research and social policy.

Depending on the definition used, the assumptions made, and the reference populations, estimates of the environmental contribution to the total avoidable global burden of disease span a wide range. In the first systematic use of a metric—the disability-adjusted life year (DALY; Murray & Lopez, 1996), which combines morbidity and mortality data in a manner suitable for international comparisons—the World Bank (1993) concluded that about 50% of all global DALYs were due to diseases associated with environmental (including microbiological) exposures in the household and an additional 30% were due to diseases associated with the community environment. However, it was considered that only a small proportion of these DALYs were amenable to feasible preventive interventions (World Bank, 1993). A reassessment conducted for the fifth anniversary of the Rio "Earth Summit" (WHO, 1997) estimated that about 25% of global DALYs were caused by environmental hazards, including the workplace environment. Smith, Corvalan, and Kjellstrom (1999) in a recent and comprehensive analysis estimate that 25–33% of the global burden of disease and premature death is attributable to direct environmental risk factors. Even higher percentages emerge if factors such as active tobacco smoking are included (Pimentel et al., 1998).

The largest environmental health burdens are borne in low- and middle-income countries with significant household-level risks, which also tend to affect young children particularly. Figure 8–1 illustrates the estimated percentages of several important environmental risk factors in the national burdens of disease in the two largest countries, India and China. It compares the burden imposed by dirty air and water, lack of sanitation, and occupational risks with burdens from other important risk factors.

## ENVIRONMENT: ENCOMPASSING BOTH "HAZARD" AND "HABITAT"

Most analyses of environmental health effects focus on specific, direct-acting hazards within a localized setting. Exposure is assessed either at the individual or group level, health outcomes are assessed, and dose-response relationships are estimated, usually by fitting statistical models. Where data are sparse, model-fitting

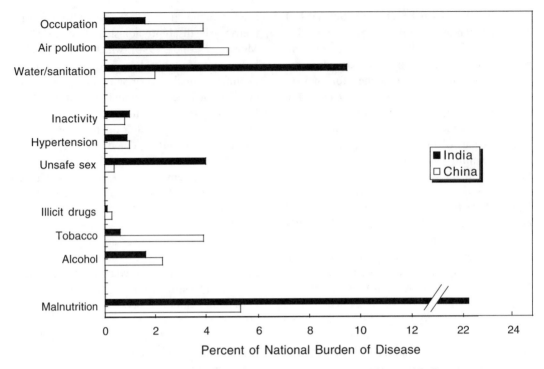

**Figure 8–1** Impact of Major Risk Factors on National Burden of Disease in China and India

may be guided by theoretical considerations. Once dose-response relationships have been satisfactorily estimated, and if the causal interpretation is convincing, then the results can be used to guide environmental policy. However, exposures have often been higher in workplaces than in the ambient environment, and many of the published dose-response relationships are based on occupational epidemiologic studies.

During recent decades this mode of environmental and occupational health research, culminating in formal risk assessment (Samet, Schnatter, & Gibb, 1998), has prevailed in industrialized countries. Ambient and workplace environmental exposure standards have thereby been set for several hundred specific environmental exposure agents. There are currently more than 80,000 man-made chemical substances in commercial use worldwide, and 4,000 of these are in widespread use. Further, thousands of naturally occurring chemicals are in general use, including

many in low- and middle-income countries. Evidently there are insufficient epidemiologic and toxicological data to evaluate the potential health effects of most of these chemicals (Moochhala, Shahi, & Cote, 1997).

Meanwhile, a larger scale of environmental hazard to human health began to emerge in the final decades of the twentieth century. With increased emissions of greenhouse gases and various ozone-destroying gases, the composition of the world's lower and middle atmospheres is, for the first time, being altered. The world's great geochemical cycles of sulfur and nitrogen are changing. Human-induced environmental changes are also causing worldwide depletion of soil fertility, aquifers, ocean fisheries, and—perhaps most serious—biological diversity. These human-induced changes are beginning to weaken the world's life-supporting systems and change the conditions of the biosphere—our habitat. Various serious consequences for human health must be expected, such as changes in the pattern of infectious diseases and in regional agricultural yields, and in the impacts of economic hardship or demographic displacement.

Therefore, the scope of our "environmental health" framework must be extended to include the impairment of our habitat. Meanwhile, our hazard-oriented environmental health research must also be maintained. As the environmental impact grows larger, so do the dimensions of our research, risk management, and policy development tasks.

## ENVIRONMENTAL HEALTH RESEARCH, RISK ASSESSMENT, AND MONITORING

### Research Scope and Strategies

Environmental health research seeks to elucidate causal relations between environmental exposures and impaired states of health, prioritize and develop appropriate interventions to reduce risks to health, and evaluate the effectiveness of such interventions. Epidemiology is the basic quantitative science of environmental health research. In essence, epidemiologic research describes and explains variations and temporal changes in the pattern of illness and disease between and within populations. Most environmental epidemiology is observational (that is, nonexperimental)—and this introduces some important issues in research design and data interpretation (Morgenstern & Thomas, 1993). However, where health benefit is anticipated from exposure-reducing interventions, experimental studies may be carried out.

Historically, epidemiology has played a crucial and largely self-sufficient role in identifying the environmental health hazards posed by relatively high levels of exposure—such as to severe air pollution (for example, the London smog of 1952), to heavy metals in water and food, and to solar ultraviolet radiation (UVR). Those studies were mostly done in industrialized countries, where research expertise existed and

where technical and information resources were available. Increasingly, studies of physicochemical environmental exposures are being done in low- and middle-income countries, as well as in the former territories of the Soviet Union where extensive environmental pollution and degradation often occurred. Meanwhile, many of the environmental health questions now being addressed in industrialized countries refer to more subtle exposures, such as electromagnetic fields and chemical exposures that act cumulatively over decades upon fertility and reproduction (especially the interest in "endocrine disrupting" chemicals), and the functioning of the central nervous system and the immune system.

Many environmental exposures occur at levels that are low by comparison with occupational exposures and personal habits, such as cigarette smoking. For example, in terms of the inhalation of fine particulates and various noxious gases, living in a heavily air-polluted city entails exposures equivalent to smoking no more than several cigarettes per day. Yet most of the convincing epidemiologic studies of cigarette smoking and disease have depended on comparing persons smoking 10-plus cigarettes per day with nonsmokers. This typically lesser level of ambient environmental exposure renders difficult the task of detecting modest increments in risk. Yet the importance of such environmental exposures is threefold: (1) they typically impinge on many persons, perhaps whole populations, thereby causing a large aggregate health impact (that is, an economic-political criterion); (2) they are encountered on an essentially involuntary, and often unequal, basis (that is, an ethical criterion); and (3) they are often amenable to control at the source (that is, a practical criterion).

The epidemiologist faces two other recurrent difficulties. First, these real-world exposures are likely to be accompanied (that is, confounded) by various other exposures or risk factors—some of which may be unknown to the investigator, or indeed to science. Second, the exposure-effect relationships often entail long-term, chronic, and sometimes subtle causal processes.

Because of these complexities, environmental health research must often be tackled in a multidisciplinary fashion, in order to attain a sufficiently broad basis of evidence for causal inference. For example, causal inferences about the effect of low-level environmental lead exposure on the cognitive development of young children has required the integrated consideration of the results of epidemiologic studies, animal experimental research, and neuropathological and molecular toxicological studies.

Extra leverage may be gained via interdisciplinary research in which the techniques of several disciplines are combined within one (usually epidemiologic) study. For example, the development of molecular biology over the past several decades has yielded many new techniques for measuring "internal" exposure, especially in relation to carcinogenesis. Molecular biological markers may also elucidate the biological mechanism, thus strengthening the basis for causal inference. Further, these epidemiology-based research approaches, focusing on cause-effect relationships and underlying biological mechanisms, should be complemented by technical/engineering, behavioral, and policy research in order to develop feasible interventions. In the environmental health arena, the contribution of these "nonhealth" disciplines may be crucial for developing effective health protection.

## Causation and Other Methodological Issues

Etiological studies examine associations between exposure and health outcome, assess the causal nature of the association, and, where possible, estimate the quantitative variation in risk as a function of variation in exposure. Epidemiologic research, predominantly nonexperimental, seeks research settings and study designs that can maximize the signal-to-noise ratio, since studies of disease etiology in free-living populations, with heterogeneous exposures and circumstances, usually entail substantial background "noise." The quality of the measurement of exposure and of health status is often much less than in controlled clinical trials or laboratory-based studies. There may be many potential confounding variables (such as sex, age, and smoking habit), statistically associated with the exposure variable of interest and also predictive of the health outcome, that must be controlled for by study design or analysis. The sample of persons studied may not be a random sample of the source population with respect to the relationship that the sample either *actually* displays (selection bias), or *apparently* displays (classification bias), between exposure and outcome.

Once a sufficient number of studies have been done, in diverse settings and with adequate attention to minimizing the sources of random error (a property of a stochastic universe), systematic error (procedural bias), and logical error (confounding), then causation can be assessed. Causation is not an entity in itself; it is an inference, an interpretation, that is made about the observed conjunction of two variables (exposure and health status). There is therefore no "final" proof of causation. The eighteenth-century Scottish philosopher David Hume pointed out that causation is induced, not observed; we cannot therefore absolutely "know" that exposure X causes disease Y. In the twentieth century, the philosopher Karl Popper offered a solution to this problem of reliance on induction by stressing that science progresses by rejecting or modifying causal hypotheses, not by actually proving causation. Meanwhile, over recent decades epidemiologists have developed a set of criteria specifically suited to their predominantly nonexperimental, bias-prone, confounding-rich research—with particular emphasis upon the temporality of the relationship, its strength, the presence of a plausible dose-response relationship, the consistency of findings in diverse studies, and coherence with other disciplinary findings and biomedical theory (Beaglehole, Bonita, & Kjellstrom, 1993).

Etiologic research in environmental epidemiology entails several distinctive methodological issues. They include

- Choice of the appropriate level of comparison (population, local community, or individual). Many environmental exposures (such as ambient air pollution or drinking-water fluoride levels) impinge on whole communities, with minimal exposure difference between individuals.

- Definition of "exposure" and choice of the mode of exposure assessment.
- Choice of the relevant "reference exposure" (the theoretical minimum exposure level that a society could achieve).
- Dealing with multiple coexistent, potentially interacting, environmental exposures.

These and other issues are discussed in the following sections.

## Study Design Options

The same basic set of study designs used in general epidemiology are also used in environmental epidemiology. The studies can be descriptive, analytical, or experimental (Beaglehole et al., 1993).

### Descriptive Studies

In descriptive studies the pattern of variation in a population's environmental exposure or health status is described, usually in relation to time, place, or category of person. No formal analysis of the relationship between exposure factors and health status is made. Such studies aid in identifying research priorities and guiding the design of etiologic studies. For example, they may show that the exposure levels are not high enough to warrant more detailed epidemiologic study. The time-trend of exposure may influence how further studies are designed. The spatial distribution of exposure may indicate how to define subgroups with different exposure levels within the population.

### Correlation Studies

With planning, and sufficient variation in exposure, it is possible to examine the correlation, over time or space (or both), between the "descriptive" population-level measures of exposure and health. Usually, such studies cannot yield definite conclusions about etiology—most often because there may be inadequate informa-tion on confounding factors or because an association observed at the population level does not necessarily exist at the individual level (the so-called ecologic fallacy). Note, however, that the latter problem is much less important for exposures that impinge relatively homogeneously throughout a specified population. Thus one can reasonably compare the acute respiratory symptom prevalence rates between Beijing and Singapore in the knowledge that all Beijing dwellers are exposed to high levels of ambient air pollution while all Singaporeans are not. Such a correlation analysis would be much improved by increasing the number of observation units (populations), maximizing the variation in exposure between them and adjusting for important confounders (for example, age distribution and cigarette smoking prevalence).

For microecologic studies that examine exposure-related variations in health status between small, usually contiguous, groups of people or households, "small-area" study designs are used. A substantial body of theory has evolved recently for this type of study, and various statistical techniques for "smoothing" the data and adjusting for autocorrelation between adjoining spatial (and temporal) units have been developed. These designs are useful for examining relationships such as the variation in respiratory disease rates in relation to residential distance from major highways, or the variation in congenital anomaly rates in relation to residential distance from high-temperature incinerators. Whether working at the small, medium, or large spatial scale, there are increasingly sophisticated techniques for spatial analysis.

Time-series studies have a special role in environmental epidemiology. Some environmental exposures vary on a short-term basis, especially levels of urban air pollution and weather conditions. There are intrinsically interesting questions about the acute health impact of fluctuations in air pollution or temperature, such as whether asthma attacks increase on high-pollution days or daily death rates increase on days of extreme temperature. The statistical analytic techniques for time-series analyses have been acquired variously from econometrics and engineering research. They include sophisticated adjustments for lower-frequency (for example, seasonal) cyclical variations, background secular trends, and autocorrelation. Time-series studies benefit from the fact that ongoing characteristics of the study population, such as age distribution, socioeconomic profile, and smoking habits, remain essentially constant over time. Further, since the comparison is made entirely within the chosen population, there can be no problem of interpopulation confounding.

### Analytic Studies

Analytical studies examine formal statistical associations between an exposure variable and a health outcome variable at the level of the individual or small homogeneous exposure group (Beaglehole et al., 1993). Are individuals with higher exposure to indoor air pollution more likely to develop respiratory disease than those with low exposure? Are individuals who develop diarrheal disease in a coastal city more likely to have been swimming in contaminated sea water recently than individuals without such disease? The studies can be designed to "start" from exposures (cohort studies—for example, the indoor air pollution example above) or from the health effect (case-control studies—for example, the diarrheal disease example above).

The study of the relationship of early-life environmental lead exposure to child cognitive-intellectual development began with various types of cross-sectional studies in the 1970s. However, it was not possible to establish from those studies the temporal relationship between occurrence of exposure and occurrence of intellectual or behavioral deficit. Cohort studies were required, in which infants and children were followed from birth, with systematic documentation of their early-life lead exposure history and cognitive-intellectual development. The largest of these, carried out in and around the lead-smelting town of Port Pirie, South Australia (Tong, Baghurst, Sawyer, Burns, & McMichael, 1998), provided the type of data (see Figure 8–2) necessary to resolve this important public health issue and to estimate the magnitude of the risk (see also Exhibit 8–1).

An important issue in environmental epidemiology studies is how to deal with the problem of confounding by factors that are statistically associated with the exposure variable and, also, are independently predictive of the health outcome. If, in the above example, those people with high indoor air pollution exposure also smoke more on average than people with low exposure, then smoking habits would confound the assessment of the relationship between indoor air pollution and respiratory disease. The higher rates of disease in the more polluted households may actually be due to the greater amount of smoking. Similarly, in the above-mentioned case-control study, if the people with diarrheal disease (cases) are more likely to have eaten contaminated shellfish than people without diarrhea (controls), then shellfish consumption would confound the assessment of the relationship between diarrhea and having swum in contaminated sea water. The issue of confounding is pervasive in epidemiologic research, reflecting the nonrandom distribution of risk factors in real-world populations. It is usually more amenable to control in analytic individual-level studies than in population-level correlation analyses.

### Experimental Studies

Experimental studies (or intervention studies) begin with sets of reasonably similar populations or groups, which can then be allocated, preferably randomly, to "intervention" or "control" categories. The statistical analysis compares outcome rates in the two or more groups (the intervention may be applied at more than one level). The clinical randomized controlled trial is the model for this type of design.

Some types of environmental epidemiologic questions can be addressed experimentally at the individual level—for example, testing if the installation of household humidifiers reduces the prevalence of respiratory symptoms, or if the provision of masks to reduce workplace exposure to fumes reduces headaches. However, comparisons are more usually made at the supra-individual level—for example, testing the effectiveness of the broadcasting of safety promotion advertisements on television. A well-known

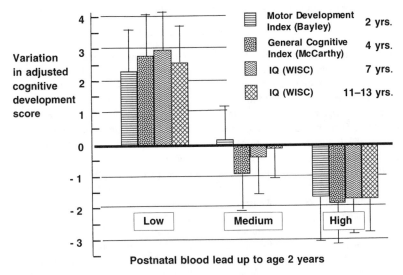

**Figure 8–2** Lead Exposure and Cognitive Development in Childhood. One point approximates to a 1% change. Low, medium, and high lead exposure categories have mean blood lead concentrations of 12.5, 18.5, and 25.9 µg/dl respectively.

historical example from the 1940s was the experimental addition of fluoride to the drinking water of four towns in North America, while not in four other similar towns, thereby allowing subsequent comparison of dental decay prevalence in children. For ethical reasons experimental studies cannot be carried out with exposures that might be harmful to those who are exposed—although it may be ethical to test experimentally the short-term, reversible, effect of annoyance factors (such as the acute effect of loud noise on blood pressure or of odors on mood).

A less rigorous approach to testing an environmental intervention is to carry out a before-and-after approach within a single group or population. However, it is often difficult to be sure that nothing else of relevance changed between the timing of the two periods.

**Exposure and Dose Assessment**

*Definitions*

Paracelsus, the sixteenth-century German physician/alchemist who is often credited with being the founder of environmental health and toxicology, wrote: "Poison is in everything, and nothing is without poison. The dosage makes it either poison or remedy" (Deishmann & Henschler, 1986). This statement lies at the heart of environmental health science as illustrated in the environmental pathway in Figure 8–3. Although some idea of the health effects of an environmental contaminant can be obtained by measuring the quantity of toxin at the *source* or in *emissions* or as environmental *concentrations*, these can be misleading measures because they do not directly indicate how much actually reaches the population. There is a huge amount of toxic mercury in the oceans, for example, but little reaches people in normal circumstances. Volcanoes emit vast amounts of toxic gases, but fortunately few persons are usually nearby to breathe them. Far more precise for predicting health effects would be measurements of *dose* itself, that is, the amount of toxins that has actually reached the vulnerable parts of the body. Unfortunately, it is difficult to measure dose directly for most toxins, either because it involves sophisticated, expensive, and invasive procedures (such as extracting and analyzing blood samples) or, for many toxins, because it is beyond our current scientific abilities. In ad-

**Exhibit 8–1** Environmental Lead Exposure and Childhood Development

Lead is the most abundant heavy metal. Lead may have been the first metal smelted, dating from 7000 to 6500 BC. The ancient civilizations of Phoenicia, Egypt, Greece, Rome, China, and India used lead for vessels, roofs, water ducts, utensils, ornaments, and weights. There was a great resurgence in its use during the Industrial Revolution. The subsequent development of the automobile hugely increased lead usage, in lead-acid batteries and as an "anti-knock" additive in gasoline. The lead content of Greenland ice layers shows a strong rise over the past thousand years, reaching 100 times the natural background level in the mid-1990s. The natural (preindustrial) blood lead concentration of humans is estimated to be much lower than the lowest reported levels in contemporary humans living in remote regions.

Lead has adverse effects on various organ systems, most importantly the central nervous system, kidneys, and blood. Epidemiologic evidence indicates that low-level lead exposure in early childhood causes a deficit in cognitive development during the immediately ensuing childhood years (Tong et al., 1998). Evidence from animal experimental studies and neuropathologic analyses corroborates this causal interpretation. Meta-analyses indicate that a doubling in blood lead concentration from 10 to 20 ug/dl—a range of lead exposure typically found between high and low tertiles in poorly controlled urban environments—is associated with a deficit in intelligence quotient of 1–3 points (Pocock, Smith, & Baghurst, 1994).

Many high-income countries, including the United States and Australia, have recently set new, lower standards on environmental lead levels, to protect young children. However, childhood lead poisoning is an increasing problem in many low- or middle-income countries. For example, the lead content of gasoline sold in Africa is the highest in the world and is associated with high lead concentrations in atmosphere, dust, and soils. Many other exposures in Africa result from industrial, cottage industry, and domestic sources. In recent surveys, more than 90% of the children in the Cape Province, South Africa, had blood lead levels over 10 ug/dl (Nriagu, Blankson & Ocran, 1996). In Dhaka, Bangladesh, the airborne lead concentration is one of the highest in the world, and the mean blood lead concentration in 93 randomly chosen rickshaw-pullers was 53 ug/dl—5 times higher than the acceptable limit in high-income countries. A recent study in six Indian cities found that more than 50% of children had blood lead concentrations higher than 10 ug/dl, and more than 12% of the children tested had concentrations higher than 20 ug/dl. In China where industrialization and motor vehicle usage are rapidly increasing, childhood exposure to lead is becoming a significant public health issue.

In developing a policy on environmental lead, two key questions arise. First, does the neurodevelopmental deficit persist over time? The currently available epidemiologic evidence suggests that the deficit persists through late childhood and early adulthood. Second, because few data are available in the very low exposure range, it remains uncertain if there is an exposure level below which no neurotoxicologic effect occurs. Overall, there is a strong case for public health measures to prevent exposure in early childhood. Because lead exposure tends to be ubiquitous within a population, a modest health impact upon each individual would yield a substantial aggregate impact for the total population. Assessments of population attributable burden are given in Ostro (1994) and Schwartz (1994). Phasing out leaded gasoline is the most effective way to reduce population exposure to lead. However, about 100 countries are still endangering their populations by allowing use of leaded gasoline (World Resources Institute, 1998).

dition, in a sense it is too late because once the toxin has entered the critical body organs the options for mitigation are limited.

Thus scientific and policy attention has increasingly focused on the intermediate portion of the environmental pathway, *exposure* (Figure 8–3), which lies directly at the interface of the environment and the body. "Exposure" is the amount of toxin actually encountered by humans in the course of their activities. More explicitly,

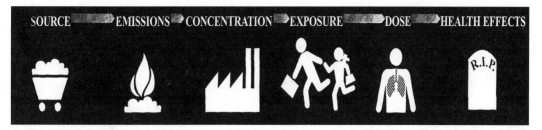

**Figure 8–3** Environmental Pathway

it is the amount of material or energy in the air, water, food, and soil that reaches the body's protective barriers of the respiratory and digestive systems, skin, eyes, and ears (see Figure 8–4). Exposure differs from dose in that it does not encompass any of the body's internal mechanisms for absorption, transformation, excretion, and storage of the toxin. Exposure differs from concentrations by incorporating not only measures of the levels of the pollutant in the environment but also who experiences them and for how long. Thus, *exposure* integrates information about where the pollution is and also where the people are.

### Total Exposure Assessment

Another important concept is that of total exposure assessment (TEA). To understand the full impact of a pollutant, it is necessary to examine all the ways it might reach people and not just rely on measurements made in the most convenient places. This is especially important for pollutants that can reach people through several different routes. For example, airborne lead pollution, arising mainly from vehicles, can spread through the environment to reach vulnerable groups, particularly children, not only through the air but also through water, soil, and food. Even though the original emissions are only to air, attention only to the air route would greatly underestimate the actual total exposure (see also Exhibit 8–1). It is total exposure, of course, that determines the risk to health.

The idea of TEA also applies to pollutants that only contaminate one medium. Consider, for example, the woman with the daily pattern of activities shown in Figure 8–5. What would be her health risk due to exposure to particulate air pollution? She lives in an urban slum of a low-income country where outdoor air pollution levels are fairly high. Her total exposure, however, is higher still because she spends considerable time in locations where particulate concentrations are higher than the outdoor levels. During the working day she works as a sweeper on busy streets, where particulate levels are higher than the average outdoor level because of proximity to traffic. In the morning and evening, she experiences even higher levels as household cook because her family can only afford poor-quality cooking fuels that produce much air pollution, such as briquettes made from coal dust. In the evening, she is exposed to the environmental tobacco smoke (ETS) from her husband's cigarettes. Her total exposure over the day is best estimated by the daily sum of the pollutant concentration in each major *microenvironment* where she spends time, weighted by the fraction of time she spends in it (see Figure 8–5).

The TEA approach can cause profound changes in the ranking of pollution sources. Consider, again, the category of persons represented by the woman in Figure 8–5. Although power plants and factories produce by far the most emissions and thus affect outdoor concentrations most, they do not produce the most exposure for those persons. Poorly maintained cars and motorbikes add significantly to outdoor concentrations of air pollution, but they have an even greater impact on actual exposure because they release their pollution in places where people spend time. Household stoves add little to the outdoor air pollution, but they profoundly

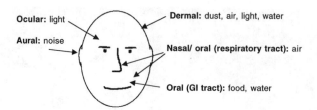

**Figure 8–4** Routes of Exposure

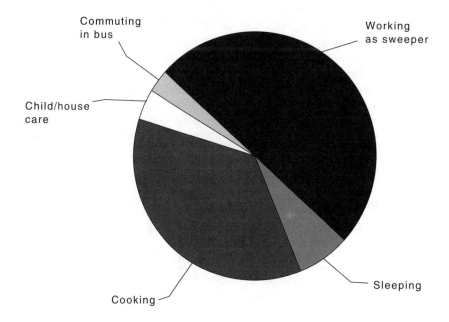

| Activity | Hours/Day | Particulate Concentration (ug/m³) | Daily Exposure Equivalent (ug/m³) | Proportion of Total Exposure |
|---|---|---|---|---|
| Sleeping | 7 | 100 | 29.2 | 0.07 |
| Cooking | 3 | 1,200 | 150.0 | 0.36 |
| Child/house care | 3 | 120 | 15.0 | 0.04 |
| Commuting in bus | 1 | 300 | 12.5 | 0.03 |
| Working as sweeper | 10 | 500 | 208.3 | 0.50 |
| Total | 24 | mean = 415 | 415 | 1 |

**Figure 8–5** Total Particulate Exposure for Woman in Urban Slum

affect exposure because their pollution is released when and where people are present. Finally, even though the total ETS emissions are negligible compared to those from outdoor sources, their contribution to the personal exposure of nonsmokers can be considerable.

The importance of TEA is thus severalfold. It can change the relative importance of sources of pollution, and it can uncover important new sources of personal risk, such as ETS, that may not appreciably affect environmental concentrations. It also reveals a new dimension of potential control measures. For example, chimneys for household stoves that would not change emissions at all—and may even increase outdoor concentrations—can lower exposures substantially by separating the people from the pollution. Laws to reduce smoking in public places can lower ETS exposure with no actual changes in total smoking emissions. In some cases, the cost-effectiveness of such exposure-control measures can be much higher than exposure reduction through generalized control of outdoor sources. Although ideally all pollution sources should be controlled, in reality there is always a limit to the resources available. Choosing the most cost-effective control measures first will ensure that the most public health protection is achieved with whatever resources are available.

The central task in most environmental epidemiologic studies is to estimate the quantitative link between ill health and a particular environmental exposure. Risks can be estimated in relation to a number of possible exposure indexes that refer to (1) ambient environmental exposure (for example, average level of air pollution within district), (2) microecological exposures (for example, neighborhood quality of housing), (3) personal-behavioral characteristics (for example, time spent exposed to indoor air), or (4) actual measurement of TEA. The choice of which to use depends on the accuracy needed and, as always, the resources available.

### Biological Markers of Dose

As shown in Figure 8–3, some measure of dose is likely to be even more closely related to health effect than any measure of exposure alone. Although not available for all situations, many types of biological markers (dose indexes) are possible, such as heavy metals in hair, nails, and blood; metabolites in urine; chlorinated organic chemicals in adipose tissue; radionuclides in bone; and antibody titers in relation to infectious agents. The advent of increasingly specific and sensitive laboratory assays—including modern fluorometric methods, atomic absorption spectroscopy, high performance chromatography, immunosorbent assays, and the development of various molecular biological markers—has greatly expanded the possibilities of measuring dose.

For all such measures, it must be remembered that a biological assay estimates the integrated outcome of a sequence of physiological and metabolic processes. Since individuals vary, for constitutional reasons, in such things as the efficiency of intestinal absorption, the profile of hepatic metabolic pathways, deposition in peripheral tissues, excretion, and tissue repair mechanisms, whatever interindividual variation exists in external exposure will be randomly amplified by these interindividual biological differences. Therefore, the rank ordering of individuals on the external exposure and internal dose measures will necessarily differ somewhat. However, with sufficiently large numbers of individuals in a study, external exposure levels will be reflected, on average, in the measure of dose. If the quality of that internal measure is high, and if its relevance to the putative causal relationship under investigation is specific and high, then it may well be preferable to a measurement of external exposure. However, a critical assessment should always be made in advance.

The field of molecular epidemiology has become prominent during the 1990s, as an approach to studying the causes—especially the environmental causes—of cancer (McMichael, 1994). This same field has also become important in modern infectious disease epidemiology, particularly for the determination of environmental sources and transmission pathways for infections such as Legionnaires' disease, tuberculosis, influenza, cholera, and food-poisoning organisms. Molecular assays make use of the variation in structure of macromolecules, particularly DNA. One example where DNA measurement has assisted the conventional epidemiologic study of causation has been in studies of dietary aflatoxin as a cause of liver cancer (McMichael, 1994). Aflatoxin is a biotoxin produced by the *Aspergillus flavus* mold in stored foods in warm humid environments. Because, previously, it was not possible to determine directly an individual's level of aflatoxin intake, epidemiologists were limited to demonstrating ecologic correlations, in eastern Africa and within China, between average aflatoxin concentrations in local diets and rates of liver cancer mortality. However, it is now possible to measure the concentration of excised, excreted, aflatoxin-DNA adducts in urine and to use this as a measure of recent individual exposure. Note, however, that the concentration of excised DNA-aflatoxin adducts in urine is an index that integrates across the following metabolic steps: absorption of aflatoxin into bloodstream, metabolic activation of aflatoxin, passage of aflatoxin into the cell nucleus (where adducts with DNA form), efficiency of DNA repair mechanism, and efficiency of excretion in urine. Because of this metabolic variation between individuals, it is necessary to study very large numbers of persons in order to be able to see an effect that is distinguishable from all the background metabolic "noise." This particular measure was used successfully in a cohort study of 18,000 Chinese men in Shanghai, followed for liver cancer incidence. The study revealed a positive association, at the individual level, between initial adduct level and cancer occurrence.

### Exposure Assessment at Individual and Population Levels

In studies of the health effects of ETS, for example, it has been common to classify exposures according to whether an adult has a smoking spouse or a child has a smoking parent. Clearly, someone living with a smoker is more likely to experience greater ETS levels than someone who does not, but this does not guarantee that this is so in every case. A child with no smoking parent, for example, may have four smoking grandparents who visit every day. Another child may have smoking parents who are careful to refrain from smoking anywhere near their child. In these cases, classification of these children by the smoking status of their parents would lead to exposure misclassification and a consequent attenuated estimate of the true effect. The risk of such exposure misclassification can be reduced by careful questionnaire design and by exposure-verification techniques, such as checking a sample of the children's urine for specific metabolites of nicotine. These validation procedures require additional resources.

The population-level classification of exposure, of whole subpopulations classified according to ecologic indicators such as location within a city, is often inexpensive and convenient. However, it can yield exposure misclassification if not done carefully. It is common, for example, to conduct air pollution epidemiology by dividing urban populations into exposure classes according to the measurements made at the nearest outdoor air pollution monitoring station or even to use one or a few monitors to represent the exposure of an entire city for comparison to other cities. This is much easier than trying to measure the total exposure of each individual according to his or her daily activity pattern. Since most outdoor pollutants penetrate to some extent indoors, people in cities are never free from them, even when not actually outdoors. On the other hand, as discussed above, local pollutant sources can sometimes overwhelm the contribution of outdoor levels. If the prevalence of local exposure sources (dirty household fuels, heavily trafficked roads, and others) differs in different parts of the city or in different cities, much exposure misclassification could result. Indeed, this problem is one of the main reasons why time-series studies have become more popular in recent decades (see also "Correlation Studies," above).

## Health Outcome Assessment

The issues pertaining to health outcome assessment are the same as for other realms of epidemiologic study. It is important to decide which type of outcome is the most relevant (and feasible). For example, many studies of the health impacts of air pollution have examined associations with mortality. Yet the underlying pyramid of nonfatal health effects is very broad-based; there is much to learn about the impacts of air pollution on hospitalizations, primary care consultations, existence of chronic conditions, impaired lung function (which requires testing of individuals), and self-assessed symptoms.

There is a natural tendency for researchers and data-collection agencies to prefer "hard" endpoints that are well defined clinically and amenable to clear-cut counting or measurement. Yet community surveys or consultations often indicate that the main perceived health impacts of environmental factors have to do with social, behavioral, and psychological disruptions, such as the mental stress of noisy environments, headaches or nausea from unpleasant odors, or underexercised overweight children who are constrained by traffic and lack of neighborhood facilities.

Having decided on the category of outcome, a formal case definition must be made. For those outcomes that enjoy preexisting population-based case registration—for example, cancers and congenital anomalies—case definition is relatively simple. However, when working anew from medical records, questionnaires, or test results, clear and stringent criteria must be specified.

If population-level research is being done, care is needed in acquiring and evaluating the data on frequency (prevalence or incidence) of occurrence of the health outcome. Issues of data incompleteness and, therefore, bias arise. Further, if health status is to be compared be-

tween populations, then it is usually necessary to make adjustments for differences in basic demographic characteristics such as age distribution, sex ratio, ethnic composition, and socioeconomic profile.

How useful are preclinical changes as health outcomes? In principle, such "outcomes" would enable earlier answers to be obtained to urgent problems or in relation to newly introduced exposures. For example, can early evidence of an effect upon skin cancer risk due to increased ultraviolet irradiation be gleaned because of the recent quarter-century of stratospheric ozone depletion? If UVR-specific mutations in skin could be identified and assayed, then that would speed up the research process.

## Data Analysis and Interpretation

Each study design described above has its own usual methods of analyzing the associations between exposures and health outcomes. In correlation studies the data are assembled at a group or population level and associations are based on comparing average exposure levels and the rates or levels of health outcomes in the different groups. Depending on the data sources the health outcomes can be expressed as prevalence rates (for example, health survey data on blood pressure) or incidence rates (for example, mortality data or cancer registration data). The comparison may involve just two groups at different exposure levels or a series of groups for which a dose-response relationship can be analyzed (for example, see Figure 8–6, Bobak and Leon, 1992).

In correlation studies dependent on the use of preexisting aggregated data, the lack of data on potential confounding factors may weaken the analysis. In analytic or experimental studies the observed association between exposure and health outcome is generally thought to be more valid because of the readier control of confounding, the observable conjunction of exposure and health outcome at the individual level, and knowledge of the temporal relationship be-

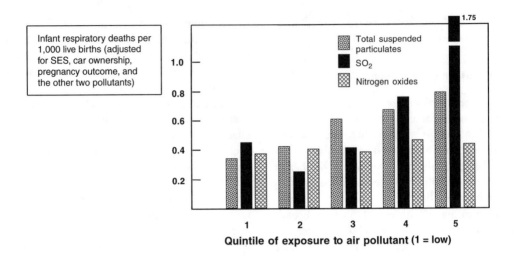

**Figure 8–6** Air Pollution and Infant Respiratory Disease Mortality in Eastern Europe

tween those two variables. Nevertheless, if information about a potential confounding factor has not been recorded in the study, or if the data have been collected or classified in biased fashion, the interpretation of the results may still be misleading.

The presentation of the results is important for effective risk communication. The statistical analysis may have shown that the mortality rate within a community for a particular disease has gone up by a factor of 1.3, with a 95% confidence interval of 1.1 to 1.6. What does this "relative risk" of 1.3 really mean? If the disease in question is rare, the 1.3-fold increase of the "absolute risk" may represent a few cases per million exposed people per year. If on the other hand the disease is quite common, a relative risk of 1.3 may imply a major public health impact. Risk estimates can also be presented in the form of the number of exposure-attributable cases per year, or as the number of cases that would occur in a longer time period (for example, a lifetime) within a community; these are sometimes called public health impact estimates. These measures are the most intuitively understandable to the lay person (for example, 27 persons dying each year due to the environmental exposure, against a "background" expectation of 90 deaths), and they may assist decision makers more than

would the more abstract epidemiologic measures of health effects. Ideally, for risk communication purposes, all three ways of expressing health risk associated with an exposure situation should be used.

Thus it is important to consider whether the results of a study are of "public health significance," in addition to being "statistically significant." The analysis and presentation of the results can highlight the public health significance of that particular problem by a combination of risk estimates as mentioned above, comparing the absolute risk estimates and public health impact estimates to the corresponding estimates for other health problems. This will provide an impression of the importance of the health effects identified. A problem in such comparisons is that it is difficult to measure the total health impact of an environmental exposure in a way that combines impacts on mortality and morbidity. In recent years various approaches have been proposed, such as the loss of quality-adjusted life years (QALYs), of health expectancy (an extension of the concept of life expectancy, the latter being confined to mortality data), or of DALYs. The DALY combines years of life lost from premature death and years lived with nonfatal conditions (assigned a disability weighting) (Murray & Lopez, 1996). The DALY was designed for comparative risk assessment and for economic impact analysis, and therefore it incorporates discount rates for the future value of healthy life. This measure has been promoted by the World Bank (1993) as a tool for priority setting in health sector investments (see Chapter 1).

These different ways of expressing the health risk of an environmental exposure may lead to different interpretations of the results of environmental epidemiology studies. No standardized approach is available yet. Note, however, that in the first published ranking of the different determinants of global burden of disease (Murray & Lopez, 1996) occupational health hazards and outdoor air pollutants were included in the top 10.

## Environmental Health Indicators and Monitoring

Environmental health issues are increasingly recognized as being part of a broader development-environment-health perspective. To achieve a lasting, sustainable impact leading to improved public health, the intervention must address underlying processes that create the exposure in the first place. In epidemiologic studies, the more direct the associations under study, the less likely are confounding and other complexities to cloud the interpretation. However, for effective decision making the relationships between underlying factors and health outcomes may be more important than acquiring detailed information about the exposure-effect relationships. The dramatic contamination of the human food chain by dioxins in animal feeds, in Belgium in 1999, raised "upstream" questions about the monitoring and regulation of feed production, and the social and economic pressures that heighten the risk of such episodes occurring. This more inclusive view of the causal chain is becoming increasingly prominent in monitoring environmental health protection.

Most industrialized countries have established a range of environmental performance indicators based on this approach. The most widely used "scheme" is that developed by the Or-

ganization of Economic Cooperation and Development (1993): the Pressure-State-Response Model (PSR). In order to analyze human health risks of environmental conditions, an expanded framework that better represents the cause-and-effect relationships between human activities, environmental change, and human health has been developed (Corvalan, Briggs, & Kjellstrom, 1996; Kjellstrom & Corvalan, 1995). This framework includes *driving forces* that lead to *pressures*; those pressures then affect the environmental quality (*state*), resulting in *exposures* (to humans) and then *effects* (in humans). The response has been labeled *actions* to highlight an active role of society rather than a passive response. The framework was termed the DPSEEA model (Figure 8–7).

Environmental indicators include the three first levels of the DPSEEA schema: driving forces, pressures, and state.

Driving force indicators are likely to be qualitative and are often expressed as yes/no answers. For example:

- Is there a policy to redirect all storm water to treatment plants?
- Are sedimentation dams in operation upstream in potentially cadmium-contaminated rivers?
- Are safety regulations for nuclear power stations adhered to?

Pressure indicators are usually quantitative. For example:

- amount of sewage-contaminated storm water entering a beach or river after heavy rain
- amount of cadmium transported via river water to paddy fields
- amount of radio nuclides released from a nuclear power station accident

The most common indicators are direct measurements of the environmental state—the concentration of a hazard in some environmental medium. For example:

- enterococci concentration in beach water or drinking water

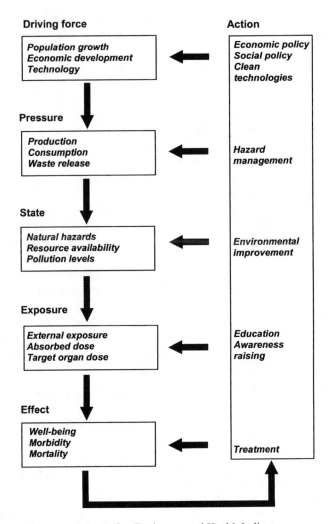

**Figure 8–7** The DPSEEA Framework To Define Environmental Health Indicators

- concentration of cadmium in rice paddy soil or rice
- level of radioactive strontium in lichens or reindeer meat

Exposure indicators may be based on exposures calculated from state indicators, as described in "Exposure and Dose Assessment," above. Biological indexes add individual-based information and can be used to monitor both exposure (for example, blood lead concentration, or DNA-adduct level) and effects (for example, enzyme assays for liver function, blood

pressure). The marked decline in breast milk concentrations of dichlorodiphenyltrichloroethane (DDT), around the world, is illustrated in Figure 8–8 (Smith, 1999). The most commonly used materials are blood and urine, although hair, nails, saliva, exhaled air, breast milk, and biopsy (or autopsy) materials from internal organs are also used in special circumstances. The material of choice for biological monitoring of exposure depends on the environmental hazard to which the person is exposed.

Ideally, an indicator of health effects should identify early effects that precede irreversible

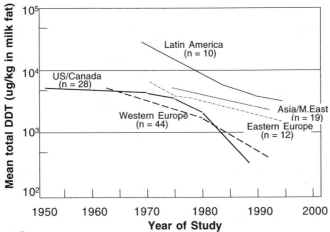

*Note:* n = number of studies.

**Figure 8–8** Worldwide Trends in DDT Levels in Human Breast Milk

health damage. Examples include free erythrocyte protoporphyrin (FEP) measurements in blood of lead-exposed people and temporary threshold shift (TTS) in hearing acuity after noise exposure. The next level of indicator includes early pathological change that may be reversible. An example is early tubular proteinuria after cadmium exposure (WHO, 1992). In some situations clinical symptoms or disease can be used in the monitoring, particularly after interventions to reduce environmental exposures. It would also be appropriate to use such indicators when there is disagreement about the actual existence of an environmental health problem. Even mortality monitoring may usefully complement other indicators. For particulate air pollution and other common air pollutants, for example, mortality monitoring may be useful, as the pathogenesis underlying increased mortality at relatively low levels of PM10 (particulate matter of less than 10 microns diameter) and carbon monoxide remains uncertain.

## Assessment of Environmental Health Impacts and Risks

### Distinguishing Impact Assessment from Risk Assessment

The related techniques of environmental health impact assessment (usually part of environmental impact assessment—EIA) and environmental health risk assessment (usually just called risk assessment [ERA]) constitute an important pair of tools for environmental policy and regulation. However, the latter is still under development in several important respects. EIA is often one of the first regulatory tools applied in low- and middle-income countries seeking control over environmental hazards, but having few economic and other resources to apply to the problem. Nevertheless, with accompanying governmental, legal, and media involvement, it can be highly effective for dealing with many gross problems. ERA, which requires more sophisticated databases and analyses, is becoming an important tool for use at every level of development because it can provide comparisons among a wide range of alternative actions.

The distinction between impact and risk assessments can be better understood by consideration of the concept of risk. Like many terms that are used in both common and technical parlance, *risk* is difficult to define precisely. In common parlance, risk refers loosely to actions or situations that involve an increased probability of adverse or undesirable outcomes. More formally, risk is a composite entity that entails three categories (two qualitative, one quantitative) of information. Sometimes called the risk triplet, those three elements are:

1. The scenario—what *could* happen (for example, a chemical plant might explode)
2. The consequence—what *type of health consequence* might ensue (for example, 10 people may be killed)
3. The probability—what *likelihood* of death is involved (for example, once per thousand years of operation)

The scenario is an imagined, plausible, occurrence and is the assumed starting point. The consequence is a foreseeable category of health outcome. The probability of that particular health outcome is estimable from research, experience, or, perhaps, theory. Only that third item entails estimation of a formal statistical probability. (The overall risk, in this hypothetical example, is 0.001 deaths per year of operation from accidents of this type.)

A simple way of distinguishing impact from risk assessment is that the former addresses only the first two components of the risk triplet, scenarios and consequences. Risk assessment addresses all three. Many types of activities with environmental health consequences are adequately understood through a fairly straightforward impact assessment. For example, the consequences of different routes for building a highway through a forest can be addressed by listing for each alternative the number of acres of first-growth timber that would be destroyed, the occupational accidents to be expected based on the construction methods, and the highway accidents and air pollution emissions that would result from use of the highway. In this case, since there is much past experience with these aspects of highways there is relatively little uncertainty about the range of consequences—and no compelling need to conduct an expensive probability assessment.

Consider, however, the case of a chemical plant. Although an impact assessment might be able to list the possible consequences from building and operating the chemical plant, it would have to encompass a tremendous range—for example, from no accident over the entire 50-year lifetime of the facility to a horrible accident such as occurred in Bhopal, India, in which thousands of persons die. Clearly, there is a compelling need to go the next step to a full risk assessment, which would tell how likely these dire consequences are. Only with this information can one alternative be compared intelligently to another.

Risk assessment is conventionally viewed as a five-point sequence. This begins with the research-based identification of an environmental hazard. Subsequent studies then estimate, first, the exposure- or dose-response relationship between the hazard and the specified health outcome, and, second, the distribution of exposure (doses) within the population of interest. From these two sets of information the overall risk to the population is then characterized, and risk management strategies are formulated. Although there is now some agreement about how to calculate risks, there is no completely objective way to compare alternatives with different patterns of risk. This is illustrated in Exhibit 8–2, which presents a choice between two ways of producing electric power with different patterns of risk and explains how reasonable consumers with different views of risk could rationally choose one over the other. This difference in risk perception is why people buy life insurance (risk aversion) and why insurance companies sell it (profits based on expected-value calculations).

Many other considerations would be included in a full assessment of alternative power plants. These include various outcomes of social importance other than those directly related to health. Thus the example illustrates that a decision about how much of what kind of risk to take demands substantial scientific input but is to a considerable extent a social and political choice.

### Probabilistic Risk Assessment

Since nuclear power plant operation is a relatively new enterprise, few accident statistics are available—particularly for large accidents in modern plants. How then can overall risk be determined? For this purpose, a technique called

**Exhibit 8–2** Risk Assessments Can Provide Additional Information for Decision Making—But Are Not Substitutes for Decision Making

Consider that a proposal has been made to build a large new power plant near your community. Everyone agrees on the need for more power and that there are only two viable alternatives available: coal and nuclear (the actual case in many parts of the world). These are found to cost about the same. A full environmental health risk assessment (EHRA) is done to compare the health implications of the two plants. The results are shown in the following illustration:

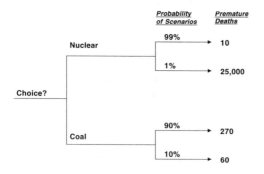

The coal plant, although of the best design, will still produce impacts because of air pollution and coal mining accidents. There is relatively little uncertainty about these factors—the EHRA finds that there is a 90% chance that 30 persons will die prematurely because of the operation of the plant over its lifetime. Because there might be a large accident at the coal mine or a fire at the coal plant during meteorological conditions that lead to severe local air pollution, there is a 10% likelihood of killing 60 persons.

The nuclear plant on the other hand is given a 99% chance of doing very little damage (that is, shortening only one person's life from the small amount of radiation released routinely). Unlike the coal plant, however, there is a small chance (here set at 1%) of a terrible accident in which 2,500

persons die from the radiation released. Which plant is safer? Which would you rather live alongside? There are at least three ways to answer, none necessarily right or wrong, but dependent on the set of values of the people making the decision:

- Maxi-min (maximize the chance of the minimum consequence): Since 99% of the time little damage is done and more may be learned in the future on how to reduce the chance of accidents, choose nuclear.
- Mini-max (minimize the chance of the maximum consequence): Since a nuclear accident would be a tragedy (cause international headlines, go down in history, destroy the community, and so on), coal should be used so as not to have any chance of such an event.
- Expected value (calculate the odds): Since the expected value of deaths from the coal plant is 33 (0.9 x 30 + 0.1 x 60) and for nuclear, 26 (0.99 x 1 + 0.01 x 2500), choose coal.

Although the particular numbers used here are fictional and real EHRAs for such facilities are much more complicated (involving hundreds of branches on the risk triplet trees shown in the figure), the overall results are often similar. Nuclear plants generally have a lower expected value of damage but carry a small probability of terrible events (much less than 1%). Coal plants produce more damage on average but do not impose anxiety about large negative events (although growing concerns about possible climate change from release of carbon dioxide from coal plants may change this perception). The fact that groups of perfectly rational people may choose different decision rules does not mean than any group is right in an absolute sense, only that they start with different values. Indeed, although there are many other factors to consider, the big difference in public acceptance of nuclear power between, say, France and Sweden, can be partially accounted to such different values.

probabilistic risk assessment (PRA) is applied to understand the potential for adverse consequences. Developed originally by NASA for assessing the risks of manned space flight, the technique basically breaks down the extremely complicated systems of large-scale technologies for which there is no overall accident information into its subsystems. These subsystems may need to be further broken down into even smaller components until a level is reached for which failure data are available. Then, the failure data for each subsystem are combined to predict the performance of the total system.

There is no information that would enable one to predict directly how a new type of nuclear plant will operate over time. However, it is made up of thousands of components for which information is available. There will be information, for example, about how often pumps of a certain size, switches of a certain voltage, or warning gauges of a particular brand will fail under various conditions. Even if a new type of component is introduced, its failure rate can be experimentally determined without putting anyone at risk, unlike testing the entire power plant.

Such PRAs, of necessity, are extremely complex and difficult for even specialists to evaluate. In particular, it is hard to tell whether all possible accident scenarios have been taken into account and whether there might be unforeseen events, such as human sabotage, that could circumvent many subsystems at once. It also assumes that the context in which each component was originally tested is not materially different in critical respects (for example, temperature or vibration) from the working context of the assembled plant.

Where an assessment reveals a potential or actual exposure to a chemical for which there is no human exposure history, a similar dilemma results. It would be dangerous and unethical, not to mention time-consuming, to deliberately expose enough people to the chemical to discover its true risk. Various techniques have been developed to estimate the risks of human exposures in this situation. The most common is to expose laboratory animals, usually rats and mice, to high enough doses of the chemical to observe effects within their relatively short life spans. When effects, such as tumors or reproductive failure, are observed, then there is legitimate concern that such effects might also be seen in humans. To quantify that risk, however,

requires extrapolating from high doses in animals to (usually) low doses in humans. This involves using a mathematical model that, ideally, is based on knowledge of metabolism, tumor induction, and other often poorly understood biological processes. Frequently, though, alternate animal models that are equally plausible biologically predict very different human risks for the same dose of the same chemical. (Had the antinausea-of-pregnancy drug thalidomide been tested in rats, not rabbits, the tragedy of limbless babies would probably have been averted.) It is necessary, therefore, to establish standard conventions for which model will be used in which circumstances so that consistent risk estimates are made. At present, many of the model choices depend more on scientific intuition than actual demonstrated knowledge. Finding more reliable and scientifically valid ways of doing such assessments is a very active research arena.

It might seem best to establish the convention of always using the most conservative model, that is, the model that predicts the largest risk. This would seem to fit the classic public health dictum that, in cases of uncertainty, it is better to err on the side of caution than to underestimate potential risk. Indeed, for this reason, such a conservative approach is used in formulating official policy by some regulatory agencies. Unfortunately, and perhaps counterintuitively, if this approach is taken for each chemical independently it can lead to the opposite effect, that is, exposing the public to unnecessary risks. This is because the degree of conservatism (or the size of the "safety factor") for specific chemicals can be quite different, depending on how well their observed animal or human impact actually compares with the predictions of the mathematical model employed. Thus society may end up spending much to control one chemical based on a risk assessment that uses a conservative safety factor of 1,000 because it appears to be more dangerous than another that is in reality more dangerous, but for which its estimated risk is based on a safety factor only 10 times its true value. Since it is rarely necessary to protect the population from only one hazard at a time, it is preferable to make judgments based on the best estimate of the actual risks rather than incorporating large, but varying, safety factors. In the real world of limited resources and time to deal with many possible hazards, an overly cautionary approach might be described as "too safe is unsafe."

### Measures of Ill Health for Risk Assessment Purposes

As discussed in Chapter 6, various measures of ill health have been proposed to take into account, separately or in combination, the degree of prematurity of death and the time lived with nonfatal disease. There are several choices to be made in such calculations—for example, whether to use different life expectancies for men and women or for different regions, how to weigh the severity of different kinds of disease, and whether to discount the value of lost life years in the future (as is the practice in economics). Whatever choices are made, it seems clear that measures of lost healthy life years, due both to death and disease, are useful as a primary indicator of ill health. Indeed, even more than money, time is a universal asset among humans in all societies. Unlike money, time is also something shared approximately equally—or it would be if all people were not differentially burdened by risk factors such as malnutrition, vaccinations, medical care, and environmental pollution. Thus the extent to which someone is denied a full healthy life span is arguably the best measure of the value lost, not only in practical terms but also in philosophical terms.

Such measures of forfeited healthy person-time, such as the disability-adjusted life year used by WHO for burden-of-disease estimates, are coming into increasing use. However, to date few current epidemiologic studies or risk assessment methods have directly applied them. More specifically, better estimates are needed of how much of the global burden of disease is due to environmental factors.

As the environmental "risk transition" progresses, and as the time between creation of a risk factor and its expression as disease tends to lengthen, the need for risk assessment increases (Smith, 1997). For evaluating measures to control diarrhea, it is reasonable to monitor diarrhea rates, for the diarrhea today is due largely to environmental exposures within a few preceding days. For controlling environmental carcinogens or greenhouse gases with their decades-long latency periods, however, waiting until ill effects start to occur would be far too late. It is thus necessary to conduct risk assessments as best we can to predict well in advance, so that appropriate measures can be taken in time. As a result, these actions—sometimes difficult and expensive actions—will have to be taken without confirmation that they will really be needed. Indeed, in some cases, confirmation may not even be attained in retrospect. However, society will usually gain collateral public health, social and often economic benefits, from expending resources to reduce longer-term risks.

### Assessing Risk: Compared to What?

Risk assessments, done in isolation, can be misleading. The following two examples are illustrative.

Determining the risk imposed by an activity requires, explicitly or implicitly, choosing an appropriate baseline. In discussing the health effects of smoking, the appropriate baseline is arguably zero. It is possible for people to quit or not take up smoking. For air pollution, however, the choice is not as clear. There are natural sources of many pollutants and human sources that are so difficult and expensive to control that a zero baseline is not feasible for many. What level is then appropriate? The national standard or the WHO guideline value? The level of the cleanest city? It is necessary to choose something in order to calculate the risk of the incremental pollution above the baseline.

Most human endeavors subject to risk assessment (technologies, industries, chemicals, regulations, and others) actually result in risk lowering as well as risk raising. A new factory in a low-income country, for example, might impose pollution on the public and accident risk on the workers, but it may provide jobs, housing, training, security, and other benefits that could lead to substantial improvements in health. Just because these effects are less direct than the accident risk does not mean they are small. Indeed, the overall impact of industrialization must be risk lowering—otherwise it would be the industrialized countries that would be unhealthy rather than the low- and middle-income countries without industry. Such risk lowering also occurs in industrialized countries as well. Consider, for example, a pesticide residue on vegetables. Looked at in isolation it may appear unacceptably risky. Looked at in terms of the overall impact on food cost and intake for low-income people, occupational risks to farm workers, and other factors, however, it may actually lower the overall risk compared to alternatives. This is not to say that all polluting activities will lower risks, but that all technologies should be judged on both their risk lowering as well as risk raising. There are also often important equity and justice issues relating to who experiences the raised and who the lowered risk. However, our current risk assessment methods are not well developed for determining risk lowering, and this potentially biases the results.

In both these cases, to be fair and done well, assessment needs to be grounded, that is, the assessor should explicitly answer the question "Compared to what?" and inform the reader why this particular comparison has been chosen. An example might be a risk assessment of the small cancer risk created by chlorinating drinking water (from the chemicals produced by reaction of chlorine and organic compounds in the water). In a place where the microbiological risks in drinking water remain high, the small incremental cancer risk may be well worth the trade-off.

## Some Special Considerations in Environmental Health Research

Various other considerations have recently acquired increasing importance in environmental health research and practice. There is a greater emphasis upon seeking "upstream" explanations of environmental health hazards, particularly because "downstream" (end-of-pipe) solutions are often ineffective (see also the discussion of the assessment of drivers, pressures, and environmental-state changes in the earlier section, "Environmental Health Indicators and Monitoring"). Meanwhile, advances in biomedical science have yielded a better understanding of how various body systems function as complex, dynamic, adaptive systems and of how their integrity might be affected, subclinically, by diverse environmental exposures. Finally, the understanding of the determinants of population and individual vulnerability to environmental stresses is improving.

### Specific Observable Toxicity versus Subclinical Organ System Effects

Most toxicological and environmental epidemiologic studies aim to characterize effects and risks associated with specific exposure agents. When such exposures yield specific avoidable disease outcomes (for example, bronchitis or bladder cancer), then this approach makes good sense. However, the functioning of certain organ systems can be cumulatively affected by multiple and continuing repeated exposures over time, resulting in immune system suppression, endocrine disruption, or cognitive impairment.

Both the immune system and the endocrine system entail complex interactive networks of organs, cells, and chemical messengers. It is not surprising that many exogenous organic chemicals can cause metabolic disturbance of these systems. Those are not so much *toxic* as *pharmacologic* effects. A growing body of evidence implicates pesticide exposures in suppression of the human immune system (Repetto & Belagi, 1996). This is also the case for other environmental exposures, such as air pollution and ultraviolet radiation. There is suggestive, but inconclusive, evidence of an environmentally induced decline in human sperm count in industrialized countries over the past half century, although the constituent data sets are neither representative nor standardized. Supportive evidence comes from observations of impaired fertility and reproduction in other mammals, birds, and fishes due to endocrine-disrupting chemicals released by human societies (Colborn, Vom Saal, & Soto, 1993).

### Determinants of Population Vulnerability

In general, low- and middle-income populations are the most vulnerable to the health impacts of environmental degradation and change. They are typically more exposed, in terms of residential and occupational location, and have fewer resources for taking protective or adaptive action. The various social, cultural, and political influences on population vulnerability to environmental change include poverty, environmentally destructive growth, political rigidity, dependency, and isolation (Woodward, Hales, & Weinstein, 1998). Changes in the age structure of populations also affect vulnerability. As average life expectancies increase, so populations become more vulnerable to many environmental stressors because of the increasing proportion of elderly persons.

More than 460 extra deaths were attributed to the effects of the extreme heat wave in Chicago in July 1995. The rate of heat-related death was much greater in Blacks than in Whites, and in persons bedridden or otherwise confined to poorly ventilated inner-city housing. In the correspondingly severe 1995 heat wave in England and Wales, a 10% excess of deaths occurred in all age groups. In greater London, where daytime temperatures were higher and there was lesser cooling overnight, mortality increased by around 15%. The excess mortality risks were generally greater in socioeconomically deprived groups. Similar patterns probably apply in low- and middle-income countries, although little such research has yet to be done.

The impact of regional changes in food and water availability will be greatest in potentially vulnerable regions where population growth is pronounced and food insecurity exists. Interactions between local environmental degradation and larger-scale environmental changes are likely to be important in determining the net impacts on human health. For example, local deforestation due to population pressure may directly alter the distribution of vector-borne diseases and the likelihood of flooding, both of which are also liable to increase because of global climate change.

### Determinants of Individual Susceptibility

Constitutional characteristics frequently influence an individual's susceptibility to environmental exposures. Ready examples include skin pigmentation modulating the risk of solar-induced skin cancer, and age modulating the efficiency of intestinal absorption of lead. Many physiological and biochemical functions of the human body—such as kidney function, liver function, eyesight, and hearing—decline with age after early adulthood. Individual variations in metabolic phenotype, substantially determined by genotype, are also important. There are many enzyme pathways known to be involved in the activation or deactivation of potentially carcinogenic or other toxic chemicals—such as the various oxidizing enzymes of the mitochondrial P450 system, the acetylation pathway (yielding phenotypically "fast" and "slow" acetylators), the glutathione transferase pathway, and the alpha-antitrypsin pathway. There has been a steady accrual of epidemiologic evidence that these polymorphisms modify the disease-inducing impact of an external environmental exposure; that is, a gene–environment interaction is observable at the individual level.

This raises important opportunities for higher resolution research. When study subjects are stratified on a metabolic polymorphic characteristic relevant to the external exposure, then the effect within the susceptible subgroup will become more evident than when the effect is diluted (averaged) across the susceptible and nonsusceptible subgroups.

This, of course, also creates new possibilities for future environmental risk management. The possibility of genetic screening in the occupational setting raises some particular dilemmas, in terms of ethics, social priorities, and public health strategies. Are we going to refocus on assessing individual susceptibility and give less emphasis to reducing the occupational or ambient environmental exposure that is the external trigger for the increase in risk?

## HOUSEHOLD EXPOSURES

Because it is where much human activity takes place, the potential for damaging exposures in households is high if pollutants are present. Unfortunately, two of the most fundamental and mundane human household activities—defecation and cooking—produce significant volumes of health-damaging waste products. When human waste is not removed completely from the household environment and isolated from drinking water supplies, it leads to outbreaks of diarrhea and other waterborne diseases. When the smoke from cooking fires fueled with wood, coal, and other low-quality fuels is released into households, it leads to respiratory diseases and other health impacts. Indeed, together, these two environmental health impacts account for the largest environmental burden of ill health globally and probably account for a larger burden than any other major risk factor, environmental or not, except malnutrition.

### Sanitation and Clean Drinking Water

Ever since hunter-gatherers turned to cultivation and settled living, sanitation has been a public health problem for human societies. Further, as urban populations have increased in size, the pressure on local sources of fresh drinking water has increased. Today, these two perennial difficulties remain widespread health hazards in the world, particularly in low- and middle-income countries in semiarid regions. Approximately 40% of the world's population does not have ready access to clean safe drinking water and approximately 60% does not have satisfactory facilities for the safe disposal of human excreta.

Water shortage amplifies the risk of many "water-washed" infectious diseases, such as chlamydia and scabies. Water shortage in combination with local fecal contamination increases the likelihood of transmission of waterborne diarrheal diseases, cholera, campylobacter, and other infections. Every year, several million children die from diarrheal diseases, contracted from infectious agents in drinking water and on food (see Chapter 4).

### Solid Household Fuels

The oldest of human energy technologies, the home cooking, fire using, wood or other biomass remains the most prevalent fuel-using technology in the world today. Indeed, in more than 100 countries household fuel demand makes up more than half of total energy demand.

A useful framework for examining the trends and impacts of household fuel use is the "energy ladder." It ranks household fuels along a spectrum running from the simple biomass fuels (dung, crop residues, and wood), through the fossil fuels (kerosene and gas), to the most modern form, electricity. In moving up the ladder, the fuel–stove combinations that represent the higher rungs increase the desirable characteristics of cleanliness, efficiency, storability, and controllability. On the other hand, capital cost and dependence on centralized fuel cycles also tend to increase with upward movement. Although there are local exceptions, history has generally shown that when alternatives are affordable and available, populations tend to naturally move up the ladder to higher quality fuel–stove combinations. Although all of humanity had its start a quarter of a million years ago at what was then the top of the energy ladder, wood, only about half has moved to higher quality rungs. The remaining half is either still using wood or has been forced down the ladder by local wood shortages to crop residues, animal dung, or, in some severe situations, to the poorest quality fuels, such as shrubs and grass.

Throughout history, in places where it was easily available, shortage of local wood supplies led some populations to move to coal for household use. This occurred in the early 1800s in the United Kingdom, for example, although it is relatively uncommon there today. In the past 150 years, such transitions occurred in eastern Europe and China, where household coal use still persists in millions of households (Figure 8–9). In terms of the energy ladder, coal represents an upward movement in terms of efficiency and storability. Because of these characteristics and its higher energy densities, coal can be shipped economically over longer distances than wood and efficiently supply urban markets. In this regard, it is like other household fossil fuels. Unlike kerosene and gas, however, coal often represents a decrease in cleanliness as compared to wood.

The two characteristics of fuels that most affect their pollutant emissions when burned are physical form and contaminant content. Generally it is difficult to premix solid fuels sufficiently with air to ensure good combustion in simple small-scale devices, such as household stoves. Consequently, even though most biomass fuels contain few noxious contaminants, they are usually burned incompletely in household stoves and produce a wide range of health-damaging pollutants (HDPs). Exhibit 8–3 lists some of the many hundred HDPs emitted as products of incomplete combustion from a range of household stoves in India. Even though biomass fuels would produce little other than carbon dioxide and water when combusted completely, in practice as much as one-fifth of the fuel carbon is diverted to products of incomplete combustion, many of which are important HDPs. Coal, on the other hand, is not only difficult to burn completely because of being solid, but it also often contains significant intrinsic contaminants. Most prominent among such emissions from coal, as shown in Exhibit 8–3, are sulfur oxides. Coal in many areas also contains arsenic, fluorine, lead, mercury, or other toxic elements that lead to serious HDPs.

Petroleum-based liquid and gaseous fuels, such as kerosene and liquid petroleum gas, can also contain sulfur and other contaminants, but in much smaller amounts than in many coals. Further, their physical forms allow much better premixing with air in simple devices, thus assuring substantially higher combustion efficiencies and lower HDP emissions. In addition, kerosene and gas stoves tend to be much more energy efficient. Hence, the HDP emissions per meal from these fuels are at least an order of magnitude less than those from solid fuels.

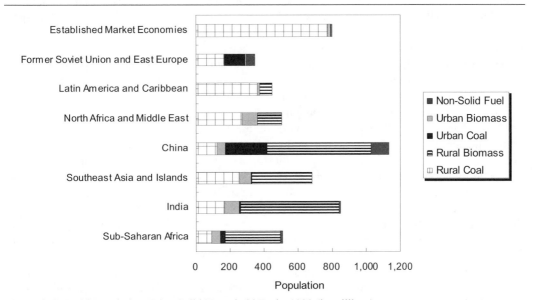

**Figure 8–9** World Population Using Solid Household Fuels, 1990 (in millions)

**Exhibit 8–3** Pollutants in Solid Fuel (Biomass and Coal) Smoke from Household Stoves in India

- Small particles, CO, $NO_2$
- Formaldehyde, acrolein, benzene, 1,3-butadiene, toluene, styrene, and others
- Polyaromatic hydrocarbons, such as benzo(alpha)pyrene
- Coal has all the above plus $SO_2$ + toxic elements, that is, As, Pb, Hg, and Fl
- Biomass and coal produce significant non-$CO_2$ greenhouse gases, such as methane

Unfortunately, not only do solid fuel stoves produce substantial HDPs, a large fraction also lack chimneys for removing the emissions. Consequently, indoor HDP concentrations can reach very high levels for various important HDPs, including fine particulates and carbon monoxide. Fine particulate levels often reach 20–40 times WHO guideline levels set to protect health. Even in households with chimneys, heavily polluting solid fuel stoves can produce significant local outdoor pollution. This is particularly true in dense urban slums where such "neighborhood" pollution can greatly exceed the urban average levels.

Pollution from household stoves is released in every household every day. This is the setting for high pollution exposures: significant amounts of pollution frequently released in poorly ventilated spaces at the times when people are present. Moreover, because they are usually responsible for cooking, women and their accompanying youngest children generally are most exposed. Thus, although the total amount of HDP pollution released from stoves worldwide is not high compared to that from large-scale use of fossil fuels, the total human exposures to a number of important pollutants are actually much larger than those created by outdoor pollution. As a result, the health effects can be expected to be higher as well.

Despite the sizes of the exposed populations and the HDP exposures involved, there has been relatively little scientific investigation of the health effects of indoor air pollution in low- and middle-income countries compared to studies of outdoor air pollution in urban populations (McMichael & Smith, 1999). Nevertheless, enough has been done to enable estimates of the magnitude of their impact, at least for women and young children who receive the highest exposures. The impacts of the high concentrations experienced by a larger number of people with generally lower overall health status exceed those for outdoor air pollution (see Exhibit 8–4).

## Housing Quality

General housing quality involves such factors as ventilation, drainage, crowding, dustiness, materials that resist pests, and insulation from sun, wind, and cold. All these factors have a significant influence on health. Indeed, much of the improvement in health that occurred in western Europe and North America during the latter part of the nineteenth and early part of the twentieth centuries is attributable to improved housing—although it is difficult to separate the relative benefits of improved housing from those due to concurrent changes in nutrition and personal hygiene behavior. Studies in some communities in low- and middle-income countries, however, indicate that health gains require improvements in a mix of factors, including general "housing" quality, rather than in just one factor at a time.

Good quality housing for low- and middle-income communities can protect health in various ways. It provides shelter from cold, hot, or wet weather conditions. Incremental improvements of traditional designs that are basically adapted to the local conditions would be the most cost-effective means of improving shelter. A factor of importance is the structural integrity of the housing in the face of typhoons, floods, or earthquakes. The location of the house is also of importance. The houses of many persons injured or killed in floods are in low-lying areas prone to flooding.

The risk of physical injuries is another important aspect of housing quality. Children and elderly need to be protected from falls. Animals, machinery, vehicles, and cooking stoves and

**Exhibit 8–4** Health Impacts of Indoor Air Pollution in Low- and Middle-Income Countries

Three main categories of health effects are thought to occur, based on studies in solid fuel households and corroborated by studies of active and passive smoking and outdoor air pollution. They are:

- infectious respiratory diseases, such as acute respiratory infections and, perhaps, tuberculosis
- chronic respiratory diseases, such as chronic bronchitis and lung cancer
- adverse pregnancy outcomes, such as stillbirth and low birth weight in infants born to women exposed during pregnancy

In addition, there is some evidence that the household use of solid fuel increases the risks of blindness, asthma, and heart disease.

The best available estimates of the range of potential health effects within the low- and middle-income country setting come from studies in India. These indicate that about 500,000 premature deaths in women and children under 5 years of age may be attributed annually to household solid fuel use. This is 4–7% of the total national burden of ill health, or 6–9% of the burden for these two population groups. This makes indoor air pollution a bigger cause of current ill health in India than from HIV/AIDS, alcohol, tobacco, malaria, vehicle accidents, or tuberculosis—although, fortunately, it is probably not increasing like several of those other health problems.

Given that India contains about one-quarter of the world's solid-fuel cooking stoves, the global impact of this exposure source could be expected to be about 4 times larger, that is, approximately 2 million deaths annually in women and children. This is roughly compatible with WHO estimates of about 2.5 million, which were generated by extrapolation of outdoor pollution studies in developed-country cities to indoor developing-country conditions (WHO, 1997).

Although it is tempting to promote technical fixes for household environmental health problems in low- and middle-income countries, alone they are often of only limited success. Provision of improved biomass-burning cooking stoves with chimneys often fails to reduce indoor air pollution because of poor maintenance and lack of consideration of local cooking practices. Promoting the use of cleaner fuels is difficult among populations that have little disposable income but have free access to local biomass resources. In general, reducing the risks related to such activities as cooking, defecation, and hygiene requires both technical and behavioral changes. Finding effective ways to achieve this is an important research task.

---

heaters need to be separated from areas to which small children have access.

Another factor of importance in tropical countries is the avoidance of breeding sites for insect vectors of disease. Good drainage around the home and elimination of any sites where water can stagnate and mosquitoes can breed are of great importance to prevent malaria and dengue fever. In parts of Latin America the prevention of Chagas disease (South American sleeping sickness) and the elimination of its vector, the triatomine bug, depends on the use of solid ceiling and wall materials without cracks.

## THE OCCUPATIONAL ENVIRONMENT

The workplace environment is generally more dangerous to health than the ambient external environment. Machinery, chemicals, dusts, ergonomic hazards, and the fact that much work is carried out with the body at its peak performance all contribute to the overall level of risk. Nevertheless, many of the same specific hazards occur in the workplace and the general environment, and hence there are many similarities in how their effects can be monitored and managed (Yassi & Kjellstrom, 1998).

There are various textbooks on occupational health/medicine describing the many workplace hazards to health (for example, Rosenstock & Cullen, 1994; Stellman, 1998). The issues in low- and middle-income countries have been highlighted by Kjellstrom (1994), and a detailed treatise is given by Herzstein et al. (1998). The following text only summarizes several key areas.

An important phenomenon in the workplace environment of low- and middle-income countries is the specific problems occurring at the time of rapid industrialization. Agricultural societies are transformed often without the infrastructure for environmental and workplace health protection that was built up in industrialized countries over decades of industrial development. Sometimes the new industries replace existing cottage industries, and the conditions may improve. In other cases industries with outmoded dangerous technology are moved from developed countries, creating new hazards in the receiving country. The term *export of hazards* has been used to describe this problem (LaDou & Jeyaratnam, 1994).

## Agriculture

Agriculture is the most common occupation in rural areas of low- and middle-income countries, where most of the world's population lives. Most workers are engaged in subsistence agriculture, in which the boundaries between work and other aspects of daily life are fluid. Workplace hazards in this type of situation include the generally poor and unhealthy living environments, with unsafe drinking water, poor sanitation, and inadequate shelter.

Further, there are specific hazards, such as injury hazards from tools used in tilling the soil, vector-borne diseases related to walking in water or mud, bites from insects and animals, and falls or drownings from working on hillsides or riversides. The health risks are further increased because subsistence farm work involves the whole family, including children and the elderly. Epidemiologic evidence of these types of health risks is scanty.

As the planting and harvesting processes become more advanced and farmers develop cash crop production, new hazards emerge. The tools involved become more mechanized and this creates new types of injury risks, particularly as the use of these tools is unfamiliar to many of the workers. Pesticides are introduced, often without full equipment and training

(WHO, 1990). It has been estimated that each year at least 1 million cases of unintentional pesticide poisoning occur among agricultural workers in low- and middle-income countries (WHO, 1990). In addition, there may be as many as 2 million suicide attempts annually, using pesticides, in these countries.

Agricultural work hazards are not only related to planting and harvesting food crops. An important activity is the collection of fuel wood for cooking and heating. Wood and agricultural waste is often collected in local forests by women (Sims, 1994). An analysis of time use for these activities, along with water collection and cooking, in four low-income countries showed that women spent 9–12 hours per day doing this, whereas men spent 5–8 hours. Firewood collection may be combined with harvesting of wood for local use in construction and small-scale cottage industry manufacturing. A number of health hazards are associated with the basic conditions of the forest, including insect bites, stings from poisonous plants, cuts, falls, and drowning. In countries with tropical heat and humidity, great strain is placed on the body, whereas the cold is a potential hazard in temperate countries. In countries with a high sunshine level, ultraviolet radiation can be another health hazard, increasing the risk of skin cancer and cataracts (WHO, 1994). All forestry work is hard physical labor, with a risk for ergonomical damage, such as painful backs and joints as well as fatigue, which increases the risk of injuries from falls, falling trees, or equipment (Poschen, 1998). Women carrying heavy loads of firewood are common in areas with subsistence forestry (Sims, 1994). Further, the living conditions of forestry workers are often poor, and workers may be spending long periods in simple huts in the forest with limited protection against the weather and poor sanitary facilities.

Urbanization leads to the development of a commercial market for firewood and larger scale production of firewood from logs or from smaller waste material left over after the logs have been harvested. Energy forestry then becomes more mechanized, and workers are exposed to additional hazards associated with commercial forestry (Poschen, 1998). Motorized hand tools (for example, the chain saw) become more commonly used, which leads to high injury risk, as well as noise-induced hearing loss and "white finger disease" caused by vibration of the hands. In addition, fertilizer and pesticides become a part of the production system with the potential for pesticide poisoning among sprayers. As the development of forestry progresses, more of the logging becomes mechanized with large machinery, reducing the direct contact between worker and materials. Workers in highly mechanized forestry have only 15% of the injury risk of highly skilled forestry workers using chain saws (Poschen, 1998). However, firewood production continues to require manual handling and may therefore remain a hazardous operation.

## Mining and Extraction

Mining is inherently dangerous to the mine workers, and most countries, including low- and middle-income countries, have recognized this by developing specific legislation and systems to protect mine workers (Stellman, 1998). There are two major types of mining with somewhat different patterns of health hazards: underground mining and open-cast mining. Ergonomic hazards and physical (accident-inducing) hazards occur in both, but underground work includes the added hazards of being crushed by falling rock, poisoned by gas or dust build-up, or affected by heat or radiation. Each type of mine entails specific hazards associated with the rock from which the ore is excavated. Most types of rock contain high levels of silica, leading to high levels of silica dust in the air of a mine and the risk of silicosis in workers. Certain types of rock (particularly uranium ore) contain radioactive compounds that emanate as the gas radon, which increases the risk of lung cancer. Other types of rock contain metals that are inherently poisonous (for example, lead and cadmium), and which in certain conditions can cause dangerous exposures.

According to various United Nations' *Demographic Yearbooks,* miners constitute a large occupational group in the international statistics. They represent up to 2% of the economically active population in some countries. Although 1% of the global work force is engaged in mining, it contributes 8% of the global fatal occupational accidents—about 15,000 per year. A detailed review of occupational health and safety issues in mining is available in Armstrong and Menon (1998).

Mining is thus a particularly dangerous occupation. Table 8–1 (Kjellstrom et al., 1992) highlights the high overall occupational mortality rates in low- and middle-income countries where reported rates are around 10 times higher than in industrialized countries, despite considerable "underreporting."

In low- and middle-income countries, coal mining employs millions of people. Coal is a major global energy source, contributing 24% of total energy consumption (WHO, 1997). It was the primary source between 1900 and 1960, but subsequently has been overtaken by oil. Coal can be produced through surface mining ("open cast") or underground mining. Both operations are inherently dangerous to the health of the workers.

Underground coal miners are exposed to the hazards of excavating and transporting materials underground. This includes injuries from falling rocks and falls into mine shafts, as well as injuries from machinery used in the mine. There are no reliable global data on injuries of this type from low- and middle-income countries (Jennings, 1998), but in industrialized countries miners have some of the highest rates of compensation for injuries. In addition, much of the excavation involves drilling into silica-based rock, creating high levels of silica dust inside the mine. Pneumoconiosis silicosis is therefore a common health effect in coal miners (Jennings, 1998). In addition, it has been shown that coal miners with silicosis have an increased risk of lung cancer.

Other health hazards specific for underground coal mining include the coal dust, which can

**Table 8–1** Occupational Death Rates in Selected Countries and Relative Rates for Miners and Construction Workers

| Country | Crude Death Rate, All Occupations (Deaths per 1,000 workers per year, 1980s) | Ratio of Crude Death Rate in Mining Relative to Rate in All Occupations | Ratio of Crude Death Rate in Construction Relative to Rate in All Occupations |
|---|---|---|---|
| Guatemala | 0.54 | 3 | 2 |
| South Korea | 0.33 | 13 | 1 |
| Zimbabwe | 0.28 | 4 | 1.5 |
| Hong Kong | 0.075 | 23 | 12 |
| United States | 0.060 | 5 | 3 |
| Sweden | 0.036 | 6 | 2 |
| Japan | 0.020 | 19 | 4 |
| United Kingdom | 0.017 | 10 | 6 |

cause "coal workers pneumoconiosis" or anthracosis often combined with silicosis. The coal dust is explosive and explosions in underground coal mines are an ever-present danger for coal miners. Fires in coal mines are not uncommon and once started may be almost impossible to extinguish. Apart from the danger of burns, the production of smoke and toxic fumes will create great health risks for the miners. Even without fires, the coal material will produce toxic gases when it is disturbed: carbon monoxide, carbon dioxide, and methane. Carbon monoxide binds to hemoglobin in the blood, blocking oxygen transport and causing "chemical suffocation." It is a colorless and odorless gas and therefore gives no warning before the symptoms of drowsiness, dizziness, headache, and unconsciousness occur. Carbon dioxide displaces oxygen in the underground air and can cause suffocation. Another health hazard is exhaust fumes of diesel engines used in machinery or transport vehicles underground. These contain very fine particles, nitrogen oxides, and carbon monoxide, all of which can create serious health problems.

Surface coal mining avoids the hazards of working underground, but still involves risk from machinery, falls, and falling rocks. In addition, coal mining is very energy-intensive work, similar to forestry, and heat, humidity, and other weather factors can affect the worker's health. The machinery used is noisy, and hearing loss is a common effect in miners. Another health hazard is the often squalid conditions under which many coal workers in low- and middle-income countries live, creating particular risks for the diseases of poverty.

A special type of mining is the extraction of oil and gas to supply the energy needs of industrializing societies. Oil and gas exploration, drilling, extraction, processing, and transportation involve a number of the hazards mentioned above: heavy workload, ergonomic hazards, injury risk, noise, vibration, and chemical exposures (Kraus, 1998). This type of work is often carried out in isolated geographic areas with inclement weather conditions. Long-distance commuting may also be involved, causing fatigue, stress, and traffic accident risks. The ergonomic hazards lead to risk of back pain and joint pain. Injuries include burns and those caused by explosions. Skin damage from exposure to the oil itself and from chemicals used in the drilling processes creates a need for well-designed protective clothing. In addition, many oil and gas installations have used asbestos for heat insulating cladding of pipes and equipment. This creates the hazard of inhalation of asbestos dust in the installation and repair of such equipment, which increases the risk of lung cancer, asbestosis, and mesothelioma (WHO, 1998).

Much exploration and drilling for oil and gas now occur offshore. This involves underwater diving work, which is inherently dangerous. In addition, the weather-related exposures can be extreme, particularly as the work often requires continuous operations around the clock (Kraus, 1998).

## Construction

Construction work is another dangerous occupation with potential exposures to a variety of hazards (Weeks, 1998). This includes injuries from falls and falling objects, and injuries from machinery or related to excavation or underground work. As much construction work is carried out in the open, weather conditions create hazards of heat, cold, UVR, and dust storms. Construction work involves heavy lifts of materials and activities in awkward body positions leading to ergonomical hazards. Injuries, strains, and sprains are common. Many injuries are severe, leading to the high rate ratio of construction workers in the occupational mortality statistics (see Table 8–1).

Construction work also involves exposures to noise, chemicals, and biological hazards. Much of the machinery used is noisy, and this problem has increased with increasing mechanization of the industry. Demolition is a common aspect of construction work and demolition activities are inherently noisy. Noise-induced hearing loss is therefore common among construction workers. Another aspect of the noisy environment is the increased safety problems due to masking of warning calls or other alarms.

Chemical and dust exposures are related to the composition of the building materials. Asbestos, which was used as insulation and as a component of asbestos-cement pipes and sheets, has been a prime example of a hazardous material. Asbestosis (a form of pneumoconiosis), lung cancer, and mesothelioma (another cancer) have been found in many construction workers (WHO, 1998). The use of asbestos has been reduced in most industrialized countries and banned in some, but asbestos-cement building products are still widely used in low- and middle-income countries because these materials have attractive technical qualities and alternatives may be more costly.

Other chemical and dust exposures include cement dust among bricklayers and concrete workers. This dust causes dermatitis. Sand-blasting or rock drilling creates silica dust in the air, which can lead to silicosis in the exposed workers. Construction work often involves welding, which adds further health hazards such as inhalation of welding fumes that lead to bronchitis. Paint fumes often contain organic solvents that may cause neurologic disorders. The hazards of dusts and fumes are increased inside confined spaces, where these concentrations can reach extremely high levels.

Because of climate change, work in the construction industry is often seasonal, and contract workers therefore rely on other work during parts of each year. The intermittent character of the work creates problems in maintaining efficient prevention programs to protect workers against these hazards (Weeks, 1998). This is particularly so in low- and middle-income countries. Subcontracting or informal employment relations often reduce the responsibility taken by the main employer or contractor on a construction site. The responsibility for health and safety is dispersed among many individuals, so the protection against hazards may become insufficient. In construction work it is therefore important that contracts include the necessary safety provisions, and that there are systems for monitoring and enforcing these provisions.

## Manufacturing

Manufacturing workplaces can involve any of a textbook list of occupational hazards, some of which were mentioned in previous sections. A recent review of the various hazards is included in the *Encyclopaedia of Occupational Health and Safety,* published by the International Labor Organization (Stellman, 1998). Manufacturing involves ergonomical and injury hazards from improper work positions, heavy lifts, and dangerous machinery; physical hazards, such as noise, heat, poor lighting, and, occasionally, radiation; and chemical exposures of many kinds. However, as in the history of today's industrialized countries, the major chemical exposure problems in low- and middle-income countries include lead, chromium, mercury, other metals, organic solvents, and welding fumes. Increasingly, the most hazardous industries and processes are exported from industrialized to low- and middle-income countries (LaDou & Jeyaratnam, 1994), without the technological improvements that have reduced workers' exposures in the industrialized countries. In addition, stress and other psychosocial hazards of long work hours and shiftwork are common in an industry that has large investments in machinery, from which economic benefit only accrues when it is in operation.

Of the various manufacturing industries, some with particular health risks are worth highlighting. In electrical appliance manufacturing (Stellman, 1998) a major problem is lead-acid battery manufacture, which produces batteries for cars. Since such batteries are too heavy to transport over long distances, local production is usually established at an early stage of the "motor car society." The operation of these factories typically involves many workers who receive unacceptably high lead exposures. The usual approach is to monitor workers' blood lead levels; if the levels exceed the national standard, the worker is excused for a few weeks. Indeed, this type of risk management is enshrined in occupational health law in many countries. This approach displaces the exposure problem to the individual rather than analyzing the workplace environment as a whole.

Another manufacturing industry common in industrializing countries is metal processing and metal working. Smelting and refining of any metal provides a major potential for occupational exposures to many types of hazards, and a particular risk of exposure to toxic metal dusts, sulfur dioxide, and other fumes. As these industries are often of very large scale, even small concentrations of toxic compounds in the processes can yield substantial emissions into the workplace and the surrounding environment. The experience from lead smelters in many countries is similar: high lead exposures to workers and contamination of the local environment. Often the workers and their families live in the vicinity of the industry, and high lead exposures in children from dust emissions are found. These exposure situations have been studied in detail in the United States and Australia, and epidemiologic research there has produced some of the most valuable quantitative data on the health risks of lead in children and workers (see also Exhibit 8–1).

## Service Occupations

Many service industries involve important occupational hazards. The services reviewed by the International Labor Organization include those with specialized and sometimes severe hazards, such as emergency and security services (for example, fire fighting and law enforcement), public and government services (for example, garbage collection and hazardous waste disposal), and health care services (Stellman, 1998). The review also includes those likely to have less severe hazards, such as retail trades, banking, administrative services, telecommunications, restaurants, education, and entertainment.

Fire fighting involves exposure to carbon monoxide and toxic fumes, as well as the heat from the fire itself. Injuries from falling debris, falls, or working in awkward positions are also of concern. Protection of workers depends on protective equipment, which in low- and middle-income countries may be in short supply. Law enforcement is another high-risk occupation, which involves hostile contacts with other persons who may be armed.

Garbage collection exposes workers to risks of cuts and other injuries from the garbage itself, as well as heavy lifts. A particular risk group in low- and middle-income countries is the people who scavenge on garbage dumps for recyclable materials from which to glean a meager existence. Sometimes these scavengers actually live on the garbage dump, with the associated risks of infectious disease, bites from rats and dogs, and other dangers. Hazardous wastes are not always separated and therefore add to the risks of the garbage collectors and scavengers. In areas where hazardous wastes are separated, the storage and handling of these requires sophisticated protective equipment, detailed information about the hazards, and efficient management systems. These are often missing even in industrialized countries.

Health care workers face other hazards, such as infections from patients, transmission of HIV or hepatitis from needle pricks, allergies to drugs given patients or to cleaning and disinfection chemicals. However, the most common problem is ergonomic hazards, from lifting or moving patients, leading to back injuries. This creates great problems for nurses and nurse aides, and in many cases curtails their careers.

One special hazard for people in service trades that involve continuous work at computer keyboards is the development of repetitive strain injury, or as it is also called, *occupational overuse syndrome*. The repetitive keyboard finger work, or the repetitive fine movement of the computer mouse, creates a wear-and-tear reaction in tendons and muscles that can lead to chronic pain. As with the situation for bad backs, these painful conditions are not always accompanied by measurable anatomical or pathological changes, which has caused substantial arguments among medical practitioners as to the genuineness of the disease. However, as many people using modern computers attest, the short-term pain after intensive use of a keyboard or a mouse is real. The ergonomical design of a computer work station and the provision of regular work breaks are essential for preventing this occupational hazard. The height of the keyboard should be adjusted to the individual user. These conditions may be difficult to achieve in low- and middle-income country situations.

## Other Occupations

Among the other occupational exposure situations of particular importance, especially in low- and middle-income countries, are cottage industries of various types. At an early stage of industrialization, small-scale operations based on family members may be the mainstay of certain industries. This may be in the form of work contracted out from a larger enterprise, or it may arise directly in relation to the local market. The production of handicrafts, clothing, and consumer items for local households may be the starting point. However, more hazardous activities, such as recycling car batteries, may also develop initially as a cottage industry. This may entail extreme exposures to toxic chemicals, with little or no protection either for the workers or other family members. Ergonomic hazards, injuries, noise damage, and all other occupational hazards are likely to be a greater danger in these cottage industries than in more organized enterprises.

## COMMUNITY-LEVEL EXPOSURES

This is the level at which much environmental epidemiologic research has concentrated, particularly in relation to ambient air pollution, industrial emissions, the problems associated with urban transport systems, contamination of local drinking water and local food supplies, and waste management. Difficult methodological choices often confront researchers at this level, particularly whether to attempt to measure exposures and make comparisons at the individual, small-group (microecologic), or community level.

### Outdoor Air Quality

Urban air pollution has, in recent decades, become a worldwide public health problem (World Resources Institute, 1998). In the industrialized countries, the earlier industrial and household air pollution from coal burning has been replaced by pollutants from motorized transport that form photochemical smog, including ozone (a strong irritant that affects eyes, upper airways, and lungs) in summer and a heavy haze of particulates and nitrogen oxides in winter. Although many industrialized cities do not yet meet annual standards for every pollutant, conditions are generally much better than in the past. Nevertheless, air pollution has become a renewed concern in various industrialized cities where it was believed that the historic problems had been solved. The experience of severe air pollution incidents around midcentury, most famously in London in 1952 when the daily mortality was doubled during a 2-week period, finally led to a political agreement to act against air pollution. During that episode the daily peaks were several thousand ug/m$^3$ for each of the pollutants. Those earlier problems were caused mainly by the industrial and household burning of coal without efficient emission controls, leading especially to high breathing-zone concentrations during temperature inversions. During the subsequent decades the annual average and daily peak levels of particulate matter and sulfur dioxide were decreased tenfold or more in most cities of industrialized countries.

In low- and middle-income countries, urban air pollution has recently attained alarming levels in many cities. In New Delhi, Beijing, and several other Indian and Chinese cities, for example, the annual average concentrations of particulates have been 5–10 times greater than the WHO air quality guideline. In China the main source of pollution is combustion of coal. Industrial, neighborhood, and household sources all contribute, however, and emissions from automobiles are increasing sharply (Florig, 1997). The estimated morbidity and mortality in Chinese cities due to air pollution is now increasing markedly (see Exhibit 8–5). Meanwhile, in many of the cities of central and eastern European countries the mix of industrial emissions and car exhausts has caused increases in air pollution. In eastern Germany and in southern Poland in the late 1980s, winter concentrations of sulfur dioxide from coal burning were even higher than those in London, during the infamous 1952 smog episode.

Studies relating ambient air pollution levels to health risks were, until the 1970s, largely confined to examining the health impacts of particular extreme episodes of very high outdoor air pollution levels. Subsequent studies, based on daily mortality time series, have elucidated the role of respirable particulates, ozone, and nitrogen oxides in acute mortality (Schwartz, 1994). The advantages and attractions of daily time series statistical analysis have been discussed in "Study Design Options" above. However, this acute component of mortality due to daily fluctuations in air pollution levels needs to be carefully distinguished from the long-term effect of chronic exposure at an elevated level (McMichael, Anderson, Brunekreef, & Cohen, 1998). Long-term follow-up studies of populations exposed at different levels of air pollution, especially particulates, indicate that the higher the background levels of exposure the greater the mortality risk.

Asthma, which has been increasing in industrialized countries for 3 decades, has a still unresolved relationship to external air pollution. Although some studies indicate a contributory role of air pollution as trigger, if not as initiator, in this marked rise in asthma rates, other studies are less conclusive. The apparent increasing susceptibility of successive modern generations of children to asthma may well derive from changes in human ecology that have altered early-life immunological experiences—such as reduced exposure to common childhood infections (due to smaller family sizes) or allergenic household exposures (for example, house-dust mites or fungal spores), or to modern vaccination regimes.

Epidemiologists have developed a diverse and increasingly sophisticated set of methods for assessing the health impacts of air pollution. Nevertheless, the issue remains bedeviled by difficulties in exposure assessment, the uncertain differentiation of acute and chronic effects, the need to sort out independent and interactive effects between air pollutants that are often highly correlated, and the fact that the profile of air pollution keeps evolving as human activity patterns change. Although there are many uncertainties, there is general agreement that significant health effects occur at pollutant concentrations that

**Exhibit 8–5** Urban Air Pollution and Health in India and China

The two largest countries in the world share an unfortunate characteristic: they rely on dirty coal for large fractions of their commercial energy. In addition, being low-income, they have not been able to devote significant resources to either cleaning the coal before it is burned or capturing the emissions in the smokestacks before they are released into the environment. Furthermore, they have many relatively small coal-burning sources, including small factories, commercial activities such as restaurants, and, in China, boilers for heating buildings and cookstoves, from which the pollution is difficult to control. The result is high air pollution levels in many cities in both countries.

Data show, for example, that the average annual outdoor concentration of PM10 (airborne particulate matter of diameter less than 10 microns) in large Indian cities is about 190 ug/m$^3$. This is 6–7 times the levels in U.S. and European cities. The worst city in India, and probably in the world, is

Calcutta, which annually averages twice as much. Recent WHO global air pollution guidelines indicate that the Indian urban average exposure may cause an extra 15–20% mortality within the urban population. Mean PM10 levels in large Chinese cities are similar, perhaps 180 ug/m$^3$, but, unlike India, China's coal also contains significant amounts of sulfur, and thus sulphur dioxide levels are also markedly elevated.

Although estimations in this context are difficult, it appears that the resulting burden of disease in each country is high, perhaps 100,000–200,000 premature deaths annually in each country from chronic lung disease, pneumonia, lung cancer, and heart disease (Florig, 1997). However, in addition to other uncertainties, such calculations depend on what baseline is assumed, i.e., how low could pollution levels realistically become? Given natural background environmental factors, a level of zero is simply not feasible.

---

used to be considered benign. In the case of small particulates, which can penetrate deeply into the respiratory system, there is no evidence of a threshold exposure below which no effect occurs. This absence of a "safe level" complicates the development of guidelines and standards. Recently, WHO decided instead to publish a table of exposure-response relationship functions. Policy makers are thus forced to decide what level of health risk is acceptable in order to determine an appropriate exposure standard.

**Traffic and Transport**

As cities grow in size, urban transport systems expand and evolve. In particular, private car ownership and travel have increased spectacularly over the past half century, creating new opportunities and freedoms—and new social and public health problems (Fletcher & McMichael, 1997). Currently, there seems to be no agreed

vision of an urban future that is not dominated by privately owned vehicles.

Transportation is one of the key polluters in the process of economic development, urbanization, and industrialization. In traditional subsistence agricultural societies, the community's basic needs could be met within a relatively localized distance. Increasing population size and density means that specialized resources for the community, such as firewood, must be acquired from increasingly distant sources, and this creates transportation needs. Modern economic development has accelerated this process, by further specialization of economic tasks and dependence on resources from distant areas. Energy sources, such as coal, have had to be transported from afar to sustain local cottage industries; this was also the case with food items to sustain people in places where little could be grown or gathered for much of the year.

Initially, transportation by waterways was favored, requiring no investment in tracks for vehicles. During the twentieth century, railways and roadways dominated. Motorcars and trucks, with internal combustion engines, have subsequently had a significant impact on the environment and health. Combustion of petroleum fuel produces various toxic emissions: particulate matter (dust), carbon monoxide, nitrogen oxides, hydrocarbon remnants from the oil, and a variety of complex hydrocarbons. The health effects of these pollutants range from minor respiratory symptoms to asthma attacks, lung cancer, and death from heart or lung disease. In addition, some of these pollutants react with oxygen in strong sunlight to form ozone.

Today, the automobile has become the dominant source of air pollution in many cities (World Resources Institute, 1998). Current technical solutions to this problem include making car engines more energy efficient and using pollution control devices, such as catalytic converters. The obvious, more radical solution is to reduce dependence on car traffic by encouraging people to walk and to travel by trains, buses, or bicycles. Such measures, carried out as part of a clean air implementation plan, as shown in certain towns in the United States and Germany (WHO, 1997), can significantly reduce automotive air pollution. However, in low- and middle-income country cities the problems have grown even faster. Whereas in Europe a local transport infrastructure based on railways, trams, and buses was already in place when the car boom emerged in the 1960s, low- and middle-income countries often have negligible transport infrastructure. Hence, with increasing affluence and urbanization, the automobile is seen as the best solution for the individual families. Cities such as Mexico City have, consequently, experienced a rapidly deteriorating air pollution situation (WHO, 1997). However, the recent experience of Mexico City also provides a case study of an effective reduction of car-generated air pollution (see Exhibit 8–6).

Since the first oil crisis in the 1970s, the average fuel efficiency of the world's automobiles increased substantially, largely through major improvements in North America up to the mid-1990s that brought efficiencies nearly to European levels. Emissions of air pollutants have also been greatly reduced, partly through combustion modifications and partly through extensive application of "end of pipe" controls, in the form of catalytic converters. It is clear, however, that if the number of automobiles in low- and middle-income countries continues to grow as it has in recent years, unacceptable air pollution levels will persist for many decades even with the best current auto technology. Fortunately, several near-commercial technologies promise much better efficiency and lower emissions. Electric cars will probably have increasing, but still specialized, applications. However, because of weight, capacity, cost, and lifetime limitations of batteries, they show no sign of being able to serve the main market. Hybrid cars that are now becoming available, however, combine the best features of both fuel and electric drive systems, and can significantly increase efficiency and lower emissions without the changes in fuel delivery systems required by all-electric vehicles. Even more promising, although not yet commercially available, are cars powered by fuel cells. These can be extremely efficient and produce only tiny amounts of pollution when powered by clean fuels such as methane or hydrogen. Both hybrid and, particularly, fuel-cell cars would also reduce the emission of carbon dioxide, the main anthropogenic greenhouse gas contributing to climate change (see "Climate Change," below).

The motor car-based transport system poses several other health risks. Most obvious is the great and increasing burden of disease due to car crash injuries (Murray & Lopez, 1996). Much of the additional future health impact will occur in the currently low- and middle-income countries. Road fatality rates, per thousand vehicles, are around 30 times higher in Africa than in Norway, the United Kingdom, and the United States, for example. These differences highlight the injury risks at an early stage of motorization when roads are still undeveloped, pedestrians and drivers are not adjusted to one another, drivers have poor driving skills, and the vehicles are not

**Exhibit 8–6** Case Study: Automobile Air Pollution in Mexico City—Thinking Things Through

Mexico City has often been cited as having some of the worst urban air pollution conditions in the world, although, from a health perspective, the large Asian coal-burning cities probably create higher risk for their residents. The pollution in Mexico City has been so intense because a large industrializing population lives within a bowl-shaped valley with frequent meteorological conditions that limit circulation of clean air from outside. (Indeed, having nearly 20 million persons living in such an arrangement has been termed a serious "topological error.") The rapidly growing number of automobiles in the city is a major cause not only of the pollution, but also of serious traffic congestion with consequent negative impacts on economic and social interactions.

In the late 1980s it was proposed to reduce vehicle pollution in the city by imposing the "A day without a car" (*hoy no circula*) program in which all cars would be prohibited from driving one weekday every week, the day depending on the last digit on each car's license plate. The reasoning was that pollution emissions and congestion would thus be reduced approximately 20% by forcing people to carpool or use public transit more often.

For the first few weeks, data show that there seemed to be a drop in pollution and congestion. The response of the population over the longer term, however, was different than anticipated. Many thousands of persons purchased second cars with a different license plate number so that they could still drive every day. Of course, once they had a second car they tended to drive more than they would have with just one. In addition, many of these second cars were older used cars, which tend to have higher emissions levels. Thus one unintended result of the regulation was to draw older, more polluting cars into Mexico City from other parts of the country.

When proposing new pollution regulations, it is important to consider the full ramifications. This is particularly so when dealing with pollution caused by behavior at the individual level, such as use of private vehicles. Economists and other social scientists need to be involved from the start, and household surveys and pretesting are needed to gauge impacts before full implementation is attempted.

To address this issue, a new scheme was implemented in 1996 by the local authorities. Cars were assigned to three broad categories according to age, pollution control technology, and emission levels:

- 1993 and newer cars, which all have a three-way catalytic converter, can obtain a verification sticker with a number 0 if they emit less than 100 ppm of total HC and less than 1% of CO. This sticker means that they have "zero" restrictions and can be driven every day.
- Cars without a three-way catalyst but with an electronic fuel injection system could obtain a sticker number 1 if they emit less than 200 ppm of HC and less than 2% of CO, the city standards. These must comply with the "day without a car" (DWC) constraint.
- If these vehicles exceed the city standard but comply with the more lenient federal standard, they receive a number 2 sticker and must comply with the DWC as well as with additional restrictions during high pollution episodes. Cars without catalysts and without electronic fuel injection systems can only obtain a sticker number 2 if they pass the federal limits.

The differential treatment of cars according to such criteria is probably the best approach. One reason is that it gives the opportunity to combine this measure with other policy instruments. For instance, the triggering point (ambient ozone levels) for the application of the episode alert can be lowered over time without changing stickers. In 2000 a car with a sticker number 1 stops 52 days a year, and a car with a sticker number 2 might stop 60–70 times. In the future the number of days of stoppage by the more-polluting 2 cars could be increased considerably by lowering the triggering point, thus putting increasing pressure on people to move to more modern and less-polluting cars.

Such an approach recognizes the now well-demonstrated fact that most car pollution comes from a small fraction of the cars. Pollution regulations that focus on the few heavy polluters can be more effective and less economically and administratively burdensome that those that apply to all cars.

properly maintained (see Chapter 6). Car traffic also creates a major noise hazard. This greatly impairs quality of life for millions of people living close to busy roads—especially in countries with tropical climates where windows of dwellings are seldom closed. Traffic noise disturbs sleep and impairs communication (of particular importance in schools). The proliferation of roads and highways can disrupt social interactions within communities. Unless town planning attends to the needs of pedestrians, cars and roadways tend to dominate the built-up landscape. In Britain the proportion of primary school children walking to school has fallen over the past 2 decades from a clear majority to a shrinking minority, as traffic has become more intense and walking along roads less safe.

Road building and the resultant large land area covered in tar-seal constitute yet another form of environmental hazard by greatly increasing the storm water runoff during heavy rains. Storm water drains are needed and, further, these will be contaminated by road dust and other surface contaminants. Often the storm water drains are connected to the community sewerage system, creating sewage overflow during rains.

### Industry and Manufacturing

Industrialization brings many benefits in the form of income and jobs, but, unless regulated in some fashion, can lead to significant occupational and public health hazards. The public hazards may be in the form of releases of toxic or potentially toxic material—as in the notorious cases in postwar Japan (see Exhibit 8–7). Some industrial facilities carry the risk of large-scale accidental releases of toxic materials. The biggest such release in world history occurred in Bhopal, India, where an explosion at a pesticide manufacturing plant resulted in some 3,000 deaths caused by the chemical methyl-isocyanate and significant health impairment in many tens of thousands. The impact of this accident at the facility was exacerbated by the lack of urban

zoning controls, with hundreds of households having been built directly adjacent to the plant. There was also inadequate planning for alerting and evacuating the public once the accident had occurred.

### Waste Management

Few issues in environmental health have generated such attention and controversy as the management of hazardous wastes, whether chemical or radioactive. This has come about through a strong sense of public outrage about numerous publicized cases in which hazardous materials have been dumped indiscriminately or clandestinely, thus leaving expensive and dirty waste sites for others to handle. Both industry and governments have been responsible for creating such sites, which, in industrialized countries, have become very expensive to clean up. Indeed, in today's dollars the Superfund program of the United States has spent to date at least $50 billion to clean up chemically contaminated industrial sites (U.S. Congress, 1998). The cost of cleaning up the chemical and radioactive contamination left as remnants of a half century of cold war nuclear weapons development and manufacture will be much higher.

Perhaps surprisingly, in spite of the large public concern in industrialized nations as evidenced by the resources devoted to cleanup, the actual health impact of hazardous waste is not significant in most areas. Although there are egregious examples of highly contaminated sites that impose notable risks on local communities, as a societal health issue hazardous waste lies far behind more mundane forms of air and water pollution. One exception, however, is hazardous waste from the military activities (including weapons manufacture) of the former Soviet Union; this waste is at such a scale that it significantly affects the health of tens of thousands of persons today. There also seem to be cases in China of widespread contamination of aquifers by chromium and other wastes, for example. Even in these countries, however, societal envi-

**Exhibit 8–7** Minamata and Itai-Itai Disease: Classical Environmental Health Disasters

Environmental health disasters have been important triggers for national and international action to prevent environmental pollution. The best-known such disaster may be Minamata disease, which struck the small coastal town of Minamata, Japan, in 1956 (WHO, 1990). Hundreds of people were seriously affected by methylmercury poisoning, and many victims died. This type of poisoning affects the nervous system, with symptoms ranging from slight numbness of fingers to loss of ability to talk and walk. The source of the methylmercury was a chemical production factory that used mercury as a catalyst in one of its processes. Surplus mercury was discharged via spill-water into a nearby bay, and this mercury accumulated in bottom sediments. Microbes in the sediments converted the mercury to methylmercury, which eventually entered the food chain of fish and caused very high methylmercury levels in the local fish. Minamata had a substantial population of small family fisheries, and these families were the most affected.

The outbreak of disease developed over several months, and it was initially thought that a new type of infectious disease affecting the nervous system was occurring. It took months of detailed epidemiologic research to conclude that the cause of the disease was associated with the consumption of fish. Further toxicologic and epidemiologic research over many years eventually identified the specific chemical involved. A second outbreak of similar methylmercury poisoning, in Niigata, Japan, intensified the search for a definite cause. In 1968 the Japanese government committee responsible for elucidating the cause finally incriminated methylmercury—12 years after the disease was first reported.

A similar story can be told about Itai-Itai disease, a form of chronic cadmium poisoning that developed in farmers in Toyama, Japan, at about the same time as the first outbreak of Minamata disease (WHO, 1992). Painstaking research identified that the consumption of cadmium-contaminated rice and drinking water was the cause. The cadmium, from a mining area and a lead/zinc ore concentration plant, had reached the affected community via a river that they used to irrigate their rice fields. The farming families in the contaminated area had small subsistence farms, providing for all their family needs. Thus, if a family's farm was contaminated, the family members ended up with very high daily cadmium intake. Cadmium is a cumulative poison that eventually damages the kidneys, indirectly leading to bone deformities and fractures because of severe osteomalacia and osteoporosis.

At the time when these two disease outbreaks occurred, Japan was a low-income country trying to recover from the disastrous economic effects of World War II. The living conditions were not dissimilar to those in today's low-income countries undergoing rapid industrialization. Rural populations consumed mainly locally produced food. Health care services were basic, and the environmental pollution situation was not closely monitored or managed. Local industry discharged waste into air, rivers, or sea without much pollution control equipment. A country with similar conditions to erstwhile Japan is China, with lead, zinc, and copper mining; rice farming; and high local food content in the diet. Indeed, cadmium-polluted areas have been found in China (Cai, Yue, Shang, & Nordberg, 1995), and environmental epidemiologic studies have discovered exposures and effects similar to the polluted areas of Japan.

ronmental health risks are dominated by more traditional water and air pollutants and occupational hazards.

It is interesting to speculate why hazardous wastes attract so much more attention than the actual health risk warrants. It is partly due to what has been called the *outrage factor*, that is, the understandable violation felt because of the inexcusable negligent and criminal behavior of industries and governments in the past. It is also due to a natural human tendency to treat "waste" with a high degree of suspicion. In reality, however, people show relatively little apparent concern for exposure to the same chemicals at much higher levels while using household and agricultural chemicals, vehicle fuel, and other toxic solvents. From the perspective of the human body, there are no differences in the ill effect of, for example, benzene molecules from one source or another. Finally, and more important, by its high attention to waste, society may be expressing a type of concern not well captured by formal health risk analyses, that is, that the incremental health gains and other benefits of the activities that produce the waste are no longer worth the incremental risks, even if those risks are relatively small.

Globally, the less exotic forms of waste generated by household garbage, mine tailings, and vegetation cuttings undoubtedly cause the most pervasive health damage year in and year out. Uncollected garbage breeds disease-carrying pests of many sorts, including rats and flies. Leached toxic materials and floods from unmanaged mine tailing ponds create health hazards as well. The spontaneous and purposeful burning of garbage, coal mine tailings, and vegetation cuttings is a major source of health-damaging air pollution worldwide, although largely controlled in industrialized countries. As discussed in the following section, garbage collection is also a significant source of occupational hazards in low- and middle-income cities.

The related problem of the export of hazardous wastes, from the more to the less industrialized countries, is addressed in "The Export of Hazard," below.

## Microbiological Contamination of Water and Food

Diarrheal disease from contaminated water and food remains one of the world's great public health problems, as discussed above. Although the hazard is in a sense generated at the household level, failure to initiate community controls can lead to large-scale outbreaks.

An important example is cholera, which spread worldwide during the 1990s. The seventh, and largest ever, cholera pandemic is now causing cases throughout Asia, the Middle East, Europe (occasionally), Africa (where the dis-

ease has become endemic for the first time), and Latin America, where it spread widely during the 1990s, causing more than 1 million cases and 10,000 deaths. Meanwhile, an apparently new epidemic of cholera was detected in the early 1990s, appearing first in southern India and caused by a new strain (number 0139) of *Vibrio cholerae*. The spread of cholera has been greatly enhanced by the increasing number of slum dwellers in low- and middle-income countries, the speed and distance of modern tourism, and an apparent increase in extreme weather events—such as the massive El Niño-associated floods in Kenya in 1997 that caused epidemics of cholera in two regions of the country (see Chapter 4).

In the villages and slums of low- and middle-income countries, poor household water quality and sanitation often lead to food contamination. The widespread and unregulated commercial street-food sector in cities offers additional opportunities for exposure. Food contamination remains a concern even in industrialized countries where food is supplied to most of the population via long agriculture, processing, and distribution chains.

The reported rates of food poisoning have increased in industrialized countries during the past 2 decades—and almost doubled in the United Kingdom during the 1990s. The spread of the potentially lethal toxin-producing *E. coli* in North America and Europe in the mid-1990s appears to have accompanied beef imported from infected cattle in Argentina. As long-distance trade expands, as commercial supply lines lengthen in large cities, as people more frequently opt for convenience or fast foods, so the opportunities for food-borne illness increase. The intensification of meat production is another hot spot for infectious disease problems, as recently evidenced by Mad Cow Disease in Britain and its human counterpart (a variant of Creutzfeld-Jacob Disease), by the outbreak of a new strain of influenza in 1998 in Hong Kong in chickens, and by the surprise appearance in 1999 of the newly named (and often fatal) Nipah virus in intensively produced Malaysian pigs and in several hundred human contacts.

## Chemical Contamination of Water and Food

The sources of chemical contamination are industrial wastes and emissions; household and agricultural chemicals (see Exhibit 8–8); chemicals that form during storage and handling of food, such as the biotoxin aflatoxin; and natural chemical contaminants. Several major episodes have occurred in Europe over the past 2 decades. In 1981 the toxic Spanish oil episode occurred, in which edible vegetable oil was adulterated with industrial oil, causing several hundred deaths and several thousand severe illnesses. In 1985 batches of Austrian and Italian wine were found adulterated with alcohol-containing antifreeze, a toxic compound. In both those episodes, the hazardous substances were added surreptitiously, for commercial gain, by persons ignorant of or indifferent to the potential risks to public health. In 1999 in Belgium dioxin-contaminated fats entered the animal feed-manufacturing process, leading to the contamination of pigs, poultry, and dairy cattle on 1,500 Belgian farms and to thousands of tons of contaminated food products. The potential for the rapid globalization of such environmental problems in the modern free-trading world became quickly apparent (McMichael, 1999): countries in the Middle East, the Americas, and Southeast and eastern Asia quickly declared a ban on Belgian food imports.

Similar problems can afflict the quality of drinking water. The widespread problem with arsenic in local drinking water supplies in various communities around the world, particularly in Bangladesh and West Bengal, India, is illustrative (see Exhibit 8–9).

## Urbanization

A spectacular shift of human populations into the world's cities is occurring. The urbanized proportion of the world's population has grown from around 5% to 50% in the past 2 centuries and is still rising. This urban migration reflects, variously, the advent of industrialization, the contraction of rural employment, the flight from food insecurity and other forms of insecurity, and the search for jobs, amenities, or a stimulating environment.

The urban environment, physically, confers various benefits upon human health and well-being. There is readier access to education and health, financial, and social services. The urban environment is rich with new opportunities. Yet big cities are often impersonal and sometimes menacing. Noise, traffic congestion, and residential crowding are stress-inducing. The air quality is poor in many cities around the world.

The mortality impact of heat waves is typically greatest in urban centers, where temperatures tend to be higher than in the leafier suburbs and the surrounding countryside, and the relief of nighttime cooling is lessened. This "heat island" effect is due to the large heat-retaining structures and treeless asphalt expanses of inner cities and the physical obstruction of cooling breezes. Each population has a middle temperature range to which it is well adapted physiologically, behaviorally, and technically. As temperatures become colder, daily death rates gradually increase. As temperatures rise above that middle comfort zone, daily deaths increase—and they often do so rather abruptly once a threshold temperature is exceeded. This threshold is much more evident in some populations than in others. In China there is a clear threshold at 34°C (93°F) in Shanghai, but no evident threshold in warmer and more humid Guangzhou. Little is known about the health impacts of extremes of heat and cold in low- and middle-income urban populations.

Urban populations play a dominant role in the mounting pressures that today jeopardize the sustainability of current human ecology. Cities have increasingly large "ecologic footprints" (Rees, 1996). There are undoubted ecologic benefits of urbanism, including economies of scale, shared use of resources, and opportunities for reuse and recycling. Equally, though, urban populations depend on the natural resources of eco-

**Exhibit 8–8** Case Study: Learning from Bitter Experience—The Banning of Methylmercury Fungicides

The infamous methylmercury poisoning catastrophe in Minamata, Japan, in 1956 highlighted the severe public health problems that could occur after environmental pollution with organic chemicals. The same chemical was used in the 1950s and 1960s as a fungicide to prevent fungal growth, which impaired crop-seed viability or caused mold damage in paper pulp. The use in the paper industry caused increased concentrations of mercury in the factories' wastewater and methylmercury contamination of fish. In the late 1960s Swedish ornithologists had identified both this and the use of fungicide-treated seeds as a potential cause of infertility in wild birds. A major environmental pollution debate followed, and eventually these fungicides were banned, not only in Sweden but in most countries with functioning regulatory systems.

In 1971 Iraq received a large consignment of fungicide-treated wheat seeds from USAID. They arrived when much of rural Iraq was suffering from severe drought, and farming families had little food. The seeds for planting had been dyed red in order to indicate that they should not be eaten, but the farmers soon found out that washing the seeds in water eliminated the dye. Unfortunately, the fungicide stayed in the seeds. The farmers then used the seeds to make bread, and about 2 months later a major epidemic of serious neurological diseases began. Eventually 500 people died and about 5,000 were hospitalized.

This was the largest known epidemic of this type. Previously some smaller outbreaks had occurred in Africa from the same seed fungicide. After the disastrous Iraq epidemic a new level of awareness arose about such problems, and the use of this fungicide was subsequently banned in most countries. This is an example of successful chemical safety management, based on the scare caused by a major epidemic.

systems that, in aggregate, are vastly larger in area than the city itself. The highly urbanized Netherlands consumes resources from a total surface area 15 times larger than itself. The estimated consumption of resources—wood, paper, fibers, and food (including seafood)—by 29 cities of the Baltic Sea region—and the absorption of their wastes depend upon a total area 200 times greater than the combined area of the 29 cities (Folke, Larsson, & Sweitzer, 1996). The scale of these externalities of urbanism is growing, and includes massive contributions to global greenhouse gas accumulation, stratospheric ozone depletion, land degradation, and coastal zone destruction. The urbanized developed world, with one-fifth of the world population, currently contributes three-quarters of all greenhouse gas emissions (Intergovernmental Panel on Climate Change, 1996).

## REGIONAL EXPOSURES: TRANSBOUNDARY PROBLEMS

As the scale of human economic activity has increased, environmental problems have increasingly spilled over beyond local community boundaries. Regional watersheds become contaminated from multiple sources; radioactive wastes and emissions spread regionally; land-use practices affect infectious disease patterns; and the industrial emissions of sulfur and nitrogen oxides acidify the regional atmosphere. Via these enlarged pathways, environmental changes can impinge adversely on human health.

### Atmospheric Dispersion of Contaminants

Following the surge of industrial growth in the third quarter of the twentieth century, the transboundary problem of acid deposition (commonly referred to as "acid rain") became increasingly problematic. It featured prominently at the 1972 UN Conference on the Human Environment in Stockholm as, by that time, eastern Canada was experiencing problems from acidic emissions traveling northeast from the United States, and Scandinavia was being exposed to emissions from the United Kingdom and highly industrialized areas of West and East Germany. More recently, the strong increase in China's

**Exhibit 8–9** Arsenic in Groundwater

The concentration of various elements, such as fluorine and arsenic, varies naturally in groundwater supplies around the world. In countries such as Taiwan and Argentina the high levels of arsenic in the drinking water have been recognized as a health hazard since the mid-1900s, causing keratoses, hyperpigmentation, and skin cancer. High levels also exist in Chile, Inner Mongolia, parts of the United States, Hungary, Thailand, and China. More recently the exposure has assumed epic proportions in Bangladesh and neighboring West Bengal, India, where several million persons in recent decades have been drinking arsenic-contaminated water obtained via tubewells, and where the number already manifesting toxic effects, especially skin lesions, probably number in the hundreds of thousands (Khan et al., 1997).

The prolonged consumption of arsenic causes a succession of toxic effects, typically appearing 5–10 years after first exposure. There is some evidence that these are greatest in low-income rural villagers with malnutrition, but this may be coincidental rather than causal. Early manifestations include keratosis and skin pigmentation, followed by dysfunction of kidneys and liver, and, perhaps, peripheral neuropathy. With continued exposure the arsenicosis progresses to liver failure and may cause gangrene and cancer. It is well established that arsenic in drinking water increases severalfold the incidence of cancers of the bladder, skin, lung, and kidney (Smith, Goycoleam, Haque, & Biggs, 1998); indeed, arsenic appears to be the most widespread cancer hazard in drinking water in the world. In Chile, for example, 5-10% of all deaths over age 30 have been attributed to arsenic-induced cancers (Smith et al., 1998). A cross-sectional study in Bangladesh has compared the prevalence of diabetes mellitus in persons living in areas with high water arsenic levels and areas without arsenic contamination of drinking water (Rahman, Tondel, Ahmad, & Axelson, 1998). Diabetes prevalence was clearly higher in the exposed population. However, there were no historical time-trend data on water arsenic concentration for either population.

West Bengal shares with Bangladesh a subterranean geologic continuity, with arsenic-rich sediments. Much of the drinking water comes from the several hundred thousand tubewells sunk over the past 2 decades to provide villagers with safe drinking water, thus avoiding the hazard of fecally contaminated surface water. The problem was first identified in Bangladesh in 1993. It is thought that the "aeration" of the deep sediment by the many bore holes leads to oxidation of the natural arsenopyrite and mobilization of arsenic into water. Many of the tubewells yield water with arsenic concentrations 10–50 times higher than the WHO guideline (0.01 mg/liter). In the village of Samta (population 4,800), in the Jessore district on the Bangladesh and West Bengal boundary, approximately 90% of the 265 tubewells had arsenic concentrations above 0.05 mg/l and 10% exceeded 0.5 mg/l (Biswas et al., 1998).

Mitigation of the problem can be complex and costly. Various chemical treatments of the water remove arsenic by absorption onto activated salts and elements, reverse osmosis, ion exchange, or oxidation. Cheaper physical methods involve sand filtration and clarification. The simplest physical solution, where possible, is to drill the tubewells deeper—in conjunction with rapid field testing able to identify contamination above 0.05 mg/l. This is being done in parts of Bangladesh and West Bengal. Meanwhile, tubewells with very high contamination should be identified and, as soon as an acceptable alternative is found, closed. The practical solution includes restricting the use of arsenic-contaminated water to washing only and to avoid using it for cooking or drinking.

industrial production has subjected Japan to acid deposition from that source. Acid levels are rising in other parts of Asia as energy use grows. The hazards to human health are neither extreme nor direct. However, the acidification of waterways and soils has demonstrably increased the mobilization of various elements—particular heavy metals and aluminum—enabling them to enter the drinking water and food chain. Human exposures to these elements have thus increased in several regions.

Another type of regional air pollution was the release of radionuclides from the Chernobyl nuclear power plant in the 1986 disaster (WHO,

1996). Much of this radioactive material was deposited within a 125-mile radius of the plant, but significant radionuclide contamination also resulted from dispersal by winds to areas several thousand miles away. About 4 million persons in the most contaminated adjoining areas were significantly exposed, via the food chain, or were otherwise affected by restrictions on the use of their land for farming. A great increase in the incidence of child thyroid cancer was found in the most polluted areas during the decade after the disaster. Further afield, such as in northern Finland, Sweden, and Norway, health protection measures had major economic impacts. Reindeer farming is the major economic enterprise in these areas, and thousands of reindeer had to be slaughtered and discarded because of high radiation levels in their meat.

The impact of regional climatic variations on human well-being and health has created great recent research interest. There is new understanding about the regional pattern of storms, floods, cyclones, and droughts in response to these quasiperiodic cycles. Indeed, advance warning of interannual variations in rainfall and drought conditions (with their implications for regional food production and outbreaks of certain infectious diseases) is now becoming possible. An interesting example of a regional impact occurred in the United States, where the El Niño event of the early 1990s was associated, initially, with drought conditions in the Southwest (in the "four corners" region where Arizona, Colorado, Utah, and New Mexico meet). This led to a drop in vegetation and in animal populations, including the natural predators of the deer mouse. When heavy rains occurred in 1993, with resultant profuse growth of piñon nuts, there was an uncontrolled proliferation in the deer-mouse population. These rodents harbor a virus, transmissible to humans via dried excreta, that causes hantavirus pulmonary disease—first described at that time (Duchin et al., 1994). This disease has subsequently spread to many contiguous states and to western Canada and much of South America.

The El Niño of 1997–1998 created unusually strong drought conditions in Southeast Asia, which exacerbated the size and duration of forest fires originally set to clear land. Such widespread use of forest-clearing fires during drought periods is a manifestation of poor government land management. The result, in addition to extensive damage to the forests, was regional air pollution in the form of wood smoke plumes that extended over thousands of miles and could easily be seen by satellites. The forest fires actually raised outdoor particulate levels to several times the acceptable upper limit in a number of large cities in the region for a period of days to weeks, apparently with significant accompanying adverse health effects. Although larger than in previous years, the same phenomenon has been occurring for decades in the region, and is likely to be repeated often unless land-use practices are modified.

## Land Use and Water Engineering

Regional tensions over freshwater supplies are increasing in many locations, as population pressures increase and an increasing proportion of agricultural production comes to depend on irrigation (Gleick, 1998). Water is essential for domestic hygiene, communal sanitation, and economic vitality. The problems in the West Bengal region, where freshwater availability is declining as the hydrologic cycle is perturbed by human interventions and where surface water is widely fecally contaminated, are illustrated in Exhibit 8–9.

During the third quarter of the twentieth century it became clear that large-scale human interventions in the natural environment—dams, irrigation schemes, land reclamation, road construction, and population resettlement programs—often affected infectious disease patterns. In particular, the composition of vector species generally changes following alterations in environmental conditions. Such large-scale developments in the Eastern Mediterranean, Africa, South America, and Asia have been consistently associated with increases in vector-borne diseases, especially schistosomiasis and filariasis. In the Sudan in the 1970s, for example, schistosomiasis appeared soon after the start of the Gezira scheme, a large irrigated cotton project; the prevalence of malaria also increased markedly in this region (Fenwick, Cheesmond, & Amin, 1981; Gruenbaum, 1983). In Africa the building of large dams in the Sudan, Egypt (the Aswan High Dam), Ghana, and Senegal all caused the prevalence of schistosomiasis in the surrounding populace to increase from very low levels to more than 90% (WHO, 1997). (See Chapter 4.)

An example of a disastrous land use decision, with major regional environmental health consequences, is the fate of the Aral Sea in Central Asia. This inland sea is dependent on the inflow of water from two major rivers. Until about 1960 the sea level was constant, and large populations in the countries surrounding the Aral Sea sustained their economies through fishing and agriculture. In the 1950s large-scale cotton farming was developed along the two major rivers based on irrigation water diverted from those rivers. This farming used large amounts of pesticides, which contaminated the water and the soil. Signs of environmental damage began emerging in the 1960s. The level of the Aral Sea sank, the irrigated farm soils became salinated, and soil erosion by wind became an increasing problem. Since then the Aral Sea has continued to shrink, the fishing industry has collapsed, and agriculture has been increasingly impaired. Adverse health impacts in the regional population of 30 million persons have been reported—although not yet satisfactorily confirmed—apparently in association with direct toxic pesticide exposures and with the socioeconomic decline caused by the environmental disaster.

Deforestation has had variable effects on malaria mosquito vectors. In some parts of Southeast Asia, deforestation has enabled malaria-transmitting *Anopheles punctulatus* species to become established. In contrast, several *Anopheles* species, including *Anopheles dirus* in Thai-land and *Anopheles darlingi* in South America, have disappeared following deforestation that removed the flora and fauna upon which they depended for feeding. Forest clearance in South America during recent decades to extend agricultural land has mobilized various viral hemorrhagic fevers that previously circulated quietly in wild animal hosts. For example, the Junin virus, which causes Argentine hemorrhagic fever, naturally infects wild rodents (the mouse, *Callomys callosus*). However, extensive conversion of grassland to maize cultivation in recent decades stimulated a proliferation of this species of virus-bearing mouse, thus exposing human farmworkers to this "new" virus. In the past 35 years, the land area carrying this new human disease has expanded sevenfold, and the average annual number of infected persons is of the order of several hundred, up to one-third of whom die (WHO, 1997). (See Chapter 4.)

Because changes in land-use patterns are typically accompanied by changes in population density, population mobility, pesticide usage, and regional climate, it is difficult to assign specific causal explanations. Indeed, many of the health outcomes result from interactions between these various change processes.

## GLOBAL ENVIRONMENTAL CHANGE AND POPULATION HEALTH

A major consequence of the increasing scale of the human enterprise is the potentially important health impact of global environmental changes. Humankind is now disrupting some of the biosphere's life-support systems—the natural processes of stabilization, production, cleansing, and recycling that our predecessors were able to take for granted in a less human-dominated world (Daily, 1997; McMichael, 1993). We no longer live in such a world. The composition of the lower and middle atmospheres is changing. There is a net loss of productive soils on all continents; most ocean fisheries have been overfished; aquifers upon which irrigated agriculture depends have been depleted; and whole species and many local populations are being extinguished unprecedentedly fast. These large-scale environmental changes pose long-term, and unfamiliar, risks to human population health.

## Climate Change

The United Nations' Intergovernmental Panel on Climate Change (IPCC, 1996) assesses that "the balance of evidence suggests a discernible human influence on global climate." Further, trends in greenhouse gas emissions will, in IPCC's estimation, cause an increase in average world temperature of approximately 1–3°C over the coming century. Rainfall patterns will also change, as, probably, will the variability of weather patterns. All these changes would vary considerably by region (see Exhibit 8–10). The health effects of climate change would encompass direct and indirect, and immediate and delayed effects (McMichael & Haines, 1997). While some health outcomes in some populations would be beneficial—some tropical regions may become too hot for mosquitoes, for example, and winter cold snaps would become milder in temperate-zone countries where death rates typically peak in wintertime—most of the anticipated health effects would be adverse (IPCC, 1996; McMichael, Haines, Slooff, & Kovats, 1996).

Direct health effects would include changes in mortality and morbidity from an altered pattern of exposure to thermal extremes; the respiratory health consequences of increased exposures to photochemical pollutants and aeroallergens; and the physical hazards of the increased occurrence of storms, floods, or droughts, in at least some regions. Intensified rainfall, with flooding, can overwhelm urban wastewater and sewer systems, leading to contamination of drinking water supplies. This is most likely in large crowded cities where infrastructure is old or inadequate—as illustrated by an outbreak of typhoid in Tajikistan in 1994 when the city wastewater system flooded during unusual torrential rains.

Indirect health effects are likely to have a greater aggregate impact, over time. They would include alterations in the range and activity of vector-borne infectious diseases (for example, malaria, dengue fever, and leishmaniasis). These diseases are spread by vectors (for example, mosquitoes) that are very sensitive to climatic conditions (see Figure 8–10), as is the parasite's development while incubating in the vector. Predictive mathematical modeling has suggested that the geographic zone and seasonality of potential transmission of malaria or dengue fever will increase in many parts of the world (IPCC, 1996; McMichael & Haines, 1997). In temperate Europe and North America, climate-sensitive, vector-borne infections include tick-borne encephalitis and Lyme disease. Other indirect effects would include altered transmission of person-to-person infections (especially summertime food- and waterborne pathogens). Of great potential importance to population health would be the adverse nutritional consequences of the likely regional declines in agricultural productivity, estimated at around 10–20% by the latter half of the twenty-first century in many already food-insecure populations in low-latitude regions. Finally, there would be inevitable adverse physical and psychological health consequences resulting from population displacement and economic disruption due to rising sea levels (for example, small island states, coastal Bangladesh, and the Nile Delta), agroecosystem decline, and freshwater shortages.

## Stratospheric Ozone Depletion

Stratospheric ozone depletion is essentially a separate phenomenon from greenhouse gas accumulation in troposphere. Ozone depletion is causing an increase in ultraviolet irradiation at Earth's surface. This increase in ultraviolet exposure is expected to peak sometime within the next 2 decades and then decline slowly over several decades, in response to the phasing out of the major ozone-destroying industrial and agricultural chemicals. For the first half of this century, increases are expected in the severity of sunburn and in the incidence of skin cancers in

**Exhibit 8–10** Modeling the Future Impacts of Climate Change on Malaria

Mosquitoes, the vector organisms for malaria, are very sensitive to temperature and humidity. Further, patterns of rainfall, river flow, and surface water affect their opportunity to breed. Scientists therefore anticipate that a change in world climatic conditions during the coming century will affect the pattern of potential transmission of malaria. Temperature and humidity affect the growth, biting rate, reproductive cycle, and longevity of the mosquito. Mosquitoes are most "comfortable" in the temperature range 20–30°C and at around 60% humidity. The malarial parasite, a single-celled sexually reproducing plasmodium, is also affected by temperature during the extrinsic phase of its complex life cycle when forming sporozoites within the mosquito. The two major species of plasmodium have minimum temperature requirements—for *Plasmodium vivax* a minimum of 16°C is required, whereas for the potentially fatal *Plasmodium falciparum* a temperature of approximately 18°C is required. Within the above-mentioned comfort range, the higher the temperature the more rapid the incubation—and hence the sooner the opportunity for transmission to another mosquito-bitten human.

From studies done during the 1980s and 1990s it is clear that malaria outbreaks are closely related to interannual climatic variations in many countries. In Venezuela, for example, the incidence of malaria consistently surged upward throughout the twentieth century in the year following an El Niño event. This is most probably due to the combination of above-average rainfall in the post-Niño year and the drop in acquired immunity in the population because of the low malaria incidence during the dry El Niño year. Studies in India, Pakistan, and Sri Lanka all display similarly strong associations with El Niño events and the associated monsoonal changes. A correspondingly strong correlation with interannual variations in temperature and rainfall has been recently reported for dengue fever—a mosquito-borne infectious disease—occurrence in the Pacific island populations.

The science of forecasting climatic fluctuations 3–6 months in advance is steadily improving. Indeed, there is considerable economic incentive to improve the forecasting of El Niño and La Niña events, as these have global repercussions on regional agricultural yields. With sufficient advance warning, farmers can switch to more appropriate crops. The equivalent approach will soon be possible for the forecasting of malaria outbreaks, enabling public health interventions (for example, activated population-based surveillance, surface water control, insecticide-impregnated bed-nets, and antimalarial prophylaxis).

Longer-term global and local forecasting are being facilitated as information accrues about the way malaria has responded to the generalized warming that has occurred since the 1970s. Forecasts on this decadal scale are relevant for inclusion in the estimation of aggregate burden of adverse health impacts that could accrue if climate change were to occur as predicted. Mathematical models are required for this type of long-range forecasting of changes in the potential transmission of malaria. The models integrate, for units of time (typically months) and units of surface area (for example, 100 kilometers square), the emission scenario-based climate change process, the mosquito and parasite "system," and the human population characteristics (size, age distribution, prior immunity). Because other determinants of malaria occurrence will also change over coming decades (for example, vaccine efficacy, human demography, land-use patterns, or parasite resistance to drugs) the modeling of climate change impacts may only indicate changes in potential transmission (for example, see Figure 8–10). This, nevertheless, is an important consideration in the formulation of long-term priorities and policies. In the future, more comprehensive modeling will undoubtedly be able to take these other covariables into account.

fair-skinned populations and of various disorders of the eye (especially cataracts). Some UVR-induced suppression of immune functioning may also result, thus increasing susceptibility to infectious diseases and perhaps reducing vaccination efficacy (UNEP, 1998; WHO, 1994).

Persistence of the ozone losses of the 1979–1992 period for several decades would

Change in Seasonality

- 3 to 5 months
- 1 to 2 months
- −2 to −1 months
- −5 to −3 months

(A)

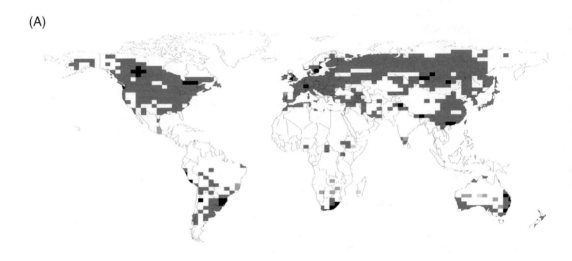

(B)

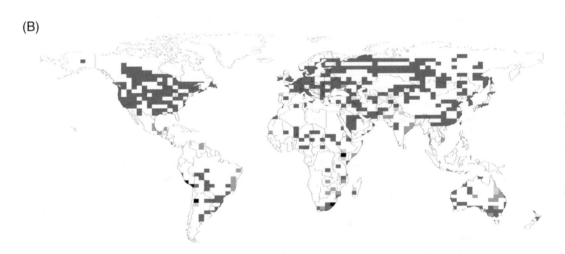

**Figure 8–10** Future Changes in Seasonality of Potential Transmission of Malaria, 2080s versus Present. (A) Change in number of transmissions per year under a future scenario of unconstrained emissions of carbon dioxide. (B) Change in number of months of potential transmission per year, under a future scenario of constrained emissions of carbon dioxide (such that atmospheric concentration stabilizes at 550 parts per million).

cause the annual incidence of basal cell carcinoma (the dominant skin cancer type) to increase by an estimated 1–2% at low latitude (5°), 14% at 55–65° in the northern hemisphere (for example, the United Kingdom), and 25% at that latitude in the south (Madronich & de Gruijl, 1993). The estimated percentage increases for squamous cell carcinoma would be twice as great. More sophisticated mathematical modeling indicates that nonmelanoma skin cancer rates would rise to a peak excess incidence of approximately 10% in the United States and Europe around the middle of this century (Slaper, Velders, Daniel, de Gruijl, & van der Leun, 1996).

A potentially more important, although much more indirect, health detriment could arise from ultraviolet-induced impairment of photosynthesis on land (terrestrial plants) and at sea (phytoplankton). Although such an effect could reduce the world's food production, few quantitative data are yet available.

### Biodiversity: Losses, Invasions

Through humankind's spectacular reproductive and technological "success," the natural habitats of many other species have been occupied, damaged, or eliminated. Biologists estimate that this fastest mass extinction may cause around one-third of all species alive in the 1800s to be gone before the end of this century (Pimm, Russell, Gittleman, & Brooks, 1995). The loss of various key species would weaken whole ecosystems, with consequences that would often be adverse to human interests, such as disturbing the ecology of vector-borne infections and food-producing systems that depend on pollinators and the predation of pests, and impairing the cleansing of water and the circulation of nutrients that normally pass through ecosystems. A rich repertoire of genetic and phenotypic material would also be lost. To maintain the hybrid vigor and environmental resilience of "food" species, a diversity of wild species needs to be preserved as a source of genetic additives. Similarly, a high proportion of modern medicinal drugs in western medicine has natural origins, and many defy synthesis in the laboratory. Scientists test thousands of novel natural chemicals each year, seeking new drugs to treat HIV, malaria, drug-resistant tuberculosis, and cancers.

The other side of this coin is the accelerating spread of "invasive" species, as long-distance trade, tourism, and migration increase in intensity. Several examples with public health consequences are given in "Environmental Hazards Resulting from Forms of Globalization," below. There are many others: the vast proliferation of water hyacinth (a decorative plant from Brazil) in Lake Victoria, eastern Africa, has extended the breeding grounds for the water snail that transmits schistosomiasis. The planting of *Lantana camerata* as a garden border shrub, with subsequent dispersed spread within Uganda, has increased the habitat for the tsetse fly that transmits African sleeping sickness.

### Land Degradation, Food, and Malnutrition

The increase in land degradation has implications for food supplies and therefore for nutrition, child development, and health. During the 1980s the combination of erosion, desiccation, and nutrient exhaustion, plus irrigation-induced water-logging and salination, rendered unproductive one-fifteenth of the world's 1.5 billion hectares of readily arable farmland (World Resources Institute, 1998). The "Green Revolution," which fed much of the expanding human population during the 1960s to the 1980s, depended on laboratory-bred, high-yield cereal grains, fertilizers, groundwater, and arable soils. In retrospect, those productivity gains appear to have come substantially from using up exhaustible ecologic "capital"—especially topsoil and groundwater. As greater food yields to feed evermore people are pursued, almost one-tenth of the world population is malnourished in ways that impair health. Meanwhile, at sea, many of the world's great fisheries are now on the brink of being overexploited. The United Nations' Food and Agriculture Organization (FAO) estimates that the sustainable fish-catch limit has been neared—around 100 million tons per year (FAO, 1995).

### Persistent, Organic Pollutants

Various chemical pollutants, particularly the many chlorinated organic chemicals such as the polychlorinated biphenyls (PCBs), are persistent and have become globally pervasive. They are referred to as *persistent organic pollutants* (POPs) (Watson, Dixon, & Hamburg, 1998). The semivolatile members of this class of chemicals undergo a type of serial distillation process in the atmosphere, as they pass from low to high latitudes, ultimately impinging at higher concentrations in the circumpolar regions. Some of these chemicals are likely to affect neurologic, immune, and reproductive systems in humans, who feed at the top of the increasingly contaminated food chain. Weakening of ecosystems may also occur, with various knock-on environmental health effects in human populations (Colborn et al., 1993).

## PATHWAYS TO THE FUTURE IN AN UNEQUAL WORLD

Sometimes low- and middle-income countries are criticized for not imposing stricter environmental and occupational standards. Too often, there are indeed situations where minimal efforts could achieve great reductions in health risks. In addition, given the likely increase in public willingness to pay for stricter standards as development continues, the early imposition of reasonable standards can often be quite cost-effective using standard economic criteria. On the other hand, most large low- and middle-income countries today have standards that are much stricter than those in the industrialized countries at the corresponding level of development. Indeed, although there are cases of the export of environmental hazard and the degradation of local environments by exploitative and destructive commercial practice (see "The

Export of Hazard," below), the overall impact of globalization may be a net export of environmental health. That is, through education, political and public pressures, technology transfer, trade agreements, and other initiatives, low- and middle-income countries have, on average, better environmental quality than would otherwise be the case.

### Setting Standards: Too Safe Can Be Unsafe

Setting and enforcing environmental standards for protection of the public and workers is a difficult exercise, even in industrialized countries with substantial resources. In low- and middle-income countries, which face a number of critical needs with few resources, the process is even more troublesome. Although official rhetoric in standard setting often states that the only concern is protection of health, in reality there are always economic and other trade-offs involved. It is too expensive and there are too many other demands on resources to bring every pollutant under the maximum control quickly. Politically, however, it is often difficult for governments in low- and middle-income nations to set standards that are significantly less stringent than those in industrialized countries. As a result, sometimes standards are unrealistically strict and cannot be met. This leads to graft, cynicism, apathy, and, too often, to exposures and ill-health above what could be achieved by more realistic approaches.

One way out of this dilemma is to emphasize environmental health protection and standard setting as dynamic and evolutionary processes, rather than static "one-time-forever" efforts. In this way a country might set 20-year goals for its standards that are as strict as any in the world, while establishing interim objectives that become progressively more strict. Thus, pollutants and industries that pose the most risk can be emphasized first, while control over other pollutants and industries (of the kind that now attract attention in industrialized countries) can be postponed to a later period. No hazard is ignored, but merely put into a rational order of priority. Industrial interests are likely to be more willing to accept stricter standards under such a scheme because they tend to have shorter-term financial goals, facilitated by clarity of the regulatory environment, whereas they are unsettled by longer-term uncertainty. A recurring problem, however, is attaining sufficient stability within governments to implement such a long-term approach.

### The Export of Hazard

In recent years there has been concern about the potential export of environmental hazard that may be occurring as part of the globalization of the world economy (LaDou, 1992). Since environmental and occupational standards and enforcement tend to be less strict in low- and middle-income countries, polluting activities may tend to migrate to those countries, thereby imposing excess risk on workers and public. Studies of international industrial trends, however, have identified few cases where differences in environmental and occupational standards have been the critical determinants of such shifts, compared to labor costs, tax regimes, and other business factors. Indeed, locally owned industries tend to have higher emissions and occupational hazards than do facilities owned by multinational corporations, which often feel considerable pressure to maintain higher standards. Besides, the mere fact of a difference in standards does not necessarily mean that an injustice exists. As noted above, nations at different stages of development may quite rationally choose different trade-offs between standards, job creation, and infrastructure development. The most outrageous examples of injustice arise where decisions about such trade-offs are made by a small oligarchy without considering the needs and wishes of the population as a whole. In these cases, perhaps the only way to protect the interests of those in the low- and middle-income countries would be to establish international norms.

Flagrant examples of the problems created by the exporting of hazard exist along borders between industrialized and low- and middle-income countries. On the Mexican side of the long U.S.-Mexican border, for example, there are many highly polluting industries with poor occupational safety and health conditions relative to standards on the U.S. side of the border. Because of the proximity, both the pollution and health problems tend to cross the border, frustrating attempts by U.S. border communities to maintain acceptable conditions. Attempts to impose U.S. standards on Mexican facilities, however, understandably create friction. There have been some encouraging successes in joint efforts by neighboring Mexican-U.S. communities to address these issues jointly in a way that takes into account the need for jobs and for clean working and living conditions on both sides.

The political and moral dilemmas are manifest. Today's industrialized world followed a path to development and wealth that put economic gains ahead of human welfare and environmental conservation for most of the nineteenth century. Today's low- and middle-income countries are dissuaded, if not formally barred, from following the equivalent pathway because (1) their populations have access to more information and hence have higher expectations; (2) the industrialized world has a moral obligation to assist via the transfer of knowledge, wealth, and technology; (3) it is now clear that the integrity of the biosphere at large is jeopardized by the prospect of huge populations in these countries accruing wealth via environmentally damaging behaviors; and (4) there is pressure from public opinion in industrialized countries to achieve higher standards.

### Environmental Hazards Resulting from Forms of Globalization

A dominant trend in the global economic environment over the past 50 years has been the rapid growth in international trade in goods, services, and human resources. The globalizing processes of the past quarter century have transformed patterns of connectedness around the world and have created new power relations among countries, international and national governance, and the public and private sectors (see Chapter 14).

In traditional agrarian-based societies that produce, consume, and trade on a local basis and with relatively low-impact technologies, the impacts on the environment are predominantly local. Few such societies remain today, in the face of strong and pervasive economic, techno-logic, and cultural influences. The industrialization of the past century and the more recent globalizing processes have altered the scale of contact between societies, intensified environmental impacts, and extended the public health impacts of one society upon another. In the name of economic development and free markets, low- and middle-income countries have come under pressure to grant unrestricted access to their resources, work forces, and consumer markets. This process has been associated with increasing poverty in many parts of the world, widening inequalities between and within countries, expanding pressures to reduce the power of the state, and subordinating national programs of social welfare and environmental protection to the agenda of economic growth.

Following the international debt crisis of the early 1980s, many struggling low- and middle-income countries were obliged to accept the economic stringencies of the World Bank's "structural adjustment program." This entailed a reduction in spending on health throughout the 1980s and into the 1990s. There is evidence that these policies adversely affected the public health capacity of those countries, with some serious health implications (Hoogvelt, 1997). This included, in many countries, a diminished capacity to respond to the resurgence of tuberculosis, maintain environmental controls on vector-borne infectious diseases, and provide basic primary family health care. In its current form, the world's globalizing economy operates to the general disadvantage of low- and middle-income countries. The exacerbation of land degradation, rural unemployment, food shortages, and urban crowding all contribute to health deficits for the rural dispossessed, the underfed, and the slum dweller.

Many features of today's globalizing world contribute to the spread of infectious diseases (Wilson, 1995). Human mobility has escalated dramatically, in volume and speed, between and within countries. Long-distance trade facilitates the geographical redistribution of pests and pathogens—well illustrated in recent years by the HIV pandemic, the worldwide dispersal of rat-borne hantaviruses, and the rapid dissemination of a new epidemic strain of bacterial meningitis along routes of travel and trade. Likewise, there has been ship-borne introduction of the Asian tiger mosquito, *Aedes albopictus*—a vector for yellow fever and dengue—into South America, North America, and Africa (Morse, 1995) and of the cholera bacterium into South American coastal water (Colwell, 1996). In a recent analysis of cholera outbreaks since 1817, Lee and Dodgson (2000) argue that the current, seventh, pandemic is clearly different from earlier ones, reflecting the unprecedented scale of social and environmental change in the world over recent years, the exacerbation of urban poverty, and the rapidity and intensity of intercontinental contacts.

An aspect of globalization that may have negative effects on environment and health is the harmonization of trade-related rules and legislation via the World Trade Organization (WTO). Particular attention has been paid to "nontariff trade barriers," which comprise any national regulation or legislation that hinders trade and is not a financial levy on the trade itself. For instance, if country A legislates that the maximum level of mercury in fish sold in that country should be 0.5 mg/kg, another country B cannot sell fish with higher mercury level to country A. If in country B, fish with levels up to 1 mg/kg can be freely sold, then country B can claim that the fish-mercury regulation of country A is a nontariff trade barrier. However, country A may have made a health risk assessment based on the local fish consumption patterns and decided that 0.5 mg/kg is the maximum acceptable. How should this be resolved? Current (1999) WTO practice means that only internationally agreed health guidelines can be implemented in this situation, and, if no such guidelines exist, country A is not allowed to have a stricter environmental health rule than country B.

Similar situations develop with the banning of hazardous products such as asbestos. If, for example, there is no international health guideline banning the use of asbestos, then any country taking a unilateral decision to ban asbestos use would risk trade sanctions from other countries wanting to export asbestos. If the trend in international environmental and occupational health guidelines went toward stricter prevention, this harmonization via trade rules could be good for health and the environment. However, the intense lobbying from commercial groups and countries that would benefit from lax rules makes it likely that the opposite is going to happen. Compromises toward less protection will be made (LaDou, 1992).

### Population Health: Index of Social-Environmental Sustainability

Current models of government reflect the compartmentalization of knowledge and policy that grew out of the classical development of scientific disciplines in the nineteenth century. In order to deal with a multifaceted world, our predecessors defined sectors of knowledge, policy, and social action—environment, industry, agriculture, transport, health, social welfare, and education. Subsequently, however, one of the great lessons to emerge from twentieth century science, with its origins in the realm of physics (the 1920s debate about quantum mechanics and uncertainty), is that the complexities of the real world require us to think in more integrative ways, across disciplines and topics, elevating holism (or ecological thinking) above mechanistic reductionist thinking.

It is within that type of integrative framework that population health can be understood as part of the total social experience, a manifestation of how well the social and natural environments are being managed. Population health should therefore be a primary criterion for all social policy making, particularly in relation to achieving the

"sustainability transition." Health is therefore not just a type of sideshow in the policy arena. Rather, it is affected by the social, environmental, and (in the longer term) the ecological consequences of policies in all sectors. Population health should therefore be an integrating index of social policy across all sectors.

### CONCLUSION

The perceived importance of environmental exposures as health hazards—at local, regional, and global levels—has increased steadily over the past several decades. Currently, scientists estimate that from one-quarter to one-third of the global burden of disease and premature death is attributable to ambient (including domestic) environmental risk factors.

In the developed world during much of the past 4 decades, the generally greater ease of measurement of specific "exposures" relating to individual lifestyle (eating, smoking, and sexual behaviors) and the workplace, compared to the more diffuse lower-concentration exposures in the external environment, resulted in that latter topic area attracting less attention and having lower credibility. More recently, improvements in exposure assessment, the harnessing of time-series analyses, the advent of spatial analytic techniques, the recognized legitimacy of population-level analyses, and the extra leverage afforded by molecular biological indexes of exposure, susceptibility, and biological damage have all helped reveal the range and extent of ambient environmental risks to health.

Meanwhile, in developing countries, the age-old scourges of diarrheal disease, acute respiratory infections, tuberculosis, and vector-borne infections have remained the dominant health problems. The ascendancy of specific health system interventions for those problems—sanitation, domestic hygiene, vaccination, pesticides, and drug treatment—has led to their wider ecological dimensions being somewhat overlooked. Many problems of environmental contamination have their origins in poverty; deficient regulation of mining, industry, and agriculture; and mismanagement of surface and ground water supplies. Domestic exposure to indoor air pollution reflects division of labor (women are mostly exposed), low-grade technology, and the biomass fuels of poverty. Infectious disease are often spread by environmental encroachments—land clearing, water damming, irrigation, and expanded trade.

The environmental health agenda is becoming ever broader. Today the burden of human numbers and aggregate consumption and waste generation is beginning to overload various of the planet's great natural systems. The resultant global environmental changes, signifying that the biosphere's human population carrying capacity is being exceeded, pose yet further risks to human health. Therefore, even as environmental health scientists strive to improve their research methods for characterizing the health risks associated with local physical, chemical, and microbiological hazards, they must also extend their ideas and methods to encompass larger-scale environmental hazards and the health consequences of disrupted ecosystems. Policy makers, in many sectors, must understand the tendency of human-wrought changes in the social, built, and natural environments to affect health—if not immediately then in the longer term, and sometimes via pathways with which we yet have little familiarity.

## DISCUSSION QUESTIONS

1. What should be the scope of the term *environment*?
2. What methodological problems are particularly characteristic of environmental epidemiology?
3. How can the differences be explained in the profile of environmental health problems between industrialized and low- and middle-income countries? Are the differences a function of history, demography, wealth, knowledge, or something else?
4. What are the characteristics of particular environmental health problems that render them more, or less, tractable to amelioration or elimination?
5. As the scale of human impact on the global environment increases, people become more concerned about the consequences of disruption of our "habitat." What does this signify?

## REFERENCES

Armstrong, J., & Menon, R. (1998). Mining and quarrying. In J. M. Stellman, *Encyclopaedia of occupational health and safety* (4th ed., Vol. III, ch. 74). Geneva, Switzerland: International Labor Office.

Beaglehole, R., Bonita, R., & Kjellstrom, T. (1993). *Basic epidemiology*. Geneva, Switzerland: World Health Organization.

Biswas, B.K., Dhar, R.K., Samanta, G., Mandal, B.K., Chakraborti, D., Faruk, I., Islam, K.S., Chodhury, M.M., Islam, A., & Roy, S. (1998). Detailed study report of Samta, one of the arsenic-affected villages of Jessore District, Bangladesh. *Current Science, 74,* 134–145.

Bobak, M., & Leon, D.A. (1992). Air pollution and infant mortality in the Czech Republic, 1986–1988. *Lancet, 340,* 1010–1014.

Cai, S., Yue, L., Shang, Q., & Nordberg, G. (1995). Cadmium exposure among residents in an area contaminated by irrigation water in China. *Bulletin of the World Health Organization, 73,* 359–367.

Colborn, T., Vom Saal, F., & Soto, A. (1993). Developmental effects of endocrine-disrupting chemicals in wildlife and humans. *Environmental Health Perspectives, 101,* 378–384.

Colwell, R. (1996). Global climate and infectious disease: The cholera paradigm. *Science, 274,* 2025–2031.

Corvalan, C., Briggs, D., & Kjellstrom, T. (1996). Development of environmental health indicators. In D. Briggs, C. Corvalan, & M. Nurminen (Eds.), *Linkage methods for environment and health analysis.* Document WHO/EHG/95.26. Geneva, Switzerland: World Health Organization.

Daily, G.C. (Ed.). (1997). *Nature's services.* Washington, DC: Island Press.

Deishmann, W., & Henschler, D. (1986). What is there that is not poison? A study of the Third Defense by Paracelsus. *Archives of Toxicology, 58,* 4, 207–213.

Duchin, J.S., Koster, F.T., Peters, C.J., Simpson, G.L., Tempest, B., Zaki, S.R., Ksiazek, T.G., Rollin, P.E., Nichol, S., & Umland, E.T. (1994) Hantavirus pulmonary syndrome: A clinical description of 17 patients with a newly recognized disease. *New England Journal of Medicine, 330,* 949–955.

Fenwick, A., Cheesmond, A.K., & Amin, M.A. (1981). The role of field irrigation canals in the transmission of Schistosoma mansoni in the Gezira Scheme, Sudan. *Bulletin of the World Health Organization, 59,* 777–786.

Fletcher, T., & McMichael, A.J. (1997). *Health at the crossroads: Transport policy and urban health.* Chichester, England: John Wiley & Sons.

Florig, K. (1997). China's air pollution risks. *Environmental Science and Technology, 31,* 276–279.

Folke, C., Larsson, J., & Sweitzer, J. (1996). Renewable resource appropriation. In R. Costanza & O. Segura (Eds.), *Getting down to earth.* Washington, DC: Island Press.

Food and Agriculture Organization. (1995). *State of the world's fisheries, 1995.* Rome, Italy: Author.

Gleick, P.H. (1998). *The world's water: The biennial report on freshwater resources 1998–1999.* Washington, DC: Island Press.

Gruenbaum, E. (1983). Struggling with the mosquito: Malaria policy and agricultural development in Sudan. *Medical Anthropology, 7,* 51–62.

Herzstein, J.A., Bunn, W.B., Fleming, L.E., Harrington, J.M., Jeyaratnam, J., & Gardner, I.R. (1998). *International occupational and environmental medicine.* St. Louis, MO: Mosby.

Hoogvelt, A. (1997). *Globalisation and the post-colonial world.* London: Macmillan.

Intergovernmental Panel on Climate Change (IPCC). (1996). *Second assessment report: Climate change 1995* (Vols. I–III). New York: Cambridge University Press.

Jennings, N.S. (1998). Mining: An overview. In J. M. Stellman, *Encyclopaedia of occupational health and safety* (4th ed., Vol. III, ch. 74, pp. 74.2–74.4). Geneva, Switzerland: International Labor Office.

Khan, A.W., Ahmad, A., Sayed, M.H.S.U., Hadi, A., Khan, M.H., Jalil, M.A., Ahmed, R., & Faruquee, M.H. (1997). Arsenic contamination in ground water and its effect on human health with particular reference to Bangladesh. *Journal of Preventive and Social Medicine, 16,* 65–73.

Kjellstrom, T. (1994). Issues in the developing world. In L. Rosenstock & M. Cullen (Eds.). *Textbook of clinical occupational and environmental medicine* (pp. 25–31). Philadelphia: W.B. Saunders Co.

Kjellstrom, T., & Corvalan, C. (1995). Framework for the development of environmental health indicators. *World Health Statistics Quarterly, 48,* 144–154.

Kraus, R.S. (1998). Oil exploration and drilling. In J.M. Stellman, *Encyclopaedia of occupational health and safety* (4th ed., Vol. III, ch. 75). Geneva, Switzerland: International Labor Office.

LaDou, J. (1992). The export of industrial hazards to developing countries. In J. Jeyaratnam (Ed.), *Occupational health in developing countries* (pp. 340–360). Oxford, England: Oxford University Press.

LaDou, J., & Jeyaratnam, J. (1994). Transfer of hazardous industries: Issues and solutions. In J. Jeyaratnam & K.S. Chia (Eds.), *Occupational health in national development.* River Edge, NJ: World Scientific Publications.

Lee, K., & Dodgson, R. (2000). Globalisation and cholera: Implications for global governance. *Global Governance, 6.*

Logie, D.E., & Benatar, S.R. (1997). Africa in the 21st century: Can despair be turned to hope? *British Medical Journal, 315,* 1444–1446.

Madronich, S., & de Gruijl, F.R. (1993). Skin cancer and UV radiation. *Nature, 366,* 23.

McMichael, A.J. (1993). *Planetary overload: Global environmental change and the health of the human species.* Cambridge, England: Cambridge University Press.

McMichael, A.J. (1994). "Molecular epidemiology": New pathway or new traveling companion? *American Journal of Epidemiology, 140,* 1–11.

McMichael, A.J. (1999). Dioxins in the Belgian food chain: Chickens and eggs. *Journal of Epidemiology and Community Health, 53,* 742–743.

McMichael, A.J., Anderson, H.R., Brunekreef, B., & Cohen, A. (1998). Inappropriate use of daily mortality analyses for estimating the longer-term mortality effects of air pollution. *International Journal of Epidemiology, 27,* 450–453.

McMichael, A.J., & Haines, A. (1997). Global climate change: The potential effects on health. *British Medical Journal, 315,* 805–809.

McMichael, A.J., Haines, A., Slooff, R., & Kovats, S. (Eds.). (1996). Climate change and human health: An assessment prepared by a task group on behalf of the World Health Organization, the World Meteorologic Organization and the United Nations Environment Programme. Geneva, Switzerland: World Health Organization.

McMichael, A.J., & Smith, K.R. (1999). Air pollution and health: Seeking a global perspective (Editorial). *Epidemiology, 10,* 1–4.

Moochhala, S.M., Shahi, G.S., & Cote, I.L. (1997). The role of epidemiology, controlled clinical studies, and toxicology in defining environmental risks. In G.S. Shahi, B.S. Levy, A. Binger, T. Kjellstrom, & R. Lawrence (Eds.), *International perspective on environment, development and health: Toward a sustainable world* (pp. 341–352). New York: Springer.

Morgenstern, H., & Thomas, D. (1993). Principals of study design in environmental epidemiology. *Environmental Health Perspectives Supplement, 101,* 23–38.

Morse, S.S. (1995). Factors in the emergence of infectious diseases. *Emerging Infectious Diseases, 1,* 7–15.

Murray, C.J.L., & Lopez, A.D. (1996). *The global burden of disease: A comprehensive assessment of mortality and disability from diseases, injuries, and risk factors in 1990 and projected to 2020.* Cambridge, MA: Harvard University Press.

Nriagu, J.O., Blankson, M.L., & Ocran, K. (1996). Childhood lead poisoning in Africa: A growing public health problem. *Science of Total Environment, 181,* 93–100.

Organization of Economic Cooperation and Development (OECD). (1993). *OECD core set of indicators for environmental performance reviews.* Environmental Monograph No. 83. Paris: Organization of Economic Cooperation and Development.

Ostro, B. (1994). *Estimating the health effects of air pollutants.* Policy Research Working Paper 1301. Washington, DC: World Bank.

Pimentel, D., Tort, M., D'Anna, L., Krawic, A., Berger, J., Rossman, J., Mugo, F., Doon, N., Shriberg, M., Howard, E., Lee, S., & Talbot, J. (1998). Ecology of increasing disease. *Bioscience, 48,* 817–826.

Pimm, S.L., Russell, G.J., Gittleman, J.L., & Brooks, T.M. (1995). The future of biodiversity. *Science, 269,* 347–354.

Pocock, S.J., Smith, M., & Baghurst, P. (1994). Environmental lead and children's intelligence: A systematic review of the epidemiological evidence. *British Medical Journal, 309,* 1189–1197.

Poschen, P. (1998). General profile (forestry). In J. M. Stellman, *Encyclopaedia of occupational health and safety* (4th ed., Vol. III, ch. 68, pp. 68.2–68.6). Geneva, Switzerland: International Labor Office.

Rahman, M., Tondel, M.J., Ahmad, S.A., & Axelson, O. (1998). Diabetes mellitus associated with arsenic exposure in Bangladesh. *American Journal of Epidemiology, 148,* 198–203.

Rees, W. (1996). Revisiting carrying capacity: Area-based indicators of sustainability. *Population and Environment, 17,* 195–215.

Repetto, R., & Belagi, S.S. (Eds.). (1996). *Pesticides and the immune system: The public health risks.* Washington, DC: World Resources Institute.

Rosenstock, L., & Cullen, M. (1994). *Textbook of clinical occupational and environmental medicine.* Philadelphia: W.B. Saunders Co.

Samet, J.M., Schnatter, R., & Gibb, H. (1998). Invited commentary: Epidemiology and risk assessment. *American Journal of Epidemiology, 148,* 929–936.

Schwartz, J. (1994). Low level lead exposure and children's IQ: A meta-analysis and search for a threshold. *Environmental Research, 65,* 42–45.

Shahi, G.S., Levy, B.S., Binger, A., Kjellstrom, T., & Lawrence, R. (Eds.). (1997). *International perspective on environment, development and health: Toward a sustainable world.* New York: Springer.

Sims, J. (1994). *Women, health and environment: An anthology.* Document WHO/EHG/94.11. Geneva, Switzerland: World Health Organization.

Slaper, H., Velders, G.J.M., Daniel, J.S., de Gruijl, F.R., & van der Leun, J.C. (1996). Estimates of ozone depletion and skin cancer incidence to examine the Vienna Convention achievements. *Nature, 384,* 256–258.

Smith, A.H., Goycoleam, M., Haque, R., & Biggs, M.L. (1998). Marked increase in bladder and lung cancer mortality in a region of northern Chile due to arsenic in drinking water. *American Journal of Epidemiology, 147,* 660–669.

Smith, D. (1999). Worldwide trends in DDT levels in human milk. *International Journal of Epidemiology, 28,* 179–188.

Smith, K.R. (1997). Development, health, and the environmental risk transition. In G. Shahi, B.S. Levy, & A. Binger (Eds.), *International perspectives in environment, development, and health* (pp. 51–62). New York: Springer.

Smith, K.R., Corvalan, C., & Kjellstrom, T. (1999). How much global ill-health is attributable to environmental factors? *Epidemiology, 10,* 573–584.

Stellman, J. M. (Ed.). (1998). *Encyclopaedia of occupational health and safety* (4th ed.). Geneva, Switzerland: International Labor Organization.

Tong, S., Baghurst, P.A., Sawyer, M.G., Burns, J., & McMichael, A.J. (1998). Declining blood lead levels and cognitive function during childhood—the Port Pirie Cohort Study. *Journal of the American Medical Association, 280,* 1915–1919.

U.N. Environment Programme (UNEP). (1998). *Environmental effects of ozone depletion.* Nairobi: Author.

United Nations. (Annual). *United Nations Demographic Yearbook.* New York: United Nations.

U.S. Congress, Subcommittee on Finance and Hazardous Materials. (1998, February). *Status of the Superfund Program.* Washington, DC: Government Printing Office.

Watson, R.T., Dixon, J.A., & Hamburg, S.P. (Eds.). (1998). *Protecting our planet, securing our future: Linkages among global environmental issues and human needs.* Nairobi: UNEP/USNASA/World Bank.

Weeks, J.L. (1998). Health and safety hazards in the construction industry. In J. M. Stellman, *Encyclopaedia of occupational health and safety* (4th ed., Vol. III, ch. 93, pp. 93.2–93.8). Geneva, Switzerland: International Labor Office.

Wilson, M.E. (1995). Infectious diseases: An ecologic perspective. *British Medical Journal, 311,* 1681–1684.

Woodward, A., Hales, S., & Weinstein, P. (1998) Climate change and human health in the Asia Pacific region: Who will be the most vulnerable? *Climate Research, 11,* 31–38.

World Bank. (1993). World development report 1993. Investing in Health. Washington, DC: Author.

World Health Organization. (1990). Public health impact of the use of pesticides in agriculture. Geneva, Switzerland: Author.

World Health Organization. (1992). Cadmium. Environmental health criteria. No. 134. Geneva, Switzerland: Author.

World Health Organization. (1994). Ultraviolet radiation. Environmental health criteria. No. 160. Geneva, Switzerland: Author.

World Health Organization. (1996). Health effects of the Chernobyl accident. WHO document WHO/EHG/96.X. Geneva, Switzerland: Author.

World Health Organization. (1997). Health and environment in sustainable development. Document WHO/EHG/97.8. Geneva, Switzerland: Author.

World Health Organization. (1998). Chrysotile asbestos. Environmental health criteria. No. 190. Geneva, Switzerland: Author.

World Health Organization. (1999). *World Health Report 1999. Making a difference.* Geneva, Switzerland: Author.

World Resources Institute. (1998). *World resources 1998–99.* Oxford, England: Oxford University Press.

Yassi, A., & Kjellstrom, T. (1998). Environmental health hazards. In J. M. Stellman, *Encyclopaedia of occupational health and safety* (4th ed., Vol. II, ch. 53, pp. 53.1–53.33). Geneva, Switzerland: International Labor Office.

# CHAPTER 9

# Complex Humanitarian Emergencies

*Michael J. Toole, Ronald J. Waldman, and Anthony B. Zwi*

This chapter focuses on public health emergencies that arise from complex political crises. Terminology changes frequently, and different definitions emphasize different aspects of a concept. For example, complex humanitarian emergencies (CHEs) have been described by the Centers for Disease Control and Prevention (CDC) as "situations affecting large civilian populations which usually involve a combination of factors including war or civil strife, food shortages, and population displacement, resulting in significant excess mortality" (Burkholder & Toole, 1995). Goodhand and Hulme (1999) define "complex political emergencies" as conflicts that combine a number of features: they often occur within but also across state boundaries; they have political antecedents, often relating to competition for power and resources; they are protracted in duration; they are embedded in and are expressions of existing social, political, economic, and cultural structures and cleavages; and they are often characterized by predatory social formations. This latter definition clearly locates the causes and effects in the political sphere, a point echoed by numerous other writers, as this has considerable implications for those working in these settings with a primarily public health agenda.

While recognizing that the roots of complex emergencies lie firmly in the political sphere, the term *complex humanitarian emergency* is used in order to maintain simplicity and consistency. The chapter grapples with current understanding

of CHEs and their political causes and considers their impact on populations and health systems.[*] It highlights current knowledge in humanitarian assistance and indicates that effective technical interventions are possible to help alleviate suffering and limit the adverse effect on the health of populations. Attention is drawn to current efforts by the humanitarian community to improve the effectiveness, efficiency, and equity of humanitarian responses; to how the pattern of early responses may influence the longer-term survival of populations and systems; and to the nature of any post-conflict society. It is clear, however, that the solutions to CHEs are political and not humanitarian, and that it is in the political sphere that both upstream and downstream responses to complex emergencies must receive priority.

In the period from the end of World War II to the end of the Cold War, most conflicts took

---

*Acknowledgments:* The authors wish to acknowledge the advice provided on food and nutrition by Professor Michael Golden of Aberdeen University.

[*]The emphasis in this chapter is on complex political emergencies and not on more traditional forms of interstate conflict and war. Further, although other forms of intrastate conflict and repression, such as torture and disappearance, are commented on, these forms of violence are not the focus of this chapter. Where possible, these issues are briefly highlighted either through the presentation of an exhibit or through reference to the literature.

439

place in the developing regions of the world, primarily in Africa, the Middle East, Asia, and Latin America. (Figure 9–1 presents the numbers of armed conflicts by world region from 1989 to 1997.) The end of the Cold War, the breakup of the Soviet Union, and the pace and intensity of globalization have led, at the turn of the millennium, to major conflicts in Europe and the former Soviet Union, notably in Tajikistan, Chechnya, former Yugoslavia, and Nagorno Karabakh. In addition, conflicts have reignited in several areas that seemed on the verge of peace, such as Angola, Ethiopia-Eritrea, and the Democratic Republic of Congo. After decades of relative stability and increasing prosperity, violence and civil unrest exploded in many areas of Indonesia in 1998–1999, culminating in the widespread destruction, killings, and forced migration that occurred following the vote by East Timorese for independence.

Modern-day conflicts are increasingly internal rather than between states and often have as a prime objective, alongside the quest for economic and political power, the undermining of the lives and livelihoods of civilian populations associated with opposing factions. Up to 90% of those affected in recent conflicts have been civilians, with all ages and both sexes affected. The distribution of impact and health outcomes will vary substantially, however, and will depend on the nature of the conflict and its history, extent, form, and prior health and health systems status.

Many CHEs have attracted considerable media attention and have sought to promote availability of at least a basic degree of humanitarian assistance, even if fundamental political solutions are not sought. However, other ongoing crises, despite causing massive loss of life, population displacement, and infrastructure destruction, are not necessarily explicitly recognized as CHEs and as a result attract few resources and attention. These "hidden emergencies" nevertheless pose fundamental challenges to the health and well-being of affected populations. Ongoing conflicts in Burma, Colombia, Sudan, Algeria, and West Africa seem to attract little attention and resources; such discrepancies are likely to result from geopolitical concerns, media interest, and economic factors. The role of the media may be particularly powerful in "anointing" a country as a complex emergency worthy of attention, such as the BBC in Ethiopia in 1984, which subsequently focused world attention and popular demands for action.

Refugees and internally displaced persons (IDPs) typically experience high mortality in the emergency phase following their migration. In children, deaths result from malnutrition, diarrhea, and infectious diseases; in adults, communicable and noncommunicable diseases, injuries and violence, and psychological distress probably contribute most to their burden of disease.

Some wars *are* still fought primarily between competing armies, such as the 1980–1988 Iran-Iraq conflict in which an estimated 450,000 military personnel died (Sivard, 1996); the Gulf War of 1991; and the Eritrea-Ethiopia and India/Pakistan conflicts of 1999. But the vast majority now take place within states. The more traditional form of warfare between uniformed military forces of different countries will not form the main focus of this chapter.

Notwithstanding the Holocaust itself, the post-World War II experience has highlighted numerous episodes of massive human rights atrocities and genocide committed against particular groups: Pol Pot's killing fields in Cambodia; the Guatemalan government action against indigenous Mayan communities; use of chemical and biological weapons against the Kurds in Halabja, Iraq, and the genocide against Tutsis in Rwanda. Recent conflicts, such as that in Kosovo during 1999, highlight the nature of internal wars, including the use of repressive techniques to evict people from their homes and to undermine their sense of security and safety, accompanied by the targeted use of force to destroy social, political, and economic structures. A particularly insidious development is the targeting of violence toward individuals and groups on the basis of their ethnicity or religion. Such conflicts have been frequent enough that the term *ethnic cleansing* has entered the language.

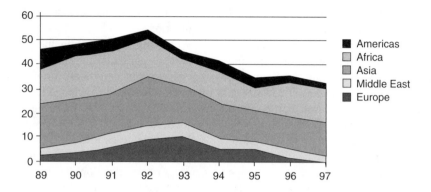

**Figure 9–1** Armed Conflict, 1989–1997

However, the reality has been that opportunistic politicians have often inflamed the perceived differences between groups, especially during times of economic and political uncertainty, resulting in open warfare.

In the same conflict, evidence of other key features of modern-day CHEs can be seen, such as:

- the willingness of powerful segments of the international community to intervene in internal conflicts and to do so in a way that minimizes their exposure to risk
- the changing nature of humanitarian assistance that increasingly forms only one dimension to the management of conflicts alongside political, economic, and military responses
- the changing role of the private sector, as well as the increasingly important role of local and global media
- trends in globalization that integrate peripheral areas within the global economy but contribute to their fragmentation as elites compete for access to the economic and political resources associated with integration in the global political economy

One consequence of the targeting of entire communities and their livelihoods has been the dramatic rise in numbers of forcibly displaced people. In 1997 there were estimated to be 30 million IDPs and 23 million refugees (those seeking refuge across international borders) (Reed, Haaga, & Keely, 1998), the vast majority fleeing conflict zones. Those displaced within countries have less access to resources and services supported by the international community, may be at ongoing risk from violence perpetrated by the state and other powerful local actors, and have their needs more hidden than those displaced across borders (Hampton, 1998).

Although refugee numbers are typically assessed in order to plan and provide relief, relatively little attention has been devoted to developing the most appropriate methods for establishing the precise composition of refugee and IDP populations, whether in terms of age, sex, religion, local geographic origin, or ethnicity. This imposes constraints, given the differing needs and roles of groups within populations, and may make it easier for the more complex issues of dealing with gender, equity, and ongoing intergroup rivalry to be overlooked. Particular groups, such as older adults, refugees not in camps, and internally displaced persons (IDPs) may neither be identified nor receive the required attention for their differing needs.

The changing pattern of conflict has been accompanied by significant changes in the delivery of humanitarian assistance. The number of agencies operating in these complex settings has increased dramatically; for example, there were more than 240 nongovernmental organizations

(NGOs) working in and around Rwanda in the aftermath of the genocide and more than 100 agencies working with the Kosovar Albanians during 1999. On the other hand, lower profile CHEs may be as severe and life threatening to large populations, such as that in Sierra Leone in 1999, but attract much lesser media, intergovernmental, and humanitarian responses, the latter all integrally related. New NGOs established in response to a specific conflict may be short-lived, inexperienced, and unable to cope with the challenges they face in providing services in complex political environments: ensuring one does more good than harm must underlie all interventions.

Every conflict has winners and losers; predators identify opportunities amidst the turmoil to further enrich themselves and entrench their political position. These players may therefore have an interest in perpetuating the conflict. Humanitarian aid itself may become a resource over which groups compete, and such assistance and resources may directly or indirectly stoke the conflict. In some distressing circumstances, humanitarian aid was used unwittingly to attract populations that were subsequently targeted by combatants, as in the Democratic Republic of Congo. Humanitarian workers have increasingly been directly targeted in latter-day conflicts, and this has led to increased efforts to work closely with the military and security sector. Despite some benefits, such as in improving logistics support, this trend may bring negative consequences, additional dangers, and threaten the neutrality and impartiality to which many agencies aspire.

NGOs are not a homogeneous community. Although some are highly professional and have given considerable thought to the development of humanitarian and technical policies and programs, there have been some negative consequences for the way in which humanitarian assistance has been provided. Recognition by the humanitarian community of these problems has led to a great deal of evaluation and introspection and measures to improve practice, including the development of codes of conduct for humanitarian agencies, the promotion of minimum standards for service provision, and debate regarding enhancing accountability to affected populations.

Promoting the derivation and uptake of good practice is particularly difficult in humanitarian agencies given rapid staff turnover, unwillingness to publicly acknowledge failures and limitations because of the possible funding consequences, and a culture of doing rather than reflecting. Interventions are often not evidence-based, and despite most agencies valuing the concept of coordination, few wish to be coordinated. Poor-quality services have significant adverse consequences: increased morbidity, mortality, disability, further spread of communicable diseases, community dissatisfaction and breakdown, and psychosocial distress. Clear policy objectives for interventions are often lacking, and mechanisms for working with new players such as the military and the private sector remain inadequately developed. Despite recognition that the accountability of relief efforts to affected populations should be enhanced, mechanisms to ensure this are in their infancy.

Ongoing humanitarian challenges include understanding how best to upgrade host population health services alongside efforts to improve those available to refugees, how to provide good quality services most humanely and efficiently, and how to maintain the role of communities in structuring both the determination of priorities and the pattern of service provision. A key issue relates to how and whether to bolster and support resilient health and social systems and individual adaptations to conflict. Our level of knowledge regarding these responses, and the potential to further support them, is weak. A persistent challenge to humanitarian workers is to institutionalize a sensitive and inclusive evidence-based culture and to build sustainable mechanisms for crystallizing policy advice from the vast and valuable foundation of field experience (Banatvala & Zwi, in press).

## DIRECT PUBLIC HEALTH IMPACT OF WAR

Measuring the impact and hidden costs of conflict is complex for a variety of reasons.

These include methodological and theoretical shortcomings, inconsistencies in definitions and terms, restricted access to areas of conflict and sources of information, the rapid evolution of many emergencies, political manipulation of data, resource constraints, and the hidden or indirect nature of the impact. One consequence of the data limitations is the difficulties in identifying more precisely which sections of the population are at greatest risk in order to develop more appropriate responses. Most low-income countries lack reliable health information and vital registration systems; their absence increases the difficulties of determining the conflict-associated costs in terms of morbidity, mortality, and disability. Further, complex emergencies may seriously disrupt surveillance and information systems.

Lack of consistency in definitions used makes it difficult to compare within and across populations. Different agencies may define refugees and IDPs in different ways; case definitions for particular conditions vary; and techniques for estimating nutritional deficiencies, for example, may vary among different agencies working with the same population. Data are at times incomplete because impartial observers who attempt to provide more accurate figures may not have access to witnesses or other reliable sources of information. On other occasions entire communities and detainees in camps may have been exterminated, leaving no witnesses.

Although innovative techniques may be used to try to build a picture of what transpired during a particular complex emergency, what were the needs and the nature of the response, the sources of data may be biased as may the ways in which information has been collected. Despite this, innovative groups, often NGOs without a political agenda linked to any of the key players in the conflict, may be able to play a valuable role in documenting precisely what occurred and the nature of present needs.

Even where huge numbers of people are involved, agreement on the magnitude of impact varies. Estimates of the number of victims of the Rwandan genocide are still imprecise and vary from 500,000 to 1 million (the best estimate is

800,000). Gulf War deaths remain disputed; so too are likely to be the number of deaths experienced in Kosovo and East Timor. In Sudan a nutrition and mortality assessment in 1993 acknowledged that reliable census data were not available for any of the four assessment sites and that the size of the populations near airstrips where food was unloaded fluctuated according to the deliveries. Each party to the conflict has its own reasons for presenting data in a particular way; unless some more "objective" source is established, we will have to continue to be extremely cautious in the use of such figures.

Particular affected populations may also be difficult to assess precisely (Ugalde, Zwi, & Richards, 1999), as in the case of war orphans or unaccompanied child refugees and IDPs. Unaccompanied children may account for 2–5% of the refugee population in camps, although this will clearly vary in different contexts. Massive population movements may occur over very short periods of time, such as the 1 million or more Hutu refugees who fled from Rwanda over a period of days. Even when the time scales are longer, considerable problems remain: approximately 500,000 Liberian refugees fled to Guinea over a period of 5 years into an area that had a population of 1.2 million inhabitants (Van Damme, 1998). Such population flows present considerable challenges in terms of assessing health status, determining needs, and developing context-appropriate responses.

Political interests greatly affect which data are released, how and when this is done, and with what accompanying analyses. In the Kosovar conflict, NATO and the Yugoslav government tussled over a number of events in which civilian casualties occurred, each side seeking to obtain maximum political and public relations benefits. Certain events such as allegations of the use of systematic rape only appeared at times when NATO was under pressure to justify its role and nature of engagement in the war.

Data on numbers of IDPs and refugees may be manipulated by states and organizations in an attempt to make a political point or to maximize access to resources. It has been alleged that some refugee camp administrators and refugees report fewer deaths than actually occur in order to maintain levels of international assistance. In Nepal, in an attempt to encourage reporting of deaths among Bhutanese refugees, free funeral shrouds were offered to relatives of the deceased together with assurances that the reporting would not result in decreases of rations (United Nations High Commissioner for Refugees [UNHCR], 1993).

## Physical Impact

Political conflicts earlier this century were mostly waged between armies and trained combatants. The main direct results, in the form of deaths, morbidity and disability, reflected the nature of the conflict; the level of technology, and nature of weapons used; the prior preparation and protective clothing available to military personnel; and the quality of emergency medical care and evacuation facilities (Garfield & Neugat, 1991).

In the vast majority of latter day conflicts, however, the entire population is often targeted, in part directly but also with massive and sustained effort at reducing the viability and integrity of the affected community. In Mozambique the anti-government forces killed approximately 100,000 persons in 1986 and 1987, a massive proportion in a relatively small country. Injuries and disabilities may follow the use of firearms, but it is notable that technology levels need not be high to achieve terrible levels of destruction. The Rwandan genocide was largely committed with a combination of guns and machetes. Antipersonnel land mines are also responsible for significant population burdens especially in a small number of heavily infested countries such as Angola, Cambodia, and Afghanistan.

Numbers and types of war-disabled are not well known because only a few countries such as Zimbabwe, El Salvador, and the Tigrayan region of Ethiopia have attempted censuses of war-related disability. In Zimbabwe in 1981–1982, 13% of all disability was assessed as being war-related; in El Salvador in the mid-1990s the census identified 12,041 war-disabled, 82% of whom were combatants and the rest civilians. About one-third of the 300,000 soldiers returning from the front at the end of the war in Ethiopia had been injured or disabled. By 1984, well before the end of the war in 1991, more than 40,000 people had lost one or more limbs in the conflict.

Estimates of mine-related disabilities are sobering: 36,000 in Cambodia (one in every 236 persons has lost at least one limb), 20,000 in Angola, 8,000 in Mozambique, and 15,000 in Uganda. In former Yugoslavia more than 3 million mines were laid, and in late 1994 mine laying was occurring at a rate of 50,000 per week, with much of this unmarked and unmapped. The costs are both physical and social and affect all age groups. Between February 1991 and February 1992, approximately 75% of the land mine injuries treated worldwide were in children aged 5–15 years. Others affected may be aware of the dangers of mines but have to enter the mined areas in search of food or to continue their agricultural and pastoral activities. Many of the severely disabled will require permanent medical and social services and strain the health resources of the country for many years. UNICEF estimates that there are about 4 to 5 million war-disabled children.

For years to come, the antipersonnel land mines and munitions will constitute a health hazard and contribute to thousands of deaths and severe disabilities, including many children. As the Soviets withdrew in defeat in Afghanistan, it is alleged that a Soviet officer told the mujahideen forces that "we are leaving but our mines will kill your grandchildren" (McGrath, 1994, p. 156). It has been estimated that one person will die and two will be injured for every 5,000 inactivated mines.

### Sexual Violence

Rape is increasingly recognized as a feature of internal wars, but it has been present in many different types of conflicts. In some conflicts, rape has been used systematically as an attempt to undermine opposing groups: this was noted in a high profile way in relation to the conflict in the former Yugoslavia where Bosnian women were systematically abused (Stiglmayer, 1994), as well as in the Rwandan conflict. It has been argued that the more extensive development of women's organizations helped to ensure that these events were made more visible and that support for survivors mobilized. It has also been suggested, however, that some forms of sexual abuse such as male rape, for example, have as a result been poorly recognized if at all. A study in Uganda found that despite widespread rape, few women spoke of their victimization (Giller, Bracken, & Kabaganda, 1991).

Rape, sexual violence, and exploitation may also be widespread in refugee camps, although the extent of its recognition is limited, and widely varying estimates of the numbers of victims have been reported. Violence against Somali women in refugee camps in Northern Kenya attracted worldwide condemnation. Despite being relatively few in number, these incidents had a profound effect as they challenged the extent to which UN agencies, such as United Nations High Commissioner of Refugees, were effective in ensuring the protection of refugee populations against further abuse. In the former Yugoslavia, estimates of the number of rape survivors have ranged from 10,000 to 60,000 (Swiss & Giller, 1993) and have firmly placed the issue of systematic use of rape on the international agenda. Indirectly, such events have also highlighted the need for agencies working with conflict-affected populations to more widely consider their reproductive health needs (Palmer, Lush, & Zwi, 1999). Efforts to establish a permanent international criminal court, in which war crimes would be prosecuted, have clearly identified systematic use of rape in war time as an issue to be addressed. Although sexual violence is most typically perpetrated by men against women, males and children of both sexes may be targeted and warrant attention, especially given the additional taboos and stigma associated with these circumstances.

In addition to long-lasting mental health disorders, rapes have resulted in the transmission of the human immunodeficiency virus (HIV). Wars and political conflict present high-risk situations for the transmission of sexually transmitted infec-

tions (STIs), including HIV infection (Zwi & Cabral, 1991). There are various ways in which war predisposes to STI and HIV transmission, such as:

- widespread population movement, causing increased crowding
- separation of women from partners normally providing a degree of protection
- abuses and sexual demands by military personnel and others in positions of power
- weakened social structures, thereby reducing inhibitions on aggressive behavior and violence against women.

Aside from these additional exposures, access to barrier contraceptives, to treatment for STIs, to the prerequisites for maintaining personal hygiene, and to health promotion advice are all compromised in conflict situations.

Women who are on their own may find it more difficult to ensure their safety and that of their children. They become targets of violence from three sides—the opposing army, the armed forces in the country to which they have fled, and finally sometimes from their own community (Palmer & Zwi, 1998). They may be forced to provide sex in exchange for food, shelter, or other necessities for self and family survival. The experience of Afghan refugees (Amnesty International, 1995) is illustrative: "In the camps in Pakistan, most of which are controlled by one or other of the warring Afghan factions, women have been attacked, particularly those who are unaccompanied by men. If they refuse sexual favours, they are often denied access to vital rations." In Somalia, fear of rape and shooting prevented women from leaving their homes.

Women's use of health care facilities may be severely reduced if males dominate service provision. Burmese Muslim women who fled to Bangladesh, many of whom had been raped, had difficulties in accessing health care due to the predominance of male providers, highlighting the importance of a gender-sensitive analysis to conflict (UNHCR, 1992). The issue of safety of women should be carefully considered when planning camp and other facilities: the placement of cooking fuels, water, and sewage removal facilities could be undertaken in such a way as to reduce risks of abuse and violence.

## Human Rights Violations

Article 25 of the Universal Declaration of Human Rights, proclaimed by resolution 217 A(III) of the United Nations General Assembly on December 10, 1948, states clearly that "[e]veryone has the right to a standard of living adequate for the health and well-being of himself and of his family, including food, clothing, housing and medical care...." In times of war, this declaration and other laws, covenants, declarations, and treaties that constitute the body of human rights law are complemented by international humanitarian law. The latter is "a set of rules aimed at limiting violence and protecting the fundamental rights of the individual in times of armed conflict" (Perrin, 1996, p. 381). These rules are intended to govern the conduct of war by banning the use of certain weapons and by minimizing the effects of armed conflicts, whether international or internal, on noncombatants. The protection of the rights of noncombatants in wartime is based primarily on the Geneva Conventions of 1949 and the two Additional Protocols of 1977. Yet, despite the existence of both of these bodies of international law, complex humanitarian emergencies are consistently associated with serious infringements of the dignity of individuals and, more specifically, with a major impact on the health status of affected individuals and populations.

General practices that can be considered to be clear violations of international humanitarian law include the intentional targeting of civilian noncombatants, medical personnel, and civilian health facilities. Protection is also conferred upon prisoners of war, wounded and ill combatants, and military medical installations. Violations by states and individuals occurred with great frequency during the second half of the twentieth century. Some of the most prominent included the murder of civilians by the government of Guatemala during the 1980s (Yamauchi,

1993); the intentional destruction of health facilities by the rebel forces, known by their Portuguese acronym RENAMO, seeking to bring down the government of Mozambique (Cliff & Noormahomed, 1988); and the genocidal activities perpetrated upon the Tutsi population of Rwanda in 1994. In the final decade of the twentieth century, the governments of Serbia and Croatia pursued "ethnic cleansing" policies (more accurately termed *ethnic repression*); against the populations of neighboring republics of the former Yugoslavia, and, in the case of Serbia, the province of Kosovo.

Violations of human rights law and international humanitarian law that target individuals can take many forms. Torture of civilians has been increasingly documented. More than 2,000 Bhutanese refugees in Nepal, about 2% of the total refugee population, reported having been tortured prior to their flight (Shrestha et al., 1998). Torture has also been reported as a frequently used weapon by China against Tibetans (Physicians for Human Rights, 1997), and by Turkish authorities against dissenters to its regime (Iacopino, Heisler, Pishevar, & Kirschner, 1996). Sexual violence is also of increasing concern, as noted earlier in this chapter. The UNHCR has noted the "widespread occurrence of sexual violence in violation of the fundamental right to personal security as recognized in international human rights and humanitarian law" (UNHCR, 1993).

The consequences of wartime human rights violations can be enduring. The physical and psychological consequences of bodily harm to individuals do not end with the cessation of hostilities. Most societies require years of reconstruction and redevelopment in order to restore viable and effective health systems to serve their surviving populations. At the turn of the century, one can only speculate as to how countries like Cambodia, Somalia, Rwanda, Liberia, Sierra Leone, the republics of the former Yugoslavia and the former Soviet Union, and newly independent East Timor will emerge from the gross abuses of human rights that occurred on their soil.

Although violations of human rights law and international humanitarian law are crimes, the legal systems for punishing the perpetrators and compensating the victims are grossly inadequate. To date, two international tribunals have been established to prosecute war criminals from the former Yugoslavia and from Rwanda, respectively. While these courts help to move the punishment of war criminals from theory to practice, they have been slow to act and expensive to implement. At least conceptually, the establishment of an International Criminal Court, a permanent standing body dedicated to the trial and punishment of individuals accused and convicted of violations of human rights law, is another step toward strengthening what has in many respects been a legal system without law enforcement capability.

Reporting and responding to reports of human rights violations pose major problems. Although wars and internal conflicts have been proximate causes of most humanitarian emergencies, few of the individuals and agencies who have been involved in providing relief to the individuals affected are trained in the recognition of human rights violations or know where and how to report them. Until more widespread attention is paid to these crimes against humanity, the victims will continue to suffer from preventable acute and chronic morbidity and the perpetrators will go, for the most part, unpunished. It would be most useful to treat human rights violations as a major cause of morbidity and mortality during wars and their aftermath and to establish the epidemiologic characteristics of their distribution (Spirer & Spirer, 1993).

## INDIRECT PUBLIC HEALTH IMPACT OF CIVIL CONFLICT

This section focuses in detail on the impact on the health of populations that is not directly the consequence of violence. Although the chapter focuses on the public health consequences of armed conflict, there is a phased evolution of public health effects as a country or region moves from political disturbances, economic

deterioration, and civil strife through armed conflict, population migration, food shortages, and the collapse of governance and physical infrastructure. Thus this section attempts to frame the indirect consequences of civil conflict in the changing context of evolving humanitarian emergencies.

### Food Scarcity

As political disturbances evolve in a country, there is generally a significant effect on national and local economies. In some cases, an economic crisis may initiate political turmoil where there have been underlying tensions between political factions, ethnic or religious groups, or disadvantaged geographic areas. Under such scenarios, especially in low-income countries, one of the first health effects is undernutrition in vulnerable groups, which is in turn caused by food scarcity (for example, see Exhibit 9–1). Local farmers may not plant crops as extensively as usual, or may decrease the diversity of their crops due to the uncertainty created by the economic or political situation. The cost of seeds and fertilizer may increase and government agricultural extension services may be disrupted, resulting in lower yields. Distribution and marketing systems may be adversely affected. Devaluation of the local currency may drive down the price paid for agricultural produce, and the collapse of the local food processing industry may further diminish demand for agricultural products.

In the Democratic People's Republic of Korea (North Korea) during the late 1990s, a food crisis occurred without any change in the political situation. Although exacerbated by drought, the major cause of the food shortages was economic collapse linked to the loss of markets after the collapse of the Soviet bloc. In 1997 the country was able to produce only 58% of its food requirements and imports or food aid covered only half the deficit (Burkholder, 1997).

If full-scale armed conflict occurs, the fighting may damage irrigation systems, crops might be intentionally destroyed or looted by armed

**Exhibit 9–1** Turmoil in Indonesia

In Indonesia, the fourth most populous country in the world, an economic crisis occurred in 1997 at a time when dissatisfaction with the ruling oligarchy was high; within several months widespread riots led to the resignation of the president. Prior to the crisis, economic growth rates had been high and food security was at its best level since independence. In 1997 and 1998 there was a dramatic flight of capital out of the country, an abrupt drop in foreign investment, widespread unemployment, and rising tensions within cities. The proportion of the population below the poverty line increased from 11% in 1996 to 14% in 1998, and unemployment increased from 4.7% to 20.3% within 1 year. By late 1999 there was secessionist violence in Aceh and Irian Jaya provinces, religious conflicts in the eastern provinces of Maluku and West Timor resulting in the loss of hundreds of lives, ethnic violence in West Kalimantan, and mass killings in East Timor. The nation faced near total collapse. Health budgets were halved, and existing health programs deteriorated in quality and coverage. Rice imports increased from 633,000 metric tons in 1994 to more than 3 million metric tons in 1998; with the greatly devalued currency, this led to the price of rice increasing threefold between 1997 and 1999. The price increases disproportionately affected the low-income Indonesians, who spent 25% of their incomes on rice, compared with only 5% among high-income households. Studies during 1998 showed decreases in the consumption of fish, eggs, and meat; increases in iron and vitamin A deficiency, the prevalence of low body mass index among women, and increased reported cases of severe wasting and nutritional edema among children.

soldiers, distribution systems may collapse completely, and there may be widespread theft and looting of food stores. In countries that do not normally produce agricultural surpluses or that have large pastoral or nomadic communities, the impact of food deficits on the nutritional status of civilians may be severe, particularly in sub-Saharan Africa. If adverse climatic factors intervene, as often happened in drought-prone countries such as Sudan, Somalia, Mozambique, and Ethiopia during the 1980s and 1990s, the outcome may be catastrophic famine (see Exhibit 9–2).

Famine may be defined as high malnutrition and mortality rates resulting from inadequate availability of food. Lack of food availability may result from either insufficient production or inadequate or inequitable distribution.

In eastern Europe, when economic and political turmoil followed the collapse of the Soviet Union and its allies during the 1990s, currencies devalued and the price of staple foods increased dramatically. Persons on fixed incomes, especially elderly pensioners and families with unemployed adults, found that their purchasing power decreased. This resulted in a large proportion of the population subsisting on inadequate diets. In industrialized countries affected by armed conflict, urban residents may be at higher risk than rural communities. For example, the 380,000 citizens of besieged Sarajevo in 1992 required approximately 270 metric tons (MT) of external food aid per day. However, in late 1992, an average of 216 MT of food was delivered daily, providing approximately 2,024 kcal per person per day, or 75% of the minimum average winter energy requirements (Toole, Galson, & Brady, 1993). In countries subject to sanctions or blockades, such as Armenia and Iraq during the 1990s, urban families were at particularly high risk of nutritional deficiencies.

When food aid programs are established, there may be inequitable distribution due to political factors, food stores may be damaged or destroyed, food may be stolen or diverted to military forces, and the distribution of food aid may be obstructed (Macrae & Zwi, 1994). The resulting food shortages may cause prolonged hunger and eventually drive families from their homes in search of relief. There have been many examples of food aid diversion, including Mo-

**Exhibit 9–2** Famine in Ethiopia

One of the worst famines in the late twentieth century occurred in northern Ethiopia in 1984–1985. While the famine was blamed by the then-government on drought, the real causes were related more to politics than climate. At the time, the central government was engaged in fierce armed conflict with opposition groups in the northern provinces of Tigray and Eritrea. Smaller conflicts were occurring in other provinces such as Wollo. These provinces were the worst famine-affected provinces in the country. The central government called for international assistance but then obstructed efforts to distribute the food aid equitably. In the midst of the famine, hundreds of thousands of people fled to neighboring Sudan, fearing both conflict and hunger. At the same time, the central government forcibly moved hundreds of thousands of northerners to inhospitable regions in the south where thousands died of malaria and other diseases.

zambique and Ethiopia in the 1980s and southern Sudan and the former Yugoslavia in the 1990s. Indeed, in latter day CHEs, targeting of relief assistance and the use of humanitarian aid as a resource that enables the warring parties to continue their violence is an ongoing challenge for humanitarian agencies.

## Population Displacement

A common response by families and communities to civil conflict is to flee the violence. Individuals may flee because they fear persecution due to their particular political beliefs, ethnicity, or religion. In some societies, migration of part of the family to a safer area may be a traditional coping mechanism, with adult males staying behind to care for their land and animals. Some of these men may also be directly involved in the conflict. Mass migration and food shortages have been responsible for most deaths following civil conflicts in Africa and Asia.

*Refugees* are defined under several international conventions as persons who flee their country of origin through a well-founded fear of persecution for reasons of race, religion, social class, or political beliefs. The number of dependent refugees under the protection and care of the UNHCR steadily increased from approximately 6 million in 38 countries in 1980 to almost 20 million in 1990. By 1998 the number declined to about 12 million due to a number of large repatriations of refugees to their homelands

(UNHCR, 1999). In March 1999 the number increased to approximately 14 million, largely due to mass exoduses from Sierra Leone and Kosovo (see Table 9–1). In addition, some 3 million Palestinian refugees, assisted by the UN Relief and Works Agency, are to be found on the West Bank, Gaza, and other parts of the Middle East.

Several of the world's largest mass migrations took place in the last decade of the century. For example, in 1991, as many as 1 million Kurdish refugees fled Iraq for Iran or Turkey following the Gulf War. More than 600,000 refugees fled Burundi for Rwanda, Tanzania, and Zaire during a 2-week period in late October and early November 1993. By early 1993 there were at least 1.5 million refugees or displaced persons within the republics of former Yugoslavia. Between April and July 1994 an estimated 2 million Rwandan refugees fled into Tanzania, eastern Zaire, and Burundi, provoking the most serious refugee crisis in 20 years. In the late 1990s hundreds of thousands of refugees fled war and civil conflict in southern Sudan, Sierra Leone, Guinea-Bissau, Liberia, Chechnya (Russian Federation), northeast India, and Indonesia.

Between March and June 1999 approximately 780,000 ethnic Albanians fled the Serbian province of Kosovo in one of the most dramatic examples of "ethnic cleansing" in the series of Balkan conflicts. This represented more than 50% of the Albanian population of the province

**Table 9–1** Origin of Ten Major Refugee Populations in 1999[a]

| Country of Origin[b] | Main Countries of Asylum | Estimated Number |
|---|---|---|
| Afghanistan | Iran/Pakistan/India | 2,562,000 |
| Iraq | Iran/Saudi Arabia/Syria | 572,500 |
| Burundi | Tanzania/D.R. Congo | 525,700 |
| Sierra Leone | Guinea/Liberia/Gambia | 487,200 |
| Sudan | Uganda/Ethiopia/D.R. Congo/Kenya/C.A.R./Chad | 467,700 |
| Somalia | Ethiopia/Kenya/Yemen/Djibouti | 451,600 |
| Bosnia-Herzegovina | F.R. Yugoslavia/Croatia/Slovenia | 448,700 |
| Angola | Zambia/D.R. Congo/Congo | 350,600 |
| Eritrea | Sudan | 345,600 |
| Croatia | F.R. Yugoslavia/Bosnia-Herzegovina | 340,400 |

[a]An estimated 3.5 million Palestinians who are covered by a separate mandate of the U.N. Relief and Works Agency for Palestine Refugees in the Near East (UNRWA) are not included in this table. However, Palestinians outside the UNWRA area of operations such as those in Iraq or Libya, are considered to be of concern to UNHCR.

[b]Statistics reflecting the countries of origin of a large number of refugees in more developed countries are not available. Also, many refugees have acquired the citizenship of the asylum country—for example Vietnamese in the USA— and therefore are not included in the refugee statistics.

prior to the war. An unknown number of Kosovars were internally displaced within the province. In June 1999 approximately 400,000 Kosovars spontaneously repatriated to their homes within 2 weeks of the end of the NATO bombing campaign. Another mass migration took place amid the violence and destruction that followed the August 1999 referendum on independence in East Timor; approximately 300,000–400,000 people were displaced (almost 50% of the population), of whom approximately 260,000 were forcibly moved into Indonesian-controlled West Timor.

In addition to those persons who meet the international definition of refugees, millions of people have fled their homes for the same reasons as refugees but remain *internally displaced* in their countries of origin. It has not proven easy to ascertain the number and location of the world's IDPs. This is due not only to definitional difficulties, but is also the result of several institutional, political, and operational obstacles. Unlike the collection of refugee statistics, a task undertaken by UNHCR, no single UN agency has assumed responsibility for the collection of figures on internally displaced populations. The question of internal displacement is also a politically sensitive one. Governments are often

unwilling to admit to the presence of such populations on their territory, indicative as they are of the state's failure to protect its citizens. IDPs may themselves be reluctant to report to or register with the local authorities. Indeed, there is evidence to suggest that a large proportion of the world's IDPs live not in highly visible camps, but mingled with family members and friends, often in urban areas where they can enjoy a higher degree of anonymity.

Finally, there are some obvious obstacles to the collection of data in areas affected by ongoing armed conflicts. In the combat zones of Liberia, Somalia, Zaire, and Kosovo, for example, the international presence has been minimal or nonexistent, making it extremely difficult even to provide rough estimates of the number of people who have been displaced. Thus in Sierra Leone the statistics have been based on food aid beneficiary lists and probably reflect only a fraction of the displaced population. In other situations, such as Chechnya, IDPs are highly mobile, again making it very difficult to determine their exact numbers at any moment in time.

Despite all these difficulties, there was a broad international consensus that the global population of IDPs stood somewhere in the region of 27–32 million in 1999: up to 16 million in Africa, 6–7 million in Asia, approximately 5 million in Europe (predominantly former Yugoslavia and the Caucasus region), and up to 3 million in the Americas.

IDPs lack the international protection afforded by the international conventions and protocols on refugees. Nevertheless, the Geneva Conventions and certain articles of the United Nations Charter afford some protection to IDPs. During the 1990s the United Nations took some extraordinary measures to protect these populations in southern Sudan, northern Iraq, the republics of the former Yugoslavia, and Somalia.

Prior to 1990 most of the world's refugees had fled countries that ranked among the lowest-income in the world, such as Afghanistan, Cambodia, Mozambique, and Ethiopia. However, during the following decade, an increasing number of refugees have originated in relatively more affluent countries, such as Kuwait, Iraq, the former Yugoslavia, Armenia, Georgia, and Azerbaijan. However, the reasons for the flight of refugees generally remain the same: war, civil strife, and persecution. Hunger, although sometimes a primary cause of population movements, is all too frequently only a contributing factor. For example, during 1992, although

severe drought in southern Africa and the Horn of Africa affected food production in all countries in those regions, only in war-torn Mozambique and Somalia did millions of hungry inhabitants migrate in search of food.

The World Bank estimates that 90–100 million persons around the world have been forcibly displaced over the past decade as a result of large-scale development initiatives, such as dam construction, urban development, and transportation programs. An unknown number have also been uprooted by lower-profile forestry, mining, game park, and land-use conversion projects. The scale of such displacement seems unlikely to diminish in the future, given the processes of economic development, urbanization, and population growth that are taking place in many low- and middle-income countries (United States Committee for Refugees, 1999a).

The most common response to mass population movements, either across international boundaries or within countries, is to establish camps or settlements. In eastern Europe many refugees and IDPs have been housed in hotels, resort camps, schools, and hostels where environmental conditions have been relatively good. However, in low-income countries most refugees and displaced persons have been placed in camps

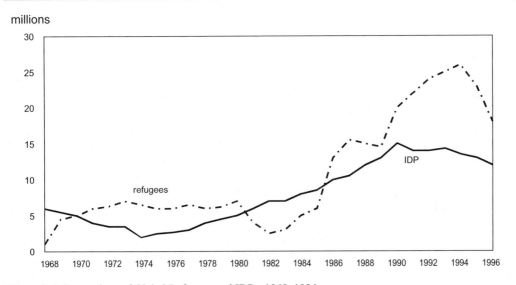

**Figure 9–2** Comparison of Global Refugees and IDPs, 1968–1996

located in inappropriate border areas. Exceptions include Mozambican refugees in Malawi in the 1980s, Liberian refugees in Guinea in the early 1990s, and Kosovar Albanians in Macedonia and Albania in 1999. In all three situations at least 50% of refugees were housed in local villages. Conditions in camps have varied enormously; in general, camps with fewer than 20,000 residents have had more favorable environmental conditions than larger camps. For example, camps for Rwandan refugees in eastern Zaire in 1994 contained up to 300,000 persons; they were poorly planned and laid out, had inadequate sanitation, and had poor access to clean water. Relief program managers found it difficult if not impossible to establish equitable systems of commodities, such as food and shelter materials, and there was a high frequency of violence and other crimes. By contrast, smaller refugee camps in Burundi were more easily managed and suffered fewer health consequences related to environmental conditions.

In addition to poor environmental conditions, crowded camps promote the spread of many communicable diseases, such as measles and acute respiratory infections (ARIs). The overwhelming nature of these large camps also tends to promote a sense of loss of dignity and independence among mostly rural refugees and induces mental health disorders, such as anxiety and depression.

**Destruction of Public Utilities**

Wars often involve the intentional or accidental destruction of public utilities, such as water and sewage systems, electricity sources and distribution grids, and fuel supplies. Although these mainly affect urban areas, local water supplies have also been destroyed in rural conflicts such as in Somalia during the early 1990s. Land mines have also intentionally been laid close to public water outlets. During the long internal conflicts in Mozambique and Angola, large cities and towns were targeted by guerrilla forces, resulting in nonfunctioning public utilities for many years. During the last 2 decades of the twentieth century, cities in Lebanon, Bosnia and Herzegovina, Chechnya, Somalia, Sudan, Kuwait, Iraq, Serbia, and Kosovo were perhaps the most severely affected. In September 1999 Dili, the capital of newly independent East Timor, was virtually destroyed in the ensuing violence.

Between 1992 and 1995 in Sarajevo, the capital, and other large cities in Bosnia and Herzegovina, municipal water supplies were destroyed by shelling; similar breakdowns in sewage systems and cross-contamination of piped water supplies led to widespread contamination of drinking water. These problems were compounded by the lack of electricity and diesel fuel needed to run generators. In the summer of 1993 residents of Sarajevo had on average only 5 liters of water per person per day, compared with the minimum of 15–20 liters recommended by the World Health Organization (WHO) and UNHCR. Although widespread epidemics of diarrheal disease were avoided, local health department data showed that the incidence of communicable diseases increased significantly after the beginning of the war. For example, between 1991 and 1993, the incidence of hepatitis A increased sixfold in Sarajevo, 12-fold in Zenica, and fourfold in Tuzla CDC, 1993a). The incidence of dysentery caused by *Shigella sp* increased 12-fold and 17-fold in Sarajevo and Zenica, respectively, during the same period.

Lack of electricity adversely impacts urban health services, in particular, hospital and clinic curative services. During a conflict, hospital generators are often able to supply only operating rooms and emergency rooms, thus further promoting a concentration of services in the area of trauma management. Routine surgical procedures; inpatient medical care; and pediatric, obstetric and gynecological, and perinatal care services deteriorate. In addition, the cold chain (a series of freezers, refrigerators, and ice-lined vaccine carriers) required to maintain immunization programs is not sustainable.

Sanctions and blockades also have a similar effect on public utilities without any physical destruction. During the winter of 1992–1993,

Armenian cities, such as the capital Yerevan, were deprived of imported fuel, including petrol, coal, kerosene, and gas. Consequently, there was practically no electricity or cooking and heating fuels available to private homes while temperatures averaged well below zero. The cold increased caloric requirements of individuals at a time when there were severe food shortages. Other health effects included increased rates of ARIs.

During the Gulf War allied bombing damaged Iraqi sewage treatment plants and water supplies; available potable water declined to 1.5 million cubic meters per day. Shortages of chemicals to monitor water quality contributed to typhoid, cholera, and gastrointestinal diseases. Even in very poor settings, available local infrastructure may be specifically targeted. The Sudanese army deliberately destroyed hand water pumps in rebel areas, and the insurgency did likewise in government-held territory (Dodge, 1990). At the beginning of the twenty-first century, the Russian army pounded Grozny, the capital city of Chechnya, with mortars and tanks in order to defeat the separatist movement based in the territory.

## Effects of Armed Conflict and Political Violence on Health Services

The model presented in Figure 9–3 offers a framework for describing the health service impact of conflict and complex emergencies. The focus of this is on the health services within the countries affected by complex emergencies; there are also related pressures and constraints on the health services of host countries to which refugees may flee.

### Access to Services

The impact of conflict on health facilities and services depends on their prior availability, distribution, and use patterns. Where services were originally available, as in Iraq (prior to 1991) or former Yugoslavia (prior to 1992), the conflict may cause rapid deterioration as a result of infrastructure and distribution systems damage,

resource constraints, declining health personnel availability and morale, and reductions in access. The prewar Iraqi health system was extensive, accessible to 90% of the population, and reached 95% of the children requiring immunization (Lee & Haines, 1991). By the end of the war, many hospitals and clinics had been severely damaged or closed, those operating were overwhelmed with work, and damage to infrastructure, water supplies, electricity, and sewage disposal exacerbated population health and health services activity.

Use is determined by geographic (that is, they are not too far away), economic (the services are affordable), and social access (there are no psychological or other barriers preventing use of services), all of which may be disrupted during complex emergencies (Zwi, Ugalde, & Richards, 1999). Peripheral services may be directly targeted as in Mozambique (Cliff & Noormahomed, 1988) or Nicaragua (Garfield & Williams, 1992) during the 1980s. Service access may be limited by fear of physical or sexual assault, physical restrictions on access as a result of antipersonnel land mines, curfews, and, in some cases, the encirclement of areas. In Afghanistan the Taliban, the victorious faction in the civil war that formed a national government, imposed constraints on women accessing services that were previously available to them. In other settings access may be restricted as a result of fear, insecurity, or lack of confidence in service providers. People injured in civil or political conflict may avoid using public services that carry a risk of security force surveillance. For example, in South Africa, the Philippines, and the Occupied Palestinian Territories, NGOs established alternative health services to allow those injured during uprisings against repressive regimes to seek care without fear of detection and detention.

Conflict may seriously disrupt links between services operating at different levels: referrals will be disrupted by logistical and communication constraints, as well as physical and military barriers to access. Towns and cities may be besieged, with entry and exit controlled by

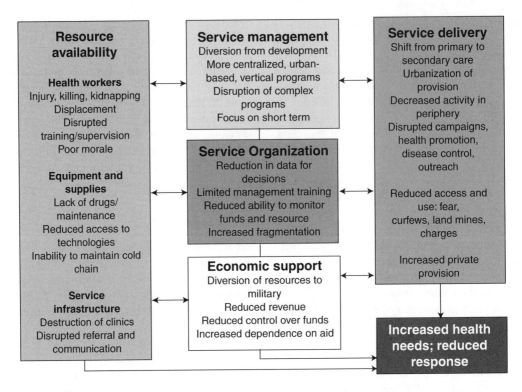

**Figure 9–3** The Health Service Impact of Conflict and Complex Emergencies

militia as in Beirut, Sarajevo, and Juba (Sudan). Health workers may move to urban areas to seek protection, other opportunities to make a living, or opportunities to provide health services privately with greater financial returns.

### Health Services Adaptations

Health services may be affected in a variety of ways. For example, systems within conflict areas may shift away from primary and community-based care to secondary, hospital-based services. This is a reflection of the movement of health care providers to urban areas; increased efforts to respond to the most serious injuries and adverse health effects; and the greater difficulty of maintaining peripheral services. Even in situations where preventive care was identified as important, such as in the struggle for liberation in the Tigrayan province of Ethiopia, priority was given to dealing with the war wounded

and maintaining the health of fighters (Barnabas & Zwi, 1997).

Emphasizing care and rehabilitation for war injuries indirectly deemphasizes longer term health development and community-based activities, including those focusing upon disease control. Malaria control activities may be seriously compromised; vector control, house spraying, environmental programs, information and education, training and supervision may all be disrupted. Disease treatment may become nonstandardized, haphazard, incomplete, and uncoordinated with considerable risk of the emergence of resistant organisms. These factors are especially important in relation to malaria, STIs, and tuberculosis control. Impaired surveillance and health information systems undermine the ability to detect unusual or exacerbated patterns of disease occurrence, and to respond to them. Public health action, such as partner notification, screening, and community education efforts, may all be compromised. Activities may become increasingly limited to small areas or specific districts and populations, and service provision may be increasingly organized through vertical programs that allow control over activities to assess needs, deliver services, monitor performance, and track finances. The gap between better funded vertical programs and the general health services may widen substantially, both during and in the aftermath of major conflicts.

Adaptation occurs and other actors attempt to fill the gaps caused by retreating and contracting public sector services. Indigenous health care providers may become more important both in their role as "healers" more generally and as health care providers. The private health care sector expands, both through the provision of services by nonprofit NGOs and through the hemorrhage of public sector workers into the private sector, whether officially or unofficially.

### Infrastructure

Direct targeting of clinics, hospitals, and ambulances may be against international humanitarian law but has frequently been experienced in latter-day conflicts. In the siege of Vukovar in eastern Slavonia during the civil war on the former Yugoslavia, the hospital was seriously damaged and much of it destroyed. Related facilities such as those necessary for water and sanitation, sewage removal, and electricity have been directly targeted; the latter in Iraq and Serbia. In Nicaragua the insurgency destroyed the main pharmaceutical storage facility of the country in Corinto, creating a severe shortage for months.

The destruction of nonhealth physical infrastructure such as roads, electrical plants, and communication systems has indirect health consequences. In Cape Town, South Africa, transport difficulties prevented health workers from attending work; experiences in the occupied Palestinian territories and other regions of active ongoing conflict have been similar. In some Iraqi hospitals, elevators did not work during energy blackouts and patients could not be moved to surgical theaters, so emergency interventions had to be delayed or take place in suboptimal

conditions. The impact on health services of electricity supply disruption, instituted by NATO bombing in Serbia and Kosovo, is unknown, as are the longer term environmental and economic consequences.

### Equipment and Supplies

Access to medicines and supplies is typically disrupted during conflicts. Drug shortages, especially where they were previously available, may lead to an increase in medically preventable causes of death, such as asthma, diabetes, and infectious diseases. Disruption to the Ugandan Essential Drugs Management Program, organized in the early 1980s, resulted in many rural dwellers who had gained access to modern medicines and vaccines being once more deprived of basic drugs. Quality of care available may suffer greatly; in Somalia amputations performed without intravenous antibiotics led to higher rates of infection, and in the former Yugoslavia operations were performed with inadequate anesthesia. Health care technologies, including x-rays and laboratories, are undermined through lack of maintenance, spare parts, skilled personnel, chemicals, and other supplies.

Additional problems may emerge as a result of the humanitarian response. Drug donations, if poorly coordinated and standardized, may lead to a large number of expired and inappropriate drugs being off-loaded in countries. These may be unable to be used, but must be safely and efficiently disposed of, placing an additional burden on the recipient country's pharmaceutical services. Another problem that typically arises results from the poor standardization of treatments with different NGOs, host government, and other services all treating similar problems using different drugs, oftentimes with inappropriate treatment regimes, raising the risk of multiresistant organisms emerging.

### Budgetary Impact

The conflict against the ruling Ethiopian clique, the Derg, led to increases in military expenditure from 11.2% of the government budget in 1974–1975 to 36.5% by 1990–1991 and to declines in the health budget from 6.1% in 1973–1974 to 3.5% in 1985–1986 and 3.2% in 1990–1991 (Kloos, 1992). The deterioration of the economy typically leads to reduced public expenditure as funds are shifted into supporting the war. In Uganda the public health budget in 1986 was only 6.4% of what it had been in the early 1970s. In El Salvador the proportion of the national budget allocated to health during the civil war plummeted from 10% in 1980 to 6% in 1990, and the budget available to the ministry of health, as a percentage of the gross national product, declined from 2% to 0.9%. Prior to 1980 the health budget had been higher than the defense budget, but during the first year of the civil war more funds were allocated to the military than to health. At the peak of the conflict in 1986, even the official figures indicated that the military received about four times more than the health sector.

### Human Resources

Injury, killing, kidnapping, and exodus of health workers are common during complex emergencies. There is evidence of targeting health workers in many recent conflicts; this has been particularly well documented in Mozambique and Nicaragua. Even if not directly targeted, health workers may flee in search of safety and security. In Uganda, 50% of the doctors and 80% of the pharmacists left the country between 1972 and 1985 (Dodge & Wiebe, 1995); in Mozambique, only 80 of the 500 doctors present before independence remained after 1975 (Walt & Cliff, 1996). In Cambodia, Pol Pot's killing fields were directed at professional and educated people, among others, with brutal and long-lasting effects; there is some as yet unconfirmed evidence of professionals being similarly targeted in Kosovo. Administrative and planning capacity may be seriously undermined by the lack of data, lack of personnel, and lack of consensus-building opportunities through which policies can be negotiated, strategies developed, and planning undertaken. In the period leading up to the referendum on independence in East Timor, there was an exodus of trained health personnel. The number of doctors in the province decreased from approximately 200 in 1998 to 69 in April 1999 (4 months before the referendum) to only 20 in February 2000.

### Community Involvement

In many latter-day conflicts and those of the Cold War period, which were described as "low intensity," community leaders and social structures were frequently targeted. Those who waged war against the Marxist Frelimo state in Mozambique attempted to reduce access to health care and educational services that the state had prioritized as a symbol of its commitment to promoting more equitable development. A similar process took place in Nicaragua where opposition forces targeted health and education services, a reflection of state commitment. Local systems of democracy and accountability are often seriously disrupted and involvement in community affairs discouraged; in some conflicts quite the reverse occurs, however, in some documented struggles, notably those in Mozambique, Vietnam, Eritrea, and Tigray.

Organizational or political responses to conflict may be positive, facilitating opportunities for health system and societal development. In the popular conflict against the Ethiopian Derg, community-based political movements in Eritrea and Tigray promoted community participation and control in decision making and facilitated the development of multisectoral health promotion strategies. The Tigrayan People's Liberation Front trained health workers and established mobile services and innovative community-financing systems. Elected local governments, the *baitos*, were established, which played a significant role in mobilizing and distributing resources to ensure that drugs and adequate services were available despite considerable constraints (Barnabas & Zwi, 1997). A recent study in Tigray and North Omo, Ethiopia, showed that although the involvement of women in local government and political activity was actively promoted during the war, their ongoing involvement in the postwar period appeared to be declining (Barnabas, 1997).

## Policy Formulation

Violent political conflict undermines capacity to make decisions rationally and accountably. A key problem in conflict-affected settings is the wide range of actors operating and the confused lines of accountability. In typical health systems, peripheral level services are accountable, usually within the health sector, to district or provincial health authorities; these, in turn, are responsible to central health authorities. Conflict may lead to greater degrees of centralization of decision making, whereas the need is for increasingly decentralized decision making so as to ensure that peripheral services can respond appropriately to their local context.

The policy framework, within which providers and purchasers of services operate, may be compromised or nonexistent, leading to an inability to control and coordinate service provision. There may be a serious lack of data upon which to make important health policy decisions. Ongoing conflict may impede learning from experience, the build-up of institutional memory, and the stimulation of ongoing critical debate around health and social policies, both locally and in relation to current international debates (Zwi, Ugalde, & Richards, 1999). Locally available fora for debate, such as the media and professional organizations, may be controlled or at any rate less accessible. In the post-conflict setting, a key challenge is to reestablish these fora for debate and to facilitate the exchange of ideas between the range of important stakeholders operating in the health environment.

## New Actors

During internal conflicts, due to scarcity of resources and government difficulties in accessing populations under the control of insurgents, NGOs usually fill part of the vacuum left by the public sector. In recent conflict-related emergencies, various military forces have played a direct role in providing relief (for example, northern Iraq, 1991), as have private companies contracted by government or UN agencies (Albania and Macedonia, 1999). The entry of these new players has further complicated the response to CHEs. The role of NGOs is extremely important both during and in the aftermath of ongoing conflict. During conflicts, indigenous NGOs and church groups may be among the few service providers who continue to operate during the conflict, especially in rural areas and those more directly affected by violence. A key problem, however, is that these NGOs often provide a patchwork of services that are relatively independent of the state and that do not necessarily fit in with other service provision approaches or priorities. They may communicate poorly with one another, adopt different approaches and standards of care and health worker remuneration, and focus attention mostly at a local level with some impact on the equity of service availability across large regions.

Health-related peace-building initiatives may provide avenues for reconnecting people and social structures, lives, and livelihoods. Evidence for the extent and limitations of such approaches is slowly emerging; but further critical analysis and debate are required. A key research challenge is to understand how health systems adapt and respond to conflict and to determine whether positive developments can be further reinforced and sustained. WHO assisted the Bosnian and Croatian health care systems to register and respond to the needs of disabled people during the war. These could be extended in the postwar period to ensure access to rehabilitation and social support services. Surgery services developed in response to antipersonnel land mine injuries should be extended to other forms of injury surveillance and treatment. Mechanisms to protect and maintain key elements of service provision and functioning, including information systems and supplies, are crucial to ensuring ongoing system functioning. How best to promote this requires further exploration.

## SPECIFIC HEALTH OUTCOMES

### Mortality

In this section, the impact of civil conflict and humanitarian emergencies on mortality rates will be confined to indirect causes, such as food scarcity, population displacement, destruction of health facilities and public utilities, and disruption of routine curative and preventive services. Mortality directly caused by the violence of war is discussed elsewhere.

The most severe health consequences of conflict—population displacement, food scarcity, and siege situations—have occurred in the acute emergency phase, during the early stage of relief efforts, and have been characterized by extremely high mortality rates. Although the quality of the international community's disaster response efforts has steadily improved, death rates associated with forced migration have often remained high, as demonstrated by several emergencies during the 1990s. For example, the exodus of almost 1 million Rwandan refugees into eastern Zaire in 1994 resulted in mortality rates that were more than 30 times the rates experienced prior to the conflict in Rwanda.

Crude mortality rates (CMR) have been estimated from burial site surveillance, administrative, hospital, and burial records; community-based reporting systems; and population surveys. The many problems in estimating mortality under emergency conditions have included

- poorly representative or inaccurate population sample surveys
- failure of families to report all deaths for fear of losing food ration entitlements
- inaccurate estimates of affected populations for the purpose of calculating mortality rates
- lack of standard reporting procedures

In general, however, mortality rates have tended to be underestimated because deaths are usually underreported or undercounted, and population size is often exaggerated. Early in an emergency, when mortality rates are elevated, the CMR is usually expressed as deaths per 10,000 population per day (CDC, 1992). In most low-income countries, the baseline annual CMR in nonrefugee populations has been reported between 12–24 per 1,000, corresponding to a daily rate of approximately 0.3–0.7 per 10,000. A threshold of 1 per 10,000 per day has been used

commonly to define an elevated CMR and to characterize a situation as an emergency (CDC, 1992). In one of the most severe refugee emergencies of the 1990s, the CMR among Rwandan refugees during the first month after their arrival in eastern Zaire was between 27–50 per 10,000 per day (Goma Epidemiology Group, 1995).

The most reliable estimates of mortality rates have come from well-defined and secure refugee camps where there is a reasonable level of camp organization and a designated agency has had responsibility for the collection of data (see Table 9–2). The most difficult situations have been those where IDPs have been scattered over a wide area and where surveys could take place only in relatively secure zones (see Table 9–3). These safe zones may have sometimes acted as magnets for the most severely affected elements of a population. For example, in 1998 a survey in Ajiep, southern Sudan, found that the CMR increased from 17.8 per 10,000 per day during the period June 3 to July 11 to 69.7 per 10,000 per day between July 12–20 (Brown, Moren, & Paquet, 1999). The increase may have been due to an influx of displaced persons in poor condition reaching Ajiep or by a decrease in the food available within the town.

On the other hand, it is possible that the worst affected communities have been in areas that have been inaccessible by those performing the surveys. In either case, it has proved difficult to extrapolate the findings of surveys on mortality conducted in specific locations to broader populations in conflict-affected countries. Extensive differences in mortality survey methods have been identified; for example, an evaluation of 23 field surveys performed in Somalia between 1991–1993 found wide variation in the target populations, sampling strategies, units of measurement, methods of rate calculation, and statistical analysis (Boss, Toole, & Yip, 1994).

Trends in death rates over time have varied from place to place. In refugee populations, such as Cambodians in eastern Thailand (1979) and Iraqis on the Turkish border (1991) where the international response has been prompt and effective, death rates have declined to baseline

**Table 9–2** Estimated Daily Crude Mortality Rates (Deaths per 10,000 per Day) in Selected Refugee Populations, 1991–1999

| Period | Country of Asylum | Country of Origin | Mean CMR for Period |
|---|---|---|---|
| June 1991 | Ethiopia | Somalia | 2.3[a] |
| March–May 1991 | Turkey | Iraq | 4.7[b] |
| March–May 1991 | Iran | Iraq | 2.0[c] |
| March 1992 | Kenya | Somalia | 7.4[a] |
| March 1992 | Nepal | Bhutan | 3.0[d] |
| August 1992 | Zimbabwe | Mozambique | 3.5[e] |
| December 1993 | Rwanda | Burundi | 3.0[f] |
| August 1994 | Tanzania | Rwanda | 19.6–31.3[g] |
| May 1999 | Albania | Yugoslavia (Kosovo) | 0.5[h] |
| November 1999 | Indonesia (Tuapukan camp, West Timor) | East Timor | 2.1[i] |

*Note:* CMR = crude mortality rate
[a]Toole & Waldman, 1993.
[b]CDC, 1991b.
[c]Babille, de Colombani, Guerra, Zagaria, & Zanetti, 1994.
[d]Marfinet et al, 1994.
[e]CDC, 1993b.
[f]CDC, 1994.
[g]UN ACC/SNN, 1994.
[h]UN ACC/SNN, 1999.
[i]WHO (HINAP), 1999a.

**Table 9–3** Estimated Crude Mortality Rates (Deaths per 10,000 per Day), Internally Displaced Populations, 1990–1998

| Period | Country | CMR for Period |
|---|---|---|
| January–December 1990 | Liberia | 2.4[a] |
| April 1991–March 1992 | Somalia (Merca) | 4.6[b] |
| April–November 1992 | Somalia (Baidoa) | 16.9[c] |
| April 1992–March 1993 | Sudan (Ayod) | 7.7[d] |
| April 1992–March 1993 | Bosnia and Herzegovina (Zepa) | 1.0[e] |
| April 1993 | Bosnia and Herzegovina (Sarajevo) | 1.0[f] |
| May 1995 | Angola (Cafunfo) | 8.3[g] |
| February 1996 | Liberia (Bong) | 5.5[h] |
| May 1998 | Burundi (Cibitoke) | 3.3[i] |
| June 3–July 20, 1998 | Sudan (Ajiep) | 26.0[j] |

[a]CDC, 1992.
[b]Manoncourt et al., 1992.
[c]Moore et al., 1993.
[d]CDC, 1993c.
[e]Toole, Galson, & Brady, 1993.
[f]CDC, 1993a.
[g]UN ACC/SCN, 1995.
[h]UN ACC/SCN, 1996.
[i]UN ACC/SCN, 1998.
[j]Epicentre and MSF France (in ACC/SCN, 1999).

levels within 1 month. Among refugees in Somalia (1980) and Sudan (1985), death rates were still well above baseline rates 6 to 9 months after the influx of refugees occurred (Toole & Waldman, 1990). In the case of 170,000 Somali refugees in Ethiopia in 1988–1989, death rates actually increased significantly 6 months after the influx. This increase was associated with elevated malnutrition prevalence rates, inadequate food rations, and high incidence rates of certain communicable diseases. Although initial death rates among Rwandan refugees in eastern Zaire were extremely high, they declined dramatically within 1 to 2 months (Figure 9–4).

Most deaths have occurred among children under 5 years of age; for example, 65% of deaths among Kurdish refugees on the Turkish border occurred in the 17% of the population less than 5 years of age (Yip & Sharp, 1993). However, in some refugee situations, such as Goma during the first month after the refugee exodus, mortality rates were comparable in all age groups because the major cause of death was cholera, which is equally lethal at any age. Among IDPs in countries affected by severe famine, high adult mortality has been reported. For example, in the Somali town of Baidoa, 59% of 15,105 deaths reported from August 1992 to February 1993 were among adults. In Ajiep, southern Sudan, the CMR among IDPs in August 1998

was equal to the under-five mortality rate. In most reports from refugee camps, mortality rates have not been stratified by sex; however, the surveillance system for Burmese refugees in Bangladesh estimated sex-specific death rates, demonstrating considerably higher death rates in females. Gendered analyses that take into account differences in the sociocultural position of women have been rare in emergency settings.

The major reported causes of death among refugees and displaced populations have been diarrheal diseases, measles, ARIs, and malaria, exacerbated by high rates of malnutrition. These diseases consistently account for between 60–95% of all reported causes of death in these populations. Measles epidemics caused high death rates among refugees during the 1980s. Epidemics of severe diarrheal disease have been increasingly common and contributed to high mortality. Cholera case fatality rates (CFRs) in refugee camps have ranged between 3–30%, and dysentery CFRs have been as high as 10% among young children and older adults.

In eastern European conflicts, a high proportion of mortality among civilians has been caused by trauma associated with the violence. Nevertheless, there has also been increased mortality in these conflicts due to the collapse of the public health system. Chronic conditions, such as cardiovascular diseases, cancer, and renal

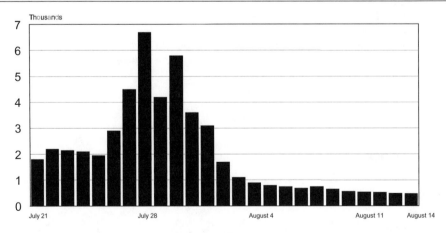

**Figure 9–4** Number of Deaths per Day, July 21–August 14, 1994, Rwandan Refugees, North Kivu Camps, Zaire

conditions, have been inadequately treated because the health system has focused on the management of war-related injuries. Medical services in most parts of Bosnia-Herzegovina were overwhelmed by the demands of war casualties. The major hospital in Zenica reported that the proportion of all surgical cases associated with trauma steadily increased following the beginning of the war in April 1992, reaching 78% in November. Preventive health services, including childhood immunization and antenatal care, ceased in many areas. Hospitals were systematic military targets in some areas, and in Sarajevo 38 of the original 42 ambulances were destroyed (Toole et al., 1993).

The collapse of health services in Bosnia-Herzegovina had significant public health effects. For example, perinatal mortality increased in Sarajevo from 16 deaths per 1,000 live births in 1991 to 27 per 1,000 during the first 4 months of 1993. The rate of premature births increased from 5.3% to 12.9%, the stillbirth rate increased from 7.5 per 1,000 to 12.3 per 1,000, and the average birth weight decreased from 3,700 gm (8.2 lb.) to 3,000 gm (6.6 lb.) during the same period (CDC, 1993a).

Recently, complex emergencies have occurred without excess mortality being reported among displaced populations. For example, although mortality rates among Kosovar refugees in Albania and Macedonia remained below 1 per 10,000 per day, significant threats to the health of the affected populations were present. It is important to continue to monitor the changing epidemiology during the emergency phase and to be prepared to provide assistance targeted at those problems that are of highest priority.

## Nutrition

Nutritional deficiencies are often the first public health effects of an evolving CHE. Economic and political turmoil leads to food scarcity among vulnerable groups, as described earlier in this chapter. In many countries experiencing political and economic crises, certain ethnic groups are disadvantaged, as well as the unemployed,

institutionalized individuals. In Africa and Asia nomadic communities are often forced to sell their animals and other food reserves. Among refugees and IDPs, there are many factors that might lead to high rates of nutritional deficiency disorders, including prolonged food scarcity prior to and during displacement, delays in the provision of complete rations, problems with registration and estimation of the size of an affected population, and inequitable distribution systems.

Two broad types of nutritional deficiencies have been suggested (Golden, 1991). Type I involves a reduction in tissue nutrient concentrations, an identifiable metabolic defect, and the demonstration of specific clinical symptoms and signs. Meanwhile, overall body growth continues normally. Deficiencies with these characteristics include iron, iodine, selenium, and both water and fat-soluble vitamins. Type II deficiencies result in primary growth failure while tissue nutrient concentrations remain normal and clinical signs are nonspecific. Deficiencies manifested in this way include zinc; the amino acids that make up tissue proteins, which have no identified body stores; and energy, which is stored in adipose tissue. When access to food is acutely deprived, the most immediate threat is the consumption of body energy stores. In the intermediate term, inadequate intake of the Type I nutrients may lead to so-called clinical micronutrient deficiency syndromes, and inadequate intake of the Type II nutrients may lead to growth faltering.

In the emergency phase, acute energy depletion is a life-threatening condition and will lead to excess mortality. A critical factor is the synergy between malnutrition and infection; thus, malnutrition prevalence may be increased by high rates of infectious diseases, such as measles, diarrhea, dysentery, ARI, malaria, and helminth infestation. Infections, on the other hand, lead to decreased appetite and increased metabolic rate, exacerbating acute malnutrition. These factors may differentially affect certain demographic groups within the population. The most common vulnerable groups include children less than 5 years of age, pregnant and lactating women, older adults, unaccompanied children, individuals with disabilities, individuals with chronic illness (for example, tuberculosis patients), households lacking an adult male, and disadvantaged ethnic or religious groups. In the later stages of famine, there may be a high prevalence of acute malnutrition among adolescents and adults. In industrialized countries, older adults are often most vulnerable, especially those living alone on fixed incomes.

### Malnutrition

In estimating the prevalence of acute malnutrition in a population, the prevalence among children between 6 months and 5 years is usually used as a surrogate. This is because the relationship between weight and height in this age group is generally similar in all ethnic groups, provided those children have access to adequate food. International reference tables may be used to define various degrees of acute malnutrition.

The prevalence of moderate to severe acute malnutrition in a random sample of children between 6 months and 5 years of age (or 110 cm [43 inches] in height) is generally a reliable indicator of this condition in a population. Because weight is more sensitive to sudden changes in food availability than height, nutritional assessments during emergencies focus on weight-for-height measurements. Moderate to severe acute malnutrition is defined as a weight-for-height more than 2 standard deviations below the mean of the U.S. Centers for Disease Control and Prevention/National Center for Health Statistics/World Health Organization (CDC/NCHS/WHO) reference population (Z-score less than –2) (WHO, 1995). Severe acute malnutrition is defined as weight-for-height more than 3 standard deviations below the reference mean (Z-score less than –3). All children with edema are classified as having severe acute malnutrition. As a screening measurement, the mid-upper arm circumference (MUAC) may also be used to assess acute malnutrition, although there is not complete agreement on which cutoff values should be used as indicators. Field studies indicate that

a MUAC of 12.0–12.5 cm (4.7–4.9 inch) correlates with a weight-for-height Z-score of –2; the lower figure is more appropriate in children less than 2 years of age (WHO, 1995). Acute malnutrition without edema has been termed wasting or *marasmus* and acute malnutrition with edema has been termed *kwashiorkor*; however, a combination of the two may occur in some children. Both are associated with anemia; however, this is often more severe in children (or adults) with kwashiorkor. The anemia may be exacerbated by local conditions, such as malaria and hookworm infection.

Malnutrition in adolescents may be assessed using an extended weight-for-height chart developed by Action Contre la Faim (ACF). Moderate acute malnutrition is defined as a weight-for-height value that is 70–79% of the reference median (Z-scores are not used in this age group); severe malnutrition is less than 70% of the median (Golden, 1999a). Adults have been assessed by the body mass index (BMI), which is the weight in kilograms divided by the height (in meters) squared ($w/h^2$). Genetic differences between ethnic groups are probably more significant among older age groups than among children less than 5 years of age. Therefore, the use of an international BMI reference poses considerable problems. For example, UNHCR and the Centers for Disease Control and Prevention conducted a nutrition survey of adolescents aged 10–19 years in four camps in Kenya housing Sudanese and Somali refugees. Comparing the BMI of the sampled adults to the WHO BMI-for-age reference population and using the recommended cutoff, the prevalence of acute malnutrition was between 57–61%. However, morbidity and mortality data did not support these high estimates. The researchers strongly suggested that the WHO reference might not be appropriate for comparisons of all adolescents worldwide (Bhatia & Woodruff, 1999). Therefore, BMI-for-age is not currently recommended as a screening index (Golden, 1999a). Studies are underway in Burundi looking at both BMI and MUAC as predictors of mortality in nonedematous adults in order to develop thresholds that might be used to admit adults to therapeutic feeding programs (TFPs); however, these studies are incomplete (Golden, personal communication, June 1999).

At present the most reliable approach is probably to use MUAC values as thresholds for screening adults under food scarcity conditions. It has been proposed to use a MUAC <23 cm (9.6 inches) in men and <22 cm (8.7 inches) in women as indicating moderate undernutrition (corresponding to BMI values of <17). MUAC values of <20 cm (7.9 inches) in men and <19 (7.5 inches) cm in women were proposed as indicators of severe wasting, corresponding to BMIs of <13 (Ferro-Luzzi & James, 1996). Nevertheless, one reliable clinical sign of severe malnutrition commonly observed in adults is "inability to stand."

In some settings, refugee children who were adequately nourished upon arrival in camps have developed acute malnutrition due either to inadequate food rations or severe epidemics of diarrheal disease (see Exhibit 9–3). In the Hartisheik refugee camp in eastern Ethiopia, for example, the prevalence of acute malnutrition increased from less than 10% to almost 25% during a 6-month period in late 1988 and early 1989 due to inadequate food rations (Toole & Bhatia, 1992). Although the prevalence decreased in mid-1989, following improvements in the ration distribution system and supplementary rations for all children under 5 years, 6 years later the situation again deteriorated. Surveys in March 1995 in Hartisheik found an acute malnutrition prevalence of 13.7% (United Nations Administrative Committee on Coordination, Sub-

Committee on Nutrition [UN ACC/SSN], July 1995).

In early 1991 the prevalence of acute malnutrition among Kurdish refugee children aged 12 to 23 months increased from less than 5–13% during a 2-month period following a severe outbreak of diarrheal disease (Yip & Sharp, 1993). Surprisingly, the malnutrition prevalence among children <12 months of age was less than 4%; however, a survey revealed that the diarrhea-associated death rate in this age group was 3 times higher than the death rate among children 12–23 months of age. Thus it is likely that many malnourished infants died, resulting in deceptively low malnutrition prevalence among the survivors.

North Korea experienced several years of severe food shortages between 1996 and 1999. In September 1998 UNICEF, the World Food Programme (WFP), and the European Community Humanitarian Office (ECHO) conducted a nutritional survey covering 61% of the counties and 71% of the country's population. The prevalence of wasting (low weight for height) was 15.6%, which was the highest in any country in East Asia that year. The prevalence was highest among children 12–35 months of age and tended to be higher in boys than girls.

Prevalence of acute malnutrition among the internally displaced has tended to be extremely high. In southern Somalia during 1992 the prevalence of acute malnutrition among children less than 5 years in displaced persons camps in Marka and Qorioley was 75%, compared with 43% among town residents (Manoncourt et al., 1992). The prevalence of acute malnutrition

---

**Exhibit 9–3** Malnutrition in Rwandan Refugees in Eastern Zaire, 1994

In Rwandan refugee camps in eastern Zaire, the prevalence of acute malnutrition was between 18–23% following the severe cholera and dysentery epidemics during the first month after the influx (Goma Epidemiology Group, 1995). Children with a history of dysentery within 3 days prior to the survey were 3 times more likely to be malnourished than those with no history of recent dysentery. Also, children in families with no adult male present were at significantly higher risk of malnutrition than those children in households headed by an adult male.

among children less than 5 years of age in various displaced populations is presented in Table 9–4.

## Micronutrient Deficiency Diseases

High incidence rates of several micronutrient deficiency diseases have been reported in many refugee camps, especially in Africa. Frequently, famine-affected and displaced populations have already experienced low levels of dietary vitamin A intake and, therefore, may have very low vitamin A reserves. Furthermore, the typical rations provided in large-scale relief operations lack vitamin A, putting these populations at high risk. In addition, those communicable diseases that are highly incident in refugee camps, such as measles and diarrhea, are known to rapidly deplete vitamin A stores. Consequently, young

refugee and displaced children are at high risk of developing vitamin A deficiency. In 1990 more than 18,000 cases of pellagra, caused by food rations deficient in niacin, were reported among Mozambican refugees in Malawi (CDC, 1991a). Numerous outbreaks of scurvy (vitamin C deficiency) were documented in refugee camps in Somalia, Ethiopia, and Sudan between 1982 and 1991. Cross-sectional surveys performed in 1986–1987 reported prevalence rates as high as 45% among females and 36% among males; prevalence increased with age (Desenclos et al., 1989). The prevalence of scurvy was highly associated with the period of residence in camps, a reflection of the time exposed to rations lacking in vitamin C. Outbreaks of scurvy and beriberi were also reported among Bhutanese refugees in Nepal during 1993 (UN ACC/SSN,

**Table 9–4** Prevalence of Acute Malnutrition among Children <5 Years of Age in Internally Displaced and Conflict-Affected Populations, 1992–1999

| Date | Country (region) | Population Affected | Prevalence of Acute Malnutrition |
|------|------------------|---------------------|----------------------------------|
| 1992 | Southern Somalia | 3,000,000 | 47%–75%[a] |
| 1994 | Sudan (Bahr-el-Ghazal) | 345,000 | 36.1%[b] |
| 1994 | Afghanistan (Sarashahi) | 163,000 | 18.6%[c] |
| 1995 | Angola (Cafunfo) | 10,000 | 29.2%[d] |
| 1995 | Liberia (Goba town, Margibi) | N/A | 11.7%[e] |
| 1995 | Sierra Leone (Bo) | 250,000 | 19.8%[f] |
| 1996 | Zaire (Masisi) | 100,000 | 31.0%[g] |
| 1998 | Burundi | N/A | 14%[h] |
| 1998 | Panthou and Toch, Northern Bahr-el-Ghazal, Sudan | N/A | 40.8% (April); 11.7% (Nov)[i] |
| 1998 | Yirol, Eastern Bahr-el-Ghazal, Sudan | N/A | 17.7% (Sept); 33.4% (May)[j] |
| 1999 | Malange & Huambo, Angola | N/A | 11–14.7%[k] |
| 1999 | West Timor, Indonesia | N/A | 24%[l] |

*Note:* Acute malnutrition is defined either as weight-for-height 2 standard deviations below the reference mean or less than 80% of the reference median. N/A = not available.

[a]Toole & Waldman, 1993.
[b]Médecins sans Frontières (MSF) Belgium (in RNIS), UN ACC/SCN,1994.
[c]MSF Holland (in RNIS), UN ACC/SCN, 1994.
[d]Action contre la Faim (ACF) (in RNIS), UN ACC/SCN, 1995.
[e]MSF Holland (in RNIS), UN ACC/SCN, 1995.
[f]ACF (in RNIS), UN ACC/SCN, 1995.
[g]MSF Holland (in RNIS), UN ACC/SCN, 1996.
[h]Concern International (in RNIS), UN ACC/SCN, 1998.
[i]World Vision (in RNIS), UN ACC/SCN, 1999.
[j]Concern/Medair (in RNIS), UN ACC/SCN, 1999.
[k]MSF Holland and Save the Children Fund [UK] (in RNIS), UN ACC/SCN, 1999.
[l]WHO/HINAP, 2000.

1995). Iron deficiency anemia has been reported in many refugee populations, affecting particularly women of childbearing age and young children (UN ACC/SSN, 1995).

## Impact of Communicable Diseases

In most CHEs the high rates of excess preventable mortality have been attributed primarily to communicable diseases. The specific causes of mortality, and their age and gender distribution, do not differ from those that prevail in nonemergency conditions. Accordingly, measles, diarrhea, ARI, and malaria have been most frequently cited as proximate causes. Substandard conditions found in camps do not change the diseases that account for most of the morbidity and mortality in humanitarian emergency settings, but they do alter epidemiologic patterns in two important ways: the incidence, or attack, rates of commonly occurring and potentially fatal diseases are increased, and the CFRs are higher than usual.

## Measles

Measles has traditionally been among the most feared of communicable diseases in emergency settings. During the 1970s and 1980s measles epidemics were common, and it was not unusual for measles to be the major cause of mortality in large, displaced populations. High incidence rates (particularly in populations with low levels of vaccination prior to displacement), high mortality rates, and unusually high CFRs are typical of measles outbreaks in emergencies. In an epidemic that occurred in the Wad Kowli refugee camp in eastern Sudan in 1985, the overall measles-specific mortality rate was 13 per 1,000 population per month and the under-five mortality was 30 per 1,000 per month. CFRs in this outbreak reportedly reached an extraordinarily high level of 33%, probably due to a combination of underlying malnutrition, including widespread vitamin A deficiency, and inadequate medical services.

In well-vaccinated populations, such as Bosnian and Kosovar refugees in the Balkans, Kurds in northern Iraq (1991), and Rwandans in Tanzania and Eastern Zaire (1994), measles has been a less prominent public health problem. However, where unvaccinated populations reside in the midst of better protected ones, measles can still be an important problem. For example, indigenous populations living on the slopes of Mount Pinatubo, Philippines, who had not benefited from health services largely available to neighboring populations, were devastated by a measles epidemic that struck during their displacement following the eruption of the volcano in 1991.

### *Diarrhea*

Unlike measles, which can be easily prevented, diarrheal diseases remain one of the top three causes of mortality in humanitarian emergencies. In Somalia (1979–1981), Ethiopia (1982), Sudan (1985), Malawi (1988), northern Iraq (1991), and Goma (1994), diarrheal diseases were responsible for between 25–85% of all mortality and accounted for a major share of all clinic visits as well (70% in northern Iraq). Although most often a condition of young children, cholera and dysentery—the major epidemic forms of diarrhea—affect people of all ages. Of all disease conditions, diarrhea is the most closely linked to poor sanitation, inadequate water quantity, and contaminated water.

Cholera epidemics have occurred frequently in emergency settings. Although deaths due to noncholera watery diarrhea have been far more numerous, cholera, in addition to being able to cause death rapidly from dehydration, incites fear and even panic in many populations. Its ability to affect other relief activities and to divert health personnel and supplies from other activities may even contribute to higher death tolls due to other diseases. Outbreaks of cholera have occurred in all parts of the world; large outbreaks were recorded in India (1971), Thailand (1979), Sudan (1985), Somalia (1985), Ethiopia (1984), Malawi (1988–1991), northern Iraq (1991), Goma (1994), and Rwanda (1996).

In many of these settings, cholera was a recurrent problem, and in Malawi at least 20 separate outbreaks were recorded among Mozambican refugees during a 5-year period. Investigations of these outbreaks have documented numerous modes of transmission and risk factors, including contaminated water, shared water containers, inadequately heated leftover food, insufficient soap, and funeral gatherings for cholera victims. One of the most lethal cholera epidemics ever recorded occurred in 1994 among refugees in Goma, Zaire, when it was estimated that 45,000 people (about 9% of the total population) died in a 3-week period. The source of contamination is believed to have been Lake Kivu, the principal source of water on which the population depended. Epidemics due to *Shigella dysenteriae* type 1 have also been reported from a number of emergency settings and contributed to the high mortality in Goma.

### Acute Respiratory Infection

Acute lower respiratory infection (ALRI), or pneumonia, has been an important cause of morbidity and mortality in emergency settings and was recorded as one of the top three causes of mortality in Thailand (1979), Somalia (1980), Sudan (1985), and Honduras (1984–1987). Risk factors have included crowded conditions, inadequate shelter, vitamin A deficiency, and indoor air pollution, especially in societies that cook indoors (such as Nepal). ALRI is undoubtedly a major cause of morbidity and mortality in cold climates, such as northern Iraq, the Balkans, and the war-torn former Soviet republics. ALRI is the leading cause of death among children in low-income countries, but it has been less consistently reported and investigated than many other communicable diseases in emergency settings.

### Malaria

In endemic areas, including Southeast Asia, the Indian subcontinent, and most of Africa, malaria is consistently among the leading causes of morbidity and mortality. It has been responsible for incidence rates as high as 1,034 per 1,000 per month (Thailand, 1984) and for as many as 30%

of all deaths in displaced populations. It was the leading cause of mortality among Cambodian refugees in Thailand in 1978, Ethiopian refugees in Sudan in the mid-1980s, and Mozambican refugees in Malawi in the 1980s. It has been well established that populations that are displaced to areas of higher malaria endemicity than their place of origin have higher incidence rates and higher mortality. Following the collapse of health services during and following the conflict in East Timor, along with mass population displacement, the incidence of malaria increased significantly. In October 1999 approximately 30% of all morbidity in East Timor was attributed to malaria, compared with 10% the previous year (WHO/HINAP, 2000). The occurrence of epidemic malaria has also been more frequent in these circumstances. There is, however, little risk of displaced populations from areas of high malaria incidence causing increases in the diseases in areas to which they are displaced, because transmission is largely vector-dependent.

Major risk factors for malaria in emergency settings include the lack of adequate housing, poor siting of refugee camps (especially when they are placed in marshy areas), overcrowding, proximity to livestock (which may be the primary targets of mosquito vectors), and a general lack of competently trained health personnel. Although it has not been clearly documented in emergencies, the association of malaria with low birth weight (especially in the offspring of first and second pregnancies) and with iron-deficiency anemia may cause increases in incidence and CFR from a variety of causes, especially in children.

### Meningitis

Although not a consistent problem in emergencies, the threat of meningococcal meningitis is a formidable one. Overcrowding, especially during the drier seasons of the year, can be an important risk factor for this disease, which is transmitted via the respiratory route. In the Sakaeo camp in Thailand in 1980, a large outbreak of Group A meningococcal meningitis had an attack rate of 130 per 100,000 population and an overall CFR of 28% (50% in children less than 5 years old). Other epidemics have occurred in Sudan (1989), Ethiopia (1993), Guinea (1993), and in Goma, where attack rates ranged from 94–137 per 100,000 population over a period of 2 months. Outbreaks of meningitis tend to be protracted, lasting from 1 to 2 months. Unless they are detected and controlled at an early stage, they can be directly responsible for high mortality; in addition, they can be resource-intensive and detract attention from other high-priority health programs.

### Hepatitis E

Like meningitis, outbreaks of hepatitis E have not been frequent occurrences in emergencies but have had major consequences when they occurred. An enterically transmitted disease, usually linked to contaminated drinking water, especially when water quantity is compromised, hepatitis E is associated with a particularly high CFR in pregnant women. Clinical attack rates appear to be higher in adults, with children relatively spared. In Somalia in 1985 an outbreak of more than 2,000 cases was associated with an overall attack rate of 8% in adults. The overall CFR of 4% was more than quadrupled in pregnant women (17%). Outbreaks of similar magnitude occurred in Ethiopia (1989) and among Somali refugees in Liboi Camp, Kenya, in 1991. In the latter, the overall case fatality rate was 3.7%, but CFR in pregnant women was 14%.

### Tuberculosis

Tuberculosis is one of the most important communicable diseases to control in the postemergency phase. Its reemergence as a public health problem in many parts of the world is characterized by its close association with immune deficiency disorders, especially HIV/ acquired immune deficiency syndrome (AIDs), and with the identification of multiple drug-resistant strains. Tuberculosis can be quite common in some postemergency situations. It is highly prevalent during the emergency as well, but because of the difficulties in developing programs

to control its transmission, to diagnose and to reliably treat for adequate periods, other more acute conditions are appropriately accorded priority. In Somalia in 1985 more than one-quarter of all adult deaths were attributed to tuberculosis, which was the third leading cause of death overall. Tuberculosis has also figured prominently in Sudan in the mid-1980s and Pakistan throughout the protracted displacement of Afghan refugees.

### Other Important Communicable Diseases

HIV/AIDS and other STIs are major problems among emergency-affected populations from areas where there is a high prevalence of these conditions. They are discussed in the section on reproductive health. Other communicable diseases that have occurred in emergency or postemergency settings have had a relatively minor impact. In the individual setting in which they occur, however, they command an important allocation of resources and may be important contributors to morbidity and mortality. Yellow fever, typhoid fever, relapsing fever, Japanese B encephalitis, dengue hemorrhagic fever, typhus, and leptospirosis are all real threats. Nevertheless, morbidity and mortality in CHEs have been shown time and again to be due to the same conditions that are responsible for the bulk of the disease burden in low-income countries in nonemergency settings. Important aspects concerning the control of these major communicable disease problems are presented later.

### Injuries

Injuries are widespread in all populations and are responsible for significant mortality, morbidity, and disability. Conflicts typically conjure up images of firearm-related morbidity and mortality, but other types of weapons—from high-tech laser-guided missiles and chemical and biological warfare agents to low-tech machetes—can cause substantial morbidity and mortality. Injuries, aside from those that are directly war- and conflict-related, are typically neglected in preference to an emphasis on communicable diseases. This is unfortunate, given the widespread occurrence of intentional (homicide, war, suicide) and unintentional (falls, traffic injuries, drowning, poisoning) injuries in many populations affected by conflict. Given exposure to firearms and other weapons, rapid and forced population movement, poor environmental conditions, and compromised safety and security, injuries of all sorts are bound to occur in these settings. In situations where injuries are shown to be major causes of morbidity and mortality, they should be addressed as vigorously as communicable diseases.

Most attention has been focused on land mine injuries, an area in which notable international successes have been achieved. The Ottawa Process has led to the effective banning of the production and distribution of antipersonnel land mines, although a number of key countries, including the United States, have thus far refused to sign the relevant treaties. Evidence of the harmful effects of antipersonnel land mines and their concentration in the world's lowest-income countries, such as Angola, Ethiopia, Cambodia, and Afghanistan, has led to a dramatic increase in press and media interest and a related public policy response leading into the Ottawa Process.

The spontaneous repatriation of refugees to Kosovo in mid-1999 was associated with a large number of land mine deaths and injuries. Aside from evidence of deaths and disability, the costs to the health services of caring for and supporting disabled community members through the health services and in the longer term within the community are considerable. The opportunity costs are similarly important: staff and equipment devoted to war surgery and specifically the treatment of injuries resulting from antipersonnel land mines could be devoted to other activities. Indeed, extending war surgery facilities introduced by organizations like the International Committee of the Red Cross (ICRC) into resource-poor countries to facilitate the provision of a much wider range of treatment and rehabilitation services that would be available to those with any sort of injury is currently being promoted by WHO.

Aside from the direct health problems associated with antipersonnel land mines, they create a wide range of other problems—fear and insecurity, as well as limited access to areas affected by mines, which, consequently, become unavailable for agriculture and animal husbandry. Despite community knowledge of the sites of concentration of antipersonnel land mines, community members are often forced to enter into these unsafe areas in order to collect firewood, water, or animals that have gone astray. The widespread availability of antipersonnel land mines has also led to their use for personal security with community members, in some cases using them to protect their homes at night or when they are away. In some situations, mines have been used to assist with tasks such as fishing, and children have been known to play with them. The long-term effects of land mines are serious: high levels of surgical skill and resources are required and repeated refitting and modification of prostheses are necessary if disability is to be minimized.

## Reproductive Health

Unfortunately, reproductive health services for refugees and displaced persons have often been considered to be secondary priorities. While there is no doubt that the provision of food, water, sanitation facilities, and shelter is the highest priority during a complex humanitarian emergency, steps should be taken to ensure that other critical health needs of women, men, and adolescents are met as quickly as possible. Women are a particularly vulnerable subset of the population because the gender-based discrimination that is all too common in stable societies is frequently exacerbated in times of societal stress and meager resources. Uncontrolled violence and its aftermath are characterized by a number of specific features that impact negatively on reproductive health. These include the breakdown of family networks and the consequent loss of protection and safety, as well as channels of information to adolescents and women of reproductive age.

Loss of revenue within the family can result in a restricted ability to make appropriate reproductive health choices and may predispose women and adolescents to risk through, for example, engagement in commercial sex work. Increased sole responsibility, as manifested by an increase in the proportion of female-headed households, also changes the way women spend their time and money as they seek increased security and well-being for their families. Finally, as with all members of the affected population, women tend to pay more attention to securing health services for lifesaving interventions than for nonemergency reproductive health services.

A minimum initial service package of essential reproductive health services has been developed and is recommended by the major relevant international agencies. They are described later in this chapter. Interventions beyond this essential package require major investments of time and personnel that should not be diverted from the principal task of reducing excessive preventable mortality as rapidly as possible. In all cases, special care must be taken to ensure that women heads of household are being given equitable quantities of food and nonfood commodities for themselves and their families.

## Mental Health

War and political violence have direct and indirect mental health consequences for victims, relatives, neighbors, and communities. The severity and type of mental health problems relates to the nature, intensity, and form of the violence; the relationship of the assessed person to others affected (self, family, and community members); the cause of the conflict; and the affected person's relationship to participation, victimization, or causation of the conflict. Anxiety, uncertainty, and fear about the future, and about whether family members and homesteads remain alive and intact, are a substantial cause of distress for affected individuals and communities. Among those who are forced to flee either as refugees or as internally displaced people, lack of knowledge about relatives and property left behind can cause high levels of stress and distress. Despite ongoing challenges of maintaining lives and livelihoods, life as a refugee, especially in a camp situation, may be monotonous and conducive to stress, anxiety, and depression.

The extent of mental health "trauma" experienced during and in the aftermath of war and conflict is controversial, with some analysts identifying significant proportions of affected populations suffering from posttraumatic stress disorder (PTSD), while others argue that this term and the response to it is medicalizing an essentially social phenomenon. The former school calls for large-scale counseling and mental health support structures, while the latter, represented by Bracken, Giller, and Summerfield (1995), argues that reconstituting a sense of community and humanity, and reestablishing livelihoods and community structures, are far more important interventions than trauma centers and counseling. It is clear, and little disputed, that some individuals who experience particularly horrific experiences as a victim of torture or gross human rights abuses during conflicts may well suffer from PTSD. However, the debate centers around the extent to which this label can be applied to whole populations, rather than to the minority whose experiences have been particularly extreme. A key problem remains the difficulty of articulating the experiences suffered and of facilitating community and individual-oriented systems of support. Women who had been raped during the civil war in Uganda benefited from opportunities to share their experiences with other women who had similarly been abused during wartime; in the absence of any health-related interventions, such experiences may well have remained bottled up and cause for continuing distress. A key issue is to learn not only from those who succumb to the stresses placed upon them, but also to understand and learn from the resilience of survivors. What mechanisms do they use to protect themselves and their mental health, and can others benefit from learning about such strategies?

Few national surveys of the mental health impact of conflicts are available, and, even if such studies could be conducted, prior measurement of the distribution of mental health status within the population would be required to assess impact. A number of small and focused studies on particular subgroups of conflict-affected populations have been conducted, but their biomedical biases make them open to challenge. Little is known about the etiology of the symptoms of multiple trauma, the mental health consequences suffered by those who victimize, and the role of coping mechanisms. Anecdotal data indicate the serious mental strain, substance abuse, and high risk of suicide among some groups, such as South African policemen from the apartheid era and Vietnam veterans. The effects of personal experience of extreme violence, such as torture or rape, may be long-lasting and may impede normal sexual and other social relationships.

Torture is a common practice in many conflicts, especially during the Cold War when ideological factors were central to ongoing conflicts. The impact of torture has been extensively documented in Latin America and South Africa, in particular. Between 1973 and 1983, the Uruguayan state used torture widely to extract information, instill fear, and engender a feeling of worthlessness in those detained, and to frighten family and colleagues. In so-called dirty wars of state-perpetrated internal repression, common in Latin America in the mid-1980s, torture was used systematically as a means of attempting to maintain societal structures, through fear and intimidation. Mental health workers have identified "disintegration" as one of the consequences of torture and political repression: the destruction of the person as an autonomous subject with norms and values that inspired his or her political and social activities (Barudy, 1989).

Combatants who participate in brutal events in situations over which they have limited control may also suffer. Posttraumatic stress disorder, a recognized mental health condition following exposure to massive stress, has been diagnosed among Vietnam veterans in a general community survey conducted in the United States. Among wounded veterans up to 20% had full blown PTSD, while 60% had one or more of the associated symptoms. Children and adolescents who are forced in some contexts to mutilate, rape, or murder friends and family may be similarly affected by their extreme experiences. In many settings, including Uganda, Liberia, and Sierra Leone, a great deal of attention must be paid to programs whose objectives include working with ex-combatants of all ages on issues surrounding disarmament, rehabilitation, and reintegration into functional roles in society.

Mental conditions of persons who moved to other countries or are exiled vary according to specific circumstances. While some political refugees and asylum seekers in industrialized nations have access to comprehensive health care, even these relatively more fortunate exiles are likely to experience cultural and language barriers when they attempt to access services. Uncertainty and guilt for relatives left behind, legal restrictions to employment, and ethnic discrimination are common causes of stress among exiles in advanced industrial nations.

Persons who have not been exposed to combat may also suffer mental health distress. An examination of distress in three communities in El Salvador (one that had not been exposed to combat and two others that had experienced different levels of conflict intensity) found that 3 years after the conflict many people still suffered from anxiety, depression, sleep disturbances, suicidal tendencies, trembling, dizziness, fears, and flashbacks. The proportion affected by symptoms varied according to the level of intensity of the exposure to conflict, but were present even in those that had not directly experienced the conflict (Ugalde et al., 1999).

## Noncommunicable Diseases

Responding to the health needs of refugees and IDPs has traditionally emphasized the direct causes of ill health, such as firearms and other weaponry, as well as communicable diseases, which have been shown to pose a major problem in many CHEs. In light of the aging of the population generally, and of the changing geographic distribution of conflicts to include areas previously well served by health care, such as the former Yugoslavia, new problems are emerging.

Noncommunicable diseases are widespread in all populations of older adults worldwide. In those situations where medical care was at some stage available, the withdrawal or destruction of medical facilities, drug distribution mechanisms, and health workers from areas of active conflict all impact upon the treatment and care available for noncommunicable diseases. Recent examples of reductions in the quality and availability of care for noncommunicable diseases come from Iraq in the aftermath of the Gulf War, from Sarajevo during its siege in the Yugoslav civil war, and from the Kosovar Albanians, especially those internally displaced who lost access to services and care.

Conditions such as cardiovascular disease (including hypertension), diabetes, asthma, and cancers may deteriorate given the lack of access to medical care, which typically occurs in conflict settings. Maintaining diagnostic and treatment services, drug supplies, and access to care are extremely difficult given destruction of infrastructure, targeting of health services, disruption of logistics and supply systems, and absolute resource constraints. In some conflicts, the imposition of sanctions may play some role in reducing access to technologies and drugs necessary for diagnosis, treatment, and care of noncommunicable disorders.

## Impact of Economic Sanctions and Embargoes

The imposition of economic sanctions has become a more common means of punishing nations and is increasingly considered as an alternative to war. The penalties and restrictions that constitute economic sanctions vary widely. Usually, trade is limited or prohibited in certain products ranging from agricultural products to high-technology instruments, to military equipment. At times, international travel, sporting events, and cultural exchanges can be curtailed. Assets held in foreign banks can be frozen. In each case, no matter what form the economic sanctions take, the goal of those imposing them is to achieve political objectives while avoiding

the cost and destruction of war. Indeed, the popularity of economic sanctions parallels trends in military strategy. As governments appear to become increasingly hesitant to commit troops to fight foreign wars in which casualties may occur, they seek alternative ways of achieving political objectives. Sanctions tend to be used when diplomacy fails and when the costs and potential destruction that accompany military intervention are deemed to be excessive.

Sanctions can be imposed and administered by a single nation, a group of allied nations, or by the United Nations. The United States has used unilateral economic sanctions more than any other country and has been associated with imposing sanctions more than 100 times during the twentieth century. More than one-third of those came during the 1990s. Also during that decade the United Nations Security Council instituted multilateral economic sanctions against nine countries (Burundi, Haiti, Iraq, Liberia, Libya, Rwanda, Somalia, the Sudan, and the former Yugoslavia) and against two nonstate parties (the Khmer Rouge in Cambodia and the National Union for the Total Independence of Angola [UNITA]).

Although economic sanctions as an instrument of foreign policy are aimed at pressurizing the targeted governments, experience has usually demonstrated that they are far from a benign weapon. They are rarely successful in achieving their desired political objectives and they frequently take a heavy toll on civilian populations. In fact, although the Geneva Conventions provide wartime protection to civilians, by prohibiting the destruction of crops, livestock, sources of drinking water, and the like, few if any international standards protect civilians from the unintended consequences of broad economic sanctions imposed on their governments during peacetime. This is the case even when humanitarian exemptions are stipulated in the terms of the embargo. For example, although importation of measles vaccine intended for childhood vaccination programs in Haiti was allowed under the terms of the sanctions imposed upon that country in 1992, kerosene was not. As a result, refrigerators required to maintain the potency of the vaccine were unable to function and a large epidemic occurred.

Nowhere has the devastating effect of economic sanctions on a civilian population been better documented than in Iraq. It has been estimated that the sanctions imposed on that country were associated with the deaths between 1991 and 1997 of as many as 200,000 children less than 5 years old). Dramatic increases in rates of malnutrition and preventable infectious diseases such as childhood diarrhea have occurred. The prices of basic food items such as flour, rice, oil, meat, and milk have soared out of proportion to wage increases as a result of trade restrictions. Distribution systems for food and other essential commodities have been severely disrupted. In addition, by 1995, 4 years after the war, national water distribution was estimated to be only 50% of prewar levels and a UNICEF survey in that year found that 50% of the population had no access to potable water. Wastewater facilities and solid waste disposal systems were destroyed during the war, and sanctions have contributed to an inability to restore them. The lack of adequate quantities of food, water, and acceptable sanitation has contributed to increased mortality in most segments of the population. The causes of mortality resemble those of a developing country more than those that occurred previously in a country with a relatively advanced health care system. Indeed, the number of deaths attributable to the imposition of economic sanctions following the war far exceeds those that occurred as a result of the war itself. Moreover, throughout it all, the government against which severe sanctions were imposed remained in power.

Sanctions can be effective: they are felt to have played an important role in pressuring the pro-apartheid government of South Africa to relinquish power. For the most part, however, sanctions, in the form in which they have most frequently been applied, have not been able to produce their desired effect and have exacted an inappropriately severe toll on the most vulnerable elements of society, including children, women (especially pregnant women), and older adults. In this sense, the imposition of economic

sanctions has been a blunt instrument of foreign policy. Critics have called for the development of "smart sanctions," penalties on travel and on the assets of the wealthy and powerful elements of a targeted nation that will not have the destructive effect on social sectors, such as public health systems. Sanctions seem to be a good idea gone wrong; it is inappropriate to negatively affect the health status of a nation's civilian population when the objective is to bring about a change in its leadership.

## PREVENTION AND MITIGATION OF CHEs

The prevention of CHEs is primarily the prevention of the conflicts that cause them; thus the task is largely political. Since 1990, most CHEs have had their roots in ethnic and religious conflicts within sovereign states. The United Nations Charter is ill equipped to intervene in issues deemed to be "internal" by member states. Chapters 6 and 7 of the charter allow the Security Council to authorize appropriate action, including the use of force, in situations that threaten international peace and security. During the Cold War, these provisions were rarely used because such action was likely to be vetoed by one of the five permanent members of the Security Council (China, France, Soviet Union, the United Kingdom, and the United States). However, Security Council resolutions supported intervention by the international community to protect civilians in conflicts in Somalia, Bosnia and Herzegovina, Haiti, Iraq, Angola, and East Timor during the 1990s.

In general, however, the international community has had little success in resolving internal conflicts. Certain private organizations, such as the Carter Center in Atlanta, have attempted to facilitate the resolution of conflicts in Sudan, Haiti, Somalia, Afghanistan, the former Yugoslavia, and other countries. However, in these situations, the cessation of hostilities if attained at all has tended to be temporary. Sometimes, health campaigns have been used to seek a temporary halt to armed conflict, most commonly to implement child immunization programs. Such initiatives, like the "Corridors of Tranquility" and "Health as a Bridge to Peace" have not addressed the root causes of the conflicts nor led to permanent, peaceful resolution.

The United Nations has a poor record in conflict resolution. The internal conflict in Somalia was allowed to evolve over 5 years into the total disintegration of the nation state. Only when famine reached appalling levels in 1992 did the Security Council authorize extraordinary action to ensure the protection and care of the civilian population. Within 6 months of their arrival, UN troops became embroiled in the conflict itself, taking sides with or against certain armed factions. This led to heavy loss of life and the eventual withdrawal of the UN forces. In Bosnia and Herzegovina, between 1992 and 1995, the UN mobilized peacekeeping troops to safeguard the delivery of humanitarian supplies. However, these forces were not authorized to intervene to protect civilians from the violence intentionally directed at various ethnic groups; as a result, the international community's armed representatives were forced silently to witness gross abuses of human rights. This dilemma has been termed the "humanitarian trap." One of the notable failures occurred when approximately 7,000 Muslim men in the so-called safe haven of Srebrenica in Bosnia were massacred by Bosnian Serbs despite the presence of UN peacekeeping forces in the area. When the genocide began in Rwanda in 1994, several Belgian peacekeepers already in the country with a UN contingent were killed by extreme Hutu nationalists. Instead of increasing the level of UN presence, the entire peacekeeping force was withdrawn, leaving civilians defenseless against these extremists. Eventually, more than 500,000 Rwandans were killed. It is likely that this string of UN failures led to NATO taking unilateral action in the form of a massive bombing campaign against Serbia to protect ethnic Albanians in 1999. While appearing to be well-intentioned, this action seemed to accelerate the pace of atrocities and ethnic cleansing instigated by the Serbs against the Kosovar Albanians.

The basis of protection of civilians in time of conflict is the Geneva Conventions of 1949 and the Additional Protocols of 1977. In addition, the Convention on the Prevention and Punishment of the Crime of Genocide, in 1951, was intended to protect civilians from the type of slaughters that occurred in Cambodia in the 1970s and Rwanda in 1994. UN General Assembly resolutions in 1971, 1985, and 1986 also elaborated on the protection of civilian populations. However, international human rights and humanitarian (armed conflict) laws are only as good as their enforcement. The United Nations Commission on Human Rights (UNCHR) in Geneva is one of the primary official bodies that oversees this sometimes overwhelming task and relies on the documentation and testimony provided by accredited NGOs. Eleanor Roosevelt was instrumental in giving birth to the commission, along with the Frenchman Rene Cassin, who received the Nobel Peace Prize for authoring the Universal Declaration of Human Rights. Today UNCHR passes influential resolutions on human rights abuses in member states and is the subject of intense lobbying by governments and NGOs. It is thanks to the efforts of a number of human rights advocacy groups that resolutions continue to be adopted by the commission condemning human rights violators. Such resolutions occasionally lead to action by the General Assembly and Security Council, which may dispatch peacekeeping forces to a troubled region (for example, Central America in the 1980s and East Timor in 1999) in order to settle the conflicts giving rise to the violations in the first place.

The United Nations Office for the Coordination of Humanitarian Affairs (OCHA), based in New York and Geneva, is the UN office responsible for coordinating efforts in early warning, prevention, mitigation, and response to disasters, including CHEs. Its Relief Web project's purpose is to strengthen the capacity of the humanitarian relief community through the timely dissemination of reliable information on prevention, preparedness, and disaster response. Like many other similar projects, the information is available on the Internet site Relief Web (http://www.reliefweb.int).

Given the difficulty in preventing or resolving armed conflicts, what else can be done to prevent or mitigate the worst consequences of such conflicts on civilian populations? Although not yet tested, it may be possible during the early phase of national disintegration to focus development efforts on activities that strengthen the capacity of local organizations to implement lifesaving programs. Accelerated training of health workers in emergency preparedness and response, support to local food production activities, and adaptation of health information systems to the priorities of an emergency assistance program may all help to minimize the eventual impact of the CHE. Given the frequency of CHEs in the past decade and the likelihood that they will continue to occur, donor governments should support pilot projects to examine what can and cannot be done to prepare for such emergencies.

### Early Warning and Detection

Efforts to prevent and mitigate the impact of CHEs on populations must rely on accurate and timely information in order to be effective. Given the enormous cost of military intervention (US$100 million a day in Kosovo, in 1999), major relief, and rehabilitation programs, it is surprising that so little has been invested in early warning, emergency detection, preparedness, and mitigation projects. In the 1980s United States Agency for International Development (USAID) funded a Famine Early Warning System that focused on famine-prone countries, mainly in Africa. Most of the indicators routinely collected by the system related to agricultural and climatic conditions, economic conditions, nutritional indexes, and population migrations. Although data on political factors were collected, there was no mechanism by which the world would respond if a certain "threshold" of instability or conflict was reached. The system accurately predicted a food shortage in southern Africa in 1992, but this was largely due to drought conditions rather than political instability.

In the late 1990s there were a number of "systems" that collected, aggregated, and disseminated information on a number of indicators relevant to CHEs. Most systems relied on information collected by other agencies, such as governments, UN agencies, and NGOs. Relief Web, a project of OCHA, has already been mentioned. The news wire service Reuters is supporting AlertWeb, another Internet-based data dissemination project. A relatively new project is the Health Information Network for Advanced Planning (HINAP), which is based at WHO headquarters in Geneva. HINAP's major objective is to consolidate, sort, edit, organize, and redistribute background information and other existing sources of data to the right people, at the right time, in the right format. HINAP does not collect primary data but relies on information already produced by other parts of WHO and external organizations for general use. The system aims for the early detection of negative trends in key health and medical indicators that would assist governments and relief organizations in mounting more timely, targeted interventions. It focuses on country situations where latent or low-level tensions have not yet attracted significant attention but could escalate.

It is perhaps too early to evaluate the impact of such information systems as HINAP on the effectiveness of preparedness planning and the quality of humanitarian responses. The lack of preparedness for the mass exodus of hundreds of thousands of Kosovar refugees into neighboring countries in early 1999 by both UN agencies and NGOs seems surprising given the knowledge since 1989 that there was the potential for a major conflict in Kosovo province. This lack of preparedness was also evident in 1994 when more than 1 million Rwandan refugees crossed the border into eastern Zaire within 1 week.

Unlike natural disaster early warning systems and preparedness programs, monitoring and detecting CHEs is fraught with political obstacles. The common adage that the first casualty in war is truth applies to attempts to collect accurate data on the health outcomes of war. The existence of armed conflicts is no secret; the political response is still inadequate. What would be valuable as CHEs evolve would be a more accurate picture of which health interventions are going to be the highest priorities and most effective in preventing excess mortality and morbidity. In European wars, the most important public health priorities have been the direct effects of violence. Stopping the violence is a public health issue that can only be addressed by the world's leaders. In low-income countries, the priorities are most likely to be nutrition and communicable disease control. Thus key indicators to monitor in early warning systems include food availability, nutritional status, immunization coverage, incidence of vaccine-preventable diseases, and antenatal program coverage.

In the late 1990s, as Indonesia went through economic and political turmoil, at least 20 different centers and institutes maintained information systems on economic and social indicators. However, few were able to provide reliable information on health and nutrition outcomes. Systems of early warning, preparedness, and mitigation of the health effects of CHEs are in their infancy. They should receive generous donor support if future humanitarian responses are to be based on science rather than instincts.

## RESPONSES TO CHE

### Primary Prevention

Primary prevention is the basic strategy of public health, and epidemiology is one of its essential tools. In situations of armed conflict, however, epidemiology can be practiced safely and reliably in few areas. Hence, the traditional documentation, monitoring, and evaluation elements of disease prevention may be ineffective in this situation. The provision of adequate food, shelter, potable water, sanitation, and immunization has proved problematic in countries disrupted by war. Primary prevention in such circumstances, therefore, means stopping the violence. More effective diplomatic and political mechanisms need to be developed that might resolve conflicts early in their evolution prior to

the stage when food shortages occur, health services collapse, populations migrate, and significant adverse public health outcomes emerge.

### Secondary Prevention

Secondary prevention involves the early detection of evolving conflict-related food scarcity and population movements, preparedness for interventions that mitigate their public health impact, and the development of appropriate public health skills to enable relief workers to work effectively in emergency settings. Preparedness planning needs to take place both at a coordinated international level and at the level of countries where complex emergencies might occur. Relief agencies need resources to implement early warning systems, maintain technical expertise, train personnel, build reserves of relief supplies, and develop their logistic capacity. At the country level, all health development programs should have an emergency preparedness component that should include the establishment of standard public health policies (for example, immunization and management of epidemics), treatment protocols, staff training, and the maintenance of reserves of essential drugs and vaccines for use in disasters.

### Tertiary Prevention

Tertiary prevention involves prevention of excess mortality and morbidity once a disaster has occurred. The health problems that consistently cause most deaths and severe morbidity, and the demographic groups most at risk, have been identified. Most deaths in refugee and displaced populations are preventable using currently available and affordable technology. Relief programs, therefore, must channel all available resources toward addressing measles, diarrheal diseases, malnutrition, ARIs, and, in some cases, malaria, especially among women and young children. The challenge is to institutionalize this knowledge within the major relief organizations and to ensure that relief management and logistical systems provide the necessary resources to implement key interventions in a timely manner.

Initially, both refugees and displaced persons often find themselves in crowded, unsanitary camps in remote regions where the provision of basic needs is highly difficult. Prolonged exposure to the violence of war and the deprivations of long journeys by refugees cause severe stress. Upon arrival at their destination, refugees—most of whom tend to be women and children—may suffer severe anxiety or depression, compounded by the loss of dignity associated with complete dependence on the generosity of others for their survival. If refugee camps are located near borders or close to areas of continuing armed conflict, the desire for security is an overriding concern. Therefore, the first priority of any relief operation is to ensure adequate protection, and camps should be placed sufficiently distant from borders to reassure refugees that they are safe.

To diminish the sense of helplessness and dependency, refugees should be given an active role in the planning and implementation of relief programs. Nevertheless, giving total control of the distribution of relief items to refugee "leaders" may be dangerous. For example, leaders of the former, Hutu-controlled Rwandan government took control of the distribution system in Zairian refugee camps in July 1994, resulting in relief supplies being diverted to young male members of the former Rwandan Army.

In the absence of conflict resolution, those communities that are totally dependent on external aid for their survival because they have either been displaced from their homes or are living under a state of siege must be provided the basic minimum resources necessary to maintain health and well-being. The provision of adequate food, clean water, shelter, sanitation, and warmth will prevent the most severe public health consequences of complex emergencies. It would seem that the temporary location of refugees in small settlements or villages in the host country would have fewer adverse public health consequences than placement in crowded, often unsanitary camps. Public health priorities include a rapid needs assessment, the establishment of a health information system, measles vaccination, the control of diarrheal and other communicable diseases, maternal and child health services, and nutritional rehabilitation. Critical to the success of the response is coordination of the many agencies involved in the relief effort.

## Rapid Assessment

Displacement is the final, desperate act of a threatened population. Wherever possible, assessments of the public health needs of the population should be conducted prior to the act of migration or resettlement, whether it is within the country of origin or beyond its borders. Impending disasters, even the development of complex emergencies, can frequently be predicted. Knowing the size of the population and its age and gender distribution, having baseline data concerning its health status and the level of health services available to it, and being aware of the characteristics of the place or places to which they are most likely to move can be of immense help in knowing what relief supplies will be needed and what kinds of health programs should be implemented. Needless to say, such predisplacement assessments have been rare.

Early assessments can be made by a variety of means. Technology-dependent methods such as satellite surveillance can provide information regarding crop growth, population densities, and even troop movements, although such technology is often unavailable to those agencies that need it the most. Reviews of existing documents and other information provided by a variety of UN agencies, bilateral governments, NGOs, and national authorities familiar with the situation can be helpful. On-the-ground economic evaluations, including a description of trends in market prices for food and essential commodities to food-basket analyses, can be very helpful. More detailed information can frequently be obtained from visual inspection of the affected area, including mapping, key informant interviews, and observation of the affected population. For complex emergencies, however, where political instability and increased violence are almost always compounding factors, more direct means of assessment prior to displacement are often impossible, and the earliest assessment can only be conducted after the displaced have reached a relatively safe area of resettlement.

The purposes of early, rapid assessments are multiple. They can provide important information regarding the evolution of the emergency, identify groups and areas at greatest risk, evaluate the existing local response capacity, determine the magnitude of external resources required, and indicate which health programs will be required in the short- and medium-term. Every complex emergency is characterized by a different set of causes and consequences and each should be assessed for its impact on the health of the population affected.

For complex emergencies, early assessment should include both a description of the conflict and its sequelae, in terms of the affected areas and populations, and a characterization of the health consequences of displacement. In some cases, affected populations may not have migrated but might be trapped in a siege-like setting, such as in Sarajevo and Beirut. For the conflict, variables of particular significance include the duration of the conflict, the progress of negotiations (and the likelihood of an early return for the displaced), the patterns of violence, the size and location of inaccessible areas and populations, and the state of remaining available health services.

The highest priorities for early assessment are the availability and adequacy of drinking water, food, and shelter. Minimum standards described later in this chapter must be met. Regarding the health status of the population, perhaps the most important and most sensitive indicator is the mortality rate. Early documentation of mortality will establish an indispensable baseline and allow for the monitoring of trends that will attest to the overall effectiveness of the relief program. In an emergency, crude mortality rates are expressed as deaths per 10,000 per day. A CMR of greater than one has been used to define the

existence of a public health emergency; a CMR of greater than two indicates a critical situation. Whenever possible, age- and gender-specific mortality should be assessed in order to identify population groups at highest risk.

Rates of diseases commonly associated with high rates of preventable mortality should be assessed as early as possible. These include diarrheal illnesses, ARIs, and diseases with high epidemic potential, such as cholera, dysentery, measles, and meningitis. Where appropriate, the occurrence and risk of locally endemic diseases like malaria and dengue should also be analyzed.

Complex emergencies are usually accompanied by food shortages that can lead to malnutrition. Assessment of protein-energy malnutrition among children should be undertaken as soon as possible. A variety of methods are available for doing so. Mass screening of all children is optimal, but an initial random sample of the population can establish the prevalence of malnutrition and indicate the need for targeted screening and feeding interventions. Vaccination coverage of children should also be assessed in order to determine the urgency of mounting vaccination campaigns.

Rapid assessments require detailed planning and may fail because of the inadequacy of transport, maps, communications equipment, and fuel. In addition, attention needs to be given to the security situation in the affected area, and necessary travel permits are usually required by local authorities. An assessment is of limited value unless its results are communicated in a timely and effective manner to those who can act upon them. Presentation of the findings should be organized and clear, and recommendations of the assessment team should clearly indicate which actions are of highest priority, what a reasonable time frame for action would be, and what resources will be required. Without these, essential information required for the survival of large populations of displaced individuals may not be acted upon in time to prevent high levels of excess preventable mortality. The potential usefulness of rapid assessment should not be underestimated. However, in the past there have often been *too many* assessments done by different agencies in an uncoordinated manner. It is essential that a designated lead agency coordinate rapid assessments, ensuring that sectoral assessments (for example, water, medical services, food) are integrated and that the findings are used to inform program policies and planning.

## Health Information Systems

Epidemiologic surveillance is the ongoing and systematic collection, analysis, and interpretation of health data. This information is used for planning, implementing, and evaluating public health interventions and programs. Surveillance data are used both to determine the need for public health action and to assess the effectiveness of programs. In complex emergencies, after the response to an initial rapid assessment has been instituted, the development and implementation of ongoing health information systems immediately becomes a high-priority activity. Although data on many of the subjects included in the rapid assessment will continue to be collected on a regular basis, routine health information systems will allow for the monitoring of a significantly larger number of other potentially important health conditions and health programs.

### Characteristics of Effective Health Information Systems

In order to be useful, surveillance systems must be relevant, especially in complex emergencies where time and resources are frequently in short supply. Data collection should be restricted to the most important actual and potential public health problems. Equally important, data should only be collected if it will be useful in stimulating and guiding a response; if no intervention is feasible, there is little need to encumber the system with information on the problem.

The best health information systems are the simplest. In a number of complex emergencies,

difficulties have arisen in explaining the importance of the data to local staff responsible for its collection as well as to decision makers who frequently do not appreciate the limitations of data of variable accuracy collected under the most difficult of circumstances. Case definitions must be clear, consistent, and suited to the local capacity to make accurate diagnoses. Where there are no microscopes, for example, malaria may have to be represented by "fever and chills." The data generated from simple systems must be represented for what it is worth and should not be overinterpreted. Representativeness is another essential element of health information systems that is related to the quality of the data. Careful interpretation of data collected from a surveillance system is required before extrapolations can be made to the general population. For example, in southern Sudan, nutrition and mortality assessments are hard to interpret because health information has been collected and reported from food distribution centers to which the displaced and most severely malnourished elements of the population were drawn. Mortality and malnutrition rates derived from these sites are not necessarily representative of the population of the region.

The organization and implementation of health information systems should be made the responsibility of one individual or agency that ensures widespread cooperation and coordination. It is important for the interpretation and response to the data that there be standardized case definitions, data collection methods, and conditions of reporting. This would avoid the problems described earlier in Somalia when different agencies used different data collection methods.

In emergencies, reporting must be timely. When the goal is to prevent excess mortality, undue delays between any two links of the surveillance chain—from the peripheral data-collection level, to the more central policy-making level, and back to the periphery where action needs to be taken—can result in an unnecessary loss of life. Depending on the nature of the data, especially when an epidemic illness is deemed likely or is occurring, daily reporting of select information is not necessarily excessive. For other conditions, data are generally reported and analyzed on a weekly basis during the emergency period and monthly during the less acute phases of the crisis. Of course, data needs may change rapidly as an emergency evolves. For this reason, information systems must have a high degree of flexibility, and their response to new demands should be achieved with minimal disruption.

### Methods

As long as they possess the qualities mentioned above, surveillance systems may combine active and passive reporting mechanisms. Active reporting can include randomized population-based surveys aimed at gathering data on one or a selected few parameters such as vaccination coverage or nutritional status. Alternatively, it can involve the hiring of personnel for the specific purpose of monitoring important health events that might occur outside the bounds of the health care system itself, such as hiring grave-diggers to report on mortality. Passive reporting generally refers to the routine collection and relaying of health statistics within the system itself, whether it be from community-based health posts, primary care clinics, or hospitals. Because access to the health care system may be limited and use may be low because of a variety of factors, such as fear or mistrust of the health care providers, unfamiliarity with the system, and other reasons that are frequently unrecognized by relief agencies, it is especially important that emergency health information systems be regularly evaluated for the characteristics described above.

### Content of Health Information Systems

Trends in crude mortality remain an important feature of surveillance throughout the emergency phase and beyond. In many cultures, death is a family and religious matter, and deaths are not normally brought to the attention of the health care system. In fact, severely ill patients in hospitals are frequently taken home to die. For this reason, active surveillance is best for es-

timating mortality. Grave watchers, often those who dig the gravesite, can be hired on a 24-hour basis to report new burials and, if possible, to ascertain age and gender of the deceased. In some cultures, the free distribution of burial shrouds or other materials used for burial or funerals can provide a useful incentive for reporting. At times, mortality can be determined by means of a population-based survey, but the data derived from these surveys are subject to different sorts of bias and are frequently dated.

Health information systems should collect morbidity data on commonly occurring diseases and on diseases of epidemic potential. Diseases that have been prominent in all complex emergencies include watery diarrhea, ARIs, malaria and other important endemic conditions, and malnutrition. Measles, cholera, shigellosis (dysentery, or bloody diarrhea), and meningitis have all been responsible for major epidemics in emergency settings, and sensitive thresholds for the occurrence of each need to be established. The detection of an epidemic should trigger an immediate and aggressive response.

In addition, at least two health programs—treatment of malnutrition and vaccination—need to be regularly monitored. Indicators of the numbers of patients in intensive or supplementary feeding programs need to be regularly tracked. Vaccination coverage rates also need to be estimated and measles vaccination should be offered to all children aged 6 months to 12 years regardless of prior vaccination status as soon as resources permit. Routine vaccination with the six antigens of the WHO Expanded Programme of Immunizations (see Chapter 4) should be established when feasible. Other vaccines may be offered after careful consideration by public health authorities of the epidemiology of the target diseases, logistical implications, and national policies.

Two areas that have been relatively neglected in complex emergencies are those of reproductive and psychosocial health. Ample evidence has accumulated to show that in emergencies women of reproductive age, and especially pregnant women, need special attention and their health conditions, including pregnancy, should be carefully monitored by surveillance mechanisms. Forced migration is itself a traumatic event and, when compounded by the ethnic strife and violence that frequently accompanies complex emergencies, close attention should be paid not only to individuals who might be seriously affected by posttraumatic stress disorders, but also to the reestablishment of community structures. Finally, when the emergency has subsided (when CMRs drop below 1 per 10,000 per day), increased attention can be paid to dealing with more chronic or less fatal diseases such as tuberculosis, STIs (including HIV), diabetes, hypertension, and elective surgical conditions.

In all emergencies, it is difficult to respond to the immediate needs of the population and impossible to plan for the future without some health information having been put in place. The establishment of a useful health information system, with all the characteristics described above, is an essential function of the health services. Without one, programs will be developed by guesswork, and the effectiveness of program implementation will remain a matter for conjecture.

## Shelter and Environment

As mentioned earlier, the placement of refugees and IDPs in small settlements or integrated into local villages is preferable to the establishment of large camps. Health outcomes are probably better in these small settlements because environmental conditions are more favorable and there is less crowding. However, the provision of relief assistance to a large number of scattered settlements may pose a difficult management challenge and may provoke resentment in the surrounding communities. In Guinea in the early 1990s food aid and other relief items were provided to communities for distribution to both Liberian refugees and local inhabitants. This system worked well, perhaps because the refugees and locals were of the same ethnic origin and many were related.

When camps are unavoidable, three key determinants of location should be the safety of residents, access to adequate quantities of clean water, and all-weather access by vehicles. In many instances local politics determines the site, and the location is often less than desirable. For example, in 1988 the Ethiopian government placed Somali refugees in a large camp of 180,000 persons on a site that had no local supply of drinking water. The nearest source with an adequate quantity of water was situated in a town 100 km (62 miles) from the camp. For many years, water was delivered daily in convoys of trucks at enormous cost to the relief agencies. The Ethiopian government refused to move the refugees closer to town for fear of exacerbating political problems that it was experiencing with local ethnic Somalis. In 1981–1982, many camps for Ethiopian refugees in the central region of Somalia were flooded in the wet season, and food trucks were unable to reach them for weeks at a time.

Sites should be chosen with ease of water drainage in mind, though sometimes drainage systems have to be created at the time of camp construction. This is critical to ensure access by vehicles, limitation of disease vector breeding, and ease of access by refugees to services, such as health clinics and food distribution. When hundreds of thousands of refugees fled ethnic cleansing in Kosovo in 1999, spontaneous camps were established near the border of Macedonia where up to 45,000 refugees were camped on a muddy, snowy field sheltered only by their vehicles and makeshift tents. An added hazard was the large quantity of land mines laid by Serb forces along the border; these mines killed several refugees. In Albania a chaotic situation was created when tens of thousands of refugees arrived, many with tractors that clogged access to the point that it was almost impossible to deliver services and establish shelters. Kosovar refugees were forcibly removed by bus from areas in Macedonia where the government did not want them located. Other inappropriate locations have included the swampy, malarious areas on the Thai border where Cambodian refugees were housed and the Rwandan refugee camps in eastern Zaire that were placed on volcanic rock that precluded both latrine construction and burial of the deceased.

Ideally, the size of camps should be limited to 20,000 residents for reasons of security and ease of administration. Such camps should be further divided into sections of 5,000 persons for the purpose of service delivery. Shelter is an urgent priority. On average, the covered area provided per person should be 3.5–4.5m$^2$ (Steering Committee for Humanitarian Response, 1998). In warm, humid climates shelters should have optimal ventilation and protection from direct sunlight. In cold climates, shelter material should provide adequate insulation combined with sufficient clothing, blankets, bedding, space heating, and caloric intake. Ideally, houses should be built using a traditional design and local materials. This may pose environmental problems so building materials should be trucked in from areas remote from the camp. Waterproofing is essential and may be achieved with plastic sheeting or tarpaulins. Tents may provide temporary shelter; however, they deteriorate in rain and wind and should be replaced with local materials as soon as possible. To limit further environmental damage through deforestation, cooking fuel, such as charcoal, wood, oil, or kerosene, should be brought to the site from remote areas and fuel-efficient stoves provided or constructed. Camps may easily become fire hazards, and fire prevention should be an objective of proper camp design.

## Water and Sanitation

When refugee camps are unavoidable, proximity to safe water sources needs to be recognized as the most important criterion for site selection. The Sphere Project minimum standard for water quantity is 15 liters of clean water per person per day for domestic needs—cooking, drinking, and bathing. Other standards include at least one water point per 250 people and a maximum distance from shelter to the nearest water point of 500 meters. Ideally, both the quantity and quality of water provided to refugees and displaced persons should meet international standards; however, in many cases this is not possible. In general, ensuring access to adequate quantities of relatively clean water is probably more effective in preventing diarrheal disease, especially bacterial dysentery, than providing small quantities of pure microbe-free water. Nevertheless, there have been some important exceptions to this rule (see Exhibit 9–4).

The usual options for supplying water to refugees and IDPs include surface water (such as lakes, rivers, streams), shallow wells, springs, bore wells, and water trucked in from remote sources. Although surface water is often abundant in quantity, it needs to be treated, usually through a system of sedimentation and chlorination, and sometimes with filtration. A system of piped distribution and outlet taps needs to be developed to avoid crowding and drainage problems. Shallow wells and springs need to be protected and provided with a mechanism for drawing water, such as pumps. Deep bore wells provide clean water at the source; however, it may take some time to bring in the necessary equipment.

In addition, measures to prevent post-source contamination need to be implemented, including treatment at the source (for example, "bucket chlorination"), sufficient collecting and storage containers (at least three 20-liter containers per family), and containers with narrow openings should be made available. A study in a Malawian refugee camp in 1993 demonstrated a significant reduction in fecal contamination of water stored in such buckets compared with standard buckets (Roberts, Chartier, Malenga, Toole, & Rolka, 1999). In addition, the incidence of diarrhea among children under 5 years of age in the households with the improved buckets was considerably lower than in control households.

Adequate sanitation is an essential element of diarrheal disease prevention and a critical component of any relief program. While the

**Exhibit 9–4** Cholera in Goma, Zaire, Despite Large Quantities of Water Available

Between July 14–17, 1994, large numbers of ethnic Hutus fled Rwanda and sought refuge in the North Kivu region of neighboring Zaire; initial estimates ranged as high as 1.2 million. Many refugees entered through the town of Goma, at the northern end of a large body of deep water, Lake Kivu. Following the influx into Goma, many of the refugees were located near Lake Kivu, whose water flows very slowly, is carbonated by a volcanic bed, and is alkaline. These are favorable conditions for maintaining live cholera vibrio, which were endemic in the region. At the time there were no available means to purify and transport sufficient quantities of water to distribute to refugees. Although efforts were made by some agencies to chlorinate water in containers as refugees removed it from the lake, coverage was inadequate and most refugees consumed untreated water.

After 5–7 days, the refugees were moved to camps with no easy access to any water at all. Advisors to the relief program, especially the U.S.

military, opted for a high-technology approach, namely a large purification plant that was flown in after 1 week, with distribution of clean water to the camps by tankers.

A few days after arrival, a diarrhea epidemic occurred among the population and was confirmed as being due to cholera. This epidemic had already peaked before July 29, when the relief operation was able to provide an average of only 1 liter of purified water per person per day. At least 58,000 cases of symptomatic cholera occurred in this population. Given the usual high ratio of asymptomatic to symptomatic infections (up to 10:1), it is likely that most refugees in the Goma area were infected with *Vibrio cholerae*, and that few infections were prevented (Goma Epidemiology Group, 1995). In a subsequent evaluation of the epidemic, concerns regarding failure to adopt best treatment practice and poor coordination between agencies were highlighted.

eventual goal of sanitation programs should be the construction of one latrine per family, interim measures may include the designation of separate defecation areas and the temporary provision of neighborhood latrines. The Sphere Project minimum standard is a maximum of 20 persons per latrine. Toilets should be segregated by sex and be no more than 50 meters from dwellings. To achieve maximal impact, these measures should be complemented by community hygiene education and regular distribution of at least 250g of soap per person per month. Hygiene education has been shown to significantly increase the impact of sanitation programs. An analysis of data gathered in the Malawi study cited above demonstrated that the presence of soap in households significantly reduced the risk of diarrhea (Peterson, Roberts, Toole, & Peterson, 1998). The objective of post-emergency sanitation measures should be to restore the predisaster levels of environmental services rather than attempting to improve on the original levels.

The provision of water and sanitation in emergency-affected populations in urban and rural areas of eastern Europe has posed different challenges. The problems caused by the destruction of public utilities in cities such as Beirut, Sarajevo, and Grozny have already been discussed. In general, the goal is to repair existing systems; however, interim measures may be required, such as rehabilitating old wells; providing generators to pump water from distant sources, such as rivers; and providing containers and security for residents to collect water at available sources.

### Food Rations and Distribution

The quantity and quality of food rations are critical determinants of health outcomes in emergency-affected populations. During the early evolution of CHEs, measures should be taken to increase access to food without forcing people to leave their homes. The establishment of "feeding camps" may act as a magnet for hungry fam-

**Exhibit 9–5** The Sphere Project

Perhaps the largest single effort to establish minimum standards of care in emergency settings has been the Sphere Project (*www.sphereproject.org*). Launched in 1997 by a group of private humanitarian agencies, Sphere recognized that humanitarian relief would be increasingly required for many years and that the existing capacity to respond with high-quality interventions was, for the most part, lacking. To address this situation, a large consortium (more than 228 private humanitarian organizations) from around the world participated in the development of the Sphere Humanitarian Charter and Minimum Standards in Disaster Response. These standards are intended to govern the overall conduct of relief NGOs and to provide benchmark levels of performance in the areas of water supply and sanitation, nutrition, food aid, shelter and site management, and health services. First published in 1999, the charter did not intend to establish new standards. Instead, it sought to consolidate and reach agreement based on existing information. Standards will continue to be developed and existing standards will be modified in accordance with new findings, both from research and from experience gained in the field following the initial dissemination and pilot-testing of the charter.

ilies and lead to the spontaneous establishment of settlements and camps with the subsequent health problems described earlier in this chapter. Subsidized food shops; food-for-work or cash-for-work programs; emergency support for home food production, such as the distribution of fast-growing seed varieties; agricultural tools; and other measures may be effective prior to the onset of armed conflict.

Once armed conflict has commenced, either forcing people to flee their homes or be trapped in siege-like conditions, it is usually necessary to distribute food. General food rations should contain at least 2,100 kilocalories of energy per person per day as well as the other nutrients listed in Table 9–5. Rations should take into consideration the demographic composition of the population, the specific needs of vulnerable groups, and access by the population to alternative sources of food or income. In cold climates, the minimum energy value of the ration should be adjusted upward. Pregnant women require on average an extra 285 kcal per day and lactating women an extra 500 kcal. These extra requirements should be provided through distribution of rations within the household; however, this may need to be monitored, perhaps indirectly via the prevalence of low birthweight babies.

Food should be distributed regularly as dry items to family units, taking care that socially vulnerable groups, such as female-headed households, unaccompanied minors, and older adults, receive their fair share. This requires an accurate registration system listing all residents in family groups. If a refugee or displaced population is organized in well-defined communities, food may be distributed to community leaders who then divide it further to the heads of households in quantities based on the number of family members. In other situations, food is distributed directly to heads of households, based on a ration card system. In low-income countries, food rations usually comprise a staple cereal, such as rice, wheat, or maize; a source of dense fat, such as vegetable oil; a source of protein, such as beans, lentils, groundnuts, or dried fish; and extra items, such as salt, tea, and spices. Experience has shown that women are fairer than men in distributing each food item in the correct quantity. Standard serving containers based on a known weight or volume of food are essential for distribution centers. Guards are often necessary to maintain crowd control. Because of the indignity of being counted and the fact that many refugees are afraid to have their identities known and precise locations reported, attempts at registration for the distribution of humanitarian aid should be carried out with the security and cultural concerns of the population taken into careful consideration (see Exhibit 9–6).

**Table 9–5** Minimum Nutritional Requirements of Emergency-Affected Populations (for Planning Purposes during the Initial Stage of an Emergency)

| Nutrient | Mean Requirements (per person per day)[a] |
|----------|------------------------------------------|
| Energy | 2,100 kcals |
| Protein | 10–12% total energy (52–63 gm) |
| Fat | 17% of total energy (40 gm) |
| Vitamin A | 1,666 I.U. |
| Thiamine | 0.9 mg (or 0.4 mg per 1,000 kcal intake) |
| Riboflavin | 1.4 mg (or 0.6 mg per 1,000 kcal intake) |
| Niacin | 12.0 mg (or 6.6 mg per 1,000 kcal intake) |
| Vitamin C | 28.0 mg |
| Vitamin D | 3.2–3.8 micrograms calciferol |
| Iron | 22 mg |
| Iodine | 150 micrograms |

[a]Based on standard age and sex distribution (WFP/UNHCR, 1997).

There is a widespread belief that currently available refugee rations, especially those distributed in non-European populations, are inadequate for nutrient requirements, which may be higher than the traditional recommended daily allowances. The best way to combat depletion of essential nutrients is to take active steps to increase the variety of the diet. This is not possible with relief foods that have to be capable of bulk storage and shipment—cereal, legumes, sugar, oil, and salt. Thus there should be positive encouragement to barter food items for local produce; market facilities should be set up, supported, and controlled by camp leaders. Seeds for leaf vegetables should be distributed as part of all relief activities, even in the acute phase. Every effort should be made to provide spices and herbs, used traditionally by the population, with all food baskets. There is no need for a special food basket for children or pregnant and lactating women—only a sufficiently varied diet for the whole family (Golden, 1999b).

In addition to food, adequate cooking fuel, utensils, and facilities to grind whole grain cereals need to be provided to all families. Fuel-efficient stoves, often made of mud, may lead to more efficient use of scarce fuel. In children less than 2 years of age, breastfeeding will provide considerable protection against communicable diseases, including diarrhea. Thus attempts to introduce or distribute breast milk substitutes and infant feeding bottles should be strongly opposed in an emergency situation. The evidence that vitamin A deficiency is associated with increased childhood mortality and disabling blindness is now so convincing that supplements of vitamin A should be provided routinely to all refugee children under 5 years of age at first contact and every 3 to 6 months thereafter (Nieburg, Waldman, Leavell, Sommer, & DeMaeyer, 1988).

In eastern Europe, the same principles have been followed; however, the types of food have varied and have included cheese, meat, dried orange juice, and fruit. In some industrialized countries experiencing economic and political instability, ration vouchers that can be redeemed for food at designated stores have been distributed to vulnerable persons, such as older pensioners.

One of the main problems in Africa, and in some parts of Asia, has been providing refugees and IDPs with foods containing adequate quantities of micronutrients, especially niacin, riboflavin, thiamine, iron, and vitamin C. Epidemics of pellagra, scurvy, and beriberi have not been

**Exhibit 9–6** Food Distribution in Somalia

During the civil conflict and famine in 1992–1993, dry food rations distributed to families in Mogadishu, Somalia, were often stolen as families returned to their homes. Thus relief agencies were sometimes forced to establish feeding centers where cooked meals were served to people of all ages. This was an unusual exception from the general rule of providing dry food that families prepare at home, thus preserving some independence and dignity.

uncommon in African refugee camps. For many years, this was a "blind spot" in emergency food and nutrition planning; however, in recent years the problem has been acknowledged but solutions are still inadequate. In southern Africa, niacin has been added to maize flour during the milling process. However, vitamin C is water soluble and very sensitive to heat, light, and bruising; thus the transport, storage, and distribution of large quantities of foods such as citrus fruit has been problematic. One solution to this problem is to allow and encourage people to swap some of their ration items in local markets for foods containing vitamin C, such as tomatoes, onions, potatoes, green chili peppers, and other fruits and vegetables. In addition, the provision of seeds to enable refugees to grow small amounts of vegetables in kitchen gardens is an effective measure. The provision of fortified blended cereals has also been proposed as a vehicle for ensuring adequate micronutrient intake. Studies in Ethiopia, Nepal, and Tanzania have shown that these cereals are generally acceptable; however, overcooking and consequent depletion of the vitamin C content may be a problem in some communities (Mears & Young, 1998).

A food ration monitoring system is important to ensure that families are receiving fair and adequate quantities of food. On a food ration distribution day, monitoring teams can establish themselves at several points not far from the distribution center. They should be equipped with weighing scales and food composition tables. Families should be stopped randomly as they return to their homes and asked to participate. Each of the items in their ration should be weighed and converted to calories, and other nutrients using the tables. The total weight of each food item (in grams) and the total nutrients provided should be divided by the number of family members and the number of days until the next distribution day. This will provide the average quantity per person per day and may be compared with the official ration and with standard tables of recommended daily allowances of nutrients.

Although much work has been done to develop standard nutritional guidelines, the complicated UN system of food procurement, transport, and distribution and the inconsistent generosity of donor governments has meant that many emergency-affected populations have received rations quite inadequate in both quantity and nutritional content. As mentioned earlier, food distribution may be targeted by parties to the conflict, and various measures to avoid this have been taken, such as that described above in Somalia. Some of these measures, such as giving food aid to military forces, raise serious ethical dilemmas. For example, in southern Sudan, the major rebel group demanded that all aid agencies working in areas under their control sign a memorandum of understanding, essentially providing the rebel force with inappropriate credibility and control over the distribution of food and other resources.

### Nutritional Rehabilitation

In general, the goal of an emergency feeding program is to provide adequate quantities of nutrients through the general household distribution of food rations. However, due to the many factors described earlier, there may be population subgroups who may either already be acutely malnourished or at high risk of becoming malnourished. These groups may require targeted feeding, or what is termed *selective feeding*. Figure 9–5 demonstrates the various kinds of selective feeding; however, these programs should be seen as additional to, not a substitute for, the general feeding program. They need clear objectives and criteria for opening, admission, discharge, and closure that should be based on population-based anthropometry surveys and agreed upon nutritional indexes. In general, children are defined as acutely malnourished according to their weight-for-height index. Adolescents and adults may be defined according to their MUAC, BMI, or according to clinical signs. Selective feeding programs should be complemented by measures to improve the food ration distribution system, provide adequate clean water and sanitation, and control measles and other communicable diseases. These programs should be integrated into community health programs that offer other prevention and care services.

Supplementary feeding programs (SFPs) provide nutritious foods in addition to the general ration, attempt to rehabilitate moderately malnourished individuals, and aim to decrease the population prevalence of acute malnutrition. There are two kinds of SFPs—targeted and blanket. Each type may provide food supplements either as on-site, precooked ("wet") or take-home ("dry") rations. Take-home rations are usually considered preferable because they require fewer resources, carry lower risks of cross-infection among recipients, and retain the family's primary responsibility for feeding. On-site feeding may be justified when the security situation is poor, the general ration is inadequate (thus food would be shared within the household), and when cooking fuel is scarce.

A targeted SFP aims to prevent the moderately malnourished from becoming severely malnourished and to rehabilitate them. The focus is generally on children <5 years of age and pregnant and lactating women. Care should be taken not to apply strict guidelines for the opening of selective feeding programs. Like all decisions taken in an emergency, it should be based on a review of both current public health priorities and available resources.

Current guidelines suggest that a targeted SFP should be implemented when one or more of the following situations occur:

- The prevalence of acute malnutrition among children <5 years is 10–14%.
- The prevalence of acute malnutrition among children is 5–9% in the presence of aggravating factors (for example, inadequate general food ration, CMR greater than 1 per 10,000 per day, epidemics of measles or pertussis, and high incidence of ARI and diarrheal diseases).

Criteria for admission should include:

- children under 5 years with a weight-for-height Z-score between –3 and –2
- older children, adolescents, and adults moderately malnourished according to their BMI, MUAC, or clinical condition
- referrals of children whose weight is increasing from TFPs
- selected pregnant women and nursing mothers, for instance, using a MUAC less than 22 cm

Blanket SFPs are meant to provide extra nutritious food to all members of groups at risk of malnutrition. They are started under the following conditions:

- at the onset of an emergency when general food distribution systems are not in place
- problems in delivering and distributing the general ration
- prevalence of acute malnutrition equal or greater than 15%
- prevalence of acute malnutrition of 10–14% in the presence of aggravating factors

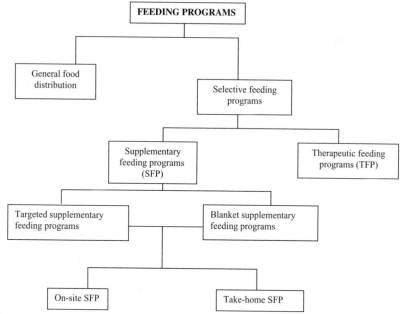

**Figure 9–5** Overall Feeding Program Strategy

- anticipated increase in acute malnutrition rates due to seasonally induced epidemics
- in the case of micronutrient deficiency disease outbreaks, to provide micronutrient-rich supplements to target population

The primary recipients of blanket SFPs are all children younger than 5 years, pregnant women and nursing mothers (up to 6 months after delivery), and other groups such as older adults or the medically ill.

Therapeutic feeding programs aim to rehabilitate severely malnourished persons, the majority of whom are children with severe wasting or nutritional edema. A TFP should be commenced when the number of severely malnourished individuals cannot be treated adequately in other facilities. Although current guidelines for opening a TFP are based on population malnutrition prevalence, the decision should largely be based on an assessment of the public health needs and the resources available. In a large camp, the percentage of children malnourished may not be an appropriate basis for this decision. A more

practical guide might be the presence of, say, 50 potential beneficiaries in a settlement. The following criteria are used for admission (UNHCR/WFP, 1999):

- children <5 years with weight-for-height Z-score less than –3 or with edema
- severely malnourished children >5 years, adolescents, or adults assessed by other means
- low birthweight babies (less than 2,500 g)
- orphans younger than 1 year of age when traditional caring practices are inadequate
- mothers of children <1 year with breast-feeding failure where relactation counseling has failed

Rehabilitation of severely malnourished individuals is a medical procedure demanding careful attention to detail; therefore, well-trained staff are essential. TFPs usually have two phases:

1. The intensive care phase includes 24-hour care with medical treatment to control

infection and dehydration, correction of electrolyte imbalance, and nutritional treatment. Very frequent feeds with therapeutic milk (known as F-100) are essential to prevent death from hypoglycemia and hypothermia. This phase usually lasts 1 week.

2. The rehabilitation phase provides at least six meals per day along with medical and psychological support, including mothers of malnourished children. This phase usually lasts 5 weeks.

Details of the quantity and types of food recommended, discharge criteria, and reasons for stopping SFPs and TFPs are provided in two reference manuals (Médecins Sans Frontières, 1995; UNHCR/WFP, 1999). In addition, detailed information on the management of severe malnutrition is provided in a recent WHO manual (WHO, 1999a). However, it should be noted that there is not general consensus on the adequacy of therapeutic foods currently recommended and provided by WFP and UNHCR. Those who support the classification of nutrients into two types stress the need to provide all Type II nutrients in order to promote growth recovery and have proposed a "precooked porridge" containing essential minerals and other micronutrients as an alternative to the traditional high energy milk-based preparations (Golden, Briend, & Grellety, 1995). Saharawi refugee populations provided with the formula have achieved catch-up height and eliminated anemia within 6 months (Golden, personal communication, June 1999). Nevertheless, this approach has not yet been adopted as standard practice.

## Health Services: Response to CHEs

CHEs severely disrupt normal health care service activity (see Figure 9–3). In developing appropriate responses to this disruption, it is worth considering the impact and response by at least three different sets of services:

- service provision in the country directly affected by the CHE

- service provision in countries to which refugees have fled
- service provision by multilateral organizations and NGOs

### Service Provision in Countries Directly Affected by CHEs

The main challenge in these settings is to minimize the direct and indirect adverse impact of the conflict on the health services, personnel, and resources available. In many conflicts, as highlighted earlier, health services may be specifically targeted, as may health service providers. In such situations it may be extremely difficult to maintain services due to absent or fleeing health personnel, lack of drugs and equipment, disruption of referral systems, and destruction of physical infrastructure including hospitals and clinics. Even if the "official" health system is destroyed, however, the health workers who previously worked within it may still be present within the community (unless they have themselves fled to safer areas) and may still be able to offer services and advice. The extent to which services can be maintained is in part dependent on earlier disaster preparedness activities—both in terms of training and the prepositioning of drugs and other supplies in areas where logistic support was predicted to be vulnerable to disruption.

In some situations it has been possible to ensure that services likely to be disrupted have received prior stocks of drugs and equipment so as to maintain services despite the disruption of linkages to normal supply chains. Although this might be possible for certain forms of equipment and drugs, others such as immunization facilities, which are dependent upon maintaining the cold chain, and support activities such as training and supervision, are invariably disrupted. Nevertheless, local level responses are possible. In Afghanistan, despite the war disrupting medical school activity in Kabul, the medical school was able to relocate itself in another city in order to continue its training activities. In relation to availability of drugs for treatment, prior distribution of necessary drugs to responsible community members (for example, community and other health workers, teachers, and in some cases patients with chronic conditions) may ensure their availability despite the population having to move suddenly. Patients with chronic conditions such as leprosy or tuberculosis could be issued with drug supplies for extended periods, assuming the drugs can be mobilized and that patients with these conditions will be able to adhere to the treatment regimes recommended to them. The potential to distribute impregnated mosquito nets to populations on the move might be an option in areas of high malaria risk; some experience in this approach has been gained among the highly mobile Burmese refugees on the Thai border.

### Service Provision in Countries to Which Refugees Have Fled

When refugees flee their country and cross borders, their normal sources of health care are no longer available to them. Therefore, they may be dependent on what they can provide for themselves, which is often desperately little if they have been forced to flee suddenly, such as the Kosovar Albanians in 1999. Alternatively, refugees depend on what can be provided in the host country to which they have fled either through existing host country services or through additional services mobilized through NGOs and other organizations. Host government services may rapidly become overwhelmed if large numbers of refugees suddenly move into an area and seek to use local health services. Their absolute numbers may pose a large burden on local health services; in addition, their health condition may be poor, especially if their journey has been traumatic and unplanned or if their prior state of health was poor.

In most cases, at least in the short term, these local host country services will not receive additional resources and will therefore have to cope as best they can with the additional service load. This may disadvantage local community members who ordinarily use such services, as the supply of drugs and usual access to health workers may be compromised. Communities will typically be willing to accept these compromises, but if they are long-lasting and ultimately lead to a decline in services available to the local population this may cause friction and tension between the host and refugee communities. Another point of friction occurs when refugees are offered access to host services at no cost, while local community members may be required to pay user charges, both informal and formal, to obtain care. Devoting attention to issues of equity and to ensuring that host and refugee communities gain similar access to services will be in the longer-term best interest of both groups.

A key challenge to the host community is to use opportunities presented by the influx of refugees, along with other organizations and resources, to ensure that their services are developed further and capacity strengthened. Unfortunately, this happens rarely in such circumstances, although increasing awareness of these problems has begun to highlight the need for more capacity-strengthening responses. When the Kosovar Albanians fled into Macedonia and Albania in 1999, for example, there were widespread calls for funds and other support to the health and welfare systems of these countries. This was in contrast with the lack of additional support provided to Tanzania in building a more appropriate system in response to the influx of Hutu refugees following the Rwandan genocide in 1994.

Even in circumstances where the international community, through UNHCR and a wide range of international NGOs, is providing services to the refugee community, an impact on local health services may be felt. This may result from the recruitment by these agencies of local health workers, thus depleting indigenous systems of their usual human resources. Moreover, additional needs may be placed on other levels within the health system, such as referral, rehabilitation, and chronic disease services that the NGOs may be ill-prepared or unwilling to address. Therefore, it is important to anticipate and provide support to the host health system to ensure that it is best able to respond to the increased needs without collapsing under the pressure of greater demands upon the services provided.

### Service Provision by Multilateral Organizations and NGOs

The key challenges for these organizations are, in the short term, to reduce excess loss of life and to reestablish an environment in which maintaining and promoting health is possible. Many of the subsequent sections deal with the nature of the health-related interventions that are necessary in these settings. A much-debated issue is the extent to which these interventions should focus solely on immediate and short-term needs, or should have longer-term objectives in mind. Many relief and humanitarian organizations see their primary role as saving lives that have been placed at risk as a result of extraordinary events. In such situations, doing whatever is necessary, within the available resources, is deemed appropriate even if some of what is done cannot be replicated or sustained over the longer term.

In camp settings, health services should be organized to ensure that the major causes of morbidity and mortality are addressed through fixed facilities and outreach programs. An essential drug list and standardized treatment protocols are necessary elements of a curative program. It is not necessary to develop totally new guidelines in each refugee situation; several excellent manuals already exist, from which guidelines can be adapted to suit local conditions. Curative services should be decentralized in a camp system of community health workers (CHWs), health posts, central outpatient referral clinics, and a small inpatient facility to treat severe emergency cases. Patients requiring surgery or prolonged hospitalization should be referred to a local district or provincial hospital, which will require assistance with drugs and other medical supplies to cope with the extra patient load. Camp medical services need to ensure that women and children have preferential access, and specific programs need to provide an integrated package of growth monitoring, im-

munization, antenatal and postnatal care, the treatment of common ailments, and health promotion.

Organizations that typically espouse a development- rather than relief-oriented approach have sought to place the issue of "developmental relief" onto the agenda, arguing that early attention to the difficult issues of efficiency, effectiveness, sustainability, equity, and local ownership will be beneficial in the longer term. If the latter approach were adopted, greater effort would be given to activities such as training, building local capacity, and keeping costs down, rather than seeing these as desirable but not practical given the acute needs faced in relation to saving lives.

An additional key concern facing the range of organizations offering services in response to humanitarian crises is the importance of coordination. Organizations need to work together closely if they are to reinforce each other's actions, maximize the use of available resources, minimize duplication and overlap, and enhance effectiveness, equity, and efficiency. The Code of Conduct for Humanitarian Organizations, developed under the leadership of the International Federation of Red Cross and Red Crescent Societies and endorsed by the vast majority of NGOs worldwide, highlights the need for effective coordination, usually under the aegis of a lead organizations such as the UNHCR, or in some cases another UN agency, such as UNICEF in relation to Operation Lifeline Sudan, a multi-agency relief program in southern Sudan established in 1988 and coordinated from Kenya by UNICEF.

In addition, there has been considerable unease in recent years regarding the quality of much of the service provision by NGOs operating in complex emergencies. A key problem is the lack of transparency and accountability of such services, and the fact that, despite meaning well, some organizations may do more harm than good. Recent initiatives, such as the Sphere Project, seek to establish guidelines and minimum standards to which agencies operating in these environments will be asked to adhere. Along with mechanisms of enforcement, or at least encouragement to adopt such evidence-based standards, various other forms of incentive may emerge that will ultimately push or pull agencies in this direction. The professionalization of humanitarian workers, as described below, similarly reflects these trends toward improving practice and accountability.

### Refugee Health Workers

CHWs were seen in many countries as the mainstay of primary health care promotion, although some critiques have questioned their value when promoted as a national program (Walt, 1988). In refugee and displaced person settings, the selection and training of refugee health workers has been considered as one key mechanism by which health programs can interface more closely with affected communities.

According to Ververs (1997), the principal advantages of refugee health workers are related to their role as intermediaries between the affected community and services provided by humanitarian agencies, which are often dominated by expatriate staff. They are likely to understand the cultural, behavioral, and environmental influences on health status; contribute to a growing potential for self-care and refugee provided services within the community; share the health service provision workload; build capacity and skills that will potentially be available after repatriation; and enhance the dignity of both the community and the health care providers themselves. CHWs who are relatively unskilled and trained within the community may be the mainstay of service provision. However, it is important to recognize that the presence of trained health workers within the affected community—whether these be traditional birth attendants (TBAs), nurses, doctors, or others—represents an extremely valuable resource whose role should be facilitated in whatever services are developed with expatriate agency support.

The role of CHWs in refugee settings will depend on the public health needs, the availability of host country and NGO-provided services, the prior level of skill of the workers, and the extent and quality of training received. In many cases, refugee health workers have worked outside of health center settings and have performed a range of tasks including:

- identifying sick and malnourished community members and assisting them in obtaining assistance
- collecting and reporting health-related data, such as births and deaths
- providing first aid and basic primary care, such as oral rehydration for children with diarrhea
- encouraging participation in health campaigns and disease control programs
- ensuring that the needs and perspectives of refugees are taken on board in the development of health programs (Simmonds, Cutts, & Dick, 1985).

In many conflicts, notably those in Vietnam, Mozambique, Tigray, and Eritrea, liberation movements trained various cadres of CHWs, who played a valuable role in establishing core health care services. These initially focused on basic curative care, but they also played a role in preventive health and health promotion. In a number of these struggles, such health workers also played a role in community mobilization and in laying the foundations for primary care-oriented services.

One of the first refugee programs that systematically trained large numbers of CHWs as the basis of health service delivery was in Somalia in the early 1980s. At that time, almost 1 million refugees from Ethiopia were housed in 35 camps scattered throughout three regions of the country. The Ministry of Health's Refugee Health Unit coordinated the training of approximately 2,000 CHWs and 1,000 TBAs with the help of NGOs working in the country. The training curriculum was standardized, as were treatment protocols, essential drugs, salaries, and working conditions. As NGOs gradually withdrew from the country, health services were largely provided by CHWs and TBAs, supervised by Somali Ministry of Health nurses, trainers, and doctors.

Despite a range of potential advantages to developing and working with a cadre of refugee health workers, there are also numerous problems (Ververs, 1997). It may be difficult to recruit health workers, especially in unstable settings or if potential workers have other pressing priorities and they will require training and ongoing supervision. Their selection may be highly political, and identifying the political and other affiliations of potential health workers may be difficult for agencies with a limited history in the area. There is potential to stimulate rivalry and exacerbate perceptions of inequity if an inappropriate mix of workers from different areas and backgrounds is selected. In the presence of adequately resourced host country services, especially those with sufficient numbers of trained staff, establishing a cadre of CHWs with more limited skills may not be seen as a priority.

Among the prerequisites for effective CHW training programs are a clear description of the tasks at hand and an explicit job description, an adequate level of logistic and supervisory support, a transparent system of selection, remuneration, and the consent and involvement of the affected and, where relevant, host communities.

## Maternal and Child Health Care Services

Children and women, especially pregnant women, have been repeatedly shown to be the most vulnerable elements of refugee and displaced populations, especially during the emergency period. Among Rohingya refugees in Bangladesh (1992–1993), women and girl children were seen less at health facilities than men and boys, but had much higher mortality (see Figure 9–6).

In Goma, households headed by women were found to have substantially less food and nonfood commodities that had been issued at general distribution points by international relief officials than those in which an adult male was present. For these reasons, health services oriented to the specific needs of children and women are essential in reducing morbidity and mortality within a population to a minimum level. Maternal and child care should begin within the community, at the household level, and not depend entirely on established health facilities. Often, community members, such as traditional birth attendants or others previously trained as community health workers, can be recruited from within the affected population itself to provide basic services.

For children, routine screening and preventive services are important. Growth monitoring and the identification of children whose growth is faltering, with referral to supplementary feeding programs when indicated, are essential functions of maternal and child services. Such a program will also ensure that all children are vaccinated on schedule and are receiving regular supplements of vitamin A. When curative care is required, as for diarrhea and ARI, it can be offered at the household by trained CHWs or the child can be referred to peripheral health facilities.

Pregnant women (who can constitute 3% of the population) should be regularly monitored. At least three prenatal examinations should be conducted to identify high-risk pregnancies. All women should be vaccinated with tetanus toxoid to prevent neonatal tetanus in their newborn. Iron and folic acid should be distributed (and their ingestion monitored, if possible). Malaria chemoprophylaxis, if appropriate, should also be undertaken. In the postnatal period, counseling services addressing a variety of issues, from family planning to child care, and especially about breastfeeding, should be offered. Finally, although many elements of maternal and child health care can be instituted in the postemergency phase, a critical service that must be provided during the earliest stages of a relief effort is the establishment of emergency obstetrical care for dealing with any complications of term pregnancies. Caesarean section and transfusion facilities are essential if maternal mortality is to be kept low. Provisions for emergency delivery are part of an overall minimum initial service package (MISP), which is discussed below.

## Reproductive Health Measures

UNHCR, WHO, and the UN Population Fund (UNFPA) state that while food, water, and shel-

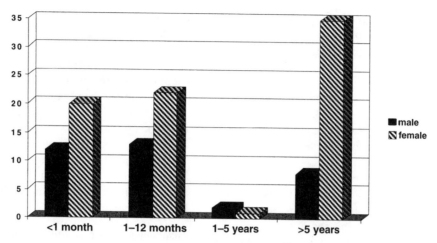

**Figure 9–6** Number of Deaths among Burmese Refugees, by Age and Sex, Gundhum II Camp, Bangladesh, May 6–June 26, 1992

ter remain priorities in an emergency assistance program, reproductive health care is among the crucial elements that give refugees the basic human welfare and dignity that is their right (UNHCR, 1999). The response to reproductive health problems during emergencies consists of a constellation of assessment, services, and regular monitoring that addresses the implementation of the following programs:

- a minimum initial service package
- safe motherhood
- prevention and treatment of sexual and gender-based violence
- prevention and care for STIs
- family planning
- reproductive health needs of adolescents

### Minimum Initial Service Package

Although resources should not be diverted from attempts to control the diseases that have traditionally been the leading causes of death in complex emergencies, there are five interventions related to reproductive health that should be implemented even in the acute phase. In addition, a reproductive health coordinator should be designated to ensure that these measures are adequately addressed.

***Emergency Contraceptives.*** Forced migration is frequently accompanied by sexual vio-

lence (see above). To prevent unwanted pregnancies resulting from rape, emergency postcoital contraception supplies should be available to women who request them. Although the extent of this problem has never been adequately documented, and although it is likely to vary from one situation to the next, the current recommendation is to have sufficient supplies immediately available for 1% of women of reproductive age. Two methods of emergency contraception are currently available: the combined oral contraceptive (two formulations are available), which must be taken within 3 days of unprotected sexual intercourse, or the copper intrauterine device, which must be implanted within 5 days of unprotected intercourse.

***Universal Precautions.*** To prevent the transmission of human immunodeficiency virus, universal precautions must be respected from the outset of an emergency. Although chaotic conditions are frequently prevalent and although health services are implemented under very stressful conditions, the threat of HIV infection can and must be minimized. Universal precautions include:

- washing hands with soap and water after contact with body fluids or wounds
- wearing gloves for procedures involving contact with blood or other body fluids

- using protective clothing when exposure to large amounts of blood is likely
- practicing safe handling of sharps
- disposing of waste materials safely (by burning or burial)
- disinfecting of or sterilizing medical equipment
- wearing gloves when handling corpses and washing with soap and water afterward

*Contraceptive Availability.* Little is known about sexual behavior during times of emergency. To prevent unwanted pregnancies and to minimize the transmission of preventable diseases, including AIDS, an adequate supply of condoms should be available on request to all members of the target population.

*Delivery Services.* All populations affected by complex emergencies will include women in the later stages of pregnancy or who are at high risk for complicated deliveries. These women need services even during the acute phase of the emergency. In a population of 2,500 with a crude birth rate of about 3%, there will be five to eight births per month. In order to deal with these deliveries, simple supplies must be made available. Simple delivery kits and midwife kits are both readily available from UNICEF and other suppliers of health supplies. Although it is not traditionally part of the MISP, sites where complicated delivery can be treated should be established as early during an emergency as possible. Caesarean section for obstructed delivery, transfusion for excessive hemorrhage, and intravenous antibiotics for the treatment of sepsis are the only ways to reduce maternal mortality, and these measures should be available and easily accessible from the onset of a relief operation.

*Comprehensive Reproductive Health Services.* The last element of the MISP is planning for the provision of comprehensive reproductive health services as rapidly as is feasible. To do this, reproductive health indicators should be included in health information systems to allow for the collection of baseline data on maternal, infant, and child mortality, prevalence of STIs, and population contraceptive prevalence rates. Suitable sites for the delivery of reproductive health services should be identified but need not be separate from other health facilities. The sites should be secure and allow for safe passage of women between their home and the clinic. They should be easily accessible to all who wish to use them, guarantee privacy and confidentially, and have access to clean water and latrines. In addition, an adequate referral system should be identified or established to provide care to women with obstetrical complications or other health emergencies.

### Postemergency Reproductive Health Programs

When adequate food, water, sanitation, and shelter have been provided, programs to address the initial emergency health priorities have been implemented (for example, measles vaccination), and mortality rates have declined, the range of reproductive health services should gradually be expanded. In the postemergency phase, health care would be incomplete unless the entire range of programs aimed at maintaining or improving reproductive health was included. The key to successful reproductive health programs is soliciting active participation of as many adolescents and women of reproductive age as possible. Although training female health workers (including traditional birth attendants) is usually the focus of such programs, male health workers should also be trained in the basic principles of reproductive health care. In addition, because adequate reproductive health services are frequently unavailable to the local, nonrefugee population, it is a good idea to try to extend to women and adolescents in the host population whatever programs expatriate relief workers are providing to refugees and displaced persons.

### Communicable Disease Control

Concern for the potential impact of communicable diseases has dominated the public health response in many emergency settings. As discussed above, this attention has been frequently warranted. Although many of the technical interventions and public health programs used in emergencies draw heavily from their counterparts in stable settings, a few important differences should be considered. Most important among them include addressing the needs of the local, nondisplaced, population; maintaining respect for national health policies when dealing with refugees; and promoting substantial community involvement as early as is feasible.

## Measles

Because of the devastating impact that measles has had in many emergencies, it has become almost universally accepted that mass measles vaccination, regardless of vaccination history or place of provenance, should be instituted as early during an emergency as possible. Leading reference publications (CDC, 1992; Médecins Sans Frontières, 1997; Steering Committee for Humanitarian Response, 1998) accord measles immunization the highest priority of all interventions and recommend that it be undertaken immediately after an initial rapid assessment regardless of the circumstances. If children cannot be vaccinated upon arrival or registration, a mass vaccination campaign should be undertaken. In general, this rule should be followed, although any mass vaccination program must be planned carefully if it is to be implemented successfully. Sufficient vaccine should be on hand (with a reserve in case of excess wastage) and stored in a functioning cold chain of adequate capacity. Only autodestruct syringes should be used, and safety boxes must be available for their storage and disposal.

The target population for measles vaccination in emergencies is usually children aged 6 months to 12–15 years. WHO recommends reducing the usually recommended minimum age for measles vaccination from 9 months to 6 months because high attack rates and high CFRs have occurred in younger children, especially in large displaced populations living in relatively crowded conditions. Still, because vaccine ef-

ficacy in children 6–9 months may be lower than optimal because of the persistence of maternally transferred passive antibodies to measles virus, children in this age group should be vaccinated again at the age of 9 months. The upper age limit for mass vaccination is more flexible and depends, to a large extent, on the amount of measles vaccine, injection equipment, and health personnel available, and the pressure of competing health care priorities. Because age and undernutrition are such important risk factors for complicated measles and for high CFR, all children up to 12 years old who are eligible for selective feeding programs or who are hospitalized with other illnesses should be vaccinated against measles on a priority basis. Then, depending on the factors mentioned above, all children less than 2 years old should be considered for vaccination, followed by all children less than 5 years old. Finally, if the circumstances allow, the target population can be expanded. A common recommendation is to vaccinate all children between the ages of 6 months and 12 years, when feasible. In any case, a mass vaccination campaign should seek to achieve at least 95% coverage of the target population.

Because a mass vaccination campaign can reach such a high proportion of the most vulnerable population, there are frequently demands to attach other services to it. Vitamin A, for example, can be offered to the same target group during the course of the campaign. There have been suggestions to provide polio vaccination along with measles vaccine, although the logistical burden of doing so must be carefully considered because complicating the mass measles vaccination campaign by adding other interventions may interfere with the primary objective of the program. In any case, a routine vaccination program for all children using the standard antigens recommended by WHO should be established during the postemergency period. Other vaccines, such as yellow fever and meningitis, are effective in interrupting transmission after an epidemic has been detected, but should not be offered routinely at the time of measles vaccine. Cholera vaccination has also been recommended at the time of measles vaccination. But the most commonly available cholera vaccine, a killed whole cell/B subunit vaccine, cannot interrupt transmission during an outbreak (unlike measles vaccine), because it requires two doses 1 week apart and does not induce immunity until at least 1 week after the second dose. In areas where cholera is endemic and there are recurrent outbreaks, vaccination of the entire population, including new arrivals, should be carefully considered. The early detection of measles cases when they occur is an important feature of an effective community-based surveillance system. Measles treatment includes the administration of two doses of vitamin A and the appropriate treatment of common complications such as pneumonia, diarrhea, malnutrition, and meningoencephalitis. Children with measles should be closely monitored in regard to their nutritional status and, if indicated, should be enrolled in supplementary feeding programs during their convalescence.

Measles remains an important threat to the health of children in many emergency settings. However, as vaccination programs in many parts of the world have progressed and as vaccination coverage levels increase, measles vaccination should be considered alongside other priority interventions. In northern Iraq, Rwanda, and the Balkans, measles vaccination was delayed in order to address other more urgent problems. In spite of the clear threat that measles poses to the health of populations in emergency settings, it is always appropriate to weigh the public health needs in light of the available resources and to order priorities accordingly.

## Diarrheal Diseases

The importance of diarrhea as a contributor to morbidity and mortality in emergency settings cannot be underestimated. The detection and reporting of diarrhea should be part of the routine surveillance system in emergencies. Acute watery diarrhea and bloody diarrhea should be reported separately by age (under 5 and over 5 years old are minimum age groups).

All health personnel should be sensitized to the potential impact of diarrhea and should be skilled in most aspects of prevention and treatment. The key to prevention lies in providing adequate sanitation facilities and at least the minimum recommended quantity of water of acceptable quality (see above). The mainstay of diarrhea case management is oral rehydration therapy (ORT). Although any fluids can be used to prevent the development of dehydration, oral rehydration solution (ORS) can be used in all cases and is the treatment of choice for all levels of dehydration (see Chapter 4). In fact, the first large field trial of ORS took place in a refugee camp in West Bengal, India, where it was shown that cholera patients treated with what was standard treatment at the time were 3.8 times as likely to die from dehydration as those treated with ORS.

Rehydration facilities should be available in all health facilities, including health posts and outreach sites within the community. Keys to the success of ORT in emergencies, where the caseload can be substantial, include careful organization of ORT centers and the presence of concerned and skilled staff. Mothers or other caretakers are important contributors to ORT and must be instructed as to the quantity of fluid that their children require. Breastfeeding should be continued, and the nutritional status of children recovering from diarrhea must be carefully monitored. Rehydration of unaccompanied children should be carefully overseen and appropriate follow-up ensured (see Chapter 4).

### Cholera

Early detection of possible cases of cholera is essential to the effective management of an epidemic. Although noncholera diarrhea is a far more common cause of morbidity and mortality in children, the death of an adult from dehydration should raise suspicions of cholera. Attack rates can be higher in refugee camps than in noncamp situations. Laboratory confirmation should be obtained as quickly as possible at the start of a suspected epidemic, but need not be continued. Whenever cholera is suspected, aggressive attempts to educate the community should be made, in order to limit the panic that frequently accompanies this disease. During the course of an epidemic, cases and deaths should be reported on a daily basis through the institution of an active surveillance mechanism.

The need to establish rehydration facilities at multiple sites within the community has been dramatically highlighted by the occurrence of epidemics of cholera. In an outbreak in Somalia in 1985, a new camp with only a centralized treatment facility and no trained CHWs reported a CFR of 23.3%. In contrast, in seven camps in which peripheral ORT corners with trained personnel had been established in the framework of a primary health care system, case fatality was limited to 2.4%. Even more dramatically, during the devastating outbreak in Goma in 1994, more than 90% of the approximately 45,000 deaths during a 3-week period occurred beyond the reach of the health system. Active case finding and rehydration therapy within the community, rather than reliance on overwhelmed and understaffed health facilities, may have averted a significant fraction of these deaths.

Although as many as 90% of patients during a cholera epidemic can be treated orally, intravenous rehydration will be required for the most severe cases. A referral system must be in place and cholera treatment sites should be identified and prepared with adequate bed capacity, human resources, water, drugs and other supplies, and disposal facilities. The treatment of cholera is the same as is described in Chapter 4. In emergency settings, however, selective chemoprophylaxis is usually not indicated. Resources can be used more efficiently and effectively in other ways, such as establishing adequate water and sanitation and ensuring that all patients are identified and treated quickly and appropriately.

### Dysentery Due to S. dysenteriae *Type 1*

The management of epidemics of dysentery in emergency settings is very difficult. As is true of other diarrheal diseases, ensuring adequate water and sanitation facilities is essential, but because of the highly communicable nature of *S.*

*dysenteriae* type 1, its role in reducing transmission may be limited, especially in the crowded conditions of refugee camps. Nevertheless, the use of narrow-neck containers for water storage in order to reduce contamination and the distribution and use of soap for hand washing have been shown to be useful. Early case detection and prompt treatment are the keys to limiting spread. An epidemic of *S. dysenteriae* type 1 should be suspected whenever a case of diarrhea with blood in the stool is reported. Laboratory confirmation and sensitivity to antibiotics should be obtained immediately, with careful attention paid to the transport of stool specimens.

The key to dysentery case management is antibiotic therapy. However, there are severe limitations to effective case management on a large scale. These include the large caseloads that may require treatment, the resistance of organisms to first-line antibiotics, and the difficulty of ensuring patient compliance with 3–5 day courses of treatment. In the relatively sheltered environment of refugee or IDP camps or settlements, where an international relief effort may be instituted, access to sophisticated antibiotics and better patient supervision may be possible. However, because outbreaks frequently involve the surrounding, local population, careful consideration should be given to the level of care provided. During the Goma epidemic, for example, the U.S. military donated a large quantity of ciprofloxacin, then a relatively expensive antibiotic, for the treatment of refugees. The local population, also severely affected by the epidemic, had recourse only to nalidixic acid, an antibiotic to which many of the isolated strains of *S. dysenteriae* type 1 were resistant. This situation created tension between the local public health authorities and the international organizations working with the refugees.

In general, during epidemics of *S. dysenteriae* type 1 an effective antibiotic should be given to all patients, under close supervision of health staff. If supplies of an effective antibiotic are limited, patients who are severely ill or most vulnerable (children, pregnant women, older adults) should be given antibiotics and others given supportive treatment only. This would include nutritional support, rehydration when necessary, and other specific measures.

## Malaria

Malaria control in emergencies depends to some extent on knowledge of the local vectors. In any case, site planning and selection should be done with the possibility of malaria in mind and areas with swamps, marshes, and other vector-dense characteristics should be avoided. Where mosquito density is high and immunity of the population is low, periodic residual spraying of interior walls can be undertaken, although it is less effective where temporary and shoddy shelters are in use and may be damaging to the environment. Aerial spraying should usually be avoided except in special circumstances. Barrier protection methods can also be useful, and the impregnation of materials, including bed nets, curtains, and even clothing, has been effective. The level of transmission, biting habits of the prevalent vectors, sleeping habits of the population, and cost should all be taken into consideration before embarking on mass impregnation programs. In emergencies where people are displaced with their livestock, periodic permethrin sponging of the animals has been shown to reduce vector density and malaria transmission.

Although chemoprophylaxis of selected, highly vulnerable groups can be implemented in emergencies, it is logistically complicated, resource-intensive, and, when implemented, should usually be instituted in the postemergency phase. Widespread resistance of plasmodia to chloroquine is making chemoprophylaxis less attractive as a strategy, although the administration of pyrimethamine/sulfadoxine in a single dose each trimester to pregnant women (especially during their first and second pregnancies) is a potentially effective strategy that should be evaluated. Chemoprophylaxis of children attending feeding centers can also be considered, although antimalarials other than chloroquine, which can be used in areas where

plasmodia remain sensitive, are not generally recommended in children.

Whenever feasible, the diagnosis of malaria should be confirmed microscopically. The recent development of highly sensitive, highly specific colorimetric paper strips for the diagnosis of malaria may make the diagnosis of malaria considerably easier. If neither microscopes nor test papers are available to do so, malaria should be treated on the basis of a presumptive diagnosis, although other causes of fever should be suspected as well. In determining who should be treated, with which drugs, according to what dosage schedule, it is important to consider the national guidelines of the host country. Strategies for uncomplicated malaria, for severe malaria, and for treatment failures should be developed and explained to all health service personnel.

## Meningitis

The detection of outbreaks of meningococcal meningitis at an early stage is essential. During emergencies a high level of suspicion should be maintained. All cases that are clinically suspicious should be diagnosed by either visual inspection of cerebrospinal fluid or, where available, by the appropriate microscopic, serological, and bacteriological analyses. Background rates of meningococcal disease vary considerably from one area to another, and cases are highly seasonal. The detection of an epidemic therefore requires a sensitive surveillance system. It has become customary to institute epidemic control measures when a threshold incidence rate of 15 per 100,000 population per week has been exceeded for 2 consecutive weeks. In small populations, or where the population has not been accurately determined, a weekly doubling of the number of cases over a 3-week period can also signal the early stages of an epidemic.

Meningococcal vaccine (for Group A and Group C *Neisseria meningitidis*) is effective in conferring at least short-term protection to all population groups and can also contribute to reducing transmission during the course of an epidemic. Mass vaccination campaigns are an intervention of choice in areas in which an epidemic is occurring and have been implemented in Burundi (1992), Guinea (1993), and Zaire (1994), as well as in other situations. Vaccination campaigns usually target the entire population aged 1 year and older, although resource limitations may require limiting the age group to be vaccinated. As is the case with Shigella dysentery, epidemics of meningitis usually occur in both displaced and local populations simultaneously, and arrangements should be made to provide vaccine to the host population as well.

Neither mass chemoprophylaxis nor prophylaxis of household contacts has proven to be an effective intervention during outbreaks and neither should be instituted. Most cases can be effectively treated with a single intramuscular injection of chloramphenicol in oil, although intravenous penicillin remains the treatment of choice. Its use is limited at times, however, by the need for hospitalization and attentive nursing care.

**Tuberculosis**

Tuberculosis control should be instituted only after mortality rates have fallen below 1 per 10,000 per day or when an emergency situation has stabilized and it is apparent that the displaced population will remain for at least 6 months. From a public health standpoint, the objective of tuberculosis control is to treat patients so that they cannot infect others, while helping to restore health in infected individuals. For this reason, only sputum smear-positive individuals are usually included in tuberculosis control programs, although individuals who are severely ill with noninfectious forms of tuberculosis can also be included. Patients should be treated according to WHO guidelines, which stress directly observed therapy with a short course (6–8 months) of a combination of antituberculosis drugs (DOTS). Because both infec-

tion with HIV and malnutrition are associated with tuberculosis, the presence of these conditions should be determined and dealt with appropriately.

Tuberculosis programs are complicated. The decision to implement one should not be made unless there are clear written guidelines that will be followed. Laboratory facilities must be available and the regular provision of supplies ensured. Drugs, also, must be stocked and resupply guaranteed. Finally, a system for tracing those who are unable to adhere to treatment regimens must be in place in order that they can be identified and assistance provided to ensure treatment completion. Successful implementation of a tuberculosis control program requires a high level of community awareness, education, and involvement. Each of these needs to be carefully and meticulously developed and nurtured over time. Agencies that intend to implement tuberculosis control programs in postemergency settings should have a clear commitment to continue for at least 12–15 months, have an adequate budget, and have the personnel and material resources necessary to run a successful program.

## ROLE OF INTERNATIONAL, NATIONAL, AND NONGOVERNMENTAL ORGANIZATIONS

The vast and complex array of organizations involved in the various stages of humanitarian emergency preparedness and response reflects the complexity of the international community itself. It is hard to imagine any other situation that attracts such a range of players: heads of state; diplomats; UN political, social, economic, and technical organizations; military forces; and a broad variety of NGOs, including an increasing number of commercial interests.

The UN Security Council plays a critical role in determining how and when the world will respond to the conflicts that lead to CHEs and how emergency humanitarian assistance programs will be protected from the forces that fuel the conflicts themselves. Security Council decisions are in turn determined by the leaders of its member states, in particular the permanent members. OCHA coordinates emergency preparedness and response within the UN system and is governed by an interagency standing committee of relevant UN agencies, including UNHCR, WHO, UNICEF, WFP, and UNFPA. OCHA launches joint appeals for funds to support coordinated UN agency response programs; however, these may sometimes be competing with appeals launched by individual agencies.

UNHCR is responsible for the protection and care of all refugees who cross international borders. In other emergency situations, such as the crises in the former Yugoslavia, the UN secretary-general has designated UNHCR as the lead relief agency. At other times, as was the case in Somalia and southern Sudan, UNICEF or the WFP has been the designated lead agency in the UN system. In general, UNHCR and other relief agencies need to be invited by the government of the affected country to provide assistance. In situations of internal conflict, the Security Council may authorize involvement by a UN agency without the approval of the host government (for example, in the case of the displaced Kurdish population in northern Iraq in 1991). The lead UN agency is mandated to coordinate the activities of other relief agencies, including NGOs, in cooperation with the host government where that is appropriate. However, in certain chaotic emergency settings, individual NGOs have sometimes negotiated involvement directly with government authorities and ignored efforts by the lead agency to coordinate activities.

In many emergencies, especially those involving large refugee populations, the host government has granted temporary asylum to the refugees and actively become engaged in the relief effort. Many countries have coordinating bodies, such as relief commissions, that take a lead role in mobilizing, organizing, and delivering relief services. For example, in Somalia in the early 1980s, the Ministry of Health formed the Refugee Health Unit (RHU), which coordinated public health and nutrition assistance to the 800,000 Ethiopian refugees scattered in 35 camps throughout the country. NGOs wishing to provide assistance to refugees had to agree to follow technical guidelines developed by the unit and signed a tripartite agreement with the RHU and UNHCR. In areas such as southern Sudan where rebel forces are largely in control, relief programs are implemented with little or no involvement by the national government.

The ICRC, based in Geneva, is mandated to carry out the protection and care of civilian populations during armed conflict as outlined in the Geneva Conventions. The ICRC relies on low-key and confidential negotiations with all parties to a conflict to allow it to carry out its humanitarian assistance. The ICRC is committed to carrying out its mission with independence, impartiality, and neutrality. Once the only organization to operate within areas affected by conflict, in recent years many other NGOs have joined the ICRC in taking on this challenge. Some of these NGOs, while providing relief impartially to all those in need, believe that they should also speak out in the face of gross human rights abuses and have become advocates for more effective international responses. This action may sometimes jeopardize their ability to remain in the affected area and is therefore not taken lightly. One of the most debated issues within NGOs is whether to provide humanitarian relief and remain silent about human rights abuses and the diversion of relief resources or to speak out and risk having to leave the area.

There are many NGOs engaged in providing humanitarian assistance in emergencies; they include national Red Cross and Red Crescent societies, international secular and religious agencies, and local churches and community-based organizations in the affected country. Specialized public health agencies such as the Centers for Disease Control and Prevention and Paris-based Epicentre, a nongovernment, not-for-profit technical agency, provide technical advice to a range of bilateral, UN, and nongovernmental operational agencies. The level of technical skills, experience, management, and logistics capacity of NGOs varies enormously. In an effort to promote coordination and best practice among NGOs, a number of initiatives have been taken. These include the Code of Conduct for the International Red Cross and Red Crescent Movement and NGOs in Disaster Response, and the Humanitarian Charter and Minimum Standards in Disaster Response (the Sphere Project). Most professional relief NGOs have signed onto these documents, and the impact of these codes is being monitored. In addition to relief NGOs, an increasing number of human rights advocacy NGOs have been active in recent years, including Amnesty International, Human Rights Watch, Physicians for Human Rights, and Africa Watch.

Funding for international humanitarian assistance programs generally comes from the governments of high-income countries, such as the United States, Japan, members of the European Union, and other Organization for Economic Cooperation and Development states. The generosity of such governments varies enormously and often depends more on the perceived geopolitical importance of the conflict than the actual needs of the affected populations. High profile media, such as CNN, the *New York Times,* and the BBC, often play an influential role in the size of the response to an emergency. For example, the blanket media coverage of emergencies in northern Iraq and Kosovo ensured that relief programs were adequately funded. However, the conflict in Somalia was largely ignored prior to late 1992 when President George Bush decided to promote a highly visible humanitarian relief operation in the waning months of his presidency. Until there is a consistent response to conflict-related emergencies around the world, the quality and timeliness of humanitarian responses will be unpredictable.

## REHABILITATION, REPATRIATION, AND RECOVERY

In countries emerging from conflict, the costs of reconstruction may be staggering. In the immediate aftermath of the Gulf War, it was estimated that Iraq would require $110–200 billion and Kuwait $6095 billion to repair the war damage (Lee & Haines, 1991). In comparison, implementing worldwide the goals adopted by the World Summit for Children in 1991 would require $20 billion. Estimates of the cost of rehabilitation and recovery in countries affected by the Kosovo crisis show that many billions of dollars will be required annually for a considerable period of time, not only for Kosovo but for the entire subregion if ongoing conflict is to be averted. However, it is important to note that the entire annual budget of the UN authority in postconflict Kosovo was less than 50% of the daily cost of the NATO bombing campaign.

A particularly important issue for those engaged in dealing with the aftermath of conflicts is to determine whether, and the extent to which, the prior health system will be reestablished along the lines it previously existed or if it will be greatly reformed in an effort to improve efficiency, effectiveness, and equity. The usual response is to seek to reconstruct what has been destroyed in the conflict; this apparently logical response may be deeply flawed, however. One key impediment is that the resource base available for reconstructing and operating the health system may be vastly inferior to what it was previously. In Uganda the postconflict resource base was less than 10% of that prior to the civil war, making simple reestablishment of prior services totally unfeasible. Further, much changes during the period of ongoing conflict: the range of providers, the role of the state, the attitude and demands of the community that uses services, and the approach of the international community and key donor organizations. The latter, for example, may seek to promote a radically different state, one that facilitates but does not provide services and that places cost-effectiveness and value for money at its core. During the postconflict phase, international financial institutions and donor governments may greatly influence policy direction, and frequently do so in favor of reducing state expenditure and freeing up private sector opportunities.

In the period between the commencement of conflict and resolution, which may last decades, approaches to the nature of health services and who purchases and provides them have changed. In many conflicts other providers fill the gap left by retreating and undermined state-provided health services; these include for-profit and not-for-profit providers, as well as the indigenous and traditional sector. There has been little documentation of how and why the private sector emerges to play an important role in these settings. Nor is there any clarity about how best to control and regulate such activities in the interests of ensuring that minimum standards are adhered to and that medical treatment offered by different providers does not compromise public health goals and objectives. The emergence and changing role of the nonprofit nongovernmental sector is easier to appreciate. It fills gaps resulting from the withering state services and is often supported by donor funds that ensure that humanitarian relief services are provided in acute emergencies and that development-oriented services are offered where suitable funds and partner organizations, including government, can be identified.

A major weakness of NGO-provided services is that they are often poorly coordinated, act in parallel with the state systems, have a different vision of the system they are seeking to bolster or reestablish, and compete for partners, resources, and publicity. Failing to support indigenous capacity may increase the risk of little being left behind when humanitarian agencies withdraw; increasingly, there is debate regarding how best such services could interface with host government services and policy and could reinforce the limited capacity often present.

A particularly important and difficult challenge is to establish the policy framework within which health services and the health system will operate. Some have highlighted the key issues that any government will need to address when refining or reforming its health system; these include consideration of the key concerns of solidarity and equity. Different stakeholders (politicians, professionals, donors, multilateral organizations, and the private sector) all have their own agendas, which they prioritize. A key role of government, when it functions effectively, is to provide a framework within which the different actors can operate. In many settings, including those afflicting countries emerging from major periods of conflict, the policy framework may be lacking or challenged, given its often uncertain legitimacy. In the presence of challenges to a government's legitimacy, as in Cambodia after the overthrow of Pol Pot by a Vietnamese-backed party, international donors may withdraw development funding and assistance, or where they do provide such relief and development support may choose to channel it outside of government structures (Lanjouw, Macrae, & Zwi, 1999). This may simultaneously undermine local capacity and reinforce fragmentation; at the same time, it is important to recognize that NGO-supported interventions may be extremely effective and may facilitate the emergence of good, or at least better, practice. Moreover, NGOs generally promote more genuine participation by local communities in development activities. An important role for policy makers, both locally and internationally, is to facilitate the development of consensus about broad health system direction and the policy framework within which service provision will be undertaken. The transitional authority established in East Timor by the United Nations in late 1999 faced an enormous challenge both to coordinate the activities of multiple international agencies and to help build the capacity of the newly independent East Timorese for eventual self governance (see Exhibit 9–7).

Key issues to be debated in the aftermath of periods of conflict include the financing of health services, the extent to which health services can and should be decentralized, the role of the private sector, and the priority to be accorded to issues of equity. These issues need to be seen within the broader context of promoting and consolidating the peace, reestablishing the economy, facilitating the demobilization of

**Exhibit 9–7** Transitional Authority in East Timor

The violence following the August 1999 independence referendum was stopped by a United Nations authorized international force in East Timor. In February 2000 responsibility for the administration of the territory was assumed by the UN Transitional Authority in East Timor (UNTAET), headed by a special representative of the UN secretary-general, for a period of 2 years leading up to elections and full independence for the new nation. Security was maintained by UN peacekeepers from 41 member nations.

The development of public policies and services, including health, was conducted in the framework of a National Consultative Council, which included three senior UNTAET officials; seven members of the major East Timorese political coalition known as the Council of National Resistance in East Timor (CNRT); and seven non-CNRT East Timorese representatives (from churches, human rights organizations, and so on). Given the shortage of skilled local specialists, much of the policy direction was driven by consultants from various specialized technical agencies, such as WHO and UNICEF. Although the United Nations was reluctant to work closely with CNRT, the World Bank promptly consulted with the coalition and a US$20 million trust fund was established for "community empowerment" projects that were to be implemented through local community structures.

In a country of 800,000 people, 60 international NGOs and 68 locally registered NGOs were active in the postconflict phase; however, few had a commitment to capacity building and long-term national development. Various sectoral committees (for example, health, education, and police) were formed with representation by the various players mentioned above. The role of the National Consultative Council was to consider policy recommendations made by these committees and to provide approval when appropriate and in the longer-term national interest.

troops and their absorption into the economy, and promoting the return of refugees and internally displaced people. Other key priorities include demining and establishing accountable systems of governance.

Ensuring that, to as great an extent as possible, existing inequities in distribution and access to health services are resolved in the aftermath of conflict may assist in removing tensions between groups. Such inequities are often significant contributors to conflict between communities and different social groups in society. In the postconflict period, a fundamental challenge is to analyze and seek to address those factors that contributed to the conflict. Promoting the development of a more equitable health and social system may provide an important opportunity for bringing together different groups within affected populations and may provide early opportunities to stimulate debate, exchange of ideas, and the rekindling of trust. "Health as a bridge to peace" is, however, relatively untested, and it is apparent that in some circumstances health-related interventions, if insensitively or differentially applied, may reinforce tensions and conflicts within and between communities.

Identifying opportunities to increase the availability of funds for responding to basic needs in rural, urban, and periurban poor areas will be important to ensuring a degree of public health control. Enhancing quality of both publicly and privately provided services, and identifying new partnerships between state and nonstate actors, will similarly be important to developing more sustainable systems for the future.

Gender inequalities permeate many societies; in the postconflict environment it may be possible to address these, given that the conflict itself may have changed gender relations and modified the traditional roles of men and women. Given that even in patriarchal societies men will often be absent during periods of conflict and women will absorb a multitude of usually male-dominated roles, conflict often requires women to take on a more important role in relation to making household decisions and controlling household resources. Certain countries, notably Eritrea, Ethiopia, and South Africa, clearly raised gender issues as part of the postconflict dispensation sought by many. The Palestinian conflict drew extensively on women as a major force within the political struggle. Postconflict development of civil society and good governance may reflect opportunities for positive change; if inadequate support is given to such groups, however, such as in Yugoslavia, opportunities to promote a more accountable state that seeks negotiated rather than violent means of resolving conflict may be missed.

Emphasis on reorganization of services to promote preventive and primary care should receive at least as much attention as physical reconstruction of the infrastructure. In many settings, however, emphasis appears to be mistakenly placed largely upon the rehabilitation and construction of hospitals and clinics, with little attention devoted to the more difficult tasks of improving the policy process, improving management capacity, consolidating human resources, developing the provision of preventive care, and extending services to the poor. The major international donors play a significant role in undermining more effective policy development; donors typically seek high visibility inputs, often dominated by infrastructure support or by supporting tightly controlled vertical programs.

A recent initiative to focus on the health system challenges facing countries emerging from conflict identified a number of key priorities for intervention (Zwi et al., 1999):

- maximizing the contribution of both government and donors to the formulation and development of health policy
- developing a clear conceptual framework, informed by multidisciplinary approaches, to guide health system development

- establishing inclusive processes, involving a range of stakeholders in a participatory and transparent process of identifying needs and priorities, and agreeing upon models and approaches to health system development
- appreciating the limitations and constraints operating upon the range of different stakeholders (government at the central and local levels, UN agencies, NGOs, traditional public and private sector providers) in financing, providing, and overseeing health service provision
- promoting evidence-based policy and planning to ensure that more good than harm results from interventions and that resources are used as equitably and efficiently as possible

### Donor Assistance and Coordination

As mentioned earlier, there is considerable confusion regarding the different roles played by donors and implementing agencies in relief and development contexts and little clarity regarding how these roles change in relation to financing and provision of services during periods of "postconflict" reconstruction, rehabilitation, and development. The provision of relief is dominated by attempts to secure survival, with the input of materials and support, often using NGOs as the key providers. In longer term development projects, equity and reform are key objectives, human resource and institutional capacity development are key inputs, and partnership with government dominates the form of interaction with government. The transition from one phase to another is uncertain, contested, and marked by competition and self-interest. Since the end of the Cold War, the funds allocated to emergencies have been increasing and appear to have peaked around the midpoint of the decade. At the same time, development assistance has declined, in part because of budgetary pressure, but also reflecting the changing geopolitical situation in the absence of two clear superpowers.

The United States has already announced that "it expects Europe" to pay for most rehabilitation, repatriation, and recovery in the Balkans.

## Improving Donor Coordination

Donor coordination is, at the best of times, highly contentious and disputed. Although enhanced donor coordination is clearly desirable, the mechanisms to achieve this in the highly politicized and contested postconflict settings are unclear. Although postconflict settings have heightened needs for policy coordination, they may be particularly unstable and complex, and they lessen government capacity to manage and direct the process. Innovative and sectorwide approaches based around the identification of a common basket of funds, and agreement on the key features of reform and development to be promoted, may facilitate coordination although experience of these mechanisms in weak countries emerging from conflict has been poor.

## Conceptual Framework for Health System Development

Having a clear conceptual framework for how the health system will operate is fundamental; the process of establishing this needs to be inclusive, involving a wide range of stakeholders in an open and transparent policy debate. Inputs to such processes include making available relevant literature, reports, and studies to all parties; sponsoring health-related media work; promoting policy fora in which participants from different institutions and organizations could exchange views and develop trust; and developing the roles of professional organizations to promote peace-building and more equitable services.

Defining the policy framework is often contested by different parties and groups. Any proposed structure will have winners and losers. In the presence of a functional state, the government at central and especially local levels should play a key role in policy formulation and implementation. Analysis to inform the development of appropriate frameworks needs to be conducted by credible groups that can assist state capacity to manage the period of negotiation and policy formulation.

Experience from Mozambique highlights the value of early preparation and commitment to postwar health system development. Such plans need to be flexible and adaptable to new conditions, but having in place a broad policy framework for planning was valuable in guiding human resource development as well as capital and recurrent expenditure decisions in the immediate postwar period.

## Decentralization and Participation

Promoting more widespread participation in highlighting needs and influencing policy decisions regarding health matters was raised. In particular, local civil society organizations and local government structures could play a valuable role in contributing to policy debates. Working closely with decentralized systems could help ensure more effective targeting, the directing of resources to what and where they were most needed, and facilitating intersectoral planning and decision making.

## DEVELOPMENT OF HUMAN RESOURCES

The maintenance and development of human resources is a fundamental challenge in postconflict settings. The lack of staff (numbers and quality), inability to retain staff, difficulty of attracting longer-term funding to support an appropriate human resource strategy, and the lack of skills available due to the lack of continuity and decline in infrastructure are all key impediments. Attention needs to be devoted to both public and private sectors, at local and central levels, and in relation to management and technical functions. Improving standards of care and developing a range of training approaches sensitive to different constraints and capacities, including short courses, distance-based learning, and on-the-job training, may all be valuable; facilitating ongoing commitment to local institutions and their development is a key pillar of such interventions.

### Promoting Evidence-Based Policy

Key inputs to the promotion of evidence-based policy are information about needs and about the perspectives of different actors, especially affected communities, concerning the nature and form of the future health system. Health policy should be based on evidence, not only of effectiveness and efficiency, but also of equity, sustainability, satisfaction, local ownership, and leadership. Information needs include assessments of human, material, and financial resources; donor aid flows and activities; private contributions to health sector activity; distribution and condition of health facilities and logistic supports; capacity and quality of available human resources; and availability of drugs and equipment. Assessing health needs requires examination and analysis of baseline information on mortality, morbidity, and disability. Routine surveys such as the Demographic and Health Surveys or UNICEF's Multiple Indicator Surveys conducted regularly in some countries could provide useful data. Qualitative data on community perceptions and priorities are similarly extremely important although often lacking. Making more data available would help promote accountability, transparency, and democracy; collected data should routinely be made available in the public domain. Such measures should clearly be undertaken within a framework that seeks to build local capacity to undertake and further develop their applied research and information system management capabilities.

### Attention to Particular Disease Burdens

Specific disease burdens may be exacerbated by conflict and demand attention. The spread of STIs and HIV may be intensified, as may other communicable diseases such as malaria, tuberculosis, and a variety of water-related conditions. Psychological distress may be widespread, demanding efforts to reestablish communities and livelihoods. Injuries, violence, and specifically violence against women may be widespread and require attention and collaboration across and between different sectors.

## CURRENT ISSUES

With each new complex emergency, new problems arise that must be addressed. In addition, the response to each emergency has led to a reconsideration of previously encountered problems. Although countless issues can be considered to be at the forefront of contemporary thought in this field, three are consistently debated and deserving of special attention: the role of new humanitarian actors, improving the quality of NGO programs, and the role of research in developing more effective responses.

### The Role of the Military and Other Humanitarian Actors

Traditionally the domain of international agencies and not-for-profit nongovernmental humanitarian organizations, complex humanitarian emergencies have evolved into major geopolitical theaters in which many diverse and disparate actors have sought to define new roles. Since an increasing number of CHEs have been precipitated by armed conflict within and between nations, third-party military forces, especially those of Western nations, have been prominently involved in recent relief operations.

Following the Gulf War of 1991, an extensive international humanitarian effort for the Kurdish population of northern Iraq was coordinated by the United States military, which operated under the auspices, but not the command, of the United Nations. For almost the first time, NGOs were to a large degree dependent upon Western military forces (including Germany, the United Kingdom, France, and Holland, in addition to the United States) for security, transportation, and logistics. The establishment of a secure operational area and the delegation of the delivery of relief services to the humanitarian community were important elements in bringing about a rapid response to the plight of the internally displaced Kurds. However, many NGOs, including the ICRC, were uncomfortable with working closely with the military and were forced to confront and reassess their notions of political neutrality. In addition, although their presence was positive in a number of ways, the military authorities proved to be novices when it came to humanitarian relief. They were ignorant of its basic principles, unfamiliar with appropriate relief services, and unable to promptly deliver essential supplies, such as measles vaccine, to meet the public health needs of a civilian population where maternal and child health problems were the main priority.

The military intervention in Somalia in 1992 by Allied armed forces, including those of the United States, was launched for humanitarian reasons, with the assent of the UN Security Council. In the chaotic situation of generalized lawlessness, severe factional combat, and the total collapse of governance, compounded by crop failure and ensuing famine, the only way to secure the delivery of essential relief was with the protection of armed forces. From a military standpoint, the intervention was felt to be a fiasco. However, many humanitarian organizations felt that the military operation contributed to decreasing the high mortality rate, at least initially. Prior to this episode, the military had steadfastly maintained that its role should be limited to providing security for humanitarian supplies; following its Somali experience, it began to review in earnest the broader role of the military in humanitarian relief.

The war over Kosovo, fought between NATO and Serbia, was associated with a complex emergency in which the military forces exercised control over the relief operation. A general lack of coordination between UN organizations, NGOs, and the military commanders resulted in information gaps, confusion regarding roles and responsibilities, and a generally chaotic situation. Fortunately, morbidity and mortality levels among the refugees in Macedonia and Albania remained low, but the potential for a humanitarian disaster in the face of a military victory was clearly present.

The increasingly constant presence of armed forces in CHEs has raised a number of issues within the relief community. There is a need to reconsider whether the fundamental principles of neutrality and impartiality held so dearly by most humanitarian agencies are compatible with such close involvement with the military, which is trained to wage war. At a time when deaths of civilian relief workers outnumber those of peacekeeping forces, there is a need for increased personal security in areas where conflict is occurring. Finally, a serious review of the roles and responsibilities of the military, the United Nations, bilateral governmental agencies, and private humanitarian organizations should be undertaken. All these players should strive to develop a mode of operating in complex emergencies that will work to relieve—not prolong—the suffering of those in greatest need of humanitarian relief. If military involvement is going to be useful, then commanders may have to relinquish certain decision-making roles to those more experienced in the effective delivery of public health services.

In addition to the military and other participants listed earlier in this chapter, other important agencies have emerged in recent years. Organizations that specialize in monitoring, detection, and advocacy around human rights abuses and the prosecution of their perpetrators have become increasingly active during CHEs. These include the Office of the UN High Commissioner for Human Rights: regional organizations, such as the Office for Security and Cooperation in Europe; private organizations, such as Amnesty International, Human Rights Watch, Physicians for Human Rights; and national committees supporting the International War Crimes

Tribunals. In some situations where human rights abuses were extremely common, such as Rwanda in 1994 and Kosovo in 1999, these organizations have helped ensure that public health assistance programs addressed the sequelae of these abuses.

Finally, there has been increasing criticism of existing relief organizations because of their perceived inability to implement relief programs on the scale that is frequently necessary. Some have suggested that the rapid construction, maintenance, and management of large refugee camps; global logistical support; organization of health care services to large populations; and even the provision of security services might be done more effectively, rapidly, and efficiently by commercial companies contracted by governments or the UN. This challenge to the existing relief mechanisms, based as they are on the humanitarian motive, has yet to be resolved. In many ways it could lead to the transformation of humanitarian relief into a business enterprise, one that might inevitably become more closely linked to the donor agencies and used by them as agents of foreign policy. This has been the experience of bilateral development programs.

## Professionalization

Partly to stave off this challenge, and partly to correct perceptions of incompetence and amateurism, efforts have been made to establish certain minimum standards of performance for relief workers. Due to the transient nature of NGO relief programs and the high personnel turnover both in the field and at headquarters, experiences are not easily institutionalized and lessons need to be learned repeatedly. Limited field experience, a poor understanding of the public health priorities of emergencies, and inadequate skills to carry out the most essential tasks such as organizing large-scale vaccination and ORT programs have been frequently observed problems. After what is widely regarded as an initially ineffective relief effort in Goma in 1994 (see above), major efforts were undertaken

to improve the technical abilities of relief workers in the public health sector.

A number of short-term training courses have been developed and implemented by schools of public health, government disaster relief agencies, and the NGOs themselves. Master programs in humanitarian assistance and public health in complex emergencies have been established in schools in the United States and Europe. Although emergency public health workers are not yet required to have accredited qualifications, the quality of health care may improve as more of these training courses become available.

## Research

The acquisition of new knowledge relevant to public health practice in displaced populations has been scant. Although most emergency public health programs rely on the safe and effective interventions that already exist—for example, vaccines, ORS, water purification, essential drugs, and the like—their implementation in emergency settings may be affected by the size of the populations and the urgency of the circumstances. Little is known about the impact of rapid, forced migration on human behavior, disease transmission, and the delivery of effective services in emergency settings. For many years it had been considered unethical to conduct research of any kind among emergency-affected populations, who could be characterized as the most vulnerable members of the world's population. However, it is increasingly acknowledged that it will be difficult to reduce morbidity and mortality levels from their current, excessively high levels without applied research studies designed specifically to address operational issues in the context of emergencies.

Existing standards are largely based on field experience; few are based on rigorously designed and evaluated observational field trials. Although policies in some areas, such as measles vaccination and aspects of food and nutrition, are based on field research, this is not the case in other important public health areas (for example, reproductive health and the control of STIs). Similarly, little reliable information is available on which to base policies and programs to promote psychosocial health despite its rapid emergence as a consistent major public health problem. However, research is only useful where there is genuine concern for improved performance. Unfortunately, emergency relief has been largely guided by short-term concerns.

Much of what is learned in humanitarian response is rapidly lost from view. Of the many people who have worked in the field, few forge careers in humanitarian assistance. Data that are collected and reported by field workers are often either discarded or filed in internal agency reports and never seen again. There is no professional society for humanitarian public health workers and no peer-review journal in which the results of high-quality studies can be published. Although the number of people affected by CHEs continues to grow, a solid body of research on which to base policy and practice is still sadly lacking. Without this database, relief policies will remain relatively uninformed and mistakes will continue to be made.

## CONCLUSION

Significant progress has been made during the past 2 decades toward the provision of effective, focused, needs-based humanitarian assistance to conflict-affected populations. Greater emphasis is now placed on the impact, including health outcomes, of international aid. The quantity of aid delivered is no longer considered a valid indicator of effectiveness; its relevance, quality, coverage, and its equitable distribution are now accepted as more pertinent. As public health in emergency settings has developed as a specialized technical field, a number of relief agencies, especially NGOs, have developed technical manuals, field guidelines, and targeted training courses. Ability to meet the standard performance indicators developed recently by the Sphere Project and adherence to the international NGO code of ethics are arguably valid

criteria to assess the quality of specific agencies.

Although a considerable body of knowledge has accumulated specifically relating to the health needs of emergency-affected populations, there remain many areas that require further development. Donor agencies should acknowledge the need to support applied health research in emergency settings if more effective interventions are to be developed against old problems, such as cholera, and emerging issues, such as HIV/AIDS, tuberculosis, and mental and, reproductive health. The recent process of identifying applied health research priorities in emergencies, sponsored by WHO, and the creation of research and ethical advisory committees are steps in the right direction.

In planning for responses to future humanitarian emergencies, it must be recognized that improving the technical and management capacity of operational agencies will not be good enough. Recent experience has dramatically demonstrated that those in need will not benefit unless the international community ensures that there are mechanisms to permit secure access by those agencies. The means by which this access is provided is critical and most likely to be the central focus of international policy dialogue. The varied nature of responses to emergencies in northern Iraq, Somalia, Bosnia, Rwanda, Kosovo, Sierra Leone, and East Timor demonstrates the lack of consistency and predictability.

The issue of primary prevention remains. The perceived differences between communities are generally tolerated in prosperous societies; conflict and all its consequences generally arise in times of economic distress and political instability. Although programs in good governance proliferate, the reality is that governments everywhere today are perceived to have failed to provide for the basic needs of their peoples. Unless these root causes of conflict are seriously addressed, all that will be accomplished is the perpetuation of a millennial relief industry that inevitably will experience only patchy success.

## DISCUSSION QUESTIONS

1. What are the major objectives in the initial management of a refugee emergency?
2. What does the word "complex" as used in the term "complex emergency" imply?
3. What is the best indicator of the general health of a refugee population during an emergency?
4. Why are female-headed households in refugee camps at special risk of food scarcity?
5. What are the minimum standards in emergency relief operations for the provision of water and latrines?
6. What roles do general rations, supplementary, and therapeutic feeding programs play in maintaining population nutrition?
7. At what age should children in emergency-affected populations be vaccinated against measles?
8. What are the immediate measures that can be taken in an emergency-affected population to prevent HIV/AIDS?
9. How adequate are the existing international legal statutes in protecting internally displaced persons?
10. What roles may community health workers play in an emergency public health program?
11. What are the immediate interventions that should be in place to address reproductive health needs of women and men?
12. What population-based interventions have been developed to address the mental health needs of emergency-affected populations?

## REFERENCES

Amnesty International. (1995). *Women in Afghanistan: A human rights catastrophe.* Anonymous. London: Amnesty International.

Babille, M., de Colombani, P., Guerra, R., Zagaria, N., & Zanetti, C. (1994). Post-emergency epidemiological surveillance in Iraqi-Kurdish refugee camps in Iran. *Disasters, 18,* 58–75.

Banatvala, N., & Zwi, A.B. (in press). Public health and humanitarian interventions: Developing the evidence base. *British Medical Journal.*

Barnabas, G.A. (1997). Local government, equity, and primary health care in Ethiopia. Unpublished doctoral dissertation, University of London.

Barnabas, G.A., & Zwi, A.B. (1997). Health policy development in wartime: Establishing the Baito health system in Tigray, Ethiopia. *Health Policy and Planning, 12*(1), 38–49.

Barudy, J. (1989). A programme of mental health for political refugees: Dealing with the invisible pain of political exile. *Social Science and Medicine, 28,* 715–727.

Bhatia, R., & Woodruff, B. Ngonut Internet discussion group (ngonut@abdn.ac.uk). Accessed 11 February, 1999.

Boss, L.P., Toole, M.J., & Yip, R. (1994). Assessments of mortality, morbidity, and nutritional status in Somalia during the 1991–1992 famine. *Journal of the American Medical Association, 272,* 371–376.

Bracken, P.J., Giller, J.E., & Summerfield, D. (1995). Psychological responses to war and atrocity: The limitations of current concepts. *Social Science and Medicine, 40*(8), 1073–1082.

Brown, V., Moren, A., & Paquet, C. (1999). *Rapid health assessment of refugee or displaced populations.* Annex 3. Paris: Epicentre and Médecins sans Frontières.

Burkholder, B.H. (1997, April 10). Trip to the Democratic People's Republic of Korea (DPRK), April 2–8, 1997. Trip report. Atlanta, GA: Centers for Disease Control and Prevention.

Burkholder, B.T., & Toole, M.J. (1995). Evolution of complex disasters. *Lancet, 346,* 1012–1015.

Centers for Disease Control and Prevention. (1991a). Outbreak of pellagra among Mozambican refugees—Malawi, 1990. *Morbidity and Mortality Weekly Report, 40,* 209–213.

Centers for Disease Control and Prevention. (1991b). Public health consequences of acute displacement of Iraqi citizens: March–May 1991. *Morbidity and Mortality Weekly Report, 40,* 443–446.

Centers for Disease Control and Prevention. (1992). Famine-affected, refugee, and displaced populations: Recommendations for Public Health Issues. *Morbidity and Mortality Weekly Report, 41,* RR–13.

Centers for Disease Control and Prevention. (1993a). Status of public health in Boznia and Herzegovina, August–September 1993. *Morbidity and Mortality Weekly Report, 42,* 973–977.

Centers for Disease Control and Prevention. (1993b). Mortality among newly arrived Mozambican refugees, Zimbabwe and Malawi, 1992. *Morbidity and Mortality Weekly Report, 42,* 468–469, 475–477.

Centers for Disease Control and Prevention. (1993c). Nutrition and mortality assessment—Southern Sudan, March 1993. *Morbidity and Mortality Weekly Report, 42,* 304–308.

Centers for Disease Control and Prevention. (1994). Health status of displaced persons following civil war—Burundi, December 1993–January 1994. *Morbidity and Mortality Weekly Report, 43,* 701–703.

Cliff, J., & Noormahomed, A.R. (1988). Health as a target: South Africa's destabilization of Mozambique. *Social Science and Medicine, 27*(7), 717–722.

Desenclos, J.C., Berry, A.M., Padt, R., Farah, B., Segala, C., & Nabil, A.M. (1989). Epidemiologic patterns of scurvy among Ethiopian refugees. *Bulletin of the World Health Organization, 67,* 309–316.

Dodge, C.P. (1990). Health implications of war in Uganda and Sudan. *Social Science and Medicine, 31,* 691–698.

Dodge, C.P., & Wiebe, P.D. (1995). *Crisis in Uganda: The breakdown of health services.* Oxford: Pergamon Press.

Ferro-Luzzi, A., & James, W.P. (1996). Adult malnutrition: Simple assessment techniques for use in emergencies. *British Journal of Nutrition, 75*(1), 3–10.

Garfield, R., & Neugat, A.I. (1991). Epidemiologic analysis of warfare: A historical review. *Journal of the American Medical Association, 226,* 688–692.

Garfield, R., & Williams, G. (1992). *Health care in Nicaragua: Primary care under changing regimes.* New York: Oxford University Press.

Giller, J.E., Bracken, P.J., & Kabaganda, S. (1991). Uganda: War, women and rape. *Lancet, 337,* 604.

Golden, M.H. (1991). The nature of nutritional deficiency in relation to growth failure and poverty. *Acta Paediatrica Scandinavia,* Suppl., *374,* 95–110.

Golden, M.H. (1999a, June 22). Indicators for adolescent malnutrition. Ngonut Internet discussion group (*ngonut@abdn.ac.uk*).

Golden, M.H. (1999b). Preventing nutritional deficiency in emergencies. In Enhancing the Nutritional Status of Relief Diets. Workshop Proceedings. April 28–30, 1999. Washington, DC.

Golden, M.H., Briend, A., & Grellety, Y. (1995). Meeting report: Supplementary feeding programmes with particular reference to refugee populations. *European Journal of Nutrition, 49,* 137–145.

Goma Epidemiology Group. (1995). Public health impact of Rwandan refugee crisis: What happened in Goma, Zaire, in July 1994? *Lancet, 345,* 339–344.

Goodhand, J., & Hulme, D. (1999). From wars to complex political emergencies: Understanding conflict and peace building in the new world disorder. *Third World Quarterly, 20*(1), 13–26.

Hampton, J.D. (Ed.). (1998). *Internally displaced people. A global survey, 1997.* London: Earthscan and Norwegian Refugee Council.

Iacopino, V., Heisler, M., Pishevar, S., & Kirschner, R.H. (1996). Physician complicity in misrepresentation and omission of evidence of torture in post-detention medical examinations in Turkey. *Journal of the American Medical Association, 276*(5), 396–402.

Kloos, H. (1992). Health impacts of war in Ethiopia. *Disasters, 16,* 347–354.

Lanjouw, S., Macrae, J., & Zwi, A.B. (1999). Cambodia and post-conflict rehabilitation of health services: Coordination in chronic political emergencies. *Health Policy and Planning, 14*(3), 229–242.

Lee, I., & Haines, A. (1991). Health costs of the Gulf War. *British Medical Journal, 303,* 303–306.

Macrae, J., & Zwi, A. (Eds.). (1994). *War and hunger: Rethinking international responses to complex emergencies.* London: Zed Books.

Manoncourt, S., Doppler, B., Enten, F., Nur, A.E., Mohamed, A.O., Vial, P., & Moren, A. (1992). Public health consequences of civil war in Somalia. *Lancet, 340,* 176–177.

Marfin, A.A., Moore, J., Collins, C., Biellik, R., Kattel, U., Toole, M.J., & Moore, P.S. (1994). Infectious disease surveillance during emergency relief to Bhutanese refugees in Nepal. *Journal of the American Medical Association, 272,* 377–381.

Mears, C., & Young, H. (1998). *Acceptability and use of cereal-based foods in refugee camps: Case studies from Nepal, Ethiopia, and Nepal.* Oxford: Oxfam.

Médecins sans Frontières. (1995). *Nutrition guidelines.* Paris: Author.

Médecins sans Frontières. (1997). *Refugee health: An approach to emergency situations.* London: Macmillan.

Moore, P.S., Marfin, A.A., Quenemoen, L.E., Gessner, B.D., Ayub, X.X., Miller, D.S., Sullivan, K.M., & Toole, M.J. (1993). Mortality rates in displaced and resident populations of Central Somalia during the famine of 1992. *Lancet, 341,* 935–938.

Nieburg, P., Waldman, R.J., Leavell, R., Sommer, A., & DeMaeyer, E.M. (1988). Vitamin A supplementation for refugees and famine victims. *Bulletin of the World Health Organization, 66,* 689–697.

Palmer, C.A., Lush, L., & Zwi, A.B. (1999). The emerging international policy agenda for reproductive health services in conflict settings. *Social Science and Medicine, 49,* 1689–1703.

Palmer, C.A., & Zwi, A.B. (1998). Women, health and humanitarian aid in conflict. *Disasters, 22*(3), 236–249.

Perrin, P. (Ed.). (1996). *War and public health.* Geneva, Switzerland: International Committee of the Red Cross.

Peterson, E.A., Roberts, L., Toole, M.J., & Peterson, D.E. (1998). Soap use effect on diarrhea: Nyamithutu refugee camp. *International Journal of Epidemiology, 27,* 520–524.

Physicians for Human Rights. (1997, October). *Striking Hard: Torture in Tibet.* Boston, MA.

Reed, H., Haaga, J., & Keely, C. (Eds.). (1998). *The demography of forced migration: Summary of a workshop.* Washington, DC: National Academy Press.

Roberts, L., Chartier, Y., Malenga, G., Toole, M., & Rolka, H. (1999). Keeping clean water clean in a Malawi refugee camp: A randomised intervention trial. Unpublished.

Shrestha, N.M., Sharma, B., Van Ommeren, M., Regmi, S., Makaju, R., Komproe, I., Shrestha, G.B., & de Jong, J.T. (1998). Impact of torture on refugees displaced within the developing world: Syptomatology among Bhutanese refugees in Nepal. *Journal of the American Medical Association, 280*(5), 443–448.

Simmonds, S., Cutts, F., & Dick, B. (1985). Training refugees as primary health care workers: Past imperfect, future conditional. *Disasters, 9*(1), 64–69.

Sivard, R.L. (1996). *World military and social expenditure 1996* (16th ed.). Washington, DC: World Priority Review.

Spirer, H.F., & Spirer, L. (1993). *Data analysis for monitoring human rights.* Washington, DC: American Association for the Advancement of Science.

Steering Committee for Humanitarian Response, InterAction. (1998). The Sphere Project: Humanitarian charter and minimum standards in disaster reponse. Geneva, Switzerland: The Sphere Project.

Stiglmayer, A. (Ed.) (1994). *Mass rape: The war against women in Bosnia-Herzegovina.* Lincoln: University of Nebraska Press.

Swiss, S., & Giller, J.E. (1993). Rape as a crime of war. *Journal of the American Medical Association, 270,* 612–615.

Toole, M.J., & Bhatia, R. (1992). A case study of Somali refugees in Hartisheik A camp, eastern Ethiopia: Health and nutrition profile, July 1988–June 1989. *Journal of Refugee Studies, 5,* 313–326.

Toole, M.J., Galson, S., & Brady W. (1993). Are war and public health compatible? Report from Bosnia-Herzegovina. *Lancet, 341,* 1193–1196.

Toole, M.J., & Waldman, R.J. (1990). Prevention of excess mortality in refugee and displaced populations in developing countries. *Journal of the American Medical Association, 263,* 3296–3302.

Toole, M.J., & Waldman, R.J. (1993). Refugees and displaced persons: War, hunger, and public health. *Journal of the American Medical Association, 270,* 600–605.

Ugalde, A., Zwi, A., & Richards, P. (1999). Health consequences of war and political violence. In L. Kurtz (Ed.), *Encyclopaedia of violence* (pp. 103–121). New York: Academic Press.

United Nations Administrative Committee on Coordination, Sub-Committee on Nutrition (ACC/SCN). (1994, August). *Refugee Nutrition Information System* (Vol. 6). Geneva, Switzerland: Author.

United Nations Administrative Committee on Coordination, Sub-Committee on Nutrition (ACC/SCN). (1994, October). *Refugee nutrition information system* (Vol. 7). Geneva, Switzerland: Author.

United Nations Administrative Committee on Coordination, Sub-Committee on Nutrition (ACC/SCN). (1995, July). *Refugee Nutrition Information System* (Vol. 11). Geneva, Switzerland: Author.

United Nations Administrative Committee on Coordination, Sub-Committee on Nutrition (ACC/SCN). (1995, November). Report of a workshop on the improvement of the nutrition of refugees and displaced people in Africa. Machakos, Kenya. December 5–7, 1994. Geneva, Switzerland: Author.

United Nations Administrative Committee on Coordination, Sub-Committee on Nutrition (ACC/SCN). (1996, April). *Refugee Nutrition Information System* (Vol. 15). Geneva, Switzerland: Author.

United Nations Administrative Committee on Coordination, Sub-Committee on Nutrition (ACC/SCN). (1998, June 15). *Refugee Nutrition Information System* (Vol. 24). Geneva, Switzerland: Author.

United Nations Administrative Committee on Coordination, Sub-Committee on Nutrition (ACC/SCN). (1999, March). *Refugee Nutrition Information System* (Vol. 26). Geneva, Switzerland: Author.

United Nations High Commissioner for Refugees. (1992). Bangladesh social services mission 22–31 March 1992. UNHCR Program and Technical Support Section. Internal Report. Geneva, Switzerland: Author.

United Nations High Commissioner for Refugees. (1993). Refugee protection and sexual violence. Executive Committee conclusion No. 73 (XLIV), preamble. Geneva, Switzerland: Author.

United Nations High Commissioner for Refugees. (1995a). *Reproductive health in refugee situations. An inter-agency field manual.* Geneva, Switzerland: Author.

United Nations High Commissioner for Refugees. (1995b). *Sexual violence against refugees. Guidelines on prevention and response.* Geneva, Switzerland: Author.

United Nations High Commissioner for Refugees. (1999). *UNHCR by Numbers.* Geneva, Switzerland: Author.

United Nations High Commissioner for Refugees World Food Programme (UNHCR/WFP). (1999, February). Guidelines for Selective Feeding Programmes in Emergency Situations. Geneva, Switzerland: Author.

United States Committee for Refugees. (1999). *World refugee survey, 1998.* Washington, DC: Author.

United States Committee for Refugees. (1999, June 21). Crisis in Kosovo update. (http://www.refugees.org/).

Van Damme, W. (1998). *Medical assistance to self-settled refugees: Guinea 1990–96.* Antwerp, Belgium: ITG Press.

Ververs, M. (1997). CHWs in health care for refugees and displaced people: Their role and their training. Unpublished manuscript.

Walt, G. (1988). CHWs: Are national programs in crisis? *Health Policy and Planning, 3*(1), 1–21.

Walt, G., & Cliff, J. (1996). The dynamics of health policies in Mozambique 1975–1985. *Health Policy and Planning, 1*(2), 148–157.

World Food Programme (WFP)/UNHCR. (1997). *Joint WFP/UNHCR guidelines for estimating food and nutritional needs in emergencies.* Rome: Authors.

World Health Organization. (1995). *Physical status: The use and interpretation of anthropometry.* Report of a WHO Expert Committee. WHO Technical Report Series 854. Geneva, Switzerland: Author.

World Health Organization. (1997). *Tuberculosis control in refugee situations: An inter-agency field manual.* WHO/TB/97.221. Geneva, Switzerland: Author.

World Health Organization. (1999a, Dec. 8). *Health Information Network for Advanced Planning (HINAP).* Health situation report—West Timor. Geneva, Switzerland: Author.

World Health Organization. (1999b). *Management of severe malnutrition: A manual for physicians and other senior health workers.* Geneva, Switzerland: Author.

World Health Organization. (1999c). *Rapid assessment guidelines.* Geneva, Switzerland: Author.

World Health Organization. (1999d). *Rapid health assessment protocols for emergencies.* Geneva, Switzerland: Author.

World Health Organization. (2000, Jan. 5). *Health Information Network for Advanced Planning (HINAP).* Health situation report—West Timor. Geneva, Switzerland: Author.

Yamauchi, P.E. (1993). Patterns of death: Descriptions of geographic and temporal patterns of rural state terror in Guatemala, 1978–1985. *PSR Quarterly, 3*(2), 67–78.

Yip, R., & Sharp, T.W. (1993). Acute malnutrition and high childhood mortality related to diarrhea. *Journal of the American Medical Association, 270,* 587–590.

Zwi, A., & Cabral, A.J. (1991). Identifying "high risk situations" for preventing AIDS. *British Medical Journal, 303,* 1527–1529.

Zwi, A.B., Ugalde, A., & Richards, P. (1999). The effects of war and political violence on health services. In L. Kurtz (Ed.), *Encyclopaedia of violence* (pp. 679–690). New York: Academic Press.

# CHAPTER 10

# The Design of Health Systems

*Anne J. Mills and M. Kent Ranson*

Health systems are the means whereby many of the programs and interventions discussed in earlier chapters are planned and delivered. They are a crucial influence on the extent to which countries are able to address their disease burden and improve overall levels of health and the health of particular groups in the population.

A health system has been defined as "the combination of resources, organisation, financing and management that culminate in the delivery of health services to the population" (Roemer, 1991). Health systems vary greatly from country to country. Unlike the study of disease, there is little standardized terminology or methodology for studying and understanding health systems. Each country's health system is the product of a complex range of factors, not least historical patterns of development and the power of different interest groups. Nonetheless, it is possible to identify common features, and knowledge is increasing on what design features are associated with what outcomes, thus facilitating cross-country learning.

It is extremely important to study and understand how health systems function and how they can be changed. Total expenditure on health care was around 5.4% of world gross domestic product (GDP) in 1994, or 4.5% of the GDP of the low- and middle-income countries, which contain 84% of the world's population (Bos, Hon, Maeda, Chellaraj, & Preker, 1998). Health services are thus one of the largest sectors in the world economy. However, countries at similar income levels differ greatly in how effectively they look after the health of their populations. The health-related differences between countries of similar income can be enormous, as shown in Figure 10–1. While a variety of factors affect health, as discussed in depth in Chapter 11, it is clear that the health system is an important determinant.

Gro Harlem Brundtland, the new director general of the World Health Organization (WHO) appointed in 1998, emphasized that "in many parts of the world, health systems are ill-equipped to cope with present demands, let alone those they will face in the future" and that "there is a need to develop more effective health systems" (WHO, 1999). Understanding health systems and how they can be changed is an endeavor that can benefit from the insights of a number of disciplines, most notably economics, sociology, anthropology, political science, and management science. In recent years, not least because concerns of resource scarcity, cost inflation, and efficiency have been uppermost in policy makers' minds, the discipline of economics has had a dominant influence on the study of health systems. This chapter therefore draws primarily on economics to review key features of the design of health systems.

The section that follows provides a conceptual map of the health system and its key elements. The historical development of health systems is then briefly reviewed, followed by a section addressing the fundamental and controversial

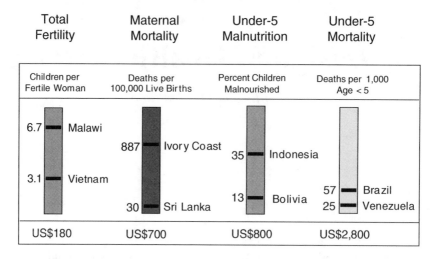

Approximate Income Levels (US$ per capita per year)

**Figure 10–1** Outcomes at Similar Income Levels

question of the role of the state. Subsequent sections then consider each of the key functions of health systems in turn: regulation, financing, resource allocation, and provision. Current trends in health system reform and what lessons emerge on reform policies are then reviewed. Throughout, the text is illustrated by country examples, but a core set of illustrations is drawn from Zambia, India, Mexico, and Thailand, which have been chosen to illuminate key differences in health systems across the world.

## CONCEPTUAL MAPS OF THE HEALTH SYSTEM

Since the seminal study of Kohn and White in 1976, an expanding body of literature has been attempting both to systematize the discussion of the various elements of health systems and to categorize health systems into a limited number of different types (Kohn & White, 1976; McPake & Machray, 1997; Roemer, 1991). These two issues are taken in turn.

### Elements of Health Systems

Roemer (1991) identifies five major categories that enable a comprehensive description of a country's health system to be made (Figure 10–2):

- Production of resources (trained staff; commodities such as drugs; facilities; knowledge)
- Organization of programs (by government ministries, private providers, voluntary agencies)
- Economic support mechanisms (sources of funds, such as tax, insurance, user fees)
- Management methods (planning, administration, regulation, legislation)
- Delivery of services (preventive and curative personal health services; primary, secondary, and tertiary services; public health services; services for specific population groups, such as children, or for specific conditions, such as mental illness)

This categorization is helpful for describing health systems; indeed, Roemer (1991, 1993)

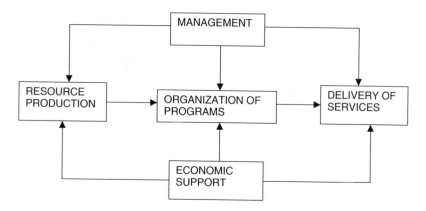

**Figure 10–2** The Elements of Health Systems

applies it in his books to a very large number of countries. However, it is not helpful for understanding how health systems behave in terms of efficiency and equity. This would require much more detailed subcategories and greater elaboration of the relationships, not just within each category but particularly between categories (for example, between economic support mechanisms and organization of programs).

The Organization for Economic Cooperation and Development (OECD) has developed a categorization that is helpful for understanding not only the economic dimensions of health systems in OECD countries, but also the directions that reforms are taking them in (OECD, 1992). The key categories are:

- whether the prime funding source consists of payments that are made voluntarily (as in private insurance or payment of user fees) or are compulsory (as in taxation or social insurance)
- whether services are provided by direct ownership (termed the integrated pattern, where a Ministry of Health or social insurance agency provides services itself), by contractual arrangements (where a Ministry of Health or social insurance agency con-

tracts with providers to deliver services), or simply by private providers (paid by direct out-of-pocket payments)
- how services are paid for (prospectively—where financial risk is transferred to providers, or retrospectively—where the cost of care is reimbursed)

These various arrangements are explained further below in the relevant sections.

## Typologies of Health Systems

In order to make comparisons of how different types of health system perform, it is necessary to group countries into a manageable number of types. There have been various attempts to do this. Countries can be classified according to:

- the dominant method of financing (for example, tax, social insurance, private insurance, out-of-pocket payments)
- the underlying political philosophy (for example, capitalist, socialist)
- the nature of state intervention (for example, to cover the whole population or only the poor)
- the level of gross national product (GNP) (for example, low, middle, high)

• historical or cultural attributes (for example, industrialized, nonindustrialized, transitional)

A key difficulty, however, is that countries do not fit neatly into these categories. Roemer (1991), for example, uses two dimensions:

1. economic level (with four categories: affluent and industrialized, developing and transitional, very poor, resource-rich)
2. health system policies (again with four categories: entrepreneurial and permissive, welfare orientated, universal and comprehensive, socialist and centrally planned)

While some of these categories are less relevant than they were at the time (for example, centrally planned), it is also the case that the second dimension does not classify well the health systems of low- and middle-income countries, which tend to be fragmented, with different arrangements for different population groups (McPake & Machray, 1997). For example, Roemer (1991) classifies Thailand as "entrepreneurial and permissive," and Mexico and India as "welfare orientated." Yet, as shown in Exhibit 10–1, which summarizes the structure of the health systems in these three countries plus Zambia, these four countries cannot be clearly categorized into such neat categories.

Since a typology suitable for low- and middle-income countries has yet to be worked out, the content of this chapter is based on a simple framework (shown in Figure 10–3) that identifies four key actors:

1. the government or professional body that structures and regulates the system
2. the population, including patients, who as individuals and households ultimately pay for the health system and receive services
3. financing agents, who collect funds and allocate them to providers or purchase services at national or lower levels
4. the providers of services, who themselves can be categorized in various ways, such

as by level (primary, secondary, tertiary), function (curative, preventive), ownership (public; private, for-profit; private, not-for-profit), degree of organization (formal, informal), or medical system (allopathic, ayurvedic)

and four key functions required in any health system:

1. regulation
2. financing (through taxes, premiums, and direct payments)
3. resource allocation
4. providing services

**Evaluation of Health Systems**

The criteria frequently used to judge health systems are efficiency and equity. Efficiency has a number of different dimensions:

• Macroeconomic efficiency refers to the total costs of the health system in relation to overall health status; countries differ in how efficiently their health systems convert resources used into health gains.
• Microeconomic efficiency refers to the scope for achieving greater efficiency from existing resources. It is of two types:
  –allocative efficiency: devoting resources to that mix of activities that will have greatest impact on health (that is, is most cost-effective)
  –technical efficiency: using only the minimum necessary resources to finance, purchase, and deliver a particular activity or set of activities (that is, avoiding waste)

Equity refers to the distribution of the costs of health services and the benefits obtained from their use between different groups in the population. It is inherently a question of values; however, indicators of who pays for health services and who receives benefits provide evidence on the degree of equity achieved by particular health systems. Equity can be expressed

**Exhibit 10–1** Illustrations of the Structure of Health Systems

| | |
|---|---|
| **Zambia** (per capita GNP $380) | **India** (per capita GNP $390) |
| The health system is made up of a large public sector, covering all levels from primary to tertiary, which until recently has been very centralized. There is an extensive network of industrial (concentrated in urban areas) and mission (church) services (generally rural), subsidized by the state. Private doctors practice in the main cities, and there is a large informal sector of traditional practitioners and drug sellers. There are only a handful of private hospitals (0.2% of beds are in the private-for-profit sector and 25% in the mission sector). An executive agency has been created to take over management responsibility from the Ministry of Health at national level, and the role of health districts has been strengthened. | The public sector is large in absolute terms, providing all levels of care. Health care is in general a state function, with central government involved mainly in overall policy and specific disease control programs. There is a large formal private sector, providing both ambulatory and inpatient care, and an even larger informal sector consisting of unlicensed and unqualified practitioners and drug sellers. There is limited formal interaction between public and private sectors. A compulsory state insurance system covers lower paid, formal-sector workers, and there is another scheme for government workers. There are numerous community-based health schemes, some with an insurance component. |
| **Mexico** (per capita GNP $3,680) | **Thailand** (per capita GNP $2,800) |
| Public and private sectors play an important role in financing and provision. The health sector is highly segmented. Formal sector employees (roughly 60% of the population) are covered by various social insurance institutions (Fundacion Mexicana para la Salud, 1995). The poor receive care through government facilities or private providers (allopathic and traditional). There is little interaction between public and private sectors, either in the form of regulation or contracting for service delivery. There is much duplication and waste of resources between the three "sub-systems"—social security, other government, and private. Mexico's health sector reform plan is based on decentralization and managed-market ideas.<br><br>*Note:* GNP is in 1997 prices. | Both public and private sectors are large, providing all levels of care. There is widespread use of the private sector, especially for outpatient care. Different population groups have different rights to care, and there are an increasing number of public and private arrangements. Compulsory social insurance covers those in formal employment and finances care provided by public and private hospitals (chosen by the insured). Civil servants have their own medical benefit scheme that pays for care at public and private hospitals. A prepayment scheme (voluntary health card) is available in rural areas. The poor can obtain a low-income card, which exempts them from fees charged in public facilities. |

in two different ways (Donaldson & Gerard, 1993):

1. *Horizontal equity refers to the equal treatment of equals.* With respect to financing and resource allocation, this implies that the charge levied by all agents or providers for a particular good or service should be the same for households with equal ability to pay (regardless of gender, marital status, and so on). Horizontal equity is therefore assessed by the extent to which there is variation in contribution levels among those with similar ability to pay. With respect to provision, horizontal equity means that individuals with the same health condition should have equal access to health services.

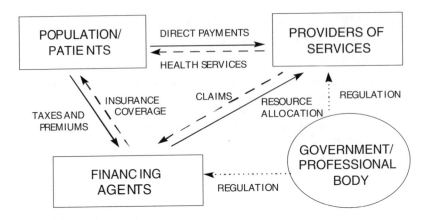

**Figure 10–3** A Map of the Health System

---

2. *Vertical equity is based on the principle that individuals who are unequal in society should be treated differently.* Vertical equity in the financing and purchasing of health services means that consumers should be charged for the same good or service according to their ability to pay.

Table 10–1 demonstrates how equity and efficiency criteria can be used to set goals for the financing, allocation of resources, and provision of health services, and for evaluating their performance.

## HISTORICAL DEVELOPMENT OF HEALTH SYSTEMS

As indicated by archaeological evidence, medicine has had its role in all cultures and civilizations (for example, in ancient Mesopotamia and Egypt). It has also been a concern of the state: the law code of Hammurabi (1792–1750) specified the fees for an operation to be paid to a healer on a sliding scale, depending on the status of the patient, and also specified penalties for failure. The Romans built hospitals for domestic slaves and soldiers in permanent forts in occupied territories such as England. However, the real development of the hospital derived from the spread of Christianity and of ideas of Christian charity and caring for all who might be in need after the conversion of Constantine (died

AD 337) made Christianity an official imperial religion (Porter, 1996a). Hospitals developed in the main cities of the Christian world, often associated with churches or monasteries. The Islamic world also developed hospitals, and by the eleventh century there were large hospitals in every major Muslim town. Hospitals were for the sick who lacked families or servants to care for them—the poor, travelers, and those working away from home (Abel-Smith, 1994).

In Europe by the Middle Ages, a multiplicity of institutions and organizations had developed with pretensions to authority over medicine: the church, guilds, medical colleges, town councils, and powerful individuals. In Brussels, for example, a board of clergy, doctors, and midwives licensed midwives in the fifteenth century. The arrival of the plague—the Black Death—which in its first wave killed around 25% of Europe's population, stimulated growing state involvement to protect health through measures such as imposing quarantine and isolating the sick.

From the early nineteenth century, the scientific basis of medicine was increasingly established, with scientific training becoming essential for the practice of medicine (Porter, 1996b). The eighteenth and nineteenth centuries also saw a vast expansion of hospitals in Europe and the United States, supported by philanthropy and also by public funds especially for hospitals for infectious diseases and the mentally ill (Porter, 1996a). The charitable and voluntary basis for

**Table 10–1** Equity and Efficiency Goals for the Financing, Purchasing, and Provision of Health Care

| Functions | Efficiency | | Equity | |
| --- | --- | --- | --- | --- |
| | Allocative | Technical | Horizontal | Vertical |
| Financing | — | Maximize the proportion of resources raised that are actually available for purchasing health care (for example, reduce the overhead costs of collecting taxes) | Equal payment by those with equal ability to pay (for example, same insurance premium for same income group) | Payment in relation to ability to pay (for example, progressive income tax rates) |
| Allocating resources | Purchase that mix of interventions that provides the greatest health gains | Maximize the proportion of resources spent by agents that are actually available for providing health care | Services purchased for similar groups (for example, the elderly) should be the same in different geographical areas | Services purchased should reflect the different needs of different groups (for example, the elderly versus children) |
| Providing services | Provide those interventions that return the greatest value for money (for example, in a poor country, antenatal care should be provided before radiotherapy for cancer) | Make the best use of resources in providing interventions deemed worthwhile (for example, have nurses as opposed to doctors provide most antenatal care) | Equal access for equal need (for example, equal waiting time for treatment for patients with similar conditions) | Unequal treatment for unequal need (for example, unequal treatment of those with trivial versus serious conditions) |

the funding of hospitals in many countries faced a crisis as medicine became more elaborate and expensive. The enormous increase in surgery, and the development of technology, led both to much greater numbers of patients and to much higher costs per patient. Voluntary hospitals ran into financial difficulties. In the United States hospitals developed business strategies based on insurance that could attract the well-off. In the United Kingdom, where insurance was much less well developed, hospitals were eventually brought into public ownership. In Scandinavia local authorities had had responsibility for pro-

viding hospital services since the late nineteenth century and so they developed largely as a public service (Abel-Smith, 1994). The strong development of the discipline of public health in the nineteenth century was a response to the disease hazards of the urban environment. In England and Germany public health measures focused on safe water supply and drains.

Over the eighteenth and nineteenth centuries, modern forms of medical regulation developed. Countries in which medicine was dominated by free markets (such as the United States) converged with countries in Europe with strong state control (such as Germany) to produce the closely regulated medical markets that exist today. However, the degree of state involvement in the provision of health services varied enormously between countries, as it still does.

A key development was the increase in collective arrangements for funding health services. State services developed in all Western countries to provide health services for those who could not afford to purchase it themselves. In addition, mutual insurance schemes developed in Europe and the United States to protect workers against financial losses, and these often included medical care (Abel-Smith, 1994). These schemes were encouraged by the German states and developed into a national program of health insurance. In the United Kingdom, in contrast, they were nationalized as part of the expansion of state welfare. Other European countries also saw the development and expansion of compulsory financial arrangements for health services, whether through the extension of insurance arrangements for medical care (the Bismarck model—named after the German chancellor who introduced the first compulsory insurance scheme) or through general taxation (the Beveridge model—named after the British minister of health who is regarded as the founder of the United Kingdom National Health Service). Since World War II, all high-income countries, with the exception of the United States, have extended mechanisms for protection against the financial risks of ill health to the point where they can be said to have achieved "universal coverage."

Another key development in the creation of the modern health system was the development of organized systems of medical care, as opposed to fragmented and competing individual doctors and hospitals. World War I marked a turning point in Europe, when the need to organize medical care on a massive scale highlighted the advantages of a large, coordinated system. In the United Kingdom the Dawson report in 1920 designed a system of district health services based on general practitioners and health centers, with referral upward to hospital (WHO,

1999). The later development of the philosophy of national economic plans, and a strong government role in many sectors of the economy, also supported the development of organized health systems. Even in those countries with less of a tradition of a strong state role in health services, cost escalation in recent decades has forced greater state involvement.

In the late nineteenth century Western medicine spread around the world, often as part of the process of colonial expansion (Zwi & Mills, 1995). Medicine acted in part as an agency of Western imperialism, and organized health services were a component of British, French, German, and Belgian colonization. These were initially intended for the military, settler, and civil service communities, but it rapidly became apparent that protecting the health of expatriates required addressing health needs among the colonized. In addition, health services were introduced by commercial interests if they felt economic returns would improve, and by the church as part of missionary activities. To a much greater extent than was the case in the home countries of the colonizers, the provision of health services became associated with the state. This was accentuated in the postcolonial era by the prevalent ideologies of state-led growth and state responsibility for the welfare of all inhabitants. This was seen in its most extreme form in socialist countries such as Tanzania, China, and Vietnam, which banned private practice. However, more generally in Africa and Asia, attention of policy makers focused on publicly financed and provided services, neglecting the often large private sector. The aim was to extend public services to cover the whole population, even if the reality was very different.

Developments in Latin America were somewhat different. As in Africa, the earliest Western health services were developed by the colonists, especially for the armed forces and the police. Major employers provided health services, especially where enterprises were remote from urban centers. Some religious hospitals were built to care for the poor (Abel-Smith, 1994). These hospitals were later supplemented by government hospitals and clinics, especially in areas without charitable hospitals. A key difference with most of Africa and Asia was the early development of compulsory insurance arrangements for workers in the formal sector. Since medical care infrastructure was lacking, the insurance agencies often built and ran their own services, thus contributing to the parallel health systems seen today in many Latin American countries.

The historical development of health services in many countries resulted in a health infrastructure that was biased toward hospitals. Attempts to reorientate services culminated in 1978 in the Declaration of Alma Ata, which emphasized the importance of primary health care, involving the delivery of curative and preventive services at community level. This encouraged strong emphasis on the building up of integrated health services, involving community-based health workers. Nonetheless, a rival approach argued in favor of selective primary health care, to include those interventions that addressed the greatest disease burden and were most cost-effective (Walsh & Warren, 1979). Services for children were a key priority in this approach, and, together with the emphasis on family planning that resulted from the preoccupation of many donors with world population growth, meant that peripheral health services in many low-income countries were targeted primarily at women and children. Only recently has there been greater emphasis on achieving a more integrated approach to the delivery of health services at peripheral levels.

A marked development in recent years in low- and middle-income countries has been the increasing questioning of the government's role. The most radical changes have occurred in countries formerly under strict communist rule, where a market economy has been introduced and market forces allowed to influence health services (see Saltman & Figueras, 1997, for such developments in eastern and central Europe). Social insurance arrangements are being introduced for those in formal employment, health professionals allowed to do private practice, private markets encouraged in pharmaceuticals,

and much greater costs are falling directly on household budgets. In China, for example, in 1981 approximately 71% of the population—including 48% of the rural population—had some insurance protection; by 1993 overall insurance coverage had dropped to 21%, with 7% coverage of the rural population (WHO, 1999). Although changes have been less radical in other parts of the world, governments have been forced by economic crisis to consider how they can best prioritize what they do and ration services to those most in need; many have introduced revenue generation schemes, such as user fees. This reconsideration has also been forced by rapidly growing private markets in medical care.

## THE ROLE OF THE STATE

This brief historical review indicates that one of the key issues in the design of health systems is the role assigned to the state. This section examines the economic arguments commonly put forward to specify the state's role in health, and then considers other explanations for the roles observed in practice.

The first main economic justification lies in explanations of market failure. The efficient outcomes of private markets depend on a number of conditions being met. Because of the particular characteristics of health and health services, this may not be the case.

First, the presence of externalities means that the optimal amount would not be produced or consumed. Externalities are costs or benefits that are not taken into account in the transactions of producers or consumers. For example, an individual's decision on whether to be immunized will be related to the value of the protection to that individual, not to protection that may be accorded to others by reducing the pool of susceptible individuals.

Second, for goods that are "public goods," the market may fail to produce them at all. Such goods are those where consumption is "nonrival" (consumption by one person does not reduce the consumption of another) and nonexcludable (a consumer cannot be prevented from benefiting from the good—for example, through requiring payment). Control of mosquito breeding sites to reduce malaria transmission is an obvious example: all living in the area will benefit regardless of whether they have paid. Information can also be seen to be a public good since it is nonrival; it is not nonexcludable, but the cost of providing information to extra people is often very low. This applies to knowledge gained through research, for example.

Third, monopoly power can lead to market failure, because it enables the provider to charge more than if the market were competitive. Monopoly power may be held by a hospital in a particular geographical area, by a pharmaceutical firm, or even by a profession as a whole (such as the medical profession).

These arguments provide a rather weak justification for state intervention in the entire health system since the range of services they apply to is quite limited. The arguments are most relevant to public health services and preventive care, and less relevant to the bulk of curative services. Moreover, problems such as monopoly are not unique to health and are commonly dealt with by regulation rather than state provision. A more powerful argument for a large state role lies in the asymmetry of information between provider and consumer. Medical consultations are often sought precisely because patients do not know what is wrong with them: they are therefore ill-informed, in contrast to the normal assumption in economics of perfectly informed consumers. Hence in medical care, providers are in an unusually strong position. While they may act as perfect agents for the consumer, it is also possible, especially when income is related to care provided, that the personal interests of the providers may enter into decisions made on treatment. The poor and less well educated are particularly vulnerable to unscrupulous profit-seeking by private providers.

Another characteristic of health care is its uncertain nature, and the potential for very high costs. This makes it an obvious candidate for insurance, but it is generally accepted that private insurance markets do not work well (World Bank, 1997a). Individuals who purchase insurance may indulge in activities that put their health more at risk than if they were not insured, or once ill may consume more health care. This phenomenon is known as moral hazard and will raise the cost of insurance, making it unaffordable for some. Another problem is that those who are at greatest risk of needing care will be more likely to seek insurance, but due to asymmetries of information between insurer and insured, it is often difficult for the insurer to tailor the premium charged to the nature of the risk. This process, known as adverse selection, means that the insurer ends up with a more costly risk pool, premiums rise, and the more healthy opt out. In addition, insurance becomes more expensive, excluding many who cannot afford the increased premiums. Although the result is clearly inequitable, it is also inefficient because there will be people unprotected who would be willing and able to purchase insurance if the market worked well.

There are also arguments in favor of state involvement that are distinct from those of market failure. One is the argument that some types of health services are "merit goods": goods that society believes should be provided, but that individuals, if left to themselves, might underconsume because they are not the best judge of what is in their own or the public's interest. This argument is strongest for health services for children and the mentally ill.

The other argument is founded on equity principles: that even with perfectly operating private markets for health services and health insurance, there will be individuals too poor to afford to access them. Although it could be argued that this problem could be taken care of by income redistribution policies, equitable access to health services is of concern, and hence it can be argued that providing benefits in kind is appropriate.

Although these are the standard arguments used to explore the appropriate role of the state in health services, the judgment on their significance differs enormously between economists, leading to radically different policy prescriptions. Even though much of this debate has focused on the relative merits of the United States versus the Canadian or British health systems, it has influenced the nature of the debate concerning the reform of health systems in low- and middle-income countries, as noted later in discussion of health reform trends. Underlying this debate are alternative views on the ethical basis of a health system. One view sees access to health services as similar to access to other goods and services, and dependent on an individual's success in gaining or inheriting income. The other sees access to health services as a right of citizenship that should not depend on individual income or wealth. According to the first view, the state's role in health would be confined to regulation of the market, public health measures, and public welfare for the poor to provide a minimum acceptable level of service, but nothing like the level of service available to those better off. According to the second view, the role of the state should be to ensure equal access to health services that does not differ depending on economic or social status.

It is important to note that while economic arguments provide justification for state involvement, they provide little guidance on the precise nature of intervention, and in particular they do not necessarily imply that the state should itself provide health services (as opposed to contracting others to provide it). A key change in recent decades in thinking about public management has been the recognition that the state need not provide services itself directly, but instead could play an "enabling" role (Walsh, 1995).

An important influence on this position is a recognition that in many countries the state has failed in its policies to provide public services, including health services, for everyone. These arguments derive from a number of strands of economic thinking, notable among which are public choice theory and property rights theories. The former is concerned with the nature of decision making in government. It argues that government officials are no different from anyone else in pursuing their own interest. Thus politicians will be concerned to maximize their chances of being reelected, and bureaucrats will

serve their own interests (for example, maximize their budget because their own rewards [salary, status] are related to that). The result is that the public sector is wasteful because politicians and bureaucrats have no incentive to promote allocative or technical efficiency.

Property rights theorists argue that the source of inefficiency in the public sector is the weakening of property rights. In the private sector it can be argued that the entrepreneur, or the shareholders, have a strong interest in the efficient use of resources. In the public sector there is little obvious threat to the enterprise if staff perform poorly; hence incentives to efficient performance are weak.

These theories underlie what has been termed the "new public management," which seeks to expose public services to market pressures, without necessarily privatizing them (Walsh, 1995). Such approaches change the nature of state involvement, with policies of opening up services to competitive tender or putting services out to contract on a competitive basis, introducing "internal markets" where public providers have to compete for contracts from public purchasers, devolving financial control to organizations such as individual hospitals, and spinning off parts of government into separate public agencies (such as an agency to manage government health services, as in Zambia).

Although theories justifying particular roles of the state feature prominently in writings on health systems, it is clear in practice that the actual role of the state in any particular country is shaped by a wide variety of influences. Most notable are the history of state involvement in health services and the rationale for its involvement over time, the extent to which private providers and insurers developed early in the history of the development of the health system and thus were able to play a prominent role, and the attitude of the medical profession to an increased state role (Mills et al., in press). One key issue has been the extent to which the state took on itself the responsibility for providing services to the whole population, or instead concerned itself only with the poor and indigent.

Exhibit 10–2 summarizes the role of the state in four countries. In Zambia and India, the state's aims have historically been to provide services free at the point of use to the whole population. In contrast, both Mexico and Thailand have had specific schemes that cater to the poor and indigent.

## REGULATION

Regulation is the role that all governments must carry out, regardless of their degree of involvement in health service provision. It occurs when government exerts control over the activities of individuals and firms (Roemer, 1993). Its traditional rationale relates to the arguments of market failure outlined above and also to the desire of governments to meet other social objectives, such as equity. Market failure creates the need either to regulate to make the market work better (for example, to limit the control any one pharmaceutical firm may have over the market) or to prevent harmful effects (for example, to ensure minimum quality standards

---

**Exhibit 10–2** Illustrations of the Role of the State

| Zambia | India |
|---|---|
| Health services for the whole population have traditionally been seen as the responsibility of the state (2.6% GDP; 78% of total health expenditure (Bos et al., 1998); 75% of hospital beds). Independence brought in a government that was anti-private sector and, until recently, the private health sector was ignored in government policy. Reforms have decentralized public management and introduced fees for public services. Management reforms specify a purchasing role for district authorities. The poor are reliant mainly on state services and the informal private sector. | The historical emphasis was on a strong state role, but resources were never provided to make this a reality (1.2% GDP; 22% of total health expenditure (Bos et al., 1998); 68% of total hospital beds). Public services are often of poor quality and are adversely affected by the private practice of government doctors. People in general distrust the state. Charging policies for public facilities vary by state, but income from fees is very small. There is widespread use of the private sector by all sections of the population, including the poor. |
| **Mexico** | **Thailand** |
| The public health sector makes up 2.8% of GDP, 57.3% of total health expenditure (Fundacion Mexicana para la Salud, 1994), and 80% of hospital beds (Fundacion Mexicana para la Salud, 1995). The government's primary role is as owner of social security institutions, which account for some 44% of all health expenditures, and cover approximately 60% of the total population. Ministry of Health and municipalities play a residual role in caring for the poor and uninsured. There is dissatisfaction with the quality of both MOH and social security services, with those who can afford it preferring to use private services. | The public health sector is 1.7% GDP, 49% of total health expenditure (Tangcharoensahien et al., 1999); and 77% of total hospital beds. There is a tradition of strong central government and laissez-faire economic policies. Public hospitals charge substantial fees, with exemption schemes for the poor and vulnerable groups. Government policies have encouraged the private sector to grow through tax exemptions and public funding for private care for specific groups. Public services are of generally good quality; their main problem is a lack of consumer orientation. |

for private clinics). While regulation is often thought of as action involving control, sanctions, and penalties, it can also take the form of incentives to encourage appropriate behavior. In health services, where outcomes are difficult to observe (that is, it can be difficult to relate treatment to change in health), it can be argued that incentives are particularly appropriate and are currently the subject of much interest, with consideration of what is termed "incentive regulation" (Kumaranayake, 1998).

In practice, regulatory action seeks to influence:

- market entry and exit
- remuneration of providers
- quality and distribution of services
- standards and quality

Key mechanisms used in the health system to regulate the provision of health services are summarized in Table 10–2. Controls over market entry and exit are not shown separately since they also serve to influence quantities and quality.

Licensing of professionals to provide services is one of the key regulations, with professional councils usually being empowered to carry out this function. As new professions arise or become more important, eventually they are brought within the scope of laws. While such laws dictate entry into the market, their prime rationale from a government perspective is to maintain quality and protect the consumer. However, actual experience demonstrates that licensing on its own is not adequate to ensure quality.

A second key regulation is licensing or registration of facilities, which is required before they can open. Legislation often specifies the requirements particular categories of facility should meet, covering such aspects as trained staff, availability of equipment and supplies, and buildings. Because of the cost-enhancing capabilities of high technology, some countries have an approval process for the purchase of equipment such as computed tomography scanners. Entry to medical school may also be controlled

with the same aim: controlling costs by limiting supply. In a normal market such action might be expected to raise costs, but it is considered justified in health because of the power physicians have to generate their own income or to prevail on government to employ greater numbers than the country can really afford.

Often countries are concerned about the geographical distribution of providers, and controls and incentives are used to influence where new providers can set up. For example, South African provinces can control the creation and expansion of private hospitals, depending on the number of private beds already existing. Certificate of need legislation has been used for many years to control the construction of new buildings and investment in new equipment in the United States (Kumaranayake, 1998).

Control of prices and reimbursement levels may have several purposes: to restrict incomes in the private sector so that remuneration differences between public and private professionals do not get too great; to ensure that health services remain affordable for the not-so-wealthy; and to restrict the financial burden placed on risk-pooling arrangements, such as social insurance or employer medical benefit schemes. However, given the power of the medical profession, there is a risk that price control operates more in the interests of the profession than the public; in addition it can be difficult to enforce or monitor.

Control of quality is one of the prime concerns of regulation. Licensing and registration have this as an aim, as well as control of quantity. For example, in Kenya a private clinic must be kept in good order and state of repair, not be a residential building, and keep essential drugs and accurate drug records.

Regulations often seek to control the nature of services provided, to ensure that services are within the competence of a particular type of provider and to limit the scope for excessive service provision. Regulations usually lay down what type of health professional can prescribe what type of drug, limiting, for example, the

**Table 10–2** Examples of Regulatory Mechanisms for Health Care Provision

| Variable | Mechanism | Examples from Low- and Middle-Income Countries |
|---|---|---|
| Quantities/ Distribution | • licensing providers<br>• licensing facilities | • universal for main professional groups<br>• increasingly common for hospitals and clinics |
| | • controls on number and size of medical schools | • common (for example, Latin America) |
| | • controls on practicing in overprovided areas | • South Africa, for private hospitals |
| | • controls on introduction of high technology | • being considered by Malaysia and Thailand |
| | • incentives to practice in underserved areas and specialities | • many countries for doctors, often in form of compulsory rural service |
| | • requiring capitation or case-based payment to control supply of services | • social insurance in Korea (case payment) and Thailand (capitation) |
| Prices | • negotiation of salary scales | • Zimbabwe nursing salaries; Argentina doctors |
| | • fixing of charges (for example, for lab tests, drug mark-up) | • South Africa: drug mark-up for reimbursement by medical schemes |
| | • negotiation of reimbursement rates | • many social insurance schemes (for example, Chile) |
| Quality | • licensing of practitioners<br>• registration of facilities | • universal for main professions<br>• increasingly common; specifies structural standards |
| | • control on nature of services provided | • restrictions on drug dispensing by general practitioners (for example, Zimbabwe); range of procedures (clinical officers, Kenya) |
| | • accessibility | • hospitals legally obliged to provide emergency care irrespective of patient financial status (Thailand, Malaysia) |
| | • required complaints procedures<br>• required provision of information for monitoring quality | • consumer laws applicable (India)<br>• many countries |
| | • control of training curricula<br>• requirements for continuing education | • many countries<br>• increasingly being introduced |
| | • accreditation | • increasingly being introduced; existing in Taiwan and pilot schemes in Brazil and Thailand |

range of drugs that can be given by low-level health workers. It is quite common for private practitioners to be allowed to dispense medicines only if there is no pharmacy nearby. Where this rule does not exist, drug dispensing is often a major source of the income of private doctors, leading to predictable concerns about overprescribing.

Control of training curricula is fundamental to ensuring quality, and is often one of the functions given by law to professional bodies. A trend in high-income countries, which is also becoming apparent elsewhere, is the requirement for professionals to receive regular refresher training if they are to continue to be licensed. Such a provision, however, is demanding on regulatory bodies, since it requires the introduction of monitoring procedures, training programs, and relicensing arrangements.

Accreditation is a process of certifying that a facility meets a certain standard, and is usually applied as a self-regulating procedure that is voluntary and managed by an independent body. However, in practice it may act more as a regulatory device than as a peer review process, especially when accreditation is required for hospitals to be eligible for reimbursement from a social insurance scheme, as in Taiwan.

There are also other markets with considerable relevance to health services that governments regulate. These include the health insurance and pharmaceutical markets. Both have features unique to themselves. In the case of insurance, regulations may impose a particular approach to risk pooling (for example, require schemes to give lifetime coverage, or use community rather than risk-rating). In the case of pharmaceuticals, regulations may establish which drugs can be imported and which will be sold over the counter or require a doctor's prescription, and may specify quality control procedures for imported and locally made drugs.

Separate consideration may also be given in regulatory structures to not-for-profit providers. On the one hand they may be treated more strictly: for example, their fee structures may be regulated, they may be required to provide a certain amount of free care to the poor, and requirements to provide information may be stricter. On the other hand they may benefit from their not-for-profit status: for example, tax exemptions are often available to them.

In practice, regulation encounters a number of key problems, as highlighted in Exhibit 10–3 (Mills et al., in press). One is that laws are frequently out of date and also difficult to change. For example, many low-income countries have laws they inherited from colonial regimes that have not kept pace with the development of the private sector, resulting in whole categories of facility that may be completely unregulated. Private laboratories are often a case in point.

Another problem is that regulation requires substantial knowledge on the part of the regulatory bodies. However, it is common in low- and middle-income countries for even basic information, such as lists of providers and facilities, to be incomplete. Moreover, the poorer the country the greater the proportion of providers who are small and informally organized, making it difficult to require any regular provision of information.

A third problem is that of "regulatory capture": the body meant to be doing the regulating in practice operates in the interests of those being regulated, not in the public interest. This is a common problem in the case of regulation of professional groups, which is often done by the profession itself, leading to the very slow processing of complaints and consideration of professional negligence. India has had the interesting experience of introducing a consumer rights law, which the courts have ruled applies to government health services as well as those that are privately provided, and which is providing an alternative channel for pursuing complaints. However, India is also a country where the overlap of public and private interests makes it extremely difficult to introduce new regulations or change existing laws. In India, as in a number of countries, it is common to find government-employed doctors doing private practice—with or without legal sanction—and senior Ministry of Health officials, as well as politi-

**Exhibit 10–3** Key Regulatory Problems

| **Zambia**[a] | **India** |
|---|---|
| • Antiquated laws<br>• Rapidly increasing private sector that is largely self-regulated<br>• Private physicians are required to register with government; otherwise there is really no infrastructure for collection of data on the private sector, or enforcement of laws and regulations | • In 1997 only three states required any registration and inspection of private hospitals<br>• Widespread practice by unqualified "doctors"<br>• Widespread unethical practices (for example, payments between hospitals and general practitioners to encourage referrals)<br>• Lack of database of private providers<br>• Inability to enforce regulations<br>• Regulatory bodies lack resources |
| **Mexico**[b] | **Thailand** |
| • Private hospitals are not subject to a strict process of accreditation that verifies their capacity to provide an acceptable standard of care<br>• Lack of control on pharmacists prescribing and selling most drugs<br>• Use of public facilities for treating private patients<br>• Resistance from the private sector to providing epidemiologic and other information<br><br>[a]Sally Lake, personal communication.<br>[b]Miguel Betancourt, personal communication. | • Insufficient information on activity in private sector<br>• Difficult to control unethical practices (for example, turning away emergency cases)<br>• Professional council regulation ineffective<br>• Regulatory bodies lack resources |

cians, having financial interests in private sector health services (Mills et al., in press). Thus a clear distinction between the regulators and those being regulated is absent.

A fourth problem is the inadequacy of the resources provided to the regulatory bodies to apply the laws effectively. Quality monitoring in particular requires regular inspection to ensure laws are being followed. This places great demands on the limited staff capacity of regulatory agencies, especially for drugs and clinics where outlets are numerous and widely dispersed. It also creates further difficulties when low-paid staff seek illicit payments in place of carrying out their job effectively. An extreme form of this is in China, where because government subsidies to public health activities have been severely cut, environmental health units are dependent on revenue generation for much of their income, and hence may inspect those firms that are more able to pay their fees. Those that are less profitable, and hence likely to have worse safety and hygiene practices, go uninspected.

A final problem is a lack of institutional structures to back up the regulatory process. Strong consumer groups, media, professional associations, and insurance agencies all have important roles to play (Kumaranayake, 1998). The consumer role is particularly important since consumers can identify problems through complaint procedures and legal action, and also levy pressure more broadly through consumer groups. However, the common imbalance in power and access to resources between consumers and professionals suggests that complementary pressures are also important: one source of these can be the purchasing agencies considered further below.

## FINANCING

This section establishes a conceptual model for describing the system for financing health services, defines and evaluates the major sources of health financing in developing countries, describes trends in health financing across countries, and presents the national health account (NHA) methodology that is increasingly being used to collect health financing data.

## Conceptual Model

Financing refers to the raising or collection of the revenue to pay for the operation of the system. Financing agents are those entities that collect money to pay providers on behalf of consumers. Financing agents may be publicly or privately owned, and may provide health services directly (for example, the Ministry of Health through public hospitals and health centers) or purchase health services from providers (for example, a private insurer may purchase inpatient care from a variety of hospitals).

There is some disagreement in the literature as to the definition of sources of financing. Sources may be defined as the *entities* who provide funds to financing agents (Berman, 1997). Individuals and firms can be thought of as the primary sources of funds. Individuals generate income in the form of wages or salaries, while businesses may earn profit on capital investments or rent on properties owned. Resources may pass through several levels of sources before reaching the agents. For example, the Ministry of Finance can be thought of as a secondary level source insofar as it generates funds by taxing the incomes of households and businesses, and then transfers these resources to other government agencies to purchase health services. A single entity may act both as a source and an agent of financing. For example, households commonly pay for health services both indirectly (through taxation, contributions to social and private insurance, donations to charities, and so on) and directly (through out-of-pocket payments).

More often, however, the term *source* is applied to the *method* whereby an agent mobilizes or collects resources. For example, the sources of financing to the Ministry of Health include personal and business taxes, and donations, loans, and grants from domestic and foreign

agencies. The sources of financing for private insurance agencies are premiums paid by the enrollees in these schemes. In this chapter, the term *source* is used with this definition in mind, unless otherwise indicated.

## Description and Evaluation of Predominant Sources

This section defines the most commonly used sources of financing and briefly discusses the efficiency, equity, and revenue generating ability of each source. Table 10–3 summarizes the relative merits of each source. The relative advantages of differing sources in pooling financial risks is dealt with in detail in Chapter 12, where a more detailed review of evidence on their efficiency and equity implications is also provided.

Efficiency with respect to a source of financing involves a number of elements, including administrative (or technical) efficiency, stability, and flexibility (Zschock, 1979). Administrative efficiency relates to the cost of the management of the system and is the difference between gross yield (all funds that are collected) and net yield (that portion of gross yield that is actually available for the purposes of health service delivery). This difference results from the costs of revenue collection, allocation, and distribution; advertising and promotion; and funds lost to corruption and fraud as well as the cost of fighting corruption and fraud. The stability of an agent is determined by the degree to which revenue raising varies with changes in economic or political conditions. Finally, for a financing agent to be efficient, there must be flexibility in terms of the allocation of funds to different expenditure categories. Least flexible are those sources of financing pledged to a specific activity. Public sector sources tend to be less flexible than private sector sources due to the stringent rules and regulations that are often applied to government spending, as well as the political constraints to reallocation.

The concepts of horizontal and vertical equity of financing were introduced earlier. With respect to vertical equity, a progressive system

**Table 10-3** Evaluation of Health Financing Sources

| | Efficiency | | | Equity | | Revenue Generation |
|---|---|---|---|---|---|---|
| | Administrative Efficiency | Stability | Flexibility | Horizontal | Vertical | |
| Public sources | | | | | | |
| general tax revenues | high | low | low | high | progressive | high |
| retail sales taxes | high | high | low | high | regressive | low |
| lotteries and betting | low | high | low | high | regressive | low |
| deficit financing | low | low | low | depends | depends | depends |
| external grants | low | low | low | high | progressive | low |
| social insurance | low | high | low | high | regressive | depends on size of formal sector |
| Private sources | | | | | | |
| households | low | high | high | low | regressive | high |
| employers | low to medium | high | variable | low | depends | low |
| private insurance | low | high | high | low | regressive | low |
| voluntary organizations | high | variable | variable | high | progressive | medium |

is one in which lower income groups pay a lower proportion of their income than higher income groups. A regressive system is one in which lower income groups pay a higher share of income than higher income groups. A proportional or neutral system is one in which all income groups pay the same percentage of their income.

Apart from problems of inefficiency and inequity, health systems in many low- and middle-income countries face the difficulty of simply not being able to generate sufficient funds to ensure that the entire population has access to a minimal package of health services. Thus a goal of the financing function of health systems is to increase the availability of funds for the purchase and provision of health services. As countries become richer and the demand for high-technology, hospital-based interventions increases, the goal generally shifts from generating funds to constraining the financial flow through the health system (that is, cost containment).

### Public Sources of Financing

Direct taxes are paid directly by individuals or organizations to government and include personal income tax, taxes on domestic business transactions and profits, duties on imports and exports, and property taxes. Some portion of these resources may then be allocated to the annual budget for health services. The best-known examples of general tax financing for health services are in the United Kingdom and other Commonwealth nations (Hsiao, 1995a).

Direct tax revenues should have relatively high net yields, but this will depend on the overhead costs of the government bureaucracy needed to collect, allocate, and disburse them. They may not be a particularly reliable or stable source, as the health sector must compete directly with other social and economic programs for a portion of the government's budget; as such, this source may fluctuate, depending on the economic and political climate. Furthermore, this source of financing is likely to be inflexible, as it is controlled by public sector agents that

are constrained by rules and regulations and the political feasibility of reallocations.

Direct taxation achieves horizontal equity insofar as taxes on individuals are generally not related to characteristics other than income. Income tax is generally the most progressive form of revenue raising, as income tax rates usually rise as a person's taxable income increases (Doorslaer, Wagstaff, & Rutten, 1993). For example, in Cote d'Ivoire income taxes range from 26% for the lowest income groups to 32% for the highest, and in Peru from 8% for the lowest income groups to 45% for the highest (Baker & van der Gaag, 1993). The ability of taxation to redistribute resources from the rich to the poor is hindered when the wealthy are able to evade the payment of taxes.

Ability to mobilize resources is another strength of direct taxation. Although most developing countries are restricted in their ability to collect income taxes and indirect taxes (due to limited infrastructure and small formal sectors), the government has many other options for generating tax revenue, including property, business, and import and export taxes. As a group, low- and middle-income country governments derive about 30% of their revenue from trade taxes (World Bank, 1997b).

Indirect taxes pass through an intermediary en route to government coffers. Indirect taxes are incorporated into the selling price of a good or service; these include sales and value-added taxes (taxes on a broad variety of items) and excise duties (imposed on the sale of specific items, such as tobacco products, beer, and liquor). Revenues generated in this manner are often allocated to finance specific programs. Taxes that are pledged to a specific sector or activity are termed *hypothecated*, and the practice is known as *earmarking*.

As with direct sales taxes, the net yield of indirect taxes will vary, depending on the efficiency of the government agency responsible for collecting them. Indirect taxes are likely to be reliable when they are earmarked for the health sector, or even specific projects within the health sector. The flexibility of this source may be constrained by the government rules and regulations that guide revenue allocation.

Indirect taxation, and excise duties in particular, are generally regressive, as poorer households often spend a higher percentage of their income on the goods being taxed (for example, alcohol and cigarettes). In the Philippines, for example, overall financing through the Ministry of Health is regressive as the bulk (60%) of public funds for health care is collected from indirect taxes. The effective (indirect and direct) tax rates for the lower, middle, and highest income classes are 27%, 32%, and 18%, respectively (WHO, 1993, p. 18).

Lotteries and betting may also serve as sources of earmarked income for health services, although these methods are not often used. They have low net yields as they are costly to administer. As with indirect taxes, the resulting revenues are likely to be reliable as they are earmarked, but inflexible as they are administered by public agents. As with retail sales taxes, lotteries and betting tend to fall particularly heavily on the earnings of the poor (because of their popularity among lower income groups).

National authorities can augment general tax revenues through domestic and international deficit financing. Funds are borrowed for a specific project or activity and have to be paid back to the source over some future period of time. Domestic deficit financing is usually achieved through the issue of debt certificates, or bonds, with guaranteed interest rates. International borrowing is typically in the form of loans from bilateral and multilateral organizations.

The largest single international financier of health services in low- and middle-income countries is the World Bank (1999). Two types of loans are provided by the World Bank. The first type is for developing countries that are able to pay near-market interest rates. The second type of loan goes to the poorest countries (GNP per capita below an established threshold, currently US$930). These loans are free of interest, carry a low 0.75% annual administrative charge, and are very long term (35 or 40 years including 10 years grace). Loans that bear an interest rate substantially below market interest rates are termed *soft loans*.

The costs of processing and administering loans in the health sector are usually quite high, resulting in poor administrative efficiency. Stability is limited insofar as these loans are typically of short duration with no guarantee of renewal. The flexibility of loan financing is variable. At one time, it was common for loans to be made for specific, free-standing health projects. With such loans, decisions on expenditure are usually made prior to disbursement. Increasingly, donor assistance is being made to sector investment programs (SIPs), whereby government and donors agree to a public-expenditure program that incorporates both domestic and foreign resources. Under SIPs there may be more flexibility over time in the spending of donor funding. On the other hand, the process of shifting funds from one expenditure category to another may be more complicated under SIPs, as both government and donors must agree on reforms.

The equity of deficit financing will depend entirely on how the loan is ultimately paid back. If, for example, funds generated through direct taxation are used to pay back a loan, then their impact may be progressive. Domestic and international borrowing are generally minor sources of health financing in low- and middle-income countries.

External grants are charitable donations (to governments), by foreign governments or organizations, that do not have to be repaid. Efficiency of external grants is the same as for deficit financing. External grants should be equitable as they are provided by wealthy nations and are commonly used to establish and run projects in remote or underserved areas. However, the extent to which they actually achieve a progressive redistribution of resources will depend on the extent to which the government shifts spending as the result of the grants. Only limited resources are generated through external grants except in the very poorest countries: donations (both public and private) are estimated to account for less than 1% of total spending in both India and Thailand.

Social insurance premiums are mandatory insurance payments made by employers and employees in the formal sector, usually as a percentage of wages, and hence often termed payroll taxes. Social insurance payments can have relatively low net yields due to the cost of processing claims. According to WHO (1993), administrative costs in western European insurance funds amount to approximately 5%, compared to an upper limit of 28% among social insurance schemes in Latin America, and potentially higher costs in Africa. The monies generated are likely to be stable as they are earmarked for the health sector; however, they may not be flexible, again related to government restrictions and requirements.

Social insurance is usually horizontally equitable as the value of premiums is based on income alone, but it tends to be a regressive method of raising revenue. This is because contributions are typically subject to a ceiling, although in some countries the marginal contribution rates themselves decline as earnings rise. Social insurance premiums may be progressive, for example, if ceilings can be eliminated or if low-income groups are exempt from contributions. Occasionally, contributions are levied at a flat rate for administrative simplicity, in which case the scheme is regressive.

Coverage achieved by social insurance schemes in many low- and middle-income countries has been limited, as premiums can only easily be collected from formal sector employees. This has given rise to much criticism of the equity of social insurance arrangements, since a relatively small proportion of the population has access to better services than much of the rest of the population, and in addition sometimes benefits also from government subsidies to the social insurance program. However, some countries, including Costa Rica, the Republic of Korea, and Taiwan, have achieved universal or near-universal coverage through combining funds from social insurance with general tax revenues, in order to ensure that all population groups have access to similar types and levels of care (Mills, 2000).

## Private Sources

Direct household expenditure includes all out-of-pocket payments or user fees paid by the consumer of health services directly to the provider (including private practitioners, traditional healers, and private pharmacists). Even services provided by the government or an insurance program may include some element of copayment, which may take a variety of different forms. Coinsurance means that the consumer is responsible for paying for a certain percentage of all services received. Limited indemnity means that the insurer only covers health service costs up to a prespecified absolute amount (or ceiling) above which the consumer is responsible for paying. A deductible is a specific amount that must be paid by the consumer above which reimbursement starts.

The administrative efficiency of direct household expenditure is low, due to the labor-intensive task of collecting fees from individuals. The stability of household spending on health will vary according to household income, but it is likely to be fairly stable unless economic crisis causes widespread poverty. Household spending is extremely flexible and will be allocated to the most pressing health needs as they are perceived by members of the household. Household spending is horizontally inequitable, as it varies according to factors such as distance lived from health facilities and individual preferences. Out-of-pocket payment is the most regressive modality of financing (Doorslaer et al., 1993).

Direct employer financing occurs when firms pay for, or directly provide, health services for their employees. Employers as agents are likely to be more efficient than households, though less efficient than compulsory purchasers of care (such as social insurance schemes) due to their fragmentation. Employer financing is likely to be reliable (in the absence of economic crisis) but relatively inflexible as employers are biased toward specific types of health services (for example, curative care). Direct payment by employers contributes to horizontal inequity in the health system as a whole, as employed workers are disproportionately young and healthy. Because the benefits of employer financing are generally restricted to employees of the formal sector, it is likely to have little impact on the redistribution of resources among different income groups. The quantity of resources mobilized by employees is high in some countries; for example, in Zambia financing provided by parastatal copper mines accounts for roughly 13% of all health resources (Department of Economics, University of Zambia, 1996). As governments implement social insurance schemes, these replace employer financing of health services.

Private health insurance premiums are regular, voluntary payments to private insurance companies in return for coverage of prespecified health service costs. Private insurance typically does not cover the costs of frequent, predictable events (such as pregnancies). Experience rating means that premiums are based on an individual's actuarially determined likelihood of illness. Community rating means that the premium is based on the pooled risk of a defined group of people (for example, inhabitants of a geographic area or employees of a firm).

Private health insurance tends not to be an efficient method of mobilizing funds for the health sector. Net yield is low because of the costs of marketing, claims processing, handling of reimbursements, and fraud detection. In unregulated markets, administration costs plus profits may account for up to 35–45% of the premiums. Private health insurance is a stable agent of financing, as it is not subject to political allocation processes and must be flexible in order to respond to consumers' needs and to attract clientele.

Private health insurance premiums are a perfect example of a horizontally inequitable source. Experience rating means that premiums will vary according to factors that are considered by the insurer to be related to risk of illness, such as age, sex, and occupation. Private insurance tends to be regressive because rates are adjusted for risk, and the poor are at highest risk of falling ill. The ability to mobilize resources through private insurance is limited in poorer countries, as these schemes are targeted at a very small

(although well-off) segment of the population— less than 2% of the population in most cases.

Charitable contributions are contributions made in cash or in kind. Examples include cash contributions from wealthy families, business enterprises, or religious organizations; community labor for construction and maintenance of local health facilities, including clinics as well as environmental sanitation projects; and local help in specific disease eradication campaigns. Voluntary organizations (or nongovernmental organizations [NGOs]) have high net yields, although they may be unpredictable in their ability to generate funds. The flexibility will vary from one voluntary organization to another, but generally they prefer to fund specific types of health services, not necessarily those most suitable for the community being served. Voluntary organization funding should be progressive in that they raise revenue from the better-off, although their ability to mobilize resources is limited.

### Mixes of Financing Sources

No one source of financing stands out as being superior in terms of all the outcomes considered. Nor is there an optimal mix of sources that can be prescribed for all countries. Countries vary in terms of the number of different financing agents and methods that are used, and the mix can change over time within a country. The mix of sources used will depend in part on the relative importance that policy makers place on the various objectives described above and in part on the mix of sources historically used in that country. Most low- and middle-income countries have more pluralistic health financing structures than are found in high-income countries. Low-income countries typically finance the bulk of their health care expenditures from (1) direct household expenditure, (2) taxation, and (3) deficit spending. The most important financing agents are typically the Ministry of Health (and other government agencies), households, and firms.

Although using a variety of sources may increase the resources available for health care and may allow better adaptation to the diverse social and economic conditions that may exist within a country, it makes the pursuit of health policy goals more complex than in a single-source system (WHO, 1993). The greatest risks in a pluralistic health financing system are those of "duplication and overlap in function and coverage" (WHO, 1993, p. 13). According to Mach and Abel-Smith (1983, p. 13), "in many countries the different financial sectors of the national health effort operate in watertight compartments even when there are monetary flows between them." This adversely affects both efficiency, because of duplication, and equity, because of limited risk-pooling and cross-subsidies between income groups.

Another complex but important issue relates to the displacement effect that one source of finance may have on others (termed *fungibility*). The introduction or expansion of one source of financing may impact on the efficiency, equity, or revenue-generating ability of other sources. This may be especially important when large external grants or loans are introduced into a health sector. For example, it might seem that a large external grant earmarked for the treatment of tuberculosis among the rural poor would be equitable. However, in response to such a grant, the Ministry of Health may shift resources that would have been spent on this activity toward high-technology, hospital-based services. Thus the positive impact that the new source of funding has on equity might be counterbalanced by the negative equity impact of displacement. Fungibility is one of the rationales for SIPs.

### Health Financing Innovations

Certain approaches to raising finance recently have gained popularity as means of improving efficiency, equity, or resource-generating ability. These approaches include community financing, medical savings accounts (MSAs), and a variety of targeted user fees.

Community financing does not refer to a special source of financing, but rather to programs where the community manages the collection of resources and the purchasing of health services (that is, the community acts as the financing

agent). Resources for community financing may be generated through voluntary contributions, user fees, or insurance premiums. Community management can potentially improve the efficiency, equity, and revenue-generating ability of these sources of financing, although experience is quite varied (McPake, Hanson, & Mills, 1992; Stinson, 1982).

MSAs involve prepayment for health care, but there is no pooling of resources and thus no risk sharing. Generally, individuals are compelled to deposit a fixed portion of their earnings in the MSAs. Withdrawals can only be made to pay for hospital services and selected (typically expensive) outpatient services. Individuals may choose from public and private caregivers. MSAs may be used in combination with a risk-sharing scheme (for example, social insurance) to cover especially expensive services (as is the case in Singapore). Upon death, any balance left in an MSA becomes part of a person's estate and may be willed to family, friends, or charity (Hsiao, 1995b). MSAs were first implemented in Singapore and have created widespread interest, particularly in their emphasis on the responsibility of the family to finance the lifetime health care needs of its members. By making individuals responsible for managing their health care funds, the Singapore government hoped that MSAs would provide incentives for consumers to be more cost-sensitive in their demand for health services; evidence suggests that this aspect of the scheme has not been very successful (Hsiao, 1995b).

Abel-Smith (1994) provides examples of how direct spending by households and firms can be made more equitable through targeted user fees:

- charges levied on employers to recoup the full cost of treating accidents at work
- fees charged to cover the cost of treating motor accident cases and claimed from the insurance policies of the victims
- full cost charges for patients who bypass the referral system by going directly to hospitals without being referred or being a genuine emergency

- charges for private rooms at government hospitals that cover the full costs
- pay clinics at government facilities outside normal working hours for those who are willing to pay and want to avoid queues

Historically, many of these charges have been opposed within the public system, as acknowledging the existence of two-tier services (different facilities for paying and nonpaying patients). However, economic realities and the need to exploit all possible sources of revenue for public services are changing these attitudes.

## Compiling Financing Data: National Health Accounts

The development of improved financing policies is limited by the availability of good information on financial flows. This hampers both national analysis and also cross-country comparisons:

> cross-country comparisons of health financing data are often difficult because of the lack of reliable data on out-of-pocket expenditures. Where these exist at all, estimates are often incomplete and prone to measurement errors. Furthermore, private health expenditures are rarely disaggregated into different forms of payments, such as direct fees for service, insurance premiums or other forms of prepayments, and cost-sharing payments (Bos et al., 1998, p. 6).

Emphasis recently has been placed on creating a national health account, which is a statement that provides information about the flow of health funds between sources (here referring to the entities that provide funds), agents, and uses in a country (Berman, 1997). The NHA is intended to give a comprehensive picture of both public and private health spending. It requires calculation and presentation of national estimates through a "sources and uses" matrix. Table 10–4 provides such a matrix for national

health expenditure in India, and Exhibit 10–4 highlights the findings of NHA studies carried out in Zambia, India, Mexico, and Thailand (caution is required in comparing the NHAs in these four countries; despite using similar methodologies, strikingly different categories and data sources were used).

The main objective of NHAs is to provide the key pieces of information required by decision makers. By systematically bringing together data on sources, agents, and uses of health funds, the NHA can provide answers to many different questions. Data contained in the NHA include:

- total health expenditures
- proportion of funds from different sources, including out-of-pocket payments
- health expenditure by level of care

An NHA enables concrete answers to be given to questions such as the extent to which expenditure is biased in favor of hospitals, and to what extent the burden of paying for care falls on out-of-pocket payment by households. In addition, the NHA provides a framework for modeling reforms and monitoring the effects of changes in financing and provision.

Establishing an NHA generally involves four steps (Griffiths & Mills, 1983):

1. define what criteria distinguish "health expenditure" from other expenditures
2. define categories of sources, agents, and uses into which the NHA can be divided
3. collect the data
4. present the results, usually using a sources and uses matrix, and identifying policy implications

Although this four-step process sounds quite simple, complications can arise at almost every step.

It is widely accepted that NHAs should be limited to expenditures with the primary intention of improving health. This excludes expenditures that have health effects, but whose primary goal is not health (for example, housing, food subsidies, and urban water supply proj-

**Table 10–4** India: An Estimated "Sources and Uses" Matrix for National Health Expenditure in 1991 (as a Percentage of Total Expenditure)

| | Sources | | | | |
|---|---|---|---|---|---|
| Uses | Central Government | State and Local Government | Corporate/ Third Party | Households | Total |
| Primary care | 4.3 | 5.6 | 0.8 | 48.0 | 58.7 |
| curative | (0.4) | (3.0) | (0.8) | (45.6) | (49.8) |
| preventive and public health | (4.0) | (2.7) | (NA) | (2.4) | (9.0) |
| Secondary/tertiary inpatient care | 0.9 | 8.4 | 2.5 | 27.0 | 38.8 |
| Nonservice provision | 0.9 | 1.6 | NA | NA | 2.5 |
| Total | 6.1 | 15.6 | 3.3 | 75.0 | 100.0 |

*Note:* Totals may not add due to rounding. NA = not available.

ects). There are, however, many areas of uncertainty. NHAs often fail to capture private expenditures on traditional or nonallopathic providers, such as faith healers, midwives, and practitioners of herbal medicine. Further, it may be difficult to determine when activities performed under the auspices of the education, agriculture, or labor ministries are performed with the primary intention of improving health. Zschock (1979), for example, suggests that the cost of practical training of practitioners be included while the cost of formal medical training (often funded in the education sector) be excluded. Where there is uncertainty, researchers should indicate clearly what has been included in a definition, and, where possible, expenditures should be recorded as separate line items (Berman, 1997).

Defining categories of sources, agents, and uses can also pose difficulties. For example, substantial differences between two health expenditure studies in Thailand were attributed in part to differences in categorizing medical benefits provided by state-owned firms. One study considered these benefits to represent income transfers to household members and classified them as private health sector expenditures. The other considered the state-owned firm to be the agent, and classified the expenditures as public (Tangcharoensathien et al., 1999).

Data for NHAs are collected from a great variety of sources, including spending records, records of social and private insurance institutions, sample surveys of firms, national consumer expenditure surveys, and more focused household health utilization and expenditure surveys. In countries where similar data may be collected from more than one source, comparison and triangulation from the different sources helps to improve the accuracy of the results. Perhaps the biggest problem in collecting data on government expenditures is finding data on funds spent as opposed to budgeted. Far more significant problems occur in estimating private health expenditures, specifically the expenditure size and composition of firms and households. Where secondary data are not available, primary data may need to be collected through firm and household surveys.

## RESOURCE ALLOCATION

The significance of processes of resource allocation in a health system has been clearly acknowledged only in the past decade or so. Financing agents, such as government bodies at various levels (ministries of health and provincial offices), social insurance agencies, and private insurers, have always been one of the components of a health system, channeling funds

**Exhibit 10-4** Key Findings of National Health Accounts Studies

| Zambia[a] | India[b] |
|---|---|
| **Sources:** Approximately 40% of health care resources are provided by the government of Zambia. Other major sources include external donors (30%), the semiautonomous copper mines (13%), and households (11–16%). **Uses:** The Ministry of Health accounts for 61% of health care expenditures. Other "uses" include facilities owned by copper mines (14%) and missions (5%). Private clinics account for only 3% of expenditures and private chemist shops 7%. **Flows:** More than 60% of direct household spending is accounted for by private chemist stores (and more than 12% goes on traditional healers). | **Sources:** Households are the source of 75% of health care spending. Other major sources include state and local governments (16%) and the central government (6%). External donations are estimated at less than 1%. **Uses:** Curative primary care accounts for almost 50% of health care expenditure, and secondary and tertiary inpatient care almost 40%. **Flows:** Together, all levels of government spend a greater percentage of their resources on inpatient care (43%) than do households (36%). |
| **Mexico[c]** | **Thailand[d]** |
| **Sources:** The sources are households (49%), firms (30%), and the federal government (21%). The major financing agents are social security institutes (45%), private funds (firm and household, 40%), and other government agencies (12%). **Uses:** 44% of total health expenditures are on social security services, 43% on private services, and roughly 13% on services provided by other government agencies. **Flows:** Very little money flows from social security institutions into the private sector (only 1% of spending by these institutions). Funds from other government agencies are spent exclusively on public services. Only a small percentage of private spending is on government services (roughly 1%). | **Sources:** Households and central government both account for approximately 40% of health care resources. Smaller sources (each accounting for 2–4%) include local governments, the social insurance scheme, private firms, and private insurance companies. Donors are estimated to account for only 0.23% of spending. **Uses:** Roughly 6% of total expenses are administrative. Public and private providers both account for roughly 40% of total health care spending. **Flows:** Only 8% of spending by public agents flows to private providers. Approximately 29% of spending by private agents flows to public providers. |

[a]Department of Economics, University of Zambia and Swedish Institute for Health Economics, 1996.
[b]Berman, 1995.
[c]Fundacion Mexicana para la Salud., 1994.
[d]Tangcharoensathien et al., 1999.

from sources (taxpayers, payers of insurance premiums) to providers. What is new is an emphasis on their role as active purchasers of services rather than passive allocators of funds. For government bodies, such as the Ministries of Health, this has demanded the creation of a clear distinction between their role of purchasing health services and their role as providers of health services. For other financing agents, this requires them to take a much more active role in decisions on which services should be paid for and how they should be paid for.

## The Purchasing Role

An emphasis on the purchasing role has arisen for a number of reasons:

- Integrated systems of purchasing and provision, such as those created in 1948 in the United Kingdom national health service and existing in many similar public systems across the world, are thought to operate more in the interests of providers than the general public and to lack incentives to be technically efficient; highlighting purchasing as a separate function helps redress the balance and strengthen the power of managers.
- Patients, who in markets for other goods and services would be the purchasers, are believed—for the reasons laid out earlier—to be in a weak position to be active purchasers.
- In health systems such as the United States, where there is third-party payment (that is, insurance agencies pay providers), cost escalation has been a major problem because patients chose their health provider, who was then reimbursed by the insurer. Although the insurers funded a large volume of services, traditionally they did not use this power to influence either the quantity or price of services provided. The development of ideas of "managed care" (Witter, 1997) has led to an emphasis on the role of the purchaser as "managing" the provision of health services and ensuring that there are incentives for efficiency and cost containment (and also for equity where the purchaser has public responsibilities).

Purchasers may be of different types and sizes. The most limited role would be that assumed by an insurance agency whose concerns are solely the patient group it cares for and ensuring it maintains its position in the marketplace. The most extensive role is where a purchaser has responsibilities for the health services of the population of a defined geographical area,

and hence can plan services on a population basis. This is the position of public purchasers in health systems that were previously integrated but where the roles of purchaser and provider have been distinguished. Exhibit 10–5 sets out the main stages in purchasing for this type of purchaser. In many ways this is no more than a traditional planning cycle; what marks it as different is that the concern of the purchaser is not to maintain a network of services but to purchase services to meet the needs of its population. The contracts that are agreed upon with providers may be formal legal contracts (and would need to be where providers are private bodies) or may simply be management agreements. As discussed below in "Health System Reform," contractual relationships have become one of the key features of health reform plans in a number of countries.

A key issue in the design of a purchasing role is whether there should be a single purchaser or a number of purchasers who compete among each other for clients. Private insurance agencies compete for clients, and it can be argued that this ensures that there are pressures for efficiency and services that meet client preferences. It remains an open question for tax and social insurance funded health systems whether a single purchaser or multiple purchasers is desirable. There is much caution about encouraging competition among purchasers:

- If the system of allocating funds does not provide adequate compensation for meeting the costs of the health risks covered, the purchaser will have an incentive to avoid enrolling the more expensive risks; this problem is known as "cream-skimming." In reality, it is difficult to predict the health service needs of a given population and compensate purchasers appropriately.
- It can be difficult for individuals to choose between competing purchasers: the more superficial aspects of the promised package of health services may influence them, rather than technical quality, which is more

**Exhibit 10–5** Stages in Purchasing

1. Assess needs of population.
2. Identify cost-effective strategies to meet needs.
3. Relate strategies to existing services to identify scope for change.
4. Consult public/patients/professionals on their values and priorities.
5. Draw up health service objectives and priorities.
6. Draw up contract specifications.
7. Verify contracts with providers, including service quantity, quality, and cost.
8. Monitor performance of providers directly and through surveys.
9. Feed this information back into next round of needs assessment, priority setting, and contracting.

difficult to judge. This would then lead purchasers to compete on the superficial aspects.

- If there are economies of scale in purchasing, these may be lost.
- Transactions costs—the costs of agreeing arrangements for purchasing services—may be higher.

Whatever the number of purchasers, information systems are crucial in enabling purchasers to carry out their role. Government health systems traditionally have poor information on cost and quality, and hence new systems have to be developed to underpin the purchasing function. Insurance agencies often have much information since they are paying for services, but commonly do not exploit these data to monitor providers. Purchasers need information in order to act as active purchasers; this includes information on provider performance (for example, waiting times, specific health outcomes where this can clearly be related to services provided) and adherence to standard treatment protocols (for example, with respect to use of antibiotics).

## Payment Mechanisms

A key influence on the success with which the purchasing role is carried out is the method chosen to pay providers, whether these be bodies responsible for services for specific populations, individual providers, or specific facilities. Although financial remuneration is not the only influence on provider performance, it is a powerful one.

Authorities responsible for the provision of services to a specific population can be provided with a global budget. A key issue is how that budget is determined. There has been increasing interest in using a resource allocation formula to calculate the budget appropriate to the populations of different geographical areas. The most well-known example is that of the United Kingdom, where funds have been allocated from the national level to regions using a formula that reflects the "need" for health services of each region, as proxied by indicators such as size of population and standardized mortality ratios (Department of Health and Social Security, 1976). Similar formulas are being used in South Africa and Zambia to allocate funds geographically. This approach will be combined with various means of paying individual providers and facilities within each geographical area.

Individual providers can be paid by salary, fee-for-service, or capitation. Salary represents a fixed annual payment unrelated to work load. Salary scales allow an individual's remuneration over time to be increased. While in theory this can be done on the basis of performance, in practice it is common for years of service alone to determine pay increases and promotions, thus undermining incentives to work hard. Another problem with salary payment that is not inherent in the method is the level of the salary. In low-income countries this is often very low, further weakening the incentive to work hard or to work the required number of hours, and encouraging staff to find additional ways of generating income, such as demanding informal payments from patients.

Additional elements can be added to salary payments to encourage good performance. These can be financial, as when an element of performance-related pay is included (for example, a pay increase or end-of-year bonus can be based on a performance assessment), or nonfinancial (award of certificates or other ways of giving recognition to high performers). Salary is the basis for remuneration in public systems, especially in hospitals and in privately owned facilities for nonmedical staff and even for physicians in some high-income countries. Although evidence is scanty, it is probably not uncommon in low- and middle-income countries for at least some of the physicians in private hospitals to be salaried.

Fee-for-service has traditionally been the payment method for general physicians and specialists in a number of countries in continental Europe and in North America and Japan. It has also been adopted in some new social insurance schemes in Asia and eastern Europe. It is usually the method of payment that physicians prefer since it does not involve an employer/employee relationship, and this explains its persistence despite known problems. Where a financial agent pays the bill, there will be agreement on the fee schedule, which is usually negotiated with the medical association.

From a patient's perspective—particularly a patient covered by insurance—fee-for-service is attractive. It readily permits free choice of doctor, since payment can follow the patient. It encourages the doctor to be responsive to the patient, and there is no incentive to under-provide. However, from a purchaser's perspective, fee-for-service payment encourages doctors to provide more consultations and more expensive procedures. Visit rates in countries using fee-for-service payment are often double those that use capitation, and more tests and drugs are also prescribed (Ensor, Witter, & Sheiman, 1997). Surgical rates are also often higher (Abel-Smith, 1994). Administrative costs are higher because of the need to monitor claims, and some degree of fraudulent claims is inevitable. When financ-

ing agents try to hold down costs by not increasing fee rates, there is good evidence that doctors respond by increasing the volume of service, as in Taiwan.

Some adjustments can be made to fee-for-service methods of payment to address some of these problems. For example, the overall budget can be fixed, as in Germany, so that volume of services in excess of that budgeted for will cause the fee per item of service to fall. Or copayments can be required from patients, although there is little good evidence that these act as a constraint on physicians' behavior, and they may simply render care unaffordable for lower-income groups in the population.

Capitation is most common for primary care services and involves a fixed payment per year per person registered with the provider. It may differ depending on the nature of the patient—for example, the elderly and children may attract a higher payment, reflecting their greater needs for health services. Capitation payment has been the traditional form of payment for general physicians in much of Europe, sometimes supplemented by extra payments to encourage particular aspects of primary care services (such as primary care teams) or priority services (such as preventive care).

This payment system supports continuity of care and an emphasis on preventive services—and not just curative care; it makes the general physician a gatekeeper for hospital care, thus encouraging the provision of services at the lowest possible level. It leaves the doctor substantially free to practice medicine and to organize the primary care service with little interference and with minimum administration. From the patient's point of view, capitation can ensure a personal relationship with a doctor and a personal medical record, although changing doctors may be difficult. However, since payment does not depend on the number of times a patient is seen, it can encourage doctors to minimize the volume of services given to patients and to refer patients to the hospital unnecessarily, subject only to the need to keep patients sufficiently satisfied that they do not change doctors. Doctors may also try to avoid registering the more demanding and expensive patients. The extent to which this is a problem will depend on how much of the cost of services is covered by the capitation fee (for example, whether drugs are paid for separately) and to what degree the capitation fee is risk-adjusted.

Hospitals may be paid a fixed annual budget (often called a "global budget") or in a variety of ways that reflect workload. Fixed budgets have traditionally been paid to public hospitals, but some countries have introduced them even for private hospitals that are paid by an insurance fund. Budgets are a highly effective means of cost containment and can provide a manager with great flexibility if discretion is allowed on line-item expenditure. However, there can be little incentive to have a high turnover of patients (since this increases costs) or to provide good quality service. These problems can be addressed by good monitoring systems.

Payments to hospitals that reflect workload can be by itemized bill, daily rate (including all recurrent costs), average cost per patient, case adjusted for diagnosis, types of services, or block and volume contracts. These range from the most detailed—and, therefore, the most demanding and costly to administer—to the least detailed and the simplest to administer. All have their own particular advantages and disadvantages.

Payment by itemized bill has the same inherent problems as fee-for-service for doctors: it encourages excessive procedures and hospital stays. Per diem rates discourage excessive procedures but encourage unnecessary stays. Average cost per patient discourages long length of stay but does not encourage technical efficiency. Case-based payment, particularly developed in the United States with the diagnosis-related group approach, reimburses hospitals for the "average" case but provides an incentive to classify patients in more expensive groups or to shift patients out of the hospital earlier. Case-based payment is also information intensive and hence costly to administer.

The introduction of contracts into the United Kingdom health system was accompanied in the early years mainly by block and volume contracts. In the former, a provider is contracted to deliver one or more services (for example, acute hospital services) to a given population for a fixed sum—it is hence, in effect, a capitation payment. It transfers financial risk to the provider and may thus encourage cream-skimming and the provision of too few services. This type of payment, often risk adjusted to a certain extent, is increasingly being used in managed care arrangements and between social insurance agencies and providers, as in Thailand. Volume contracts are appropriate where the purchaser wishes to limit the number of procedures paid for (for example, elective surgery). Purchasers can use these contracts to take advantage of economies of scale that can be achieved by larger units with high volume.

This list of payment methods provides a confusing range of options. The key issues relate to what incentives each payment method creates for providers. These are summarized in Table 10–5. In particular:

- What are the incentives to overprovide or underprovide services to patients within the facility? A key issue is who bears the financial risk—purchaser or provider.
- What are the incentives to be technically efficient?
- What are the incentives to exclude altogether certain types of patient?
- Given these incentives, what are the administrative costs of the payment system together with the monitoring required to prevent abuse?

This provides a rather crude basis for evaluating methods, however, not least because financial remuneration, although important, is not the only factor affecting the behavior of providers. The effects of a method in practice will also depend on the system and context within which it is introduced, for example the extent to which:

**Table 10–5** Key Payment Methods and Their Incentives to Providers

| Payment Method | Unit of Paid Services | Key Financial Incentives for Providers |
|---|---|---|
| Salary | usually one month's work | restrict number of patients and services provided |
| Fee-for-service | individual acts or visits | expand number of cases seen and service intensity; provide more expensive services and drugs |
| Capitation/block contract | all relevant services (for example, primary care, hospital care) for a patient in a given time period | attract more registered patients (especially the healthier); minimize contacts per patient and service intensity |
| Fixed budget | all services provided by a facility in a given time period | reduce number of patients and services provided; keep patients in hospital longer |
| Daily rate | patient day | expand number of bed days (through longer stays or more admissions) |
| Case payment | cases of different types | expand number of cases seen (especially the less serious); decrease service intensity; provide less expensive services |

- purchasers or patients can change provider
- strict ethical standards are adhered to and monitored by the medical profession (thus limiting cream-skimming and both under- and overprovision)
- the media is active in publicizing cases of medical negligence
- consumers are well informed and able to exercise choice effectively

Since each payment approach has its advantages and disadvantages, which depend also on the context in which it is introduced, it is difficult to be prescriptive. In practice, some of the problems with any one method are addressed by combining methods (for example, using capitation payment but with additional fees for certain procedures). Perhaps the strongest conclusion that can be drawn is that fee-for-service payment should be avoided as the main payment approach. Studies have suggested that providing care on a fee-for-service basis costs one-third more than using capitation, without substantial differences in health outcomes, and that fee-for-service payment for outpatient care is associ-

ated with 11% higher expenditures in OECD countries (Ensor et al., 1997). A further conclusion is that no payment method will work well if providers think they are seriously underpaid.

## PROVISION OF SERVICES

Health service providers in low- and middle-income countries can be categorized into seven main groups:

1. government-run health services for the general public (these include the services of the Ministry of Health and those services coming under other government ministries, such as local government and education)
2. services run by social insurance agencies for the insured and their dependents
3. nongovernmental organization services, including those run by church organizations and charitable groups
4. occupational health care providers (medical services provided by employers for their employees); this includes services

for the armed forces and police, which come under government ministries; universities may also run services for their own staff

5. private, for-profit allopathic providers, both individuals and facilities
6. traditional systems of medicine, such as Ayurveda, homeopathy, and Chinese medicine; and traditional healers of various types, including traditional birth attendants
7. the informal sector of drug peddlers and unqualified practitioners

In general, the richer a country, the more organized and structured and the less diverse the system of health service provision. For example, over time government-run services may be brought within a single structure, as they were in the United Kingdom under successive rounds of reorganization; services of the Ministry of Health and social insurance agency may be amalgamated, as they were in Costa Rica. As government services and services for the insured improve, there is less reason for occupational health services to provide general medical care; as regulatory structures strengthen, the informal sector becomes much smaller.

Information on the supply of health services in low- and middle-income countries is sorely lacking, and indeed is much weaker than information on the demand side. Hence it is difficult to summarize the relative significance of these different sources of services. Most studies focus on what is called the "public-private mix"—that is, the relative numbers of providers in public and private sectors. McPake (1997) suggests that there may be at least three different patterns. Among the lowest-income countries, the formal private, for-profit sector is small, but especially in Africa there is a rather larger NGO sector. The informal sector is large, consisting of unregistered allopathic providers, drug sellers, and a variety of traditional practitioners. For example, in Zambia 0.2% of beds are in the private, for-profit sector and 25% in the NGO sector, and 73% of private expenditure is on drugs.

However, in some very low-income countries, especially in Asia, the private, for-profit sector plays a much more important role; this constitutes the second pattern. For example, in India 75% of total health expenditure is paid by private households as out-of-pocket expenses (Mills et al., in press). Large and concentrated populations may be one explanation; another may be a longer history of Western health services and training of professionals, together with government health services that have never extended to provide coverage of the whole population. However, even in these countries, private provision is still concentrated at lower levels of the health system. For example, in India, although 67% of hospitals are private, this amounts to only 35% of beds (1993 data; Mills et al., in press). Much of the high expenditure on private health services in these countries still goes on informal services, ambulatory care, and drugs: 60% of private expenditure in India is on curative services at the primary level and around 35% on secondary and tertiary services (see Table 10–4).

McPake identifies a third pattern of provision, in countries with rather higher per capita GNP, which usually includes a major role for social insurance (funding services either through its own facilities, as is common in Latin America, or through mixed public and private providers, as is more common in Asia) and a private sector that is playing an increasingly important role (certainly at the secondary level and sometimes also at the tertiary level).

Hanson and Berman (1998) assembled what data they could find on private physicians and hospital beds to see if any general patterns emerged. They found extreme variability in both absolute numbers and public/private shares. The supply of both private physicians and for-profit beds was income elastic (that is, they increase at a rate that is higher than the growth rate of income). In contrast, public beds increase at a much lower rate than the rate of growth of income. Thus while it is well established that the public role in financing increases with rising income, it seems that the public share of provision (measured in this study as beds and physicians) decreases.

Since the relative roles of public and private sectors has been a key policy question, there has been much interest in whether private providers are more efficient. Those who believe in the virtues of private markets claim this to be the case, but information is scanty, of poor quality, and equivocal. A review by Bennett (1997) finds that private providers are more efficient, but she points out that all the studies refer to not-for-profit providers, suggesting that differences in efficiency are not due to the profit motive. In addition, comparisons are problematic because an increasing number of studies are finding that the nature of the patients seen by private, for-profit hospitals is different from that dealt with by public hospitals. In particular, the illness of patients in the former may be less severe and require only a short length of stay. Moreover, the structure of the payment method for their patients will affect whether they have an incentive to be efficient. For example, in South Africa medical benefit schemes pay private hospitals a fixed per diem for hotel-type services, which encourages hospitals to organize these as efficiently as possible. However, drugs and supplies are reimbursed with a percentage mark-up, encouraging use of the most expensive drugs.

Another difficulty in drawing conclusions stems from the fact that there is a tendency to make an overall judgment on all private providers. However, there is ample evidence of highly diverse types of providers. In India, for example, at one end of the spectrum there are private hospitals delivering services of international standard; at the other end are unlicensed and unqualified practitioners using Western prescription drugs. In between there are trained physicians and Western-style hospitals whose quality of care can be extremely poor (Bennett, 1997). Private clinics, although in theory run by doctors, in practice often depend on staff with little training; this is because, in many countries, doctors will also have a public post where they spend at least some part of their time, as well as in several clinics. Financial relationships between different types of facility are also a concern in a number of countries; hospitals, laboratories, and diagnostic centers may pay general practitioners to refer patients to them or may pass them a share of their fee.

Absolute lack of resources can place a limit on the costliness of public facilities. Nevertheless, there is ample evidence of poor resource use, such as very low staff productivity and waste of drugs and supplies (Mills, 1997). However, the evidence is by no means conclusive; it comes from a relatively small number of country-specific studies, and the evidence of greatest inefficiency comes from the lowest-income countries in Africa, making it difficult to know to what extent the conclusions can be generalized. In addition, there are examples of highly efficient public health centers and hospitals (World Bank, 1993).

As in the case of private facilities, there are a variety of explanations for observed public provider inefficiencies, some of which do not relate to ownership per se (Mills, 1997). In particular, decision making may be centralized and staff at hospital level given little power to control resource use. Very low salaries also contribute to poor performance, because they reduce staff motivation, and staff may need to spend time generating income in other ways in order to ensure an income adequate for survival.

The clearest area where private facilities outperform public ones is in their acceptability to patients. People commonly complain that the staff of public services are rude and unhelpful, in contrast to private providers. The latter are also open longer hours, especially in the evening, and do not run short of complementary resources, such as drugs. However, people generally make shrewd judgments of the motivations of providers. Patients may use private providers for the convenience and the available resources, but they are aware that it is the profit motive that drives the private providers' behavior and influences the care given, rather than any humanitarian ethic (Mills et al., in press).

## PERFORMANCE OF DIFFERENT TYPES OF SYSTEMS

The above sections have demonstrated that the design of health systems varies greatly between countries, particularly with respect to:

- the sources of funding (for example, balance between tax, insurance, and out-of-pocket payment)
- the degree of integration of financing agents and providers (are there large numbers of financing agents or one major one, such as a Ministry of Health or single social insurance agency; are financing agents and providers integrated or separated?)
- the ownership of providers (public; private, not-for-profit; private, for profit)
- the extent to which the whole population of a country has access to the same services, or different groups in the population have different entitlements and use different providers.

These marked differences have led not surprisingly to intense debate over whether any one design can be shown to perform better, in terms of criteria such as efficiency and equity, than any other. Attention has particularly focused on differences between the U.S., Canadian, and British systems. The United States relies heavily on voluntary insurance organized largely through employers, plus publicly funded programs for the low-income and older adults; Canada has a compulsory national insurance system; and the United Kingdom relies largely on general tax revenues. Whereas most services in the United Kingdom are government owned, privately owned services play an important role in Canada and especially the United States. Table 10–6 shows some key comparative indicators for the United States and Canada for 1988 or nearby years. Canada had substantially lower per capita spending on health and GNP share than the United States, despite physician and beds per population ratios that were greater than those in the United States. The United States spent approximately 27% more per capita than Canada, even though 13% of the population had no health insurance. Health status indicators such as infant mortality and life expectancy were better in Canada. Study of waiting times and physician practice patterns show that in some instances Canadians got less health care or had

to wait longer, but there were few observable effects on mortality and other outcome indicators.

Analysis of explanations as to why Canada spent less highlights two key differences (Folland, Goodman, & Stano, 1997). One is that physician fees and hospital costs were significantly lower in Canada, no doubt because these are regulated. Physician fees are negotiated between physician associations and provinces, and hospital budgets are set by the provinces. Another reason is substantially lower administrative costs, which were approximately $300 higher per capita in the United States than Canada (amounting to 23.9% of health care expenditure in 1987). Studies comparing expenditures in a larger number of rich countries have found that countries in which health services are financed primarily by private payments have the highest expenditures, and that there is no evidence that this is reflected in better health status. Health systems where there is comprehensive risk pooling based on compulsory insurance or tax finance, covering the whole population, appear to be more cost-effective (WHO, 1999).

Similar, detailed comparisons have not been done for low- and middle-income countries. They can take two key lessons from richer countries:

1. a significant public share in financing enables greater control of expenditure, meaning that higher population coverage can be achieved at lower cost
2. the greater the fragmentation of the health system and the greater the reliance on private insurance, the greater the proportion of total health expenditure taken up by administrative costs

However, rich countries demonstrate that there are a variety of ways in which a strong public role and coordinated health system can be achieved, and that the traditional model prevalent in many low- and middle-income countries of an integrated public system financed from general taxation is only one approach.

**Table 10–6** Comparative Data on U.S. and Canadian Health Systems for 1988 (Financial Data in $US)

| Indicators | Canada | United States |
|---|---|---|
| % of population with no insurance (1985) | 0.0 | 13.3 |
| Population per physician | 486 | 418 |
| Beds per 1,000 population | 7.1 | 5.4 |
| Occupancy rate | 83.8% | 68.4% |
| % of gross national product on health care | 8.7% | 11.1% |
| Per capita health expenditure (1985) | $1,556 | $1,973 |
|    publicly funded | 75.9% | 41.1% |
|    physician sector | 15.7% | 19.6% |
|    hospital sector | 40.4% | 39.6% |
| Hospital occupancy rate | 73.9% | 64.3% |
| Hospital length of stay | 8.1 | 7.1 |
| Expense per hospital stay | $2,014 | $3,532 |
| Expense per hospital day | $243 | $500 |

## HEALTH SYSTEM REFORM

Widespread dissatisfaction with the performance of health systems in rich and poor countries alike has encouraged what has been described as a worldwide movement of health sector reform. The term *reform* is used deliberately, in the sense of "a sustained process of fundamental change in policy and institutional arrangements, guided by government, designed to improve the functioning and performance of the health sector, and ultimately the health status of the population" (Sikosana, Dlamini, & Issakov, 1997).

The key problems that reforms are designed to address have been referred to at various points in the above text, and can be summarized as follows:

- In many low-income countries, resources and funds are grossly inadequate to provide even a basic level of care for the population, with many governments spending less than $10 per capita on health services.
- Levels of health produced by health systems are often lower than what is technically possible—in particular:
  —Many activities funded by the public sector are not very cost-effective, and coverage is inadequate of interventions that are highly cost-effective (World Bank, 1993); conversely, too high a share of the budget is spent on hospital care, especially higher levels of hospital care.
  —Health systems operate with low or very variable levels of technical efficiency: studies of facility costs invariably show great variation in costs across similar types of services, to an extent that is not easily explained by differences in quality but is more likely to be due to problems of managing resources (Mills, 1997).
- Quality of services is poor in public facilities, especially in the poorer countries where funds are very limited, health service inputs are in short supply, equipment is poorly maintained, and staff are poorly paid and hence poorly motivated; staff are often criticized for their lack of courtesy to patients and lack of responsiveness to their needs. Many private services are also often of very low quality and almost completely unregulated.
- The possibilities for health interventions created by technological developments place ever-increasing demands on limited funds, accentuating the need for govern-

ments to consider ways of setting priorities and defining limits to what can be provided.

- New problems, such as HIV/AIDS, and the growing importance of chronic diseases are putting even greater pressure on services.
- Most low- and middle-income countries fare poorly in terms of both equity of access to health services and equity of payment for services, with a few notable exceptions. Poorer households commonly use health services less frequently, especially in rural areas where access is more difficult and expensive, and spend a much higher proportion of their income on health services, partly because public subsidies do not meet their needs well.

The goals of health sector reform follow from this list of key problems, namely increased efficiency, equity of access, and consumer satisfaction. The means of reform are being significantly influenced by shifts in beliefs about the appropriate role of the state and appropriate means for the delivery of public services. Current ideologies favor a slimmed down state, increased efficiency in the provision of public services through mechanisms such as contracting-out and competition, and an extension in the role of the private sector. While these ideas are being applied to the government's role in general, they are influencing reforms in the health sector. Current thinking emphasizes the following key roles of the state:

- setting and enforcing standards, including minimum quality standards
- monitoring the behavior and performance of providers and insurers (where they exist), including ensuring information is available to do so
- defining an appropriate package of services and benefits
- regulating to encourage efficient and equitable financing and delivery of services and to constrain cost inflation

- financing health services as a last resort for those unable to contribute to insurance arrangements

Reforms are considered below following the same headings of the key health system functions used earlier, namely regulation, financing, resource allocation, and provision. Exhibit 10–6 lists the key reform areas under each heading.

## Regulation

As part of health sector reforms, many countries have been amending out-of-date legislation and seeking to ensure that new private activities are brought within the scope of the law. Countries that previously banned or strictly controlled the private sector, such as countries in eastern and central Europe, some countries in Africa, and Vietnam and China, now allow and even in some cases encourage it through tax subsidies. However, much of the expansion of the private sector has taken place without deliberate planning, and often with little regulation.

These changes have increased the need to strengthen regulations, but attempts to tighten regulations are frequently opposed by powerful interest groups. Moreover, regulation of a private sector that consists of numerous small-scale providers is inherently difficult, and few countries have the administrative capacity to do this effectively. Few lessons are yet available on the success of different approaches to strengthen the regulatory role of the state.

## Financing

Reform of health financing has been at the top of the policy agenda in many countries, particularly the introduction (or raising) of user fees and compulsory insurance. User fees were at one time argued to offer a significant source of additional revenue, with their harmful effects on access to be countered by exemption policies. Expectations are now less sanguine: administrative difficulties of fee collection have been sig-

**Exhibit 10–6** The Main Areas of Health Sector Reform

> **Regulation**
> - liberalizing laws on the private health sector and introducing incentives for improved efficiency and equity
> - updating regulatory structures
>
> **Financing**
> - user fees
> - community financing, including community-based insurance
> - social health insurance
> - restructured external assistance arrangements
>
> **Resource Allocation**
> - creation of purchasing agencies
> - specification of essential packages
> - introduction of contractual relationships and management agreements
> - reforming payment systems
>
> **Provision**
> - decentralization of health service and hospital management
> - encouraging competition and diversity of ownership
> - strengthening primary care
> - evidence-based medicine
> - quality improvement measures
> - improved accountability to service users and population

nificant; ability to pay has been a significant barrier to use, and exemption schemes have not been effective; and even if there is ability to pay, people have been unwilling to pay if service quality does not improve.

User fees have also been introduced in the form of copayments in compulsory insurance schemes as a means of restraining demand. However, evidence suggests that copayments have to be very high to have this effect, and even then it is not clear that they will deter "unnecessary" as opposed to "necessary" demand.

In Europe it is generally held that measures to restrict the volume of care provided are more effectively applied to providers than to patients (Saltman & Figueras, 1997).

Partly because of the increased concern over the equity effects of user fees, attention has switched to the scope for locally based insurance schemes. Although a number of such schemes exist in various countries, there is as yet little experience of how they can be encouraged to grow in size and scope. Historically, they were an important stage in the development of universal coverage of health services in Europe and Japan, but no low- and middle-income countries have schemes that are yet sufficiently developed to offer this sort of promise for the future—with the possible exception of Thailand, which instituted the voluntary health card scheme that covered around 14% of the population in 1997.

The introduction of compulsory insurance has been a component of reform policies in the rapidly industrializing countries of Southeast Asia and in central and eastern Europe. Compulsory insurance has been of considerable interest in a number of African countries and in the Caribbean, and a number of Latin American countries have sought to reform their existing schemes. According to Mills (2000), key issues have been:

- Should compulsory insurance be introduced when the proportion of the population in formal employment is still rather small?
- Should the insured have a choice of competing schemes or should there be a single fund?
- Is there any role for private insurers?
- What should be the relationship between the insurance agency and providers: what form of contract and what payment method?
- As schemes cover a higher proportion of the population, how can they be integrated with arrangements for other groups of the population, in order to diminish inequalities between those in the scheme and those outside?

These questions concern the nature of the purchaser and the provider, rather than of the funding source itself. They are discussed further in subsequent sections.

Changing relationships between multilateral and bilateral donors and countries are affecting the way in which external funds are channeled in an increasing number of countries. Donors are favoring sector-wide approaches including the development of a sector investment program, which is funded by a combination of local and external resources. This replaces donor funding of specific projects for those donors who join the SIP.

## Resource Allocation

One of the most common features of sector-wide reforms has been the introduction of a purchaser-provider split in public systems that were previously integrated. Planned management reforms in South Africa, Zimbabwe, and Zambia all envisage a purchasing role for local health authorities. In Thailand the social security office acts as a purchaser on behalf of the insured and accredits and monitors the hospitals that they use. Along with the specification of the purchaser's role has come an emphasis on contractual arrangements between purchasers and providers. At one extreme, these arrangements may be seen as no more than the formalization of a management relationship, as where annual contracts are agreed between the Ministry of Health and an executive agency (Zambia) or the Ministry of Health and a regional health authority (Trinidad), or between a province and a district (South Africa, Zambia, Zimbabwe). At the other extreme, the contracts may be awarded on a competitive basis and may be legally binding (as in New Zealand).

The specification of essential packages of health services, which purchasers require providers to make available, has been a key feature of many reform programs. *The World Development Report 1993*, on the basis of analyzing the burden of disease and the cost-effectiveness of interventions, proposed a package of essential health services that governments should ensure is universally available (World Bank, 1993). In low-income countries, this would comprise:

- public health services for children, such as immunization and school health services; tobacco and alcohol control; health, nutrition, and family planning information; vector control; sexually transmitted infection (STI) prevention; and monitoring and surveillance
- clinical services, such as tuberculosis treatment, treatment for sick children, prenatal and delivery care, family planning, STI treatment, treatment of infection and minor trauma, and pain relief

The initial global analysis has been followed by many country studies, to identify country-specific packages. However, ensuring reallocation of public subsidies away from lower priority services such as tertiary hospital care has proved politically difficult, and there is as yet inadequate evidence of the successful implementation of this approach to priority setting. There is, however, increasing recognition of the need to involve the general public in priority-setting processes in order to ensure acceptability and use of the package.

Also linked to the relationship between purchaser and provider is the payment mechanism: the basis on which funds are allocated from purchasers to providers. Health sector reforms commonly involve changes to traditional modes of payment, although the nature of the reforms depends on the starting point and is severely constrained by powerful interest groups; hence a great variety of reforms are apparent in practice. Although, in general, fee-for-service methods of payment are seen to be undesirable, countries such as those in eastern and central Europe that previously provided salaries to primary care providers have sought to raise remuneration levels and encourage greater productivity by using a mix of salary, fee-for-service, and capitation. Indeed, capitation appears to be one of the areas where there is most experimentation worldwide. Traditionally an approach for paying primary care providers, capitation has been extended to pay for hospital services as well (for example, in Thailand), and is the basis for payment in many managed care arrangements.

Global budgets for hospitals have been a feature in Europe under different funding regimes. Concern that they do not provide incentives to efficiency has led to the introduction of mechanisms that relate payment to measures of hospital activity, such as bed days or cases, or even specific services. Some similar reform trends can be seen elsewhere; Thailand, Taiwan, Korea, and Mexico are all considering the widespread introduction of case-based payments to hospitals.

In those countries introducing compulsory insurance, and those engaged in reforming existing systems, a key and controversial issue has been whether to encourage competition between insurance funds and to encourage choice of insurer. In Western Europe countries have proceeded very cautiously. In contrast, there is an active exploration of arrangements that would permit competitive pressures to be felt by financing agents in some countries in Latin America and in central and eastern Europe. A model of reform has been proposed for Latin America that involves the social insurance agencies competing with private insurers to enroll individuals and being compensated by a risk-adjusted capitation payment (Londono & Frenk, 1997). This approach is, for example, being implemented in Colombia, Argentina, and Peru. However, there is as yet little evidence of how well it works and whether cream-skimming is as much a problem as some fear.

A trend for the future is the increasing prominence of managed care companies anxious to break into low- and middle-income markets. While managed care can take a variety of forms, key features are prepayment by those who choose to enroll (or are compulsorily enrolled as part of employment benefits); agreement with a limited number of health providers, on whom some element of financial risk is often placed (for example, through full or part capitation payment); and active management of the services provided (for example, through medical care review procedures and standard treatment protocols). Latin America already has a large number of people enrolled in managed care type arrangements, and American companies, keen to expand, are actively exploring markets in Latin America, South Africa, and Asia. Options for involvement include contracting with governments or social insurance agencies to manage health programs for particular population groups or covering groups allowed to opt out of social insurance arrangements. These possibilities require a strong regulatory framework to be put in place.

**Provision of Services**

Key reform themes affecting providers have been decentralization, competition and diversity of ownership, strengthening primary care services, evidence-based medicine, and quality improvement.

Even in health systems that maintain a strong public role in provision, decentralization has been an almost universal theme. At the national level, decentralization has taken the form of restructuring the role and functions of the Ministry of Health, with some countries creating executive agencies to take over management responsibility at the national level (for example, Zambia, Ghana), leaving the ministry to concentrate on regulation, policy, and monitoring. Some form of decentralization to intermediate and local levels is also a common theme, with most countries choosing to decentralize services within a hierarchical structure with the Ministry of Health at the top, although there are a few notable examples of devolution of health to local government (for example, the Philippines). Finally, decentralization even further, to hospital level, is a common trend in countries with centrally funded, public systems of health provision (Mills et al., in press). In the lowest-income countries, because of limits on management capacity, this reform may be confined to teaching hospitals, but in some countries such as Indonesia a wider range of hospitals is being made "autonomous" or "corporatized."

Competition between providers is similarly being widely promoted as a means to encourage efficiency, though with rather more caution and doubts about its effects than in the case of decentralization. Diversity of ownership is also promoted as a means to increase competitive pressures, especially on poorly performing public systems of provision. African governments have been urged to give greater emphasis to NGOs. In a number of Southeast Asian countries, tax incentives have been provided for the construction of private hospitals (for example, India, Philippines, Thailand), though from the perspective of the health sector as a whole, there are considerable doubts about the desirability of this policy (Mills et al., in press).

Strengthening the role of primary care has long been a theme in reforms in many countries, although often without substantial changes in resource allocation patterns. The United Kingdom reforms, which gave funds to primary care doctors to purchase other services, have aroused much interest, although efforts to create high-quality primary care services, with a gatekeeper role for the primary care provider, do not as yet appear to feature strongly in reforms in most low- and middle-income countries.

Included in many reform packages have been measures to improve the quality of the services provided. In rich countries a range of approaches is being used, including evidence-based medicine, technology assessment, clinical guidelines, medical audit, and quality assurance methods. These are beginning to be featured in less wealthy countries, but in the lowest-income countries more basic problems have been addressed, such as availability of drugs and supplies, improvement of staff skills, and maintenance of equipment.

Health reform policies usually include mention of the need for improved accountability to service users and the general public, but there are few concrete examples. Some reforms include the introduction of health or hospital boards with citizen representation, although there has been little evaluation of experience. In many of the poorest countries, local government structures are weak, ruling them out as an immediate means for ensuring local representation. Often community involvement is seen to occur via NGOs rather than government health services. Similarly, little attention has been paid to patient rights, and patients tend to appear as the object of reforms, rather than as the subject.

## CONCLUSION

This chapter has outlined the main components of health systems in low- and middle-income countries. It has focused on the health system itself, with little attention, due to lack of space, given to the sectors that supply resources to the health system (such as education and training institutions; pharmaceutical, medical supplies, and medical equipment industries) or to broader influences on health, such as government policies on smoking, alcohol consumption, and transport—all of which have major impacts on health.

In terms of the health system, this chapter has identified its key functions as regulation, financing, resource allocation, and provision, and the key actors as the government, populations, financing agents, and providers. Although these core elements can be identified in all systems, the number of bodies involved in each one, and the way they relate to each other, differs enormously in practice, making it difficult to draw clear conclusions on whether any one arrangement of functions and actors is better than any other.

This chapter has also reviewed the most common reforms being proposed and implemented to deal with weaknesses of the current health systems. A number of agencies are suggesting that reform policies are converging and include the following features:

- an emphasis on the regulatory and enabling role of the state
- an emphasis on increasing public control over sources of funding (although not necessarily increased funding from general taxation)
- more explicit prioritization of what services can be financed and provided, especially

by the public sector (it is often argued that this should be driven by consideration of cost-effectiveness)

- greater targeting of public subsidies to those most in need
- a greater involvement of the private sector, especially in the provision of health services
- greater decentralization of the management of provision within the public sector
- creation of arrangements that encourage competition between providers, in order to improve efficiency and quality
- greater emphasis on the role of consumers, both as informed purchasers and as citizens to whom providers should be accountable (Mills, in press)

However, there is a tendency for ideology rather than empirical evidence to drive these reform policies. These types of reforms are much reviewed and discussed, but there is little empirical evidence of how well they work and whether systems reformed along these lines will perform any better than unreformed ones. Because country health systems differ greatly, so should reform policies, and there is no ideal blueprint for reform. Evidence from countries suggests that reform is more rhetoric than reality, not least because it uses the fashionable language of current reform ideology, but reforms affect the position of powerful interest groups, which mobilize to block change. Far greater understanding is needed of the best ways to introduce reforms and manage these various interests.

---

## DISCUSSION QUESTIONS

1. How can the concepts of efficiency and equity be used to assess the performance of a health system?
2. Access to health care can be viewed as similar to access to other goods and services, that is, dependent on an individual's success in gaining or inheriting income, or as a right of citizenship that should not depend on individual income or wealth. Debate the relative merits of these two positions.
3. What should be the respective roles of the government and the private sector in the health systems of low- and middle-income countries?
4. Imagine that you live in a formerly socialist country, and that the health system is soon to be opened to private investment. What kind of regulatory mechanisms might be put in place in order to optimize efficiency and equity?
5. What are the relative strengths and weaknesses of the main financing sources in a low- and middle-income country context?

---

## REFERENCES

Abel-Smith, B. (1994). *An introduction to health: Policy, planning and financing*. London: Addison Wesley Longman Ltd.

Baker, J., & van der Gaag, J. (1993). Equity in health care and health care financing: Evidence from five developing countries. In E. van Doorslaer, A. Wagstaff, & F. Rutten (Eds.), *Equity in the finance and delivery of health care: An international perspective* (pp. 357–394). Oxford, England: Oxford University Press.

Bennett, S. (1997). Health-care markets: Defining characteristics. In S. Bennett, B. McPake, & A. Mills. (Eds.), *Private health providers in developing countries* (pp. 85–101). London: Zed Books.

Berman, P. (1995). Financing of rural health care in India: Estimates of the resources available and their distribution. International workshop on Health Insurance in India, Bangalore, India.

Berman, P.A. (1997). National health accounts in developing countries: Appropriate methods and recent applications. *Health Economics, 6,* 11–30.

Bos, E., Hon, V., Maeda, A., Chellaraj, G., & Preker, A. (1998). *Health, nutrition, and population indicators: A statistical handbook.* Washington, DC: World Bank.

Department of Economics, University of Zambia, and Swedish Institute for Health Economics. (1996). *Zambia health sector expenditure review, 1995.* Lusaka, Zambia: University of Zambia.

Department of Health and Social Security (1976). Sharing resources for health in England. Report of the Resource Allocation Working Party. London: HMSO.

Donaldson, C., & Gerard, K. (1993). *Economics of health care financing: The visible hand.* London: Macmillan Press Ltd.

Doorslaer, E., Wagstaff, A., & Rutten, F. (Eds.). (1993). *Equity in the finance and delivery of health care: An international perspective.* CEC Health Services Research Series. Oxford, England: Oxford University Press.

Ensor, T., Witter, S., & Sheiman, I. (1997). Methods of payment to medical care providers. In S. Witter & T. Ensor (Eds.), *An introduction to health economics for eastern Europe and the former Soviet Union* (pp. 97–114). Chichester, England: John Wiley & Sons.

Folland, S., Goodman, A.C., & Stano, M. (1997). *The economics of health and health care.* Englewood Cliffs, NJ: Prentice Hall.

Fundacion Mexicana para la Salud. (1994). *Las Cuentas Nacionales de Salud y el financiamiento de los servicios.* Mexico: Fundacion Mexicana para la Salud.

Fundacion Mexicana para la Salud. (1995). *Health and the economy: Proposals for the progress in the Mexican health system.* Mexico, Fundacion Mexicana para la Salud.

Griffiths, A., & Mills, M. (1983). Health sector financing and expenditure surveys. In K. Lee & A. Mills (Eds.), *The economics of health in developing countries* (pp. 43–63). Oxford, England: Oxford University Press.

Hanson, K., & Berman, P. (1998). Private health care provision in developing countries: A preliminary analysis of levels and composition. *Health Policy and Planning, 13*(3): 195–211.

Hsiao, W.C. (1995a). A framework for assessing health financing strategies and the role of health insurance. In D.W. Dunlop & J.M. Martins (Eds.), *An international assessment of health care financing.* Washington, DC: World Bank.

Hsiao, W.C. (1995b, Summer). Medical savings accounts: Lessons from Singapore. *Health Affairs, 14*(2), 260–266.

Kohn, R., & White, K.L. (1976). *Health care: An international study.* London: Oxford University Press.

Kumaranayake, L. (1998). *Economic aspects of health sector regulation: Strategic choices for low and middle income countries.* London: London School of Hygiene and Tropical Medicine, Health Policy Unit, Department of Public Health and Policy.

Londono, J.L., & Frenk, J. (1997). Structured pluralism: Towards an innovative model for health system reform in Latin America. *Health Policy, 41,* 1–36.

Mach, E.P., & Abel-Smith, B. (1983). *Planning the finances of the health sector.* Geneva, Switzerland: World Health Organization.

McPake, B. (1997). The role of the private sector in health service provision. In S. Bennett, B. McPake, & A. Mills (Eds.), *Private health providers in developing countries* (pp. 21–39). London: Zed Books.

McPake, B., Hanson, K., & Mills, A. (1992). *Implementing the Bamako Initiative in Africa.* London: London School of Hygiene and Tropical Medicine, Health Economics and Financing Programme, Health Policy Unit, Department of Public Health and Policy.

McPake, B., & Machray, C. (1997). International comparisons of health sector reform: Towards a comparative framework for developing countries. *Journal of International Development, 9*(4), 621–629.

Mills, A. (1997). Improving the efficiency of public sector health services in developing countries: Bureaucratic versus market approaches. In C. Colclough (Ed.), *Marketizing education and health in developing countries: Miracle or mirage?* (pp. 245–274). Oxford, England: Clarendon Press.

Mills, A. (2000). The route to universal coverage. In S. Nitayarumphong and A. Mills (Eds.), *Achieving universal coverage of health care: Experiences from middle and upper income countries* (pp. 283–299). Thailand: Ministry of Public Health, Office of Health Care Reform.

Mills, A. (In press). Reforming health sectors: Fashions, passions and common sense. In A. Mills (Ed.), *Reforming health sectors.* London: Kegan Paul.

Mills, A., Bennett, S., Russell, S., Attanayake, N., Hongoro, C., Muraleedharan, V.R., & Smithson, P. (In press). *The challenge of health sector reform: What must governments do?* Basingstoke, England: Macmillan.

Organization for Economic Cooperation and Development (OECD). (1992). Sub-systems of financing and delivery of health care. In OECD, *The reform of health care* (pp. 19–29). Paris: Author.

Porter, R. (1996a). Hospitals and surgery. In R. Porter, *The Cambridge illustrated history of medicine* (pp. 202–205). Cambridge, England: Cambridge University Press.

Porter, R. (1996b). Medical science. In R. Porter, *The Cambridge illustrated history of medicine* (pp. 154–201). Cambridge, England: Cambridge University Press.

Roemer, M.I. (1991). *National health systems of the world* (Vol. 1: *The countries*). Oxford, England: Oxford University Press.

Roemer, M.I. (1993). *National health systems of the world* (Vol. 2: *The issues*). Oxford, England: Oxford University Press.

Saltman, R.B., & Figueras, J. (1997). *European health care reform: Analysis of current strategies*. Copenhagen, Denmark: WHO Regional Office for Europe.

Sikosana, P.L.N., Dlamini, Q.Q.D., & Issakov. A. (1997). Health sector reform in sub-Saharan Africa. A review of experiences, information gaps and research needs. Geneva, Switzerland: World Health Organization.

Stinson, W. (1982). Community financing of primary health care. *Primary Health Care Issues, 1*(4), 1–90.

Tangcharoensathien, V., Laixuthai, A., Vasavit, J., Tantigate, N., Prajuabmoh-Ruffolo, W., Vimolkit, D., & Lertiendumrong, J. (1999). National health accounts development: Lessons from Thailand. *Health Policy and Planning, 14*(4), 343–353.

Walsh, J.A., & Warren, K.S. (1979). Selective public health care: An interim disease control strategy in developing countries. *New England Journal of Medicine, 301*, 967–974.

Walsh, K. (1995). *Public services and market mechanisms: Competition, contracting and the new public management*. London: Macmillan Press Ltd.

Witter, S. (1997). Purchasing health care. In S. Witter & T. Ensor, *An introduction to health economics for eastern Europe and the former Soviet Union* (pp. 81–94). Chichester, England: John Wiley & Sons.

World Bank. (1993). *World development report 1993: Investing in health*. Oxford, England: Oxford University Press.

World Bank. (1997a). *Sector strategy: Health nutrition & population*. Washington, DC: World Bank Group.

World Bank. (1997b). *World development report 1997: The state in a changing world*. Oxford, England: Oxford University Press.

World Bank. (1999). What is the World Bank? *http://www.worldbank.org/html/extdr/about.htm*.

World Health Organization. (1993). Evaluation of recent changes in the financing of health services. Geneva, Switzerland: Author.

World Health Organization (1999). *The world health report 1999: Making a difference*. Geneva, Switzerland: Author.

Zschock, D.K. (1979). *Health care financing in developing countries*. Washington, DC: American Public Health Association.

Zwi, A., & Mills, A. (1995). Health policy in less developed countries: Past trends and future directions. *Journal of International Development, 7*(3), 299–328.

# CHAPTER 11

# Health Systems Management

*William A. Reinke*

Should management be classified as art or science? Some observers have taken the position, implicitly at least, that managers are essentially problem solvers who face a series of unique challenges that cannot be easily codified and met through the use of ready-made management techniques. Rather, these challenges must be attacked one by one, through the application of common sense molded by years of experience. Support for this position is weakening as management methods covering a wide array of circumstances have been developed, successfully applied, and incorporated into the formalized body of knowledge known as management science. Truly management is both art and science, and competent managers are noted for their skillful blending of technical knowledge, common sense, and experience.

A carpenter without tools is helpless. At the same time, those who own an expensive toolkit but don't know how to use its contents can hardly be called carpenters. Possession of the tools, as well as knowledge of how and when to use them, is needed. Although the truth of the statement regarding carpentry is readily accepted, its applicability to the field of management is less clear, especially in the health sector where advanced medical knowledge and skills seem paramount. Our task is to provide understanding of important management concepts, principles, and methods, to cite requisites and instances of their successful application, and thereby to provide convincing evidence of the

value of the "management toolkit." The common sense and experience needed to select appropriate tools and use them successfully, however, must remain with the manager.

As multipurpose and multidisciplinary endeavors, health service enterprises require coordinated efforts among numerous individuals and units, making efficient and effective systems of management essential. Increasingly, the effort involves collaboration with external bodies. Private hospitals and public health departments must deal with health sector regulatory agencies, government officials in other sectors, social security and insurance offices, professional organizations, community groups, media organizations, and a host of other interests. This broadened perspective emphasizes the importance of collaborative relationships in contrast to direct control (Korten, 1979). The notion that management involves simply the hierarchical directive and controlling relationship between managers and subordinates is certainly unrealistic in the present climate if, indeed, it ever was relevant.

## MANAGEMENT FRAMEWORK

Although it is essential that we maintain the perspective of the entire health system, the main focus in this chapter will be on management of the individual institution, or in some cases a unified network of organizations, such as primary care and referral facilities. The institution, of course, must be prepared to respond to external influences and seek to influence and collaborate with other interests appropriately.

## Management Scope

Within this context, management is defined as the organized effort to achieve the entity's purpose(s) in an effective, efficient, equitable, and sustainable manner. The effort involves the development and use of *human resources* within an *organizational framework* of appropriate authority and responsibility relationships; provision of adequate *physical support* (for example, equipment, drugs, and supplies) that allows personnel to use fully their knowledge and skills; making available *financial resources* in a timely manner; and operation of an *information system* that permits effective oversight of the services operations and support activities.

## Management Functions

Management functions are most easily described as logical sequences of activities, although in practice they are carried out in whatever order is appropriate (McMahon, Barton, & Piot, 1992). Thus managers may shift attention from planning to implementation and monitoring, then back to planning.

### Statement of Mission

The initial function of management is to establish the organization's basic mission and direction. For example, should the organization provide specialized care in certain areas in which it has acknowledged expertise, or should its mission be to provide comprehensive services to a defined population?

### Policy Setting

In order to move expeditiously in the desired direction, the entity should be able to function in as favorable a climate as possible. Policy setting encompasses efforts to create a favorable climate for pursuing organizational goals. Organizational subunits should be encouraged to act in ways that enhance the mission and prohibited from actions that might detract from the basic purposes that have been set forth. To improve coverage of antenatal care, for example, a policy may be adopted to provide these services on demand, rather than at clinic sessions held only on Tuesday afternoons. Or, to ensure that health care decisions are made at the appropriate level, patients going directly to a specialty clinic might be charged a higher fee than is assessed for those who are referred appropriately from a primary care center.

### Planning

Planning is a third important function of management in which alternative courses of action are formulated and evaluated, often requiring management to shift attention back and forth among various management functions. The aim here is to identify the most cost-effective means of achieving desired objectives. To illustrate, the cost and expected coverage of a clinic-based immunization program might be compared with a program based upon outreach through mobile units and another that relies upon annual National Immunization Days. In the course of planning, management sometimes finds that resources are inadequate to achieve initially desired objectives by any means. In this case more modest objectives might have to be set, or existing policy altered to place higher priority on the program of interest and to assign more funds to it.

### Scheduling and Budgeting within the Plan Framework

Planning is essentially strategic. Tactical considerations relate to the scheduling of personnel effort in the form of a work plan and the budgeting of requisite funds. Planning and scheduling are clearly interconnected; indeed three interrelated levels of health planning are worth noting: long term, intermediate, and short term. Intermediate-range plans, which look forward 5 to 7 years, are most common, but the timeframe is of limited relevance. Basic changes in the design of services and the consequent mix of facilities and personnel require many years to implement; therefore, documents that present broad visions of the future, known as perspective plans, with time horizons of 15 to 20 years, are recommended. Intermediate-range plans can then be formulated with the longer-term goals in mind. Even 5-year plans are not adequately operational, however, unless accompanied by annual work plans and budgets. Because those documents reflect actual resources made available, they tend to determine where principal effort is in fact placed. Too often 5-year plans are not adequately related to longer-term considerations, because intermediate-range plans are little more than unrealistic "wish-lists," and perspective plans provide only a broad vision of the future. Proper integration of planning time horizons is therefore an important function of management.

### Decision Analysis

Plan implementation requires sound decision making every step of the way. Future uncertainties inevitably make the task more difficult, and decisions in the health field are further complicated by the need for making value judgments regarding intangible "quality of life" outcomes, along with more tangible economic considerations of resources use and cost. Methods of decision analysis developed in recent years have become indispensable tools for the modern manager and receive further attention later in the chapter.

### Problem Solving and Process Improvement

Decision making is closely associated with problem solving, which has long been recognized as a key function of management. A more dynamic view in recent years, however, has shifted emphasis from problem solving to process improvement (Berwick, Godfrey, & Roessner, 1991). The view is, in effect, that if all workers could become 10% more productive, the overall gain would be greater than if the few laggards who are only half as productive as they should be were identified and removed or brought up to standard. This revision in man-

agement thinking has brought about substantial changes in management practice. In place of the vision of the boss charged with the responsibility for controlling and disciplining weak subordinates, we now envision the work team itself as best able to identify areas where improvements can be made and jointly to devise appropriate courses of action. Of course team members must see a clear link between organizational interests and personal needs for recognition and fulfillment. The poor motivational climate in many bureaucracies makes this understanding difficult, a factor that deserves further attention in considering the execution of management functions in practice.

### Development and Use of Information Systems

Sound decision making requires the application of reasoned judgment to both quantitative and qualitative information that has been made available in a timely manner. A well-functioning health and management information system (HMIS) is therefore essential to effective management. Vitally important is integration of the "health" and "management" elements. Health information systems that report morbidity and mortality rates, hospital admission rates, and other indicators of health status are commonplace. Likewise, management systems for tracking staff disposition and vacancies, budgets and cash flow, and drug inventories are in use. But information regarding the availability and use of resources must be directly related to the epidemiologic data, so that a determination can be made of the extent to which health needs are being met effectively, efficiently and equitably.

### Organized Coordination

The conversion of sound decisions into effective action requires the coordinated efforts of numerous participants in the organization. Some organizational units generate information and advice that form the basis for decisions made by those same units or others; the decisions are then transmitted to still other units for action. Thus, the separate roles of data gathering, standard setting, information dissemination, decision making, implementation, monitoring, and evaluation must be smoothly coordinated.

Difficulties arising from lack of proper coordination are well known. Central authorities who are unaware of specialized needs at local implementation sites pass on unrealistic instructions to those sites. Local officials are assigned responsibility for certain actions but are not granted the requisite authority and resources to carry it out. For example, a hospital may have responsibility for the performance of personnel whose selection and training it cannot control. Workers attempting to follow standard operating procedures formulated by technical experts in "staff" positions receive conflicting orders from "line" supervisors in the direct chain of command. Means of achieving effective coordination are discussed later under the heading "Organization Structure and Relations."

### Implementation Functions

To many, the essence of management is in the oversight of planned activities in the course of program implementation. Although a broader view of management is described in this chapter, clearly the supervision and training functions of personnel management, cost accounting and control in financial management, and logistical considerations associated with stock control and transport management are critically important. Later sections will address modern management methods in these areas. For example, the superiority of performance budgeting over traditional methods of line-item budgeting will be pointed out.

### Monitoring and Evaluation

Although it is cited as the final function, the monitoring and evaluation function represents a set of tasks to be carried out continuously throughout the process of managing. Ongoing monitoring of progress is at least as important as end-stage retrospective evaluation. After all, travelers driving from Paris to Frankfurt would refer frequently to a map to make sure they were following the desired route, rather than waiting until the end of their journey to determine whether they recognized the Frankfurt skyline in the distance.

### Central Principles of Management

Two basic principles of management practice provide the foundation for carrying out the functions described. The first principle, management by objectives, requires that the organization define its aims clearly and explicitly. Recent management thinking further emphasizes the importance of a democratic process in which those who are to be responsible for achieving the objectives are involved in setting them in the first place (Drucker, 1974). It is thought that as a consequence the objectives will be realistic and widely understood. In addition, members of the organization who gain a sense of ownership and function as a team are expected to be more highly motivated and productive.

The second principle, management by exception, recognizes that management effort is too valuable to be squandered on oversight of routine activities; attention should be focused instead on areas of exceptional concern, such as an individual worker or health unit that has an especially high absentee rate. Obviously, application of the management by exception principle requires advance specification of objectives and standards if meaningful departures from expected levels of conduct are to be identified. This in turn requires a reliable information system to signal the emergence of problems.

Although these two principles are generally accepted as reasonable, some authors have questioned their practicability (Suchman, 1967). Circumstances are cited, for example, in which the external environment is so uncertain and/or volatile that adherence to predetermined objectives is problematic. To illustrate, failure to achieve expected results could be due to a deterioration of economic conditions and consequent budget cuts, for which the project manager should not be held accountable. Such external considerations suggest adoption of a systems approach in which managers respond optimally to a dynamic external environment and "to do the best that can be expected under the circumstances," rather than to be judged against predetermined static objectives that may become irrelevant. Then the difficulty is in defining the "best" that circumstances permit.

The principle of management by exception carries a problem-solving connotation somewhat at variance with the notion of continuous process improvement cited earlier. In practice, of course, good managers seek to improve overall standards of performance at the same time that they identify and take remedial action against those who perform unsatisfactorily according to current standards. In this connection, the criterion of greater uniformity and dependability is applied with increasing frequency (Ryan, 1989). Suppose, for example, that one hospital experiences an average infection rate of 3% among its patients, but the rate is subject to month-to-month variation that ranges from 1% to 8%. In contrast, experience at a second facility is consistently between 3% and 5%, with an average of 4%. It might be argued that the first facility's variance in performance should attract at least as much management concern as the second facility's inferior average performance.

## Presentation Format

With the broad scope and numerous functions of management now outlined, what follows is a discussion of important features of the management process and methods that have been devised for dealing with them. The field of management science has gone well beyond the view that management is merely the application of experience and common sense in problem solving. At the same time, it involves more than the mechanistic application of modern techniques expounded in academic halls of management training. Rather, management practice demands the thoughtful and intelligent use of appropriate tools and techniques in unique settings. Thus, the challenge in sound management

is the establishment of a proper blend of art and science. It would be foolhardy to provide an exhaustive listing of circumstances encountered and decisions to be made by managers. Likewise, a comprehensive course in management methods cannot be presented here. What shall be offered, however, is generalized commentary on certain important issues, principles, and methods of management as follows: first, the organizational context for management will be established; next, selected methods applicable to management functions generally will be addressed; and in conclusion, specific features of personnel, physical resources, and financial management will be presented.

## ORGANIZATION STRUCTURE AND RELATIONS

Organizations are independent, lifelike entities that have defined purposes, functional capabilities, and unique personalities. Young organizations, for example, tend to be vigorous and oriented to change, much like youthful individuals. As organizations mature they are prone to conservatism and protection of the resources and authority they have acquired, much like persons who reach middle age. Thus, a significant management concern is how to remain dynamic and innovative through continuous infusion of "new blood" and ideas without sacrificing hard-won prior accomplishments.

The individuals comprising an organization have their own interests, ideals, aims, capabilities, and personalities. Effective organizations are sensitive to these characteristics and strive to establish congruence between organizational and individual goals and motivations. To illustrate, considerations of efficiency led industry in the past to form highly specialized job assignments, leading to the stereotype of the auto assembler devoting his entire day to the insertion of certain bolts into an engine mounting. At last recognizing that this arrangement is at odds with individual desires for fulfillment and a sense of accomplishment, some manufacturers have shifted to a team approach in which work teams are responsible for completing a larger assignment as a group. The apparent loss of efficiency is more than offset by increased motivation and productive effort from individual members of the organization. In the same way, job descriptions in health facilities need to balance quality benefits achieved from repetitive application of certain skills and the contributions to employee morale and patient satisfaction available from a more holistic view of patient care (McKee, Aiken, Rafferty, & Sochalaski, 1998). Thus, arterial bypass surgery should be performed at a limited number of sites where the volume of work is sufficient to maintain skills, whereas primary care functions may be more productively performed by multipurpose workers.

While the organization is an independent, purposeful entity composed of individuals, it is not a closed system; it must relate effectively to its external environment. The enterprise is sometimes called upon to respond appropriately to externally imposed changes; for example, the introduction of fee schedules where services were formerly free requires action to ensure that high levels of use are maintained, and those with low-incomes are not denied access to needed services. In other circumstances, change brings new opportunities to be seized. Managers and policy makers must constantly strive to maintain a proper balance between reactive and proactive postures.

The point is illustrated by the transfer of power that brought Hong Kong within the political structure of mainland China. The Hospital Authority of Hong Kong foresaw changes in management philosophy and regulations to which it should be prepared to adapt. At the same time, the Authority saw itself as part of an enlarged system with a tremendous need for trained managers in the mainland. The proactive view recognized the opportunity to tap the already existing training capacity and experience in Hong Kong to meet this broader need. As a result, negotiations for collaboration with mainland institutions were initiated prior to the transfer of authority.

## Effective External Collaborations

Some organizations have a tendency to look inward and disregard external agencies until forced to deal with them in their day-to-day affairs. A more useful approach is to acknowledge explicitly the presence of significant outside "actors," and to determine their interests and agendas. The list will undoubtedly include other formal public and private service agencies, as well as the informal sector comprised of indigenous healers and others that may be important to the public, though largely ignored by other professions. Financial interests will also be noted as reflected in ministries of finance, social security agencies, and other funding bodies within government, along with international donors and private insurers.

National and international nongovernmental organizations often represent significant sources of financial support for services and may be direct providers of care as well. In the latter respect they are frequently considered to offer the advantage of innovative flexibility independent of government bureaucratic procedures and regulations. This advantage, however, must be weighed against the feasibility of later replication on a wider scale where conformity to usual practices is required.

Professional organizations are in many respects part of the system, but they may have particular interests that differ from those of other "actors" in the system. Health departments have been thwarted in the introduction of less expensive paramedical providers of primary care by professional associations fearful of the loss of authority, status, and revenue.

Finally, community groups form increasingly vocal and organized sources of discontent and cooperation. Providers must clearly distinguish between genuine partnerships with community groups and the mere co-opting of community resources. Too often individuals selected and trained to work in their own communities serve in effect as poorly paid government workers but without the usual civil service benefits. Such arrangements are convenient in the short run but do not foster the sense of local ownership and participation required for long-term sustainability.

When an organization identifies significant external players, it must assess their roles in relation to its own interests. Which agencies are likely to oppose a particular program of interest to the subject organization? What is the force and nature of the opposition? How can it be overcome? At what cost, tangible and otherwise? Which agencies are mutually supportive of subject organization endeavors? How can coalitions be formed to strengthen the mutuality of interests?

The method of force field analysis (Mayo-Smith & Ruther, 1986) offers a visual means of conducting these appraisals. On the left side of the force field diagram, arrows of varying thickness (force) depict the factors exerting a positive influence pointing left to right on the organization's endeavor and outcome of interest. Countervailing forces are presented in a negative direction from right to left. The balance of forces in opposite directions suggests the feasibility and likelihood of success of the proposed endeavor. Possibilities for changing the balance of factors involved are assessed from examination of the nature and magnitude of forces depicted.

Another practical means of dealing with the outside world is through members of the organization's governing board. Enterprises in which most board members are appointed from within tend to focus on the maintenance and possible improvement in efficiency of existing operations, whereas a large representation of outside interests on the board is more likely to lead to a search for innovation in recognition of a dynamic climate for change (Morlock, Nathanson, & Alexander, 1988).

## Internal Organization and Control

### Pursuit of Multiple Objectives

Organizational arrangements and decision processes within an organization should accommodate the inevitable multiplicity of objectives and interests. Some are widely accepted, though not necessarily mutually compatible. There may be a desire to improve overall service coverage in a defined target population, to ensure that the services are equitably distributed according to need, and to provide them cost-effectively. What if rural areas or ethnic minorities are more costly to reach with services than the urban elite? How is the resultant trade-off between cost-effectiveness and equity to be handled?

Other possibly conflicting aims may reflect more parochial interests. Physician providers may stress the importance of beneficial care to all comers, whereas hospital trustees may exhibit greater concern over coverage of costs incurred in providing services and avoidance of a deficit. Yet a third perspective may be offered by the ombudsman who focuses attention on patient satisfaction in general and length of waiting time in particular. Obviously, the organization structure should contain provisions for prompt and acceptable resolution of conflicting aims.

### Unity of Command

In addition to providing assurance that the organization adheres to a unified set of objectives, the principle of unity of command should be followed (Szilagyi, 1988). In its simplest form this means that each employee should have a single "boss" (see Exhibit 11–1). While acknowledging the acceptability of arrangements whereby a worker receives *technical* guidance from other sources, the unity of command principle calls for administrative authority to be clearly vested in a single *line* supervisor.

Confusion due to the absence of clear lines of authority can be especially troublesome when the jobs of those being supervised are poorly defined. Good job descriptions define what is expected from job performance and indicate the skills required and consequent training needs. Because workers are often called upon to perform tasks for which they are inadequately trained, on-the-job training is critical, and needs for such training should be clearly identified. In addition, job descriptions, combined with

**Exhibit 11–1** Who Is in Charge?

In an effort to improve service coverage, a new category of community worker was designated to perform an array of tasks related to curative care, maternal and child health, family planning, nutrition, and environmental sanitation. Workers were given approximately 1 month of training and were supervised by enrolled nurses for some of the responsibilities and by sanitarians for others. As a result of inadequate training and an impossible work schedule, the employees required considerable supervisory support. Instead of receiving this support, however, they were impelled by the enrolled nurse supervisor into giving greater attention to personal health care at the same time they were challenged by the sanitarian supervisor to fulfill their community responsibilities. The result was both unsatisfactory performance and low morale (Reinke, 1988a).

reasonable productivity standards, determine workload. The emphasis in recent years on improved coverage of primary health services has too often led to the employment of minimally trained, multipurpose community health personnel whose job descriptions include an impossible array of tasks that workers have neither the skills nor the time to perform (World Health Organization [WHO], 1998).

### Span of Control

Just as job descriptions should reflect a reasonable scope of work, supervisory arrangements should provide a realistic span of control in terms of the number of individuals for whom one supervisor has responsibility. The rule of thumb is that one manager can oversee not more than five to seven persons, but this number can vary according to individual circumstances (Szilagyi, 1988). Because individuals performing routine, repetitive work require relatively little supervisory support, the span of control over their performance can be increased. Likewise, managers of departments employing highly skilled professional or technical staff may be able to supervise large numbers of personnel

because of their ability to function quite independently. The span of control decision in other cases may depend upon the experience and stability of the work force, but apart from these exceptional circumstances, the "five-to-seven" rule usually works quite well.

### Services Integration

Efforts to improve primary health care have produced the vision of a neatly packaged mix of basic health services available to all communities, including the most remote. Current practice, in which categorical programs are centrally mandated, funded, and controlled despite local differences in needs and capabilities, is considered to be contrary to this vision. Therefore, the two strongest recommendations in recent years regarding organizational matters have called for further integration of services and greater decentralization of authority and responsibility (Araujo, 1997; Janovsky, 1988; Tarimo, 1991). These two issues are discussed in this and the next section.

Health service operations include health promotion and disease prevention, as well as curative care, which has management implications. Curative care at district level in some countries is organized separately from other health services. Typically, the district hospital superintendent or another physician manages curative care, whereas a health inspector or other nonphysician is placed in charge of preventive services. While preventive services thereby receive explicit attention, often they are assigned relatively low priority, partly because of a general lack of appreciation of their importance, and partly because they are the responsibility of a manager with lower status than the principal physician of the district.

To overcome this problem, some districts are organized to place overall authority for all health services in a single department headed by a high status medical officer. In this case, preventive services may receive inadequate attention because they represent only one of the many responsibilities of the busy chief medical officer who may be inexperienced in these matters.

A broader organizational question concerns the relationship between district health authorities and other personnel. In some places the district health officer is under direct control of the provincial or central ministry of health. In others district health officials receive technical guidance from higher-level health offices but report administratively to a district chief of local government who has multisectoral jurisdiction. The latter arrangement has the advantage of stimulating intersectoral cooperation to set local priorities and meet local needs, but provision for adequate technical support to the health sector must be ensured. In short, the importance of the proper blending of line authority and technical staff guidance is once again emphasized.

The fact that there is not an obvious solution to the dilemma of improperly balanced operations suggests that organization charts in themselves do not solve organizational problems. The organization's "personality" must provide a general climate that favors the requisite balance, regardless of how the boxes on the organization chart are arranged.

Likewise, the placement of individual boxes on the organization chart should not cause us to overlook the value of team effort. Health and other officials functioning as a district management team, along with community representatives, can be effective in prioritizing problems, formulating strategies for action, and fostering a sense of ownership and partnership in seeking health improvements. The World Health Organization has formalized the district team problem-solving approach and has assisted its application in a number of countries (Thorne, Sapire, & Rejeb, 1991).

The notion of a competent management team functioning with clearly defined roles in a rational organization forms an attractive norm to be pursued. In doing so, however, bureaucratic reality that often stands in the way should not be overlooked. The rapid turnover of ministers of health, "permanent" secretaries, and other politically appointed decision makers means that these officials spend much of their time learning the problems of their current ministry and have little left to formulate improved policies and procedures before they are assigned to posts in other sectors.

Meanwhile mid-level administrators, who provide organizational continuity, often spend their time following outmoded procedures instead of seeking results through innovative practices. They can hardly be blamed for this emphasis on form rather than substance, because the organization values loyal service above innovation. The pay is low and opportunity for advancement for merit is limited, but the position carries permanent civil service status and one can look forward to modest salary increments for seniority and, if the "right people" are befriended often enough, perhaps a more favorable post. Because the management climate is such a far cry from the ideals described, the challenge is great, but so are the possibilities for management improvement.

Implicit in the preceding discussion is the distinction between clinical expertise and management competence. Too often successful clinicians are given managerial responsibility by default, despite their lack of formal management training. It would be foolish to argue that the chief executive officer (CEO) of an industrial organization should inevitably be recruited from the ranks of production managers. Then why should the CEO of a health care institution necessarily be a medical officer? Because this question is being raised with increasing frequency, the professional manager is gaining a greater role, but this, too, is causing difficulty because of the technical nature of decision making in the health field (McMahon et al., 1992). The argument is made that it is unrealistic to expect that professional managers will become medical experts; it makes more sense, therefore, to provide adequate management training to a cadre of medical professionals. There can be no argument, however, with the fact that trained managers are needed.

A final point on integration is the link between primary, secondary, and tertiary care services. Where health centers and health posts are of poor quality, hospital outpatient departments usually serve, in effect, as relatively expensive primary care centers. As primary care at the periphery improves, greater emphasis is given to strengthening small hospitals to make them true first referral centers (WHO, 1992). In this regard more effective communication links are needed to provide feed-forward of information on patients referred, hospital feedback on continuing care needs for both acute and chronic illness, and greater involvement of hospitals generally in activities of health promotion and rehabilitation.

### Decentralization

There are obvious advantages to the decentralization of authority and responsibility, so that resource allocation decisions are adjusted to local needs, and partnerships with local communities are fostered. Consequent demands on management to make decentralization work are less evident but no less real (Cassels & Janovsky, 1996). In the first place, not all functions need to be decentralized. Most training is best carried out at provincial or national levels. Nationally established uniform standards of care also make sense, allowing for minor adaptations to local circumstances. Thus, the first management issue is to determine which functions to decentralize. The optimum balance is likely to be a combination of top-down support coupled with bottom-up initiatives systematically introduced, strengthened, expanded, and sustained (Taylor-Ide & Taylor, 1995).

Second, local authority implies local management competence. Although existing expertise is usually inadequate, it certainly can be developed in time. Personnel who have received competency-based training in primary health care can be as effective as scarce doctors in this regard. Similarly, minimally trained local managers can be a more-than-adequate substitute for nonexistent professional managers (see Exhibit 11–2).

Third, effective decentralization demands the delegation of authority as well as responsibility. National officials, pleased to add responsibilities to local portfolios, have sometimes been reluctant to give up authority over budgets and personnel assignments. Thus hamstrung, local officials have been unable to function effectively.

Decentralization of funding can be difficult, even when the will to decentralize exists, because revenues are principally generated at the national level. In Indonesia, for example, the move toward decentralization, prompted by the existence of large differences in population density and health needs among provinces on Java and the other islands, has been hampered by the fact that three-fourths of the funds available to local health departments come from the national treasury (Bossert, Soebekti, & Rai, 1991; Reinke, 1988a). Although block grants not earmarked for specific purposes are possible, decisions must be made regarding the degree of accountability to be demanded by national authorities in order to ensure the legitimacy of local fund allocations.

In the interests of both integration and decentralization in Indonesia, integrated health planning and budgeting systems (IHPB) have been developed at the district level. Yet funds continue to flow to districts from national and provincial coffers in a fragmented way through a variety of categorical development and recurrent cost accounts (Rand Corporation, 1995). Under these conditions, local revenues generated from hospital fees provide much needed flexibility in moving revenues to areas of unmet need. Indonesia is not alone in facing the dilemma; it simply illustrates the difficulties that must be overcome in balancing available resources with local needs if the benefits of decentralization are to be realized.

It is unrealistic to think of decentralization as leading to complete local autonomy, because an organization hierarchy inevitably remains. More typically, instead of local units being told in advance what to do, they decide for themselves how to act and then account for their actions after the fact. The nature of the hierarchical relationship affects information flow and span of control. Consider the hypothetical case of a country with 1,200 counties. If each of the

**Exhibit 11–2** Decentralization Dilemma in Indonesia

Districts had been granted authority to plan and budget for services in accordance with local needs. Administrative posts at district level were few in number, however, and were designed for performing clerical duties more than for carrying out management responsibilities. Authorization of new posts would require time-consuming travel through the civil service bureaucracy, and it was unlikely that the new pay scales would be commensurate with the significant management skills required. There was provision, however, for the employment of technical consultants subject to fewer administrative regulations. The best solution, therefore, seemed to be in recruiting as consultants experienced former civil servants who had reached the mandatory retirement age of 55. This stopgap measure was hardly a long-term solution to the decentralization initiative, but it was the most feasible response to bureaucratic inflexibility that was not yet attuned to policy changes.

county officers reported to the chief of state, the latter would have an unwieldy span of control. If instead the country were divided into five regions, each containing six provinces, and each province contained five districts, there would be eight counties per district. Officials at each level would now have a manageable span of control, but information passing through the many layers of authority could be distorted or acted upon inappropriately. One district officer might usurp the authority of provincial officials and take unwarranted action, while another district officer might pass on to higher authority matters that he is fully able to handle. The situation could become even worse if decentralization simply increased the number of levels at which concurrence (or possible disapproval) was required. This example could be applied to an individual institution with many departments. In any case, though simplistic and artificial, it illustrates the importance of designing organization hierarchies of appropriate "steepness," in the interests

of effective communication and reasonable span of control.

## Community Involvement

The rationale for decentralization logically extends to considerations of community involvement. If decentralized decision making makes locally relevant actions more likely, participation of the communities themselves should offer further assurance of relevance. Because both terms *community* and *participation* are ambiguous, however, the subject deserves separate attention.

### Why Community Participation

Community participation is beneficial to the extent that it contributes to usual health service objectives of effectiveness, efficiency, equity, and sustainability (Newell, 1975). One of the most successful community-based efforts, the Jamkhed Project in India (Arole & Arole, 1994), illustrates community participation in numerous ways. For example, a 40-bed hospital set up under project auspices provides quality care at low cost because village people take care of all nontechnical hotel functions, and project professional staff focus limited resources on the technical aspects of care. Functioning at the grassroots level, the project also has been able to achieve equity by, for example, concentrating the finding of water sources in low-caste residential areas, thereby making advantaged segments of the population dependent upon the disadvantaged for an important contributor to well-being.

A village health project in Somalia provides striking evidence of sustainability. According to informal reports from WHO staff closely associated with the project, community "ownership" of the enterprise was so well established when armed conflict escalated and most government services of all types were curtailed, that health care in the project villages continued virtually uninterrupted. Although the circumstances make it impossible to document the experience in detail, the anecdotal evidence is informative.

The value of community health projects is not limited to the health sector. More generally, they encourage community cohesion and empowerment. The theology of liberation movements in Latin America has been especially notable in emphasizing *conscientization*, whereby traditionally subservient individuals and groups are emboldened to demand their rightful place in society.

### Meaning of Community

It is misleading to think of community in strictly geographical terms, for those living within defined boundaries are often divided into several factions with conflicting goals. It is more useful, therefore, to define communities in terms of common culture, traditions, interests, and needs (Madan, 1987). In this sense, an association of geographically dispersed nurses is a community. Although community considerations in health services management often have a geographic base, we must bear in mind that separate community interests exist within the geographic area of concern. Leadership questions arise within this framework because designated leaders may reflect the interests of a single influential faction that is not prepared to support broader reforms. In this case the central authority that fails to serve local needs is simply replaced by an equally unrepresentative local authority.

### Meaning of Participation

The initiative for community collaboration usually comes from outside the community. This raises the question: Is the aim to enlist community support in order to satisfy project objectives? Or is project support sought to satisfy community wants and needs? Whereas the latter approach is usually specified or implied, it seems that the former is more often practiced. The meaning of partnership is colored accordingly.

Communities can contribute *physical resources* (as when a room in a village home is used as a health post), *funds* (for example, establishment of a drug revolving fund), or *personnel*. The latter can offer ideas and advice, be empowered to make decisions, or take actions, as in providing care or conducting surveys of health needs. The appropriate form of involvement depends upon what decisions are to be made and what action is to be taken, at what level, and when. These activities run the gamut from policy analysis to planning, implementation, and evaluation. If a policy of charging for drugs dispensed by community health workers (CHWs) is under consideration, should the fee schedule be established by a village health committee (VHC) with community membership (in part or exclusively), or should the CHWs merely collect the fees that have been set by district health authorities? In any case the presence of truly functional VHC decision-making bodies and respected CHW service providers has been found to be crucial to effective community participation.

Nine specific sets of activity have been identified for which community roles should be defined (Taylor, 1988). They are as follows:

1. establishing community representation
2. setting community organization objectives
3. determining community organization strategies and functions
4. determining community structures
5. identifying appropriate incentives for participation
6. managing the community organization
7. providing supervision and support
8. implementing community organization activities
9. monitoring and evaluating community performance

### Guidelines for Overcoming Obstacles

Numerous roadblocks to effective community participation must be overcome (Korten, 1981). Even in the absence of overt threats to success, certain actions can be taken to make the partnership more rewarding. Several of the more important considerations are summarized here.

Official commitment is needed at all levels to provide a favorable climate for collaboration. Because community-level decisions and actions cannot be carried out in isolation, support throughout the health system is important and takes the form of stated policy at central and district levels, as well as consequent evidence of willingness to relinquish control as necessary.

Much care is required in the formation of effective community links. Although external change agents can provide the needed initial stimulus, they must not be dictatorial. This approach requires exceptional sensitivity on their part. Leadership within the community must be established to fit the circumstances. Does the community role require democratically determined representation? Or should the leader be someone chosen because of specialized technical competence or community respect?

The evolving partnership between staff and community representatives should provide mutual learning opportunities that establish common terms of reference. Staff members should become sensitive to community needs and priorities. Community participants should become acquainted with local epidemiologic conditions and intervention possibilities. When a survey of health professionals and residents of a certain area in Nepal enumerated local health problems, it was found that half of the problems were independently recognized by both professionals and the community, indicating substantial congruence in perspective (DeSweemer, Parker, Taylor, & Reinke, 1979). Equally revealing was that, among the items initially identified by only one of the parties and later accepted by the other, the number of items contributed by the community exceeded that put forward by the professionals, making clear the value of exchange of views.

Individuals tend not to place their problems into neat categories. Moreover, the usual priorities involving food, shelter, employment, and education are not seen to have direct health implications. Health workers therefore face a challenge in entering into a dialogue with the community (Flavier, 1970). The Jamkhed project began the effort by organizing volleyball contests. These were followed by chat sessions that eventually led to formation of Women's Clubs and Young Farmers Clubs for men. When health-related projects were initiated with community support, they usually dealt at first with broad issues of safe water and nutrition. Only later were specific problems like immunization and contraception tackled. In contrast, others have found advantage in launching a clearly targeted immunization or diarrheal diseases control program capable of producing visible results in a relatively short period of time (Taylor & Waldman, 1998).

Successful as the Jamkhed project and a few others have been in expanding coverage to a relatively large population, "scaling up" efforts remain difficult. Because each community has its own needs, perceptions, and leadership characteristics, formation of local partnerships must be individualized. As more communities are enlisted, competing community groups can become a disruptive force, or, in contrast, traditional patterns of bureaucratic uniformity may be imposed, thus stifling grassroots efforts. Much remains to be learned about successful large-scale community participation.

The CHW is the critical link in providing services. Much of the program success therefore hinges upon CHW selection and training. Recruitment decisions made solely by the community can lead to the nomination of unqualified members of the headman's family. Selection by health staff, on the other hand, is contrary to the notion of community participation. A workable solution allows the community to nominate three acceptable candidates, one of whom is chosen by the health team having responsibility for the training (Were, 1982). Competency-based training then mixes considerable practice with essential theory in preparing candidates to carry out at most five or six priority tasks. Once these are consistently carried out satisfactorily, other tasks can be added. Too often in an attempt to improve coverage, CHWs are assigned responsibility for an overwhelming array of activities that they have neither the time nor the competence to undertake.

While limiting the number of activities, the importance of data gathering in the CHW job description should not be underestimated, as village-based workers are in an excellent position to track their neighbors' problems. The Jamkhed study found, for example, that whereas health center workers typically identified two or three leprosy cases in community surveys, the CHWs were able to uncover 10 times as many.

Once trained, CHWs should be fully supported in their daily activities. An attractive work site should be provided and adequate levels of supportive supervision should be provided. Although some programs try to rely on volunteer effort, experience suggests that some form of remuneration in money or in kind is highly recommended. Funding may come from government through the community, from the community directly, or from fees collected. If funds come directly from the government, the community loses control, and CHWs become in effect government workers co-opted from the community. Remuneration through collection of fees for drugs dispensed has the disadvantage of encouraging curative care at the expense of health promotion and disease prevention activities. Regardless of the financial arrangements, the risk of corruption exists. Under decentralization, special care must be taken to prevent past corrupt practices at the central level from multiplying across communities, where they can be especially damaging.

## HUMAN RESOURCES MANAGEMENT

The most important resource in the labor-intensive health sector is its personnel; they account for up to two thirds of total expenditures, and even then remuneration is often inadequate because of budget limitations. But to function effectively, personnel and organizational units must have access to drugs and supplies, medical equipment, transport, and other physical resources (WHO, 1990). These in turn require adequate funding. Problems occur when countries are forced to curtail public health budgets during periods of economic decline. When budgets were severely reduced in Nigeria, for example, it was not feasible politically to reduce staffing levels correspondingly (World Bank, 1991). Instead, nonpersonnel expenditures on such things as drugs and maintenance were dras-

tically curtailed, becoming less than 20% of the limited budget. Patients, who soon realized that they would not find necessary drugs and laboratory services at the health centers, stopped using those facilities, which in turn became increasingly inefficient as a result of enforced staff idleness. Because of the separate and combined importance of human, physical, and financial resources, the management of each is taken up in turn.

## Shifting Emphasis in Personnel Management

In the early years following World War II, principal attention was focused on training increased numbers of doctors, nurses, pharmacists, and other health personnel. This emphasis was especially evident in countries that had recently achieved independence and were bent upon making health care widely available as an essential human right (Fulop & Roemer, 1982). By the 1970s it was becoming apparent that a mere increase in the number of personnel was not sufficient to guarantee health improvement. It was also essential that personnel be used effectively, especially in view of the increasing cost of supporting fully staffed facilities. Thus attention shifted to the content of training and its relevance to subsequent practice in addressing community health needs.

Two divergent studies of national health manpower needs in the 1960s reflect the needed change in emphasis. One study found that Turkey had twice as many doctors as nurses, and two thirds of the physicians were practicing in three urban centers (Taylor, Dirican, & Deuschle, 1968). By contrast, another study found that Nigeria had approximately 10 times as many nurses and midwives as doctors, especially in rural areas. It seems unlikely that conditions in the two countries were so different that the manpower situation in each was optimal. Undoubtedly, urban doctors in Turkey were performing "nursing" tasks, and Nigerian nurse-midwives were acting as doctors, even though they were not trained to fill this role. Although Turkey evidently needed more nurses and Nigeria needed more doctors, the desired content of the training was unclear in view of existing role differences and ill-defined unmet needs.

Methods of functional analysis (elaborated below) for assessing job content have been very informative (*The Functional Analysis of Health Needs and Services,* 1976). For example, it is not unusual to find that more time is spent in recordkeeping than in providing direct services. Repeatedly it is found that paperwork, meetings, work preparation, and other activities in support of services consume 2 to 3 times as many hours of effort as the services themselves. Interesting as these findings are, their usefulness is limited, apart from specification of standards of time allocation and care, as in, for example, the average number of home visits expected per day and the educational messages to be transmitted during such visits. For this reason emphasis has further shifted in recent years from quantitative measures of activity to qualitative considerations of the appropriateness and effectiveness of that activity. Parallel to this shift, the field of quality assurance (QA) has evolved from a focus on quality control, designed to reduce errors in existing patterns of care, to continuous quality improvement (CQI), designed to achieve higher levels of, and increased uniformity in, performance (Berwick et al., 1991).

The change in emphasis from personnel numbers to job content to quality of job performance does not mean that any of the three considerations is unimportant, but that personnel assessment has become more comprehensive in scope. The following discussion of human resources management, presented from this broad base of interest, deals sequentially with determination of the size of the work force, development of the requisite skills mix and job assignments, deployment of a motivated team of employees to carry out these tasks, and monitoring and supervision of the individual and team efforts.

## Projecting Quantitative Needs

Projected personnel requirements can be satisfied in part through retention of existing personnel and in part through recruitment or training of additional staff. To understand the implica-

tions of this obvious truth, consider a district of 520,000 persons that has set a standard of two basic health workers (BHW) per 1,000 population but at present has only 880 in contrast to the stated need for 1,040.

Superficially, it appears that if 40 additional workers were trained each year, the deficit of 160 could be erased in 4 years. Realistically, however, the two effects of population growth and attrition also must be considered in projecting training requirements. Let us suppose that population is growing by 3% annually, and on average 10% of the BHWs leave service each year. Among new recruits there is a 20% dropout rate during training.

Applying formulas (see Exhibit 11–3) that recognize these factors in a projection of needs 4 years hence, we find that 173 graduates annually are needed, and allowing for dropouts during training, 216 persons must enter training each year. This is vastly different from the 40 trainees that were initially contemplated so naïvely. The difference is largely due to the dropout and attrition rates overlooked earlier.

Let us suppose that losses from service could be cut in half from 10% to 5% annually, and that the dropout rate during training could be trimmed from 20% to 10%. Using the same formulas, now 122 graduates would be needed from a yearly input of 136 trainees. At least some of the cost savings from the 37% reduction in recruitment and training effort might be used to make jobs more attractive after completion of training. Failure to appreciate this concept often causes excess attention to be paid to training programs and too little effort given to the retention of satisfied, productive workers who are already fully qualified.

## Skills Mix and Job Descriptions

Health planners from several Asian and Middle Eastern countries were asked if they could agree on the main existing gaps in information that inhibited their planning endeavors. Using the nominal group technique (described later), overwhelming consensus was reached that the primary difficulty concerned job con-

**Exhibit 11–3** Projection of Personnel Requirements

---

It can be shown that

$W_t = W_0R_t + G(1-R_t/(1-R))$, where

| | |
|---|---|
| $W_t$ is the number of workers needed by time (year) t = 4 | $[(1,040)(1.03)^4 = 1,171]$ |
| $W_0$ is the original number of workers | $[880]$ |
| R is the annual retention rate | $[0.9]$ |
| G is the annual number of graduates | |
| t is 4 years. | |

It follows that

$$G = [W_t - W_0R_t][1 - R] \div [1 - R]$$
$$= [1,171 - (880)(0.9)^4][0.1] \div [1 - 0.9^4]$$
$$= [1,171 - 577[0.1] \div [0.3439]$$
$$= 173$$

---

tent. At least in the countries represented, planners felt that they had an adequate database describing the numbers of personnel who had been trained and were registered to practice in various job categories. What the planners lacked, however, was adequate information on what those personnel were actually doing, whether they were meeting priority needs, and whether individuals had adequate skills to do the jobs they were being called upon to perform. These questions continue to be raised, albeit usually more informally and often implicitly. Methods variously known as job analysis, task analysis, or functional analysis have been developed to deal with these matters. For our purposes, the latter term is most descriptive because it directs attention to the functions that are most appropriately carried out by personnel individually and as a team.

### Framework for Functional Analysis

The conceptual framework for functional analysis is depicted in Figure 11–1. On the one hand, we have a target population with its defined demographic characteristics, health needs, and demands for care. On the other hand, human, physical, and financial resources are available or can be mobilized to meet population needs. The needs are usually defined demo-graphically and epidemiologically in terms of birth rates, disease incidence rates, and similar indicators, whereas resource levels are described in economic terms, such as health expenditures per capita, or in administrative units, such as doctor-population or bed-population ratios. One is left with the question: What is the relation between 20 doctors, 50 midwives, 200 CHWs, 10,000 cases of diarrhea and 1,500 pregnancies per year? The first task of functional analysis is the development of mutually compatible measures that link needs and resources.

Service units and associated standards of service and productivity form this link. Using the example above, if qualified midwives are expected to be present at 80% of all deliveries, this service standard calls for 1,200 units of service in the form of deliveries by qualified personnel. If 1 midwife working full time assisting deliveries (or, more realistically, 10 midwives each devoting 10% of their time to the task) can handle 200 deliveries per year, this productivity standard translates into a need for 6 full-time equivalent (FTE) midwives to assist in deliveries.

The mobilization of resources to provide needed service capacity requires development of personnel competencies and the provision of support for the appropriate use of those competencies. Service programs designed to improve

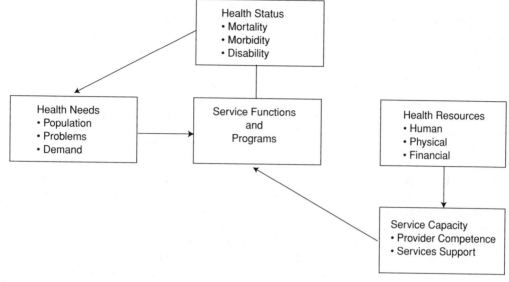

**Figure 11–1** Link between Health Needs and Resources

health status and thereby reduce the level of need can fail because (1) persons with health needs do not seek care, (2) resources to meet service needs are inadequate, (3) available resources are not organized most efficiently and effectively to address those needs; or (4) workers are not motivated or otherwise prepared to use available resources properly. The Asian and Middle Eastern health planners cited earlier were especially concerned about the third constraint. This is the focus of the methods used in functional analysis. The especially troublesome questions of motivation and quality are elaborated further in the next section, "Making Maximum Use of Personnel Capabilities."

In order to assess the vast array of needs, it is necessary to break them down into manageable categories for separate analysis. Intuitively we tend to categorize tasks according to existing job breakdowns, so that, for example, we speak of the nursing function among others. Unfortunately this approach leads to a stereotyped, inflexible view of the health system, in which certain tasks irrevocably fall in the domain of specific worker categories, and objective assessment of alternative arrangements becomes

difficult. Changes are resisted, and the relative professional status of doctors, registered nurses, enrolled nurses, technologists, and others is overemphasized.

Combining relatively homogeneous tasks into functional categories permits more objective appraisal. Hospital functions might be examined according to the urgency of attention required in emergency, intensive, normal acute, and outpatient care. Acute care in turn might be subdivided into services requiring surgical or medical procedures. One study in the Gambia focused solely on the care of acute respiratory infection (ARI) breaking this further into infections of the upper and lower respiratory tracts because of significant differences in the type of care and level of skill needed in the two cases (Meima, Peters, & Sanneh, 1992).

A more comprehensive view of primary health care might reasonably distinguish among (1) responses to patient-felt needs (mainly curative care), (2) provision of provider-initiated personal services (mainly preventive care), and (3) delivery of community-level services (such as environmental sanitation). In addition, family planning, mental health, nutrition, and other categories of service might be identified because of their special characteristics. One array found useful in practice is displayed in Exhibit 11–4.

Along with the listing of functions, the matrix of Exhibit 11–4 notes the range of personnel involved in carrying out these functions. Again, stereotyping problems can arise if specific job titles reflecting current practice are listed. Instead, the aim is to present relative skill levels from least to most extensive, left to right in the diagram. In principle then, movement of tasks as far to the left as possible without jeopardizing service quality will produce the least costly array of job assignments for a defined mix of services. Thus, for example, recognition is given that the mother and other members of the family form the important first line of care and should be enabled to perform their roles effectively.

As an idealized model, Exhibit 11–4 does not indicate how real data might be inserted into the matrix and used to improve job conditions. In contrast, Tables 11–1 and 11–2 capture actual experience from selected health centers in India. Table 11–1 reveals that the auxiliary nurse midwife (ANM), trained as a hospital assistant in curative care, was actually functioning quite independently in the field as a multipurpose worker. Clearly, either her responsibilities should have been more limited or her training broadened. In contrast, the family planning worker was functioning in a single-purpose capacity, raising the question of whether she might be given certain responsibilities for the health care of her family planning clients and their children.

Activities carried out within each functional area can involve direct provision of services, technical and administrative service support, travel (especially significant in community outreach), and personal nonproductive activities (ranging from unauthorized idle time to paid leave). Table 11–2 summarizes the overall work pattern identified in the same health centers reported in Table 11–1. (Also see Exhibit 11–5.) Supporting activities were found to account for more than twice as much time as direct service provision. In fact, time spent in recording and report preparation alone consumed more time than all direct service activity. Surprisingly, community-level services like communicable disease control, mainly malaria control, consumed twice as much time as curative care. Although the existence of an active malaria control program was well known, its dominant role had not been appreciated earlier.

### Data Requirements

It is evident that data collected purposefully, formed into meaningful management indicators, and presented clearly can contribute significantly to sound management decisions. Ways to make the data collection more purposeful are considered next.

Unfortunately, service records are inadequate sources of information about health needs. They only document the use of a particular service provider and do not reveal unmet community needs. Financial records are likewise of limited value in measuring consumption of resources, because the data usually are not organized in functional terms. Although existing record systems can and should be strengthened to better meet management purposes, a proper functional analysis usually requires special studies to obtain further documentation. Fortunately, such studies need be carried out only occasionally, yet can be very informative.

Household health surveys are the best means of assessing community health needs, as well as individual and family characteristics and existing health hazards that contribute to these needs. Households can also provide useful information on usual sources of care and reasons for choosing them. If needed information is clearly defined in advance, the surveys need not be excessively long, time-consuming, or costly. Following this principle, a national health survey conducted in Chile as a supplement to a periodic routine labor survey was carried out at less than 5% of the usual cost of a separate survey (Hall, Reinke, & Lawrence, 1975). Because only a few questions could be added to the existing labor survey, great care was taken in the selection of items to be included and in advance preparation for analysis.

**Exhibit 11–4** Idealized Model of the Measurement of Effort by Functions

| Functions | Individual Effort | | | | | Existing Functional Balance | Functional Balance Based on Need |
|---|---|---|---|---|---|---|---|
| | Family and Friends | Indigenous Practitioners | Auxiliary Workers | Nursing | Physician | | |
| Medical care | | | | | | | |
| Preventive care | | | | | | | |
| Environmental sanitation | | | | | | | |
| Etc. | | | | | | | |
| Effort by category | | | | | | | |
| Personnel capacity | | | | | | | |

**Table 11–1** Illustrative Staff Allocation of Service Time by Function in Selected Health Centers in India

| Staff Category | Medical Care | Maternal and Child Health (MCH) | Family Planning | Communicable Diseases Control (CDC) | Environmental Sanitation | Total |
|---|---|---|---|---|---|---|
| **Facility-based Care** | | | | | | |
| Doctor | 86 | 2 | 12 | | | 100 |
| Nurse | 82 | 7 | 11 | | | 100 |
| Pharmacist | 95 | | 5 | | | 100 |
| Dresser | 97 | | 3 | | | 100 |
| Lab technician | 7 | | 13 | 80 | | 100 |
| *Total Health Center* | *64* | *1* | *13* | *22* | *0* | *100* |
| **Community-based Care** | | | | | | |
| Doctor | 14 | 9 | 29 | 48 | | 100 |
| Lady health visitor | 16 | 29 | 47 | 8 | | 100 |
| Auxiliary nurse midwife | 33 | 35 | 26 | 6 | | 100 |
| Trained traditional midwife | 40 | 32 | 26 | 2 | | 100 |
| Health inspector | 6 | 2 | 8 | 69 | 15 | 100 |
| Block ext. educator | 1 | 2 | 92 | 4 | 1 | 100 |
| Family planning worker | 2 | 1 | 95 | 2 | | 100 |
| Basic health worker | | | 2 | 97 | 1 | 100 |
| *Total Field* | *12* | *12* | *22* | *53* | *1* | *100* |
| Grand Total | 23 | 10 | 20 | 46 | 1 | 100 |

This turned out to be an advantage rather than a constraint, as interviews averaging less than 15 minutes each provided a wealth of useful data that were thoroughly analyzed. Matters of survey design and sample selection are discussed more fully in a later section of the chapter.

Work activity patterns can be obtained from workers' estimates of time devoted to various tasks or from detailed diaries they are asked to maintain for a period of time. The former technique is obviously subject to reporting biases, and the latter is extremely time-consuming and error-prone. Work sampling procedures originally developed for industrial time and motion studies have usually proved to be superior in practice because they simplify both data collection and analysis (Bryant & Essomba, 1995).

In work sampling procedures, an individual representing a particular category of worker is selected for intermittent instantaneous observation at randomly selected times. To facilitate the recording of observations, a form is prepared that lists possible functions and categories of activities within them. If an individual is to be observed at 8:14 A.M., for example, the observer notes on the form what the worker is doing at that instant. Suppose the doctor is taking the temperature of a sick child while discussing with the mother the next due date for an immunization. The observer would place a tick mark

**Table 11–2** Percentage Distribution of Overall Effort in Health Centers in India

| Category of Activity | Percent of Total Effort |
|---|---|
| Direct service | |
| Medical care | 3.6 |
| Maternal and Child Health (MCH) | 1.5 |
| Family planning | 3.1 |
| Communicable diseases control (CDC) | 7.2 |
| Environmental sanitation | 0.1 |
| *Total Direct Service* | *15.5* |
| Supporting services | |
| Records, reports | 16.3 |
| Staff interaction | 7.9 |
| Meetings | 4.9 |
| Preparation, maintenance, cleaning | 4.2 |
| *Total supporting services* | *33.3* |
| Travel | 21.3 |
| Personal | 29.9 |
| **Total** | **100.0** |

under the medical care and personal preventive functions, and also under activity headings that might be labeled "diagnosis" and "advice." If the worker being observed were preparing a report on contraceptive use, the family planning function and reports activity would be ticked. If the report were a monthly submission of health center activities to district headquarters, the reports activity alone would be ticked. Time would later be allocated across all functions.

Work sampling studies focus on the providers of service; household surveys relate to service beneficiaries. A third source of information documents service encounters between the two. This is the point at which judgments are formed about the quality of care. When medicines are prescribed, for example, it is important to know whether the medication prescribed was appropriate, whether the prescription was properly filled, whether the correct dosage was noted, and whether the patient was informed about the correct procedure for taking the medication. The encounter documentation system requires iden-

**Exhibit 11–5** Judgment of Practice Patterns

The analysis does not produce an optimal set of job descriptions, but it does describe problem areas that could benefit from further investigation or application of reasoned judgment. The point was made clear in the comparison of practice patterns in two different states included in the study presented in Tables 11–1 ands 11–2. In one state the doctor saw virtually all patients on their first visit, while nurses usually handled revisits, and injections were normally given by an ANM. The results of the study were tabulated and presented without editorial comment at a meeting of top health officials from the two states. Both groups recognized that in the first state doctors were overburdened. They also agreed that the training of ANMs did not qualify them to give injections properly. It was clear, therefore, that either ANMs needed inservice training in the giving of injections, or doctors needed to reassess their time limitations and service priorities. The two groups of officials shared experiences with respect to the identified problem and then returned home to judge what was best in their local circumstances.

tification of specific stations where services are provided, preparation of checklists of possible activities at each station, determination of which activities should be carried out for an individual patient seen at the station, and a recording of whether the activities were performed satisfactorily or at all. These requirements can be fulfilled through record review or through observation. Record review is relatively unobtrusive and generally is less time consuming, but over- and underreporting can be a problem. Moreover, the record may not present clearly the need or lack of need for a certain procedure. Observation procedures, on the other hand, must rely upon trained observers whose personal judgment about the "gold standard" of care in a specific situation might be questioned. Moreover, the observed provider may behave differently while being observed than under usual circumstances.

The aforementioned Gambia study of acute respiratory infection (ARI) provides disconcerting evidence of problems of reliability and validity in assessing quality (Meima et al., 1992). CHWs were observed treating ARI cases. Because of the part-time workload of these workers, the number of ARI cases seen by each worker was small. They were, therefore, given verbal descriptions of "cases" and asked to specify actions they would take in each situation. Finally, each worker was asked to view a video that presented four ARI cases. Because workers acted independently in the "treatment" of the same four cases, a direct comparison of worker responses was possible. Findings from the three methods of quality assessment were not uniform. Workers exhibiting acceptable performance under one method sometimes fell short in the others. In general, the quality of care in actual practice was poorer than was indicated from responses to the hypothetical cases verbally presented. Apparently, workers tended to know what to do but for some reason did not always follow prescribed procedures in practice. Understandably the search for better methods of quality assessment continues.

## Making Maximum Use of Personnel Capabilities

Having the right person in the right job does not ensure that he or she will do the right thing and do it efficiently. Numerous theories have been proposed for dealing with this dilemma. In the early years of the industrial revolution, Taylor, Gilbreth, and others introduced the principles of scientific management (Szilagyi, 1988). The initial emphasis was on improvement in the physical work environment. Manual laborers were given shovels of optimum size that would permit movement of the maximum amount of raw material per hour. Materials used by assembly workers were placed to minimize the amount of reaching and other movement required, thereby increasing assembly speed. Other production activities were similarly analyzed scientifically through time and motion studies.

Although dramatic increases in productivity were achieved by these methods, the benefits were found to be limited by the failure to consider attitudes of the workers themselves. In the famous Hawthorne study that set out to improve lighting and other aspects of the work environment, it seemed that employee appreciation for the evident management interest in them had an even greater effect on morale and productivity than the improvements themselves (WHO, 1988).

Of the behavioral theories of management that began to emerge, two deserve emphasis. McGregor distinguished what he referred to as management theories x and y (Szilagyi, 1988). According to theory x, work is distasteful and will be shunned whenever possible. Therefore, supervisors must exercise tight control over subordinates to ensure fulfillment of the organization objectives, which are thought to be at odds with those of its workers. In contrast, theory y proposes that individuals gain satisfaction from worthwhile accomplishments and, therefore, are self-motivated to engage in productive effort. The supervisor's role, therefore, is to guide the energies of subordinates in directions that meet organization needs while providing a sense of accomplishment to its members.

Herzberg added further insight regarding behavioral influences by distinguishing between contextual factors and content factors of the job (WHO, 1988). He argued that worker dissatisfaction arises from contextual factors such as low pay, poor working conditions, incompetent supervision, and poor administration. Removal of these negative influences will overcome the dissatisfaction but will not produce the desired positive effects on productivity and performance. These come from motivational factors inherent in the job content. Workers can respond positively to the work itself and associated sense of responsibility, opportunities for self-improvement, recognition, advancement, and general sense of achievement gained on the job.

It is easier in many ways to remove the negative features of the job; pay can be increased or supervisors replaced. It is often more difficult to provide the positive forces that make the job interesting and challenging. Recognition of the importance of positive reinforcement, however, has led to a de-emphasis of the notions of direction and control in management and increased emphasis on teamwork and self-improvement. High priority is given to maintenance and enhancement of employee morale because this stimulates the motivation, self-actualization, and teamwork that are in the organization's interests, as well as those of its members.

### Performance Monitoring and Evaluation

A number of evaluative comments have appeared throughout the discussion of personnel management. Rather than treating evaluation as a separate endeavor, it is important to perform ongoing monitoring in the interests of process improvement. Thus evaluation is a forward-looking endeavor, not a periodic backward reflection to cast blame for past failures. Consonant with this view are the two important concepts associated with evaluation of performance: *selective supervision* and *continuing education.*

Selective supervision is based upon the principle of management by exception. Because individuals and work units inevitably experience differing degrees of difficulty in performing their tasks, supervisory attention should be focused on those units in greatest need of support. This is contrary to the conventional wisdom that declares all field units should be visited at the same regular intervals.

Application of the methods of selective supervision requires formation of certain key performance indicators that are either incorporated into reports submitted periodically or are made part of a supervisory checklist that is reviewed on field visits (Loevinsohn, Guerrero, & Gregorio, 1995). Units with indicator values below specified levels are then contacted more frequently than the others. To illustrate, selective supervision was practiced in a family planning project in Brazil that had limited transport to the field (Reinke, 1983). Minimum acceptable values were specified for the number of new contraceptive acceptors per month and the level of continued use among old acceptors. Field

units that did not meet the minimum standards were visited monthly, whereas other units received quarterly visits. The more frequent visits were not to castigate, but rather to determine causes of difficulties encountered and ways of overcoming them.

Whereas selective supervision relates to individual service units, continuing education should cover specific areas of responsibility in which units in general are performing inadequately. This distinction is shown in Table 11–3, which presents the percentage of service targets met by four hypothetical health units in three service categories. Statistical analysis would usually be applied to the results in order to identify statistically significant departures from usual practice. Apart from such statistical confirmation, it is apparent that performance in Simba is well below that of other sites, suggesting that Simba is in special need of supportive selective supervision. It is also clear that service units in general lag in meeting family planning targets. Perhaps personnel are less experienced in family planning, or it may be receiving low priority for attention. In any case, a program of continuing education directed at family planning services seems to be in order.

Continuing education often receives little systematic attention despite changing circumstances in which health workers are continually called upon to perform unanticipated tasks for which they have received little or no training (see Exhibit 11–6). When training courses or workshops are conducted, the subject is often based upon the specialized interests of a particular health officer or the availability of funds for a specified training purpose. In contrast, the data gathering and analysis underlying Table 11–3 can help identify concrete needs for training and can facilitate selective supervision as well.

### PHYSICAL RESOURCES MANAGEMENT

Much has been said about methods for developing work force capabilities and for motivating individuals to use their capabilities fully. All is for naught, however, if staff do not have the

**Table 11–3** Hypothetical Record of Performance, in Percentage of Service Targets Met

| Subdistrict | Antenatal Care | Illness Care | Family Planning | Overall |
|---|---|---|---|---|
| Tambala | 84.2 | 93.7 | 61.1 | 79.7 |
| Simba | 78.2 | 81.9 | 48.1 | 69.4 |
| Magora | 77.6 | 97.2 | 59.4 | 78.1 |
| Ogere | 102.8 | 91.3 | 53.8 | 82.6 |
| **Districtwide** | 85.7 | 91.0 | 55.6 | 77.4 |

drugs and supplies, functioning equipment, and transport needed to perform their jobs satisfactorily. Because the cost of drugs and supplies is usually second only to personnel costs, it deserves particular management attention and discussion, but first some observations are offered on the subjects of transport and equipment use and maintenance.

## Transport and Equipment Use and Maintenance

The classic example of overcentralized management is in the control of transport. Procedures that require headquarters approval to purchase fuel and spare parts increase administrative costs and result in excessive and costly downtime for ambulances and other vehicles. On the other hand, unauthorized private use of vehicles under local control is, unfortunately, commonplace. What is needed, of course, is a set of locally relevant rules and procedures that are competently enforced. It is hard to generalize how to achieve this management structure, but decentralized authority coupled with strict rules of accountability is paramount, along with a large measure of good will.

As community outreach efforts expand in an effort to satisfy the needs of underserved areas, travel time and costs mount. Unnecessary costs of a different sort are incurred when inoperative vehicles make impossible the transport of emergency cases from the periphery to the district hospital. These two considerations draw attention to the use of appropriate modes of transport. Motorized vehicles used in place of bicycles

save travel time of field personnel; hence they might be justified despite their higher cost. The benefits are lost, however, when spare parts are not locally available or mechanics familiar with the particular vehicle are not present. Again, it is difficult to generalize, but clearly considerations of appropriate technology must receive the attention they deserve.

**Exhibit 11–6** Do Workshops Provide Training?

In the interests of management improvement, the Ministry of Health in Malawi formed an administrative committee of all department heads to meet weekly. Training was the dominant issue raised by committee members during the first several meetings. Job descriptions were felt to be unclear, and incumbents were often poorly equipped to carry out necessary tasks, many of which were related only vaguely to the written job specifications. The numerous workshops that were held did little to satisfy training needs because they usually gave only a broad overview of the subject and contributed little to specific skills development.

Workshops were mainly seen as sources of additional remuneration through per diem allowances. Department heads admitted that they usually attended internationally sponsored sessions themselves because of the generous allowances, whereas other staff members were selectively chosen as a reward for loyal service to attend workshops where more modest government per diems were provided. Participation in neither case was based specifically on training need.

In the usual situation where funds are severely limited, there is a temptation to postpone needed maintenance in order to satisfy more immediate budgetary demands, despite the clear implications for increased costs in the long run. It is often more rational to move in the opposite direction by performing early preventive maintenance. Because of the potential cost savings in this regard (not unlike the benefits from preventive health care), mathematical models have been developed to determine optimum preventive maintenance policies. The models themselves are beyond the scope of concern here, but the principle behind them is worth noting (Morse, 1958).

Take the classic case of lightbulb replacement. When a bulb failure is reported, maintenance personnel must make a special trip to the failure site. Once there, they can replace other bulbs that are about to fail at relatively little additional cost. The question is: Which ones are about to fail? The answer cannot be determined precisely, but appropriate recordkeeping can yield a probability distribution of survival times from which the cost of early replacement can be ascertained. Specifically, one must weigh the added cost of lightbulb purchases due to more frequent replacement against the reduction in personnel costs obtained from the simultaneous replacement of multiple units.

## The Logistics Cycle

An even richer potential for gain is available from the mathematical modeling of drug usage because of the costs involved. Before elaborating on this point, however, the four basic elements of the logistics cycle must be outlined: selection of items to stock, procurement of those items, their distribution to the sites of use, and actual disbursement and replenishment (Management Sciences for Health, 1997).

With regard to selection, the value of a limited list of essential drugs is well established. Considering price and efficacy, the list should contain only materials shown to be cost-effective. Where several varieties serve essentially the same purpose and are similarly cost-effective, the choice of a single item can result in a price advantage gained from large volume purchases and can simplify administrative stock control procedures as well.

Procurement decisions are important, but may be beyond the control of local institutions and agencies. The decision might be made to (1) manufacture drugs domestically, (2) import raw materials and process them domestically, or (3) purchase the finished product in the international market. Although the decisions are sometimes made on political grounds (see Exhibit 11–7), they should be based on considerations of manufacturing capacity, price, quality control, and foreign exchange requirements.

Procurement decisions at the district or institutional level can relate to purchase locally in the open market versus procurement through the national depot system. This issue is then closely tied to questions of distribution. To secure price advantages and other controls from volume purchasing, items are often procured at the national level, then distributed to regional warehouses and on to local institutions such as hospitals for further reallocation. The longer the chain of distribution, the more opportunity there is for bottlenecks and shortages to develop. For this reason, the flexibility of local purchase is sometimes preferred even at the expense of higher prices.

The increasing number of drug revolving funds (DRFs) further complicates the matter. The funds are designed to broaden the distribution base by making commodities available for sale to all patients, even those at the periphery, and using the revenues thus generated to replenish the initial supply. If the DRF serves to extend the national network to one lower level, the shortage problems described above can be made worse. If, on the other hand, the DRF is strictly a local enterprise, different concerns arise with respect to price, availability, control, and corruption. These funds have enjoyed considerable success and have served a useful purpose, but their management is a matter of continuing concern.

**Exhibit 11–7** Can Drugs Be Managed Efficiently?

Scientific management methods are especially advanced in connection with drug procurement and stock control. Essential drug lists and national formularies can be readily produced and stock replenishment rules can be established with mathematical precision. Unfortunately, the field is also one in which departure from optimal practice is commonplace. Deals with drug distributors are tempting. Fake drugs are manufactured and widely distributed in some countries. Importation of foreign pharmaceuticals is often subject to an elaborate, time-consuming bureaucratic process and foreign exchange restrictions. Local distribution practice frequently favors hospitals, leaving health centers unable to meet primary care needs. In short, political realities are often of greater relevance to managers than are the principles and methods of modern management science.

## Stock Replenishment Decision Rules

Effective procedures are essential for the selection, procurement, and distribution of drugs and supplies, but drug availability ultimately depends upon stock control procedures employed at the point of usage. Shortages can cause costly interruptions in service delivery, but excessively high inventory levels can also be costly, especially when the items stocked are perishable. Because of these cost implications in the industry, mathematical models prescribing optimal stock replenishment decision rules were among the earliest contributions of operations research to management practice (Morse, 1958). Inventory cost-saving rules are available in the health field as well.

The simplest model recognizes two conflicting costs requiring trade-offs, as shown in Figure 11–2. First a restocking cost, $C_r$, is incurred every time replenishment takes place. Because the cost of placing the order and transporting the stock to the site where it is dispensed is essentially the same regardless of the amount ordered, restocking costs can be minimized if orders are

placed infrequently, say annually. Such a decision, however, requires a large investment in inventory and storage facilities and increases the risk and cost of pilferage and spoilage. These holding costs, $C_h$, must be weighed against the restocking costs, $C_r$. The optimal balance depends on the ratio of these costs and usage levels, U. Specifically, the optimal *economic order quantity* is determined to be the square root of the expression $2UC_r/C_h$ (see Exhibit 11–8).

In the typical case where many items with different usage rates are stocked, there are obvious advantages to joint replenishment regardless of the reorder frequency dictated by the above formula. The mathematically derived $S,s$ decision rule achieves these advantages without loss of the benefits from the single-item replenishment model. Its application is illustrated in Figure 11–3.

The rule specifies that stock levels be reviewed periodically (say monthly) in order to identify items that have fallen below their individually determined minimum (order trigger) value, $s$. Orders are placed for these items to bring their stock levels up to the maximum value $S$ established for each. Minimum and maximum values are determined by frequency of review, lead time needed between placement of the order and actual replenishment, average usage during the lead time, variation in usage, and economic order quantity considerations.

**Exhibit 11–8** Economic Order Quantity Example

Considering that the optimal economic order quantity is the square root function of $2UC_r/C_h$, we find that if 800 vials of a certain drug are needed annually, the cost of restocking each time is $50, and the cost of holding a vial for 1 year is $2, one is advised to order 200 vials on each of four occasions during the year. Because of the square root function, a quadrupling of demand would only double the size of the order, and the frequency of replenishment would increase correspondingly.

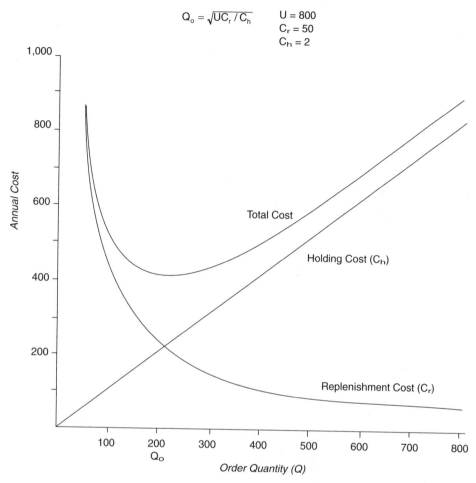

$$Q_o = \sqrt{UC_r / C_h}$$

$U = 800$
$C_r = 50$
$C_h = 2$

**Figure 11–2** Economic Order Quantity

Other mathematical models developed to accommodate additional realities are beyond the scope of present discussion. The point here is that cost trade-offs can be assessed objectively with the aid of mathematical representations of the circumstances, and these models have been found to be especially useful in connection with stock control.

## FINANCIAL MANAGEMENT

The financial management of an enterprise first requires appraisal of alternative strategies for allocating the limited resources available. Once a preferred strategy is identified, a de-

tailed budget is prepared to carry it out. Then in the course of implementation, expenditures are monitored in relation to budgeted levels (Mills, 1990a, 1990b). Financial management practice, therefore, is discussed under three headings: (1) resource allocation decisions, (2) performance budgeting, and (3) cost analysis.

### Resource Allocation Decisions

The fundamental aim in the design of health programs is to achieve desired results at minimum cost. This is the essence of cost-effectiveness analysis (CEA) (Reynolds & Gaspari, 1985). In recognition of the special importance

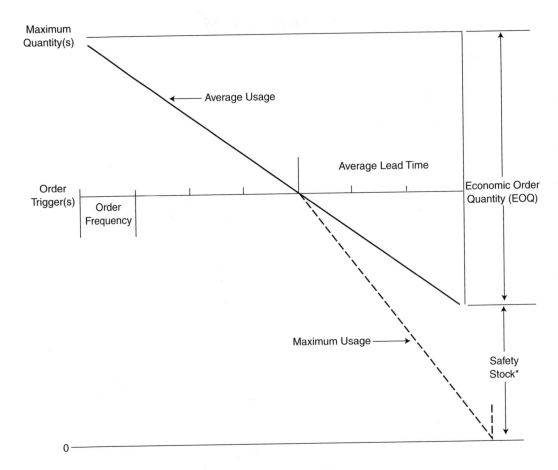

**Figure 11–3** Periodic Reorder Inventory Model

of intangible benefits in connection with health and other social services, the economic orientation of CEA has been broadened to form cost-utility analysis (CUA) (Gold, Russell, Siegel, & Weinstein, 1996; Torrance, 1986). The notion of health for all has further directed attention to the distribution of benefits along with overall levels of achievement. Thus equity has become a prime concern (Musgrove, 1986). More recently we have come to appreciate the labor-intensive nature of health care and its effect on recurrent costs. One-time development costs

incurred with donor support to improve service coverage leads to an ongoing recurrent cost commitment normally borne by the host country government to maintain the capability that has been developed. Issues of program sustainability and affordability have, therefore, come to the forefront (Abel-Smith & Creese, 1989; Bossert, 1990; Lafond, 1995; Olsen, 1998; Prescott & De Ferranti, 1985). This interest has been heightened by growing concern over quality issues, which can be costly. The question is raised whether improved quality, achieved at a cost, carries with it a level of client satisfaction that results in a willingness to pay for the added costs. Thus issues of cost recovery (see Chapters 10 and 12) enter the equation (Creese & Kutzin, 1995; Kanji, 1989; Knippenberg, Reinke, & Hopwood, 1997).

These multiple desires are not necessarily mutually compatible. For example, the most cost-effective strategy in a given situation might focus on a readily accessible urban population, but this approach would be unlikely to satisfy even minimum criteria of equity. Sound and reliable appraisals of the trade-off between cost-effectiveness and equity require explicit comparisons of each evaluative indicator. Although cost-effectiveness measures have been well defined, the meanings of equity, quality, and sustainability are still somewhat vague. Financial analysis methods must be refined to clarify the various evaluative measures and to facilitate integrated analysis of the trade-offs required among them.

### Review of CEA and CUA

Although cost-effectiveness measures are quite well defined, we need to consider one possible ambiguity that is important for present purposes (Reinke, 1994). Because evaluations relate inputs (IP) to outputs (OP) and outcomes (OC), the ambiguity arises over whether to focus on the cost per unit of output or per unit of outcome. To illustrate, should the focus be on the cost per child immunized against measles, or the cost per measles death averted? The answers will differ, of course, according to program emphasis, but a general clarification of terms is helpful. If efficiency is defined as OP/IP, and impact is defined as OC/OP, then cost-effectiveness is defined as OC/IP, and we have

Cost-effectiveness = Efficiency x Impact

$$OC/IP = OP/IP \times OC/OP$$

Distinguishing the two components of cost-effectiveness can be useful in making equity comparisons. Usually an underserved population is hard to reach (physically or culturally)

and, therefore, commands a high cost per unit of service. It is inefficient, therefore, to serve such a population (OP/IP low). On the other hand, service provided to members of this especially needy group is likely to have considerable impact (OC/OP high). Whether the product of efficiency times impact for the underserved is fully cost-effective depends upon whether inefficiency is outweighed by impact. If not, a trade-off between cost-effectiveness and equity is required.

CUA extends CEA thinking to recognize quality of life as more than an economic value. Program benefits are typically measured as *quality-adjusted life years* (QALYs) gained. The utility associated with a specified state of well-being is judged by standard gamble and other techniques of decision analysis, which are described in a later section of this chapter. The QALY concept has been modified to produce *disability-adjusted life years* (DALYs) in connection with national comparisons of the burden of disease (Murray, 1994). An important feature of DALYs is that life (of whatever quality) lived at younger and older ages is considered less valuable than a year of life at, say, age 25. The rationale is that because persons in their 20s and 30s usually have relatively high family and social responsibilities, disability at that age is especially burdensome to family, community, and society generally (see Chapter 1).

Both CEA and CUA methods include the discounting feature, which assigns less value to the future than the present. This feature, combined with the DALY assumption that child years are of relatively little current value, leads to the assignment of less priority to efforts to reduce child mortality, as the future years of productive life lost are discounted, and near-term years are not worth much anyhow. Lives saved at older ages are given relatively little value for somewhat different reasons. These attitudes toward the young and older adults seem contrary to societal views and raise the question of whether evaluative measures should reflect societal values, or be more "objectively" derived and society educated to accept the professional judgments.

## Equity Considerations

Reference to inequity suggests that there is a maldistribution of resources between a relatively advantaged segment of the population and a disadvantaged group. The precise nature of the maldistribution, however, is seldom made explicit (Montoya-Aguilar & Marin-Lira, 1986; Musgrove, 1986; Reinke, 1994). Is the problem an inequity in the distribution of the resources (budgets) themselves, in the benefits derived from the resources (outcomes), or according to some other criteria? Suppose that the infant mortality rate in urban areas is 60, while the rural rate is 80. Would a strategy of resources allocation that produces a reduction of 20% in both areas be considered equitable, even though the two rates remain unequal at 48 and 64? The dilemma is compounded, as indicated earlier, when the cost of producing a specified effect in rural areas exceeds that of producing a similar benefit in urban areas.

## Quality and Satisfaction

Service quality considerations are receiving increasing independent attention, but realistically they should be incorporated into CEA, because quality improvement presumably enhances effectiveness and changes the cost structure. As with equity, the meaning of quality improvement in a given situation must be clear (Reinke, 1995, 1999). Is the goal a higher level of performance, or greater dependability at existing levels?

The extensive experience and documented success in industrial quality control has largely resulted from increasing *product dependability* under the assumption that reductions in wastage and rework would produce substantial cost savings. Costs incurred in the massive recall of automobiles and other products to repair or replace unsafe or inoperable components provide ample evidence of the wisdom of quality improvement.

Corresponding cost savings are undoubtedly available in connection with health care. Concerns about quality are perhaps more related, however, to matters of *service improvement* by means of advanced technology that, more often than not, increases cost. Health care management attention is, therefore, directed at the recovery of the added costs. If consumers are willing to bear them, everyone is pleased; if not, additional pressures on limited public resources will be felt unless the higher cost per unit of service is offset by a decline in the volume of services. Neither outcome is satisfactory.

Figures 11–4, 11–5, and 11–6 help conceptualize the introduction of quality dimensions into health services evaluation. Figure 11–4 presents a typical provider-oriented input-process-output-outcome evaluation model with quality improvement explicitly added to the linked relationship. Available resources are organized to provide a service capability that is partially or fully used to produce an impact on health. Quality improvement alters the mix and amount of resources provided and thereby affects services capacity, use, and impact.

Figure 11–5 offers the beneficiary's perspective of the system. Service capabilities offered by the provider (Figure 11–4) are acted upon according to willingness and ability to pay and generate overt demand for care that yields a degree of satisfaction. From the client perspective, quality improvement efforts potentially modify the level of satisfaction derived and consequent willingness to pay for services. Willingness and ability to pay are distinguished because willingness is directly related to level of satisfaction envisioned, whereas economic and other factors intervene to affect ability to pay and, therefore, effective demand.

Improved technical quality is expected to enhance client satisfaction, but the two are by no means the same. The client is likely to be interested, for example, in the way services are delivered (location, timing, and so forth), as well as in the health benefits derived from them. Hence quality is depicted separately from satisfaction in Figure 11–6, which is a composite of Figures 11–4 and 11–5. In bringing the two prior figures together in the composite, certain modifications are appropriate. Available resources are broken

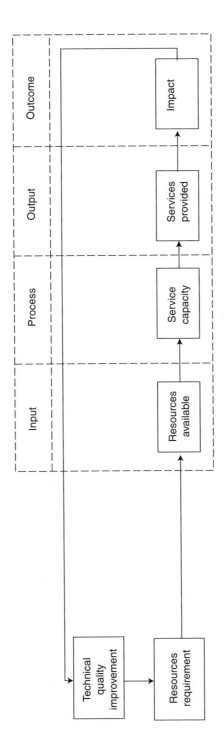

**Figure 11–4** Provider-Oriented Evaluation Model

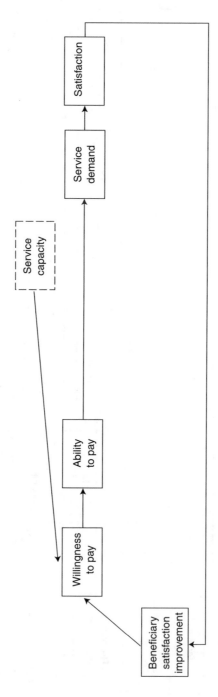

**Figure 11–5** Beneficiary Perspective on Evaluation

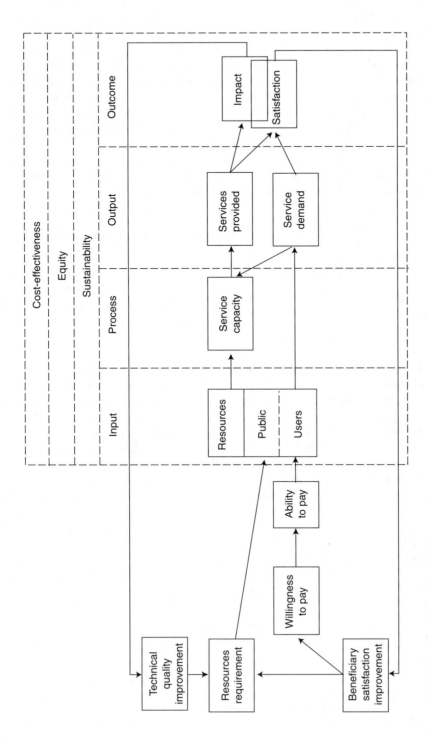

**Figure 11–6** Composite Evaluation Model

down into two categories to reflect cost recovery considerations (see Exhibit 11–9). Some costs are borne by public agencies; others are in the form of user fees based upon willingness and ability to pay. It may also be useful to distinguish between services sought (demanded) and those actually offered and provided. The latter produce a health impact and degree of patient satisfaction. Though these terms have a somewhat different meaning, as previously suggested, they are not mutually exclusive. It is to be hoped that providers have concern for patient satisfaction, and patients seek health benefits. Therefore, the two concepts are shown as overlapping in Figure 11–6. Also noted in the figure is that evaluative indicators of input, output, and outcome, as well as quality and satisfaction, must be formed in a manner that permits comparative appraisal of cost-effectiveness, equity, and continued sustainability.

### Sustainability

Suppose that a reasonable balance has been established between cost-effectiveness and equity in the provision of quality health care, and this balance is sufficiently satisfying so that users share enough of the cost to make the program affordable to the government. Can this level of success be indefinitely maintained? Effectiveness, quality, and affordability undoubtedly contribute to sustainability, but the matter deserves closer scrutiny. Once again the difficulty of clear definition arises. Which aspects of the program *should* be continued?

Even programs considered to be generally effective usually have some dead wood in them that needs to be pruned. One primary care program, for example, trained medical assistants at health center level, village-level volunteers, and health communicators, several of whom were to function within each village (Reinke & Wolff, 1983). The first two categories were used effectively, but because the role of the communicators was unclear, they were felt to be superfluous. A good monitoring system was needed to identify and distinguish useful program components from unnecessary features.

Other aspects of sustainability likewise require definition (see Exhibit 11–10). Is it enough simply to continue essential inputs such as training programs? Must the inputs continue to be productive (services usage maintained)? Should the program piloted in one district be adopted by others? Should the program be self-supported by the community, or is it acceptable for government support to replace donor funding? What if support from one donor is replaced by aid from another donor? In short, future desires for continuity should be made explicit so that the evaluation of program status can produce unambiguous results.

### Integration of Performance Measures

There are six steps in program planning and evaluation that might be followed to integrate the many desired aspects of program performance. To summarize the discussion of resource allocation, these steps are outlined here.

*1. Define improvements in health outcomes sought and the activities and services that should be initiated, maintained, extended, and/or expanded in order to achieve the outcomes.*

Projects are not launched in a vacuum; they are initiated under circumstances that are more or less satisfactory in some respects and unacceptable in others. Decisions are to be made, therefore, regarding new activities to be undertaken, current endeavors to be maintained or strengthened, and present efforts to be abandoned.

*2. Determine, or at least form a judgment about, incremental levels of resources to be made available for the coming project period.*

Desired objectives may seem to be unachievable because of resource limitations. On the other hand, if it can be shown what inputs are required to achieve desired results, the necessary resources might be made available. Thus, the planner must move back and forth between objectives specification and resources determination until a realistic relationship between the two is established. "Ballpark" budget estimates can help focus attention on reasonable amounts

**Exhibit 11–9** Provider Incentives

The argument is made that revenues generated from cost recovery should be retained by the institution providing the services and receiving the payments. Funds will then be available for the purchase of drugs, making other quality improvements, offering staff refresher training, or augmenting low salaries. Although seemingly reasonable, this arrangement could be ineffective under circumstances in which public providers also engage in private practice. They might resist implementation of practices that make public services more attractive, thereby jeopardizing private practice income. Even if fees collected are used directly to augment provider income, it is doubtful that public service remuneration will come close to matching the financial rewards of private practice. The effect of cost recovery on staff motivation is therefore questioned. Much remains to be learned about the practical implications of proposals for revenue enhancement that in principle have considerable merit.

**Exhibit 11–10** What Is a Fair Wage?

An HIV/AIDS program was to be introduced in Malawi with donor agency support. In the interests of long-term sustainability, the program was to be set up as a unit of the Ministry of Health (MOH) with in-country leadership. An energetic, competent young MOH physician was identified to head the program, and her salary was budgeted at about 3 times the level of other department heads. However, an international-scale salary for this position was considered inequitable, unsustainable, and generally unacceptable to the donor agency. The candidate refused to accept the position at a usual government salary level and joined an international agency assigned to another country. Thus the HIV/AIDS program was left without the creative leadership needed, and the MOH lost one of its most valued young professionals. What is an equitable, sustainable solution to such a dilemma?

of effort to be contemplated for project fine-tuning.

*3. Determine the cost of prospective new services and the marginal cost of service improvements, along with expected use levels for the new and improved services package.*

Total cost depends upon volume of use, and use is affected by cost. Despite this dilemma, a rough appraisal of market demand is usually feasible. To illustrate, demand is low in many clinics because of uncertain drug availability. Because staff are already budgeted and present but underemployed, quality improvements in the form of dependable supplies of drugs could be made at small incremental cost of the drugs. Recognizing drug shortage as the principal bottleneck and noting patient willingness to pay for drugs, substantial increases in demand could be anticipated at small increase in total cost and actual reduction in unit costs.

*4. Estimate how the anticipated costs might be borne.*

This requires establishment of a clear, quantitative link between quality and cost, association of quality with patient satisfaction, and implications regarding willingness and ability to pay. On the basis of cost recovery estimates thus derived, the consequent budget needs of government can be determined and "affordability" established. To the extent that budgetary requirements are excessive, the planner must return to steps 1 and 2 and modify projections arising from them accordingly.

*5. Within the framework of realistic budget limitations, identify the most cost-effective mix of activities and services.*

Once limits are established on what is affordable, that is, having fixed the amount of input anticipated, the mix of outputs that is expected to maximize outcome is determined.

*6. Ascertain trade-offs between cost-effectiveness and equity considerations in order to derive an acceptable balance between the two.*

Explicit measures of equity must be introduced to determine the extent of incompatibility, if any, between cost-effectiveness and equity aims. Although the optimal trade-off cannot be mathematically prescribed, quantification of both dimensions permits sound subjective judgments to be made.

The six-step approach suggested is deceptively simple. In practice, one cannot simply move from step 1 through step 6 in linear fashion. Planning requires dynamic movement back and forth among the various steps until the results at each are mutually compatible. Further, the present state-of-the-art is such that quantification and integration of the entire evaluative process are not yet entirely straightforward. Considerable judgment remains to be exercised in bringing together the various dimensions of evaluation cited. Nevertheless, it is hoped that clearer, more explicit, measures of cost-effectiveness, equity, quality and satisfaction, and affordability and sustainability can help unite the various components into a single, comprehensive strategy for evaluation.

## PERFORMANCE BUDGETING

Too often budgeting is merely an exercise in which planners take last year's allocation and project a certain percentage increase this year as reasonable or feasible. Or perhaps, a 15% increase in the personnel budget is considered necessary, while a 10% increase in the transport budget would be satisfactory. Budgets based upon line item inputs like personnel, transport, drugs, and maintenance, apart from the outputs expected, are necessarily arbitrary and not easily justified.

Program budgets are somewhat more satisfactory because the inputs are related to areas of activity. Thus, the judgment might be made to give higher priority to family planning and increase that program budget by 20% while holding the budget for communicable disease control to last year's level. Still, as a budget of resources only, albeit for selected purposes, the program budget is of limited value to program managers for tracking performance during the budget period. Suppose that halfway through the budget year, family planning expenditures have consumed 40% of budgeted funds for family planning, or 80% (40/50) of expected levels for the period. Perhaps cost savings have accrued as a result of efficient use of resources; but what if only 30% of planned contacts for the year have been made during the first 6 months. This presents a picture of relative inefficiency, in which 40% of budgeted resources were consumed in providing 30% of intended services. For management action purposes, it is clearly preferable to relate inputs and outputs explicitly. The performance budget permits this relationship, as described in the following example, which is simplified for purposes of exposition (Reinke, 1988b).

A certain health center has established two cost centers, one for clinical care, the other for community outreach. These service units are each directed by a manager who is responsible for providing the targeted level of services at budgeted cost. Apart from fixed costs, which must be incurred regardless of the level of operations and which are not under the service managers' control, budgetary provision must be made for personnel and expendables (drugs and supplies). Based upon past experience and estimated needs of its target population, the center envisions provision of 50,000 clinic services and 35,000 outreach visits for the coming year.

Whether this level of performance is realistic depends upon the availability of requisite resources, which in turn must be based upon reasonable unit cost standards. The clinic personnel team costs $90 per hour, and a standard of six patients per hour has been set. Therefore, the standard personnel cost per patient is $15. The average cost of expendables is $5 per clinic patient. Similar calculations for outreach services have produced standard unit costs of $10 and $4 for personnel and expendables respectively, as shown in Table 11–4. Thus, cost center budgets must provide $1 million for the 50,000 clinic services to be rendered and $490,000 for 35,000 outreach services to be provided. If this level of funding is not available, more modest service objectives need to be set, or productivity must be increased. Because the performance budget directly links inputs and outputs, realistic and justifiable budgets may be set. The budgets are

**Table 11–4** Preparation of Performance Budget

|  | Clinical Care | Community Outreach |
| --- | --- | --- |
| Standards ($ per unit of service) |  |  |
| Personnel | 15 | 10 |
| Expendables | 5 | 4 |
| Performance Budget |  |  |
| Service Objectives | 50,000 | 35,000 |
| Budget ($000) |  |  |
| Personnel | 750 | 350 |
| Expendables | 250 | 140 |
| Total | 1,000 | 490 |

based upon cost centers in which managers have both the authority and the necessary resources to perform defined tasks for which they are held accountable (see Exhibit 11–11).

Table 11–5 shows actual experience during the budget year in question. On the face of it the savings of $174,600 is attractive, resulting from underexpenditures of $81,700 in the clinical cost center and $92,900 in community outreach. Because, however, service performance fell well below targets in both areas, it is not so surprising that fewer resources were consumed than were budgeted. Clearly, both cost centers were relatively ineffective. The clinical center achieved only 87% of its target and the outreach unit reached 76% of its goal. What is unclear is the degree of efficiency present in each center, as the budget surpluses are a mixture of efficiency and effectiveness factors. All that can be said for sure is that the clinic center spent 92% of its budget to accomplish 87% of its service objective, whereas the outreach unit consumed 81% of its budget to provide 76% of targeted services. Both units were therefore inefficient overall, the clinical unit somewhat more so.

To examine questions of efficiency more closely, an adjusted budget can be prepared that accepts observed levels of effectiveness as given and determines the amount of resources that *should have been used* to achieve these levels of performance. The adjusted budget of Table 11–6 is obtained by applying the unit standards of Table 11–4 to the actual service volumes of

Table 11–5. The comparison of adjusted and actual figures reveals that personnel costs were excessive in relation to the volume of services, but the underexpenditure in drugs and supplies remains, though not at the same level as before.

Although the performance budgeting procedures and subsequent cost analysis are informative, care must be taken in interpretation. The low level of drug expenditure could mean that wastage was kept to a minimum. It could also mean there were frequent stockouts. The latter possibility may explain the reduced volume of services provided. Perhaps the uncertain availability of drugs served to curtail health center

**Exhibit 11–11** Cost Control Limitations

The Jordanian hospital director was under pressure because his unit costs had increased markedly. Last year his hospital had performed approximately the same number of surgical procedures as in recent earlier years, but his costs were substantially higher. Upon closer examination, it was found that a number of Jordanian physicians had recently returned from advanced training overseas. Under terms of the training they returned to government employment, and several had been assigned to the hospital in question. Thus the hospital's indicators of cost relative to performance suffered for reasons beyond the director's control.

**Table 11–5** Actual Experience Compared to Budget

|  | Clinical Care | Community Outreach |
|---|---|---|
| Budget (from Table 11–4) |  |  |
| Service Objectives | 50,000 | 35,000 |
| Budget ($000) |  |  |
| Personnel | 750.0 | 350.0 |
| Expendables | 250.0 | 140.0 |
| Total | 1,000.0 | 490.0 |
| Actual Experience |  |  |
| Services Provided | 43,620 | 26,480 |
| Expenditures ($000) |  |  |
| Personnel | 734.6 | 294.6 |
| Expendables | 183.7 | 102.5 |
| Total | 918.3 | 397.1 |
| Variances from Budget |  |  |
| Services | –6,380 | –8,520 |
| Expenditures ($000) |  |  |
| Personnel | 15.4 | 55.4 |
| Expendables | 66.3 | 37.5 |
| Total | 81.7 | 92.9 |

use, so that personnel were forced to remain idle part of the time. The continuing personnel costs were then distributed over fewer services, thus increasing the cost per unit of service.

Despite the advantages of performance budgeting, standard government procedures are often different and must be followed. Hence the Ministry of Health (MOH) faces the prospect of keeping two sets of accounts if it is to adopt performance budgeting. Although such duplication is probably unwise, the MOH can still enjoy many of the benefits of performance budgeting by establishing cost standards and periodically reviewing actual expenditures in relation to levels of achieved performance.

## Cost Analysis

### Costing for Different Purposes

Although cost analysis techniques comparing actual experience with budgeted expectations

have been introduced, further elaboration of costing methods is needed. First it is necessary to understand how costs are interpreted differently at various stages of budgeting and cost accounting (Creese & Parker, 1994). To illustrate, consider a presently used piece of equipment that is to be replaced by a more automatic labor-saving instrument. Specifically, the old equipment was purchased 2 years ago for $48,000 and was expected to last for 6 years, and the new instrument costs $70,000 and is expected to remain serviceable for 5 years.

In the *resource allocation* decision to purchase, the capital cost of the new equipment enters into the calculation, but not the initial cost of the existing instrument, as this expenditure has already been expended and is not subject to reversal. At issue in the allocation decision is whether either the new capital cost will be offset by personnel and other cost savings, or whether the superior performance of the new device justifies its purchase.

If purchase of the new equipment requires full payment in advance, the next *budget* must include the entire cost of the new equipment, but nothing for the old. In contrast, the *accounting records* will show entries for both instruments. One-sixth ($8,000) of the original cost of the old equipment is to be accounted for during each year of its expected life, and now $14,000 will be added during each of the 5 years that the new instrument is expected to be in use. The thinking behind this procedure is that because the equipment is anticipated to produce service benefits over time, its cost should be similarly allocated in order to permit determination of cost per unit of service. Cost calculations, then, must suit the purpose for which the determination of cost is being made. In particular, accounting records are of limited value in analysis of cost-effectiveness.

### Cost Allocation among Programs

In discussing budgeting procedures it was noted that line-item costs for personnel, drugs, and so forth are not very meaningful until they are related to specific programs or cost centers.

**Table 11–6** Actual Experience Compared to Adjusted Budget

|  | Clinical Care | Community Outreach |
|---|---|---|
| **Adjusted Budget ($000)** | | |
| Personnel | 654.3 | 264.8 |
| Expendables | 218.1 | 105.9 |
| Total | 872.4 | 370.7 |
| **Actual Experience ($000)** | | |
| Personnel | 734.6 | 294.6 |
| Expendables | 183.7 | 102.5 |
| Total | 918.3 | 397.1 |
| **Adjusted Variances ($000)** | | |
| Personnel | −80.3 | −29.8 |
| Expendables | 34.4 | 3.4 |
| Total | −45.9 | −26.4 |

Methods are needed, therefore, to allocate line-item amounts among various programs. Greatest care is necessary in the assignment of personnel costs, for these represent the largest line-item component. The simplest way to handle these costs is in terms of services provided. If a nurse sees 200 patients in the clinic and makes 100 home visits, two-thirds of her salary and fringe benefits would be assigned to clinical services and one-third to home visiting. This method of allocation is not very accurate, however, when there are substantial differences in the amount of time and effort needed to render different types of service. Functional analysis, which provides such a picture of time allocation, serves the multiple purposes of determining how staff are, or should be, employed, assessing training needs, establishing standards of performance for budgeting and program evaluation purposes, and for allocating actual costs.

Allocation of drug and supply costs is usually more straightforward. Vaccines are clearly attributable to preventive services, whereas antibiotics usually go for curative care. Because other cost categories are less significant, simple approximations are generally adequate. Suppose that a nursing station occupies 30% of the floor area in a health center, and staff working at the station spend half their time on family planning. It seems reasonable, then, to assign 15% of the building cost to the family planning program.

### Definition of Terms

Financial analysts use terms from economics and accounting that are not in the usual vocabulary of lay managers. Because a conceptual understanding of their meaning is useful, this section closes with brief commentary on some of the more important terms. First, *economic* and *accounting* costs must be defined and differentiated. Because the discipline of economics concerns resource allocation, it follows that economic costs relate to the actual allocation of resources, regardless of how their use is accounted for. In an earlier example, the economic cost of new equipment was of interest because the decision was being made whether funds were to be used for the equipment purchase or devoted to alternative uses. The economic cost of the old equipment was no longer at issue, because resources had already been allocated for that purpose and were now considered as *sunk costs*, or no longer retrievable for other purposes. In contrast, the accounting records included costs assigned to both pieces of equipment. Accounting costs are those recorded in the records of each year.

*Fixed* and *variable* costs are also to be distinguished. Fixed costs are incurred once and are unrelated to the volume of service provided. Expenditure on an X-ray unit is fixed, for example, and is incurred even if the unit stands idle. In contrast, X-ray film costs are variable since they are directly related to the volume of X-rays produced. Reference is sometimes made to semi-variable (or semi-fixed) costs that are incurred more than once but not in direct relation to the volume of services provided. To illustrate, staff assignments may be reviewed monthly and changed as appropriate. The corresponding costs are fixed periodically, not once and for all. During a given period, though, they are not affected by service volume.

*Development* and *recurrent* costs are related to fixed and variable expenditures, but each set of terms has its own special meaning. Governments usually assign initial expenditures for new projects to a development budget, whereas annual commitments thereafter to sustain the effort are allocated to a recurrent cost budget. In other words, fixed costs tend to show up in the development budget, whereas variable costs are dominant in recurrent cost budgets. The correspondence is not automatic, however. The fixed cost of a new family planning clinic set up with donor support is likely to be considered a development cost. If the donor also supplies contraceptives and pays the salary of the project director for the first 2 years, these variable (or semi-variable) costs may also be included in the development budget.

The notion of *marginal* cost also springs from the distinction between fixed and variable costs. Marginal costs are incremental, that is, they reflect the additional cost incurred as the result of an incremental change in level of effort (for example, an increase in service coverage). The cost of adding 100 new acceptors to the family planning rolls includes expenditures on supplies and perhaps on fuel needed for travel to the communities served, but it would not include the cost of a preexisting vehicle.

Where fixed costs are high and service volume is low, average unit cost will be relatively high, because the fixed cost is absorbed by relatively few services. Under these circumstances, the marginal cost of additional services is likely to be low, and the added use will bring down the average cost as well. These conditions are found when a health center is underused because of a drug shortage. If use were increased substantially by adding an ensured supply of drugs at little marginal cost, unit costs would decline as previously idle staff become more fully used.

## GENERAL MANAGEMENT METHODS

Previous sections have focused on management issues, principles, and methods associated specifically with provision and use of human, physical, and financial resources. Many management methods are, of course, more broadly applicable. These methods are the subject of the present section.

### Situation Analysis

Expressions of dissatisfaction with the present situation are commonplace. Problem statements that provide understanding of contributing factors and offer insight into possible solutions are more difficult to enunciate. Because underlying causes often lie hidden below the symptomatic condition and immediately obvious contributing factors, the appraisal has been likened to the peeling of an onion. To assist this peeling effort, a number of systematic methods for problem formulation have emerged in recent years.

Construction of a *problem diagram* begins with a notation of the specific condition considered to be unsatisfactory. Perhaps growth faltering according to defined criteria is present among many preschool children. The question is then asked: Why? Factors like high incidence of communicable diseases, absence of an effective program of growth monitoring, and lack of green, leafy vegetables in the diet might be cited as contributing factors. Then the question is raised: Why are these factors present? And the process continues; one author suggests that the probe is likely to be incomplete if the question "why" is raised fewer than five times (Berwick et al., 1991).

Each of the factors listed is connected to related factors by means of a line, an arrow showing the direction of the effect, and an indication of whether the effect is positive or negative. Preparation of a visual network facilitates identification of possible points of effective intervention. Action taken too close to the surface of the problem may be ineffective if earlier causal factors are not removed. Or the effect of change early in the process might be overturned by subsequent events. Where several points of intervention are feasible, some may be more costly than others. From consideration of each of these possibilities, the outline for an appropriate line of action should emerge.

### PRECEDE

The popular approach, Predisposing, Reinforcing and Enabling Causes in Educational Diagnosis and Evaluation (PRECEDE), is somewhat more sophisticated (Green, Kreuter, Deeds, & Partridge, 1980). As with problem diagramming, the first step in PRECEDE involves a description of the problem. But the description goes further in identifying epidemiologic and social dimensions separately. Epidemiologic evidence of growth faltering may be accompanied by poverty and lack of economic opportunities. Next, a behavioral diagnosis is made; feeding practices might be listed at this stage. At the third step of the analysis, predisposing, enabling, and reinforcing factors that contribute to the cited behaviors are noted. Predisposing factors relate to states of knowledge and value systems (for example, ignorance about the nutritional content of certain foods). Enabling factors concern such things as availability of resources (for instance, the presence or absence of a program for regular weighing of children). The attitudes and behaviors of others constitute reinforcing factors. For example, the practice of bottle feeding among respected urban elite may discourage breastfeeding in the villages. Administrative diagnosis at the next stage identifies possible points of intervention and promising strategies for altering the predisposing, enabling, and reinforcing factors and therefore modifying consequent behaviors. The final evaluative step provides for the monitoring of chosen interventions to ensure that the hypothesized effects are achieved. (See Chapter 2 for further discussion of the PRECEDE model.)

### Pareto Diagram

Pareto diagrams provide a different kind of visual aid found especially useful in directing attention to quality problems (Berwick et al., 1991). Their value lies in the common experience that the vast majority (perhaps 80%) of errors occurring in a given setting can be attributed to a few (perhaps five or six) repeated mistakes. Possible problem areas are classified, and the number of occurrences of each is tallied for a specified period of time. Thus, a list of patient complaints registered over a 6-month period might show 23 occasions on which a doctor was not present at the health center, 16 cases of rude treatment by the nurse, 12 circumstances in which waiting time was considered excessive, and so on. The tally of findings is then plotted in the form of a histogram, the most common complaint shown at the left, the next most common complaint next to it, and complaints reported less frequently recorded further to the right of the diagram. Perhaps frequently occurring difficulties were already known, but the Pareto diagram clearly highlights them and helps to focus management energies on a limited number of problem areas in which efforts can be most effective.

### Decision Analysis

Management attention should involve (1) a review of the current situation in order to identify priority areas for improvement, (2) formulation and analysis of policies that could guide the improvement, (3) a design of alternative strategies for achieving the improvement, and (4) selection of a preferred strategy as the basis for a plan of action. Methods of decision analysis have been developed to increase objectivity in the appraisal of both policy and strategy options (Bell, Raiffa, & Tverksy, 1988; Hill et al., 1986). Although strategies preferred on quantitative grounds may not always be politically acceptable, the assessment can at least acquaint decision makers with the trade-offs they face in following a political agenda. A doubling of the tax on cigarettes might not be politically viable at present, for example, but the consequent impact on disease incidence and mortality may be worth knowing. Tools of decision analysis are also used in making operational management decisions. Because of their broad applicability, the tools now form the core of management training in academic centers and are outlined in the following paragraphs.

### Decision Process Elements

The decision process consists of five essential elements. First, desired outcomes or end results are specified. Second, alternative courses of action or means are identified. Because the actions cannot be guaranteed to produce the desired results, the element of uncertainty in terms of probabilities is the third element to be included. To illustrate, a decision to add evening sessions to a clinic's operation is likely to increase costs and will produce an uncertain effect on use. In some circumstances data reflecting prior experience can be used to assess probabilities. Other situations are so unique that probabilities take the form of subjective guesstimates reflecting personal judgment. The clinic scheduling example, like many others, falls between the two extremes.

Because different outcomes are possible from the various strategies contemplated, assessment of their comparative values constitutes the fourth step in the decision process. This step is especially important and difficult in connection with health outcomes, which often have intangible features. Consider two treatments for a particular malady. The first cures the condition 60% of the time and produces no effect in 40% of cases. The second remedy has a 90% cure rate, but in 1% of cases produces a ringing in the ears that may last for up to 1 month. How are the two treatments to be evaluated, considering "quality of life," as well as economic, benefits and costs? So-called *standard gamble* and other techniques have been devised, tested, and incorporated into the procedures of decision analysis for making such value judgments (von Neumann & Morganstern, 1947).

Outcomes are traditionally measured in terms of benefits achieved or costs incurred. A third measure, *regret*, often important in practice, arises from the fact that action must be taken in the face of uncertainty. Eventually the uncertainty is removed, and a determination can be made as to whether the decision was a "good" one. Those evaluating the decision have the benefit of hindsight, which the decision maker lacked initially. For this reason, the concept of regret is of considerable importance in decision analysis.

The fifth element in the decision process is the application of specified criteria to the assembled information in order to select a preferred strategy. In the previous example, where there are two treatments for a particular malady, the doctor as decision maker, who sees many patients with the specified condition, might choose the second treatment because on average it produces the best results. To the patient as decision maker, given the same information, averages mean little. The patient is concerned only with what might happen in his or her case and, therefore, wants to avoid the possibility of adverse consequences from the second treatment regardless of the unlikelihood of occurrence. Different decision makers faced with the same prospects might rationally draw different conclusions from the data because different decision criteria make sense to them.

### Risk Aversion

Research into the decision making process is revealing peculiar relationships between uncertainties and value judgments, which, after all, are at the heart of decision making (Kahneman, Slovic, & Tversky, 1982). Consider a newly identified disease that afflicts 50 individuals and causes 20 deaths per month if left untreated. The one available drug would either reduce the case fatality rate to zero or increase it from 40% to 80%. Experts are evenly divided regarding the drug's effectiveness. Should it be employed? When prospects like this have been posed to groups of individuals in terms of deaths averted, they have overwhelmingly favored intervention. When the same scenario has been presented in terms of lives saved, however, respondents have been reluctant to support the risky action (Kahneman et al., 1982). Evidence is building that individuals are inclined to take considerable risks to avoid loss but are unwilling to take similar risks to achieve corresponding gain. In short, how we look upon the choices before us is extremely important, quite apart from the objective evidence presented.

### *Formalized Decision Processes*

Such reasoning quirks underscore the importance of attempts to rationalize the decision process. More systematic appraisal along four lines is needed. First, concrete objectives must be specified. These can take the form of reduced operating costs; higher performance levels; improved quality of performance; greater service impact; improved client satisfaction; more equitable distribution of resources, services, or benefits; or a combination of these aims. Appraisal then moves to the second stage: formation of indicators to reflect results achieved and resources consumed.

The third step, introduction of an effective Health and Management Information System (HMIS), is required to monitor indicator performance. Because data gathering is time consuming and costly, the HMIS should not be excessively cumbersome. For example, levels of patient satisfaction may be periodically sampled, rather than continuously assessed. As a result, the HMIS will provide only estimates of indicator levels.

The indicators are action oriented in that they are associated with decision rules designed to trigger management intervention when it is deemed necessary. Because indicator values are only estimates, they can lead to erroneous decisions. At the fourth step in the process, therefore, the rules should be set in a way that limits errors of commission (wastage of resources through unnecessary action) and errors of omission (costly delays in taking needed action). These errors could be reduced, of course, if more definitive data were available, but collecting the data would be costly. The management task is to balance the cost of information against the cost of inappropriate decisions. Obviously, management improvement can begin by eliminating the common practice of gathering data and preparing costly reports that are never acted upon.

### Survey Methods

The need in decision making for better, more carefully analyzed data is beyond dispute. A statement offered with respect to quality improvement is quoted here because of its broad management applicability (Berwick et al., 1991).

> [The] scientific approach to quality is, by its nature, based on data. Therefore, it is a characteristic of quality management to invest heavily in the design and deployment of measurement. . . . Unlike other approaches to improvement, however, in which measurement is used to reward and discipline people, measurement in the quality management effort is used to gain knowledge of the processes, so that they can be understood, predicted, and improved. *Measurement is used so that everyone can control and improve processes, not so that some people can control other people* [emphasis added]. (p. 41)

The requisite data can sometimes be obtained from well-organized, routine record systems. Often, however, the identified need for further investigation calls for the acquisition of new data as inexpensively as possible, or it may call for a quick sampling of existing massive records. Managers should, therefore, have a basic understanding of sampling methods and should be acquainted with some of the more common survey procedures (Cartwright, 1983; Kish, 1967; Smith & Morrow, 1991; WHO, 1993). Because sampling procedures rely on statistical principles, an introductory presentation of those principles is appropriate. The level of statistical sophistication need be only sufficient to ensure sound application of the principles and methods involved.

### *Estimation*

Representative samples inevitably produce estimates, not the definitive results available only through complete enumeration of the target population. If the estimate is adequately precise, it can be considered good enough for action purposes. The level of precision depends upon only two factors: the amount of variability among individuals in the population and the number of persons sampled. If all children in a community had exactly the same weight on their first birthday, data from a single child would be adequate to determine what that weight was. Realistically, of course, weights vary, so that several children must be weighed in order to gain a reasonably precise estimate of average weight. The more variation there is in the population, the larger the sample that will be needed to get adequate representation of the overall situation.

A certain formula to measure variation has become the standard; application of the formula therefore produces a *standard deviation* measure ($S$). A measure of *standard error* is obtained by dividing $S$ by the square root of $n$, the number of observations in the sample. The importance of the standard error is that under a wide range of circumstances the sample average will be within two standard errors of the population average 95 times in 100. Thus, if weight data from a random sample of 25 one-year-olds produced a standard error of 100 grams, it could be concluded with 95% confidence that the observed average weight was within 200 grams of the true average weight in the population sampled.

Decision makers need to specify the level of imprecision they can tolerate in sample estimates obtained for specific purposes. Thus, if a manager decided that he needed to have an estimate of average weight that was in error by less than 100 grams, a sample of 25 would be insufficient. Because of the square root function of sample size, a doubling of precision (reduction in maximum sampling error from 200 to 100 grams) would require a quadrupling of sample size from 25 to 100. We see, therefore, the importance of specifying the need for no more precision than is really required for sound decision making.

Surveys are frequently conducted to compare results in two populations, such as, for example, urban and rural residents. Here each component sample has its own degree of imprecision, so that the sample estimate of the difference between the two population averages contains errors from both sources of estimation. Because errors are additive, the estimation of population differences requires a larger sample from *each* to obtain specified precision than would be required to obtain the same level of precision from a single population.

### Inference

Often the interpretation of results is based, not on the estimates obtained, but on their comparison with a specified standard. One might seek to determine, for example, whether, in a certain district, the average weight of children on their first birthday meets or falls below the standard of 10 kg established for such children. As suggested earlier, the results could lead to the erroneous conclusion that the standard had not been met, when, in fact, sampling error alone was to blame because the children selected were by chance unusually nonrepresentative of conditions in the population. It is also possible that the sample results will lead to the conclusion that standards had been met when in reality they had not. In this case a larger proportion of high-weight children would be included, by chance, in the sample than were present in the population at large. Because two types of error must be guarded against when drawing inferences, the sample sizes necessary are larger than those needed for simple estimates.

It is beyond the scope of present discussion to go further in the development of sample size formulas (Lwanga & Lemeshow, 1991). It is necessary, however, to understand the importance of predetermining the use to which the data are to be put, the levels of imprecision that can be tolerated, and what inferences, if any, are to be drawn. These determinations are to be made by management. Then the statistician can be called in to assess the statistical implications.

### Forms of Survey

Some studies seek only to obtain *aggregate* estimates of the prevalence of a certain condition, such as the level of immunization coverage in a particular district. These are usually conducted in stages. For example, only certain subdistricts are initially chosen for inclusion in the study, then specific towns and villages in those subdistricts are selected, and finally a determination is made of households in the selected villages. Other studies are conducted to compare conditions in various population subgroups, or *strata*. Here it is important to ensure that the number of observations in each subgroup is adequate. Thus, a survey among different educational groups may need to sample a relatively large proportion of the rare college graduates in order to obtain sufficiently precise indicators of conditions in that group. In both cases, the aim is to obtain enough information promptly and at minimum cost to permit sound and timely decisions to be made (Reinke, Stanton, Roberts, & Newman, 1993).

Another distinction of importance has been made between what is known in industrial sampling circles as *lot sampling* and *process control*. Cross-sectional studies in the health field often use industrial lot sampling techniques, while ongoing health surveillance programs could profitably draw upon industrial process control sampling methods. Common examples of each of these forms of data gathering are given below (Reinke, 1991).

### Multistage Sampling

All categories of study considered thus far require randomness. That is, all members of the population studied must at the outset have an equal probability of being selected. When the survey covers a large geographic area, simple random sampling could be very costly. To obtain the aggregate estimate of immunization coverage cited above, only one or two persons might be selected in each of many villages scattered throughout the district. Placing a limit on the number of villages chosen would be desirable in the interests of survey cost reduction, provided that the principle of "equal likelihood of selection" could be retained.

Random selection is accomplished in multistage sampling by following the rule of selection with "probability proportional to size" at each stage until the final one and then selecting a constant number of individuals at that stage. Consider the case in which a sample of 300 households is to be selected from 20 villages, or 15 dwellings per village. A village with 400 households would be twice as likely to be chosen as one with 200 households, but if the larger village were chosen, its residents would each have 15 chances in 400 of being selected. In contrast, selection of the smaller village would be associated with household probability of selection 15/200, twice that in the larger village. Thus differences in the two sets of probabilities would even out.

The best known example of multistage sampling is the World Health Organization "30 clusters of 7" method (Henderson & Sundaresan, 1982), developed to produce estimates of immunization coverage that are within 10% of true values. The sample size needed with simple random sampling is approximately 100. Considering that villages, or clusters, may not be uniform in their coverage levels, and only 30 are to be chosen for administrative reasons, the total sample size is approximately doubled in order to ensure the desired level of precision. Thus, the plan recommends selection of 7 children in each of the 30 clusters, thereby providing a total sample size of 210.

### Lot Quality Acceptance Sampling (LQAS)

The size of the sample affects the level of precision obtained from sample results, but the population size is not a factor unless it is very small. Thus, the size of sample needed to assess each of various population subgroups hardly differs from the sample that would be required to draw conclusions about the overall universe. Because the requisite sample size applies to each of the subgroups, however, the total amount of sampling needed can mount up very rapidly. Recall further that comparison of results with a specified standard further increases the amount of sampling beyond what would be needed to obtain simple estimates without judging whether the results are "satisfactory."

Illustrative of these considerations, the "30 clusters of 7" approach can produce reasonable estimates of immunization levels reached in the aggregate, but it would not be useful in identifying particular sub-areas that had not reached specified levels of performance, say 80% coverage. In an effort to accomplish the latter task with minimum sampling, surveyors have discovered an industrial sampling technique introduced more than 70 years ago. The publication in which Lot Quality Acceptance Sampling (LQAS) is described lists a number of specific sampling plans that call for relatively small samples, usually 20 to 30 observations (Dodge & Romig, 1959). Unfortunately, these plans do not refute the basic laws of probability and calculation of sampling errors. Their application therefore permits detection of large departures from a standard but are unreliable in detecting smaller differences (Robertson et al., 1997). Specifically, an LQAS plan designed to identify service units with immunization coverage levels below 80% would almost always find a unit that had achieved 50% coverage to be significantly below standard. However, it would not be able to identify consistently units that were truly at the 70% level. It would be difficult in such units to distinguish chance deviations from standard due to sampling error from real departures from standard. This dilemma has led to the adoption of double sampling schemes in which a small sample is initially selected to determine whether a clear-cut determination of performance can be made. If not, a larger, second sample is called for to resolve uncertainties remaining from the first sample. In this way, additional information is obtained only as the need for it is recognized.

### Control Charts

LQAS and related methods are used for lot sampling, or assessment of conditions at a certain place and time. For the continuous monitoring of performance over time, control charts have been widely used in industry for more than 60 years (Grant & Leavenworth, 1980; Ryan, 1989). Their use has been surprisingly limited in the health sector, where performance monitoring is likewise essential.

The possible application of control charts is shown in Figure 11–7 in connection with home visiting. A certain health unit supervises five field workers who average 28 home visits per week. The difference between the best and poorest performance in a given week averages 7 visits. Simple tables have been constructed to convert these average *ranges* into standard deviation units and in turn into values that depict the limits within which observed weekly averages of a process "in control" should fall. An average below the lower control limit (LCL) suggests that performance has deteriorated significantly and should be investigated. In contrast, an average above the upper control limit (UCL) indicates that performance has improved markedly and should be examined to determine causes that might be sustained. Ranges above their UCL indicate that variability among workers has increased, perhaps because one worker (rather than the group) is performing poorly.

Control charts involve very small samples, five in this case, simple calculations, and visual displays that are readily interpreted. Trends soon become apparent. Where the process remains in control, the numerous small samples can be combined to produce overall averages that are based upon a substantial body of data and are therefore very precise. Control charts have also been devised for percentages, such as proportion of pregnant women receiving antenatal care, and for counts of events, such as number of pneumonia deaths per month.

### Establishing Group Consensus

Results obtained from the preceding survey methods are designed to be representative of conditions in the population of interest. Other methods are intended to elicit the views of especially knowledgeable persons. Group meetings in which experts on a subject participate are the most common of these methods, but meetings tend to be dominated by a few articulate or high-status individuals, so that the ideas of others never surface. The *nominal group technique* (NGT) (Delbecq & van de Ven, 1971) and the *Delphi technique* (Dalkey, 1969; University of Wisconsin, 1973) seek to obtain the views

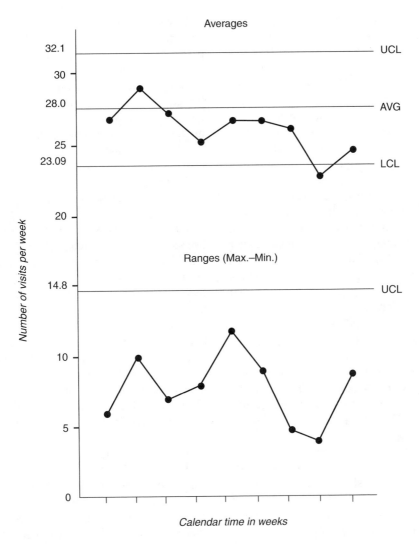

Notes: UCL, upper control limit; AVG, average; LCL, lower control limit.

**Figure 11–7** Control Charts for Home Visiting

of many while avoiding the negative interactions that often emerge when individuals express conflicting views.

In NGT a specific question is posed, such as: What are the most important management shortcomings present in our organization? Each participant then spends perhaps 15 minutes independently writing down ideas that come to mind. All of the ideas are registered on a single flipchart and discussed briefly for purposes of clarification, not advocacy. Participants then

independently vote for the five listed items each considers to be most important. All votes are combined to identify items around which consensus has been reached. Usually a few such items do emerge in an efficient manner that guarantees the participation of all present and does not involve interminable redundant discussion in support of a particular proposition.

The Delphi technique also fosters participation and does so in a way that does not require the assembly of group members in a single place. To illustrate the application, suppose that a nominal group session has identified 10 important management problems. The 10 items would be posted on a questionnaire and mailed to participants with instructions to rate on a scale from 1 to 10 the relative importance of each item listed. When a response has been obtained from each participant, the median score is determined, recorded on each form, and returned to the participant. Now everyone has a record of his or her own first-round votes and the anonymous averages from his or her peers. On the second round they can maintain their original positions or modify them as seems appropriate. Usually, stability representing consensus is obtained after three or four rounds. The author has used this technique to obtain views from pediatricians on the relative levels of disability represented by certain defined chronic conditions. In this way consensus judgments were reached about appropriate quality of life measures applicable to the conditions of interest.

*Focus group* discussions represent another popular means of obtaining insight into the attitudes and beliefs of a defined category of individuals (Eng, Glick, & Parker, 1990). A group of mothers might be assembled to determine beliefs about breastfeeding practices. Or nurses might be brought together to consider factors affecting morale. Discussion is more open-ended than with the NGT or Delphi approaches, but focus group deliberations are kept on track by trained moderators who follow a structured agenda based on a defined set of issues and questions. As with the other methods, participants are key informants with special insights to offer, not randomly selected representatives of the community.

## Research and Evaluation: The Logical Framework

The subject of monitoring and evaluation has been discussed repeatedly throughout the chapter. These discussions are appropriate because performance appraisal should be an ongoing endeavor; it should not be an ad hoc effort. A comprehensive evaluation plan should be prepared at the outset of a project. For this purpose a formally prepared logical framework *(logframe)* has been found useful in project planning; indeed, certain international donor agencies require inclusion of a logframe in proposals submitted to them for funding (Nancholas, 1998). As shown in Table 11–7, the logframe forms a matrix that incorporates both vertical and horizontal logic.

The vertical dimension presents a hierarchy of goals, purposes, outputs, and inputs. The project of interest has its own purposes that are imbedded in broader program goals. A project to reduce the case fatality rate from pneumonia, for example, may be part of a broader program to reduce mortality and morbidity rates generally among preschool children. In order to achieve project objectives or purposes, certain service outputs are required, such as, for example, the identification and appropriate treatment of pneumonia cases with antibiotics. Finally, specified inputs are needed to produce the outputs. To illustrate, antibiotics must be regularly in stock, and CHWs need to be trained in their use.

Indicators in the vertical hierarchy are linked by various assumptions. For example, prescribed antibiotics are assumed to be administered properly. If indicators are satisfactory at one level but not at the next, it should be determined whether necessary activities at the higher level were not undertaken, or whether the assumptions linking the two sets of activities were faulty.

Because inputs, outputs, purposes, and goals are closely linked, placement of indicators in the appropriate category can sometimes be difficult or arbitrary. One project may have as its purpose the production of trained personnel with specified qualifications, whereas another project may have trained personnel as an input required to achieve larger purposes. The distinction between outputs and outcomes (achievement of purposes) can be especially problematic. As a general rule, service outputs are focused on providers, whereas outcomes relate to the service

**Table 11–7** The Logical Framework

| Narrative Summary | Objectively Verifiable Indicators | Means of Verification | Important Assumptions |
|---|---|---|---|
| Program goals: broader aims to which this project contributes | Reduction in under-fives death rate to 90 per thousand | Sample vital registration | } Pneumonia is a major contributor to child mortality |
| Project purposes: intended results from service outputs | Reduction in pneumonia case fatality rate by 50% | Hospital records Household survey | |
| Outputs: service activities using project resources | 90% of pneumonia cases treated adequately with antibiotics | Quality assessment study | } Potency of antibiotics is maintained |
| Inputs: resource requirements | Antibiotics always in stock | Stock records | } Infections are bacterial in nature and treatable by antibiotics |

beneficiaries. Thus the indicator "percent of cases in which antibiotics are prescribed properly" is an output, while "percent of persons with pneumonia who recover" is an indicator reflecting outcome.

Indicators at each level of the vertical hierarchy are first presented in narrative form. To be sure that they are nonambiguous and practicable, they are subjected to a test of horizontal logic. First the indicators must be objectively verifiable. Would two observers necessarily agree that a certain purpose had been satisfied, or is this a matter of opinion? In the latter case the indicator employed is not adequately objective. To illustrate, if patient satisfaction is judged as an attitude exhibited in an interview, but the attitude is poorly defined, this indicator is probably subject to different interpretation by different interviewers and therefore cannot be considered objective. On the other hand, satisfaction measured in terms of return to the clinic for follow-up is objectively verifiable (though not necessarily valid as a true indicator of satisfaction).

The indicators should distinguish project accomplishments from those that would have occurred anyhow. Suppose that project communities and others not scheduled to receive project services both had achieved immunization coverage for 30% of children under the age of 2. This was projected to increase to 80% in project communities, but, in fact, it only rose to 65%. Meanwhile, coverage in nonproject areas spontaneously rose to 45%. The performance indicator should show that increased coverage due to the project was expected to amount to 35% (80% − 45%), whereas a project gain of only 20% was achieved (65% − 45%). Thus the project achieved 20/35, or 57% of the gain expected.

Indicators that are objectively verifiable in principle may not be measurable in practice. The indicator "percent of patients who follow prescribed treatment" is adequately objective, but because it requires accurate reporting or observation in the home, it may not be practicable. The horizontal logic therefore includes specification of the means of verification in order to confirm the feasibility of measurement. When sources for all of the indicator data have been identified, an information system can be assembled and its practicability assessed.

Finally, the subject of evaluation should be linked to health systems research, which is sometimes shunned by managers as something of academic interest only but which should become an integral part of management thinking. Sometimes problems that arise have obvious solutions. Perhaps a high absenteeism rate among nurses is due to child-care responsibilities that often interfere with work duties. Hospital-based child-care centers are identified as the solution to be implemented and monitored as a normal management function.

Nurses who leave service for child rearing and fail to return may present a more problematic situation for which no single solution is apparent. Instead, several possibilities are suggested for testing. Perhaps some could be attracted back into service if a flexible work schedule were offered. Possibly employment to do needed outreach in their own communities would be attractive. Other options might be formulated. The testing of the options requires employment of scientific methods that ensure objective appraisal. In other words, a research approach is needed, but it must be sharply focused on the problem at hand and should produce results that are prompt and can lead to timely management action, not just a journal article.

Unlike classical forms of research, health systems research is characterized by the presence of numerous variables not subject to investigator control. The testing of a certain food variety in the laboratory can use a single strain of mice as both experimental and control animals whose consumption can be closely monitored and controlled while other aspects of their diet and environment are held constant. In contrast, community interventions face the prospect of dealing with families with different socioeconomic states and feeding practices, children whose health and nutrition status varies, and workers whose relationships with their communities may not be uniformly positive. Whereas the emphasis in classical research is on the *research design*

that minimizes variation in other than the experimental variables, the focus in health systems research is on *analysis* of uncontrolled variables, along with the experimental effects. The two approaches are equally scientific and require access to consultants with requisite technical knowledge, albeit of different types (Grundy & Reinke, 1973).

## Quality Assurance

As previously shown, recognition of the importance of services quality and satisfaction has led to the explicit integration of these concerns into the evaluation framework. Indeed, quality assurance (QA) has been the central focus of some of the most successful efforts at management improvement in recent years, based on adaptation of advanced methods developed earlier and widely applied in industry (Brown, Franco, Rafeh, & Hatzell, 1998). Successful adaptations have been made in connection with hospital inpatient services (Exhibit 11–12), family planning (see Chapter 3 for information on family planning in Bangladesh), and clinic ambulatory care (Exhibit 11–13). Accordingly, the subject deserves separate attention here.

Early industrial emphasis on *quality control* was directed to the inspection and acceptance of past efforts. In contrast, current attention to *continuous quality improvement* (CQI) looks to the advancement of future performance. Because hospitals share many of the characteristics of commercial enterprises, it is not surprising that many of the earliest applications of CQI in the health sector were based in hospitals (Berwick et al., 1991). Applications have ranged from clinical practice to administration and personnel management.

The concentration on hospital services management has not been at the full exclusion of community service concerns, notably in family planning. Remarkably successful family planning programs in Indonesia have been characterized by sound management promoted through a high-level central government institution. In Bangladesh, semi-independent entities have

**Exhibit 11–12** Hospital Experience

A sampling of hospital successes in management improvement reveals the wide range of possible applications of QA methods (Hughes, 1992). Reduction of Medicare claims rejections in one institution has saved $120,000 annually. When the problem of lost medical charts was investigated in a health center, losses were virtually eliminated, and yearly costs were reduced by $200,000. Lower nursing turnover at a respiratory hospital saved $390,000 annually, and a thorough review of open heart surgery practices at a cardiology center produced better integration of clinical progressions, improved standing orders, and reduced length of stay to the tune of $2 million per year.

**Exhibit 11–13** Pediatric Practice in Armenia

Because there had not been a unified training program in pediatrics, it was felt that practice was varied and generally poor. Consensus among pediatricians was reached regarding tasks to be performed in carrying out various procedures, including the conduct of well-child visits. A checklist of such tasks was formed, and providers were trained in their use. Performance following training was assessed and compared with that at baseline. The advance hypothesis was that after training, performance would be better and more uniform. Results did show higher levels of average performance following training, but variation among providers had increased. Whereas performance was consistently poor at baseline, it improved markedly for some after training, but others exhibited little change. Further investigation showed that those who used the new structured medical record that had been introduced along with the training tended to perform very well, whereas those who continued to follow the old practice of preparing unstructured medical notes continued to perform poorly.

worked cooperatively with each other and the government in investigations to identify key factors in fertility reduction (for example, supervision of community workers and counseling of clients). Innovative techniques have then been developed and applied to improve performance in these areas (Haaga & Maru, 1996).

As suggested by its title, The Primary Care Operations Research (PRICOR) project focused on primary health care in 109 projects carried out with support from the U.S. Agency for International Development (AID) mainly during the 1980s. Through these efforts checklists were developed to highlight essential tasks to be carried out in clinical practice associated with selected diseases and in program administration. PRICOR was the forerunner of the current Quality Assurance Project (QA Project) in primary health care, which has assisted in numerous quality improvement efforts at the request of individual countries that have identified specific problems in program management.

One of the earliest of these efforts in Chile has achieved remarkable success and has led to a national commitment to systematic efforts to improve quality management (Gnecco & Brown, n.d.). Top-level Chilean MOH interest in quality improvement led to a request for external consultation and the presentation of a quality awareness workshop. These actions initiated the first phase of a three-phase project. In the first phase, problems of poor performance were identified and communicated to health service managers to stimulate their interest in taking remedial action. Training sessions were then conducted in the second phase to develop quality improvement skills. During this phase, support from senior management was further encouraged, but the main thrust was extension of interest in practical problem solving in local health units, development of process indicators, and identification of quality improvement approaches. Training continued and emphasized quality awareness as a normal part of service delivery. By the beginning of the third phase, external technical assistance had been virtually eliminated, resources for QA were incorporated into routine budgets at all levels, and quality management was further decentralized through formation of local quality committees. Moreover, the importance of quality improvement was widely recognized and QA activities were being institutionalized. A QA unit was established within the Chile Public Health Association, and the subject was included in the Annual Latin American Seminar on Maternal and Child Health.

As with hospital applications, the range of primary health care quality problems tackled was broad. The 40 specific projects initiated during the first 3 years of the QA Project included concerns for monitoring adolescent pregnancies, treatment of respiratory infections, medical records quality, laboratory practice, and supervision.

Although the QA Project has been a concerted attack on poor performance, it is by no means an isolated effort. Other projects have produced locally useful results and together have revealed important themes. A study in Nigeria, for example, showed the importance of well-structured medical records to serve as guides to obstetrical practice (Adeyi & Morrow, 1997). A subsequent evaluation of pediatric care in Armenia similarly determined that training in the performance of specified tasks in well-child care led to better results only when a structured medical record that incorporated the tasks was used (McPherson, 1999).

### Work Scheduling

After the overall design of a project endeavor has been established, detailed scheduling is necessary. Because so many interrelated activities must be carried out, coordination is not easy, and sometimes a bottleneck in one activity can delay completion of the entire endeavor. Scheduling techniques that help to anticipate and eliminate potential bottlenecks recognize two types of activities: those that can move forward simultaneously, and those that must be carried out in sequence. The *Critical Path Method* (CPM) is among the easiest to use for identifying, diagramming, and analyzing a set of activities (Levy, Thompson, & Wièst, 1963). A simple

example of its application to the planning and conduct of a meeting is given in Figure 11–8.

First, all the necessary activities are listed and numbered sequentially. The numbering is for ease in later diagramming and has no other significance, because the list is assembled as items come to mind, not necessarily in the order in which they are to be carried out. In the example, eight activities have been identified. Limitations on sequencing are then noted by designating predecessor events that must be accomplished prior to the initiation of further activity. (Note that events are defined as completed activities.) In Figure 11–8 the determination of conference room availability and ordering of refreshments can proceed simultaneously with the selection of meeting participants, but meeting time cannot be set until after participant calendars and conference room availability have been checked. Estimates of time necessary to carry out each activity are then made, assuming that all predecessor events have been concluded.

The list of activities, along with their predecessor events and times, is then converted into a network as shown in the figure. Inevitably, a number of paths must be traversed between the initial node (determining that a meeting is necessary) and the actual holding of the conference. Path 01238 includes four activities that are expected to consume 1, 4, 1, and 1 days, respectively. The total time, 7 days, exceeds that of any other path. Any delay along that path would delay the completion of the endeavor (holding the meeting); hence path 01238 is designated the critical path. Special attention is called to the avoidance of bottlenecks along that path. Focusing on a limited number of potential bottlenecks is a good example of management by exception at work.

Paths other than the critical path have slack time available; that is, some delay can be encountered in the activities involved without jeopardizing overall project completion. A detailed schedule known as a *Gantt chart* (Exhibit 11–14) is prepared, taking into account the flexibility permitted by slack time. For example, the 3 days of slack time in Activity 7 (preparation of a detailed meeting agenda) means that it can be

| Event | Predecessor Events | Time (Days) |
|---|---|---|
| 0. Need for meeting established | – | – |
| 1. Meeting participants selected | 0 | 1 |
| 2. Participants determined | 1 | 4 |
| 3. Meeting time set | 2, 4 | 1 |
| 4. Conference room available | 0 | 2 |
| 5. Refreshments ordered | 0 | 2 |
| 6. Refreshments delivered | 5 | 1 |
| 7. Agenda set | 0 | 2 |
| 8. Meeting held | 3, 6, 7 | 1 |

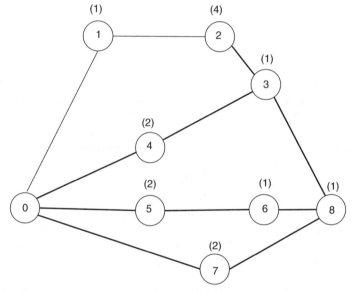

| Path | Time |
|---|---|
| 01238 | 7 |
| 0438 | 4 |
| 0568 | 4 |
| 078 | 3 |

**Figure 11–8** Example of Use of Critical Path Method

initiated anytime between Day 2 and Day 5. The Gantt chart shows it scheduled on Days 3 and 4, thereby allowing the convener of the meeting to tend to other matters on Day 2 before he or she prepares the agenda.

One would never apply CPM formally to the simple set of tasks we have described, though the thought processes of CPM would undoubtedly be applied informally. Consider, however, preparation for a 2-week workshop with par-

ticipants to be housed and fed and several speakers to be invited. In such circumstances CPM has been found to be indispensable to avoiding snarls in planning. In fact, a more sophisticated technique might be justified. The *Program Evaluation and Review Technique* (PERT) in particular has been found to be useful, in large part because it takes cognizance of uncertainties in the times required for task completion by assigning three estimates for each: expected time,

**Exhibit 11–14** Gantt Chart of Scheduled Activities

| | Day | | | | | | |
|---|---|---|---|---|---|---|---|
| *Activity* | *1* | *2* | *3* | *4* | *5* | *6* | *7* |
| 1. Participant selection | ——— | | | | | | |
| 2. Participant availability determined | | ——————————————— | | | | | |
| 3. Meeting time setting | | | | | ——— | | |
| 4. Conference room reserving | | | | ——————— | | | |
| 5. Refreshments ordering | | ——————— | | | | | |
| 6. Refreshments delivery | | | | | ——— | | |
| 7. Setting agenda | | | ——————— | | | | |
| 8. Holding meeting | | | | | | | ——— |

most pessimistic time, and most optimistic time (Merton, 1966). Thus, probability estimates can be made, along with "expected" results. Analysis might reveal, for example, that a project is expected to be completed in 18 months, but that there is a 20% probability that it will require as many as 22 months. Further, it might be determined that path x is "critical," but there is a 30% probability that delays on path y will cause that path to become critical. Therefore, principal attention should be devoted to path x, but path y should also be tracked carefully. Probability considerations in PERT make manual calculations infeasible, but computer programs are available for its application.

## CONCLUSION

It is hoped that the reader has gained a better understanding of management as a multifunctional endeavor that requires a blend of common sense, experience, and technical know-how. The manager must be able to develop needed human, physical, and financial resources and to organize them appropriately to achieve multiple, often conflicting, objectives involving considerations of effectiveness, efficiency, equity, quality, and sustainability.

Some management techniques relate to problem clarification and appraisal; others bring specific resources to bear on the solution of management problems. Management is more than ad hoc problem solving, however. The continuing aim is process improvement, to bring more services of high quality and value to a growing population, especially those in greatest need. Of overriding concern in management today is the application of modern methods of decision analysis, making maximum use of quantitative data, but not overlooking the importance of psychosocial and other qualitative aspects of well-being.

## DISCUSSION QUESTIONS

1. Decentralization of authority is recommended to enable relevant responses to be made to varying local needs. Resources are limited and unevenly distributed at district level, however. How can local control be adequately and equitably exercised under these circumstances?

2. The need is often expressed for clearer job descriptions. The importance of teamwork is also emphasized. This leads to the notion that job responsibilities should be flexible, so that personnel can take on added duties when the workload is heavy or colleagues are absent. Prepare an adequately specific job description for a health center nurse that takes both of these factors into consideration.

3. Various cost recovery mechanisms can inhibit use of needed services, contribute to or discourage overuse, and affect equity in sharing the burden of health care costs. Discuss the pros and cons of fee-for-service and prepayment schemes in these regards. Is there an optimum arrangement?

4. It is argued that Health and Management Information Systems (HMIS) do not meet management needs adequately because they are designed by computer experts and statisticians who do not understand those needs. In response the point is made that managers do not appreciate the value of quantitative information and are therefore not qualified to formulate performance indicators and design information systems. What collaborative roles should managers, statisticians, and computer software specialists play in HMIS development and use?

## REFERENCES

Abel-Smith, B., & Creese, A. (Eds). (1989). *Recurrent costs in the health sector: Problems and policy options in three countries.* Geneva, Switzerland: World Health Organization.

Adeyi, O., & Morrow, R. (1997). Essential obstetric care: Assessment and determinants of quality. *Social Science and Medicine,* 45(11), 1631–1639.

Araujo, J.L., Jr. (1997). Attempts to decentralize in recent Brazilian health policy: Issues and problems, 1988–1994. *International Journal of Health Services,* 27(1), 109–124.

Arole, M., & Arole, R. (1994). *Jamkhed.* Bombay: Archana Art Printers.

Bell, D.E., Raiffa, H., & Tverksy, A. (Eds.). (1988). *Decision making: Descriptive, normative and prescriptive interactions.* New York: Cambridge University Press.

Berwick, D.M., Godfrey, A.B., & Roessner, J. (1991). *Curing health care.* San Francisco: Jossey-Bass Publishers.

Bossert, T.J. (1990). Can they get along without us? *Social Science and Medicine,* 30(90), 1015–1023.

Bossert, T.J., Soebekti, R., & Rai, N.K. (1991). "Bottom-up" planning in Indonesia: Decentralization in the Ministry of Health. *Health Policy and Planning,* 6(1), 55–63.

Brown, L.D., Franco, L.M., Rafeh, N., & Hatzell, T. (1998). *Quality assurance of health care in developing countries* (2nd ed.). Chevy Chase, MD: Center for Human Services.

Bryant, M., & Essomba, R.O. (1995). Measuring time utilization in rural health centers. *Health Policy and Planning,* 10(4), 415–421.

Cartwright, A. (1983). *Health surveys in practice and in potential.* London: King Edward's Hospital Trust for London.

Cassels, A., & Janovsky, K. (1996). *Strengthening health management in districts and provinces: Handbook for facilitators.* Geneva, Switzerland: World Health Organization.

Creese, A., & Kutzin, J. (1995). Lessons from cost-recovery in health. Discussion paper no. 2. Geneva, Switzerland: World Health Organizaiton.

Creese, A., & Parker, D. (Eds.). (1994). *Cost analysis in primary health care: A training manual for programme managers.* Geneva, Switzerland: World Health Organization.

Dalkey, N.C. (1969). *The Delphi method: An experimental study of group opinion.* Memorandum RM-5888-PR. Santa Monica, CA: Rand Corp.

Delbecq, A.L., & van de Ven, A.H. (1971). A group process model for problem identification and program planning. *The Journal of Applied Behavioral Science, 7*(4), 466–492.

DeSweemer, C., Parker, R.L., Taylor, C.E., & Reinke, W.A. (1979). Unresolved issues in primary care in the developing world. In K.L. White & P.J. Bullock (Eds.), *The health of populations: a report of two Rockefeller conferences.* New York: Rockefeller Foundation.

Dodge, H.F., & Romig, H.G. (1959). *Sampling inspection tables* (2nd ed.). New York: John Wiley & Sons.

Drucker, P.F. (1974). *Management: Tasks, responsibilities, practices.* New York: Harper & Row.

Eng, E., Glick, D., & Parker, K. (1990). Focus-group methods: Effects on village-agency collaboration for child survival. *Health Policy and Planning, 5*(1), 67–76.

Flavier, J.M. (1970). *Doctor to the barrios.* Quezon City, Philippines: New Day Publishers.

Fulop, T., & Roemer, M.I. (1982). *International development of health manpower policy* (W.H.O. Offset Publication No. 61). Geneva, Switzerland: World Health Organization.

*The functional analysis of health needs and services.* (1976). New Delhi: Asia Publishing House.

Gnecco, G., & Brown, L.D. (n.d.). *Making a commitment to quality health care: Developing a national strategy for Chile.* Unpublished report of the Ministry of Health of Chile and the Center for Human Services.

Gold, M.R., Russell, L.B., Siegel, J.E., & Weinstein, M.C. (Eds.). (1996). *Cost-effectiveness in health and medicine.* New York: Oxford University Press.

Grant, E.L., & Leavenworth, R.S. (1980). *Statistical quality control* (5th ed.). New York: McGraw-Hill Book Co.

Green, L.W., Kreuter, M.W., Deeds, S.G., & Partridge, K.B. (1980). *Health education planning: A diagnostic approach.* Palo Alto, CA: Mayfield Publishing Co.

Grundy, F., & Reinke, W.A. (1973). *Health practice research and formalized managerial methods* (Public Health Papers No. 51). Geneva, Switzerland: World Health Organization.

Haaga, J.G., & Maru, R. (1996). The effect of operations research on program changes in Bangladesh. *Studies in Family Planning, 27*(2), 76–87.

Hall, T.L., Reinke, W.A., & Lawrence, D. (1975). Measurement and projection of the demand for health care: The Chilean experience. *Medical Care, 13*(6), 511–522.

Henderson, R., & Sundaresan, T. (1982). Cluster sampling to assess immunization coverage: A review of experience with a simplified sampling method. *Bulletin of the World Health Organization, 60,* 253–260.

Hill, P.H., Bedau, H.A., Chechile, R.A., Crochetiere, W.J., Kellerman, B.L., Ounjiàn, D., Pauker, S.G., Pauker, S.P., & Rubin, J.Z. (1986). *Making decisions.* New York: University Press of America.

Hughes, J.M. (1992). Reducing health care costs: A case for quality. *Physician Executive, 18*(4), 9–15.

Janovsky, K. (1988). *The challenge of implementation: District health systems for primary health care.* Geneva, Switzerland: World Health Organization.

Kahneman, D., Slovic, P., & Tversky, A. (Eds.). (1982). *Judgment under uncertainty: Heuristics and biases.* New York: Cambridge University Press.

Kanji, N. (1989). Charging for drugs in Africa: UNICEF's "Bamako Initiative." *Health Policy and Planning, 4*(2), 110–120.

Kish, L. (1967). *Survey sampling.* New York: John Wiley & Sons.

Knippenberg, R., Reinke, W.A., & Hopwood, I. (Eds.). (1997). Sustainability of primary health care including immunizations in Bamako Initiative programs in West Africa. *Health Planning and Management, 12* (Suppl. 1).

Korten, D.C. (1979). Toward a technology for managing social development. In D.C. Korten (Ed.), *Population and social development management* (pp. 1–42). Caracas: Population and Social Development Management Center, Instituto de Estudios Superiores de Administracion.

Korten, F.J. (1981). Community participation: A management perspective on obstacles and options. In D.C. Korten & F.B. Alonso (Eds.), *Bureaucracy and the poor: closing the gap* (pp. 181–200). Singapore: McGraw-Hill International Book Co.

Lafond, A.K. (Ed.). (1995). Research on sustainability in the health sector. *Health Policy and Planning 10* (Suppl.), 1–76.

Levy, F.K., Thompson, G.L., & Wièst, J.D. (1963). The ABCs of the Critical Path Method. *Harvard Business Review, 41,* 98–108.

Loevinsohn, B.P., Guerrero, E.T., & Gregorio, S.P. (1995). Improving primary health care through systematic supervision: A controlled field trial. *Health Policy and Planning, 10*(2), 144–153.

Lwanga, S.K., & Lemeshow, S. (1991). *Sample size determination in health studies.* Geneva, Switzerland: World Health Organization.

Madan, T.N. (1987). Community involvement in health policy: Socio-structural and dynamic aspects of health beliefs. *Social Science and Medicine, 25*(6), 615–620.

Management Sciences for Health. (1997). *Managing drug supply: The selection, procurement, distribution, and use of pharmaceuticals* (2nd ed.). West Hartford, CT: Kumarian Press.

Mayo-Smith, I., & Ruther, N.L. (1986). Force Field Analysis. In I. Mayo-Smith & N.L. Ruther (Eds.), *Achieving improved performance in public organizations* (pp. 47–68). West Hartford, CT: Kumarian Press.

McKee, M., Aiken, L., Rafferty, A., & Sochalaski, J. (1998). Organizational change and quality in health care: An evolving international agenda. *Quality in Health Care, 7,* 37–41.

McMahon, R., Barton, E., & Piot, M. (1992). *On being in charge* (2nd ed.). Geneva, Switzerland: World Health Organization.

McPherson, R. (1999). *The use of clinical practice guidelines to improve provider performance of well-child care in Armenia.* Unpublished Ph.D. diss., Johns Hopkins University.

Meima, F., Peters, D., & Sanneh, K.M.L. (1992). Quality assessment of the ARI control program in the Gambia. Unpublished report of a field study.

Merton, W. (1966). PERT and planning for health programs. *Public Health Reports, 81,* 449–454.

Mills, A. (1990a). The economics of hospitals in developing countries, Part I: expenditure patterns. *Health Policy and Planning, 5*(2), 107–117.

Mills, A. (1990b). The economics of health in developing countries, Part II: costs and sources of income. *Health Policy and Planning, 5*(3), 203–218.

Montoya-Aguilar, C., & Marin-Lira, M.A. (1986). International equity in coverage of primary health care: Examples from developing countries. *World Health Statistics Quarterly, 39*(4), 336–344.

Morlock, L.L., Nathanson, C.A., & Alexander, J.A. (1988). Authority, power and influence. In S.M. Shortell and A.D. Kaluzny, *Health care management* (pp. 265–300). New York: John Wiley & Sons.

Morse, P.M. (1958). *Queues, inventories and maintenance.* New York: John Wiley & Sons.

Musgrove, P. (1986). Measurement of equity in health. *World Health Statistics Quarterly, 39*(4), 325–335.

Nancholas, S. (1998). A logical framework. *Health Policy and Planning, 13*(2), 189–193.

Newell, K. (Ed.). (1975). *Health by the people.* Geneva, Switzerland: World Health Organization.

Olsen, I.T. (1998). Sustainability of health care: A framework for analysis. *Health Policy and Planning, 13*(3), 287–295.

Prescott, N., & De Ferranti, D. (1985). The analysis and assessment of health programs. *Social Science and Medicine, 20*(12), 1235–1240.

Rand Corporation. (1995). *Financing health care: Lessons from the Indonesia Resource Mobilization study.* Santa Monica, CA: Author.

Reinke, W.A. (Ed.). (1983). *Issues in the supervision of CBD projects.* Washington, DC: U.S. Agency for International Development.

Reinke, W.A. (1988a). Health care in Indonesia: Dealing with diversity. In I. Sirageldin (Ed.), *Public health and development* (pp. 175–191). Greenwich, CT: Jai Press.

Reinke, W.A. (Ed.). (1988b). *Health planning for effective management.* New York: Oxford University Press.

Reinke, W.A. (1991). Applicability of industrial sampling techniques to epidemiologic investigations. *American Journal of Epidemiology, 134*(10), 1222–1232.

Reinke, W.A. (1994). Program evaluation: Considerations of effectiveness, efficiency and equity. *Journal of Family and Community Medicine, 1,* 61–71.

Reinke, W.A. (1995). Quality Management in Managed Care. In H. Jolt (Ed.), *State of the art reviews* (Vol. 2, No. 1) (pp. 79–88). Philadelphia: Hanley and Belfus.

Reinke, W.A. (1999). A multidimensional program evaluation model: Considerations of cost-effectiveness, equity, quality, and sustainability. *The Canadian Journal of Program Evaluation, 14*(2), 145–160.

Reinke, W.A., Stanton, B.F., Roberts, L., & Newman, J. (1993). *Rapid assessment for decision making* (Water and Sanitation for Health Project Field Report No. 391). Washington, DC: U.S. Agency for International Development.

Reinke, W.A., & Wolff, M. (1983). The Lampang health development project: The road to health for all? *World Health Forum, 4,* 114–120.

Reynolds, J., & Gaspari, K.C. (1985). *Cost-effectiveness analysis.* Chevy Chase, MD: Center for Human Services.

Robertson, S.E., Anker, M., Roisin, A., Macklai, N., Engstrom, J., & La Force, F.M. (1997). The lot quality technique: A global review of applications in the assessment of health services and disease surveillance. *World Health Statistics Quarterly, 50,* 199–209.

Ryan, T.P. (1989). *Statistical methods for quality improvement.* New York: John Wiley & Sons.

Smith, P.G., & Morrow, R.H. (1991). *Methods for field trials of interventions against tropical diseases: A "toolbox."* New York: Oxford University Press.

Suchman, E.A. (1967). *Evaluative Research.* New York: Russell Sage Foundation.

Szilagyi, A.D. (1988). *Management and performance* (3rd ed.). Glenview, IL: Scott Foresman & Co.

Tarimo, E. (1991). *Towards a healthy district: Organizing and managing district health systems based on primary health care.* Geneva, Switzerland: World Health Organization.

Taylor, C.E. (1988). Community involvement. In W.A. Reinke (Ed.), *Health planning for effective management* (pp. 172–186). New York: Oxford University Press.

Taylor, C.E., Dirican, R., & Deuschle, K.W. (1968). *Health manpower planning in Turkey.* Baltimore: The Johns Hopkins University Press.

Taylor, C.E., & Waldman, R.J. (1998). Designing eradication programs to strengthen primary health care. In W.R. Dowdle & D.R. Hopkins (Eds.), *The eradication of infectious diseases.* New York: John Wiley & Sons.

Taylor-Ide, D., & Taylor, C.E. (1995). *Community based sustainable human development: Going to scale with self-reliant social development.* New York: UNICEF Environment Section.

Thorne, M., Sapire, S., & Rejeb, H. (1991). *District team problem solving guidelines for maternal and child health, family planning and other public health services.* Geneva, Switzerland: World Health Organization.

Torrance, G.W. (1986). Measurement of health state utilities for economic appraisal: A review. *Journal of Health Economics, 5,* 1–30.

Von Neumann, J., & Morganstern, O. (1947). *Theory of games and economic behavior.* Princeton, NJ: Princeton University Press.

Were, M. (1982). *Organization and management of community-based health care.* Nairobi, Kenya: UNICEF Regional Office.

World Bank. (1991). *Federal Republic of Nigeria: Health care cost, financing and utilization* (Report No. 8382-UNI). Washington, DC: Author.

World Health Organization. (1988). *Training manual on health manpower management.* Geneva, Switzerland: Author.

World Health Organization. (1990). *Coordinated health and human resources development* (Technical Report Series No. 801). Geneva, Switzerland: Author.

World Health Organization. (1992). *The hospital in rural and urban districts* (Technical Report Series 819). Geneva, Switzerland: Author.

World Health Organization. (1993). *Rapid evaluation method guidelines for maternal and child health, family planning, and other health services.* Geneva, Switzerland: Author.

# CHAPTER 12

# Health and the Economy

*Jennifer Prah Ruger, Dean T. Jamison, and David E. Bloom*

Health and health care systems interrelate with the economy in a number of ways, but the multiple causal mechanisms that define this relationship divide naturally into two categories. The first comprises the linkages between health and the level growth rate and distribution of income. The second concerns the relationships among health care delivery institutions, health finance policies, and economic outcomes. The two major sections of this chapter follow this division of topics.

Figure 12–1 provides a summary of these linkages and a guide to the structure of the chapter. The first major section deals with relations between the health status of populations and income levels. Health and demography affect income (arrow F) through their impact on labor

An early version of this chapter was prepared for the 1998 transition team of the then-incoming World Health Organization (WHO) Director-General Dr. G.H. Brundtland. Preparation of that version was supported by grants from the Royal Norwegian Ministry of Foreign Affairs to WHO and the World Bank. The WHO Commission on Macroeconomics and Health supported extension and revision, and discussions with the Commission's chair, Jeffrey Sachs, provided valuable ideas and feedback during preparation of this chapter. Conclusions and opinions are those of the authors and not necessarily those of any of the sponsoring agencies. David Canning, Felicia Knaul, Lawrence Lau, Pia Malaney, and Anne Mills also made valuable suggestions and comments on earlier drafts. Leslie Evans prepared the tables and graphics.

productivity, savings rates, investments in physical and human capital (education, for example), and age structure effects. The current literature suggests these effects to be more significant than previously thought, even up to the early 1990s; these issues are addressed in the section titled "Economic Consequences of Ill Health."

The other direction of causality lies in income's impact on health and demography (arrow E). An important part of the literature on the health benefits of higher income assesses the extent to which income operates through improved capacity to purchase food, to have adequate sanitation, housing, and education, and through incentives for fertility limitation. The section titled "Economic Development's Consequences for Health" briefly discusses these points. Further, health systems as a whole play an important role in improving health and are themselves greatly influenced by health finance and related policies (arrows C and D). Other chapters in this volume deal with these issues.

Finally, wealthier countries tend to spend a higher percentage of their income per capita on health and to rely more substantially on public sector finance than lower-income countries (arrow B, Figure 12–1). Conversely, health finance and delivery mechanisms affect income level and distribution (arrow A) through their effects on incentives and institutional environments. Some health finance systems are, for example, more progressive than others, favorably affecting the distribution of income, whereas

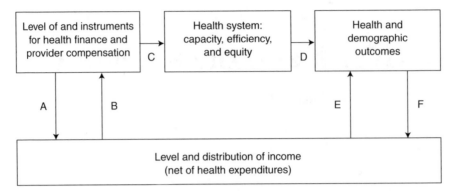

**Figure 12–1** Health, Health Policies, and Economic Outcomes

others have detrimental efficiency consequences through their effects on labor markets or on the adequacy with which financial risks are shared. The second major section of the chapter explores these linkages.

Whether the final objective of development policy is economic growth, poverty alleviation, or improved health, these domains are inextricably linked. Better information on the magnitude of the association between health and economic growth and of health systems and economic outcomes can aid academics and policy makers in understanding and devising health and development policies that will improve people's quality of life worldwide. This understanding allows the development of more balanced policy portfolios (Bloom & River Path Associates, in press).

## HEALTH AND ECONOMIC DEVELOPMENT

The evidence presented here suggests that health is closely linked with economic growth and development. Figure 12–2 illustrates the multiple pathways through which illness can have an effect. The top half shows the age-structure effects of demographic transition as seen by a change in the dependency ratio that has been a significant determinant of growth in East Asia, for example. High levels of fertility and child mortality (both in part a result of child illness), along with reductions in the labor force brought on by mortality and early retirement, can cause

an increase in the dependency ratio that ultimately reduces income. A reversal of these effects can cause a decrease in the dependency ratio, which increases per capita income. In addition, childhood health can affect adult health. Recent research points to a strong link between the health of adults and how healthy they were as children (Kuh & Ben-Shlomo, 1997). The relevant arrow in Figure 12–2 represents that additional pathway between child health and economic outcomes. The lower half of Figure 12–2 illustrates the effects of illness and malnutrition, operating through other factors such as reduced investments in human and physical capital, in reducing labor productivity. And finally, reduced labor productivity has a direct impact on reducing per capita income. Economic conditions influence health as well: the relationship between health and economic development is causal in both directions.

Progress in health and other dimensions of development during the twentieth century arguably constitute mankind's greatest achievements. Rates of progress were so high that projecting them back—or forward—in time suggests that never before and, probably, never again will so much be achieved in so short a period. Before turning to the more systematic discussion of health and economic development, it is worth touching on the broader context.

Table 12–1 provides examples of progress in five domains: health itself, fertility rates, physical growth (or nutritional status), cogni-

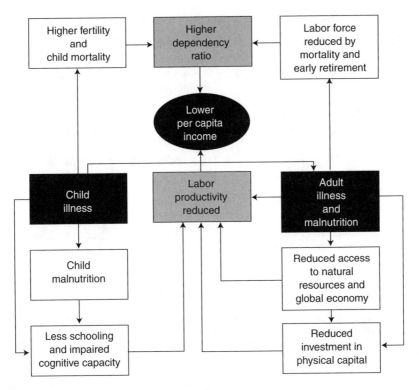

**Figure 12–2** Channels through Which Illness Reduces Income

tive growth, and income, linked in a web of mutual causation. Row 1 takes health using the life expectancy of Chilean females in the period 1909 to 1999 as an example. At the beginning of this period, their life expectancy was 33 years; it then increased at an average rate of 1% per annum over 90 years to a level of 78 years in 1999 (WHO, 1999). Had this rate been in effect for the preceding 70 years, life expectancy would have been 16 years in 1835, far lower than the actual level. If this rate were to continue, life expectancy would exceed 150 years by 2070—conceivable, but unlikely. For the other indicators, the twentieth century also stands out, in some cases more dramatically, in others less so.

The example of cognitive growth may be less familiar than the others. Evidence from an increasing number of studies around the world suggests major improvements in the average level of general, or "fluid," intelligence. The Dutch study cited in the table is particularly suggestive. All Dutch males are screened (including an IQ test) for military service at about age 20. The study matched sons (1982 cohort) with fathers (1952 cohort) and found a 21-point gain. This gain is larger than that found in most studies, but it is indicative of the general pattern. Flynn (1998) summarizes the Dutch and many similar studies (while placing caveats on how they should be interpreted.)

**Economic Consequences of Ill Health**

Microeconomic analyses that study the link between health and economic outcomes focus on household, family, and individual-level data. Such studies typically look at the relationships between human resources, particularly education and health, and labor market outcomes (em-

**Table 12–1** Human Progress in the Twentieth Century: Never Before, Never Again

| Welfare Indicator | Example | Before and After | Rate |
|---|---|---|---|
| Health (proxied by mortality) | Life expectancy, Chilean females (1909–1999) | 33 years in 1909<br>78 years in 1999 | 1.0% per annum OR .45 s.d.[a] per generation[b] |
| Total fertility rate[c] | TFR, Western Pacific Region (1950–1998) | 5.9 in 1950<br>1.9 in 1998 | −2.4% per annum OR −.53 s.d. per generation |
| Physical growth (height-for-age or BMI) | Height, 10-year-old Norwegian females (1920–1970)[d] | 130.2 cm in 1920<br>139.6 cm in 1990 | 1.9 cm/decade OR .84 s.d. per generation |
| Cognitive growth (general or "fluid" intelligence) | Dutch males IQ (1982) relative to that of their own fathers (1952) | IQ = 100 in 1952<br>IQ = 121 in 1982 | 7 points per decade OR 1.4 s.d. per generation |
| Income | Income per capita, Latin America (1913–1992), in 1990 dollars | $1,440 in 1913<br>$4,820 in 1992 | 1.5% per annum |

[a]An s.d. refers to an estimate of the standard deviation of the variable's distribution at the initial time.
[b]This defines a generation to equal 30 years.
[c]The total fertility rate (TFR) is the expected number of children a woman will have if she gave birth at the then-current age-specific fertility rates.
[d]Source for 1970: G.H. Brundtland et al., *Acta Paed Scand* 1975.

ployment, wages and productivity, and age of retirement). Although it is increasingly well established empirically that a person's health affects his or her labor performance (market and nonmarket), much of the microeconomic literature in the past has been dominated by attention to the role of education and training on labor outcomes. Recent work in this area demonstrates why the relationship between health and productivity is of special interest to low- and middle-income countries. Investments in health both contribute directly to individual productivity and complement investments in education and physical capital.

Macroeconomic studies provide evidence of a different sort by assessing the influence of health on national income in cross-country comparisons. This chapter focuses on such studies from low- and middle-income countries, although a number of examples from high-income countries are included. Thomas and Strauss (1998) provide more extensive coverage of this area, particularly with respect to household studies. Currie and Madrian (1999) cover the research

literature concerning health and labor market outcomes in the United States and other high-income countries and provide a careful discussion of problems of causality and statistical specification. This chapter notes those important issues, but does not address them in a substantial way.

### Households and Diseases

*Health, Nutrition, and Productivity.* The growing body of knowledge of the relationship between health and the earnings of individuals can be useful in designing policy interventions aimed at health improvement. These measures have the potential to enhance labor productivity, especially among those in lower income countries and among lower income groups within countries.

Much of the work in this area has examined the impact of adult anthropometric measures such as height, weight, body mass index (BMI), and patterns of illness and disability (all measures or indicators of health) on individuals' labor productivity as measured primarily by wages or earnings. Height and mortality have been found to be inversely related, implying that reductions in height can ultimately reduce an individual's number of productive working years (Schultz, 1997). Short height and low BMI have also been found to be associated with chronic morbidity in midlife (ages 20–50) and with male deaths in late life (Fogel, 1994). A number of other studies have assessed the effects of nutritional status on productivity in lower income countries (Behrman, 1993; Deolalikar, 1988; Sahn & Alderman, 1988) and the cumulative impact of parental nutrition, childhood nourishment, and health over the course of the life cycle on adult height, which ultimately affects individuals' wage and earning potential.

Sahn and Alderman (1988) found that energy intake influenced wage offers for male and female labor in rural and urban areas of Sri Lanka, suggesting that better nutrition increases labor productivity. Behrman (1993) also found, in a comprehensive literature review, that nutrition has direct effects on the labor productivity of poorer individuals in lower income countries. Working in rural south India, Deolalikar (1988) found that although neither market wages nor farm output was affected by a worker's daily energy intake, both variables were influenced by weight-for-height ratios, indicating that chronic malnutrition has a significant effect on market wages and farm output. Evidence from Rwanda described in Exhibit 12–1 does, however, show direct effects of energy consumption operating through time allocation.

Thomas and Strauss (1998) have proposed two main reasons why household production studies should focus on health as an important determinant of productivity. First, they argue that the marginal productivity of good health is likely to be higher in lower income countries than in industrialized societies because of lower absolute levels of health and different patterns of disease. In particular, the predominance of infectious diseases in lower income countries causes higher rates of infant and child morbidity and mortality. The result can be ill health consequences that are felt throughout the life cycle and not primarily at older ages, as in the case of higher income countries. Second, Thomas

and Strauss argue that because employment opportunities in lower income economies tend to depend on physical strength and endurance, the benefits of better health are likely to be greater in these settings. For example, Indonesian men with anemia were found to have 20% lower productivity than men without. In an experiment, men were randomly assigned to one of two groups, receiving either an iron supplement or a placebo. Those who were anemic initially and received the iron treatment increased their productivity to nearly the levels of non-anemic workers, and the productivity gains were large when weighed against the costs of treatment. Thus the effects of improved health are likely to be greatest for the most vulnerable, that is, the lowest income, the sickest, and those with the least education. Further, if there are thresholds of health status below which functioning and productivity are seriously impaired, policies that target those with the poorest health will yield the greatest increases in income. Bhargava, Jamison, Lau, and Murray (2000) found strong evidence to support the plausible view that the effects of health on growth rates (using adult survival rates as the measure of health) are strongest at low levels of income.

In their earlier work in urban Brazil, these individuals (Strauss & Thomas, 1995; Thomas & Strauss, 1997) analyzed the effects on wages of health indicators such as height and BMI, along with energy and protein intake, while controlling for educational variables that also contribute to earnings.[*] Including health variables in their analysis significantly reduced the effects

---

[*]It is important to maintain a sharp distinction, as Strauss and Thomas have done, between nutrient intake and malnutrition. Nutrient intake is one determinant of nutritional status (as measured by anthropometric indicators such as height-for-age, or biochemical indicators such as hematocrit for anemia). In many environments, infectious diseases will also be important determinants of malnutrition. For this reason, prevention or control of infection may often be more cost-effective for controlling malnutrition than attempts to improve diets through food transfers, food subsidies, or social marketing. (See Chapter 5 for more information on nutrition.)

of education on wages. They found that height had a significant effect on wages (taller men and women earned more than shorter men and women), that higher BMI was associated with higher wages among males, and that this effect was most pronounced for less educated men. In addition, lower levels of energy and protein intake per person were associated with reduced wages for market workers, but not for the self-employed.

In Ghana, Schultz (1996) found that height significantly affected wages; for example, a 1 cm increase resulted in an 8% increase in male hourly wages and a 7% increase in female hourly wages. In Mexico, Knaul (April 1999) studied the productivity of investments in health and nutrition for women. The author analyzed the impact of age at menarche, or first menstruation (an indicator of cumulative health and nutritional status), on female labor market productivity and found that investments in health and nutrition had significant effects on productivity. A 1-year decline in age of menarche was associated with a 25% increase in wages.*

Human energy intake and nutritional deficiencies significantly affect people's ability to work. A number of studies (Basta, Soekirman, Karyadi, & Scrimshaw, 1979; Gardner, Edgerton, Senewiratne, Barnard, & Ohira, 1975; Spurr, 1983) have demonstrated the influence of iron deficiency on oxygen consumption and the positive impact of iron supplementation on labor productivity. The effects of nutritional status on work performance are of interest to policy makers designing food and economic programs to improve energy and nutrient intake.

In summary, the literature indicates a positive relationship among earnings, productivity, and energy intake. Higher earnings give people greater ability to purchase food, improving energy, nutrient intake, and health; improved health ultimately enhances productivity. Leiben-

*See also Knaul and Parker (1998) on the patterns over time and the determinants of early labor force participation and school dropout in Mexican children and youth.

stein (1957), Mirrlees (1975), and others have espoused this set of relationships. Fogel (1994) also has done significant historical research in this area, suggesting that improvement in nutritional and health status contributed to the economic growth of England and France from about 1750.

***Disability and Income.*** In a study of the effects of illness on wages and labor supply in Côte d'Ivoire and Ghana, Schultz and Tansel (1997) found that wages were significantly lower for each disabled day; in other words, poor health in the form of disability has negative consequences for labor productivity. In examining the productivity of household investments in health in Colombia, Ribero and Nunez (1999) found that an additional day of disability in a given month decreased male rural earnings hourly by 33% and female earnings by 13%. A disability in a given month was also detrimental to urban workers' wages, decreasing hourly earnings of urban males by 28% and urban females by 14%. Height was also found to affect productivity significantly: a 1 cm increase resulted in a 6.9% increase in urban female earnings and an 8% increase in urban male earnings. (Ribero and Nunez [1999] also evaluated the effects of public and private investments in health. They found that an increase in social security coverage in rural areas could result in a lower incidence and duration of illness, whereas increases in urban areas would result in a greater propensity to report illnesses. They also found that, although basic service interventions, such as electricity and sewage or potable water, had very little effect on height and productivity, policies focused on providing adequate housing for those in need did have a positive impact on health and productivity.)

Murrugarra and Valdivia (1999) studied the returns to health for Peruvian urban adults. Employing a two-stage process, they first estimated the relationship between education and health; then they examined the effects of health on productivity (measured by wages), looking at different subsamples of the population (for example, stratified by gender, age, location in the wage

**Exhibit 12–1** Nutrient Intake and Time Allocation in Rwanda

Information on energy (calorie) intake and use can be difficult to obtain in all societies, but it is especially difficult in lower income countries. Some people are self-sufficient, working primarily on their own land and in their own homes; because they do not receive monetary compensation in the marketplace, measuring the variables necessary to test implications for health is not easy. It can also be difficult to ascertain this relationship when health effects lag behind other changes; for example, simple measures, such as changes in dietary habits through protein intake and micronutrient supplementation for children, can prevent diseases later in the life cycle (Bhargava, 1994). Hence, some scholars analyze time allocation (from time allocation surveys, which document time spent on different activities, such as sleeping, resting or sitting quietly, work involving agriculture or heavy activities, or housework), and evaluate the relationship between time allocation and nutritional status to examine the energy intake, nutritional status, and health nexus.

In a 1982–1983 study of the time allocation patterns of adult men and women in approximately 110 Rwandan households surveyed four times, Bhargava found that low incomes and high food prices reduced households' energy intakes, resulting in more time spent resting and sleeping. The study also gathered statistics on age, consumption, production, protein intake, and weight and height (used to calculate body mass index). The study found that the energy standard for active adult subsistence requires energy intakes of at least twice the basal metabolic rate.

The policy implications of this work are important. Interventions designed to improve nutrient intake and use through better health would enable individuals to carry out the activities necessary for active adult subsistence. Subsistence at higher activity levels will, in turn, enhance people's ability to purchase nutritious food in the marketplace, and dietary guidelines at a broad policy level should reflect the nutritional and energy needs for human activity.

distribution, and type of employer, either public or private, small or large, or self-employed). The authors found that schooling's effects on health were positive, strong, and increased with age for urban males. They also found a positive effect of health on wages, controlling for education and income effects, which differed for different subgroups of the population. For example, among older, self-employed males, an additional sick day resulted in a 4.3% reduction in average hourly earnings. These males experienced greater effects due to illness than other groups; for instance, those at the lowest end of the earnings distribution experienced a reduction in average earnings due to an additional sick day of 3.8%, and those in the private sector experienced the weakest effect, with a 1.8% reduction in hourly earnings due to an additional sick day. The results for females were inconclusive.

Finally, disease and disability affect individuals' retirement decisions. For example, in Jamaica, Handa and Neitzert (1998) found that individuals with chronic illness face an increased probability of retirement as compared to healthy individuals. In the United States, Dwyer and Mitchell (1999) studied the impact of mental and physical capacity for work on older men's retirement decisions. They found health variables were more influential than economic factors on the decision to retire and estimated that men in poor health would retire, on average, 1 to 2 years earlier than those in good health.

In total, these studies suggest that health is related to productivity, both through the direct effects that adult height and chronic morbidity have on adult productivity, and through the inverse relationship between height and mortality that can ultimately reduce an individual's number of productive working years. In addition, illness and disability have negative consequences on labor productivity, reducing hourly wages by as much as 33%. The studies summarized in Exhibit 12–2 provide strong evidence that the health to productivity link is causal in nature. These factors are particularly important in lower income countries, where a significant proportion of the work force is involved in agriculture and other forms of manual labor. Also,

**Exhibit 12–2** Do Health Changes Cause Income Changes?

In efforts to study the relationships among different variables (such as, for example, health and wages), it is difficult to disentangle mutual causation, that is, the strength of causation in each direction. In some studies, researchers attempt to go beyond standard statistical techniques, such as ordinary least-squares regression, in efforts to deal with both measurement error and the endogeneity of health. These studies require complicated multiple-staged statistical methods and produce results that are suggestive but seldom definitive. Three studies have used data allowing for a simpler, sharper assessment of causality and are illustrative of how data sets including nonincome-related determinants of health can resolve the causality problem. Each study confirms a strong causal link from health to economic outcomes.

A British experiment (Moffett et al., 1999) evaluated the effectiveness of an exercise program for patients with lower back pain, through a randomized controlled trial of the program compared with usual primary care management. The results indicated that at 1 year the intervention group showed significantly greater improvement on a scale of back pain, and reported in total only 378 days off work compared with 607 in the control group. The intervention group used fewer health care resources.

Another study, in the United States, traced the consequences for wealth status of a sudden health shock (Smith, 1999), evaluating the impact of the onset of chronic health problems (controlling for demographic factors, health risk behaviors, and preexisting conditions) and mild and severe new health conditions. Researchers found that onsets of even mild health problems may have lowered wealth accumulation by US$3,620. The impact of new, severe health problems on savings was found to be a mean wealth reduction of about US$17,000 or 7% of household wealth (per incident). Finally, among Americans aged 70 and over, a new health condition was found to lower wealth accumulation by about US$10,000, half of which was found to be a reduction in financial assets.

Finally, an experiment involving 6,000 households in Indonesia (Dow, Gertler, Strauss, & Thomas, 1997) studied the effect of changes in prices of publicly provided health services on labor force participation. By randomly selecting districts where fees were raised, and by holding fees in neighboring control districts constant, the authors found that some health indicators and the use of health care declined in test areas relative to controls. Higher prices were associated with more limitations in daily activities and more days spent in bed, especially among the poor and among women in households with low economic and educational status. Finally, the study found significant declines in labor force participation in the test area among vulnerable groups.

the negative effects of malnutrition during childhood can have lasting effects on human capacity, and the effects of improved health are probably greatest for the most vulnerable: the lowest income, the sickest, and the least well educated.

### Economic Costs of \Particular Diseases

The economic effect of specific aspects of health status can be assessed by evaluating the economic burden created by particular diseases. The economic costs of particular diseases typically comprise two elements: (1) the direct costs of prevention and treatment and (2) the indirect costs of labor time lost due to illness. Although empirical work in this area is limited, this section reviews economic analyses of three diseases, malaria, tuberculosis, and HIV/ADS with additional illustrative examples of the Onchocerciasis Control Program (OCP), and mental illness.

*Malaria.* Malaria, among the most significant public health problems in lower income countries, still claims about 1.1 million lives per year. In all WHO member states, the estimated total of disability-adjusted life years (DALYs) lost in 1998 due to malaria is calculated to be 39 million, or 2.8% of the total DALYs lost because of disease (WHO, 1999).* The high rates of morbidity and mortality caused by this disease suggest significant economic costs. (See Chapter 4.)

Chima and Mills (1999) and Malaney (1998) have delineated the direct and indirect economic costs of malaria as follows: the direct costs of prevention (mosquito coils, aerosol sprays, bed nets, residual spraying, and mosquito repellents) and treatment (drugs, treatment fees, transport, and costs of subsistence at a health center); and the indirect costs of labor time lost because of illness. Given these two components, malaria directly increases household and public sector expenditures and reduces labor inputs and can reduce human capital as a result of declines in school attendance, lowered school performance, and increased cognitive impairment. It has also been suggested to cause inefficiencies with respect to land use. Leighton and Foster (1993) estimate the total annual value of malaria-related production loss is 2–6% of gross domestic product (GDP) in Kenya and 1–5% of GDP in Nigeria. Malaria-related costs as a percentage of total household costs for small farmers were 0.8–5.2% in Kenya and 7.2–13.2% in Nigeria.

Microeconomic studies of malaria tend to evaluate the costs of the disease in terms of its impact within a specific economic environment. Potentially more significant, however, is the effect of disease on economic opportunities. If a factory goes unbuilt in a region because of malaria, for example, the consequences for income may be far more substantial than malaria's consequence for productivity in traditional agriculture. Gallup and Sachs (1998) advance this perspective and argue for a macroeconomic approach that uses cross-country time-series data to capture effects that would go unobserved with household data. In particular they find a significant negative relationship between malaria and GDP growth, with far greater estimated magnitude than reported in the household-level studies. Due to compounding, small changes in

the rate of economic growth can have large long-term effects. Gallup and Sachs suggest that the most important ways in which malaria affects long-run economic growth are the effect of the disease on a country's ability to attract foreign direct investment and to create an environment suitable for modern economic growth. Allowing countries to undertake new enterprises, rather than just improving productivity in traditional enterprise, may be the most economically significant consequence of malaria control programs. Although there are shortcomings in the malaria data, the findings remain suggestive, even if not definitive.

***Tuberculosis.*** Tuberculosis is a serious health threat across the globe. In 1998, the number of deaths from tuberculosis in all WHO member states was roughly 1.5 million, or almost 2.5% of all deaths. In 1997, in China alone there were 2.2 million new cases of tuberculosis with an average case fatality rate of 20% (WHO, 1999). Tuberculosis is estimated to be four times more concentrated in lower income populations than among the well-off (WHO, 1999). In addition, the considerable barriers to detecting the disease and to reducing infectiousness exacerbate the impact of tuberculosis and increase the probability of transmitting it to others. It is estimated that only half of all tuberculosis cases are detected. If a patient does receive treatment, the risk of 5-year mortality is reduced to roughly 15%. Tuberculosis is a disease that primarily affects adults, especially those in their most productive years. It is estimated that 77% of tuberculosis DALY cases and deaths occur among adults ranging in age from 15–59 years old (Murray, Lopez, & Jamison, 1994). (See Chapter 4).

This section discusses two aspects of tuberculosis that have been addressed in the literature: (1) its economic burden, which necessarily compares different treatment options; and (2) the economic benefits and the cost-effectiveness of control, comparing the relative economic merits of different interventions. Exhibit 12–3 discusses the economic benefits of a tuberculosis control program in India.

---

*The World Bank (1993) introduced disease burden measurements based on DALYs, and the initial full publication of results appears in Murray et al (1994).

**Exhibit 12–3** Economic Benefits of Tuberculosis Control in India

Tuberculosis is estimated to be one of the leading causes of ill health and death in India, where, in 1997, there were 4 million tuberculosis sufferers. The health and economic consequences of tuberculosis infection are considerable: prolonged illness and premature mortality and medical costs and indirect costs due to lost productivity. Although chemotherapy treatment options are available, these programs are often self-administered or are costly in terms of the direct medical costs of treatment in tertiary or hospital settings and in terms of the time necessary to receive care—sometimes as much as 12 months of treatment. These self-administered and long treatment programs in tertiary facilities have limited effectiveness due to high relapse rates, low cure rates, high case fatality rates, and drug resistance.

The World Health Organization developed DOTS (directly observed treatment short-course strategy) to alleviate some of the problems of existing long-course and self-administered chemotherapy. Dholakia and Almeida (1997) attempted to estimate the potential health and economic benefits of successfully implementing the DOTS program in India, based on two primary assumptions: (1) DOTS will succeed in alleviating pulmonary tuberculosis in India, and (2) DOTS will reach 100% of tuberculosis patients with full and instantaneous coverage. He found that, with a relatively high discount rate, a low percentage growth in labor productivity, and use of present value calculations for the future stream of benefits resulting from DOTS, the potential economic benefit to the Indian economy was about 4% of GDP in real terms or US$8.3 billion in 1993–1994.

Realistically, however, the DOTS strategy will probably not be immediately 100% implementable, involving a phasing-in process in which personnel are trained, the drug supply system is reformed, and organizational and management changes are made. The longer the period of phase-in, the lower the present discounted value of economic benefits associated with DOTS. Dholakia and Almeida (1997) estimated that a phasing-in of DOTS coverage in India over 10 years with a conservatively high discount rate of 16% would result in a present value of economic benefits of 2.1% of GDP (1993–1994) or US$4.6 billion with a 16% rate of return in real terms. This translates into US$750 million per year in tangible economic benefits from a successfully implemented DOTS program that costs US$200 million per year.

---

The economic impact of tuberculosis, like malaria, comprises two components: the direct costs of prevention and treatment, and the indirect costs of earnings lost due to illness or mortality. Because tuberculosis largely affects adults in the most productive stage of their lives, the indirect costs of the disease can be quite high. Ahlburg (1999) provides a cost analysis in various lower income settings.

In their study of patients presenting to a tuberculosis clinic in northwest Bangladesh, Croft and Croft (1998) found a mean financial loss to the patient of US$245, or 4 months' income (roughly 30% of annual family income based on an average annual income for a Bangladeshi family of US$780).The breakdown of the loss of income was US$115 out of US$245, while the direct medical costs totaled roughly US$130,

consisting of medicine costs of US$112, doctor's fees of US$9, and laboratory costs of US$8.50. Of the 21 patients studied, 8 were forced to sell land or livestock in order to pay for necessary treatment. Geography was a significant factor in obtaining treatment: 6 of the 21 patients were able to walk to the clinic, but of the remaining 15 patients, 5 reported that transportation costs (US$0.25–1.25) were a relatively significant amount for their family.

Saunderson (1995) compared the costs and consequences of current treatment practices for tuberculosis in Uganda with a program based on treating ambulatory patients at their nearest health unit while they lived at home. He found that the total costs per patient for the current practice was £190 versus £115 for ambulatory care. The breakdown of costs for each program showed a total cost per patient to the health service of £55 for current practice and £65 for the ambulatory program. In addition, the total costs per patient were £134 for the current practice and £49 for the alternative program. Thus, the largest difference between the two programs was patient costs: the ambulatory care program resulted in roughly one-half of the costs to the patient as compared to current practice, primarily because of reduced costs before diagnosis (halved in the alternative program due to greater access to the program), the elimination of a hospital stay, and the reduced costs due to work loss.

In a cost-effectiveness analysis* between the two programs at different levels of cure rate, the ambulatory program was found to be more cost-effective (at a total cost per cure of £230 for a 50% cure rate, £192 for 60%, and £164 for 70%) than the current practice (at a cost per cure of £380 for a 50% cure rate and £316 for 60%). In comparing the two programs, Saunderson (1995) concluded that savings from the avoidance of loss of work had the greatest effect on cost per cure. Under the current program, the average time spent away from normal activities due to illness was 9.5 months (range: 1 week to 3 years). Interviewing patients revealed that many had spent this time visiting various clinics and hospitals in search of care. The shadow price for time away from work was assumed to be the salary of a nursing aide (approximately £10 per month) for an average loss of £95. Also, 33 of 34 patients interviewed reported that their work and income had been affected by the illness. Eight out of 10 patients involved in paid employment or business reported that they had stopped work or closed their business due to illness, and 23 out of 24 farmers reported reduced work and lost production as a result of their illness. Five patients noted the need to remove their children from school because they could no longer pay school fees. The assumption was that the time

---

*For another cost-effectiveness analysis of alternative tuberculosis management strategies in South Africa, see Wilkinson, Floyd, and Gilks (1997).

away from work could be reduced by roughly 60% with ambulatory treatment.

In northeastern KwaZulu-Natal (Hlabisa health district) in South Africa, Wilkinson, Floyd, and Gilks (1997) conducted an economic evaluation of the directly observed treatment, short-course strategy (DOTS), and the conventionally delivered treatment for managing tuberculosis. They found that the total health system costs per patient in 1996 U.S. dollars were $649 for DOTS and $1,775 for conventional treatment. The total cost per case cured for DOTS was $740 and for conventional treatment $2,047, making DOTS 2.8 times cheaper overall than conventional treatment. In a scenario analysis of the best and worst cases, DOTS was 2.4 to 4.2 times more cost-effective, costing $890 per patient cured compared with either $2,095 (best case) or $3,700 (worst case) for conventional treatment. Wilkinson and Gilks attributed the reduced expense of DOTS to reduced hospital stays.

In most of these studies, costs may be underestimated in the sense that they do not always include monetary equivalents of losses in the household's production due to illness (that is, indirect costs), reduced efficiency of land use, transport, housing and food costs during treatment, human capital loss (increased absenteeism and reduced performance at school for children of a household with an adult infected with tuberculosis), and the value of pain and suffering. What is clear, though, is that costs are substantial and that cost-effective means of control are available. The case for control efforts will be strong in many contexts.

***HIV/AIDS.*** For example, a study of the impact of HIV/AIDS on the national economy of India (Anand, Pandav, & Nath, 1999) found that the estimated total annual cost of HIV/AIDS in India under low (1.5 million infected), medium (2.5 million), and high (4.5 million) prevalence scenarios was 7 billion, 20 billion, and 59 billion rupees, respectively. AIDS treatment and productivity loss were the two major components of costs. Anand et al. concluded that the estimated annual cost of HIV/AIDS (assuming 4.5 million infected) was roughly 1% of the GDP of India.

Conversely, in a study of 51 developing and industrialized countries, controlling for potentially confounding variables and correcting for simultaneity, Bloom and Mahal (1997) found that the AIDS epidemic—early in its course—had an insignificant effect on the growth of per capita income. Bloom, Rosenfield, and River Path Associates (in press), however, discuss evidence of the economic effects of AIDS on individual businesses. Over, Bertozzi, and Chin (1989) estimated direct and indirect costs attributable to a given HIV infection in the Democratic Republic of the Congo and Tanzania. Estimates of total costs per case of HIV infection ranged from US$940 to US$3,230 (1985 dollars) in the Democratic Republic of the Congo, and from US$2,460 to US$5,320 in Tanzania. Cuddington (1991) and Cuddington and Hancock (1992) estimated that, assuming AIDS treatments are entirely financed from savings, and workers sick with AIDS are 50% as productive as they would be without AIDS, the growth rate of GDP would be reduced by 0.8 percentage point in Tanzania and by 1.5 percentage points in Malawi. In 1992, Over estimated that (assuming 50% of AIDS treatment costs come from savings) GDP growth is slowed by 0.9 percentage point per year in the average country (among 34 sub-Saharan countries), and per capita growth by 0.2 point.

***Other Diseases.*** In a cost–benefit analysis of the Onchocerciasis Control Program (OCP) in West Africa, which prevents river-blindness, Kim and Benton (1995) estimated OCP's net benefits in terms of net present value (NPV) and economic rate of return (ERR) over two project horizons, 1974–2002 and 1974–2012. The NPV of labor and land-related benefits together (assuming 85% labor participation and land use) over a 39-year project horizon (1974–2012) ranged between US$3,730 million and US$485 million, in 1987 constant dollars at discount rates of 3% and 10%, respectively. The estimated ERR under the same assumptions was approximately 20%. Using a project horizon

of 29 years yielded an ERR of approximately 18%.

In their study of the impact of mental illness on employment, Ettner, Frank, and Kessler (1997) found that in aggregate, psychiatric disorders reduced the probability of employment by roughly 14–15% for both men and women. Robins and Regier (1991), in their analysis of the impact of mental health problems on income, found that 4.5% of women and 3% of men in the United States report an inability to work or assume normal activities at some point in the past 3 months due to emotional stress. In reviewing a broad range of studies from high-income countries (mostly the United States), Currie and Madrian (1999) pointed to the particular significance of mental illness.

In contrast to the findings of many other condition-specific studies, Svedberg (2000), in a broad assessment of linkages between poverty and undernutrition, concluded that the malnutrition to poverty links were probably relatively weak. In this he also differs from much of the literature cited earlier in this chapter.

### Health and Education

Health and nutritional problems can also have significant consequences for the educational success of many school-aged children. Such problems result not only in direct welfare losses, but also in losses of learning opportunities that are essential to the economic, social, and parental success of these individuals and, ultimately, their societies. The close link between health and school attendance and performance raises the question of how educational systems might intervene to improve conditions that undermine both health and educational success.

Figure 12–3 illustrates the different ways in which health, school participation, and learning outcomes are related, and how health and school quality interventions can influence educational outcomes. The evidence examining these relationships is discussed below. The figure demonstrates that school quality interventions can affect the learning rate, which, in conjunction

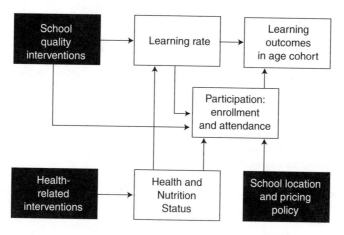

**Figure 12–3** Health, School Participation, and Learning Outcomes

with enrollment and attendance rates, can directly affect the distribution of learning in a given age cohort. The figure also illustrates that health-related interventions, through their influence on health and nutrition status, can enhance learning rates and participation, both of which contribute to learning outcomes. School location policies also have direct links to participation rates, which in turn influence learning.

Leslie and Jamison (1990) reviewed the links between health conditions and three important education problems in developing countries: (1) children who are unprepared to begin school at the usual age; (2) the failure of many students to learn adequately in school; and (3) the unequal participation of girls in schooling. Despite data limitations, their study found that several widespread health and nutritional problems clearly have negative consequences for school participation and performance. When children suffer from weakened or lower-than-expected physical capacity (and concomitant problems with cognitive ability, psychological well-being, and social competence), they may be incapable of attending school or be developmentally limited. Lack of school readiness in the form of physical and cognitive abilities and social and communication skills can result in significantly lower than average school performance as compared nationally and internationally. When children are too sick to learn in school, they fail to obtain minimal literacy and numeracy skills central not only to educational success but also to later economic and social achievements.

The authors suggest that seven categories of health conditions are likely to affect school participation or learning, and occur frequently in lower income country contexts. These conditions are (1) nutritional deficiencies, (2) helminthic infections (including intestinal parasites and schistosomiasis), (3) other infections, (4) disabilities, (5) reproductive and sexual problems (including premature fertility, sexual violence, and exposure to sexually transmitted infections), (6) injury and poisoning, and (7) substance abuse. Table 12–2 demonstrates that not all types of childhood illness and malnutrition are important for education, nor are these conditions all easily alleviated through school-based interventions. For example, in dealing with certain health conditions, such as early protein-energy malnutrition, school-based measures offer little help, whereas school is a potentially important venue for intervening against certain other conditions, such as tobacco use, that are important for health but not important for schooling.

In their summary of the relationships between the seven health conditions mentioned above

**Table 12–2** Health Conditions and the Schools

| Condition | Important for Education[a] | Potential for Intervention[b] | |
| | | Schoolbased | Other |
| --- | --- | --- | --- |
| Schistosomiasis (moderate to severe)<br>Iodine-deficiency disorders<br>Anemia<br>Short-term hunger<br>Intestinal helminths (moderate to severe) | Yes | Yes | Yes |
| Early protein-energy malnutrition<br>Diarrheal disease<br>Acute respiratory illness<br>Ill health of the parents of school-age children | Yes | Low | Moderate |
| Risk behaviors for chronic diseases (for example, tobacco use)<br>Some immunizable diseases<br>Mild schistosomiasis or intestinal helminthiasis | No | Yes | Yes |
| Serious but infrequently occurring childhood diseases<br>Cataract<br>Most cancers | No | No | Limited |

[a]Conditions that are likely to affect school participation or learning and to occur relatively frequently in some environments.
[b]Conditions for which school-based interventions are likely to offer significant help.

and the three education problems (unpreparedness, failure to learn, and unequal participation by girls), Leslie and Jamison (1990) concluded that nutritional deficiencies have the most significant negative impact on education. Such deficiencies cause reduced cognitive function in both preschool and school-aged children, and are directly reflected in poorer school attendance and achievement. Their review suggests that prenatal iodine deficiency causes permanent mental retardation, and chronic iodine deficiency can lead to less severe mental impairment among school-aged children and adults (see also Chapter 5). It also reveals that among infectious diseases, hookworm has a strong negative effect on cognitive function and Guinea worm on school attendance. Finally, although research on the links between education and reproductive health and substance abuse problems is limited, it is believed that the combined effects of early marriage, unwanted pregnancy, and concerns about sexual vulnerability at least partially influence the lower school participation rates of young females compared with those of males.

The question then arises as to how educational systems might intervene to improve the health and nutrition status of school-aged children. In a companion paper reviewing the costs and effectiveness of school-based interventions, Jamison and Leslie (1990) have concluded that, given the current state of research on the health and education relationship, and the relatively low costs of well-designed and targeted programs, increased investment in child health and nutrition will benefit education. School-based interventions with the potential to improve both learning and attendance, and to improve the participation of girls, include improvements in school location and facilities; a school health worker or teacher trained to screen for easily recognized health and nutrition problems and the ability to make referrals to local health facilities and to provide minimum first aid and basic medication; mobile health teams to deal with more extensive clinical problems such as vitamin A and iodine deficiencies and intestinal helminthic infections; school feeding to provide incentives for attendance and to address micronutrient deficiencies; and health, nutrition, and family planning education. School feeding has been the most frequently evaluated program and has had a significantly positive effect on school attendance despite limited evidence of its effects on height or weight. School feeding also was by far the most costly of school-based programs, and benefits would need to be weighed carefully against the high costs. Using evidence of a very different sort on determinants of school attendance, Knaul and Parker (1998) found school participation in Mexico to be adversely affected by indicators of fertility in the child's household.

In efforts to confront the health and nutrition problems that negatively affect girls' school participation rates, education planners can enhance sexual safety through the location and gender basis of schools, by increasing the number of female teachers, and by improving school security. Other measures include the establishment of a sex, rape-prevention, and family-planning curriculum, and the dissemination of contraceptives and abortion referrals to reduce premature fertility and the onset of sexually transmitted infections. Evaluation of a school feeding program in India found greater positive effects on girls' enrollment as opposed to that of boys. Finally, experience from Bolivia suggests that programs to provide iodine and iron to micronutrient-deficient girls can enhance their cognitive function and school achievement. In particular, the Bolivia study found that a reduction in goiter was associated with improvements in IQ scores and that this relationship was stronger for school-aged girls than for boys. From the time of puberty, the incidence and severity of both anemia and iodine deficiency in girls substantially ex-

ceeds that in boys; hence the greater intervention impact on girls is not surprising. Perhaps not coincidentally, female enrollment relative to males drops at puberty. In addition to seeking cultural explanations, low-cost nutritional intervention will, in many cases, prove relevant and more amenable to policy.

In an illustrative cost-benefit analysis, Jamison and Leslie suggested that "potential exists for benefits greatly to exceed costs for health and nutrition interventions in schools" (1990, p. 212).

### Health and the Wealth of Nations

One of the main empirical tools used to understand variation in income levels and growth rates of countries is cross-country regression of economic growth (typically measured in terms of the growth rate of per capita GDP) on the variables believed to explain that growth.[*] Among the factors that are usually explored in such analyses are: levels and patterns of educational attainment (schooling); health status (life expectancy, mortality rates, disease prevalence); population growth, density, and age structure; natural resource abundance; personal and government saving (investment rates); physical capital stock; trade policy, as in, for example, the degree of trade openness; quality of public institutions; and geography, as in, for example, the location and climate of a country (Bloom & Canning, 2000).

Research focused on the links between several specific variables, and economic growth includes both variables that directly link economic performance and health variables, such as life expectancy and mortality rates, and variables that indirectly link health with economic growth, such as geography and demography. Geogra-

---

[*]Conceptually quite distinct is a recent attempt (Cutler and Richardson, 1998) to assess the value of health in the U.S. economy between 1970 and 1990. Assuming a value for a year in perfect health, one can estimate "health capital." This has increased over time in the United States, but more so for older adults than the young.

phy, particularly tropical location, is highly correlated with disease burden, which in turn affects economic performance. Demography, on the other hand, which is determined in part by health status, has a direct effect on economic growth through age-structure effects. This section focuses on the available empirical evidence that estimates the influence of these various factors on a nation's overall level and rate of growth of income (Figure 12–2).

*Life Expectancy and Economic Outcomes.* Life expectancy has been shown to be a powerful predictor of income levels and subsequent economic growth. Studies (Barro & Lee, 1994; Bloom & Williamson, 1998; Jamison, Lau, & Wang, 1998; Radelet, Sachs, & Lee, 1997) have revealed that lower levels of mortality and higher levels of life expectancy have a statistically significant effect on income levels and growth rates. In a study of determinants across countries of 5-year economic growth rates, Bhargava et al. (2000) concluded that health's favorable impact on growth declined with a country's initial income level. The mechanisms through which this effect works are believed to be (1) the improvements in productivity that arise from a healthier work force and less morbidity-related absenteeism; (2) the increased incentive higher life expectancy gives individuals and firms to invest in physical and human capital; and (3) the increase in savings rates as working-age individuals save for their retirement years.

Jamison et al. (1998) combined their empirical estimates of the effects of adult survival rates on national income with country-specific estimates of improvements in survival rates to generate estimates of the contribution of health to economic growth. In India, for example, income per capita grew at a rate of just over 2% per annum between 1965 and 1990, and the adult survival rate improved by 20% in the same period. Their calculations suggest that 13% of total growth rate in per capita income was due to health improvements. In their sample of 58 countries, income grew at 2.4% per capita, of which 8% resulted from increases in adult survival rate.

Historical studies reached similar conclusions using very different types of data. In a study of the determinants of the economic progress in Great Britain between 1780 and 1979, for example, Fogel (1997) estimated that 30% of the per capita growth rate can be explained by health and nutritional improvements.

*Demography and Growth.* Health improvements also play a role in economic growth through their impact on demography. For example, in the 1940s improvements in health in East Asia provided impetus for a demographic transition. An initial decline in infant and child mortality prompted a fall in fertility rates somewhat later. These changes in mortality and fertility—the first phase of the demographic transition—substantially altered Asia's age distribution because the working-age population began growing much faster than the youth-dependent population, temporarily creating a disproportionately high percentage of working-age adults. This bulge in the population's age structure created an opportunity for increased rates of economic growth. By introducing demographic variables into an empirical model of economic growth, Bloom and Williamson (1998) suggest that East Asia's changing health and consequent changes in demography can explain one-third to one-half of the economic growth "miracle" experienced between 1965 and 1990.

Although this "demographic dividend" provides an opportunity for increasing wealth, it does not guarantee such results. East Asia's growth rates were achieved because government and private sectors were able to mobilize this growing work force by successfully managing other economic opportunities. Adopting new industrial technologies, investing in education and human capital, and exploiting global markets allowed East Asia to realize the economic growth potential created by the demographic transition.

The importance of demographic variables is supported by Jamison et al. (1998), who examined the role of total fertility rates in relation to economic levels using an aggregate-production function approach. They found a statistically significant negative relationship, similar to findings by Bloom and Freeman (1988), which showed that crude birth rates are negatively correlated with economic growth because they are associated with younger age distributions and lower labor force participation.[*] The link between mortality reduction and subsequent fertility reduction constitutes an important component of the total effect of health on development. This strength and causal nature of this link has been discussed, but the direction of the evidence is now fairly clear. Schultz (1997, p. 418), for example, concludes in a major review that "Whatever the cause of the mortality decline, the response of parents has been to reduce their births."

Bloom, Canning, and Malaney (in press) further developed this line of research by incorporating demography into a model of endogenous economic growth. They showed that the interaction of exogenous demographic influences with human and physical capital development can lead to a virtuous cycle of growth, enabling a country to break free of a poverty trap (in which poor health perpetuates low income that itself perpetuates poor health).

*Geography, Disease Burden, and Economic Growth.* In their cross-country growth studies, Gallup and Sachs (1999) introduced a focus on geographical factors among the empirical determinants of economic growth. They found that countries in tropical regions develop more slowly than those in temperate zones. In addition to the effects of climate and geography on soil quality, they believe that an intermediate mechanism through which this effect operates is the interaction of tropical climates and disease

---

[*]In an early paper, Myrdal (1952) raised many of the issues dealt with in health economics in the years to come. Among other points, he noted the links between age distribution, fertility, health, and economic growth.

burdens; this interaction can have a significant cost in terms of economic performance. Both high disease burdens and geographical isolation can separate countries from the global economy, denying them the benefits of trade, foreign direct investments, and technological interchange.

## Economic Development's Consequences for Health

Previous sections have discussed how health can lead to greater growth and reduced poverty. In fact, the causal relationship between health and development operates in both directions. Income influences health through a variety of intervening determinants. More distal determinants include housing, education, water, sanitation and nutrition, energy, health services, institutions, and industrial and agricultural policies. Industrial safety programs and environmental regulations, for example, have specific health objectives and are targeted at specific groups, namely, industrial workers and the general public. Housing policies aimed at subsidizing or providing housing for lower income individuals have broader social and health objectives, but may also have concrete health impacts. Empowering women through better education, among other measures, can enhance their capacity to improve their health and that of their families. Education is strongly correlated with health in many studies in industrialized countries as well, even after controlling for other factors, including income and medical care (Berger & Leigh, 1989; Farrell & Fuchs, 1982; Fuchs, 1993; Grossman, 1975; Kenkel, 1991).

The 1993 World Development Report (World Bank, 1993) provides an extensive overview of the determinants of health that are outside the health sector and their attractiveness from a policy perspective. For example, even if there were no benefits to primary education for girls except health benefits, education would still appear highly cost-effective.

There is also a growing body of information on health inequalities and the experience of relative deprivation as a cause of ill health. In Great Britain, for example, the Whitehall Study (a longitudinal study of behaviors and health status of more than 10,000 British civil servants) found that over a 10-year period males aged 40–64 in the lower grades (clerical and manual) of the civil service had an age-adjusted mortality rate 3.5 times higher than males in senior administrative grades (Marmot & Theorell, 1988; Marmot et al., 1991; Wilkinson, 1986).There was a gradient in mortality that stretched across all levels of the civil service: each status group had a higher mortality rate than the group immediately above it, which was not explainable by access to medical care or other primary goods, such as absolute levels of income, shelter, food, or education.

Other research, aimed at confirming the Whitehall Study findings on a cross-national level, revealed a similar correlation between hierarchy and health. In a study of 11 Organization for Economic Cooperation and Development (OECD) countries from 1975–1985, using two measures of income inequality, the Gini coefficient and the ratio between the percentage of income flowing to the top and bottom 30% of a country's population, Wilkinson (1990) found an inverse relationship between the level of income in a country and the average national life expectancy. Whereas nations with absolute levels of higher average income per capita will have higher average life expectancy than those with a lower level of average national income (for example, industrialized versus lower income countries), these studies suggest that greater income inequality within a country may also have a negative influence on life expectancy. Nations with a relatively flat income gradient, such as Japan and Sweden, had higher life expectancies than countries such as the United States and West Germany, which have steeper gradients. Moreover, in the United States, the sensitivity of mortality rates to socioeconomic status has increased sharply between 1960 and the early 1980s (Preston & Elo, 1995).

Recent work (Deaton, 1999; Deaton & Paxson, 1999) interprets the apparent effect of income inequality on health to result from effects of rank-

ing within a reference group that is much smaller than a country. If, for example, an academic had a low salary relative to others in her discipline, this might have a deleterious effect on health even if her absolute income were relatively high, and she lived in a country where income was relatively evenly distributed. Even if individuals' reference groups are unobserved, individual income levels will provide partial information about the individuals' standing in their reference group (the amount of information depending on the relative levels of within-group and across-group inequality). The mechanism of effect can generate the widely documented adverse effect of inequality on average health status even if there is no real effect of either within-group or between-group inequality on health. Deaton and Paxson's (1999) analyses using U.S. data support the conclusion of no effect. More research will be needed to extend the evidence base on how reference group rankings and socioeconomic inequalities influence health.*

An important question in assessing the historical determinants of health is the impact of income, in relation to other factors, on health improvements, especially during the second half of the twentieth century. Preston's (1980) work provides a broad framework for assessing income's impact, and his study has influenced subsequent work. A WHO analysis (WHO, 1999) examined these relationships. Figure 12–4 shows the results from this work and illustrates the relationship. From 1952 to 1992, mean income increased by about 66% from roughly US$1,500 to US$2,500. The curves in Figure 12–4 indicate that IMR declined more than predicted (to 55 per thousand rather than to 116 per thousand) based on the

---

*Note that the literature on inequalities in health is not, for the most part, about inequality in the univariate distribution of health but generally about the strength of the effect of inequality in other variables (for example, income) on health levels. Le Grand (1987) assessed univariate distribution of health or pure inequalities. Not surprisingly, these inequalities decline steadily with declines in overall mortality rates, even though the socioeconomic gradient may be getting steeper.

1952 relationship between income and IMR, suggesting that factors more important than income are influencing health. Historical analyses by Easterlin (1998) point to the same conclusion. The WHO study and related World Bank analyses (Wang, Jamison, Bos, Preker, & Peabody, 1999) assessed the relative impact of three key areas on health improvements: increases in average income levels, improvements in average education levels, and the generation and application of new knowledge; it found that approximately 50% of health improvements were due to access to better technology, whereas the remaining gains result from income improvements and better education. Continued work along these lines— Jamison, Sandbu, and Wang (1999)—finds that country-specific differences in application of new knowledge are large indeed and, when properly accounted for, further reduce the apparent effect of income on health.[*]

Just as health conditions at any time improve with income level so, too, might adverse income shocks adversely affect health. The major economic crisis of 1998 in Indonesia provides an example. The available evidence is mixed, but Frankenberg, Beegle, Thomas, and Suriastini (1999) conclude that children's health was no worse after the crisis. (School enrollment rates among the low-income did, however, decline significantly.) Enduring effects of long-term, income-dependent determinants of health may be countering potential adverse consequences of economic crisis.

## HEALTH SYSTEMS AND ECONOMIC OUTCOMES[**]

An important aspect of the link between health and economic development is how the

_____

[*]Even though income differences may account for only a modest amount of cross-country variations in health outcomes over a period of several decades, the situation can be quite different within a given country at a given time. Important forthcoming work by Wagstaff and colleagues at the World Bank reaches such conclusions.

characteristics of a particular health care system, especially health financing policies, affect economic performance. Health care is one of the largest sectors of the world economy, accounting for 9.9% of total global product in 1998, and has significant potential to affect economic development and growth. This influence can operate at both a macro- and a microeconomic level.

As Figure 12–5 illustrates, health finance policies can have direct economic consequences in one of four ways: the total resources withdrawn by health care systems from the economy (for example, in terms of health expenditure in relation to GDP); the extent to which these systems provide welfare gains that can be achieved from risk pooling; the incentives that health finance policies can create in terms of the labor market and consumer and provider behavior; and the extent to which health expenditures generate or perpetuate poverty. As introduced in Chapter 10 and as shown in Figure 12–5, financing policies can take a number of different forms (for example, user fees, private voluntary insurance, universal mandatory finance, public health and social insurance, and supply and demand side measures for cost control and revenue generation) depending on the type of health care system. This section reviews the relationship between health care systems and the economy, and discusses particular issues within this arena that need to be addressed. Hsiao (2000) addresses many of the same issues from a rather different perspective.

### Total Resources Withdrawn from the Economy

#### Health Expenditures and GDP

Countries tend to devote more resources and increasing shares of their national income to

_____

[**]Chapter 10 provides a description of the main financing mechanisms of health systems; this section has a more detailed presentation of specific aspects of these arrangements in terms of their economic and equity impacts.

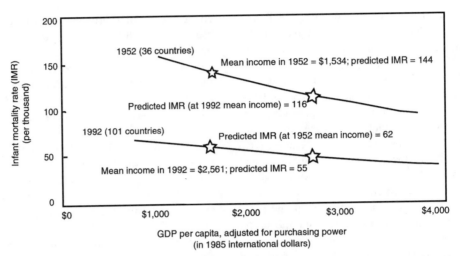

Note: Results are based on a cross-sectional time-series regression that relates, at 5-year intervals, the natural logarithm of IMR to the natural logarithm of income, the square of the natural logarithm of income, and indicator variables for time.

**Figure 12–4** The Role of Improvements in Income in Reducing Infant Mortality Rates

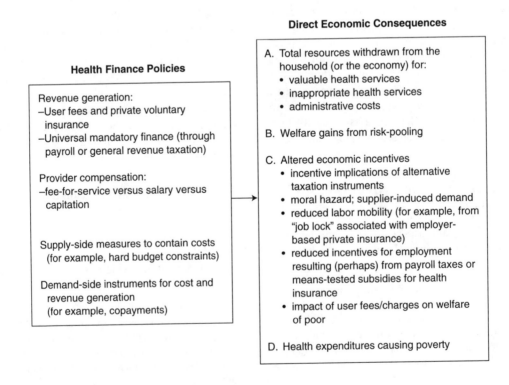

**Figure 12–5** Economic Consequences of Health Finance Policies

health care as their income increases. Lower income countries, on average, spend less than wealthier countries on health on a per capita basis, in terms of percentage of GDP and in terms of public spending on health. This leads to a lower level and a less equitable distribution of health care and public health services—and ultimately of health—in these societies. However, although health care affects health, it is not the only determinant of health. As Table 12–3 illustrates, in the mid-1990s, low-income countries spent an average of US$23 per capita as compared with US$199 for middle-income and US$2,585 for high-income countries. South Asia (US$17), East Asia and the Pacific (US$47), and sub-Saharan Africa (US$33) spent the least of low- and middle-income regions, whereas the Middle East and North Africa (US$177) and Latin America and the Caribbean (US$284) spent the most for that group of regions. In the very lowest income countries, annual health spending can be as low as US$2 or $3 per capita, and most of that spending is from private sources.

In terms of percentage of GNP, as shown in Table 12–3, low-income countries on average spend 4.4% of GDP on health, whereas middle-income countries spend an average of 6.7% and high-income countries spend an average of 10.2% of GNP on health. By region among low- and middle-income regions, South Asia (4.0% of GNP) spends the least on health, while Latin America and the Caribbean spend the most at approximately 7.4% of GNP.

Both health spending generally and the public share of health spending increase with increases in national and per capita income. As shown in Table 12–3, the public share of health expenditures (as a percentage of total health spending) was 31%, or the equivalent of 1.3% of GDP, in low-income countries, 54% (3.1% of GDP) in middle-income countries, and 63% (6.2% of GDP) in high-income countries. Among low- and middle-income countries, regions such as Eastern Europe and Central Asia have the largest public share (69%) of health spending, and South Asia has the smallest (17%). According to Schieber and Maeda (1993), the income elasticity of demand for health services (the percent-

age change in health expenditures as a result of a 1% change in income) in 1994 was roughly 1.13 worldwide, and in a range of 1.47 for high-income countries, 1.19 for middle-income countries, and 1.00 for low-income countries. This means that, for every 1% increase in per capita income, public health expenditures will increase by 1.47% in middle- and high-income countries, and by 1.19% in middle-income countries and by 1.00% in lower income countries. Thus the increase in health expenditures in low-income countries is less responsive to increases in income than it is in middle- and high-income countries. Figures 12–6 and 12–7 show the relationship between income and health spending and between income and public health spending, respectively. In addition, these authors found that private health spending (income elasticity of 1.02) is less responsive to increases in per capita income than public health spending (income elasticity of 1.21).

Some of the implications of lower levels of spending in lower income countries include lower levels of capital stock, such as clinics, hospitals, and inpatient beds; of human resources, such as physicians and providers; and of service use, such as outpatient and inpatient visits. For example, the number of hospital beds per 1,000 population in the mid-1990s was much higher in high-income (7.4) as compared to middle-income (4.3) and low-income (1.8) countries. Of the regions worldwide, Eastern Europe and Central Asia had the greatest number of inpatient beds per 1,000 in the mid-1990s, at 8.9, and South Asia (0.7) and sub-Saharan Africa (1.1) had the lowest. This pattern persists when analyzing physicians per 1,000 population in the mid-1990s: high-income countries (2.8) fare better than middle-income (1.8) and low-income (1.0) countries on this indicator of health system infrastructure. Comparing different regions of the world, the number of physicians per 1,000 population in the mid-1990s was highest in Eastern Europe and Central Asia (3.3) and lowest in sub-Saharan Africa (0.1) and South Asia (0.4).

Many have taken the evidence on the income elasticity of expenditures on health as indicative of the nature of health as a normal consumption

**Table 12-3** Health Expenditures by Income Group and Region, Mid-1990s[a]

| Region or Income Group | Population (millions) 1998[a] | Per capita GNP (1998 US$)[b] | Health Expenditures[a,c] | | Average across Countries Spent on Health[d] | | |
| --- | --- | --- | --- | --- | --- | --- | --- |
| | | | Total Health Expenditure per capita (1990–1998 US$) | Total Health Expenditure as % of GNP | Total Expenditure (% of GDP) | Public Sector Expenditure (% of GDP) | Public Sector (% of total) |
| World | 5,897 | 4,890 | 483 | 9.9 | 5.5 | 2.5 | 46 |
| Low-income | 3,536 | 520 | 23 | 4.4 | 4.2 | 1.3 | 31 |
| (Excluding China and India) | (1,295) | (370) | (14) | (3.8) | (3.1) | (1.2) | 39 |
| Middle-income | 1,474 | 2,990 | 199 | 6.7 | 5.7 | 3.1 | 54 |
| High-income | 886 | 25,480 | 2,585 | 10.2 | 9.8 | 6.2 | 63 |
| Low- and middle-income by region | 5,011 | 1,250 | 75 | 6.0 | 4.6 | 1.9 | 41 |
| East Asia and Pacific | 1,817 | 990 | 47 | 4.7 | 4.1 | 1.7 | 42 |
| Europe and Central Asia | 475 | 2,200 | 138 | 6.3 | 5.8 | 4.0 | 69 |
| Latin America and the Caribbean | 502 | 3,860 | 284 | 7.4 | 6.6 | 3.3 | 50 |
| Middle East and North Africa | 286 | 2,030 | 117 | 5.8 | 4.8 | 2.4 | 50 |
| South Asia | 1,305 | 430 | 17 | 4.0 | 4.8 | 0.8 | 17 |
| Sub-Saharan Africa | 627 | 510 | 33 | 6.5 | 3.2 | 1.5 | 47 |

[a]Data are for the most recent year available, which ranges between 1990 and 1998.

[b]GNP is calculated using the World Bank Atlas method.

[c]These figures show the total (that is, public and private) expenditures on health in the indicated regional or country group divided by the total GNP of that group. Countries with high expenditures on health are weighted heavily by this procedure.

[d]For a typical person in the indicated regional or income group, these columns show the expected percentage of GNP spent on health in that person's country. Figures are calculated by averaging across countries, weighted by population (for example, India and China weighted more heavily).

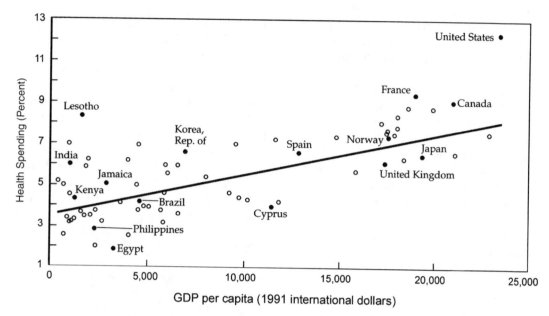

**Figure 12–6** Percentage of GDP Spent on Health

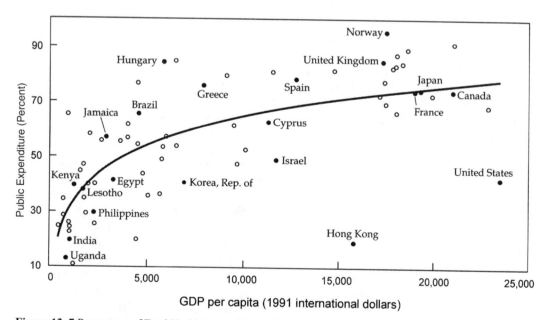

**Figure 12–7** Percentage of Total Health Expenditures That Are Public

good. More recently there has been an upsurge interest in the nature of health care as an investment good. Expenditures on health care can lead to improvements in health status that, in turn, promote income growth and the efficiency and equity of health systems in both improving health and affecting income, productivity, and the overall economy. Lower income countries in particular tend to underinvest in health, leaving their populations vulnerable to disease and disability and ultimately affecting labor productivity and growth. They also have health systems that are often highly inefficient at both macro- and microlevels, and highly inegalitarian in both financing and delivery.

### Health System Efficiency and Equity

*Macroeconomic Efficiency.* Health system efficiency at the macroeconomic level describes the relationship between aggregate health care expenditures and health outcomes. There is considerable variation in both health expenditures and health outcomes by country. For example, in 1995, life expectancy at birth for males ranged from 34 years in Sierra Leone, 37 in Rwanda, and 44 in Uganda, Guinea-Bissau, The Gambia, Burundi, and Afghanistan, to 75 in Canada, Cyprus, Greece, Israel, Macao, and Norway, and 77 in Iceland and Japan. Child mortality rates per 1,000 live births in 1995 ranged from 177 in Liberia and 159 in Afghanistan to 4 in Japan, Iceland, and Switzerland, 5 in France, Hong Kong, and Norway, and 6 in Australia, Austria, Canada, Denmark, Finland, Germany, Ireland, Luxembourg, Netherlands, Switzerland, and Taiwan (World Bank, 1999). Many factors influence health outcomes, but some countries appear to be more efficient in the use of health care resources than others.

Expenditures on health systems, however, often correlate poorly with outcomes. For example, in 1995 India spent 5.6% of GDP (48% of which was public spending) to achieve an IMR of 72 per 1,000 and a 1998 male and female life expectancy of 62 and 63 years, respectively, whereas in the same years (1995 and 1998, respectively) China spent 3.8% of GDP (54% from public spending) to achieve an IMR of 41 per

1,000, and male and female life expectancy of 68 and 72 years, respectively. In addition, in the same years Mauritius spent 4.0% of GDP (58% from public spending) to achieve an IMR of 16 per 1,000 and male and female life expectancies of 68 and 75 years, respectively. Among higher income countries the patterns are similar. For example, in 1995 the United States spent 14.0% of GDP (47% from public expenditure) to achieve a 1998 IMR of 7 per 1,000 and male and female life expectancies of 73 and 80 years, and the UK spent 6.9% of GDP (84% from public expenditure) and Japan spent 7.2% of GDP (78% from public expenditure) to achieve respective IMRs of 7 per 1,000 and 4 per 1,000, and male and female life expectancies of 75 and 80, and 77 and 83 years. Finally, in the same years, France spent 9.7% of GDP (81% from public expenditure) and Germany spent 10.5% of GDP (78% from public expenditure) to achieve IMRs of 6 per 1,000 and 5 per 1,000, and male and female life expectancies of 74 and 82, and 74 and 80 years, respectively. Wang et al. (1999) present systematic data on 115 countries for the period 1960 to 1991 on country performance relative to income (or income and education) on several health indicators. These performance measures are intended to catalyze discussion of the role of health system characteristics as partial explanations.

This evidence suggests that health systems probably vary in the efficiency with which they produce health, and, of course, health care services are only one of multiple determinants of health. Some countries obtain better health for less money; others obtain good health by spending more; some seem to be in a situation of diminishing marginal returns to increases in health care expenditures. In lower income countries it is often the case that very little health is obtained for the money spent. When total health spending is as low as it is in some lower income countries (for example, 2–3% of GDP), there are insufficient resources to cover even the minimum necessary care. This means that even the most basic package of preventative and clinical services is not available to the whole population. Inadequate allocations of public and private resources to health can lead to continued poverty and stifled development. These countries require increases in money spent (especially equally distributed public resources) on the most basic and cost-effective services. At the other end of the spectrum, countries such as the United States, France, Germany, and Switzerland, which spend more than 9% of GDP on health, have a tripartite health policy focus of increasing access and improving quality with a central emphasis on controlling and decreasing health care costs.

Although there is scant evidence of the economic impact of greater spending on health, some believe that higher health expenditures can reduce a country's relative productivity in the global economy due to the large costs of health benefits for the labor force, and due to resultant reduced investments in other sectors of the economy. While the labor market effects of certain health policies are addressed later in this section, it is less clear that overall productivity and growth are severely hindered by very high health expenditures. It is not possible to determine the most efficient level or percentage of health spending for any given economy. With this wide range of spending on health care, the challenge is to increase spending among lower income nations and analyze spending in both higher and lower income countries. The aim is to develop methods to enhance the efficient production of health within health care systems.

*Microeconomic Efficiency.* Microeconomic efficiency focuses on getting the best return on existing resources and reducing the waste and inefficiency that some systems generate. "Allocative inefficiency" occurs when resources are allocated not to activities that are highly cost-effective but to those that are costly with a low return in terms of effectiveness. It means allocating resources to the most cost-effective way of achieving given health objectives (for example, investing in cost-effective preventative measures, such as immunizations for certain diseases or behavioral modification, rather than spending extensively at later stages of the health cycle through high-cost tertiary services). A health system is allocatively inefficient when

greater gains could be achieved with a different pattern of resource use. The 1993 World Development Report (World Bank, 1993) concluded that improvements in allocative efficiency of health systems in lower income countries could be achieved through the introduction of basic cost-effective intervention packages for the most common conditions in a given country. Technical inefficiencies occur when the pattern and level of resources (human, financial, and physical) do not adequately meet the level of health (or access) outcomes possible with that degree of resource commitment. In lower income countries, scarcity of providers and basic clinic and hospital resources, in addition to poor quality and accessibility of facilities (ill-equipped and run-down infrastructure) and providers (poorly trained and unqualified) all contribute to a failure to meet the health needs of the populations. In higher income countries, the focus has been on assessing and improving the efficiency of particular aspects of health systems, including cost and use control measures on the supply and demand side of the health care market, medical care appropriateness, and health care administration. These topics are addressed in Exhibits 12–4 and 12–5, respectively. In addition, some health systems in higher income countries have begun explicitly to prioritize or ration health services to improve the allocative efficiency and public acceptability of their health systems.

*Equity.* Equity in health policy typically focuses on both the financing and the delivery of health care services. Two important dimensions of equity include vertical and horizontal equity. In terms of financing, vertical equity refers to the requirement that health care be financed by ability to pay; that is, contributions to the cost of health care must be determined by income status. Some mechanisms for raising revenues for health care expenditures are more progressive than others. Horizontal financial equity means that individuals with the same ability to pay should contribute the same amount to financing health expenditures regardless of medical need, gender, marital status, geography, age, or employment status. In terms of delivery, verti-

**Exhibit 12–4** Costs of Health Care Administration

One aspect of health system inefficiencies is the perception of some administrative expenditures as wasteful. Comparisons of different health systems suggest that administrative costs can be an important factor in the level and rate of change in health care spending.

Single-payer plans are claimed to be advantageous in that they tend to centralize and therefore reduce the costs of health care administration—a significant issue around the world. International comparisons of international health systems show that administrative costs as a percentage of total costs vary by country and financing mechanism, and these large differences suggest, at first glance, wasteful and inefficient use of resources in some countries. Several national (United States) and cross-national (OECD countries) studies have attempted to estimate such costs (Bovbjerg, 1995; Gauthier, Rogal, Barrand, & Cohen, 1992; Poullier, 1992; U.S. Congress, 1994; Woolhandler & Himmelstein, 1991, 1997; Woolhandler, Himmelstein, & Lewontin, 1993). One study found that in 1987, U.S. health care administration cost between US$96.8 billion and $120.4 billion ($400–497 per capita), equivalent to 19.3–24.1% of total health care spending (Woolhandler & Himmelstein, 1991). The same study found that in comparing the United States, Canada, and the United Kingdom, administrative costs in the United States were 60% higher than in Canada and 97% higher than in the United Kingdom.

Another study, employing OECD data from 1991 and 1992, compared costs of health care administration across 20 industrialized countries. With respect to administrative costs, the United States had the highest (and Germany the second highest) per capita spending for health administration. The authors concluded that administrative costs were higher in insurance-based systems than in direct-delivery systems. Insurance-based systems are more complex and involve multiple, decentralized payers, all of which contribute to higher administrative costs (Poullier, 1992).

Illustrating the unusual character of the health sector among sectors of the economy, the available research suggests that single-payer systems (in which a single authority processes claims and pays providers directly for services) have lower administrative costs than multiple-payer systems. Single-payer systems accrue benefits by standardizing, consolidating, and integrating functions. Single-payer systems are well situated to take advantage of efficiency gains from standardization and of technological advances in information systems, especially electronic claims transmission and magnetic card technology. Even without a single-payer system, standardization and reform could reduce costs for multiple payers. For instance, introducing a common electronic administrative system (common formats and standards) that connects multiple systems of insurance and medical information through the use of "smart cards" could improve health system performance. These technologies could bring a number of health administrative functions under common guidelines, thereby improving communication, claims processing, and use review.

Ultimately, the costs and benefits of health administrative reforms must be assessed. Although certain administrative costs might be reduced without the loss of benefits to individuals or to society, others might not. The extent to which the results of administrative reforms are categorized as benefits or costs will also depend on the value that is placed on any given economic or health-related outcome. These values might vary from one community to another. In general, administrative activities that clearly confer benefits to patients and the health system should be prioritized, and in some cases beneficial administrative activities can be provided more efficiently. For example, benefit management costs—including data collection, clinical evaluation, and statistical analysis—confer consumer benefits by improving health care quality, enhancing patients' decision-making autonomy, and reducing inappropriate care. These activities will become an increasingly valuable tool as additional information on effective and cost-effective health service delivery becomes available.

**Exhibit 12–5** Medical Care Appropriateness and Resource Allocation

While achieving a broad spread of risk, health insurance can, in principle, lead to incentives for too much medical care. When people are insured, they do not individually bear the costs of the medical services they consume, so some individuals will have an incentive to overconsume health care resources. (Countering these financial incentives are other costs of seeking care such as time, pain, and inconvenience.) This central problem of any insurance plan is called the moral hazard problem and has spawned a number of efforts to ensure medical care appropriateness and efficient resource allocation within insurance plans, both public and private. The private insurance markets have developed a number of techniques for assessing and enforcing medical care appropriateness.

The first approach is economic. Health economists endeavor to reduce overuse of health care through the use of various economic incentives on both the supply and demand side of the health care market. On the demand side, copayment plans and health insurance deductibles, which require patients to pay a portion of the price of a given medical procedure, reduce use rates. On the supply side of the health care market, price, budgetary, and salary incentives, such as prospective and capitated payment plans, and global budgets, deter physicians and hospitals from providing excess care. These incentives force physicians and hospitals to internalize costs in the process of health service delivery and therefore to provide the most cost-effective services. The rise of health care financing and delivery institutions, such as managed care organizations, is a result of these efforts.

Studies have shown that these economic devices are effective in reducing health care use. For instance, in a randomly controlled health insurance experiment, researchers found that increasing patient copayment on health insurance reduced demand for health care services, in some cases by as much as 40% (Rand Health Insurance Experiment, see Newhouse, 1993). In practice, though, copayments are eliminated for expensive procedures, thereby attenuating the usefulness of copayments in cost containment. In addition, cross-cultural comparisons of national health systems provide evidence for the effectiveness of capitation and global budgeting in reducing health care use (see, for example, Aaron & Schwartz, 1984). However, because these economic approaches are devoid of clinical input, they are blunt instruments in achieving their objective; in most cases, they reduce medically appropriate as well as inappropriate care. Without the ability to discriminate between productive and unproductive care, these tools can have deleterious health consequences and can be highly inegalitarian.

Distinguishing between types of care requires clinical input to create a system of assessing and ranking which treatments are medically appropriate for a given health condition. There is at least one existing model that attempts to do just that: the RAND/UCLA appropriateness method. The method involves multiple stages of collecting and interpreting data about specific procedures from literature and clinicians, with the goal of developing guidelines for appropriate care. Since 1986, more than 30 studies using this method have been conducted to examine the appropriateness of procedures (Table 12–4). This literature suggests that the percentage of inappropriate use across procedures ranges from 2.4–75%, whereas the percentage of appropriate care ranges from 35–91%, and the percentage of equivocal use ranges from 7–32%.[a]

Ultimately, attempts to achieve the optimal level of health status from any given amount of resources will require a joint economic and clinical solution. Social scientists and clinicians should continue to study the magnitude and determinants of inappropriate care and to harness technological advances to create effective information systems and accessible guidelines for medical care. Economic incentives should follow and complement clinical progress, but not to the exclusion of professional incentives. As the evidence on the magnitude and determinants of inappropriate care accumulates and is widely understood, economists and health policy analysts can create policy instruments that give an incentive for physicians, patients, and planners to provide productive care. Particular attention should be paid to encouraging and training physicians by rewarding the provision of appropriate care and correcting for the provision of inappropriate care.

---

[a]See also, Bernstein et al., 1993; Brook, 1992, 1994, 1995, 1997; Brook & Lohr, 1986, 1987, 1990; Brook et al., 1990; Brook, Park, & Chassin, 1990; Carlisle et al., 1992; Chassin, Kosecoff, Solomon, & Brook, 1987; Hilborne et al., 1993; and Leape et al., 1990.

**Table 12–4** Medical Appropriateness and Health Care Use

| Author(s) | Sample/Procedure | Magnitude of Appropriateness |
|---|---|---|
| Winslow, C.M., Solomon, D.H., Chassin, M.R., Kosecoff, J., Merrick, N.J., Brook, R.H. (1988b) | Random sample of 1,302 Medicare patients in three geographic areas who had a **carotid endarterectomy** in 1981. | Estimated the appropriateness of carotid endarterectomy. Found 35% appropriate, 32% equivocal, 32% inappropriate. Concluded that carotid endarterectomy was substantially overused in three geographic areas studied. |
| Bernstein, S.J., McGlynn, E.A., Siu, A.L., Roth, C.P., Sherwood, M.J., Keesey, J.W., Kosecoff, J., Hicks, N.R., Brook, R.H. (1993) | Retrospective cohort study. Random sample of all nonemergency, nononcological **hysterectomies** performed in seven managed care organizations over a 1-year period. | Roughly 16% inappropriate and only one plan had significantly more hysterectomies rated inappropriate compared with the group mean (27%, unadjusted). Age and race adjustments did not affect percentage appropriate. |
| Leape, L.L., Hilborne, L.H., Park, R.E., Bernstein, S.J., Kamberg, C.J., Sherwood, M., Brook, R.H. (1993) | Random sample of 1,338 patients from 15 different hospitals undergoing isolated **coronary artery bypass graft surgery** in New York state in 1990. | Nearly 91% appropriate, 7% equivocal, 2.4% inappropriate. Low inappropriateness rate differs significantly from 14% rate found in 1979, 1980, and 1982 studies. Rates did not vary by hospital, hospital location, volume, or teaching status. |
| Winslow, C.M., Kosecoff, J.B., Chassin, M., Kanouse, D.E., Brook, R.H. (1988a) | Appropriateness of **coronary artery bypass surgeries** performed in three randomly selected hospitals in a western state. Data obtained from medical record with 488 indications; 386 cases from years 1979, 1980, and 1982. | Found 56% appropriate, 30% equivocal, 14% inappropriate. Percentage appropriate varied by hospital, from 37% to 78%, but did not vary by patient age. |
| Kleinman, L.C., Kosecoff, J., Dubois, R.W., Brook, R.H. (1994) | Appropriateness of **tympanostomy tube surgery** for recurrent acute otitis media and/or otitis media with effusion. Random selection of subsample (6,611) of cases deemed appropriate by use review firm methodology. Represented otolaryngologists, practices from 49 states and DC. | Found 41% of proposals appropriate, 32% equivocal, and 27% inappropriate. Concluded that roughly 25% of tympanostomy tube insertions for children were proposed for inappropriate indications and 30% for equivocal ones. |

*Note:* All studies cited employed RAND/UCLA Appropriateness Method.

cal equity refers to the requirement that individuals with different needs should receive different amounts and levels of health services. Horizontal equity means that individuals with equal needs should receive equal medical treatment (Van Doorslaer, Wagstaff, & Rutten, 1993).

An alternative to concern for equity is concern for the status (health and financial) of the most disadvantaged segments of society. Improving equity and improving the conditions of the very poor may often go together, but sometimes they do not, posing tradeoffs.

In the 1990s, many countries in the OECD initiated reforms designed to improve the efficiency and responsiveness of their health systems. Hurst (2000) provides an overview of the achievements of these systems, and of their reforms, while pointing to an essential tension that increasingly confronts public policy in these countries. This tension results from upward pressures on costs (for technological and demographic reasons), core commitments to universal public (or publicly mandated) funding for reasons of efficiency as well as equity, and general reluctance to raise taxes. Feachem (2000) suggests that in the United Kingdom both radical reform of delivery institutions and increased resources will be required, while Enthoven (2000) reviews the history and lessons from the (incomplete) reforms of the U.K. National Health Services in the past decade. Preker, Harding, and Travis (2000) review these experiences from the perspective of the "new institutional economics" to reach a number of important conclusions about the evolving roles of the public and private sectors in the health sector. To quote their main findings concerning the public sector role, "Consequently, in parallel with moving out of the area of production of goods and services, in many low- and middle-income countries it may be desirable to have... greater public sector involvement in health care financing, knowledge generation, and the provision of human resources (p. 877).

## Welfare Gains from Risk Pooling

Insurance involves collective risk reduction, reduced financial risks, and increased human welfare. Insurance reduces risks in the aggregate by pooling a large number of people with similar, small, individual risks. This pooling enables insurers to increase aggregate predictability even when given health episodes remain unpredictable. The larger the risk pool, the greater the precision with which insurers can predict the probability of financial loss occurrence. Many health systems in low- and middle-income countries fail to take advantage of the economic and welfare benefits that accrue from collective risk reduction in the form of risk pooling through insurance.

### Risk Aversion

Several aspects of health insurance are rooted in the risk-averse nature of human beings. Individuals do not like, nor can they always financially afford, to pay a large amount of money for what could be an unpredictable adverse health event, such as a heart attack, the onset of AIDS, or a fractured skull. Without insurance, if a person suffers a medical catastrophe he or she may not have the financial resources to pay the large sums required for treatment of these adverse health events. Instead, a person would prefer, and could better afford, to pay a relatively small amount of money on a regular basis to avoid a large financial loss at one time. This is also known as "smoothing" or "evening-out" financial payments for adverse health events.

### Risk Pooling

By pooling a large number of people and therefore a large number of adverse health events, insurance companies (which employ statistical experts known as actuaries) are better able to predict the occurrence of these events and to spread the financial risk. Enhancing the predictability of the event reduces the financial risks associated with it. Pooling risks across people is more efficient than pooling risks within individuals but across time. For example, if the risk of an adverse health event that costs $2,000 is 1 in 1,000, and 1,000 people pooled $2 each, then the cost of the health event would be covered should it occur. In this case, each individual will have paid $2, rather than being exposed to the risk of paying $2,000. If the risk-pooling organization, such as an insurance company, has administrative costs to bear or aims to make a profit, the cost per person is increased by the additional administrative costs or profits divided by the number of people in the insurance pool.

There are other ways to pool risks, one of which is to pool risks for a given individual across time—a medical savings account—which can generate potential inefficiency even though there have been some effectively implemented examples (for example, Singapore). For example, if an individual saved $2 per year to cover a potential cost of $2,000, it would take that person 1,000 years to cover the cost; saving $20 per year would require 100 years; and saving $50 per year would take 40 years. Pooling across individuals is more efficient than pooling within individuals over time, because the same protection against the potential financial loss of $2,000 is achieved through a yearly payment of $2 versus a payment of $2 per year for 1,000 years or perhaps saving $50 per year for 40 years. Because people are risk-averse, risk pooling protects people from large financial losses that result from catastrophic health events.

### Insurance versus Direct Purchase

Given its benefits,* insurance is a preferred mechanism for financing personal health care services for high-cost, low-probability health

---

*Public insurance pools health risks through public financing from general taxes or other public revenue sources that are collected through a government mandate (for example, through a social security program, earmarked taxes, or an employer mandate). Social insurance is also a form of compulsory universal health insurance coverage that is typically implemented under the auspices of a social security-type program and is usually financed by employer and employee contributions to government or nonprofit insurance funds. Social insurance funds usually pool risks through social insurance financed from mandatory earmarked payroll taxes set aside specifically for social programs. Public and social health insurance provision can help alleviate many of the insurance market failures that occur with private insurance markets, and the dominant provision of public insurance obviates the need for health insurance regulation.

events. However, it may not necessarily be the preferred method of payment for low-cost, high-probability health events, because individuals have the ability to plan and save for such occurrences, depending on the relative expense of the event. A low-cost service (relative to income) in a higher-income country may be very costly (relative to income) for individuals in lower-income settings. If the service is relatively inexpensive and highly probable, risk pooling may be of little benefit, especially because administrative costs and expected profits associated with insurance can be high. Attempting to divide services between those that are and those that are not covered entails its own set of problems: Should individuals with different incomes have different cutoffs? Is the incentive for early (usually less costly) care reduced? Will individuals attempt to move to venues (usually hospitals) where care is free but may be less efficiently provided? For all these reasons most national health services do cover routine care, and appear to do so at modest administrative costs. The financial burden of a direct-purchase system falls disproportionately on the poor, who are more price-sensitive than the rich, and who typically have more health problems and higher health costs. As a result, the poor underutilize services (some of which are medically necessary) in such a system; direct payment can involve underutilization of necessary care. The World Health Organization's World Health Report 2000 provides a valuable discussion of these issues (WHO, 2000).

***Degrees of Risk Sharing.*** As Figure 12–8 demonstrates, different financing and provider arrangements distribute risks among patients, providers, and third-party insurers in different ways. In this context, it is important to note that government finance is one form of insurance in that it shifts the risk away from the individual (see Figure 12–8). When the patient carries the full financial risk of health care costs, he or she must pay for all services out-of-pocket, and is susceptible to significant financial loss should an expensive adverse health event occur. This type of arrangement represents the majority of health financing plans in low- and middle-in-

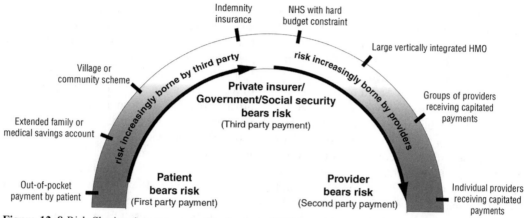

**Figure 12–8** Risk Sharing Arrangements: The Impact of Different Financing Schemes and Provider Payment Systems

come countries and tends to be the least equitable, efficient, and organized form of payment.

Private insurers pool risks to a certain extent, but because they are profit maximizers, their main strategy is risk segmentation, or insuring only the lowest risk individuals to gain the greatest profit. This practice is known as cream skimming or cherry picking, and from the perspective of society as a whole is not an efficient or equitable way to spread risk. Risk pooling in private insurance markets can be ensured through regulation. In addition, the existence of private insurance can create a two-tiered system (one in which different groups obtain different sets of benefits) and can exacerbate inequities of access without efforts to enhance the quality and equity of services (typically public) for those in lower income groups. It is also possible to have a system in which providers, such as hospitals, clinics, or practitioners, assume the financial risks of health care costs, a practice that is increasingly common in the United States.

***Informal Community Financing and Risk Pooling.*** Informal community financing can be a useful solution to risk pooling and health insurance constraints seen in low- and middle-income countries where neither government risk-sharing (that often redistributes wealth through subsidies) nor private or social health insurance exists on a large scale. These plans are typically rural, informal, and nongovernmental in nature,

and involve either voluntary or compulsory risk pooling through a community fund to which individuals contribute prepayment of premiums that entitle them to postservice payments of certain health services defined by the community. As Figure 12–8 suggests, these plans can shift risk substantially toward the collective. Some plans obtain contributions from employers and governments. Often, the community fund also manages the organization and provision of care (including immunizations and pharmaceuticals), creating a structure similar to an integrated health maintenance organization.

In their analysis of 82 health insurance plans for people outside formal-sector employment, Bennett, Creese, and Monasch (1998) found that, with the exception of China's rural medical plan, few plans covered very large populations or even high proportions of the eligible population, and many plans faced significant problems of adverse selection. In addition, nearly all the plans depended on external subsidies, but very few served the poorest households and were instead targeted toward the rural middle class. In terms of delivery, plan managers failed to focus sufficiently on efficiently delivering high quality health care, and the administrative structure and practice of plans varied widely, some focusing on insuring against primary care and others against tertiary or hospital care. Administrative costs for plans ranged from 5% to 17% of total costs, which is low compared to pluralistic systems with multiple insurers (the United States, for example, with administrative costs of 19–24%) and compared to western national health insurance systems (for example, the Canadian system, with 8–11% administrative costs). Many of the plans that were primarily based on tertiary care (for example, in Nkoranza in Ghana, Masisi in the Democratic Republic of the Congo, Korea, and Taiwan) had problems with overuse of services and cost escalation, whereas plans that were primary care-oriented employed primary care physicians as gatekeepers to control use and costs. Plan managers were found to be highly inefficient in financial planning.

In terms of equity, Bennett et al. (1998) found that, although nearly all of the insurance plans they studied had community-rated insurance premiums (whereby everyone pays the same amount), the premiums were flat-rated and therefore regressive in nature. Other taxation or payment measures that associate tax rates with income level (for example, direct taxes and higher tax rates for higher incomes on a gradient basis) are more progressive than such plans. With the exception of a few plans, there were no exemptions or subsidies for those who had difficulty affording membership in the plan, which amounted to 5–10% of annual household budget in some plans, such as that in Nkoranza district, Ghana. Because the low-income population often could not afford to begin or maintain payments in a plan, they were forced to pay user fees for health services.

The authors also assessed use patterns of different plans and concluded that households located closer to a health facility were more likely to enroll in insurance plans and had higher use rates than those farther away. Thus geography played an important role in use patterns. This geographic effect could create adverse selection problems whereby those living farther from a health facility drop out, increasing premiums and leading to further withdrawals. The authors also noted a number of structural features that contributed to poor financial sustainability: small scale; adverse selection leading to smaller risk pools and higher costs; significant administrative structures; and costs.

While risk pooling and insurance are generally preferred to direct purchase of health care due to their efficiency and welfare gains, they also have significant incentive altering effects that reduce efficiency and equity in other areas of the health system. For this reason, public and private policy is increasingly shifting risk from government (or third-party private insurers) to providers by moving clockwise around the circle in Figure 12–8. In addition, the mechanisms through which funds are obtained to finance health insurance affect our behavior. Exhibit 12–6 explains two types of health insurance market failures that result from the altered incentives of health insurance, and the next section addresses many of the incentive effects of various health-financing policies.

## Health Financing Policies and their Incentives

The evidence presented earlier suggests that lower income countries underinvest in health, and their use of already low health investments is often inefficient and inequitable. These factors contribute to lower economic growth and lead to poor health and economic outcomes. To improve these outcomes, lower income countries face the challenge of raising political support and revenues to sustain greater public investments in health and to improve efficiency in use of both public and private resources. In addition, many health systems in lower income countries fail to take advantage of the economic and welfare benefits that accrue from collective risk reduction in the form of risk pooling, and from analytical efforts to set priorities through improvements in allocative and technical efficiencies. Constraints that are particular to lower income countries include low personal income, a large informal or subsistence sector that is exempt from income taxation, and low administrative and tax collection capacity, all of which result in low levels of insurance and risk pooling, health-related capital stock, such as facilities, equipment, beds, and pharmaceutical products, and human resources, such as nurses and providers. Lower income countries, because of less-targeted and lower levels of public expenditure, are

**Exhibit 12–6** Insurance Market Failures: Adverse Selection and Moral Hazard

Insurance market failures, credit shortages, and information asymmetries and insufficiencies can inhibit individuals from realizing the economic benefits of collective risk reduction through risk pooling and efficient insurance systems. Thus a rationale exists for public financing of health care services or for strong regulation of private health insurance markets. Two commonly noted forms of health insurance market failure include adverse selection and moral hazard.

*Adverse selection* occurs when individuals who are sicker than average self-select into plans that offer better benefits than other plans. This selection increases premiums, making it more likely that the average or healthier-than-average individuals will opt out from these plans. If healthier individuals opt out, then spreading risk across the population is no longer possible, as only the sickest are left in the plan. The result is a spiraling effect in which premiums increase and risk pooling disintegrates. In just 3 years in the late 1990s, for example, the indemnity insurance option in the UCLA staff health plan rose from $200 per month to more than $1,000 per month as all but those at highest risk opted for managed care (at less than $50 per month). Insurance companies attempt to combat adverse selection by screening high-risk individuals through mechanisms such as excluding preexisting conditions from coverage, refusing coverage, requiring medical exams, and having waiting periods. These costly insurance company strategies further add to the instabilities in health insurance markets. Regulating insurers, offering insurance through groups, such as employers, and requiring mandatory public insurance can help alleviate these problems in the private health insurance market.

*Moral hazard* occurs when people are insured and thus do not have to pay the full costs of health care. They have a reduced incentive to avoid certain health care costs, resulting in behavior that may actually increase the probability of occurrence of an event that has been insured against. This feature can be present in either public or private insurance systems. To mitigate moral hazard, insurers create cost sharing, benefit limitation, frequent renewability, and use management features for the health insurance system.

*Equity.* Ill health and financial ruin resulting from catastrophic illness lead to poverty and income inequality and add to efficiency arguments for government financing of health care services for the low-income and other vulnerable groups. Equitably financed health systems raise revenues based on people's ability to pay, and equitable delivery systems allocate resources based on people's medical care needs. While often goals can be achieved only at some cost in efficiency, this trade-off is far less acute in health finance precisely because of the insurance market failures just discussed. Private health insurance markets will not ensure equitable revenue generation for health care financing, the equitable distribution of health insurance, or the equitable allocation of health resources. Regulation and public financing are required to achieve equitable as well as efficient outcomes in health finance and delivery.

sometimes characterized by greater inequality in the distribution of income compared to more developed economies.

Increasing lower income countries' overall and public investments in health—and ensuring equitable and efficient use of those resources—is essential to improving health and economic growth and to reducing poverty. However, revenue generation policies have their own economic and equity implications that must be analyzed in order to ensure that efforts to finance health investments do more good than harm. This section assesses the economic and equity consequences of various specific financing mechanisms: taxation; insurance funding, especially as it affects employment; and user fees/user charges and their effect on the welfare of the low-income. Certain choices among financing and provider compensation options can create conditions for excessive spending on health, and this appears to be an emerging problem in middle-income countries.

### Taxation

In terms of economic efficiency and revenue generation, most forms of taxation (with the exception of lump sum or poll taxes) distort the consumption and production decisions made by individuals, households, and firms, resulting in a cost (a deadweight loss) to consider when devising health financing plans involving public taxation. Lump sum and poll taxes, which avoid these burdens, are less desirable on equity grounds and are typically infeasible politically (Schieber & Maeda, 1993).

However, while taxation can be inefficient due to the deadweight loss created by distorting production and consumption decisions, it can also be effective in generating revenue; it serves as a primary mechanism for some types of investment in the economy; and it can be a means for enhancing equity through subsidies and transfers if progressive taxation is employed. A difficulty with general tax revenues in all countries, especially lower income ones, is that budget allocations by sector are dependent upon the political support that a given sector generates. In such intersectoral budgetary decisions, health care often loses out to other, more popular, sectors. This fact is especially true when budget projections are overestimated, leaving a shortfall to be made up through budget cuts, as is the case in many lower income countries. Finally, taxation capacity can be limited in lower income countries because of underdeveloped and inefficient administrations.

### Medical Care Demand Effects of Expanding Private Insurance

The economic impact of expanding private insurance is believed to be the increased demand for private, and the reduced demand for public, insurance among those with the ability to pay the increased insurance rates (higher income groups). Jamaica has recently experienced such a transition. Gertler and Sturm (1997) studied the demand for public and private medical care with the expansion of private sector insurance in Jamaica. Jamaica has a universal public health care system in which anyone can use public facilities free of charge, and access to facilities by all groups has been found to be quite good. Jamaica also has a significant private sector health care market in which higher quality services are

offered at higher prices. Gertler and Sturm (1997) found that insurance did induce individuals to opt out of the public sector in favor of higher quality private sector care, and that private insurance coverage was concentrated primarily among the upper income groups, a factor that then freed up public resources for lower income individuals (see Table 12–5 for results). This stratification also creates a two-tiered system of health care, in which upper-income groups obtain private care through private insurance companies, and lower income groups obtain publicly financed, and often publicly provided, care.

The work of Gertler and Sturm is especially relevant in the context of low- and middle-income countries because health care financed by governments in these settings often subsidizes the wealthier groups in society. For example, in Indonesia the lowest income quintile consumes less than 14% of public sector health care expenditure, while the highest income quintile consumes more than 30% (Van de Walle, 1994). Gertler and Sturm (1997) found that introducing mandated private insurance induced covered individuals to opt out of the public sector in favor of perceived higher quality services in the private sector, and that this shift reduced the total public health expenditure on health care. They also suggested that this policy shift improved the targeting of public health care services toward the low-income. Their simulations suggest that "a reduction in total public sector visits from expanding health insurance to the top half of the income distribution implies: (1) a reduction in public expenditures of about 33%, (2) an increase in the share of public expenditures captured by the poor by about 25%, and (3) a shift in the mix of subsidies away from curative in favor of preventative care" (Gertler and Sturm, 1997, p. 255). This shift could yield significant public sector cost savings and improved targeting of subsidies to the low-income and toward preventative services.

### Employer-Related Health Insurance

Some aspects of employer-related health insurance (ERHI) have economic consequences that are worthy of consideration. Securing health insurance through formal employment is typi-

**Table 12–5** The Estimated Effect of Health Insurance on the Demand for Medical Care

| | Preventive Care Visits per Month | | | Curative Care Visits per Month | | |
|---|---|---|---|---|---|---|
| | *Public* | *Private* | *Total* | *Public* | *Private* | *Total* |
| Insurance | 0.138 | 0.473 | 0.611 | 0.022 | 0.089 | 0.111 |
| No insurance | 0.191 | 0.221 | 0.412 | 0.040 | 0.065 | 0.105 |
| Difference | −0.053 | 0.252 | 0.199 | −0.018 | 0.024 | 0.006 |

cal where the formal employment sector is substantial (higher income as opposed to lower income settings) because an individual's income is higher, identifiable, taxed, and subsidized, and because organization is more feasible through formal employment. The extent to which national insurance plans are successful can depend on the size and nature of the formal employment and private insurance sectors and government administrative capacity. Employer-related (or employment-based) health insurance is primarily an American phenomenon. In the United States, approximately 90% of Americans who are covered by private health insurance obtain this coverage through their employment. Of the total compensation package for U.S. workers, health insurance coverage accounts for approximately 34% of benefits expenditures and 7% of the total compensation package (U.S. Bureau of Labor Statistics, 1994).

The link between employment and health insurance in the United States has historical roots in mid–twentieth century legislation and policies devised to deal with the excess demand for labor in the aftermath of World War II. In particular, two policy efforts confirmed the employment–health insurance link: (1) congressional efforts to restrict wage increases after World War II, which resulted in employer competition for employees on the basis of non-wage benefits such as pensions and health insurance; and (2) tax laws that exempted benefits from taxation, making them a tax-deductible expenditure of business for employers. Both measures created an incentive for employers to offer health insurance as a benefit of employment (Federal Reserve Bank of San Francisco, 1998). In reality, although employers advertise health insur-

ance as an employer-subsidized benefit, it is the employees who "pay" for the cost of these services through reduced real wages (except in cases where, like the U.S. after World War II, core wages have been artificially capped). Given the established employment–health insurance link in the United States, the market for employer-related health insurance has a number of implications for employee decisions around job mobility, retirement, and labor supply.

*Job Mobility.* Job-lock is a relatively new term used to describe the situation in which employees are reluctant to change jobs for fear of losing health insurance coverage. It might occur when an individual does not take a better job at a new company because of differences in health insurance coverage between the old job and the new one. Such health insurance differences for this individual might involve requiring a waiting period of several months before health insurance can be obtained, or it might mean that the new employer's coverage excludes health care services that treat one of his or her family's preexisting conditions. Because of the disparities between jobs in the availability and scope of health insurance, and despite potential gains in productivity and income, employees are reluctant to change jobs. Reduction of job mobility not only limits worker freedom, choice, and income, but it also has implications for the productivity of the economy if employees are reluctant to take new jobs that will enhance their individual productivity. Although it has long been surmised that job-lock exists, until recently only minimal empirical evidence existed to document the magnitude of this phenomenon in the labor market.

*Magnitude of Job-Lock.* From 1994 to 1996, at least five studies examined the effects of ERHI on job mobility, productivity, and welfare (for example, welfare loss from job-lock is the loss in productivity associated with the decline in worker mobility). A review of this literature (see Table 12–6) demonstrates that ERHI does deter worker mobility: these studies typically reported a 20–40% reduction in mobility rates due to ERHI, depending on workers' marital status, gender, and family size (Buchmueller & Valletta, 1996; Cooper & Monheit, 1993; Holtz-Eakin, 1994; Madrian, 1994; Monheit and Cooper, 1994). One study found that after controlling for pension receipt, job tenure, and spouse job change, there was strong evidence of job-lock among women, but not among men (Buchmeuller & Valletta, 1996). Another study found that reductions in job mobility due to ERHI were highest for two specific groups: (1) married men with a large family; and (2) married men with a pregnant wife (Madrian, 1994).

Fewer studies have been done on the effects of ERHI on worker productivity and macroeconomic efficiencies. However, one such study concluded that in 1987 the economic productivity loss due to job-lock accounted for approximately 0.5% of the total U.S. wage bill ($3.7 billion in annual wages out of $1.262 trillion total, assuming full-time and full-year employment) (Monheit and Cooper, 1994). The authors suggest that this figure can be explained by the fact that these effects are relatively short-lived and affect a relatively small number (1 million out of 61 million) of workers. To obtain an estimate of the net effect of ERHI on economic efficiency, these efficiency losses ultimately must be weighed against potential efficiency gains (currently not estimated) that may result from ERHI.

*Alleviating or Eliminating Job-Lock.* At least three strategies can be employed to mitigate the effects of ERHI on job mobility: (1) maintain ERHI, but ensure full portability of health insurance coverage across jobs; (2) maintain ERHI, but disallow the exclusion from coverage of preexisting medical conditions; and (3) disassociate health insurance from employment altogether.

There is limited empirical evidence of the effectiveness of these policy options, but one study did find that short-term (3–20 months) "continuation of coverage" mandates (policies that give individuals the right to purchase health insurance through their former employers for a specific period of time) had a positive effect on worker mobility (Gruber and Madrian, 1994). These results suggest that job-lock may result from short-term (as opposed to long-term) employee concerns over health insurance portability.

*Retirement.* The decision to retire or continue working is also heavily influenced by ERHI status. This is especially true because the quantity and frequency of medical expenses increase with age, as does the difference between the costs of employer-related health insurance and the insurance policies that can be purchased individually on the open market (Gruber and Madrian, 1995). In some circumstances, older individuals cannot even purchase individual market-based policies.

In their analysis of the impact of continuation of coverage laws on retirement decisions, Gruber and Madrian (1995) found that the ability to purchase an employment-based plan from a former employer at the same price as if one were employed increases the odds of early retirement (because the individual is no longer working, employees still working will be forced to pay for the subsidy provided to retired workers). The degree to which the likelihood of early retirement increases depends, the authors found, on the duration of the ability to purchase post-retirement insurance and the quality of the employer-based post-retirement and publicly offered health insurance options. More specifically, the authors found that among men aged 55–64 who are too young for Medicare (which commences at age 65), each additional year of continued coverage increases the likelihood of retiring by 30%.

*Labor Supply.* Most employers do not offer health benefits to part-time employees. In addition, many low-wage earners in service sector positions (for example, fast-food service employees) do not receive health insurance as a

**Table 12–6** Employment-Related Health Insurance (ERHI) and Job Mobility: Estimates of Job-Lock in the United States

| Author(s) | Sample/Method | Magnitude of Job-Lock |
|---|---|---|
| Madrian (1994) | 1987 National Medical Expenditure Survey (NMES). Sample of married men ages 20–55. Estimated probit equation of likelihood of job change and examined three experimental groups with difference-in-difference approach. | Estimated that mobility rates decreased by 30–31% for those with employment-provided health insurance coverage compared to those without such coverage. Mobility rates reduced by 33–37% for those married men with employment-related coverage and large families. Mobility rates decreased by 67% for those with employment-related coverage and a pregnant wife. |
| Holtz-Eakin (1994) | 1984 Panel Study of Income Dynamics (PSID). Full-time workers age 25–55. Used difference-in-difference approach. | Found no statistically significant results. For job changes during 1984–1985, mobility rates for married men declined by 1.59 percentage points and rates for single women declined by 1.06 percentage points. |
| Gruber and Madrian (1994) | Survey of Income and Program Participation (1985, 1986, 1987) | Found that state and federal policy to mandate "continuation of coverage" increased job mobility of prime-age male workers. Suggested that job-lock may result from short-run (as opposed to long-run) employee concerns over portability. |
| Monheit and Cooper (1994) | 1987 National Medical Expenditure Survey (NMES). Reviewed literature and studied the nature of welfare loss associated with job-lock. | Authors reviewed literature on job-lock and found that studies typically reported a 20–40% reduction in mobility rates due to ERHI, depending on worker marital status, gender, and family size. Examined welfare loss due to job-lock and found that the magnitude of welfare loss was $4.8 billion, less than 1% of the wage bill of those affected. |
| Buchmueller and Valletta (1996) | 1984 Survey of Income and Program Participation (SIPP). Included pension receipt, job tenure, spouse job change to estimated ERHI effects on job mobility. | Found, for dual-earner married men and women, strong evidence of job-lock among women, but weak evidence of job-lock among men. |

benefit of employment (low-wage earners typically do not receive benefits because their earnings are too low to pass on the premium costs). These factors provide an incentive for those who need or value health insurance to choose full-time over part-time employment. In their analysis of married women's decisions to work full- or part-time, Buchmueller and Valletta (1999) found that wives frequently switched from non-participation to work in order to obtain health insurance. Their estimates demonstrate a 15–36% increase in married women's labor supply associated with a lack of their husband's health insurance coverage.

### Labor Market Effects of Introducing National Health Insurance in Canada*

One of the negative economic impacts of introducing national health insurance in a given country is believed to be the deadweight loss and increased unemployment resulting from altered production and consumption decisions due to the necessary increases in payroll taxes. Economic theory predicts that increases in payroll taxes result in economic activity and deadweight losses as a result of altered production and consumption decisions in the economy. At the same time, theory points to efficiency gains from effectively implemented risk-pooling arrangements. From the early 1960s to the early 1970s, Canada moved from a primarily private insurance–based health care system to a national health insurance system financed primarily through lump sum premiums or general revenue financing, with management decentralized to the provincial level. National health insurance in Canada provides coverage to all citizens.

Gruber and Hanratty (1993) studied the effects of Canada's "natural experiment" of phasing from ERHI (roughly 70% of the population was covered by private health insurance in the mid-1960s) to national health insurance. In examining monthly data on employment, wages, and hours across 8 industries and 10 provinces over the period 1961–1975, they found that, although both employment and wages increased after the introduction of national health insurance, average hours were unchanged. These results were robust to a number of model specifi-

---

*Currie and Madrian (1999) provide an excellent overview and additional references concerning the labor market effects of health insurance, with an emphasis on the situation in the United States. See also Gruber and Hanratty (1993) and Hanratty (1996).

cations (different analyses) that controlled for the potential endogeneity of national health insurance and provincial and industry effects. The authors believe that the results might be explained by the notion that the introduction of national health insurance systematically increases labor demand across all sectors of the economy due, at least in part, to the increases in labor productivity that result from increases in job mobility or health improvements in the labor force. Despite some noted differences in the costs of medical and hospital care, the authors believe that the pre-national health insurance system in Canada is sufficiently similar to that in the United States for this Canadian experiment to offer useful evidence of the effects of a similar transition in the United States.

### The Impact of Private User Fees/Public User Charges on the Welfare of the Poor

Private user fees are part of a system in which patients pay directly out-of-pocket for health care services. These fees can take the form of payment for the whole charge, partial payment for a service, or copayment (a flat amount per visit), or coinsurance (a percentage of the cost of the service). User charges are fees paid by patients for publicly provided services and constitute public revenues. User fee/user charge financing is designed as a demand-side and revenue-generation measure to improve allocative efficiency in the health care system by making patients more cost conscious in health care decision making. In addition to use control, user charges have been designed to raise revenues and to decrease the government's financial burden in the health sector, to increase coverage and the quality of care by increasing resources for the health sector, and to increase efficiency in health service delivery.

Higher income countries promote these types of payments to reduce health care use (by making consumers more conscious of health care costs). Evidence suggests that these mechanisms have been successful in reducing use, regardless of whether reduced health care is medically appropriate (Newhouse, 1993). User fees have a greater health and income impact on the poor and medically indigent because these groups decrease their use of both necessary and unnecessary health care. Rather than employ user fees/user charges, a new system of allocative efficiency, or medical care appropriateness, has emerged to reduce inappropriate care, while ensuring that appropriate and necessary care reaches those in need. This system is currently being tested in the United States and is discussed in Exhibit 12–5.

The evidence from a number of in-country experiences with user fees/user charges demonstrates that, for the most part, such fees have not been overwhelmingly successful in raising revenue, enhancing efficiency, or improving equity. With respect to revenue generation, user charges have failed to provide more than 10% of ministry of health recurrent costs in sub-Saharan Africa (Wang'ombe, 1997). Programs in China have been much more successful in cost recovery (24–36% of Ministry of Health recurrent expenditures recovered) than have programs in sub-Saharan Africa, where an average of 5% of operating costs are recouped through user charges. This figure is probably an underestimate of the net yield because the administrative costs of collecting fees must also be considered. In many cases, it is likely that the net yield is near zero or negative for cost recovery. In addition, because systems are not raising enough revenues from user fees/user charges, there is little additional money to channel into improved quality and system reform, especially for public health services targeted at the low-income, which are especially hard hit by the lack of additional money. Funding for these efforts still must stem from the Ministry of Health budget.

A review of the literature on user financing of basic social services by Reddy and Vandemoortele (1996) further supports the conclusion that user fees and user charges generally have had negative effects on use and very little success in raising revenue to cover governmental recurrent costs. As shown in Table 12–7, recent estimates of price elasticity of demand for health care in a number of countries provide compel-

ling evidence that user fees are associated with significant reductions in use rates, especially among the low-income and children. The magnitude of revenues raised through health cost recovery in Africa ranges from roughly 0.5–20% of the recurrent budget of the Ministry of Health.

There is additional evidence that user fees/ user charges reduce use, but the overall efficiency effects are unclear given that these reductions occur with both necessary and unnecessary care. In his review of the literature on user charges, Creese (1991) found user fees decrease use, especially among the patients at greatest risk and for whom the most cost-effective preventative and treatment options are appropriate. In the Democratic Republic of the Congo, for instance, relative increases in the cost of health care (as compared to the cost of other consumer products) led to significant decreases in the demand for treatment measures, especially for prenatal care and interventions for children under age 5. The magnitude of the reduction was significant: the overall use rate fell from 37% to 31% and the coverage rate for prenatal visits fell from 95% to 84% (De Bethune, Alfani, & Lahaye, 1989). As Creese (1991) notes, these study results indicate that the demand for health care is more price elastic among lower income individuals than in higher income groups. The cost-recovery rate through user charges was insignificant.

Efficiency gains from these mechanisms have also been modest. There is some evidence that the use of graduated user charges (higher fees for hospitals and lower fees for health centers) aimed at improving technical efficiency (delivering primary care at low-level health centers and tertiary care at high-level hospitals) has been successful (Collins, Quick, Musau, & Kraushaar, 1995). Some countries, namely Côte d'Ivoire, Mali, Namibia, Zambia, and Zimbabwe, have implemented graduated user charges with some successes in technical efficiency (for example, better use of referrals, and better patterns of use for both primary care received at lower level facilities such as health centers and tertiary care received at higher level facilities such as hospi-

**Table 12–7** Recent Estimates of Price Elasticity of Demand for Health Care

| Study | Location/Year of Data | Results | | |
|---|---|---|---|---|
| Jimenez (1989) | Ethiopia (1985) | Overall | −0.05 to −0.50 | |
| Jimenez (1989) | Sudan (1986) | Overall | −0.37 | |
| Yoder (1989) | Swaziland (1985) | Overall | −0.32 | |
| Gertler and Van der Gaag (1988) | Côte d'Ivoire (1985) | *Rural Hospitals* | | |
| | | Income Quartile | Adults | Children |
| | | Lowest | −0.47 to −1.34 | −0.65 to −2.32 |
| | | Second | −0.44 to −1.27 | −0.58 to −1.98 |
| | | Third | −0.41 to −1.18 | −0.49 to −1.60 |
| | | Highest | −0.29 to −0.71 | −0.12 to −0.48 |
| Gertler and Van der Gaag (1988) | Peru (1985) | *Rural Hospitals* | | |
| | | Income Quartile | Adults | Children |
| | | Lowest | −0.57 to −1.36 | −0.57 to −1.72 |
| | | Second | −0.38 to −0.91 | −0.48 to −1.20 |
| | | Third | −0.16 to −0.37 | −0.22 to −0.54 |
| | | Highest | −0.01 to −0.04 | −0.03 to −0.09 |
| Sauerborn et al. (1994) | Burkina Faso (1985) | Overall | −0.79 | |
| | | Age Groups | | |
| | | <1 | −3.64 | |
| | | 1–14 | −1.73 | |
| | | 15– | −0.27 | |
| | | Income Quartile | | |
| | | Lowest | −1.44 | |
| | | Second | −1.21 | |
| | | Third | −1.39 | |
| | | Highest | −0.12 | |

tals) (Barnum & Kutzin, 1993; Bennett & Ngalande-Banda, 1994).

In Ghana, Creese (1991) notes, there was a sharp reduction in use as a result of large increases in health care fees. Reduced use was sustained over a 2-year period (Waddington & Enyimayew, 1990). Although the cost recovery rate of this policy (15%) was fairly high compared with some other projects, the authors believed that the demand shifted from health care sought in government facilities to rural, unlicensed sellers of drugs, which had potentially significant ramifications for health. Finally, Creese (1991) noted a sharp decrease in demand following a policy decision in Swaziland, to raise charges at government health units by 300–400% (to the same fee levels as mission providers), without raising quality. The resultant decrease in use at government facilities was 32%, but this decrease was coupled with an increase in use of 10% at mission facilities; the overall drop in use was 17%. Use continued to decrease over the course of the year following the policy change, and a disproportionate drop in use (especially for use of government services for sexually transmitted and respiratory infections) occurred among the lower income groups (Yoder, 1989).

The equity effects of user fees and user charges are not favorable. While some initially argued that equity can be improved through the use of user fees/user charges due to increased service availability and quality (from increased revenues) and better use (from price effects on demand) (De Ferranti, 1985), the subsequent evidence does not necessarily support this argument. For these factors to be equity-enhancing, the government would need to ensure that increased revenues are reinvested and targeted toward services that directly affect the low-income, and to ensure that low-income and vulnerable groups are exempted from many user fees and charges and offered public subsidies instead. Evidence from sub-Saharan Africa suggests that patients are highly sensitive to user charges and user fees (Bennett & Ngalande-Banda, 1994; Gertler & van der Gaag, 1990; Mwabu and Wang'ombe, 1995; Waddington & Enyimayew, 1990). Although nearly all sub-Saharan African user fee and user charge programs have exemptions for the poor through means testing, this method is hard to implement in many countries and can be exploited by higher income groups.

## Health Expenditures and Poverty

For those without insurance coverage, high health expenditures relative to income either can preclude treatment because of income insufficiencies or, if medical treatment options are pursued, can pose a major financial burden. While the evidence on this subject is scant, there are a few studies that demonstrate the implications both of falling ill and of facing catastrophic health expenditure. For example, in their analysis of the post-Cooperative Medical System

era in China, Liu, Hu, Fu, and Hsiao (1998) found that high health expenditures were a major cause of poverty in rural areas. Health care costs were found to be high relative to a rural farmer's income: low-income farmers often had to spend roughly 1.2 years of disposable income to pay for an episode of hospitalization at a county hospital. As Table 12–8 demonstrates, the cost of an outpatient visit as a percentage of weekly income for the lowest income households varied from 38% in a village facility to 151% at a township provider and 170% in a county facility. In addition, 18% of households using health services incurred health expenditures exceeding total household income in 1 year (1993), and of the 11,044 rural households surveyed, 24.5% borrowed or became indebted, and 5.5% sold or mortgaged properties to pay for health care. In addition, 72.6% of individuals who did not seek ambulatory care and 89.2% of individuals who did not seek hospital care made this decision based on financial difficulties. In their survey of 30 counties, the authors found that, as a result of these burdensome payments, 47% of medically indebted households suffered from hunger.

In a preliminary study of people's ability to cope with catastrophic health shocks in Indonesia, Prescott and Pradhan (1999) found that out-of-pocket health expenditures were highly skewed, suggesting that a proportion of the population faced catastrophic levels of health expenditure relative to income. Social risk management mechanisms, in the form of budget subsidies for publicly provided services and insurance for civil servants, generally benefited the better-off, whereas lower income households were forced to reduce demand (especially for inpatient services) and spend less on medical care. In their simulations of the estimated frequency and intensity of catastrophic health shocks, controlling for income, the authors found that the simulated estimate was much higher than the frequency observed from household survey data. With respect to policy measures employed to alleviate the burden on poorer households, the authors believe that efforts to ensure universal coverage through budget subsidies targeting the poor and through insurance options can sig-

**Table 12–8** The Financial Burden of Health Care Costs for Households with Different Income Levels in China's Poverty Regions

| Level of Facilities | Households with Income/Capita 200 Yuan | Households with Income/Capita 400 Yuan |
|---|---|---|
| | Cost of an outpatient visit as % of weekly income | |
| Village | 38% | 36% |
| Township | 151% | 71% |
| County | 170% | 84% |
| | Cost of an inpatient episode as % of annual income | |
| Township | 28% | 22% |
| County | 116% | 138% |

nificantly reduce, but not eliminate, the catastrophic shocks experienced by lower income households.

Finally, Fabricant, Kamara, and Mills (1999) showed that in Sierra Leone the rural low-income were disproportionately disadvantaged by user charges for health care, in that they paid a higher percentage of their incomes for health care than wealthier households. The authors concluded that greater accessibility to basic health facilities and greater reliance on additional resources generated through improved efficiency and cross-subsidization would relieve much of the financial burden placed on these lower income households. Insurance and prepayment plans also would help reduce the financial burden of health expenditure.

## CONCLUSION

The World Bank's 1980 World Development Report on human resources and poverty examined the interrelations between poverty (in terms of low income) and health, education, nutrition, and fertility levels. Table 12–1 points to the enormous progress in this century in several of these domains, progress substantially denied to the world's lowest income billion. The upper panel of Figure 12–9, reproduced (and modified) from the 1980 report, illustrates both the possible relations among these variables and the entry points for policy operating through them. Although the report indicates the importance of

public action in each domain, it concludes that expansion and improvement in primary education, particularly for girls, is the critical priority in most countries. The information presented in this chapter suggests a more central role for health, at least for low-income regions with current high levels of illness. The lower panel of Figure 12–9 places health in this central role.

The consequences of health and health policy for economic development are of major importance to policy makers in the health and development fields. This chapter has provided an assessment of the relevant conclusions from the literature available on this subject, but recognizes that the research base itself is limited. The analysis presented here suggests directions for government policy at several levels. First, it is useful to encourage policies that will accelerate the speed of favorable demographic transitions and incorporate changing age structures into government policies aimed at schooling and job creation. The changing age structure of a population that results from demographic transition provides a window of opportunity that can lead to a transitory boost in economic growth, enabling a country to break free of a poverty trap. Second, a central goal of many countries' health-sector development strategies should be to create policies to control infectious diseases, such as malaria, tuberculosis, HIV/AIDS and sexually transmitted infections, by providing information and resources necessary for avoiding, and in many cases, curing infection. Categorical con-

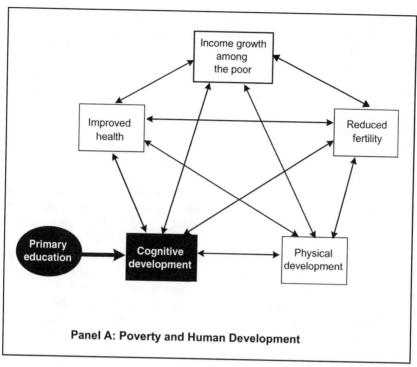

**Panel A: Poverty and Human Development**

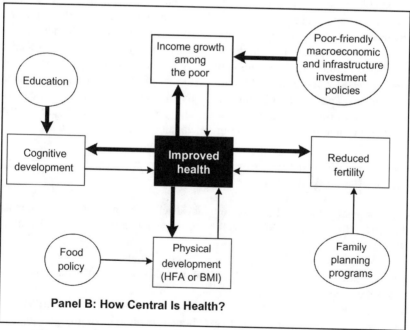

**Panel B: How Central Is Health?**

*Notes:* HFA = height for age; BMI = body mass index.

**Figure 12–9** Health and Development

trol policies against the major diseases of the low-income probably provide the most efficient means for targeting public expenditures to them. Third, improving the health of the poor is necessary to alleviate poverty. The marginal productivity of health is probably higher in low-income societies, and governments should develop policies to address the health and economic needs of the low-income population.

Efforts also must be made to assess selected health policies based on their effects on economic outcomes (as well as health). First, practitioners should promote the use of clinical protocols to improve health outcomes and enhance efficient health care spending. Economic incentives to decrease health care use (for example, copayments, deductibles, capitated payments, and global budgets) do not necessarily distinguish between types of care (appropriate versus inappropriate) and the needs of patients, and can have a disproportionate impact on the poor and medically indigent. Second, governments and policy makers should pursue sustainable health care financing to insure against health-related financial losses and to eliminate distortions in the market for health care. To spread risk and minimize insurance market failure, governments can (1) encourage universal risk-pooling through government mandates and taxes; (2) pursue health financing policies that are separate from employment, thereby preempting or reducing

labor market distortions that result from ERHI; and (3) discourage the use of user fees to generate revenue and reduce demand for health care services among the poor. Third, efforts should be taken to improve health care systems with inadequate infrastructure and access. In many societies low levels of health spending and inequitable allocation result in unacceptably low levels of capital stock, human resources, and service use that fail to meet the individuals' health needs. Fourth, health planners should promote efficient health administration policies by avoiding or reducing excessive administrative costs, especially those between hospitals and third-party payers, and by encouraging the efficient use of administrative activities to monitor and reduce the occurrence of costly and medically inappropriate procedures.

Finally, development institutions, nongovernmental organizations, and academic communities should take on a number of activities to investigate further the links between health and economic development. Primarily, they can encourage continued efforts to understand health and development links by helping low- and middle-income countries develop their own capacity to study these connections; by encouraging further generation of relevant primary data; and by ensuring that the appropriate household-level and cross-national databases are maintained, updated, and accessible to all.

---

**DISCUSSION QUESTIONS**

1. In what ways, and to what extent, do major diseases such as tuberculosis, malaria, and HIV/AIDS affect the income and well-being of people living in low- and middle-income countries?
2. What can policy makers and practitioners do in non-health-service-related settings, such as schools, to improve the health and well-being of girls and boys in low- and middle-income countries?
3. How do respective changes in fertility and mortality patterns work to influence the level and capacity of those contributing to economic production in a given society?
4. Why is the concept of risk pooling in financing health care services so important?
5. What are the health, health care service use, and economic effects of making people pay part of the costs of medical services?

## REFERENCES

Aaron, H., & Schwartz, W. (1984). *The painful prescription: Rationing hospital care.* Washington, DC: Brookings Institution.

Ahlburg, D.A. (1999). The economic impacts of tuberculosis. A Report for WHO. (In progress).

Anand, K., Pandav, C.S., & Nath, L.M. (1999). Impact of HIV/AIDS on the national economy of India. *Health Policy, 47*, 195–205.

Barnum, H., & Kutzin, J. (1993). *Public hospitals in developing countries: Resource use, cost, financing.* Baltimore: Johns Hopkins University Press for the World Bank.

Barro, R., & Lee, J.W. (1994). Sources of economic growth. *Carnegie-Rochester Conference Series on Public Policy, 40*, 1–46.

Basta, S.S., Soekirman, M.S., Karyadi, D., & Scrimshaw, N.S. (1979). Iron deficiency anemia and the productivity of adult males in Indonesia. *American Journal of Clinical Nutrition, 32*, 916–925.

Behrman, J. (1993). The economic rationale for investing in nutrition in developing countries. *World Development, 21*(11), 1749–1771.

Bennett, S., Creese, A., & Monasch, R. (1998). *Health insurance schemes for people outside formal sector employment.* (Division of Analysis, Research and Assessment Paper No. 16). Geneva, Switzerland: World Health Organization.

Bennett, S., & Ngalande-Banda, E. (1994). *Public and private roles in health: A review and analysis of experience in sub-saharan Africa* (Strengthening Health Services Paper 6). Geneva, Switzerland: World Health Organization, Division of Strengthening Health Services.

Berger, M.C., & Leigh, P. (1989). Schooling, self-selection and health. *Journal of Human Resources, 24*, 435–455.

Bernstein, S.J., McGlynn, E.A., Siu, A.L., Roth, C.P., Sherwood, M.J., Keesey, J.W., Kosecoff, J., Hicks, N.R., & Brook, R.H. (1993). The appropriateness of hysterectomy: A comparison of care in seven health plans. *Journal of the American Medical Association, 269*, 2398–2402.

Bhargava, A. (1994). Modeling the health of Filipino children. *Journal of the Royal Statistical Society, Series A, 157*, 417–432.

Bhargava, A., Jamison, D.T., Lau, L.J., & Murray, C.J.L. (2000). "Modelling the Effects of Health on Economic Growth." Geneva: World Health Organization, Global Programme on Evidence Discussion Paper.

Bloom, D.E., & Canning, D. (2000, February 18). The health and wealth of nations. *Science*, 1207–1209.

Bloom, D.E., Canning, D., & Malaney, P. (in press). Population dynamics and economic growth. *Population and Development Review.*

Bloom, D.E., & Freeman, R.B. (1988). Economic development and the timing and components of population growth. *Journal of Policy Modeling*, April, 57–82.

Bloom, D.E., & Mahal, A.S. (1997). Does the AIDS epidemic threaten economic growth? *Journal of Econometrics, 77*, 105–124.

Bloom, D.E., & River Path Associates. (in press). Social capitalism and human diversity. In *The creative society of the 21st century.* Paris: Organization of Economic Cooperation and Development.

Bloom, D.E., Rosenfield, A., & River Path Associates. (in press). A moment in time: AIDS and business. AIDS patient care and STDs.

Bloom, D.E., & Williamson, J.G. (1998). Demographic transitions and economic miracles in emerging Asia. *The World Bank Economic Review, 12*(3), 419–455.

Bovbjerg, R.R. (1995). Review essay: The high cost of administration in health care: Part of the problem or part of the solution? *Journal of Law, Medicine & Ethics, 23*, 186–194.

Brook, R.H. (1992). Improving practice: The clinician's role. *British Journal of Surgery, 79*, 606–607.

Brook, R.H. (1994). The Rand/UCLA appropriateness method. In K.A. McCormick, S.R. Moore, & R.A. Siegel, *Clinical practice guideline development: Methodology perspectives* (AHCPR Publication No. 95–0009). Rockville, MD: Public Health Service.

Brook, R.H. (1995). Medicare quality and getting older: A personal essay. *Health Affairs, 14*(4), 73–81.

Brook, RH. (1997). Managed care is not the problem. Quality is. *Journal of the American Medical Association, 278*, 1612–1614.

Brook, R.H., Kamberg, C.J., Mayer-Oakes, A., Beers, M.H., Raube, K., & Steiner, A. (1990). Appropriateness of acute medical care for the elderly: An analysis of the literature. *Health Policy, 14*, 225–242.

Brook, R.H., & Lohr, K.N. (1986). Will we need to ration effective health care? *Issues in Science and Technology, 3*, 68–77.

Brook, R.H., & Lohr, K.N. (1987). Monitoring quality of care in the Medicare program: Two proposed systems. *Journal of the American Medical Association, 258*, 3138–3141.

Brook, R.H., & Lohr, K.N. (1990). Efficacy, effectiveness, variations, and quality: boundary-crossing research. In N.O. Graham (Ed.), *Quality assurance in hospitals: Strategies for assessment and implementation* (2nd ed.). Rockville, MD: Aspen Publishers.

Brook, R.H., Park, R.E., & Chassin, M.R. (1990). Predicting the appropriate use of carotid endarterectomy, upper gastrointestinal endoscopy, and coronary angiography. *New England Journal of Medicine, 323*, 1173–1177.

Buchmueller, T.C., & Valletta, R.G. (1996). The effects of employer-provided health insurance on worker mobility. *Industrial and Labor Relations Review, 49*(3), 439–455.

Buchmueller, T.C., & Valletta, R.G. (1999). The effect of health insurance on married female labor supply. *Journal of Human Resources.*

Carlisle, D.M., Siu, A.L., Keeler, E.B., McGlynn, E.A., Kahn, K., Rubenstein, L.V., & Brook, R.H. (1992). HMO vs. fee-for-service care of older persons with acute myocardial infraction. *American Journal of Public Health, 82,* 1626–1630.

Chassin, M.R., Kosecoff, J., Solomon, D.H., & Brook, R.H. (1987). How coronary angiography is used: Clinical determinants of appropriateness. *Journal of the American Medical Association, 258*, 2543–2547.

Chima, R.I., & Mills, A. (1999). Estimating the economic impact of malaria in sub-Saharan Africa: A review of the empirical evidence. *World Health Organization Bulletin.*

Collins, D.H., Quick, J.D., Musau, S.N., & Kraushaar, D.L. (1995). Health financing reform in Kenya: The fall and rise of cost-sharing, 1989–1994. *Management Sciences for Health.*

Cooper, P.F., & Monheit, A.C. (1993). Does employment-related health insurance inhibit job mobility? *Inquiry, 30*(4), 400–416.

Creese, A.L. (1991). User charges for health care: a review of recent experience. *Health Policy and Planning, 6*(4), 309–319.

Croft, R.A., & Croft, R.P. (1998). Expenditure and loss of income incurred by tuberculosis patients before reaching effective treatment in Bangladesh. *International Journal of Tuberculosis and Lung Disease, 2*(3), 252–254.

Cuddington, J.T. (1991). *Modelling the macroeconomic effects of AIDS with an application to Tanzania* (Working paper No. 91–17). Washington, DC: Georgetown University, Department of Economics.

Cuddington, J.T., & Hancock, J.D. (1992). *Assessing the impact of AIDS on the growth path of the Malawian economy* (Working paper No. 92–07). Washington, DC: Georgetown University, Department of Economics.

Currie, J., & Madrian, B.C. (1999). Health, health insurance and the labor market. In O. Ashenfelter & D. Card (Eds.). *Handbook of labor economics,* Volume 3 (pp. 3309–3416). NY: Elsevier Science Publishing Company.

Cutler, D.M., & Richardson, E. (1998). The value of health: 1970–1990. *American Economic Review, 88,* 97–100.

Deaton, A. (1999). Inequalities in income and inequalities in health. National Bureau of Economic Research Working paper Series No. 7141: 1–37.

Deaton, A., & Paxson, C. (1999). Mortality, education, income and inequality among American cohorts. National Bureau of Economic Research Working Paper Series, No. 7140: 1–49.

De Bethune, X., Alfani, S., & Lahaye, J.P. (1989). The influence of an abrupt price increase on health service utilization: evidence from Zaire. *Health Policy and Planning, 4,* 76–81.

De Ferranti, D. (1985). *Paying for health services in developing countries: An overview* (Staff Working Paper 721). Washington, DC: World Bank.

Deolalikar, A.B. (1988). Nutrition and labor productivity in agriculture: Estimates for rural south India. *Review of Economics and Statistics, 70*(3), 406–413.

Dholakia, R.H., & Almeida, J. (1997). The potential economic benefits of the DOTS strategy against TB in India. *The Global TB Programme of the World Health Organization,* Research and Surveillance Unit, World Health Organization, Geneva, Switzerland.

Dow, W.H., Gertler, P., Strauss, J., & Thomas, D. (1997). *Health care prices, health and labor outcomes: Experimental evidence.* Unpublished paper. Santa Monica, CA: RAND.

Dwyer, D.S., & Mitchell, O.S. (1999). Health problems as determinants of retirement: Are self-rated measures endogenous? *Journal of Health Economics, 18,* 173–193.

Easterlin, R.A. (1998). *How beneficent is the market? A look at the modern history of mortality.* Unpublished paper. Los Angeles: University of Southern California.

Enthoven, A. (2000). In pursuit of an improving National Health Service. *Health Affairs, 19,* 102–119.

Ettner, S., Frank, R., & Kessler, R. (1997). The impact of psychiatric disorders on labor market outcomes. *Industrial and Labor Relations Review, 51*(1), 64–81.

Fabricant, S.J., Kamara, C.W., and Mills, A. (1999). Why the poor pay more: Household curative expenditures in rural Sierra Leone. *International Journal of Health Planning and Management 14*(3): 179–199.

Farrell, P., & Fuchs, V. (1982). Schooling and health: The cigarette connection. *Journal of Health Economics, 1,* 217–230.

Feachem, R.G.A. (2000). The future of NHS: Confronting the big questions. *Health Affairs, 19,* 128–129.

Federal Reserve Bank of San Francisco. (1998). *Economic Letter* (No. 98–12). San Francisco: Author.

Flynn, J.R. (1998). In U. Neisser (ed.), *The rising curve: long-term gains in IQ and related measures.* (pp. 25–66). Washington, DC: The American Psychological Association.

Fogel, R.W. (1994). Economic growth, population theory and physiology: The bearing of long term processes on the making of economic policy. *American Economic Review, 84*(3), 369–395.

Fogel, R.W. (1997). New findings on secular trends in nutrition and mortality: some implications for population theory. In M.R. Rosenzweig & O. Stark (Eds.), *Hand-*

book of population and family economics (Vol. 1A, pp. 433–481). Amsterdam: Elsevier Science.

Frankenberg, E., Beegle, K., Thomas, D., & Suriastini, W. (1999). Health, education, and the economic crisis in Indonesia. Paper presented at the 1999 Population Association of America meeting.

Fuchs, V.R. (1993). *The future of health policy.* Cambridge, MA: Harvard University Press.

Gallup, J.L., & Sachs, J. (1998). The economic burden of malaria. Center for International Development at Harvard: Cambridge, MA.

Gallup, J.L., & Sachs, J. (with Mellinger, A.D.). (1999). Geography and economic development. Consulting Assistance on Economic Return, Discussion Paper No. 39. Harvard Institute for International Development: Cambridge, MA.

Gardner, G.W., Edgerton, V.R., Senewiratne, B., Barnard, J.R., & Ohira, Y. (1975). Physical work capacity and metabolic stress in subjects with iron deficiency anemia. *American Journal of Clinical Nutrition, 30,* 910–917.

Gauthier, A.K., Rogal, D.L., Barrand, N.K., & Cohen, A.B. (1992). Administrative costs in the U.S. health care system: The problem or the solution? *Inquiry, 29,* 308–320.

Gertler, P., & Sturm, R. (1997). Private health insurance and public expenditures in Jamaica. *Journal of Econometrics, 77,* 237–257.

Gertler, P., & van der Gaag, J. (1988). *Measuring the willingness to pay for social service in developing countries.* Washington, DC: World Bank.

Gertler, P., & van der Gaag, J. (1990). *The willingness to pay for medical care.* Baltimore: Johns Hopkins Press.

Grossman, M. (1975). The correlation between health and schooling. In N.E. Terleckyj (Ed.), *Household production and consumption.* New York: National Bureau of Economic Research, Columbia University Press.

Gruber, J., & Hanratty, M. (1993). The labor market effects of introducing national health insurance: Evidence from Canada. *Working Paper Series* (Working Paper No. 4589). National Bureau of Economic Research.

Gruber, J., & Madrian, B.C. (1994). Health insurance and job mobility: the effects of public policy on job-lock. *Industrial and Labor Relations Review, 48*(1), 86–102.

Gruber, J., & Madrian, B.C. (1995). Health insurance availability and the retirement decision. *American Economic Review, 85*(4), 938–948.

Handa, S., & Neitzert, M. (1998). *Chronic illness and retirement in Jamaica.* (Living Standards Measurement Study, Working Paper No. 131). Washington, DC: The World Bank.

Hanratty, M. (1996). Canadian national health insurance and infant health. *American Economic Review, 86*(91): 276–284.

Hilborne, L.H., Leape, L.L., Bernstein, S.J., Park, R.E., Fiske, M.E., Kamberg, C.J., Roth, C.P., & Brook, R.H.

(1993). The appropriateness of use of percutaneous transluminal coronary angioplasty in New York state. *Journal of the American Medical Association, 269,* 761–765.

Holtz-Eakin, D. (1994). Health insurance provision and labor market efficiency in the United States and Germany. In R.M. Blank (Ed.), *Social protection versus economic flexibility* (pp. 157–88). Chicago: University of Chicago Press.

Hsiao, W. (2000). What should macroeconomists know about health care policy? A primer. IMF working paper. Washington, DC: International Monetary Fund.

Hurst, J. (2000). Challenges for health systems in member countries of the Organisation for Economic Co-operation and Development. *Bulletin of the World Health Organization, 78,* 751–760.

Jamison, D.T., Lau, L.J., & Wang, J. (1998). Health's contribution to economic growth, 1965–1990. In Health, Health Policy and Economic Outcomes. Final Report of the Health and Development Satellite WHO Director. Geneva, Switzerland.

Jamison, D.T., & Leslie, J. (1990). Health and nutrition considerations in education planning. 2. The cost and effectiveness of school-based interventions. *Food and Nutrition Bulletin, 12*(3).

Jamison, D.T., Sandbu, M., & Wang, J. (1999). Geography, technical progress and country performance in reducing infant mortality. Presented at the International Health Economics Conference, Rotterdam, June 1999, and subsequently revised.

Kenkel, D.S. (1991). Health behavior, health knowledge, and schooling, *Journal of Political Economy, 99,* 287–304.

Kim, A., & Benton, B. (1995). *Cost-benefit analysis of the onchocerciasis control program (OCP)* (Series on river blindness control in West Africa, World Bank Technical Paper Number 282). Washington, DC: World Bank.

Kleinman, L.C., Kosecoff, J., Dubois, R.W., & Brook, R.H. (1994). The medical appropriateness of tympanostomy tubes proposed for children younger than 16 years in the United States. *Journal of the American Medical Association, 271,* 50–55.

Knaul, F.M. (1999). The impact of health and health systems on economic growth and development: An overview. Geneva, Switzerland: World Health Organization.

Knaul, F.M. (1999, April). Linking health, nutrition and wages: the evolution of age at menarche and labor earnings among Mexican women. Working Paper Series R-355. Washington, DC: Inter-American Development Bank.

Knaul, F.M., & Parker, S.M. (1998). *Patterns over time and determinants of early labor force participation and school dropout: evidence from longitudinal and retrospective data on Mexican children and youth.* Paper presented at the meeting of the Population Association of America.

Kuh, D., & Ben-Shlomo, Y., eds. (1997). *A life course approach to chronic disease epidemiology.* Oxford: Oxford University Press.

Le Grand, J. (1987). "Inequalities in health: Some international comparisons." *European Economic Review, 31,* 182–191.

Leape, L.L., Hilborne, L.H., Park, R.E., Bernstein, S.J., Kamberg, C.J., Sherwood, M., & Brook, R.H. (1993). The appropriateness of use of coronary artery bypass graft surgery in New York state. *Journal of the American Medical Association, 269,* 753–760.

Leape, L., Park, R.E., Solomon, D.H., Chassin, M.R., Kosecoff, J., & Brook, R.H. (1990). Does inappropriate use explain small area variations in the use of health care services? *Journal of the American Medical Association, 263,* 669–672.

Leibenstein, H. (1957). *Economic backwardness and economic growth.* New York: Wiley.

Leighton, C., & Foster, R. (1993). *Economic impacts of malaria in Kenya and Nigeria* (Major Applied Research Paper No. 6. Bethesda, MD: Abt Associates.

Leslie, J., & Jamison, D.T. (1990, September). Health and nutrition considerations in education planning: educational consequences of health problems among school-age children. *Food and Nutrition Bulletin, 12,* 204–214.

Liu, Y., Hu, S., Fu, W., & Hsiao, W.C. (1998). Is community financing necessary and feasible for rural China? In M.L. Barer, T.E. Getzen, & G.L. Stoddart (Eds.), *Health, health care and health economics: Perspectives on distribution.* New York: John Wiley & Sons.

Madrian, B.C. (1994). Employment-based health insurance and job mobility: is there evidence of job-lock? *Quarterly Review of Economics, 109*(1), 27–54.

Malaney, P. (1998). Benefits of malaria control. Harvard Institute for International Development.

Marmot, M.G., Smith, G.D., Stansfeld, S., Patel, C., North, F., Head, L., White, I., Brummer, E., & Feeney, A. (1991). Health inequalities among British civil servants: the Whitehall II study. *Lancet, 337,*1387–1393.

Marmot, M.G., & Theorell, T. (1988). Social class and cardiovascular disease: The contribution of work. *International Journal of Health Services, 18,* 659.

Mirrlees, J. (1975). A pure theory of underdeveloped economies. In R. Reynolds (Ed.), *Agriculture in Development Theory.* New Haven, CT: Yale University Press.

Moffett, J.K., Torgerson, D., Bell-Syer, S., Jackson, D., Llewlyn-Phillips, H., Farrin, A., & Barker, J. (1999). Randomized controlled trial of exercise for low back pain: clinical outcomes, costs, and preferences. *British Medical Journal, 319,* 279–283.

Monheit, A.C., & Cooper, P.F. (1994). Health insurance and job mobility: Theory and evidence. *Industrial and Labor Relations Review, 48*(1).

Murray, C.J.L., Lopez, A.D., & Jamison, D.T. (1994). The global burden of disease in 1990: summary results, sensitivity analysis, and future directions. In C.J.L. Murray and A. Lopez (Eds.), *Global comparative assessments in the health sector: disease burden, expenditures, and intervention packages.* (pp. 97–138). Geneva: World Health Organization.

Murrugarra, E., & Valdivia, M. (1999). The returns to health for Peruvian urban adults: Differentials across genders, the life-cycle and the wage distribution. *Red de Centros de Investigacion de la Oficina del Economista Jefe Banco Interamericano de Desarrollo (BID)* (Documento de Trabaj o R-352).

Mwabu, G., & Wang'ombe, J. (1995). *User charges in Kenya: Health service pricing reforms in Kenya, 1989–1993.* A report on work in progress with support from the International Health Policy Program. Washington, DC: International Health Policy Program.

Myrdal, G. (1952). Economic aspects of health. *Chronicle of the World Health Organization, 6,* 203–218.

Newhouse, J.P. (1993). *Free for all? Lessons from the RAND health insurance experiment.* Cambridge, MA: Harvard University Press.

Over, M. (1992). *The macroeconomic impact of AIDS in sub-Saharan Africa.* (African Region/ Population and Nutrition Technical Working Paper, No. 3.). Washington, DC: The World Bank.

Over, M., Bertozzi, S., & Chin, J. (1989). Guidelines for rapid estimation of the direct and indirect costs of HIV infection in a developing country. *Health Policy, 11,* 169–186.

Poullier, J.-P. (1992). Administrative costs in selected industrialized countries. *Health Care Financing Review, 1*(4).

Preker, A.S., Harding, A., & Travis, P. (2000). "Make or Buy" decisions in the production of health care goods and services: New insights from institutional economics and organizational theory. *Bulletin of the World Health Organization, 78,* 779–790.

Prescott, N., & Pradhan, M. (1999, February). *Coping with catastrophic health shocks.* Revised draft prepared for the Conference on Poverty and Social Protection, Inter-American Development Bank, Washington, DC.

Preston, S.A. (1980). Causes and consequences of mortality decline in less developed countries during the Twentieth Century. In R.A. Easterlin (Ed.), *Population and economic change in developing countries.* (pp. 289–360). Chicago: University of Chicago Press.

Preston, S.H., & Elo, I.T. (1995). Are educational differentials in adult mortality increasing in the United States? *Journal of Aging and Health, 7,* 476–496.

Radelet, S., Sachs, J.D., & Lee, J.-W. (1997). *Economic growth and transformation* (Development Discussion

Paper No. 609). Harvard Institute for International Development, Cambridge, MA.

Reddy, S., & Vandemoortele, J. (1996). *User financing of basic social services: A review of theoretical arguments and empirical evidence.* New York: Office of Evaluation, Policy and Planning, United Nations International Children's Emergency Fund (UNICEF).

Ribero, R., & Nunez, J. (1999). *Productivity of household investment in health. The case of Columbia.* (Inter-American Development Bank, Office of the Chief Economist, Latin American Research Network, Working Paper R-354.) Washington, DC.

Robins, L.N., & Regier, D.A. (1991). *Psychiatric disorders in America: The epidemiologic catchment area study.* New York: The Free Press.

Sahn, D.E., & Alderman, H. (1988). The effect of human capital on wages, on the determinants of labor supply in a developing country. *Journal of Development Economics, 29*(2), 157–183.

Saunderson, P.R. (1995). An economic evaluation of alternative programme designs for tuberculosis control in rural Uganda. *Social Science Medicine, 40*(9), 1203–1212.

Schieber, G., & Maeda, A. (1993). A curmudgeon's guide to financing health care in developing countries. In G. Schieber (Ed.), *Innovations in health care financing.* Proceedings from a World Bank Conference, March 10–11, 1997.

Schultz, T.P. (1996). Wage rentals for reproducible human capital: Evidence from two west African countries. Yale University.

Schultz, T.P. (1997). Assessing the productive benefits of nutrition and health: An integrated human capital approach. *Journal of Econometrics, 77,* 144–158.

Schultz, T.P., & Tansel, A. (1997). Wage and labor supply effects of illness in Cote D'Ivoire and Ghana: Instrumental variable estimates for days disabled. *Journal of Development Economics, 53,* 251–286

Smith, J.P. (1999). Healthy bodies and thick wallets: The dual relation between health and economic status. *Journal of Economic Perspectives, 13*(2), 145–166.

Spurr, G.B. (1983). Nutritional status and physical work capacity. *Yearbook of physical anthropology,* 1–35.

Strauss, J., & and Thomas, D. (1995). Human resources: Empirical modeling of household and family decisions. In J. Behrman & T.N. Srinivasan (Eds.), *Handbook in development economics, Vol. 3A.* Amsterdam: Elsevier Science.

Svedberg, P. (2000). *Poverty and undernutrition.* Oxford: Oxford University Press.

Thomas, D., & Strauss, J. (1997). Health and wages: Evidence on men and women in urban Brazil. *Journal of Econometrics, 77,* 159–185.

Thomas, D., & Strauss, J. (1998, June). The micro-foundations of the links between health, nutrition, and development. *Journal of Economic Literature, 36,* 766–817.

U.S. Bureau of Labor Statistics. (1994). Employment Cost Indexes and Levels, 1975–94. Washington, DC: Author.

U.S. Congress. (1994). *International comparisons of administrative costs in health care.* (Office of Technology Assessment Publication No. BP-H-135) Washington, DC: U.S. Government Printing Office.

Van de Walle, D. (1994). The benefit-incidence of social sector public expenditures in Indonesia. *World Bank Economic Review, 8,* 115–134.

Van Doorslaer, E., Wagstaff, A., & Rutten, F. (1993). *Equity in the finance and delivery of health care: An international perspective.* Oxford, England: Oxford University Press.

Waddington, C., & Enyimayew, K. (1990). A price to pay, part 2: The impact of user charges in the Volta region of Ghana. *International Journal of Health Planning and Management, 5*(4), 287–312.

Wang, J., Jamison, D.J., Bos, E., Preker, A., & Peabody, J. (1999). Measuring country performance on health: Selected indicators for 115 countries. Washington, DC: The World Bank, Health, Nutrition, and Population Series.

Wang'ombe, J. (1997). Cost recovery strategies in sub-Saharan Africa. In G.J. Schieber (Ed.), *Innovations in health care financing: Proceedings of a World Bank conference, March 10–11, 1997* (World Bank Discussion Paper No. 365). Washington, DC: World Bank, 155–161.

Wilkinson, R.G. (Ed.). (1986). *Class and health: Research and longitudinal data.* New York: Tavistock Publications.

Wilkinson, R.G. (1990). Income distribution and mortality—A natural experiment. *Health and Illness, 12,* 391.

Wilkinson, D., Floyd, K., & Gilks, C.F. (1997). Costs and cost-effectiveness of alternative tuberculosis management strategies in South Africa—implications for policy. *South African Medical Journal, 87*(4), 451–455.

Winslow, C.M., Kosecoff, J.B., Chassin, M., Kanouse, D.E., & Brook, R.H. (1988a). The appropriateness of performing coronary artery bypass surgery. *Journal of the American Medical Association, 260,* 505–509.

Winslow, C.M., Solomon, D.H., Chassin, M.R., Kosecoff, J., Merrick, N.J., & Brook, R.H. (1988b). The appropriateness of carotid endarterectomy. *New England Journal of Medicine, 318,* 721–727.

Woolhandler, S., & Himmelstein, D.U. (1991). The deteriorating administrative efficiency of the U.S. health care system. *New England Journal of Medicine, 324*(18), 53–57.

Woolhandler, S., & Himmelstein, D.U. (1997). Costs of care and administration at for-profit and other hospitals in the United States. *New England Journal of Medicine, 336*(11), 769–774.

Woolhandler, S., Himmelstein, D.U., & Lewontin, J.P. (1993). Administrative costs in U.S. hospitals. *New England Journal of Medicine, 329*(6), 400–403.

World Bank. (1980). *World Bank Development Report.* Washington, DC: Author.

World Bank. (1993). *World Development Report 1993: Investing in Health.* New York: World Bank, & Oxford, England: Oxford University Press.

World Bank. (1999). *Health, Nutrition and Population Indicators: A Statistical Handbook.* Washington, DC: Author.

World Health Organization. (1999). *World Health Report 1999: Making a difference.* Geneva, Switzerland: Author.

World Health Organization. (2000), *World Health Report 2000.* Geneva, Switzerland: Author.

Yoder, R.A. (1989). Are people willing and able to pay for health services? *Social Science and Medicine, 29,* 35–42.

# CHAPTER 13

# Global Cooperation in International Public Health

*Gill Walt*

Why do countries cooperate in international health? This chapter explores this question, focusing on the cooperation process, the institutions and actors involved in international health cooperation, how they have changed over the past 50 years, and what implications these factors may have for future health policies around the world. A policy approach provides the theoretical framework, drawing on a number of different disciplines and focusing on the interaction among context, actors, and processes (Walt & Gilson, 1994). The chapter suggests that there has been a shift in international cooperation from *vertical representation* to *horizontal participation*. Vertical representation describes the relationship between the state and international organizations that make up the United Nations (UN) system, which was established in the mid-1940s to represent the interests of all states and promote cooperation between them. By the end of the century, international cooperation was determined less by formal vertical representation between the state and international organizations than by horizontal partnerships between many different bodies, including the state, UN agencies, industry, and nongovernmental organizations.

The chapter starts by describing briefly its analytical framework, which puts the state at the center of analysis. It goes on to describe the actors (including the state) in international health, to ask why states cooperate, and through what mechanisms. The second half of the chap-

ter analyzes the shifts in international cooperation, demonstrating how vertical representation has been replaced by horizontal participation, and what the implications of these shifts are for international health policy.

## THE POLICY FRAMEWORK

Many of the earlier chapters in this book have focused on the *content* of policy: current problems in communicable diseases (increasing rates of sexually transmitted diseases) or nutrition (lack of vitamin A leading to blindness), and what sorts of policies are employed to address these problems (training primary health workers to recognize the signs and symptoms of sexually transmitted infections, or introducing vitamin A into routine immunization programs). Some of the chapters also explore how health systems have been designed and managed to put these policies into practice, by emphasising primary health care (PHC) systems, or decentralization. This chapter provides an understanding of international health policy, by focusing on the role of *actors*, and how they are affected by, and influence, the *context* and *processes* within which policies are made and implemented.

*Actors* may be individuals (a minister of health), or groups (the National Association of Nurses), but institutions (a university or the World Bank) and even states (the United States) also are considered actors. Although actors may be involved in national or global policy, it should not be assumed that all groups, institutions, or states act with one voice, or that there are not quite different, and sometimes contending, groups of actors within institutions. The World Bank, for example, acts according to a particular mission, but is made up of individuals who do not necessarily agree with each other, or with the Bank's policy on a particular issue. The extent to which there is space to address differences, how big those differences are, and how they emerge, will influence both staff attitudes to work, and outputs from the institution. In other words, actors all have their own values and expectations, and these may not always be shared, or reflect exactly those of the institutions within which they work.

Because actors are the center of analysis in this chapter, it is helpful to differentiate ways of referring to them. Individuals can be all important, but alone are not likely to be very effective. Their influence comes because they lead social movements (bring people together, usually in protest or to promote a particular cause) or are key members of institutions. It was the combination of James Grant, as executive director between 1980–1995 and the institution, United Nations Children's Fund (UNICEF), that gave the organization its high profile and successful reputation in the 1980s. So, understanding institutions and their roles within international health is central. Institutions naturally differ in their reputations: some are strong, with high levels of influence because of their wealth, knowledge, research, professional expertise, and contribution to the economy. Such institutions (and individuals within them) are likely to have considerable access to other influential individuals in key government departments, corporations, academic institutions, and so on, and be able to influence ideas and policies. However, reputations are not set in stone, and institutions have to adapt and change with time. As will be shown later, one of the struggles that beset the World Health Organization (WHO) in the 1980s and 1990s was to retain its earlier authority and high regard.

In this chapter, then, actors are referred to as individuals, institutions such as UNICEF or WHO at the global level, but ministries of health (MOHs) at the national level, or, more broadly, governments or states also may be actors. The state is an abstract notion, but generally refers to a society within geographical borders. It is made up of all the authoritative decision-making bodies of the society, is legally supreme, and can use force to achieve its ends. The state's lawmaking occurs through government, a narrower concept, which includes the public institutions, such as parliament, the executive, the bureaucracy, and ministries or departments of state. The judiciary, which is part of government, is responsible for interpreting and applying the law. All governments are organized into different levels, and subnational bodies or local authorities may also be referred to as actors. There is a lively contemporary debate about the role of the state, and how trends in globalization are affecting it and reducing its role. However, in this chapter, the state is assumed to be a central player in international health cooperation, although, as will be shown, its role is changing.

*Context* refers to a myriad of external factors that affect the way policy is formulated and implemented. Political and economic instability in a country or region may mean that domestic policymakers are prepared to make only short-term, or incremental, changes to policy for fear of losing power; it may mean that internationally agreed upon policies on immunization campaigns, for example, cannot be executed. A newly elected government may have the legitimacy to introduce major change, as happened in South Africa in 1994 when free health services were introduced for all children under the age of 6 years. Similarly, a new leader in a UN agency may have added legitimacy to initiate new policies; for example, in 1998, after years of taking a very cautious approach on tobacco and its harmful effects on health, a high level campaign advocating tobacco control was initiated by a new director general in WHO. Multi-ethnicity, linguistic plurality, and the position of women all influence policy at both national and international levels: for example, people may not have the same trust or confidence in a health professional, a scientist, or a consultant from another ethnic or national group, or who does not speak their language. Contextual factors may be specific to particular countries, or common globally (as with world economic recessions, for example).

The *process of policymaking* will be influenced by the history and role of the different institutions of government. Policy processes can be described in different phases: how issues get on to the policy agenda (is there a role for the media?); who is consulted in the formulation and design of policy (are policies made by a handful of bureaucrats or politicians, or are they discussed with managers and interest groups, such as patients or consumers?); and how policies are communicated, executed, regulated, and assessed (is policymaking top down? are policies monitored?). Similar questions affect policy processes at the global level: do industrialized countries dominate international organizations, and decide how and where resources should be allocated?

## WHO ARE THE ACTORS IN INTERNATIONAL HEALTH?

The UN system established at the end of the World War II "to save succeeding generations from the scourge of war" (Childers & Urquhart, 1994, p.11) was conceived as a system to maintain peace and security in a world that had been torn by strife. At its center was the sovereign nation state, which could become a member of the different organs and agencies of the UN. The six principal UN organs, established by Charter in 1945, are the General Assembly, the Security Council, the Secretariat, the International Court of Justice, the Trusteeship Council, and the Economic and Social Council (ECOSOC). This last body is entrusted to supervise the work of numerous economic and social commissions and to coordinate the efforts of the specialized agencies associated with the UN. The four largest specialized agencies are the Food and Agricul-

ture Organization (FAO), the International Labor Organization (ILO), the UN Educational Scientific and Cultural Organization (UNESCO), and WHO.

The international organizations that made up the UN were established to facilitate exchange and contact between all member states and to coordinate development assistance provided collectively by some nation states to others, who would use such aid in their exercise of national sovereignty. This was a system of formal, vertical representation, with member states deciding the policies and activities of the international organizations. However, being relatively independent and having their own constitutions, the specialized agencies were not easy to coordinate.

## Actors in Health at the Global and Regional Levels

Founded in 1948, WHO is the UN's designated specialized agency in health, expected to play a leading role in coordinating international health activities. It was formed from the amalgamation of two agencies established in 1902 and 1908, respectively: the International Sanitary Bureau, which evolved into the Pan American Health Organization (PAHO) and the Office of Public Hygiene, later incorporated into the League of Nations. With headquarters in Geneva, WHO boasts an unusually decentralized structure of six regional offices plus country offices in some countries. PAHO, representing the Americas, became one of the six WHO regional offices.

Other organizations within the United Nations system also have some responsibilities in health. The more active of these are the first five in Exhibit 13–1, although some of the others, such as the World Trade Organization (WTO), may become increasingly important in the future.

Cooperation in health, however, has not been limited to collaboration through the UN and its agencies involved in health. Bilateral organizations such as the United Kingdom's (UK) Department for International Development (DFID),

**Exhibit 13–1** UN Health-Related Organizations

- World Health Organization (WHO)
- World Bank
- UN Children's Fund (UNICEF)
- UN Population Fund (UNFPA)
- UN Development Program (UNDP)
- UN Educational, Scientific and Cultural Organization (UNESCO)
- Food and Agriculture Organization (FAO)
- World Food Program
- UN High Commissioner for Refugees (UNHCR)
- International Labor Organization
- UN Environment Program
- UN Fund for Drug Abuse Control
- World Trade Organization (WTO)

the Swedish International Development Agency (SIDA), or the United States Agency for International Development (USAID), among many others, have played important roles at international and regional levels, and in many countries. These agencies are often the main contributors to international health programs through UN organizations, but they also provide assistance to lower income countries through government-to-government agreements known as bilateral aid.

International nongovernmental organizations (NGOs)—increasingly referred to as civil society organizations (CSOs)—have also made critical contributions to health development at both the international and domestic level. See Exhibit 13–2 for a discussion on definitional issues. NGOs or CSOs make up a broad group of agencies of considerable complexity, but also include church missions providing health care to isolated rural communities; agencies such as Oxfam, which may be involved in advocacy on behalf of lower income countries (for example, on debt relief) or may be working with local groups (AIDS support groups, for example); and private foundations, such as Rockefeller and Ford, which support international health programs in many different ways. Although the private sector has played only a limited role in international health over the past few years, its role is changing rapidly. Today there are increasing collaborations between public and private sectors in health, as seen, for example, in drug donation programs supported by the pharmaceutical industry.

### Linking Global and Regional Actors with Local Actors

All states take some responsibility for their own health and health services, although the resources they have available differ markedly. On average, public expenditure on health in the higher income countries is 6.9% of gross domestic product (GDP), while in the low-income countries it is 0.9% (World Bank, 1998–1999). Most resources for health are generated nationally, even in extremely low-income countries, which may also receive some aid from multilateral, bilateral, or NGOs.

While states are responsible for health policy within their own borders, they send representatives to participate in global policy discussions about health at the international level. For example, most states in the world are members of WHO. Every year they send a delegation, usually the minister of health and some officials from the health ministry, to attend the World Health Assembly (WHA) held at WHO's headquarters in Geneva. It is at the WHA that international policies on health are discussed, and ministers of health commit to programs and measures they will introduce or support when they return home. Membership in WHO entitles each state to vote on an equal basis, although membership contributions are based on population size and wealth. Even though there may be considerable consensus on policies decided at the WHA, all states are sovereign, and if they do not adhere to, or implement, recommendations agreed to at the international level, there is little that WHO can do. Its only sanctions are based on its authority and reputation.

States may serve on the boards of governors of other UN agencies, such as UNICEF or the United Nations Population Fund (UNFPA). Both

**Exhibit 13–2** What Is an NGO?

There is such a broad spectrum of NGOs that it is difficult to define them. Clark (1991) divided NGOs into six categories, reflecting their historical evolution:

1. Relief and welfare agencies, including missionary societies, providing services routinely and in emergencies
2. Technical innovation organizations, which promote new or improved approaches to problems
3. Public service contractors, which are contracted by government aid agencies to perform particular activities, such as food aid
4. Popular development agencies, which are northern NGOs and their southern counterparts and focus on self-help and social development
5. Grassroots development organizations, which are locally based, southern NGOs and may or may not receive funding from popular development agencies
6. Advocacy groups and networks, which do not necessarily have field projects, but exist primarily to educate and lobby

NGOs are often called civil society organizations (CSOs), although the latter term includes a large number of organizations not normally referred to as NGOs. Civil society refers to the sphere of interaction between the state and the household, and includes all types of organizations that are not government institutions, political parties, or individual households. CSOs, therefore, include private for-profit organizations (trade and commerce associations, for example, including multinational corporations); religious bodies; interest groups formed to promote a cause (divorce law reform) or to protect the interests of members (trade unions); and consumer, leisure, or community groups, among others. Distinguishing between NGOs and CSOs is important because the policy and power implications are different. The shift in focus from NGOs to CSOs came in the late 1980s, as ideas in development turned from service provision and program implementation through NGOs to building democratic societies through supporting civic groups with more political roles. As Van Rooy (1998, p. 35) says, "Rightly or wrongly, NGOs are often described in service-delivery roles, whereas CSOs are depicted as political agents." Although this distinction is not entirely satisfactory because both types of organizations may play multiple roles, the term NGO is used in this chapter to refer to those groups, community-based, national, or international, involved in health activities that may include lobbying, advocacy, or service delivery.

of these organizations are funds (which rely on voluntary contributions from states rather than assessed contributions, as in the case of WHO). The membership of their governing bodies changes, to allow changing country representation. States may also apply for membership in the international financial institutions (IFIs), such as the World Bank and International Monetary Fund, where membership is subject to financial subscription and other economic criteria, and voting weighted according to the number of shares held by each member. UNICEF has long supported health activities, often as a partner of WHO, and, especially at the country level, has assisted with such programs as immunization and distribution of drugs and other medical supplies. UNFPA has been a strong promoter of family planning and reproductive health programs, and in the 1990s the World Bank entered the health arena as a major financer of health programs.

States also relate to regional bodies such as the six offices of WHO, participating as members in decision making: for example, the Eastern Mediterranean Regional Office (EMRO) or the Western Pacific Regional Office (WPRO) will hold many meetings for countries in their regions, and will have considerable power and autonomy to decide policy for the region. States may also be involved in other regional bodies that have a strong economic or political focus (or both) and may or may not include health in their jurisdictions. Examples are the European Union (EU), for countries in Europe; the Organization for Economic Cooperation and Development (OECD), which includes not only all the industrialized nations, but also Turkey and Thailand, among others; the Association of Southeast Asian Nations (ASEAN); and the Southern African Development Coordination Conference (SADCC). All these organizations may provide guidance on a broad set of health-related issues, which may be binding on member states, although adherence to policies will depend on the authority and consensus on which they are based. See Exhibit 13–3 on cross-border health care in Europe, which shows the growing impact of the EU on health care in the region, and the concerns raised by governments about its implications.

While the relationship among the state, UN organizations (often called multilateral organizations), and regional bodies such as those above is important, bilateral agencies have had the potential to play a more central role in health insofar as financial resources confer power. Bilateral aid—through agreements made government to government—is more influential than multilateral aid (through the UN system). In 1996 the former provided about US$55 billion net disbursements, the latter roughly US$5 billion. Tanzania's total bilateral aid in 1988 came to US$782 million, whereas total multilateral aid received was US$196 million (Ampiah, 1996). Bilateral organizations favor some states over others, often based on historical or colonial ties and geopolitical or trade considerations. For example, until the 1990s most of Japan's aid went to countries in Southeast Asia, and 25% of the United States's aid to two countries: Israel and Egypt.

Both multilateral and bilateral agencies are often referred to as "donors" because of their roles in providing low- and middle-income countries with resources for health development— through grants, loans, or technical assistance.

Bilateral donors, in particular, play complex, multifaceted roles because they are also members of multilateral organizations, with a strong representative voice in formulating and developing policy. They provide funds directly to countries through bilateral agreements or through multilateral organizations (either through their own contributions, as members, to the regular budget, or through voluntary contributions, known as extrabudgetary funds, for particular activities). They also provide funds to NGOs for activities in low- or middle-income countries, to academic institutions for research, or to various special partnerships established to tackle particular problems, such as the AIDS Vaccine Initiative (see Exhibit 13–4) or the WHO-led Rollback Malaria Campaign.

Besides providing residence to multilateral and bilateral agencies, states also are often host to a myriad of NGOs. These NGOs may be indigenous (some of which may receive funds from organizations outside the country, such as bilateral agencies or other NGOs) or international, dispersing services themselves, employing nationals to undertake activities, or funding and supporting national groups in a variety of services and activities. International NGOs may themselves be funded by their own governments, and, when they are highly dependent on this source, may be perceived as an arm of bilateral aid. Because autonomy and independence are among the features most NGOs prize, some employ a policy of accepting only a certain proportion of their funds from their own governments.

Although there are often tensions between the state and NGOs, in many countries there is a history of considerable cooperation between them, with NGOs providing vital health services on behalf of unwilling or unable governments. Figure 13–1 illustrates the complexity of vertical representation in international health relationships between international, regional, and country levels (see also Basch, 1999; Koivusalo & Ollila, 1997).

Table 13–1, taken from a study of WHO's support to countries, demonstrates the different organizations in the health sector present at the

**Exhibit 13–3** European Court Rulings Have Made Governments Worried

" . . . Meanwhile the impact of European Union legislation continues to grow, from the 48 hour working time directive to the directive enshrining mutual recognition of professional qualifications which is spurring harmonization of professional training.

Healthcare shopping in the union may not yet be commonplace, but last year's landmark European Court rulings coupled with the price transparency that the Euro will bring will give it a boost. On the face of it the rulings were not exciting. In the first a man was given a prescription for spectacles in Luxembourg, bought them in Belgium, and when his insurance fund failed to reimburse him, took his case to the European court and won. The court upheld the view that refusing reimbursement violated the Treaty of Rome on free movement of goods. In the second, when a Luxembourg man tried to get orthodontic treatment for his daughter in Germany, he was refused on the grounds that it was not urgent and appropriate treatment was available in Luxembourg. He disputed this, took his case to the European Court, and won. The Court ruled that economic issues cannot justify obstructing the free movement of services.

Until these rulings reimbursement for reciprocal medical care between member states has hinged on individuals having to get prior authorization from their health authority or insurance fund. By doing away with this requirement in the interests of the single market these rulings have potentially opened the door to cross border healthcare shopping and put national health services under the scrutiny of Europe's consumer orientated citizens. The growing recognition that services or goods are cheaper or more readily available and reimbursable in some member states but not others is bound to provoke debate. In states where rationing is explicit and widespread, governments are likely to face growing dissatisfaction among their electorate.

Unsurprisingly several governments have been alarmed—and their fears are not misplaced. Because of differences in the perceived quality of health services patients may want to obtain treatment in another member state. The same may happen because of capacity shortages or rationing in patients' own countries. In this case, local payers will have to reimburse patients who travel abroad to circumvent this problem. Patients may also want to receive treatment in another country if it is cheaper there and they have to pay for it themselves (because it is not reimbursed under national systems). . . ."

country level in a few selected low- and middle-income countries. The table lists 12 of the most important donors to the health sector in terms of financial assistance and influence, or both, and, therefore, does not include all donors.

What this description, figure, and table suggest is that the state, as an actor, is entangled in a complexity of relationships with many different organizations at international, regional, and national levels, and that all these organizations are themselves linked to each other. But considering the state an actor, while a useful shorthand, is itself an abstraction. The state is made up of various institutions; each of those institutions can be further disaggregated into sectoral ministries, with divisions and depart-

ments at both national and subnational levels, and smaller institutions, such as hospitals, laboratories, training schools, and clinics. All of these smaller institutions are staffed by individual professionals, civil servants, politicians, technicians, managers, administrators, and others, who form networks across institutions and across borders. These networks constitute policy communities, which form the heart of policy making at national and international levels. Some of the questions explored in this chapter are as follows. What motivates these relationships? Are these policy networks largely pursuing their own self-interests? Are they disguising a complex power game in which the strong are imposing their interests on the weak?

**Exhibit 13–4** The International AIDS Vaccine Initiative (1996)

In 1998 the UK Minister for International Development said that if we leave the development of a vaccine to market forces, the strains that are killing people in Africa will not be tackled. In order to help in the development of a vaccine against AIDS, a number of donors established the International AIDS Vaccine Initiative in 1996 to ensure the development of safe, effective, accessible, preventive HIV vaccines for use throughout the world. The initiative is funded by a number of large foundations, private sector companies (including Glaxo Wellcome and Levi Strauss), the United Nations Acquired Immune Deficiency Syndrome Programme, the World Bank, and the UK's Department for International Development. In 1999 the Gates Foundation made a donation of $20 million to the initiative. Partnership is required because a single efficacy trial costs US$25 million, and product development costs up to US$250 million.

In a 1999 article titled "Bank Woos AIDS Drug Firms" the UK newspaper *The Guardian* reported that the Bank was exploring ways to end industry's reluctance to invest in vaccines for AIDS in developing countries, by guaranteeing that there would be funds to buy such vaccines, once developed. "Our message is that if a vaccine can be developed, there will be the money to buy it."

## WHY DO STATES COOPERATE?

Cooperation in health has a long history. Between 1851 and 1909, 10 international meetings were held to discuss quarantine and other measures to deal with epidemics of plague and cholera. Although most of these early meetings were ad hoc and largely limited to epidemic intelligence gathering between scientists or professionals, they led to international agreements on common approaches for the control and treatment of infectious diseases. After two world wars in the first half of the twentieth century, such cooperation expanded. The Marshall European Recovery Program of 1948–1952, in which the United States gave $13 billion to rebuild the economies of Western Europe (Basch, 1999), introduced an era of extensive global aid for many development activities, including support for health services in low-income countries.

The latter half of the twentieth century witnessed an increase in trade, travel, and improved communication, some of the factors commonly assumed to have led to the globalization of the world economy. These factors have highlighted risks that states by themselves cannot address adequately within traditional national borders. Such risks include new and emerging infectious diseases, resulting in part from the increased prevalence of drug-resistant pathogens, exposure to dangerous substances, such as contaminated foodstuffs, or banned and toxic substances; environmental exploitation, leading to pollution and such conditions as increased respiratory disorders; and violence, resulting from the huge production and sales of arms as well as chemical and biological weapons.

Although most of the direct health problems are addressed by domestic health policies decided at the national level, some depend on international collaboration. No one state can, by itself, resolve the risks and problems detailed above. Recognizing this concern, many scholars have attempted to identify *international public goods*, defined as activities countries introduce in collaboration with others, for which national action on its own is ineffective or impossible to organize or encourage. Benefits from an international public good accrue widely, and not just to the entity that pays for it. Many international meetings are held to try to reach agreement among countries on norms and standards regarding pollution levels, the trafficking of illegal drugs, nuclear tests, and other policies from which all will benefit.

However, although states may recognize the benefits of promoting international public goods, cooperation is not always easy to achieve because of conflicting interests. Bad behavior in one country that affects its innocent neighbors

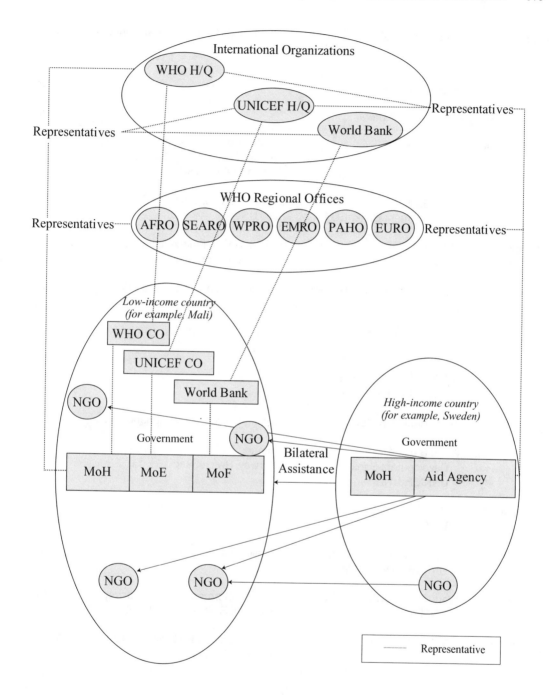

**Figure 13–1** Vertical Representation: International-, Regional-, and Country-level Interrelationships. *Note:* Afro, African Regional Office; CO, country office: EMRO, Eastern Mediterranean Regional Office; EURO, European Regional Office; H/Q, headquarters; MoE, Ministry of Education; MoF, Ministry of Finance; MoH, Ministry of Health; PAHO, Pan American Health Organization; SEARO, South East Asia Regional Office; WPRO, Western Pacific Regional Office.

**Table 13–1** The Most Influential External Donors in the Health Sector in 12 Selected Countries, 1997

| Countries | External Donors Multilateral | Bilateral | ODA[a] as a percentage of GNP |
|---|---|---|---|
| Bangladesh | World Bank, EU | Australia, Belgium, Canada, Germany, Netherlands, Norway, Sweden, UK, United States (US) | 5% |
| Cambodia | World Bank, Asian Development Bank, EU | Australia, France, Germany, Japan, UK, US | 27% |
| Cameroon | UNICEF, UNFPA, World Bank, EU | Belgium, China, France, Germany, Italy, Care International[b] | 6% |
| Ecuador | World Bank, UNICEF, UNFPA, EU, WHO | Belgium, France, Japan, Netherlands | 2% |
| Ethiopia | UNICEF, UNDP, UNFPA, WHO | Italy, Japan, Netherlands, Germany, Sweden | 23% |
| Haiti | UNICEF, UNFPA, World Bank, UNDP, EU, FAO, IDB[c], WHO | US, Canada | 5% |
| Mali | World Bank, UNICEF | Belgium, Germany, Switzerland, US | 13% |
| Mozambique | World Bank, African Development Bank, EU, UNICEF, UNDP | Denmark, Finland, Netherlands, Norway, Switzerland | 85%[d] |
| Nicaragua | UNICEF, EU, World Bank, WHO | Denmark, Finland, Germany | 24% |
| Papua New Guinea | Asian Development Bank, UNICEF, UNFPA, WHO | Australia, Japan | 8% |
| Tanzania | World Bank, UNICEF, UNDP, UNFPA | Denmark, Germany, Japan, Norway, Sweden, Switzerland, UK, US | 39% |
| Thailand | UNICEF, UNDP, UNFPA | Australia, Denmark, Germany, Japan, Sweden, Redd Barna[b] | 1% |

[a]Official development assistance (ODA) represents external resources from multilateral and bilateral sources.
[b]Cameroon and Thailand were the only countries where an NGO was named as one of the 10 most important donors to the health sector.
[c]IDB, Inter-American Development Bank.
[d]In 1997 Mozambique was recovering from war and was highly dependent on external funds.

may demand interventions that are difficult to implement. For example, excessive and indiscriminate use of antibiotics in both industrialized and low-income countries has created drug resistance, making it more difficult to treat some diseases. Concerted action is needed to combat resistance, but is complex, given that it means changing the behavior of patients who do not complete their antibiotic prescriptions or doctors who overprescribe antibiotics, or controlling and regulating the production or importation of high quality antibiotics. Similarly, getting cooperation on issues such as controlling pollution or activities that may lead to global warming are also highly problematic, as was demonstrated in Southeast Asia in 1997. The combination of unfavorable winds, drought, and forest fires in Indonesia in 1997 led to a "poison fog blanket" and an increase in respiratory disorders in several Asian neighbors, who called for closer cooperation to control pollution in the area. However, while the situation was partly due to climatic conditions, it was exacerbated by the activities of private companies clearing forests in Indonesia to provide paper and palm oil. Indonesian government policies that had promoted privatization, but employed weak regulatory controls over private sector actions, created negative externalities.

Even where there is consensus about the value of international public goods produced through international cooperation (cooperation on research to find an AIDS vaccine, for example, or campaigning to eradicate smallpox from the world), achieving international goals can be difficult, and gains may be visible only in the long run. For example, although polio is not a priority disease in many extremely low-income countries where respiratory infections, malaria, and diarrheal diseases are responsible for most mortality among children, most countries in the world are committed to the polio eradication program in the hope that future generations will save money on polio vaccines, as well as be rid of a disabling disease. When very low-income countries have been doubtful about devoting scarce resources for polio, they have been per-

suaded by protagonists, who have also provided considerable resources to help meet eradication goals. But until the disease is completely eradicated, and there is no danger that it will be reimported, all countries have to continue to immunize their children against polio. The United States, for example, has been free of the disease for 20 years, but still immunizes against polio; it will save about US$230 million annually when polio is finally eradicated globally.

States may also decide to act collectively at the international level because of the shortcomings or lack of resources in particular national health systems. Development aid, for example, aims to build and strengthen capacity in low-income countries, through technical assistance, grants, or loans. As Howson, Fineberg, and Bloom (1998, p. 586) point out, such engagement has as much relevance for high-income, industrialized countries as for low-income countries: "All developed countries have a vital and direct stake in the health of people around the world; this stake derives both from enduring traditions of humanitarian concern and from compelling reasons of enlightened self-interest. Considered involvement can serve to protect citizens, improve indigenous economies, and advance national and regional interests on the world stage."

At the extreme, states may cooperate with others because of the threat of force. This scenario is unlikely in international health, but coercion may occur in some situations. Greenough (1995) argues, for example, that at the end of the smallpox campaign in India and Bangladesh, some force was exerted on families who were reluctant (for religious reasons, for example) to have their children vaccinated. Coercion has also sometimes been used in contemporary tuberculosis (and AIDS) programs (see Exhibit 13–5). Some have suggested that the use of policy conditions attached to World Bank loans—forcing countries to introduce changes such as reducing the number of public sector health workers, introducing charges for health services, or privatizing some health services—is a type of coercion.

Most relations in health are not directly coercive, although states may have little room to maneuver because of pressure from international organizations, the media, or neighboring states. In investigating the use of policy conditions in structural adjustment programs, for example, Killick (1998, p. 11) distinguishes between "pro forma" and "hard core" conditionality. He argues that the former may well be voluntary, based on consensus, because the recipient essentially agrees with the range of measures suggested by the lender; or agreement may be based on the perceived authority of the international organization. Similarly, in conflict situations, where displaced persons have crossed borders, neighboring states may feel they have to make some response in spite of their own lack of resources or potential conflict with their own populations. Hard core conditionality, by contrast, consists of "measures that would not otherwise be undertaken or taken within the time frame desired by the lender" (Killick, 1998, p. 11) but that are accepted by recipients because they need the loans.

## HOW DO STATES COOPERATE?

States come together in many formal and informal ways that result in levels of cooperation. The UN may arrange large international meetings, attended by delegations or representatives from states, international organizations, NGOs,

private sector companies, and others. Specialized meetings may be held, such as the WHA, to which member states send representatives from MoHs, or World Bank meetings, attended by ministers of finance and national and international bankers. Or experts in a particular field may convene in small meetings. WHO, for example, uses expert committees of academics, professionals, and scientists, to decide norms and standards, such as what drugs should be included in an essential drugs list or whether hepatitis B vaccine should be included in routine infant immunization schedules. Activities in international health cooperation occur in three areas:

1. consensus building and advocacy
2. cross-learning and transfer of knowledge
3. production and sharing of international public goods (Lucas et al., 1997)

### Consensus Building and Advocacy

Many of the high-profile UN meetings that take place all over the world are exercises in building consensus on particular themes, with follow-up advocacy. UN conferences are usually agreed to by the General Assembly or the ECOSOC, and arranged outside the regular framework of the UN and its agencies, although they frequently involve inputs in the form of proposals and secretarial provision from those

---

**Exhibit 13–5** Public Health, Civil Liberties, and Tuberculosis

"The New York City epidemic of the late 1980s and early 1990s was halted and reversed through substantial investment, improvements in surveillance and infection control, and the expansion of systems to encourage treatment compliance. Coercion was also used. In 1993 a New York City health code was amended to authorize the City's commissioner of health to detain any non-infectious individual 'where there is substantial likelihood ... that he or she cannot be relied upon to participate in and/or to complete an appropriate prescribed course of medication for tuberculosis'. The authority to detain individuals was shifted from depending on an assessment of threat posed to an assessment of treatment compliance. This represented a significant shift in the balance between civil liberties and state authority. Since the amendments were adopted in New York more than 200 non-infectious patients have been detained, many for long periods, some for over two years. . . ." (Coker, 1999)

bodies (Taylor, 1993). They are highly formalized and orchestrated, with many groups holding preconference meetings to prepare background papers and recommendations. Originally, UN conferences were attended only by formal delegations representing governments, but over time they have opened to allow the participation of independent groups of NGOs, the media, and others.

In the 1990s, for example, meetings receiving a great deal of media attention were held in Rio de Janiero, Brazil, and Kobe, Japan (on the environment); in Copenhagen, Denmark (on social sector support); in Beijing, China (on women); and in Cairo, Egypt (on reproductive health). The 1994 meeting in Cairo, titled the International Conference on Population and Development, followed two earlier meetings in 1974 in Bucharest and 1984 in Mexico, and is an example of how consensus building, plus other activities, changed attitudes and approaches to population issues over 2 decades. As Exhibit 13–6 illustrates, in the 40 years of discussions on population growth, ideas changed considerably. In the 1950s and 1960s, discussion largely focused on regulating population growth through family planning programs and was highly contested, partly for religious reasons, and partly because of disagreement on the relationship between population growth and development. By the 1990s, family planning programs were universally accepted (with dispute only over the role of abortion), but the increased participation of women's groups in international discussions had broadened the emphasis from contraception to reproductive health. Over 4 decades considerable energy was expended on advocacy to change public opinion and the views of key policy makers, with Western donors exercising considerable influence on initially reluctant developing countries through policies such as generous funding of family planning programs.

## Cross-Learning and Transfer of Knowledge

Cooperation in health also occurs through exchange of experience and transfer of knowl-

edge. One of the great strengths of international organizations is that they can ignore political, geographical, or cultural barriers, and draw on "epistemic communities," networks of professionals with recognized expertise and competence in a particular domain and an authoritative claim to policy-relevant knowledge within that domain or issue area (Haas, 1992). WHO, for example, can call on a worldwide range of groups of scientists, academics, technicians, and practitioners to provide up-to-date assessment of, and consensus on, a range of health matters, from new technologies to emerging problems. From such meetings emerge consensus statements (for example, what measures health professionals can use to protect themselves when working with infectious diseases); guidelines and manuals (for example, how to treat childhood diarrheas, appropriate vaccine schedules, training community health workers) and various measures of best practice.

Cross-learning may also occur at the regional level, with regional bodies bringing states together in order to transfer information and experience. In the 1980s, PAHO set up interregional coordinating committees to assist in polio eradication in the Americas, establishing monitoring systems of immunizable diseases, and training nationals in their use. Cooperation was also promoted among these countries by PAHO's establishment of a revolving fund for the purchase of vaccines and related supplies for national immunization programs.

Scholarships, study visits, and training are all mechanisms used by international, regional, and national bodies to stimulate cross-learning.

## Producing and Sharing International Public Goods

By producing agreements on international public goods, countries all over the world agree to adopt and use technical standards, norms, and ways of tackling particular issues. Achieving global consensus occurs through the sorts of mechanisms already discussed: meetings of experts and, often, ratification by international,

**Exhibit 13–6** "Development Is the Best Contraceptive"

In the mid-1960s the U.S. government played an active advocacy role, encouraging low- and middle-income countries to adopt policies to reduce population growth, eliciting the participation of other Western donors, and mobilizing UN support for family planning (which until then had taken a cautious approach to population issues). Population activities were largely defined as family planning programs, influenced by the advent of the oral contraceptive, and from the mid-1960s, the United States was the largest funder of family planning programs around the world. In 1969 the UNFPA was established to channel additional resources to population activities and was strongly supported by the World Bank, which made its first loans for population activities in the early 1970s.

However, low- and middle-income countries were by no means unanimous about population control or even family planning. At the Bucharest World Population Conference in 1974, Karan Singh, then Minister of Health in India, said, "Development is the best contraceptive," and put population growth in the context of broader political and socioeconomic changes. Even in industrialized countries, birth control was considered a private rather than a public matter, and there was

considerable sensitivity in the media not to offend the public. By the 1980s, although family planning programs were more accepted throughout the world, the U.S. government's position changed, as right-wing pro-life interest groups and a powerful anti-abortion lobby wrung a series of major concessions on population and policy from the Reagan administration. As a result, the debates at the 1984 International Population Conference in Mexico were charged, and the U.S. aid for family planning programs decreased. The balance tipped once again in the 1990s, when President Clinton overturned the Reagan policies, and a meeting held in India to review 40 years of family planning activity was closed by Karan Singh, who reversed his Bucharest aphorism to declare, "Contraception is the best development." By 1994, when the next international conference on population was held in Cairo, a major change had taken place. With more participation in the Conference by women's groups than ever before, there was little dissension on the need for family planning. But there was a conceptual change that argued for broader reproductive health policies, which shifted the emphasis from contraception and population control to all aspects of women's health.

---

regional, or national bodies. The sorts of activities covered by such international cooperation in health include agreements on technical standards (of vaccines and drugs); the establishment of norms (for the classification and control of diseases); research on questions considered to be high priority (on AIDS, for example); and the setting up of surveillance systems (for example, to monitor antibiotic resistance). For example, WHO and the FAO together make up the Codex Alimentarius Commission, which sets food safety standards in relation to, among other things, food additives, veterinary drug and pesticide residues, contaminants, and standards of hygienic practice. When there is a failure to produce what would be an international public good, either because it is too costly (for example, new medicines for malaria), or because

industry anticipates negligible returns (for example, vaccines against diseases that affect few people, or very low-income people), partnerships may be formed between different organizations to overcome market failure (refer to Exhibit 13–4).

## THE CHANGING ROLE OF INTERNATIONAL COOPERATION: VERTICAL REPRESENTATION TO HORIZONTAL PARTICIPATION

### 1950s–1980s: Vertical Tiers of Representation

The high ideals of the UN system, which would bring peace, law, reason, and security to a war-torn world, were short-lived. As domination of membership of the UN by a few industrialized countries was challenged by newly independent nations in the late 1960s and early 1970s, the UN agenda became broader and its decisions less predictable. Growth in nation-state membership of the UN was accompanied by a considerable shift in autonomy between its component parts, and, in contradiction to original hopes, it appeared increasingly competitive and difficult to coordinate. Also, and partly because of dissatisfaction with its performance, the UN suffered financially in the last decades of the century.

In 1993 the Secretary General pointed out that halfway through the year arrears stood at $572 million, or half the year's needed resources. Only 47 (out of 186) states had fully paid their regular budget assessments—19 industrialized and 28 low- and middle-income countries. However, almost two-thirds of the total $2.2 billion outstanding to the UN was owed by the United States and the Russian Federation (Childers & Urquhart, 1994).

Such tensions within the UN in general were reflected in its specialized agencies. Because WHO was designated by the UN as the lead international organization in health, "directing and coordinating international health work," and for many years was so recognized, it is worth understanding how this organization changed between the 1950s and the 1980s. From the outset, WHO was essentially autonomous, accountable to its member states and financing and governing bodies.

### Membership Becomes More Inclusive

Most nations were eager to join WHO when it was established in 1948, and the 55 original members rapidly expanded to 189 in 1998 (Lee, 1998), with most managing to find the resources to make the requisite financial contribution. The real growth of membership occurred in the 1960s, and by the 1970s heterogeneity was evident in the different goals and strategies of different member states. What had been a largely colonized world, dominated by a few industrialized powers, was transformed into a polity of sovereign states, in which members of what was then referred to as the "Third World" formed important groupings such as the Non-Aligned Movement, or the Group of 77. After the breakup of the Soviet Union, 25 more states joined the organization, largely from the newly independent states of central and eastern Europe.

The gradual geopolitical transformation of the world led to confrontation in some specialized agencies, especially in the 1970s, with "Third World" member states calling for a reordering of the international economic order (in the United Nations Conference on Trade and Development, known as UNCTAD), or a new communications order (in UNESCO), and with the industrialized nations supporting the status quo. The consensual policy environment enjoyed by WHO in the early days (although punctuated by debates over issues such as population growth in the early 1950s) was also challenged by the growth in membership, although the debates were not as polarized as they were in UNCTAD or UNESCO. Health policies shifted from a technological, disease orientation to a more developmental, multisectoral primary health care approach in the late 1970s.

With the change in emphasis, interests and ideas about health diversified, and consensus began to break down. For example, one of the main PHC policies was to introduce the concept of an essential drugs list—a restricted list of only the most common and useful drugs to be used in the public sector, especially at primary health facility levels. Although essential drugs lists represented large savings for countries that were importing large numbers of nonessential, and sometimes even harmful, drugs, the medical profession and pharmaceutical industry generally were not in favor of this policy, which WHO promoted strongly. At one point the United States was accused of bending to pressure from its own industry to withhold its contribution to WHO (Kanji, Hardon, Harnmeijer, Mamdani, & Walt, 1992). Conflict occurred over the interpretation of PHC policies, too, between UNICEF and WHO, the two agencies that had sponsored the international meeting on PHC at Alma Ata in 1978 (see Exhibit 13–7).

**Exhibit 13–7** Competition between UNICEF and WHO

WHO and UNICEF came into conflict in the 1980s over primary health care policy. Some concern about the boundaries of the two organizations had been expressed in the late 1940s: Roscam Abbing (1979) describes the discussion about delineation of responsibilities, saying some feared that UNICEF's activities would not be confined to "medical supply" but would enter the fields that were the responsibility of WHO. A joint health policy committee was set up between the two organizations at the outset, but one observer remarked that coordination was difficult because the terms of reference between the two organizations were different: "UNICEF's approach is a comprehensive and integrated one, revolving around the 'whole' child and programs of assistance are made subject to this objective. Thus for instance, UNICEF is reluctant to assist WHO in its eradication programs, unless these are not complementary to, but part of the development of basic health services."

By the 1980s, it seemed as if the organizations had swapped roles. UNICEF had been a development agency, concerned with general areas that improved health—water and sanitation, women's education, and literacy—with grassroots, participative, policies. WHO had been technologically focused and disease-oriented. In the 1980s WHO's concerns were with preventive and multisectoral approaches to health, including nutrition, water supplies, and participation in health care. UNICEF on the other hand, searching for a role for itself in the launching of primary health care (undertaken jointly with WHO) focused on a few interventions that came to be known as the GOBI interventions: growth monitoring, oral rehydration, breastfeed-

ing, and immunization. In some countries, the way these particular programs were implemented seemed to be contradictory to the integrated approach of primary health care. Often they were run as separate projects, and even if they were incorporated into MOH programs, they were managed like vertical programs, with their own staff, vehicles, logos, and accounting systems. The then Director General, Halfdan Mahler, did not hide his irritability with what he saw as UNICEF's selective, top-down approach to PHC. In an address to the WHA, and without naming names, he said, "Honorable delegates, while we have been striking ahead with singleness of purpose in WHO based on your collective decision, others appear to have little patience for such systematic efforts . . . I am referring to such initiatives as the selection by people outside the developing countries of a few isolated elements of primary health care" (Mahler, 1983).

The public quarrel between the two agencies was short-lived, but the tensions about policies remained and were resolved by establishing a Task Force on Child Survival and Development in the mid-1980s. The original objective of the Task Force on Child Survival was to accelerate and transform the existing international immunization programs against the main six childhood diseases by getting WHO and UNICEF to work together with other agencies, such as the World Bank and UNDP, with the Rockefeller Foundation acting as a facilitator of the process (Muraskin, 1998). This was one of the early examples of the global partnerships that became a feature of international health cooperation in the late 1990s.

As newly independent states joined the organization, new delegations rapidly became more familiar with its workings and more confident about drawing attention to problems in the low-income member states, and they called for greater levels of technical cooperation. By 1966 more than half of WHO's budget was devoted to operational activities in the low- and middle-income countries, in contrast to, say, the

ILO's 8%. As technical cooperation grew from the 1960s, so differentiation between member states also sharpened: by the 1970s, the industrialized member states were increasingly seen as "donors," supporting middle- and low-income member states. And although all member states had an equal vote at the policy-determining, annual World Health Assembly in Geneva, many felt that the countries that contributed more financially had more influence in decision making.

### Funding Becomes More Exclusive

WHO's funding base changed considerably from its establishment in 1948, when it relied largely on a regular budget (US$6 million in 1950) made up of member states' contributions based on a formula of population size and gross national product (GNP). Beginning in 1960, this regular budget was supplemented by modest voluntary donations that came from other multilateral agencies or donors. For example, by 1971 the regular budget had grown to US$75 million, to which US$25 million were donated as extrabudgetary funds from the United Nations Development Program (UNDP) and UNFPA. Such extrabudgetary funds grew as particular donors (often the higher income member states, such as the European countries or the United States) gave additional funds to WHO for particular programs—an unprecedented US$100 million toward AIDS in 1989–1991, for example. By the 1990s, about 54% (as opposed to 25% in 1971) of WHO's budget came from extrabudgetary sources. WHO was by no means alone among UN agencies to experience this shift in its budget: the FAO received 58% of its total budget from voluntary sources in 1990–1991.

Extrabudgetary funds played an important supplementary role in the last decades of the twentieth century because the regular budget was under significant pressure, largely because of member states' decision to adopt a policy of zero growth in real terms of the budgets of all the specialized agencies—but partly because of the nonpayment of contributions. In 1991, the rates of collection of contributions to WHO's effective working budget amounted to just over 81%, leaving more than US$55million unpaid. Fifty member states made no contribution.

Although extrabudgetary funds supplemented WHO's budget in the short term, they increased difficulty in coordination and continuity because of changing donor interests and short-term financial commitments, and they led to dependence on a small number of donors. In the 1990s, 10 countries provided 90% of all extrabudgetary funds, and the same countries provided more than half of the regular budget through assessed contributions. "In effect, voluntary contributions increase the risk of placing institutions in the thrall of those who give them the money" (Taylor, 1993, p. 378). In the 1990s, an investigation of the role of such funds agreed cautiously that there was some truth in the assertion that a small number of donors to WHO were "driving health policy," but concluded that donor involvement had brought many advantages to the organization as a whole (Vaughan et al., 1996).

Changes in membership and funding resulted in two contradictory trajectories: On the one hand, WHO was perceived as a universalist, inclusive membership organization, with a reputation for being "neutral" in dealing with its member states (in contrast to bilateral organizations, which were seen to be partial for geopolitical or historical reasons). On the other hand, WHO was seen as increasingly dependent on a few donor member states whose interests dominated the activities of the organization. Further, where once WHO had escaped much of the criticism levied at other specialized agencies of the UN—most notably UNESCO, FAO, and ILO during the 1970s—by the mid-1980s, dissatisfaction with the organization was apparent.

### WHO's Health Policies Come under Fire

Until the beginning of the 1980s, WHO's leadership in health was unassailable. Its policies were characterized by a relatively cautious, technical approach to health problems, dominated largely by disease-oriented, vertically organized programs, tackling major disease burdens—malaria, smallpox, yaws—which could be combated with new technologies (DDT, penicillin, vaccines). Although significant advances were made during this phase, by the mid-1970s it was increasingly evident that the disease approach to health policy was problematic. For example, although malaria had largely been eradicated in southern Europe and a few low- and middle-income country areas, it had become evident that eradication of the disease was unrealistic, and even controlling malaria was complex. Not only was DDT resistance becoming apparent, but programs were unsustainable without established health infrastructures to continue detection and treatment activities. Attention shifted toward health systems and health planning, and the 1970s were witness to radical rethinking on health policies, culminating in the Alma Ata conference on PHC, sponsored by WHO and UNICEF, and forming part of WHO's major policy thrust for the next 20 years: Health For All by the Year 2000.

This second phase of health policies led to a much more politicized era, with WHO and UNICEF not always in accordance over PHC strategies, and with practitioners and academics in fierce debate over how to interpret PHC. On the one side, Walsh and Warren (1979) argued that the PHC approach was too broad and unrealistic, and that developing countries had to select certain diseases that were conducive to cost-effective interventions, a position that UNICEF and other donors supported. On the other side, WHO and others (Rifkin & Walt, 1986; Unger & Killingsworth, 1986), argued that it was health systems that needed to be supported, within context-specific economic and social development, and that PHC was as relevant to industrialized as to developing countries. This debate was played out explicitly as WHO and UNICEF competed to promote their respective interpretations of PHC, as illustrated in Exhibit 13–7.

### The World Bank: Reforming Health Systems

PHC and Health For All were developed in the 1970s, but implemented in the resource-constrained 1980s, a period dominated by neoliberal political and economic thinking. The World Bank was playing a major role in indebted countries, introducing structural adjustment programs, and it was increasingly turning its attention to the social sectors, including health. In 1980 the Bank published its *Health Sector Policy Paper* and began direct lending for health

services for the first time. At the same time, Western governments, concerned with rising costs of health care, began to review their health systems, and the era of health reforms was introduced, looking toward increased competition in delivery of health services and different forms of financing health systems, among other changes. Health reforms came at a time of considerable financial constraint—world economic recession, indebtedness among many low-income countries, disillusionment with the overextended role of the state—and rapidly became part of a wider program of economic and structural reforms sought by the World Bank and other donors in many low- and middle-income countries. By the late 1980s and 1990s, loans to low- and middle-income countries had conditions attached that called for considerable changes in health systems, especially in financing and service delivery. As the focus on health policies shifted from the delivery of PHC to concerns about financing health systems, WHO lost ground to the World Bank, which was leading the discussion on health reforms.

Some blamed WHO's waning leadership on an organizational mold, which did not fit the altered and diverse milieu of the last decades of the century. In more than 50 years the organization had not changed much, and it appeared to critics to be inward-looking, bunkered against external criticism, and disapproving of the movements of other UN organizations into health fields—movements traditionally led by itself. Attempts to reform the organization were initiated in 1992, by the then Director General (DG), Hiroshi Nakajima, but the scope, nature, and pace of change were limited and deemed to be slow: one donor withdrew 50% of its extrabudgetary funds in 1994 as a protest against the inappropriateness of the reform process. Concerns were expressed over WHO's bureaucratic procedures, costs, lack of budget transparency, and inability to decide priorities. Questions were raised openly about its effectiveness as an international organization, as well as its capacity to fulfill its leadership role (Godlee, 1994, 1995).

For example, it was argued that WHO was slow in establishing a response to AIDS; that it was UNICEF and other agencies that led the way on polio eradication and universal child immunizations; and that the organization did not identify the serious deficit in health financing during the 1980s, and so allowed the World Bank to become an important player in defining health policies for the 1990s. Discussion began on what activities WHO ought to undertake, with some taking a minimal position, others protecting an expansive role. See Exhibit 13–8.

In 1998 a new DG, Gro Brundtland, was elected to lead the organization, and, after major concerns over past leadership, the collective sigh of relief was almost audible among WHO's supporters. A first move of the new DG was a restructuring of the organization to integrate programs and to prioritize activities. Along with other organizations, WHO began to expand its links with others, looking for increased and more diverse participation in health cooperation. Instead of relying largely on its member states, WHO looked for new partnerships (Kickbusch & Quick, 1998), looking beyond the state toward civil society and the market, and leading to a shift in roles from representation to participation.

## 1990s: Horizontal and Expanding Participation

### The Role of the State

Although the extent of the state's role in the provision of services—whether health, education, or social security—has differed from country to country, there is no doubt that its size and scope expanded hugely during the twentieth century, especially in the industrialized countries. As shown in Figure 13–2, in 1960, OECD industrialized countries' total government expenditure was less than 20% of GDP, and by 1990 it was almost half. Comparable figures for low- and middle-income countries were 15% and 25% (World Bank, 1997).

Until the late 1970s, there was little challenge to the role of the state in its provision of health services, although there were differences among roles in different parts of the world. Most

---

**Exhibit 13–8** Normative and Technical Cooperation Activities

It is commonly said that WHO's activities fall into two categories: normative and technical cooperation. Normative activities have to do with the formulation of ideas, values, setting goals, standards, and advocacy, and are seen to have salience for all members of WHO; they symbolize WHO's mission to the world. Technical cooperation activities are often said to be operational, and concern assisting countries plan and implement their own health systems. They are relevant for a smaller number of countries and are assumed to be relevant largely at the country level. Although it is sometimes assumed that normative activities occur at the global level, and technical cooperation at the country level, two reviews of WHO undertaken in the 1990s suggest that WHO's functions are better characterized by differentiating between common global and country specific functions because the latter often include normative activities, such as assisting with the design of health policy goals, financing systems, or advocacy (Lucas et al., 1997; Vaughan et al., 1996). The question of what WHO's essential functions should be remains on the agenda, with very different conceptions of what would be best. They range from minimalist, a limited number of functions—only those for which international organizations have a distinct advantage over national organizations—to expansionist, where functions would be broad, and might include the redistribution of wealth among nations, or the direct management of services in particular countries.

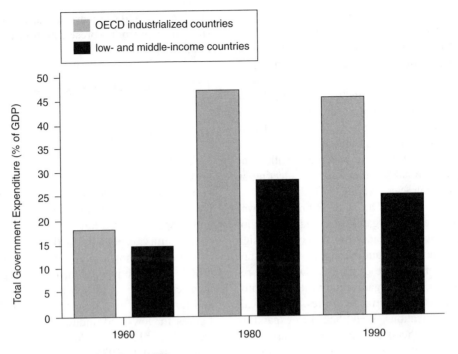

**Figure 13–2** The Growth of the State, 1997

Latin American health systems were segmented between ministries of health, which provided health services for the low-income, and better endowed institutes of social security, which provided services for workers and their families. In Asia, ministries of health functioned within very pluralistic health systems, with a flourishing private sector. In Africa, ministries of health were often the main providers of health services for urban, and with the extension of primary health services in the 1970s and 1980s, for rural populations; however, NGOs, such as missions, were also important providers in rural areas, and the informal private sector (drug sellers, traditional midwives) provided much first contact care.

By the 1980s, however, the political and economic environment began to change. Fueled partly by the rise of neo-liberal economic policies of the 1980s and partly by disillusionment with what were perceived as overextended, corrupt, inefficient, and nondemocratic states in many low- and middle-income countries, donors

began to look beyond the state and ministries of health to the private sector, and began to promote reforms to health systems that would divest ministries of some of their service roles and extend them to the private sector (see Chapter 10). To achieve such reforms, they began to attach conditions to their loans and grants to low- and middle-income countries. For example, a donor might agree to provide a grant to support the health system, but only on the condition that the MOH decentralize its authority, introduce a more robust financing system, or pass legislation encouraging private practice. Although the International Monetary Fund had always applied some policy conditionality to countries in search of assistance, the World Bank only moved seriously into policy-related funding in the 1980s. In the 2 years between 1989 and 1991, the average number of policy conditions per World Bank structural adjustment loan was 56 (up from 39 between 1980 and 1988, and minimal before). Although the bilaterals always used conditionality to some extent (for example, by tying aid to purchases of equipment to the donor country), in the 1980s they tended to "piggyback" on the conditionality of the international financial institutions, with varying degrees of enthusiasm (Killick, 1998).

Policy conditions focused on ways of reducing the role of the state, by, for example, encouraging the private sector (including NGOs) to undertake services previously provided by governments, and mobilizing additional domestic resources. Policies were not confined to the economic sphere, and attempts were made to link aid to notions of "good governance," democracy, and the growth of civil society; these attempts included, for example, promoting increased accountability in the public sector, improving procedures and the rule of law, introducing transparency in financing and other systems, promoting human rights, and encouraging multiparty democratic systems.

### The Rise of Civil Society

Although the notion of "civil society" has a long genesis, it has become common parlance in the development literature only in the past decade or so (see Exhibit 13–2, which differentiates between CSOs and NGOs). Donors have supported the notion of civil society for a number of reasons. By the 1990s, the health sector provided many examples of NGOs that had demonstrated an impact on development, as measured by mortality and morbidity in small communities, through a variety of different interventions. They were perceived to be effective, innovative, and able to reach the grassroots in a way governments and multi- or bilateral donors were not. In the 1990s the focus on NGOs broadened, and donors began funding a wider range of CSOs, whose members often participated in lobbying and other political activities. Support for such groups was seen as a way to build up democracy—by providing outlets for citizens to voice their demands—and to promote social capital, which would lead to improved economic performance. The idea of social capital came from Robert Putnam (1995), who suggested that the difference between the prosperous Ital-

ian north and the low-income south was explained by trust, family and civic responsibilities, and sharing a public spirit—all of which represent the cement that holds society together, and which were apparent in the north of Italy but not in the south. Donors saw NGOs and CSOs as ways to build up social capital, as well as to provide antidotes to the so-called bloated, autocratic, and inefficient state. By the end of the 1990s, however, there was some swing of the pendulum away from extreme antipathy to the state, with even the World Bank (1997) arguing the need for a "capable" state.

### The Role of the Market

Although some include private for-profit (or market) sector organizations within the definition of civil society, they are sufficiently distinct to be seen separately. The market sector is growing and, with trade liberalization in global markets, likely to expand further. In many countries, foreign investment in the health sector, once forbidden or heavily restricted, has begun to open up. For example, states are increasingly allowing foreign hospital management companies to invest in local hospitals and in health insurance, often as joint ventures with local, domestic partners. While some of these moves may be beneficial—for example, the entry of new insurance companies in Brazil is said to have increased coverage of the population by offering improved insurance packages and to have brought down administrative costs—foreign investment may increase inequities within and between countries because it is in their interests to invest in those areas where there is relatively high per capita income, thus improving access and services for those who can pay, but attracting workers from public into private sectors (Zarrilli & Kinnon, 1998).

While some private companies clearly are very powerful, with annual turnovers several times larger than the GNP of many lower income countries, and see as their mandates the pursuit of maximum returns for their shareholders, providing they act within the law, some observers suggest they are taking a broader view of their social responsibilities—if only out of enlightened self-interest—and partly because of the actions of CSOs pressuring for particular changes in policies. There are a number of examples where international environmental and human rights groups have managed to change companies' policies. Although not directly health related, their actions have an impact on the broader aspects of health. For example, in 1991 McDonald's Corporation bowed to the demands of environmental activist groups in the United States, and stopped using their disposable foam and plastic packaging for hamburgers. Another company ceased producing Alar, a chemical agent used on apples, after protests from environmental groups (Wapner, 1995).

There are also increasing examples of pharmaceutical companies offering large donations of drugs to help control or eradicate diseases in low-income countries. Several have followed the example of Merck (see Exhibit 13–9). For instance, in 1998 the pharmaceutical company Pfizer announced the establishment of the International Trachoma Initiative, in partnership with the United States' Edna McConnell Clark Foundation and others, to eliminate blinding trachoma. The pharmaceutical company will provide the antibiotic Zithromax free of charge initially in five countries for 2 years. Similarly, SmithKline Beecham established a partnership with a number of organizations to undertake a program to eliminate lymphatic filariasis, a disfiguring disease commonly called elephantiasis. About 20% of the world's population live in areas where they are at risk of infection from lymphatic filariasis. The program is based on the free delivery of albendazole, a drug that should help eliminate the disease, and is planned to continue for at least 20 years.

However, some companies attempt to penetrate markets by using tactics that have not always been welcomed. Dayrit (1998), for example, describes one pharmaceutical company's tactics to sell one of its new vaccines against hepatitis B in the Philippines as "unscrupulous and unethical": the company used the media to raise public fears about the disease (so that members of the public would demand the vaccine), and distributed its vaccines to the public health centers, offering special commissions to the health professionals who promoted it. The actions of the company angered public health policy makers, who introduced the vaccine to the public sector's Expanded Program so that it became generally available. However, there were fears that sustaining procurement would not be easy, given the costs of the vaccine and problems with exchange rates.

Although public sector concerns about the marketing activities of the private sector remain, the 1990s were witness to a concerted effort by the public and private sectors to negotiate ways of working together. For example, in the United States in the early 1990s, the distinguished Institute of Medicine, established in 1970 by the National Academy of Science to advise the government on policy matters pertaining to the public's health, was asked to explore ways of maximizing private- and public-sector participation in programs to advance the immunization of children. This action followed (1) the establishment of the Children's Vaccine Initiative (CVI) in 1990, a partnership between the Rockefeller Foundation, UNDP, UNICEF, WHO, and the World Bank, to harness new technologies to enhance immunization; and (2) the recognition that there was no overall strategy, guiding research, production, procurement, or distribution of vaccines in the United States. There was concern that economic factors that made vaccine research much less profitable than research on drugs were probably also responsible for the fall in vaccine manufacture in the United States: in 1985 there were 10 licensed manufacturers of human vaccines (7 commercial, 2 state laboratories, and a single university), and by 1992 there were only 5 (Lederberg, Shope, & Oaks, 1992).

During the 1990s a series of meetings between private and public sectors was held to address concerns about the lack of research and development in vaccines, and the apparent slowness of many countries to include new vaccines in their immunization programs. Such meetings

**Exhibit 13–9** Controlling River Blindness: A Win-Win Partnership

Onchocerciasis is a vector-borne disease, often called river blindness because the black flies that transmit the disease survive only within a certain distance of rivers and so infect populations living in the vicinity. It is a serious public health problem, affecting more than 17 million persons in Africa, in 27 countries. Although only a minority of people become blind as a result of the disease (267,000 in 1995, according to WHO), it causes a great deal of misery, including skin changes and itching. One of the ways of controlling the disease is by adding chemicals to rivers to prevent the fly larvae from hatching. Larvaciding was used extensively in the Onchocerciasis Control Programme (OCP) in West Africa, established in 1974 by a coalition of donors (the World Bank, UNDP, and WHO) with considerable success. However, this method of control is not appropriate to all sites where the disease exists, and in 1987, the drug firm Merck seemed to provide a better answer. Its drug, Mectizan (ivermectin MSD) needed to be taken only once a year, in tablet form. In 1987 Merck held a press conference to announce that it would supply as much of the drug as was needed for the treatment of river blindness, at no charge, and for as long as necessary. It was able to do this because the drug had been originally developed for veterinary use, and the company had made huge profits from its sale. And, although testing its usefulness for humans had generated development costs, the overall cost of production was low, and the drug would be needed for a geographically well-defined population. Further, Foege (1998) has suggested that the drug company had an ethos that allowed it to give the drug free, quoting its founder's son as saying, "We try never to forget that medicine is for the people. It is not for profits and if we have remembered that, they have never failed to appear" (p. S-7).

The Mectizan Donation Program was the largest donation program ever undertaken by a commercial company. It provided free Mectizan, not only for the West Africa OCP, but for many other programs in other countries, often through NGOs, but also through governments. In 1997 about 16 million people received Mectizan for the prevention of river blindness. This example of private-public partnership describes a win-win situation: many people in Africa formerly vulnerable to the disease were protected from it, and the program served to "enhance Merck's corporate image and increase recognition of Merck's name and helped build relationships and alliances between its key constituents" (Colatrella, 1998, p. S154). It was successful because Merck established a special program—the Mectizan Donation Program—under the auspices of an independent Mectizan Expert Committee, administratively housed at the Task Force for Child Survival and Development and chaired by a respected public health physician. According to Frost and Reich (1998), the success of this institutional arrangement was due to the transparency and open communication between Merck and the Expert Committee; because the roles and functions of each actor were clearly defined and agreed on from the outset; and because, unlike broad spectrum antibiotics, ivermectin had a specific use and had to be taken only once a year, in an easily ingestible form.

resulted in discussions of a number of new policies (such as removing price controls, or establishing a global targeting strategy and a global fund for vaccines to assist low-income countries in buying vaccines when there were significant shortfalls between what resources they had, and what they needed). As a result of some of these discussions, the International AIDS Vaccine Inititative was established (refer to Exhibit 13–4) and in late 1999 the Global Alliance for Vaccines and Immunization (GAVI) was set up to "fulfill the right of every child to be protected against vaccine-preventable diseases of public health concern." GAVI is a partnership between multilateral and bilateral agencies, the private sector, philanthropic foundations, the research and development community, and low- and middle-income countries. Its main objectives will be to (1) improve access to sustainable immunization services, (2) expand the use of all existing cost-effective vaccines, (3) accelerate the development and introduction of new vaccines, and (4) make immunization coverage an integral part of the design and assessment of health systems and international development efforts.

## VERTICAL REPRESENTATION TO HORIZONTAL PARTICIPATION: THE IMPLICATIONS FOR HEALTH POLICY

What this chapter has suggested is that states were once able to influence international health policy through their formal representation on the governing bodies or at meetings of the various organizations of the UN. However, this channel of influence no longer exists because international health policy is no longer largely decided through the UN or its specialized agency, WHO. Over the past 2 decades, international cooperation on health has expanded to include a greater diversity of actors, who are cooperating within partnerships that include the UN bodies, but do not belong to them and do not necessarily act within their rules and regulations. This shift from representation to participation has some important implications for health policy cooperation in the new century, and raises questions around five arenas: changes in the balance of power; mandates; competition and duplication; coordination; and governance. This final section of the chapter addresses those five arenas.

### Shifts in Power

As previously shown, changing trends in international health policies led to shifts in the balance of power among the different organizations involved in international health. Within the UN, WHO led the field until the 1980s, but from 1980, the World Bank played a particularly important role, and many perceived it as providing the main leadership, as well as the most funding, for health. As one writer put it, "The World Bank is the new 800 lb gorilla in world health care " (Abbasi, 1999, p. 866). From

1995 to 1996, yearly lending more than doubled from US$1.1billion to $2.3 billion, 11% of total Bank lending. By comparison, WHO's expenditure was around $900 million a year. The Bank's policy stance on health was promoted through its 1993 annual development report, *Investing in Health,* which identified four major problems with international health care systems: the misallocation of funds to less cost-effective interventions; inefficient use of funds; inequity in access to basic health care; and the explosion of health care costs, which were outpacing the growth income. Its policy recommendations included shifting the focus of government investment away from tertiary care toward public health; introducing private or social insurance plans; and fostering competition in the delivery of health services (Abbasi, 1999). Although the Bank's policies have not gone uncontested, most donors (and industry) supported them in general, and by the end of the decade, with a new DG at WHO, serious efforts were being made by both organizations to work in partnership with each other, other UN organizations, and the private sector, including NGOs as well as industry.

It is not only at the global level that the number of actors in health has diversified and power has shifted. Regional organizations such as the EU have expanded their interests in health. For example, aid disbursed through the European Commission increased from US$1.86 billion in 1987 to US$4.7 billion in 1997 (OECD, 1998), and even WHO's regional offices—particularly PAHO—act as relatively independent institutions in their own right. Bilaterals provide funds for health to regional organizations (about one-third of the UK's overseas development assistance is channeled through the EU) as well as continuing to support WHO and having a significant presence at the country level. Indeed, many expanded their activities to the country level through channeling funds through NGOs in the health field. External assistance to the health sector through NGOs grew from 13% to 23% between 1982 and 1990 (Michaud & Murray, 1994). Some bilaterals, such as USAID, made a policy decision to provide all their funding through NGOs rather than governments, so that from the 1980s on there was an explosion of NGO activity at both the country level and internationally. And the entry of actors from the corporate sector (the pharmaceutical companies, for example) into health is changing the landscape of health cooperation.

While this pluralism of activity and partnership has raised the status of health on the policy agenda and changed the balance of power, it has also led to concerns about overlapping mandates, competition and duplication of health activities, poor coordination, and more recently, about issues of governance.

## Overlapping Mandates

Lee, Collinson, Walt, and Gilson (1996) showed that many of the UN organizations' formal mandates (defined as an organization's statement of overall purpose) had evolved over time, and that what the UN organizations were actually doing—their effective mandates—had changed considerably over time. For example, UNICEF's original mandate as "a temporary body to meet the emergency needs of children in postwar Europe" (Koivusalo & Ollila, 1997) graduated from temporary relief and emergency activities to development work with children, and later included the welfare of youth and women. By the 1980s UNICEF's expenditure on health had increased by more than 120% over annual expenses of the previous decade. UNFPA, with a relatively clear formal mandate to promote population programs, did not stray far from activities around population issues, including family planning, until after the International Conference on Population and Development in 1994. It was at this conference that population activities were redefined as reproductive health activities, raising debates within UNFPA about its effective mandate. The World Bank, with a mandate to provide financial capital to assist the reconstruction and development of member states, entered the health field through its support for population policies in the

late 1960s. But as has been shown, it was only in the 1980s that the Bank began funding health programs, and since then it has had a significant influence on health policy.

Although observers have suggested that each organization has its own comparative advantage, it is not clear that in practice these always coincide or are complementary. A Bank policy maker, quoted by Abbasi (1999), suggested that collaboration with WHO was based on:

> . . . a big interface, and it builds on a comparative advantage that we have. We are generally competent across a wide range of macroeconomic and technical matters but we are not specifically competent to deal with the highest level of technical inputs, but we have a lot of money. WHO has high levels of technical competence, generally in a narrow health framework, without much money. This sounds to me like a very good complementary situation. (p. 935)

Nevertheless, some would see a contradiction between these words and the increase in technical expertise in the Bank's Health, Nutrition and Population sector, and others would argue that there are tensions between the Bank's economics framework and WHO's health framework. In attempts to reform the UN in the 1990s, there was some support for the view that the comparative advantages of UNICEF and UNFPA, as separate organizations, were not clear, and that the two organizations should amalgamate; however, it was not possible to agree on a strategy. This suggests that the defining role of an organization is dependent not only on its functions, but also on its history and culture, and that these factors differ even within the UN agencies.

It is also not clear that the various partnerships may not end up with a proliferation of arrangements that, far from building comparative advantage, actually lead to duplication and confusion. Just in the field of children's vaccines and immunization programs, there are overlapping interests among several existing organizations: WHO, the partners of the Task Force on Child Survival, and the newly established Children's Vaccine Program of the Melinda and Bill Gates Foundation, among others. A 1999 report by Brooks, Cutts, Justice, and Walt that looked at why countries were slow to take advantage of new vaccines suggested that there had been a confusion of priorities and policies at the global and country level, and this confusion had affected vaccine uptake and financing.

## Competition and Duplication

One of the recurring concerns of those in international health is the extent to which competition and duplication of health activities occur because there are so many different actors, and the effect this competition and duplication may have on domestic policy environments. MOHs, on the one hand, may experience negative cumulative effects, with multiple donors making demands on officials' time, each donor wanting its own project presentations, evaluations, accounting systems, and meetings. On the other hand, some have claimed that governments may also use competition for attention to play donors off against each other (Buse & Walt, 1997).

For example, in a few countries where WHO had the lead role among UN agencies in negotiations with the MOH about health care reforms, the World Bank was perceived as a threat and a competitor because of its standing in the country and its access to policy elites beyond the MOH. Case studies of negotiations on health care reforms in Ecuador (Lucas et al., 1997), El Salvador (Homedes, Paz, Selva-Sutter, Solas, & Ugalde, in press), and the Dominican Republic (Glassman, Reich, Laserson, & Rojas, 1999) suggest that the World Bank was sometimes seen as competing, not only with other international organizations, such as WHO, but also with certain institutions within the government. The effect was to marginalize the MOH, for example, in favor of supporting separately established reform teams. Homedes et al. (1999) suggest that in El Salvador the World Bank preferred

negotiating with a health reform group (partly financed by the Bank and divorced from the MOH) because it saw such a group to be more flexible, and able to move more expeditiously than the MOH, which was bound by civil service regulations and bureaucracy. While all three countries differed to some extent, their reform teams were regarded by those within the health sector with a degree of suspicion, and were perceived as acting secretively, and in partnership with the World Bank in competition with other agencies and the public sector.

Concerns are also sometimes expressed about duplication among agencies, or between international organizations and governments at the country level. Fryatt (1995) describes the donation of the antituberculosis drug, rifampicin, from the Japanese government to the Nepalese tuberculosis control program for 3–4 years. This generous offer raised a number of questions for managers of programs: about supply difficulties because of the resulting dependence on a single source; about erratic prescribing because of drug availability instead of best prescribing practice; and about sustainability—what would happen after 4 years, when the donor withdrew? Kanji et al. (1992) describe the establishment of a vertical program of essential drugs in Tanzania, where the donors established a drug distribution system parallel to that of the MOH; the system was ultimately not sustainable. Mayhew, Walt, Lush, and Cleland (1999), although observing that the options for alternative delivery systems are limited in countries where donors do not trust the public sector, suggest that a World Bank facility in Kenya designed to ensure the delivery of drugs to PHC facilities, specifically for the treatment of sexually transmitted diseases, may undermine the MOH system in the longer run.

## Poor Coordination

Poor coordination between organizations in health has been a problem long recognized, at both the international and country levels. The linkages that exist at the UN, such as the Administrative Committee on Coordination, chaired by the Secretary-General, are acknowledged to be very weak. The specialized agencies, funds, and financial institutions act as independent authorities, and although the United Nations Development Program (UNDP) is officially the agency that coordinates UN development aid at the country level, many of the UN agencies tend to act on their own. Coordination through committees, such as the Joint Committee on Health Policy between UNICEF and WHO, for example, have likewise been useful in some instances, but the committees are not generally held in high regard. This does not mean that collaboration between agencies does not occur, both formally and informally. At a global level, it seems to have been most effective when a particular set of agencies (which may include multilaterals, bilaterals, and private sector organizations) agreed to work together to achieve a particular goal, as in the case of the Onchocerchiasis Control Program (OCP), the Task Force on Child Survival, and the Polio Eradication Program, among others. The agencies supporting these different partnerships shared a common goal; developed clear objectives, mutual responsibilities, and means to assess achievements; and these characteristics may be all-important in ensuring their success.

Poor formal coordination mechanisms may be counterbalanced by informal collaboration, through policy communities and networks, although this type of collaboration is difficult to quantify. The professionals who work in international organizations receive postgraduate training in a handful of universities, spend time working in several international organizations, and share professional and technical interests. This network is probably most tangible on the eastern seaboard of the United States, where different nationalities tread well-worn paths between the health, nutrition, and population sectors of the World Bank, UNICEF, USAID, and Johns Hopkins and Harvard Universities, flying to and from WHO in Geneva, linking up with specific European institutions such as the London School of Hygiene and Tropical Medicine, the Swiss Tropical Institute, the EU, or European bilateral

agencies. However, such informal collaborations are also prone to competition between nationalities and institutions, and for funding.

At the country level, assistance to the health sector may come from many different donors (see Table 13–1), and, although the coordination of these donors is agreed by all to be the responsibility of the government, many studies attest to the difficulties governments—in this instance, MOHs—have in coordinating this sometimes "unruly melange" (Buse & Walt, 1997, p. 449). In the late 1990s, many donors at the country level began to promote the idea of a Sector Wide Approach program (SWAp) (see Exhibit 13–10)—as an instrument through which donors and governments agree on the broad health policy base for the management of domestic and external resources. SWAps have been perceived as the answer to competition and duplication, as well as offering a more effective way of managing resources (Peters & Chao, 1998). Few countries had fully developed and implemented a SWAp by the end of the 1990s, and although there was considerable support for the approach, observers noted a number of obstacles to SWAps' achieving their objectives (Cassels, 1997; Walt, Pavignani, Gilson, & Buse, 1999), among which are weak institutional capacity to coordinate and manage, and continuing competition among donors.

There are many reasons for the problems faced in coordination, both among and between governments and donors, including different interests, agendas, and cultures between the different actors; asymmetric power relations; and unique country contexts in which institutional capacities and characteristics play a major role (Walt et al., 1999).

## Governance

Concerns around governance arose during the 1980s, when aid was linked with "good governance," human rights, and multiparty democracy. The World Bank initially was concerned with governments that lacked accountability, transparency, predictability, and where the rule

**Exhibit 13–10** What Is a SWAp?

---

Sector-wide approaches (in the form of program aid) were promoted by the World Bank from the late 1980s, although it was only in the mid-1990s that they were more generally supported by bilateral agencies and some recipient governments. Derived from sector investment programs or sector expenditure programs, SWAps are instruments through which to deliver agreed-on health policies and to manage aid and domestic resources in a rational and optimal way.

What makes SWAps attractive is that they are perceived as being able to strengthen governments' ability to oversee the entire health sector, develop policies and plans, and allocate and manage resources. They are seen in many ways: although they are primarily a financing or organizational mechanism, because they have been introduced where health system reforms are being developed, many see SWAps as facilitating reforms. For example, some envisage a different and expanded role for MOHs, in which policy makers will look beyond the public sector to explore the potential role of other stakeholders—whether service deliverers in the private sector or financiers. Peters and Chao (1998) give the example of Ghana, where performance contracts have been developed between mission providers and government, and where, like Zambia, public providers are being moved from employment through the civil service to another public agency, with different terms and conditions of employment.

SWAps entail a number of additional implications. For one, they propose that donors will "give up the selection of which projects to finance in exchange for a voice in the process of developing sector policy and allocating resources" (Peters & Chao, 1998, p. 188). Thus, SWAps are seen as being organized around a negotiated program of work, and will only succeed if there is sufficient commitment to shared goals on the part of government and key players in the donor community. Reaching agreement on such goals may be extremely difficult, given the range of motivations driving the different organizations involved in negotiation. Most crucially, they are predicated upon national leadership and ownership, which requires that donors provide recipient authorities with the space and time to think, experiment, fail, and try again, and that recipients are able and willing to assume this risky challenge. They are seen as being implemented over the medium to long term, thus reinforcing the requirements for long time horizons, continuity, and commitment. Moreover, SWAps aspire to the use of national systems for managing resources, which will require not only significant strengthening of existing resource management arrangements but also structural and organizational reforms in the donor agencies. Finally, it is argued that SWAps will be successful only under relatively stable macroeconomic conditions (Cassels, 1997).

---

of law was weak or absent. However, as Nelson and Eglinton (quoted in Killick, 1998) observe, these concerns led to broader issues:

> . . . Transparency required not only open competition for public contracts, but adequate information on government projects and programs, and therefore the freedom of the media. Accountability entails not only effective financial accounting and auditing, but penalties for corrupt or inept politi-

cians. That in turn implies some form of elections and freedom of association and speech to make such elections meaningful. A predictable rule of law requires an independent and competent judiciary. . . . (p. 95)

Although notions of governance have been applied largely to government, they are also applicable to global institutions and corporations. Are international organizations characterized by good governance?

International organizations differ, but they are all accountable to their member states or governing bodies, which have clear mechanisms for challenging activities. Although budgets and expenditures are not always described as transparent, they are subject to annual audits, and are accessible for perusal. There are clear rules governing recruitment, selection, and behavior of those employed as international civil servants. In those organizations such as WHO, which have almost universal membership and one vote per member state, representation of different interests is ensured through the WHA—although in practice, the organization may be dominated by a smaller group of powerful members. Through their ability to draw on worldwide policy communities to provide guidance on issues and reach consensus on policies and best practices, international organizations are vested with significant authority and legitimacy. Although the highest standards are not equally adhered to in all international agencies (UNESCO, for example, was criticized for nepotism, inefficiency, and corruption in the 1980s and again in 1999), the agencies are expected to be publicly accountable.

What is not clear is how the growth in partnerships at the global level will meet the criteria of good governance, such as transparency and accountability. For example, partnerships have tended to be between powerful UN agencies, large companies, and bilateral organizations, with little representation from low- or middle-income countries or NGOs. Not only is representation of recipients or beneficiaries of partnership programs poor, but one review of four large drug donation programs observed that "consultation with recipient countries is often overlooked" (Kale, 1999). A major question for public-private partnerships will, therefore, be in the realm of "representativeness" and accountability. If partnerships are responsible to a myriad of constituencies (shareholders, governing boards, governments, beneficiaries, and consumers), will overall accountability fall between the cracks?

Achieving the governance goal of transparency may also raise difficulties. Differences in public and private ethos may create tensions or conflicts of interest for those involved. For example, sharing information may be difficult: private industry or research groups may want to protect product leads or early data from trials. There may be debates on risks, such as those around public to private subsidies (should development agencies be using public money to subsidize the research process of multinational pharmaceutical firms); or on setting norms and standards (will multinational corporations always set standards at very high levels so that local production of drugs, for example, becomes prohibitive for all but the richest countries); or on agreement between prices and profitability. In Muraskin's (1995) story of the production of the hepatitis B vaccine, some of these issues were apparent. In one of his examples, he demonstrates the conflict between the public health ethos of Albert Prince and the profit motives of Western pharmaceutical companies. Prince, whose development of a hepatitis B vaccine in the New York Blood Center led to the eventual production of an inexpensive hepatitis B vaccine by a Korean company, suffered subsequent attacks and innuendos from the pharmaceutical companies impugning his motivations, and he ultimately renounced his royalty rights as developer of the vaccine (see Exhibit 13–11).

Increasingly, those involved in global health policies are expressing concern about governance issues, and, as partnerships grow, such concerns may take precedence over other issues. Good governance may cover the roles not only of governments, but also of corporations. The OECD has recently promoted a code of practice to raise the standards of private corporations around the world. Key areas include "disclosure and transparency"; rights and equitable treatment of shareholders; and responsibilities of corporate boards.

## CONCLUSION

The profile of international cooperation in health has changed considerably since the UN was established in the late 1940s to bring peace

**Exhibit 13–11** Vaccines for Developing World Production

During the 1970s, while the pharmaceutical companies were busy on their hepatitis projects, Prince worked on his own version of the vaccine. His original motivation came directly out of his long-standing desire to prevent the disease. However, his research and that of others soon made it clear that hepatitis was more severe and destructive in the Third World than in the West. To fight hepatitis successfully, someone had to develop a technologically simple and cheap vaccine that could be directly transferred to the nations most severely affected. He knew that the drug companies working on the vaccine (e.g., Merck, Sharp & Dohme; Pasteur Vaccins) were using large and costly centrifuges, which made the process prohibitively expensive. The countries of Asia and Africa would not be able to afford such a costly technology. Though Prince worked with both French and German pharmaceutical companies on his project, his goal was the transfer of the new technology from those firms to Third World countries. Prince was committed to a basic egalitarianism that took for granted that Asians and Africans could and should acquire the skills necessary to produce the medical products they consumed (Muraskin, 1995, p. 20).

Muraskin goes on to describe that Prince's desire to develop his own vaccine became urgent when the Merck hepatitis B vaccine was licensed in the early 1980s at a cost of more than $30 a dose (with three doses required). Prince felt the price was inflated far above what even an expensive technology demanded. Knowing that hepatitis B was a major disease problem in Korea, that the country was already producing some pharmaceuticals and had the potential, and wish, to expand its biotechnology and pharmaceutical production, Prince began a prolonged process of negotiation. With a Korean-American professor of genetics in New York, a non-profit group that provided scientific assistance to the government and academic institutions of Korea, and a Korean company, he and others encouraged the production of a hepatitis B vaccine in Korea, which would some years later be sold at $1 or less a dose. This process was at times unpleasant, when, for example, Western pharmaceutical companies attacked Prince for being too closely identified with the Korean company producing the vaccine, impugning his interests in the company. Prince, whose motivation was never one of personal financial gain, renounced his royalty rights as developer of the vaccine.

and security to a world recovering from war. Years of economic growth and relative security (with important exceptions in parts of the world) facilitated a growth in overseas development assistance, and considerable consensus in health cooperation. Since the 1980s, economic growth has faltered, international insecurity has grown, and official development aid has fallen. The pace of globalization trends has changed perceptions and relationships among countries. As these changes have all taken place, so has health cooperation shifted from forms of formal, vertical representation to forms of horizontal partnership. The consequences of this shift are not clear, but will serve to focus interest and research in the new millennium. Three concluding points can be made:

First, increasing globalization will lead to different emphases in activities in health. International health cooperation is likely to focus more on issues of governance and regulation at the global level, whether it is on environmental issues, which indirectly affect health, or on transborder trade of health interventions and services, pharmaceuticals, and tobacco products. However, much of the action relating to regulation and governance will center around the WTO rather than the WHO. Juxtaposed against this global level activity, there is likely to be a continuation, or even growth in, international relief efforts at local levels, if internal, ethnic, and secessionist conflicts continue as they have since the end of the Cold War.

Second, it is likely that public-private partnerships will be an increasing characteristic of cooperation in international health at the global, national, and local levels. There is much yet to be learned about which sorts of partnerships work best, and under what conditions. And although there are clear advantages to this type of cooperation, from the input of new ideas and energy to the harnessing of new financial resources, it is as yet unclear what sorts of problems will be generated through such partnerships. For example, it may be that international health cooperation in the future will focus on much narrower programs of disease control, which lend themselves to monitoring, and neglect other important issues in health, such as developing good quality and accessible health systems, in which outcomes and impact are more difficult to measure. Partnerships may also raise issues around equity, by choosing to work in some countries with a particular disease rather than all countries. And if aid selectivity becomes a trend, so that aid is given only to those governments that demonstrate they have strong policy environments,

what will happen to the people who live in countries considered to have weak policy environments?

Third, cooperation in health will no longer be dominated by the UN or its specialized agencies such as WHO, but will be represented by a much more diverse set of actors. Aside from the private sector, there will be more activity among a range of NGOs, including consumer and professional groups, as well as large and small environmental groups and other CSOs. The revolution in communications technology, which has made it so much easier to communicate electronically across borders, will allow a relatively fluid formation of informal networks and partnerships that may come together to campaign or demonstrate on specific issues.

For all these reasons, horizontal participation is likely to be the key feature of international health cooperation in the new millennium, and although the state will still play a role, it will not be through formal vertical representation as it was in the twentieth century.

---

**DISCUSSION QUESTIONS**

1. Can you list the most important actors in international health, differentiating between international organizations, bilateral organizations, and NGOs? For each organization, characterize its strengths in terms of financial resources or technical skills. What other factors make organizations influential?
2. Give three reasons why states may cooperate, and the sorts of activities they might undertake together.
3. WHO used to dominate international health policy. Why has its position changed?
4. What are the factors that have led to the shift from vertical to horizontal representation?
5. Name three concerns about increasing public-private partnerships in health.

## REFERENCES

Abbasi, K. (1999). The World Bank on world health: Under fire. *British Medical Journal, 318,* 1003–1006.

Ampiah, K. (1996). Japanese aid to Tanzania: A study of the political marketing of Japan in Africa. *African Affairs, 95,* 107–124.

Basch, P. (1999). *Textbook of international health* (2nd ed.). Oxford, England: Oxford University Press.

Brooks, A., Cutts, F., Justice, J., & Walt, G. (1999). *Policy study of factors influencing the adoption of new and underutilized vaccines in developing countries.* Unpublished study for Children's Vaccine Initiative, USAID, Geneva, Switzerland, and Washington, DC.

Buse, K., & Walt, G. (1997). An unruly melange? Coordinating external resources to the health sector: A review. *Social Science and Medicine, 45,* 449–463.

Cassels, A. (1997). *A guide to sector-wide approaches to health development: Concepts, issues and working arrangements.* Geneva, Switzerland: World Health Organization.

Childers, E., & Urquhart, B. (1994). *Renewing the United Nations system.* Uppsala, Sweden: Dag Hammarskjold Foundation.

Clark, J. (1991). *Democratizing development.* London: Earthscan Publications Ltd.

Coker, R. (1999). Public health, civil liberties and tuberculosis. *British Medical Journal, 318,* 1434–1435.

Colatrella, B.D. (1998). Corporate donations. *Annals of tropical medicine and parasitology, 92* (Suppl.), 153–154.

Dayrit, E. (1998, April). *Current realities and practices in vaccine introduction and use in the Philippines.* Paper presented to First Asian-Pacific Regional Consultation on Economic and Policy Considerations for the Introduction and Use of New Vaccines, Chiangmai, Thailand.

Elliott, L. (1999, June 21). Bank woos AIDS drug firm. *The Guardian,* 21.

Foege, W. (1998). 10 years of Mectizan. *Annals of tropical medicine and parasitology, 92,* (Suppl.), S7–S10.

Frost, L., & Reich, M. (1998). Mectizan donation program: Origins, experiences and relationships with coordinating bodies for onchocerciasis control. Unpublished report, Harvard School of Public Health, Boston.

Fryatt, B. (1995). Foreign aid and TB control policy in Nepal [Editorial]. *Lancet, 346,* 328.

Glassman, A., Reich, M., Laserson, K., & Rojas, F. (1999). Applying political analysis to understand health reform: the case of the Dominican Republic. *Health Policy and Planning, 14,* 115–126.

Godlee, F. (1994). The World Health Organisation. *British Medical Journal, 309,* 1424–1428, 1491–1495, 1566–1570, 1636–1639.

Godlee, F. (1995). The World Health Organisation. *British Medical Journal, 310,* 110–112, 178–182, 389–393, 583–586.

Greenough, P. (1995). Intimidation, coercion and resistance in the final stages of the South Asian smallpox eradication campaign, 1973–1975. *Social Science and Medicine, 41,* 633–645.

Haas, P.M. (1992). Introduction: Epistemic communities and international policy coordination. *International Organization, 46,* 1–35.

Homedes, N., Paz, C., Selva-Sutter, E., Solas, O., & Ugalde, A. (in press). Health reform: Theory and practice. In P. Lloyd Sherlock (Ed.), *Healthcare reform and poverty in Latin America.* London: Institute of Latin American Studies.

Howson, C., Fineberg, H., & Bloom, B. (1998). The pursuit of global health: The relevance of engagement for developed countries. *Lancet, 351,* 586–590.

Jamison, D., Frenk, J., & Knaul, F. (1998). International collective action in health: Objectives, functions and rationale. *Lancet, 351,* 514–517.

Kale, O. (1999, October). *Review of disease-specific corporate drug donation programs for the control of communicable diseases.* Paper presented at the Medecins Sans Frontieres Foundation–WHO–Rockefeller Foundation meeting, Drugs for Communicable Diseases, Paris.

Kanavos, P., McKee, M., & Richards, T. (1999). Cross border health care in Europe [Editorial]. *British Medical Journal, 318,* 1157–1158.

Kanji, N., Hardon, A., Harnmeijer, J., Mamdani, M., & Walt, G. (1992). *Drugs policy in developing countries.* London: Zed Books Ltd.

Kickbusch, I., & Quick, J. (1998). Partnerships for health in the 21st century. *World Health Statistical Quarterly, 51,* 68–74.

Killick, T. (with Gunatillaka, R., & Marr, A.). (1998). Aid and the political economy of policy change. London and New York: Routledge.

Koivusalo, M., & Ollila, E. (1997). *Making a healthy world: Agencies, actors, and policies in international health.* London: Zed Books Ltd.

Lederberg, J., Shope, R., & Oaks, S. (1992). *Emerging Infections.* Washington, DC: Institute of Medicine, National Academy Press.

Lee, K. (1998). *Historical dictionary of the World Health Organization.* Lanham, MD, and London: The Scarecrow Press.

Lee, K., Collinson, S., Walt, G., & Gilson, L. (1996). Who should be doing what in international health: A confusion of mandates in the United Nations? *British Medical Journal, 312,* 302–307.

Lucas, A., Mogedal, S., Walt, G., Hodne-Steen, S., Kruse, S.E., Lee, K., & Hawken, L. (1997). *Cooperation for development: The World Health Organization's support to programs at country level.* (Report for the governments of Australia, Canada, Italy, Norway, Sweden, and UK.) London: London School of Hygiene and Tropical Medicine.

Mahler, H. (1983, May 3). The full measure of the strategy for health for all. Address to the World Health Assembly.

Mayhew, S., Walt, G., Lush, L., & Cleland, J. (1999). Donor involvement in reproductive health: Saying one thing and doing another? Paper submitted for publication.

Michaud, C., & Murray, C. (1994) External assistance to the health sector in developing countries: A detailed analysis 1972–1990. *Bulletin of WHO, 72,* 161–180.

Muraskin, W. (1995). *The war against hepatitis B.* Philadelphia: University of Pennsylvania Press.

Muraskin, W. (1998). *The politics of international health: The Children's Vaccine Initiative and the struggle to develop vaccines for the third world.* Albany, NY: State University of New York Press.

Organization for Economic Cooperation and Development. (1998). Aid and Private Flows Fell in 1997. News Release. Paris: Author.

Peters, C., & Chao, S. (1998). The sector-wide approach in health: What is it? Where is it leading? *International Journal of Health Planning and Management, 13,* 177–190.

Putnam, R. (with Leonari, R., & Nanetti, R.). (1995). *Making democracy work.* Princeton, NJ: Princeton University Press.

Rifkin, S., & Walt, G. (1986). Why health improves: Defining the issues concerning comprehensive primary health care and selective primary health care. *Social Science and Medicine, 23,* 559–566.

Roscam Abbing, H. (1979). *International organizations in Europe and the right to health care.* Amsterdam: Kluwer-Deventer.

Taylor, P. (1993). *International organization in the modern world.* London: Pinter Publishers.

Unger, J.P., & Killingsworth, J.R. (1986). Selective primary health care: a critical review of methods and results. *Social Science and Medicine, 22,* 1001–1013.

Van Rooy, A. (Ed.). (1998). Civil society and the aid industry. London: Earthscan Publications Ltd.

Vaughan, J.P., Mogedal, S., Walt, G., Kruse, S.E., Lee, K., & de Wilde, K. (1996). WHO and the effects of extrabudgetary funds: Is the Organization donor driven? *Health Policy and Planning, 11,* 253–264.

Walsh, J., & Warren, K. (1979). Selective primary health care: An interim strategy for disease control in developing countries. *New England Journal of Medicine, 301,* 967–974.

Walt, G., & Gilson, L. (1994). Reforming the health sector in developing countries: The central role of policy analysis. *Health Policy and Planning, 4,* 353–370.

Walt, G., Pavignani, E., Gilson, L., & Buse, K. (1999). Managing external resources: Are there lessons for SWAps? *Health Policy and Planning, 14*(3), 273–284.

Wapner, P. (1995). Environmental activism and world civic politics. *World Politics, 47,* 311–340.

World Bank. (1997). *The state in a changing world* (World Development Report). Oxford, England: Oxford University Press.

World Bank. (1998–1999). *Knowledge for development* (World Development Report). Oxford, England: Oxford University Press.

Zarrilli, S., & Kinnon, C. (1998). *International trade in health services.* Geneva, Switzerland: 1998 UNCTAD/WHO.

# CHAPTER 14

# Global Influences and Global Responses: International Health at the Turn of the Twenty-First Century

*Ilona Kickbusch and Kent Buse*

As we enter the twenty-first century, public health faces unprecedented challenges in a new and uncertain policy environment. Three long-term trends in particular are shaping the well-being of people around the globe: the demographic transition, the economic transition, and the governance transition. The way we live and work, how wealth is created, how we communicate, and how our societies are governed—all are subject to fundamental change. The focus of this chapter is on this changing global context for public health—particularly how globalization affects health and its determinants and how the globalization of disease affects the practice of public health.

We are, however, still very much at the beginning of trying to reconceptualize global public health, and we do not yet have a clear picture of all the implications that the present changes are having on population health. Although opinions abound, there exists little reliable research, particularly on the institutional changes and policy processes that are emerging. Public health practice at the international level has begun to understand the increased international transfer of health risks and the extreme inequalities that characterize the global health situation and is responding through new types of partnerships and alliances. The increasing number of players in the global health arena indicates a new awareness and willingness for action, but also reflects the problems inherent in the present international health system and of a state-centric approach to global health. As new mechanisms of governance emerge, the dividing line between the international and the domestic health agenda becomes increasingly difficult to draw, as does the distinction between public and private responsibilities.

This chapter uses the international relations literature as a guide for gaining an appreciation of the issues at stake in the health arena and for understanding the wider context in which public health needs to operate in order to respond to the challenges at hand. The focus will be specifically on the two key themes around which the globalization debate is presently centered: changes in *state sovereignty* and *global governance*. Both concepts are concerned with defining *the legitimate authority and ability to exercise public policy for a common purpose, be it at the global, regional, national, or local level*. For not only can the health field benefit from the discussions in other disciplines and policy arenas, but this can in turn bring much to the wider policy debate because of the special nature of health and disease.

The chapter begins with a brief overview of globalization that attempts to provide greater specificity to the concept and to illustrate the extent to which the notion and its consequences remain highly contested. This overview is followed with a consideration of how the issue of public health has been dealt with in recent discourse on globalization. Next is a substantive overview of the historical evolution of the globalization of disease, providing a number of case studies that demonstrate how modern transnational forces are changing and exacerbating global susceptibility to infectious and noninfectious diseases. The discussion of the globalization of health risks is followed by an examination of the international community's response to these hazards during the 1990s, focusing on a number of structural and philosophical inadequacies to the response from a public health perspective. The next sections deal with how transformations in state sovereignty and governance provide opportunities for a different kind of public health response. The emergence of this response toward democratic and legitimate global health governance is described as one that is characterized by networks and partnerships involving a host of new actors. The following section argues that this form of governance and its corollary in global health policy must be underpinned by a global value base, and goes on to describe its components. The chapter concludes with 10 concrete actions to take to reorient public health research, policy, and practice in light of the changes ushered in by globalization.

## THE DRIVING FORCES OF CHANGE

The revolutionary transformation of world trade and finance has long been underway, but it was the disappearance of the cold war power blocks in the early 1990s that exposed its impact on many different sectors and institutions. The term *globalization* came to express both the multitude and the magnitude of the economic, technological, political, social, and cultural changes that are emerging around the world. These changes include the dominance of market forces, the transformation of labor markets and production, increased movement of "people, information, symbols, capital and commodities" (Kearney, 1995), the speed of technological change, the media revolution and consumerism, and a

slow but steady spread of liberal democracy (United Nations Research Institute for Social Development [UNRISD], 1995).

Initially globalization was viewed as an economic phenomenon and conceptualized as the increasing interdependence of world markets. As both the social and political consequences of these economic processes became more clear, reinforced by advances in communication and increases in mobility, the responses ranged from overly optimistic scenarios of unparalleled world economic growth to scenarios of a deeply divided world economy of haves and have-nots. Held, McGre, Goldbatt, and Perraton (1999) provide an in-depth analysis of the causal dynamics, socio-economic consequences, and implications for state power and governance of the global transformations. Their definition of globalization is:

> a process (or set of processes) which embodies a transformation in the spatial organization of social relations and transactions – assessed in terms of their extensity, intensity, velocity and impact – generating transcontinental or interregional flows and networks of activity, interaction, and the exercise of power.

Globalization has spatial and temporal dimensions; it shrinks geography and increases the speed of interaction (Lee, 2000). Through global communications it also encompasses a cognitive dimension: it changes our view of the world and of ourselves. Anthony Giddens (1999) describes the processes underway as an intensification of social relations, linking distant localities in a new way. Globalization is not something "out there"; it is "in here": few areas of our lives or of the globe escape its effects. The forces of change that accompany globalization create centers of power and influence that are only partially subject to the sovereignty of the nation states within whose borders they reside. Both capital and information flow at high speed around the globe. Foreign exchange transactions alone may total more than US$2 trillion per day. World gross domestic product (GDP) will soon exceed US\$100 trillion, with foreign direct investment rising more rapidly than trade. National markets have become international; domestic production has become international production. Companies are increasingly transnational, with development centers and production lines in different parts of the world. For example, while Nestlé's headquarters resides in Switzerland, 98% of its production capacity is located elsewhere. Globalization thus creates a qualitatively new sphere of action that is independent of territory. Although proponents of globalization (Friedman, 1999) underline the benefits of these changes for the low- and middle-income countries of the world, its critics (Ramonet, 1999; Navarro, 1999) raise concerns over the concentration of wealth and power in a very small group that is not held to account for its impact.

In the health field, the debate is similarly polarized. One camp argues that globalization provides opportunities to create a renewed commitment to global health (Yach & Bettcher, 1998), whereas a critical view focuses on the damaging effects of global markets on health (Navarro, 1998). Chen, Evans, and Cash (1999) have illustrated the consequences and probable impact on health status of the major processes of global change. These processes include macroeconomics, trade, travel, migration, food safety and food security, environmental degradation, technology (including intellectual property rights), communication and media, and foreign policies. The summary (Table 14–1) provided by Chen and his colleagues highlights two facts that neither camp can contest. First, the transnational factors associated with globalization that have an impact on health are many, diffuse, and frequently interacting. Second, the control of these factors frequently and increasingly lies outside of the policy mechanisms available to both nation states and the present international system of health governance. Indeed many of the factors—or health determinants—lie outside the purview of health agencies and to modify them will require a concerted effort on the part of the global community as a whole.

Table 14–1 illustrates that public health professionals will increasingly be confronted with the consequences of globalization processes in all sectors of health policy and at all levels—local, national, and global—of public health action. At the global level, the power and decision-making structures within international health are being realigned.

## PUTTING HEALTH ON THE GLOBAL AGENDA

The impact of globalization on health and the increasing globalization of disease have only recently been gaining the attention they deserve. Although many of the issues and problems now discussed under the construct of "globalization" are not new or different from problems world health has faced for decades, the debate has enabled health to resurface as a more visible issue of global concern. Much of the global health debate, however, is taking place in industrialized countries (hereafter referred to as "the North").* The discourse has been dominated by fear mingled with enlightened self-interest, largely focusing on the threat engendered through the transborder movement of infectious diseases. The reemergence of major diseases, such as tuberculosis (TB), the increasing spread of others, such as cholera and HIV/AIDS, and outbreaks of new diseases, such as Ebola, have made politicians and decision makers in the industrialized world realize that the ill health of far removed populations could have significant ramifications for their own populations. This is forcefully expressed in the subtitle of a recent publi-

---

*Increasingly, the classification of countries as "developed" and "developing" is being replaced by other categorizations. This chapter will use the terms *the North* and *the South,* with *the North* referring to developed, industrialized countries, and *the South* referring to countries dependent on development aid. Within each of these classifications there is a wide variance in levels and speed of development. The North/South classification is frequently preferred by countries of the South.

**Table 14–1** Global Influences on Health

| Global Transnational Factor | Consequences and Probable Impact on Health Status |
|---|---|
| **Macroeconomic** | |
| Structural adjustment policies and downsizing | Marginalization, poverty, inadequate social safety nets |
| Structural and chronic unemployment | Higher morbidity and mortality rates |
| **Trade** | |
| Trade of tobacco, alcohol, and psychoactive drugs | Increased marketing, availability, and use |
| Dumping of unsafe or ineffective pharmaceuticals | Ineffective or harmful therapy |
| Trade of contaminated foodstuffs and feed | Spread of infectious diseases across borders |
| **Travel** | |
| More than 1 million people crossing borders every day | Infectious disease transmission and export of harmful lifestyles (such as high-risk sexual behavior) |
| **Migration and demographic** | |
| Increased refugee populations and rapid population growth | Ethnic and civil conflict and environmental degradation |
| **Food security** | |
| Increased demand for food in rapidly growing economies (such as those in Asia) | Structural food shortages as less food aid is available and the lowest income countries are unable to pay hard currency |
| Increase in global food trade continuing to outstrip increases in food production, and food aid continuing to decline | Food shortages in marginalized areas; increased migration and civil unrest |
| **Environmental degradation and unsustainable consumption patterns** | |
| Resource depletion, especially access to fresh water | Global and local environmental health impact |
| Water and air pollution | Epidemics and potential violence within and between countries |
| Ozone depletion and increases in ultraviolet radiation | Introduction of toxins into human food chain and respiratory disorders |
| Accumulation of greenhouse gases and global warming | Major shifts in infectious disease patterns and vector distribution, death from heat waves, increased trauma due to floods and storms and worsening food shortages, and malnutrition in many regions |
| **Technology** | |
| Patent protection of new technologies under trade-related intellectual property rights agreements | Benefits of new technologies developed in the global market are unaffordable to the poor |
| **Communication and media** | |
| Global marketing of harmful commodities such as tobacco | Active promotion of health-damaging practices |
| **Foreign policies** | |
| Policies based on national self-interest, xenophobia, and protectionism | Threat to multilateralism and global cooperation required to address shared transnational health concerns |

cation named *America's Vital Interest in Global Health: Protecting Our People, Enhancing Our Economy, and Advancing Our International Interests* by the Board on International Health of the U.S. Institute of Medicine (1997).

But increasingly the concern for equity is entering the debate on globalization and health. Accordingly, a compelling case is being made to adopt a wider perspective of global health that is based on a broader array of health determinants, revisiting a number of the initial World Health Organization (WHO) "Health for All" (WHO, 1981) concepts under another name (Berlinguer, 1999). It is now more commonly accepted that the restructuring of the world economy is shaping the patterns of health in the twenty-first century, and in turn, major epidemics and the associated levels of increased morbidity and mortality are influencing the ability of countries to participate in global economic growth (Brundtland, 1999a). The proponents of a "sustainable globalization" draw attention to the dynamic interrelationship between social justice, health, and wealth (and between the public and the private interests creating health and ill health) and see its potential to develop a new type of global public policy achieved in partnership between the private and the public sector (Chen et al., 1999). Nonetheless, some of the same forces that contribute to an increased international transfer of health risks (the knowledge and communications revolutions and unequal access to them, for example) are simultaneously at the heart of potential solutions.

The history of public health provides ample evidence of the importance of maintaining a focus on the socioeconomic determinants of health. The great strides made in population health at the turn of the nineteenth century in the then-industrializing countries of Europe and North America were due to the historically unique synergy between economic development, improved education, and living and working conditions (McKeown, 1976) on the one hand, and the large-scale institutionalization of public health measures on the other (Hamlin, 1998; Szreter, 1988). Only at a later stage was this

progress reinforced and stabilized by mass vaccination, antibiotics, and basic medical care. As a result, the twentieth century has seen an unprecedented rise in overall life expectancy in the industrialized countries. Many of the most successful strategies were implemented at the local level with local public health authorities at the forefront of change. Progress was due as much to enlightened public policies as to the constant pressure by political and social movements to improve the conditions of the poor, of the working class, and of women. Similar results can be shown for low- and middle-income countries that invested in their people's health and education (as in, for example, Kerala, Cuba, Sri Lanka, Costa Rica, and pre-reform China) (Sen, 1999). Based on this evidence, in 1978, the member states of WHO adopted and supported the first international health policy under the rubric of "Health for All." This included a set of indicators for measuring progress. By the end of the twentieth century, health indicators had become some of the most important proxy measures for human and social development. In the social arena, the progress of nation states is measured primarily in terms of infant and maternal mortality, premature deaths, and life expectancy.

The *World Health Report* of 1998 (WHO, 1998a), commemorating 50 years of the work of WHO, reiterates that the major cause of disease, ill health, and premature mortality worldwide continues to be poverty. Nearly 3 billion persons (half of humanity) subsist on less than US$2 per day. It is also estimated that 800 million persons are chronically undernourished. They cannot live "a socially and economically productive life," and they are far from benefiting from globalization. In some countries aggregate improvements in the standards of living have been reversed as global capital shifts its focus and its investments. For example, in the countries of West Asia and sub-Saharan Africa, per capita incomes have fallen below their 1970 levels. In Russia the social and economic disruption following the fall of the Soviet empire has left large sections of the population in severe socioeconomic deprivation. Between 1989 and 1994, life expectancy in Russia declined by more than 6.7 years in men and by 3.4 years in women (Shkolnikov, 1997), an unprecedented decline in the industrialized world. A new body of evidence is emerging that also establishes a correlation between relative poverty (or income and wealth inequalities) and ill health (Wilkinson, 1999). Consequently, the prevailing trend toward greater inequality among and within nations has given rise to concern. The *Human Development Report* (1999a) of the UNDP states that

> global inequalities have reached grotesque proportions: the 200 richest people in the world have combined incomes of more than the 2.36 billion people who make up the bottom 40% of the world population – the gap between the richest and the poorest quintiles of the globe has increased to 74 to 1. If the present trend continues it could well reach 100 to 1 before 2015. (p. 104)

Although health determinants and outcomes are due in part to factors that lie within the particular situation and the policy process (and choices) of the countries concerned (Walt, 1994), a significant and increasing proportion of ill health can be attributed to developments beyond the control of the nation states. Countries are faced with the fact that "although responsibility for health remains primarily national, the determinants of health and the means to fulfill that responsibility are increasingly global" (Jamison, Frenk, & Knaul, 1988). For the low-income countries still dependent on development aid (hereafter referred to as "the South") this shift represents an exacerbation of an existing impairment of health sovereignty brought about by donor influence on health policies and systems development. To some extent, resources confer power and influence. One authoritative analysis found that in 23 countries of sub-Saharan Africa, donors contributed more than 25% of public health expenditure and for 8 countries the figure

was more than 50% (Michaud & Murray, 1994). Although external funds may be marginal in many other countries, donors can nonetheless influence policy through technical assistance. Too frequently the emphasis in international public health has been oriented disproportionately toward solving health problems with "technological fixes devised by the West" (Antia & Uplekar, 1997), rather than addressing those determinants that facilitated the enormous improvement in population health in industrialized countries a century ago. The 1978 WHO Health for All strategy had attempted to shift strategies in the direction of intersectoral policies for health, but "the model of Primary Health Care as fundamental to the prevention and treatment of diseases has been hampered by the shift of power in most nations, from the Ministers of Health to the Ministers of Finance" (Berlinguer, 1999), although it could be argued that health ministers have never enjoyed much cabinet influence.

## THE GLOBALIZATION OF DISEASE

The globalization of disease is not as recent a phenomenon as it is sometimes made out to be. It is the nature of pathogens and diseases to propagate and travel. Historical exemplars include the plague epidemics of the Middle Ages, the mass death of the indigenous populations in the Americas following the colonization of the New World by the Europeans, the cholera epidemics of the nineteenth century, and the influenza epidemic that killed more than 25 million persons around the globe during 1918–1919. Jared Diamond (1997) outlines in his seminal work *Guns, Germs, and Steel* how biological agents and vectors of transmissible disease have crossed continents and influenced the course of history. It is well known that the conquest of the Inca and Aztec empires would not have been possible without the devastating impact of the diseases brought by the Europeans: smallpox, measles, influenza, typhus, and bubonic plague, to name but a few. And it has been forgotten to what extent the flu epidemic of 1918 influenced the outcome of World War I (Kolata, 1999). International public health had its origins in the first phase of global expansion, in the economics of colonization and slavery, and in the link between war, trade, and health. It was the need to protect the rapidly developing and industrializing first world and its immense commercial investments as well as its armies against the vagaries of disease and death—yellow fever, cholera, plague, malaria, syphilis—that engendered the first set of international health agreements on quarantine, control, and surveillance.

The control of disease was one of the first areas of international cooperation between sovereign nation states, and from the start it was plagued by the same perceived conflict between national sovereignty and obligations enshrined in international health agreements. The first International Sanitary Conference was held in Paris, France, in 1851, but it took numerous international meetings and until 1892 to adopt the first international sanitary convention, and until 1907 to establish a permanent secretariat and a permanent committee of senior public health officials (Fidler, 1999). This international system of surveillance, control, and governance, based on the voluntary cooperation of nation states on a limited number of diseases, continued to function along the same basic principles until very recently (Zacher, 1999). In the post–World War II era, because the industrialized world began to believe that it was no longer threatened by infectious diseases, interest in investing in the global surveillance waned, and the infrastructure was not adequately developed or maintained.

### New Patterns of Susceptibility: Mobility and Speed Facilitate Transfer of Infectious Disease

Transnational forces associated with globalization, particularly acceleration in mobility of people and goods, alter populations' susceptibilities to ill health and disease and raise the risks for countries and the global community. More rapidly than in the past, health hazards,

old and new, have significant cross border effects and contribute to the increasing international transfer of health risks. In that every infectious disease is now just a 36-hour plane journey away, reliable and timely reporting of disease outbreaks is in every country's best interest. Yet reporting a disease outbreak can place a significant economic burden on countries—often on those that can least afford it. The global media and the Internet spread the rumor of an outbreak with increasing speed, and the global community responds rapidly, but not always accurately or appropriately (Cash & Narasimhan, 1999). The economic consequences of the plague outbreak in Surat, India, in 1994 were significant; it cost the country an estimated US$1.5 billion to $2 billion through trade and travel restrictions. A cholera outbreak in 1991 cost Peru about US$800 million in trade restrictions and lost tourism. The long-term consequences for these countries have yet to be assessed.

The graph from WHO's 1999 report on infectious diseases (WHO, 1999a) shows the wide range of factors—from climate change to unavailability of health services—that affect the spread of infectious diseases (see Figure 14–1).

For its part, the industrialized world that had felt secure in having conquered infectious diseases—the U.S. Surgeon General stated in 1967, "We can close the book on infectious disease" (Fidler, 1999)—now faces HIV/AIDS, the return of tuberculosis, and the emergence of drug resistant strains of a range of diseases. High-income countries have had to reconsider their susceptibility. A WHO report on infectious disease (WHO, 1999a) presents the following picture:

- In 1995, almost 30% of San Francisco's homeless population and approximately 25% of London's homeless were reported to be infected with tuberculosis.
- New outbreaks of tuberculosis are occurring in eastern Europe, with more than a quarter of a million new cases annually. Poverty, malnutrition, and crowding are reinforcing the spread, particularly within the prison system of Russia.

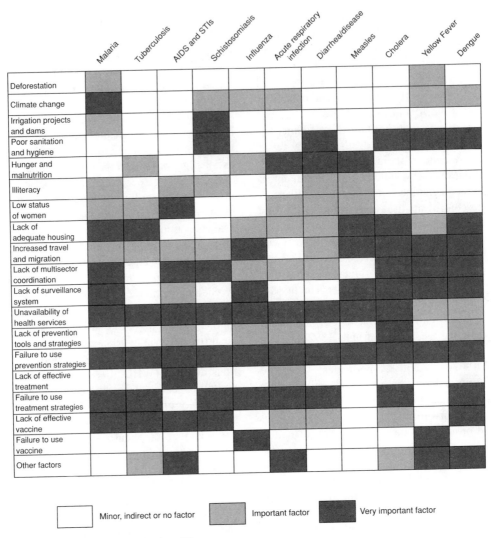

Minor, indirect or no factor    Important factor    Very important factor

**Figure 14–1** Determinants of Infectious Diseases

- Between 1987 and 1992, the United Kingdom saw 8,534 cases of imported malaria; 16% were in tourists and 50% were in persons visiting family and relatives.

These figures not only reflect the increased travel for leisure and business, but highlight other forces (economic, social, political) that drive people to live in countries other than their country of origin, as refugees, migrants for work, or immigrants seeking the opportunity for a better life elsewhere. The number of refugees, returnees, and internally displaced persons in the world has increased more than fourfold from 5.4 million in 1980 to 22.7 million in 1997 (United Nations High Commissioner for Refugees [UNHCR], 1998). Whereas the health crises associated with refugee populations are well documented (the cholera epidemic in Rwanda in 1994, for example [Kristof, 1997]), the health consequences of migration, although not as dramatic, can be just as profound. Economic migration, which disrupts social structures and introduces populations to new environmental risks, has, for example, played a major role in the transmission of HIV (Lurie, Hintzen, & Lowe, 1995).

### A Case in Point: Food Safety

The increase in foodborne diseases illustrates the transborder transfer of risk and the many factors and determinants that contribute to a global health problem. People are exposed through the food supply to pathogens from foreign countries, or acquire a foodborne disease in one part of the world and can expose others thousands of miles away. For example, in 1991 cholera returned to Latin America for the first time in more than a century. A Chinese ship had emptied its ballast tanks into Peruvian waters. It contained *vibrio cholerae*, which infected the local seafood supply. Within weeks, the first cholera outbreaks were reported in Peru, and by the end of the year the disease had spread to 11 more Latin American countries. By the end of the epidemic, more than 1 million cases were recorded and resulted in almost 10,000 deaths (Cash & Narasimhan, 1999). In 1992, 31 passengers on a flight from Buenos Aires to Los Angeles were found to have the disease, indicating the high prevalence of the disease and its potential to spread to other countries.

A range of factors converge to make food safety one of the most exemplary and challenging action areas of global health. A 300% increase in the real value of the global trade in food between 1974 and 1994 (Kaferstein, Motarjemi, & Bettcher, 1997), coupled with increased travel and changes in lifestyles and nutrition patterns, demographics and vulnerability, and microbial populations, all intertwine to create a new pattern of susceptibility. Tim Lang (1999) has eloquently described the interface between diet, health, and globalization and warns that it would be unwise to make unhedged predictions. He states, "We should not be intimidated by the challenge of globalization. Rather, we should be clear that, if the changes are as extensive as almost all observers suggest, we might need to rethink our basic assumption about the socio-economic variables that affect food and nu-

trient intake." In 1994, the Uruguay Round of the General Agreement on Trade and Tariffs (GATT) brought food and agricultural commodities under the world system of trade rules, making its successor, the World Trade Organization (WTO), a powerful actor in international food politics. The pivotal position of the WTO was exemplified by the conflict between Europe and the United States over hormone residues in American beef (Wallach & Sforza, 1999). More specifically, in 1996 the United States and Canada complained to the WTO that the European Commission's (EC) ban on imports of meat and meat products from cattle treated with any of six specific hormones for growth promotion purposes was inconsistent with WTO agreements. The WTO's dispute resolution panel weighed in favor of the complainants (and thereby free trade over public health). When the EC refused, on the basis of the precautionary principle, to lift its ban on hormonally treated beef, the WTO authorized the complainants to apply retaliatory trade sanctions against the EC worth more than US$100 million. According to Ambassador Barshefsky, leader of the U.S. trade delegation and chairperson of the Seattle Ministerial Trade round, "the United States has demonstrated a record as the most aggressive user of the WTO dispute resolution process" (United States Trade Representative [USTR], 1998). Indeed, some countries have amended domestic legislation because of the "mere" threat of a WTO litigation. For example, South Korea has bowed twice to American threats to take it to the WTO, preferring to amend domestic food safety regulations rather than incur lengthy and expensive proceedings (Magnier, 1995).

### New Susceptibilities: The Health Consequences of Social Change and Noncommunicable Diseases

The case of European concern over the safety of artificial hormones in U.S. beef belies the tendency in industrialized countries to see the impending health threat posed by increased global integration as moving mainly in one direction: as a threat from the South to the North, for example, in the potential export of infectious diseases, smuggling of illicit drugs, or bio-terrorism. It was this logic that compelled the international community to embark on the fight against HIV/AIDS in the mid-1980s and that presently drives the renewed interest in tuberculosis control—to protect "us" against "them." But threats from the North are just as serious, if not more so, because they shape the very determinants of health. Although traditional hazards related to poverty and insufficient development continue to constitute a major part of the unfinished global health agenda, a new set of hazards is quickly spreading: rapid development that lacks environmental and occupational safeguards, and brings with it both a significant change in lifestyles and increasing inequalities. The poor and the better-off in the low- and middle-income countries of the world are thus affected in different ways by the transnationalization of health risks. The health of the higher income populations is susceptible to the marketing strategies of global corporations. The WTO, with its aim of more liberalized international trade, represents one vehicle through which the so-called "nutrition transition" (Popkin, 1994)—the transfer of diets, tastes, health risks, and health profiles through commercialization, branding, and advertising—is fostered among the growing middle class of low- and middle-income countries.

> Global corporations are the first secular institutions run by men (and a handful of women) who think and plan on a global scale. . . . A relatively few companies with worldwide connections dominate the four intersecting webs of global commercial activity on which the new world economy largely rests: the Global Cultural Bazaar; the Global Shopping Mall; the Global Workplace; and the Global Financial Network (Barnet & Cavanaugh, 1994, p. 15).

This analysis of the changes in the global economy was propounded even before the explosion of the Internet and the spectacular growth

witnessed in the global financial markets in the late 1990s. The health impact—positive or negative—of each of these areas of global corporate action on specific populations and specific regions calls for careful analysis in order to devise effective strategies for public health that take us beyond the "us versus them" model still inherent in the fear of the global spread of infectious disease.

## A Case in Point: Tobacco and Firearms

The spread of the global tobacco industry into the low- and middle-income countries of the world provides a vivid illustration of the transfer of health risks from North to South. At present 4 million people die every year from tobacco-related diseases, and if current trends continue, the toll will rise to 10 million by 2030. Three hundred million of the world's smokers live in the industrialized world; 800 million live in low- and middle-income countries. According to Yach and Bettcher (1999), "the globalization of tobacco marketing, trade, research and industry influence is a major threat to public health" (p. 25). Globalization has facilitated industry's use of a "range of methods to buy influence and power and penetrate markets across the world" (Yach & Bettcher, 1999). Given the expansion of the global media and Western tobacco brands, consumers the world over are subject to the same advertisements, despite vastly different abilities among populations to appreciate and comprehend the health risks associated with the consumption of cigarettes, for example, because of poor literacy or limited health knowledge.

The tobacco industry, like a major part of the food industry, is a truly global industry, with seven companies worldwide accounting for 40% of global sales. With a decline of smoking rates in Western countries, these companies have aggressively entered low- and middle-income countries, edging out local producers and national tobacco monopolies. One third of Chinese males below age 30 will eventually be killed by tobacco, and half of these deaths will be premature. For eastern Europe it is projected that by 2020 about 22% of all deaths (many of them premature) will be related to smoking. The same nation states that are forcefully tackling tobacco smoking within their own countries are allowing these companies the trade conditions to expand into new markets. Recently, public health advocates have drawn attention to the fact that some manufacturers in the firearm industry are targeting youth in order to sustain markets (Diaz, 1999). Parallels are being drawn between the gun and tobacco lobbies' efforts to block regulations that might restrict their markets, and, as with tobacco, an increasing use of firearms by children can be identified. The United Nations Children's Fund (UNICEF) links the increase in child soldiers to the advances in arms manufacturing (Cukier, Chapdelaine, & Collins, 1999).

Other health hazards originating in the North include the export of arms, industrial wastes, and pollution, and the heavy use of energy in industrialized countries, leading to global warming, and the extensive exploitation of the environment through activities such as logging (see Chapter 8). An active global movement and a range of international protocols and regimes have created an international awareness of environmental issues, including the recent International Campaign for a Land Mine Ban. A similar broad awareness of the impact of globalization on health issues has not yet occurred. It is often easier to address viruses than the conditions that lead to higher susceptibility and spread of disease in the new urban conglomerates of the South. The global campaign against HIV/AIDS has shown repeatedly that, despite the recognition that this disease can only be contained only through determined action in the political, social, and economic spheres, very few low- and middle-income countries have been able to take the necessary steps to contain it (United Nations Acquired Immune Deficiency Syndrome Programme [UNAIDS]/WHO, 1999). It is even more difficult to address such complex and structural issues as the exploitation of women and children, the human rights violations of prisoners, the loss of social cohesion, and the growth of violence and rape through public health programs. Diseases are the symptoms of multiple

and interactive factors that build up over time in stressful and resource-poor environments. The biggest killer, now as in the nineteenth century, remains poverty; the global community will need to address the interface between global social policy (Deacon, Hulse, & Stubbs, 1997) and public health strategies in order to effect significant change.

## INTERNATIONAL COOPERATION FOR HEALTH

International public health has mainly functioned according to a model in which nation states make gains in achieving national objectives through participation in (and cooperation with) intergovernmental institutions. Readers of this chapter are encouraged to study some of the wide range of political theories of international relations that can be found elsewhere (Gilpin, 1987; Keohane & Nye, 1987; Krasner, 1983) in order to gain a better understanding of the issues at stake (see Chapter 13). One element that has been frequently undervalued but is quite clear to the actors in the international public health arena is the fact that nation states are "socialized to accept new norms, values and interests" in the context of their participation in international organizations (Finnemore, 1996). Nation states are capable of learning, and herein lies a major challenge and opportunity for the international public health system: it must continuously strive for a better understanding of the present global challenges and the need for a common response. This would not be the first time that the international public health system faces the need to reinvent itself (Kickbusch, in press). Giovanni Berlinguer (1998) has described how increased international cooperation in disease control gained a new quality, which he calls the "globalization of health" (p. 8). By this he means a process in which nation states begin to move beyond self-interest and, in recognizing the existence of common risks, move toward systems that are underpinned by shared values and joint strategies. The inclusion of health as a basic human right in Article 25 of the Universal Declaration of Human Rights adopted by the

United Nations General Assembly in 1948, the founding of WHO in 1948, and, in particular, the Health for All strategy launched by WHO in 1978—all are the crucial signposts of this striving for a new type of international public health solidarity. Yet despite the need to strengthen this global commitment, the 1990s were marked by regression. Berlinguer (1999) maintains that although risks to health have become more globalized, the capacity for global action for health has diminished.

### The Cognitive Shift: Health in the Global Marketplace

As the 50th anniversary of WHO approached in 1998, a lengthy unfinished agenda continued to loom over international public health, while inequities in health had grown both within and between countries. Indeed, as the World Health Report indicated in 1998, the world's average life expectancy was longer than ever before in human history, yet not as much by far had been achieved as had been thought possible when the Health for All strategy had been launched 20 years earlier (WHO, 1981). During the 1980s and 1990s, the international public health arena experienced three major shifts that changed the way health and development were regarded. As a result, efficiency increasingly replaced the Health for All concern with equity. These shifts are as follows:

1. Despite the exponential growth of the global economy, official development aid decreased by 17% between 1992 and 1997. The resources available to WHO also decreased considerably in the same period. In its 1993 development report (World Bank, 1993), the World Bank spearheaded a new health development paradigm for the health sector, soon to be implemented in low- and middle-income countries as an approach to "health care reform." Drawing upon its earlier analysis

(World Bank, 1987) and superior access to political and financial resources, the Bank forcefully refocused the agenda on the privatization and efficiency of health service delivery and financing (Buse & Gwin, 1998). World Bank lending to the health sector grew to more than US$2 billion in 1996 alone (World Bank, 1997).

2. Throughout the 1990s, the number of institutions and organizations with an interest in, and impact upon, health grew exponentially but became increasingly fragmented. The international public health scene came to comprise both global and regional agencies, including the regional development banks, the European Union (EU), and numerous national and international nongovernmental organizations (NGOs). WHO no longer played a leadership role and had become one player among many.

3. The health industry developed into one of the most significant growth areas of private sector activity in the global marketplace and is now one of the largest industries worldwide. It includes the pharmaceutical and proprietary industries, a wide range of goods related to hygiene and health maintenance, the insurance sector, and a range of health service industries from health maintenance organizations (HMOs) and hospitals to long-term care. The interest of this industry lies in the global market and its expansion beyond national borders. Consequently, the industry seeks to open markets within a reliable, global, rules-based system, enabling its companies to compete across a global playing field. The industry targets the potential for privatization of "foreign" public health care systems (be this the sale of assets or public decisions to rely on private sources of funding for previously public services). This represents a huge financial pool in both industrialized and low- and middle-income countries.

## A Case in Point: World Trade, GATS, and TRIPs

Access to global markets constitutes the economic core of the debate around the renegotiation of the Uruguay Round of multilateral trade agreements, the expansion of the General Agreement on Trade in Services (GATS), and on the Trade-Related Aspects of Intellectual Property (TRIPs) Agreement. Multilateral agreements, be they global (TRIPs, for example) or regional (the EU's Amsterdam Treaty), foretell the changing roles of nation states within a new system of world politics. Individual states are weaker than before and have less power than in the past to enact public policies that counteract global processes: "the reliance on international flows, however, has cost governments the ability to guarantee specific economic outcomes for their populations" (Rosecrance, 1999, p. 203).

Health globalization processes have led to increased deregulation (particularly in the former communist countries) and privatization of assets and services of national health systems in both the industrialized and the low- and middle-income countries. The corporate sector has an interest in the expansion of public resources for global health if this expansion results in the purchase of vaccines, drug treatments, and medical devices for low- and middle-income countries and public financing of biomedical research, for example, in vaccine development. At the global level this development leads to the channeling of public money into the private sector, as is the case in many of the health reforms in the industrialized world (Evans, 1996).

The TRIPs Agreement, for example, while seeking to harmonize national regulations pertaining to intellectual property, not only broadens the scope of patents to include, among other things, human and animal cell lines, genes, and umbilical cord cells, but it also extends the scope of patents to the products obtained by a patented process. It also uniformly increases the length of patents to 20 years (which varied from 0–17 years before TRIPs), thus conferring lengthy

monopolies on products such as drugs (Velasquez & Boulet, 1997). The Agreement, however, makes certain exceptions to patentability when necessary to protect, among other things, human health. Interpretation of two of the Agreement's clauses (on parallel importation and on compulsory licensing) has been highly contested. The government of South Africa, for example, asserted its rights under the TRIPs Agreement, arguing that a responsible government must be able to produce its own generic medicines at affordable prices (Bond, 1999). The pharmaceutical industry (as represented, for example, by the International Federation of Pharmaceutical Manufacturers Association [IFPMA]), reflecting a more restrictive interpretation of the Agreement, challenged the legality of South Africa's action. Because they are short on legal technical capacity, few aid-dependent, low- and middle-income countries are likely to challenge global corporate interests through the multilateral trade regime.

The influence of trade liberalization on the policies and options facing nation states is not limited to low- and middle-income countries. For example, a paper published in a prestigious medical journal on the eve of the failed multilateral Seattle Ministerial Trade Summit in 1999 outlined how the rulings of the WTO will affect domestic policies in health care in the United Kingdom (Price, Pollock, & Shaoul, 1999). Increasingly, the decisions made by the EU on the basis of the Maastricht (1992) and Amsterdam (1997) Treaties, which for the first time included public health (albeit not health services) in the EU's purview, affect the health systems of EU member states as well as those of candidate countries and their trading partners. The shifting balance of power among actors in the emerging global health arena is an area that deserves more attention as the processes that characterize globalization (structuralization and stratification, inclusion, and exclusion) determine health policies and health outcomes on a global scale. A nation state even as independent as the United Kingdom had to accept the EU ruling that placed a ban on the sale of British beef, and it was consequently forced to take ameliorative domestic measures, which it would likely have not implemented otherwise, to gain access to the European market.

### Some Political and Ethical Implications

By the late 1990s, the international public health system began to respond to the changing environment. WHO, for example, drew attention to some of the challenges arising for international public health through globalization in the "Rio plus 5" documentation (WHO, 1997b), its renewed Health for All policy (WHO, 1998a), the Jakarta Declaration on Health Promotion "New players for a new era" (WHO, 1997a), and the 1998 World Health Report (WHO, 1998a). A range of articles began to appear that further analyzed the changing situation (Kickbusch, 1997; Lee, 1998; U.S. Institute of Medicine, 1997; Walt, 1998; Yach & Bettcher, 1998). It became apparent that international public health required significant reorientation, leadership, new forms of governance, a clear agenda, and strategic creativity. The present leadership of WHO has taken up this challenge with new approaches and orientations, working through major alliances (Brundtland, 1999b) to create a new sense of global health responsibility. Some of these are discussed further below.

To date, though, there has been little systematic analysis and insufficient public debate about how the investment decisions of regional and international institutions and agencies (for example, WHO, WTO, International Monetary Fund [IMF], the World Bank, and the EU) are reached and how these affect population health in the short and the long term. The perceived lack of transparency and accountability among the many actors and organizations continues to raise concern. There is scant analysis of how policies promoted by these organizations influence the balance between public and private health services provision at the national level and local levels, or the extent to which their decisions threaten the principle of universal coverage as

well as other policy priorities in both industrialized and low- and middle-income countries. With a view to the private market in health care, Reinhardt (1999) has drawn attention to how, on the cognitive level, globalization leads to the erosion of "the governing social ethic for health care one step at a time without adequate prior debate on each step." This mind frame, which views health as a good to be purchased by individual consumers, has led to circumscribed public health investments and reduced surveillance (Zielinski-Gutierrez & Kendall, 2000).

Insufficient consideration has also been paid to issues such as the ethical implications of widely accepted global programs, such as the eradication of smallpox, the Universal Program on Immunization, or the Global Polio Eradication Campaign (Das, 1999; Taylor, Cutts, & Taylor, 1997). Antia and Uplekar (1997) have sharply criticized the ad hoc committee on health research and development (convened by WHO) as appearing "to be disproportionately influenced by the technological fixes devised (or to be devised) by the West." In their view, this influence will have the consequence of pressing even more biomedical solutions on low- and middle-income countries, which more urgently require action on the socioeconomic determinants of health. There is even less knowledge on how global policy decisions are reached and in turn affect the overall determinants of health, including housing, education, transport, welfare, and social capital (Deacon, 1999). A challenging new interdisciplinary research agenda in global public health emerges that has yet to be acknowledged by major funding agencies and research institutions.

### THE NEW REALITIES: GOVERNANCE BEYOND GOVERNMENTS

The fall of the Berlin Wall in 1989 and the failure of the Ministerial Trade Summit in Seattle in 1999 span the first decade of a new era of global policy. Within this period there was much speculation about a new organizing principle of international relations (Mathews, 1989).

Reflecting the initial optimism after the end of the Cold War, some saw a unique opportunity to strengthen the United Nations (UN) and international cooperation among nation states to deliver the peace dividend (Knight, Loayza, & Villanueva, 1996). But it soon became apparent that a much more fundamental shift was underway, a shift that was changing the power relationships that had governed international affairs during the post–World War II period. Indeed, together with the nation state, the UN system seemed to be eroding under the pressure of neoliberal ideologies, an expanding and increasingly concentrated global economy, the growing influence of NGOs, global corporations, new philanthropists, and the noncooperation of the one remaining hegemonic power, the United States (Childers, 1997).

As the number of actors pursuing disparate agendas and creating new spheres of influence in the international arena increased, the need to explore different mechanisms of governance became evident (see Exhibit 14–1). Rather than look to the UN to shape a new global order and de facto introduce some form of "world government," an approach based on global public policy networks and jointly adopted voluntary regimes has been suggested as the most realistic architecture for the politically fragmented international system (Reinicke, 1998; Young, 1997). In his analysis of the major trends that will shape the twenty-first century, Manuel Castells (1998) argues that the rise of the "network" heralds a new organizing principle of society.

These perspectives (an intergovernmental world system versus horizontal networks of differentiated actors) constitute two opposite poles of the debate on how our world will be governed in the twenty-first century, and in a final analysis they might not be as exclusive of each other as it seems at first. As much as the agenda and implementation of global public policy will be network driven, they will need a reliable and functioning framework and rules-based system within which to function. Even the organized commercial sector has acknowledged the need for and looks to the UN to provide a global

level rules-based framework. In 1999 the International Chamber of Commerce (ICC) entered into a compact with the UN. The compact "of shared values and principles will give a human face to the global market" and would focus on human rights, labor standards, and environmental practice (Cattaui, 1999). Civil society organizations (CSOs) from the North and South have, however, criticized the compact for enabling corporations to promote a positive image through association with the UN, but not binding them to observe minimum social norms. A number of groups have instead proposed a "Citizen's Compact on the United Nations and Corporations," which demands that the UN develop rules that would bind corporate behavior globally to UN-endorsed norms within a legally binding framework (Corporate European Observer [CEO], 2000).

It would be misleading to suggest that globalization is an autonomous process or some fixed end point that nation states and CSOs have no voice in determining. It is, after all, nation states that are members of the decision-making bodies of international organizations, such as the WTO, and that negotiate and ratify global agreements. A closer analysis suggests a more complex reshaping of sovereignty and governance within the context of both globalization and localization; this reshaping is defined by a growth in influence of transnational social movements (TNSM) and transnational corporations (TNC) and is thereby a redefinition of the role of the nation state in the international arena. One result of this process is the constant shifting of alliances and networks that constitute a completely new international architecture. This is as evident in the health field as in other arenas.

## Sovereignty Transformed

Sovereignty at the end of the twentieth century is characterized by what has become known as the "paradox of sovereignty." Two types of sovereignty are distinguished: "de jure," or external sovereignty, and "operational," or internal sovereignty (Bull, 1977). Although globaliza-

**Exhibit 14–1** Governance, Global Governance, and Good Governance

*Governance* is a term that is frequently misunderstood. Often, it is mistakenly equated with the far narrower concept of *government*, which constitutes merely one, albeit important, mechanism of governance (government remains unique in having legislative and coercive powers). Broadly speaking, governance can be defined as "the process whereby an organization or society steers itself" (Rosenau, 1995). In general terms, therefore, governance involves establishing and operating social institutions—such as systems of rules, norms, decision-making processes, and institutions—that guide individual behavior within social interactions. Governance is necessitated by interdependence, particularly when the actions of one group member impinge upon the well-being of another. When interdependence gives rise to conflict, governance can emerge as the basis for cooperation (Young, 1997). Governance may, therefore, include formal public authorities, but it may equally include a range of complementary and supplementary arrangements that solve collective action problems. Increasingly, governmental action is subject to nongovernmental scrutiny and pressure (for example, from organizations such as Transparency International).

Similarly, *global governance* encompasses not only the creation and operation of rules governing intergovernmental affairs (that is, between states) but also those myriad arrangements in which the creators and operators are non-state actors, working within and across boundaries. Rosenau (1995) draws attention to the various types of arrangements that increasingly coexist at different levels (subnational, transnational, and supranational), as well as the apparent shift of some power from state to non-state actors. While the role of transnational corporations in global governance is well recognized, less well recognized is the nonprofit element of civil society in governing the world of public affairs (Wapner, 1997).

Governance clearly has both normative and positive dimensions: how effective, efficient, and equitable (fair) are both the processes and results of governance? In operational terms, the World Bank suggests that governance has four components: (1) representative legitimacy; (2) accountability; (3) competency and appropriateness; and (4) respect for due process (World Bank, 1994).

---

tion leaves external sovereignty intact, it undermines internal sovereignty in that it places on the nation state limits that entail "a threat to its ability to conduct policy" (Reinicke, 1998, p. 57). Globalization, therefore, in its transformation of sovereignty, necessitates new forms of governance that ensure that the public interests remain protected—including the interest in health. On the one hand is an erosion of the operational sovereignty of the state, or its ability independently and autonomously to conduct public policy for the economy and society at large. This erosion represents a curtailment that is linked to decentralization and subnational disintegration as well as to international and regional integration. On the other hand, the external sovereignty of nation states remains the organizing principle of the international order,

and legitimate legal authority still resides in states, no matter how much power they have lost in other domains of sovereignty (Hashmi, 1997).

Although the role, influence, and raison d'être of the nation state are clearly changing, these changes do not imply that the state has become superfluous. When analyzing the major environmental regimes of recent years, Young (1997) concludes that the majority of them constitute agreements between nation states, such as the GATT, the regime for Antarctica, and the ozone regime. Yet intergovernmental agreements are not likely to have been put in place or implemented, particularly at the local level, without the active involvement of many other players and networks. Nation states are not only increasingly pressured by national and international interest groups and NGOs (for example, in the field of human rights or the protection of the environment), but they are also becoming the ambassadors for the penetration of foreign markets or for attracting foreign investment. Some analysts speak of the economization of the political state; states are trapped, says Rosecrance (1999*)*, "in the international coils of economics" (p. 203). This explains a significant amount of states' paradoxical behavior in international organizations, witnessed in the debates on the floors of WHO's decision-making bodies on essential drugs, TRIPs, tobacco control, and breast milk substitutes.

In principle, globalization does not affect the legal sovereignty of nation states over their territory and their populations, yet it requires increasing cooperation among nation states to ensure the stability and security of the global system. Because of this need for order, reliability, stability, fairness, and trust, a new set of international rules and value systems are in the making. This development does not limit sovereignty per se, but changes the rules of what is acceptable to the international community. Recent examples are the creation of an International Criminal Court, the rulings around the extradition of former Chilean dictator General Pinochet, the UN intervention in Somalia and the NATO intervention in Kosovo, the Shell/Greenpeace/BrentSpar debacle, the criticisms and attacks on the World Bank, and the Seattle Trade Summit, to name but a few. Within this context, UN Secretary General Kofi Annan regularly affirms that the rights of individuals, as enshrined in international agreements, take primacy over the sovereign authority of nation states. These events and developments are critical to the promotion and protection of individual and population health in the new global system. Yet they beg the question of how the public health community should develop consensus for appropriate responses to actions of nation states, or neglect of action, that endanger the health not only of their own population but also that of neighboring states and the global community at large.

To partially resolve this dilemma, Reinicke (1998) proposes that nation states enter into voluntary sectoral pooling of their operational sovereignty. This pooling would enable a global public policy that allows joint action against common threats and benefits all countries equally. He defines global public policy as "the pooling and collective operationalization of internal sovereignty" (p. 70), which would fall into the domain of "soft" international law and be structured around legally nonbinding international instruments, but would include a strong focus on compliance and enforcement. It is these two elements particularly that are presently lacking in most of the international health system. The first elements of such an approach can be found in the dispute settlement mechanism of the WTO and the EU. Yet, as Fox (1997) rightly indicates, the EU consists of countries that have long traditions of sovereignty and are far advanced in moving toward a new role for the nation state. Voluntarily relinquishing additional operational sovereignty is much harder for the nascent nation states in low- and middle-income regions of the world, particularly those that have only recently gained sovereign status (for example, in central and eastern Europe).

## THE NEW ACTORS IN THE GLOBAL HEALTH ARENA

According to WHO, "Issues relating to health policies, public health measures and health systems development fall under WHO governance and should not be shifted to other international forums" (Turmen, 1999, p. 9). Nevertheless, the global health system is moving toward more complex governance arrangements that can be characterized on a vertical axis by the overlapping sovereignty of different levels of governance (Kaplan, 1999) and on the horizontal axis by a wide variety of organizations, partnerships, and global public policy networks (Reinicke, 1999). Examples have already been given of how organizations such as the World Bank and the WTO are engaged in policies with significant health impact. Global health governance must now be understood as a field in flux, marked by shifts in the balance of power and influence among nodal institutions, networks, and alliances, overlapping sovereignty, and internal oppositional dynamics. As the nation state assumes a new role in the international arena, two other seminal trends are at work. Manuel Castells (1998) argues that the era of globalization of the economy is also the era of the *localization of polity* and the *age of the network*. There is both a resurgence of interest in participation at the local level and an ever-increasing activism at the global level (Kaplan, 1999). Reflecting such analysis, the 1999/2000 *World Development Report: Entering the 21st Century* outlines a "global-local development continuum" and stresses that development policies need to take into account that these two major trends occur simultaneously (World Bank, 1999).

Over the past few years, the World Bank has been at the forefront of strategic thinking with regard to policy responses to globalization. It has hosted a number of conferences exploring new forms of governance for the twenty-first century, such as public-private partnerships, knowledge management, and global public policy networks. As it becomes apparent that individual countries and single organizations cannot resolve the majority of the world's health problems, new ways of working together and new forms of governance emerge. Not only have the new actors—the TNSMs and the TNCs—become more proactive in influencing global agendas, but they also have gained increased access and unprecedented opportunities to participate in the international system. The series of major UN conferences of the past decade witnessed an increasing involvement and "professionalization" of NGOs.

## Cities

Localization refers to a set of interacting trends: the decentralization of political power from national to regional and local levels, the movement of populations and economic energy to urban areas in low- and middle-income countries, and the provision of essential services to the growing urban conglomerates. Some analysts predict a rebirth of the city states as a key organizing principle of the world of the future (Kaplan, 1999). Although the United Nations Center for Human Settlements (HABITAT) has consistently drawn attention to the importance of cities, most international bodies have not yet taken the step to involve them systematically in global governance. This negligence could have major health consequences in the twenty-first century. About 2.3 billion (45%) of the world's population now lives in urban areas, and by the year 2010, the urban population will have grown to 4 billion (56%) (United Nations World Population Prospects: 1990, 1991). The growth of urban populations is faster than overall population growth in the low- and middle-income regions of the world. The number of urban agglomerations with a population exceeding 1 million increased from 90 in 1955 to 324 in 1995 and is projected to reach 408 in 2015. While urban centers will continue to be the driving force of change, their growth—as in the late nineteenth century—will give rise to a panoply of disease threats due to poverty, socioeconomic stress, poor environments, substandard housing, homelessness, lack of sanitation, foodborne hazards, and commercial sex. Urbanization and its environmental and social consequences will constitute a core of the twenty-first century public health agenda.

With little to expect from the nation state, cities and urban conglomerates will form their own networks of governance and express their own form of sovereignty: "what local and regional governments lack in power and resources they make up in flexibility and networking" (Castells, 1998, p. 378). A range of city networks already exists and has been particularly active in the field of environment and health, as attested by a series of initiatives such as "sustainable cities," the WHO Healthy Cities Project, and in particular the many local activities around "Agenda 21" (WHO Commission on Health and Environment, 1992). The global public health community will have to place priority on involving mayors and decision makers from the local level in their programs and activities. Helping cities to deal with the public health consequences of globalization and decentralization should be in the forefront of global health agendas. Local authorities are becoming more active in calling for a voice at the global level, and the willingness of cities to be involved in international public health is clearly manifested in their committed involvement in the WHO Healthy Cities Project. It is essential that global health advocates keep the global-local development continuum in mind and develop their strategies accordingly (Kickbusch, 1999); those affected by the consequences of global policies must be involved in shaping them.

## Civil Society

It is the paradox of sovereignty, the changing role of the state, and the ensuing breakdown in trust between governments and citizens that have led to the exponential growth of NGOs as an organized response of civil society. If governance is defined as the ability to conduct policy, then the new actors are already fully involved in global health governance and are indeed sometimes more influential than some of the more established institutions. Paul Wapner (1997) argues that an international civil society has grown alongside the state-based international system and it plays just as important a role as the state system in shaping global agendas. This has been further influenced by foreign donors' lack of faith in recipient government efficiency (and, in some cases, integrity and interests as well) and has led to an ever-increasing operational role for NGOs in implementing development assistance projects.

Civil society has organized with great creativity, and, taking full advantage of modern information technology and the media, has often emerged as the voice of the global community, aiming to speak for the disenfranchised of the South as well as the enlightened, socially responsible consumers of the affluent North. Indeed, in many cases NGOs have managed to forge political alliances of very diverse groups around a specific issue. In linking locally based groups with global actors, they have placed issues such as child labor, land mines, environmental protection, and human rights on the global agenda. NGOs have formed transnational coalitions to reform the World Bank (Fox & Brown, 1997) and to resist the free trade agenda of the WTO ("The non-governmental order," 1999). Ensuring the accountability of international bodies to the global community—even though in principle they are accountable only to their member governments—constitutes a strategic breakthrough for NGOs in setting global agendas. In the public health arena, for example, NGOs were central in gaining adoption of the International Code on the Marketing of Breast Milk Substitutes (Sikkink, 1986). NGOs also act as watchdogs of the pharmaceutical industry, advocate on behalf of primary health care and women's health, and ensure that continuing attention is paid to community involvement and human rights in health matters around the globe (Keck & Sikkink, 1998).

Some NGOs occupy the gray area between being a business and an advocacy group (such as Greenpeace), whereas others are a front for commercial interests aiming to ensure a voice in the UN system. The increase in "public-private partnerships" has brought many TNCs closer to international agencies. Moreover, much is expected from the new global philanthropists in health, who come from the sectors that have profited from the markets in a globalized world, such as the capital market (for example, George Soros and the Soros Foundation Network), the global media (for example, Ted Turner and the United Nations Foundation and the Better World Campaign), and the computer software industry (for example, Bill Gates and the Bill and Melinda Gates Foundation). While funding from these philanthropists has provided significant additional resources for international public health at a difficult time, their arrival has also shifted the power balance in global health. In a relatively short period of time, many of these new actors have influenced global health priorities and strategies and prompted a number of political and ethical issues that have not yet been fully explored.

## The Private Sector

For its part, the private sector has shown increasing willingness to contribute to global health development, often through partnership with the public sector (Buse & Walt, in press-a, in press-b, in press-c). Emerging relationships often move beyond the simple philanthropy (gift giving) of the past and can be differentiated by a range of motivations, including corporate responsibility (focused on obligation), corporate citizenship (focused on rights and responsibilities), and strategic gain (Waddell, 1999). This collaboration is due to the increasing challenges to the commercial sector to show more social responsibility, to invest in the well-being of populations, to adhere to global labor and environmental standards, and to invest in research and development that benefits the lowest income populations. The Secretary General of the UN has reminded the corporate community that because "globalization is under intense pressure [a]nd business is in the line of fire," business must be "seen to be committed to global corporate citizenship" (Annan, 1999). However, as foreign investment, and particularly foreign production, increases, corporations have a heightened interest in healthy populations in low- and middle-income countries. The World Alliance for Community Health, which brings together Placer Dome, Rio Tinto, and three other mining houses, takes a broad approach to promoting health at the community level. An article in *The Economist* ("The non-governmental order," 1999) states, "Increasingly, firms realize that they cannot keep their workers productive, nor build markets, without a healthy population, particularly when the main killers such as HIV/AIDS in southern Africa or traffic accidents in Vietnam, do not respect company boundaries." Although, as Waddell (1999) points out, some public-private partnerships are proposed as priming the pump of economic globalization

in those areas of the world where the market is not well enmeshed in the global economy, partnerships are also about strategic corporate gain, and provide an opportunity to penetrate potentially important markets. The president of the medical systems unit of Becton Dickinson & Company has, for example, commented: "Of course we want to help eradicate neonatal tetanus, but we also want to stimulate the use of non reusable injection devices, and to build relationships with ministries of health that might buy other products from us as their economies develop" (Deutsch, 1999).

At the macro level, the private sector's motivation to align itself with the UN can be understood as an attempt to ensure that its interests are represented in the rules that are established to guide global interactions. For example, according to Maria Cattaui, Secretary General of the ICC,* "Business believes that the rules of the game for the market economy, previously laid down almost exclusively by national governments, must be applied globally if they are to be effective. For that global framework of rules, business looks to the United Nations and its agencies" (Cattaui, 1999). For its part, the UN seeks both resources and enhanced influence through partnership with the commercial sector. Hence, globalization brings the potential for enlightened self-interest within the commercial and public sectors, which can in turn benefit the health of populations.

The "us-them" approach in terms of public/private or state/NGO action in response to specific problems is increasingly being replaced by a series of partnerships, alliances, and networks that bring together various types of actors to discover pragmatic solutions jointly. New win-win situations are emerging as each partner contributes according to its comparative advantage and thereby meets its own, as well as collective,

---

*The ICC consists of more than 7,000 member companies and business associations in more than 130 countries.

interests. The Medicines for Malaria Venture, for example, represents a partnership to find new antimalarials, in which funds will be provided primarily by the public sector, and industry will provide the sort of support that money cannot buy: in-kind resources, such as access to chemical libraries and easier access to their technologies in the areas of genomics and pathogenomics, combinatorial chemistry, and bio-informatics (Bruyere, 1999). Jeffrey Sachs (1999) has proposed a more systematic approach to the problem of market failure in relation to vaccines to prevent diseases such as malaria, which disproportionately affect the low-income. He suggests that the industrialized countries create a market for such vaccines by pledging to purchase a specific quantity of them at guaranteed prices, should pharmaceutical manufacturers bring these vaccines to market. This arrangement, it is argued, would make malaria vaccine research and development an attractive investment option for the competitive private sector research and development community, which in turn would yield a vaccine, which in turn would contribute immeasurably to the health and economic development in low-income countries, while also benefiting the bottom line of the company concerned.

## THE MOVE TOWARD DEMOCRATIC AND LEGITIMATE GLOBAL HEALTH GOVERNANCE

How can the present patchwork of networks and alliances in health move toward a system of "legitimate global governance" (Rittberger & Bruehl, 1999) without losing its energy and creativity? Is it realistic to work toward a *global health governance network* that would build on existing organizations, common values, and accepted regimes, or is the anarchic plurality of initiatives the health network of the future? It must be conceded that at present we are in a period of exploration and experimentation. Although a range of partnerships and networks for health have been created in a very short period,

how significant and sustainable their impact will be remains to be seen.

### Partnerships, Alliances, and Networks

Partnerships can be considered at one end of a continuum with networks at the other end, and alliances somewhere in between. Partnerships involve more formalized agreements, and networks a looser grouping of parties (individuals, organizations, and agencies) organized generally on a nonhierarchical basis around some common theme or concerns. Global partnerships now exist to combat malaria and tuberculosis, to develop vaccines, and to reduce tetanus, among other things. The prototype partnership in the health sector was established by Merck & Company for the donation of its drug Mectizan (ivermectin) to treat onchoceriasis (river blindness). In addition to the manufacturer and the governments of the 11 countries of West Africa most affected by the disease, the partners in this effort include the Food and Agriculture Organization of the United Nations (FAO), UNDP, the World Bank, and numerous NGOs. The coordination of the partnership rests with an NGO—the Task Force for Child Survival and Development—which receives support from Merck to carry out this function (Frost & Reich, 1998). One of the first major alliances in the public health sector was the polio eradication network (PEN). The initiative to eradicate polio has mobilized UNICEF, the U.S. Centers for Disease Control and Prevention, Rotary International, the Bill and Melinda Gates Foundation, the UN Foundation, the governments of Australia, Belgium, Canada, Denmark, Germany, Japan, the United Kingdom, and the United States, private sector partners, and millions of volunteers. More recently crafted alliances include the Global Alliance to achieve the elimination of leprosy by the end of 2005 and a Global Alliance for Vaccines and Immunization. Similarly, many issue-based health networks are being established at all levels of governance.

Partnerships, broadly defined, may be based on diseases and issues (polio eradication), products and treatments (deworming drugs for children), product development (vaccine development), health messages and campaigns (to stop children from smoking), or knowledge sharing (surveillance networks) (Kickbusch & Quick, 1998). Partnerships for health bring together a set of actors for the common goal of improving the health of populations based on mutually defined objectives, roles, and responsibilities. Increasingly, these partnerships evolve around both vertical (from global to local) and horizontal (multitude of partners) subsidiarity.

Based on a cursory analysis, it would appear that partnerships, alliances, and networks are most effective when they address a single high profile issue; when their goals are clearly specified, time-bound, and measurable, and can be well presented in the media (possibly as a defense against a perceived threat or one with high human relations value); when roles and responsibilities are clearly delineated; when distinct benefits accrue to all partners; when there is a perception of transparency and equality among partners; when all partners regularly meet their obligations; and when partnerships comprise a manageable number of actors and include representation from civil society.

The *entente cordiale* between the public and private sectors provides significant benefits to business and undoubtedly contributes immeasurably to the welfare of those individuals and communities that benefit from improved access to drugs, vaccines, and health services. Sachs (1999) noted that "there is no escape from such public-private collaboration." Nonetheless, there is scope for more research on the governance of these new arrangements (Buse & Walt, in press-c). What, for example, will be the impact of such partnerships on agenda-setting (are recipient governments involved in decision-making?), accountability (to whom are the partnerships accountable?), equity (what happens to those populations excluded from particular programs?), and sustainability (will governments be able to continue programs when partnerships cease?). WHO has responded to these concerns by issuing provisional guidelines governing its

involvement with the commercial sector (WHO, 1999b). Although necessary, the need for regulatory oversight of these arrangements extends beyond internal scrutiny of proposed and existing partnerships by the organizations themselves (WHO, for example) and requires an independent global regulatory and accreditation system as a component of global health governance. More public debate is required on the nature and mechanisms of the governance of such partnerships to strike a balance among the need for corporate citizenship (and benefit), public sector responsibility, and programs that meet neglected public health challenges. The current climate of trust and goodwill between public and private sectors should be seized upon not only to foster new partnerships but to ensure that each partnership is truly in the interest of global public health.

## Global Democracy

In public health, as in other areas of international policy, a key challenge for the twenty-first century is to give priority to democratizing international health governance, to balance global and local priorities, and to ensure sustainability; only then can the global community respond adequately to the challenges at hand. A warning was sounded to all international organizations in 1998, when a coalition of NGOs brought down the Multilateral Agreement on Investment (MAI), which was being negotiated by the 29 members (industrialized countries) of the Organization of Economic Cooperation and Development (OECD) and the EU. The failed summit of the trade ministers from 134 member states of the WTO in Seattle in 1999 has been interpreted by some as a watershed in the conduct of global policy. A broad coalition of NGOs protested against the socioeconomic and environmental consequences of the agreements reached in the Uruguay Round and the potential accelerated negative impact of any further reduction of international trade barriers. They were successful because they were well organized, did not shy from unusual coalitions (among environmentalists, trade unions, women's groups), had a clear goal, and used the media and the Internet masterfully. But beyond the specifics, the message of Seattle was clear: the international system has a significant democratic deficit and a disregard for peoples' concerns about their livelihood and the welfare of the planet.

Charter 99—A Charter for Global Democracy (1999) is an initiative that expresses the concern for accountability in the structures of global governance in the following way:

> The United Nations has been sidelined, while the real business of world government is done elsewhere. Global policies are discussed and decided behind closed doors by exclusive groups, such as the G8 [grouping of high-income, industrialized nations], OECD, the Bank of International Settlements, the World Bank, the International Monetary Fund, the World Trade Organization and others. These agencies are reinforced by informal networks of high officials and powerful alliances such as NATO [North Atlantic Treaty Organization] and the EU. Together they have created what can be seen as dominant and exclusive institutions of world government. All too often they are influenced by TNCs which pursue their world strategies. These agencies of actual world government must be made accountable. If there are to be global policies, let them be answerable to the peoples of this world.

No international organization should believe itself secure enough to disregard the issue of democratization. WHO, the World Bank, and all agencies and alliances involved in international and global public health will need to act on this count; if not, they will be ill prepared for the conflicts around the big health issues of the near future: TRIPs and ownership of patents, genetic engineering, access to treatments, health inequalities, and human rights.

Although the pooling of internal sovereignty of nation states in public health matters seems a more probable strategy at the regional than at the global level, as the EU experience indicates, it also carries with it the danger of further increasing the distance between policy makers and citizens. Again, this risk is exemplified in the problems that the EU faces with its democratic legitimization with the peoples of Europe, despite the fact that it gives access and voice to cities and regions as well as NGOs and is controlled by an elected European parliament. In light of the European experience, it is fair to say that, although it would not solve the participation or accountability issue, some form of people's assembly on health should be explored as a mechanism to involve a wide variety of actors. The Global Health Watch that is under consideration can be a first step in this direction (Rockefeller Foundation, 1999).

## THE GLOBAL HEALTH VALUE BASE

As the role of TNCs and TNSMs becomes more pronounced in the public health arena, their systematic inclusion in global health governance becomes increasingly urgent, not least to ensure a level of accountability, which is presently weak and frequently inappropriate. The established policy mechanisms of international health institutions and agencies are not yet equipped to respond adequately to the emerging multitude of players and agendas, increasing political fragmentation, lack of authority, and lack of accountability. The international system continues to function in a state-centric and issue-specific manner, lurching from one priority health problem to the next: polio, AIDS, malaria, tobacco, tuberculosis. All the major new alliances in international public health have been created around a single disease, and it seems that many NGO initiatives and policy networks follow the same pattern. This approach risks cluttering the health agenda with the globalization of disease rather than focusing on strategies that aim for a global investment in health determinants. It could be argued, as Kaul, Grunberg, and Stern (1999) have done, that "the pervasiveness of today's crises suggests that they might all suffer from a common cause, such as a common flaw in policy making, rather than from issue-specific problems. If so, issue-specific responses, typical to date, would be insufficient—allowing global crises to persist and even multiply" (p. xxi).

This consideration of accountability and formulated strategies leads to a central issue in global public health, namely its underlying social ethic or value base that unites the global community around common goals. A shared value base has been elusive as divergent principles remain commonplace. For example, universal access to health care and affordable drugs is at odds with the ideology of market forces and privatization in health. Paradoxically, the orthodoxy of privatization exists alongside the growing recognition of the relationship among social justice, wealth, and health (Sen, 1999; Daniels, Kennedy, & Kawachi, 1999; Kapstein, 1999), and attempts to frame public health within a human rights perspective. More complex and ambiguous, though, are the ethical principles that guide the balance between global goods and goals and local priorities, the setting of global priorities, and the dilemmas posed by the establishment of vertical disease programs and their consequences for the strengthening of health systems. The ethical implications of present choices in international public health are rarely discussed. Indications are, though, that issues of universality, consent, priority setting, accessibility, equity, and fairness, which used to be part of the domestic agenda, are now critical at the global level.

### Privatization versus Social Responsibility

Price and colleagues (1999) see "huge implications" of the privatization-oriented policies of international institutions "for European traditions of democracy and community risk sharing" and (as might be added) for the principles

under which health systems in low- and middle-income nations are being established. Increasingly—so their analysis suggests—the principles of equity and universality are being replaced by the notion of consumer sovereignty within a privately managed system. As part of the global commerce of ideas, networks of consultants are consistently pushing for a globalization of the dominant American ethics in health care, which view health care as a predominantly private commodity (Reinhardt, 1999). The extent of the problem becomes clear when one considers that if the countries of Europe are finding it hard to resist this force, the situation for the low- and middle-income countries in the context of structural adjustment and debt is particularly precarious. For example, in the past 15 years structural adjustment policies for economic reform promoted by international banks have caused governments to cut health care budgets by a third to a half in most sub-Saharan countries (Evans, 1995). In many low- and middle-income countries, public sector contraction has often resulted in private sector expansion. Consequently, the private health care sector has grown significantly in these countries. In India, 78% of overall health expenditure is private, amounting to 4.7% of its gross national product (GNP) (Naylor, Jha, Woods, & Shariff, 1999). Research in developing counties demonstrates that the poor spend a disproportionate part of their income on drugs that are frequently inappropriate or harmful or provide only partial treatment. Private spending on health is encouraged in all low- and middle-income countries as a consequence of the increasing flow and availability of drugs on the global market. In many countries, quality control of private health care provision is frequently inadequate (Brugha & Zwi, 1998), and as a result, the lowest-income populations often further impoverish themselves (for example, by assuming debts) for inappropriate treatment; such treatment sometimes fosters the emergence of drug resistance that make diseases even more difficult to treat. Other problems linked to new types of global markets are appearing: for example, the ethics of an international commodification and trade in organs (for example, poor Indians selling their kidneys) (Cohen, 1999; Radcliffe-Richards, 1998).

## Social Justice

The director general of WHO has warned that "solidarity in health care financing counts among the major social achievements of the twentieth century in all but a few industrialized nations" (Brundtland, 1999b). In the face of the present inequalities in health and health care and the significant differences in the values that guide key actors in the international public health arena (Reinhardt, 1999), a global consensus on the principles of sustainable health systems will be difficult to achieve. Countries that have provided—even if they are low-income countries—access to basic health and welfare services and education (particularly of women) have made significantly more social and economic progress than those that have not (Caldwell, 1986). In terms of life expectancy, low- and middle-income countries that have invested in the social sectors compare well even with the most industrialized countries. Costa Rica, for example, by 1991 achieved a life expectancy of 76 years for its citizens, compared with an average of 77 years for the world's 22 highest income countries. It did this on a national income level of US$1,850 per capita, compared with an income level of US$21,050 per capita in the 22 highest income nations (Hertzman, 1996).

Amataya Sen (1999) takes up this issue as an argument for a new paradigm in development policy that combines development and freedom and takes as its starting point the creation of social opportunities. This investment-based approach (broadly defined as public support for the social sectors) is also championed by Ethan Kapstein (1999), who proposes to convene a new Bretton Woods Conference early in the twenty-first century to address the issue of global distributive justice and explore the impact of globalization on the least advantaged. Embedded in Kapstein's agenda is the proposal of an inter-

national social minimum, which would expect each country to define what constitutes a basic standard of living, including access to health and education. A new type of World Bank or a new UNDP (as is now being envisaged with a focus on global governance) would compile annual social policy reports, just as the IMF produces studies of macroeconomic performance.

Sen (1999) and others stress the crucial contribution public health makes to the economic well-being of societies, and from this perspective it should be high on the agenda of those promoting globalization as well as those promoting economic efficiency. Nothing can be seen as less efficient than the tragic waste of human resources that we presently witness worldwide through poverty, inequality, illness, and premature mortality. Indeed, as Hence and colleagues (1997) demonstrate, the success of South Korea and Hong Kong in rapid reduction of mortality is not due only to economic growth but to "growth mediated" policies, which allowed for the growth process to be wide and participatory and included policies such as full employment. Both support-led and growth-mediated policies run counter to the development orthodoxies of the 1980s and 1990s, which placed undue salience on sale of public assets and private finance of social services.

Health, as a resource, should be recognized as a crucial component of economic globalization because it is linked to the need for stability and security that foreign investors seek. In that "people and companies are more likely to invest in countries where health risks are manageable" (Rosecrance, 1999), a healthy population becomes a critical asset for the development of a country, enabling its participation in the global economy. Again, this principle does not apply only to the low-income countries, where it might seem more obvious. Keating and Hertzman (1999) argue that health is a crucial resource for societies that want to stay competitive in the twenty-first century, and this thought is echoed by Rosecrance (1999), who outlines how the new economy depends on a well educated and healthy work force. Health creates social opportunities; it allows individuals and communities to act. "With adequate social opportunities, individuals can effectively shape their own destiny and help each other. They need not be seen primarily as passive recipients of the benefits of cunning development programs" (Sen, 1999).

**Human Rights**

The issue of human rights is interwoven with the debate about fairness and access to opportunities and capabilities, but it brings one additional element to the international arena: human rights shifts the focus from concern with the sovereign authority of nation states to a regard for the individual. The global value system increasingly refuses to accept the infringement of certain human rights and is aiming to establish mechanisms of accountability in this domain. Fox (1997) contends that, "On or about 3 December 1992 the character of the international community changed" (p. 105). The decision of the UN Security Council to intervene in Somalia opened the door legitimately to ask the question whether decisions on humanitarian matters should be located at the national or at the international level. Fox attributes this disjuncture to a major normative change in the international system (pushed through the consistent efforts of human rights advocates). The institutional manifestation of this shift is embodied by the establishment of the Yugoslav war crimes tribunal.

This tension finds expression in the health sector in the complex balance between the public health concern with the population health and the individual human rights concern with the rights of the citizen. The tobacco industry has attempted to exploit this ambiguity in the countries of central and eastern Europe by entering into alliances with civil rights groups to promote the notion that smoking constitutes an individual right and freedom that deserves protection in the new democracies. Das (1999) draws attention to the lack of concern with citizenship and consent in the context of global immunization programs. She quotes from a UNICEF report, which attributes the success in immunization coverage to strategies that include "withholding

birth certificates (and thus denying any government child subsidies) until the child is immunized" (p. 105). Interning patients with sexually transmitted infections has been practiced in various countries. A further example involves the behavior of the international (mainly Western) media in the face of a health crisis or outbreak in low- and middle-income countries (Cash & Narasimhan, 1999). The "benign" circumvention of sovereignty and citizenship that is reflected in such well-intended global programs (such as childhood immunization) could well develop a more sinister dimension related to human rights issues.

Should there be a right to international intervention in response to disease outbreaks and concerns such as bioterrorism? Presently, the lack of health infrastructure in low- and middle-income countries makes the intervention of institutions from the industrialized countries necessary in times of crisis. Emergency humanitarian assistance has begun to overshadow the regular long-range development work that characterized the efforts of the UN during the 1970s and 1980s. The expertise to deal with an outbreak is frequently not available at country level because of lack of resources or laboratory facilities. Only a few laboratories worldwide can provide the technology and expertise to detect new viruses and other organisms. National interest, organizational reputation, and personal ambition each play a role in the efforts of agencies, institutes, and NGOs to be the first at the scene of an outbreak and to determine the cause, and to be in charge of control efforts with little regard for the coordinating role of WHO (as mandated in its constitution). The Ebola outbreak in Kikwit had the Western media competing to capture photos of people dying of the disease, with scant concern for the right to privacy or consent. Similar examples can be told from refugee camps, environmental disaster areas, and zones of civil strife. Yet can the global community continue to accept that countries cannot, or are not willing to, comply with international public health agreements? If not, who should decide whether the situation in those countries constitutes a threat to global public health, or if there have been serious breaches of human rights with regard to health? Similarly, where should the power of arbitration and legitimate authority reside?

## Health as a Global Public Good

The notions of social responsibility, justice, and human rights have been brought together in the recent proposal to conceptualize health as a global public good (Kaul et al., 1999). Global public goods are defined as outcomes (or intermediate products) that tend toward universality in that they benefit all countries, population groups, and generations (see Exhibit 14–2). At a minimum, a global public good should meet the following criteria: its benefits extend to more than one group of countries, and they do not discriminate against any population group or any set of generations, present or future. Kaul and colleagues draw attention to the two key issues that arise from this definition: (1) who defines the political agenda and sets priorities in relation to the provision of global public goods, and (2) who determines and ensures access to them.

Health belongs to the group of global public goods that are underprovided in many parts of the world despite the potential for providing them through better allocation and distribution of resources. The wealth and health of one part of the world is increasingly created at the cost of development of other parts; this imbalance results in the marginalization of many population groups and countries from the global society—and from the benefits such development brings, including access to the resources that create health. At the same time, the increased common dependence on stable financial markets, security from international crime and terrorism, and protection from environmental disasters and epidemics provide powerful incentives for creating a common cause and acting with common purpose to achieve healthy populations globally. It is this appeal to enlightened self-interest that makes Chen and colleagues (1999) optimistic about health being more easily accepted as a global public good than some of the other areas that have been proposed.

One would expect relatively little contention in accepting health as a global public good— particularly in relation to taking action that protects populations from both communicable and noncommunicable diseases. But even if eradicating a certain disease or immunizing all children is a global public good that will benefit all, decisions made at the global level for the good of the larger community are not always universally viewed in the same way. Despite the transnationalization of certain values, many contest the notion of a "global village," in which all national identity, tradition, and cultural and institutional differences are extinct (Graubard, 1999). Conflicts arose within Western countries during the nineteenth century with regard to compulsory vaccination and controls instituted by a new cadre of public health inspectors. Western experts may consider these problems "solved" and not relevant to internationally created public health campaigns. Yet societal consensus on many of these issues (such as informed consent, disclosure, patient autonomy) has yet to be established in many low- and middle-income countries. Lack of information and literacy exacerbates the challenges inherent in handling these ethical considerations, even if an awareness of them exists. The highest degree of transparency is therefore crucial with regard to, for example, the field testing of certain drugs and therapies in low- and middle-income countries.

Das (1999) draws attention to the imbalance between the very vocal ethical debate around HIV/AIDS, which is dominated by the voices of activists from the industrialized countries, and the silence around the ethical issues involved in other diseases that predominantly affect the marginalized communities of low- and middle-income countries. While the classification of a public health issue as a global priority—such as polio eradication—may provide low- and middle-income countries access to donor funding, this classification does not necessarily help them develop sustainable health systems. Moreover, the benefits of some global health campaigns may favor the industrialized countries more than the lower- and middle-income regions (Taylor

**Exhibit 14–2** Global Public Goods (and Bads)

Public goods, broadly speaking, are characterized by their benefits being "public." Pure public goods are defined by their non-excludability and non-rival consumption. These are economic concepts that have important public health ramifications. *Non-excludable* implies that once the good is produced, its benefits are available to all (for example, street names and traffic lights). *Non-rival consumption* implies that once the good is produced, it cannot be depleted through its consumption. Peace, for example, when it is obtained, can be enjoyed by all of a country's citizens (non-excludable), and its benefit by one group of citizens does not deny another group a similar benefit (non-rival). Many goods that have elements of either attribute are considered public, although impure, goods (for example, education and immunization). Public goods are generally inadequately supplied because there are no strong market incentives to provide them (market failure). Public goods (generally) depend on public provisioning (that is, collective action). Paradoxically, even when public goods are supplied, there are often problems associated with access to them (for example, the World Wide Web could be construed as a public good, yet access to it requires hardware such as a computer and phone line). The "publicness" of a good is, therefore, technically as well as socially and politically determined.

Public goods are associated with strong positive "externalities". Externalities arise when individuals and groups take actions but do not bear all of the consequences (externalities) of those actions, be they good (positive) or bad (negative). Externalities are therefore by-products of action. When such spillovers create costs for the public, they are termed "public bads." For example, the misuse of antibiotics that results in drug resistant pathogens has costs far beyond those who have mis-prescribed or mis-consumed them. Multidrug resistant microbes constitute a public bad.

The notion of public goods has been extended to those having externalities that traverse borders. With increasing interdependence, many national public goods play a strong role in producing global public goods (that is, global level goods are linked to national level action). Global public goods reach between borders and are a blend of national and international. A pure global public good (that is, ideal type) is characterized by its universality (that is, it benefits all countries, people, and generations), whereas an impure public good would simply tend toward universality. Similarly, a global public bad would have universally negative externalities (for example, greenhouse gases that lead to ozone depletion).

et al., 1997). The central questions remains unsolved: How will global goals and local priorities be balanced and what are the ethical implications of these choices? Should low- and middle-income countries spend their limited resources to reach a global goal that in the short term benefits high-income populations and has low priority for their own children?

## A REORIENTATION OF PUBLIC HEALTH PRACTICE

In order to be prepared for global health challenges, public health professionals must be able to understand

- the factors driving population health and its determinants at the beginning of the twenty-first century—particularly those related to the major transition in demography, economy, and governance
- the power shift that is presently underway in the international health system as new actors emerge and challenge existing ones
- the necessity for novel approaches to effective policy formulation and implementation required by the processes of globalization, in particular the interface between local and global health governance.

From a public health perspective, globalization presents, according to Beaglehole and Mc-

Michael (1999) "a mixed blessing" (p. 14). There is no doubt that globalization provides a unique opportunity to reinvigorate public health and bring health issues onto the global agenda, but it also has the potential to further marginalize public health as well as the values it represents. Improvements in global public health are dependent on both professional and political leadership—as demonstrated by the spread of the HIV/AIDS epidemic. Globalization has raised the stakes, and public health must respond at a new level and with innovative strategies. The health of a population can no longer be safeguarded by national policy alone; all public health is both global and local. The following 10 actions are proposed for consideration when exploring responses to globalization in public health research, policy, and practice:

### 1. Build bridges between public health and "international" health.

If we have entered a new era of public policy (Kaul et al., 1999), in which domestic and foreign policy cannot be clearly differentiated, then public health needs to work at both ends of the policy spectrum. Hence, it is essential to improve our understanding of the global consequences of local actions and to strengthen local public health practice accordingly. A clearer awareness that public health practice has both local and global ramifications will enable the public health community to put local issues into perspective and to realize the similarity of the problems that public health practitioners are tackling around the globe. This awareness constitutes the first step toward finding common solutions and identifying joint action.

### 2. Design national public health policies to promote coherence between domestic and international public health objectives and to take into consideration the need to assume national responsibility for cross-border consequences that have public health impacts.

The global public goods (and bads) framework is premised, among other things, upon the

growing acceptance that domestic policies can have global ramifications. Chen and colleagues (1999) and Zacher (1999), for example, demonstrate that ensuring global health will remain a Sisyphian undertaking until public health systems are strengthened in all low- and middle-income countries (to reduce cross-border spillovers). Based on such arguments, Kaul and colleagues (1999) make an elegant and compelling case for all countries to internalize their cross-border spillovers on the basis of the principle of "national responsibility" (p. 472). Such an approach would require that policy makers are made aware of the transborder externalities of their policies. This leads Kaul and colleagues to call for the development of "national externality profiles" (p. 467) and a reconsideration of the distinction between domestic and international policy making. In terms of public health, such an approach would require that countries harmonize domestic and global health outcomes.

### 3. Reorient public health at all levels toward an integrative strategy that addresses health equity and the broad socioeconomic determinants of health.

As McKinlay and Marceau (2000) suggest, public health is a sociopolitical activity, multisectoral in nature, and extending to all aspects and levels of society. Public health strategies have to be more firmly linked to macroeconomic development strategies at the national and global levels.

### 4. Mainstream public health.

If public health is to have an impact on the broad socioeconomic determinants of health, public health practitioners need to be ever more willing to work with other sectors and build alliances with other partners. Public health advocates need to motivate all sectors at the local, national, and global levels to be committed to "fulfilling societies interest in assuring conditions in which people can be healthy" (U.S. Institute of Medicine, 1988). Given the present marginalization of public health, bringing health-related evidence to bear on policy makers in those sectors affecting health will not be an easy task. Accordingly, it is essential for public health professionals to work in those settings where decisions affecting health are made. The presence of a health advisor in the national security council of the United States provides an exemplary innovation at the national level, and the discussion of HIV/AIDS at the UN Security Council provides a precedent at the global level.

*5. Explore more forcefully the potential for international protocols and guidelines on health issues.*

In light of the transnationalization of health risks and the diminution of national health sovereignty, the need arises for a transnational system of consumer and individual protection that addresses the broad threats to health (such as violence, firearms, drug trafficking). The present initiative of WHO to seek adoption of the Framework Convention on Tobacco Control (WHO, 1999c) could constitute a breakthrough in international health agreements that others might follow. In a similar vein, WHO has been facilitating a consultative process to revise the International Health Regulations (IHR) (WHO, 1998b) to include the obligation for member states to report information on the course of an epidemic; to empower WHO to provide other member states with information on reported outbreaks (even if the affected member state has refused to notify WHO); and to be more specific about the actions states can legitimately take in restricting commerce and travel following a reported outbreak. Making the Regulations binding has been proposed (Fidler, 1999, p. 74). The binding nature would apply equally to reporting and to ensuring that measures taken by other countries to avoid contagion are neither excessive nor punitive. The potential exists to further strengthen their enforcement by linking their compliance to dispute settlement arbitration under the aegis of the WTO Agreement on the Application of Sanitary and Phytosanitary Measures (Plotkin & Kimball, 1997).

*6. Given global mobility of goods and people, develop new strategies for global vigilance and surveillance, as*

*practically any disease can strike anywhere.*

Surveillance, asserts Morabia (2000, p. 24), "is the bedrock of public health." Without surveillance, it is not possible to set priorities and decide strategies. Presently, global epidemiologic surveillance is constrained by a variety of factors. Low- and middle-income countries are vulnerable to unfair international treatment with respect to disease outbreaks in three ways: (1) they remain more susceptible to them; (2) they are not as well equipped to report them accurately; and (3) they are more harshly treated when outbreaks are reported. In short, these countries lack the means and incentives to participate in a global surveillance system. As Fidler (1996) points out, an effective global surveillance system will have to confront the paradox that "globalization jeopardizes disease control nationally by eroding sovereignty, while the need for international solutions allows sovereignty to frustrate disease control internationally." The weakest link in the chain remains national surveillance systems in low-income countries, which lack the resources for data collection and laboratory analyses. This weakness highlights the importance of international cooperation in developing public health capacity in low-income countries. Moreover, the provisionally revised IHRs do little to provide incentives for compliance with reporting requirements. Cash and Narasimhan (1999) propose that international organizations advocate on behalf of affected nations for economic aid following an outbreak, and that consideration be given to establishing a fund to assist nations in bearing the associated economic losses.

*7. Develop new forms of governance that strengthen partnerships and networks for health and are inclusive of all actors (local, national, and international) and sectors (including public and private).*

Increasingly, many public health initiatives will be network-based. Achieving a balanced representation of interested constituencies will be critical in ensuring the legitimacy of the arrangements that govern these initiatives, as will developing novel approaches that foster trust, transparency, equality of participation, and accountability. International donors need to consider providing financial support required for such new and more flexible public health infrastructures that are partnership, and network-based.

**8.** *Complement epidemiologic skills base of public health professionals with a variety of other disciplinary approaches and skills.*

Professionals and policy makers in national public health will increasingly need skills and competence in international law, transnational negotiations, and conflict resolution. Increasingly, such skills will include mediation, boundary-spanning, and "networking." An appreciation of policy analysis, formulation, and implementation requires that public health training embrace the disciplines of political science (including organizational and institutional analysis), international relations, and law (particularly international law). Although these disciplines and skills reflect the emerging needs of the public health field, they have yet to receive the attention they deserve in schools of public health (Beaglehole & McMichael, 1999). Public health capacity building must be put back on the national and the global health agenda.

**9.** *Broaden the focus of funding and research agencies concerned with national public health issues to take into account the close interaction between local, national, and global agendas and processes.*

As the public health implications of global interdependence remain little understood, there is need to further develop a research agenda in this field (Lee, 2000). Systematically appraising the impact of globalization on the various underlying determinants of health—particularly among various populations and regions—remains a major challenge. Without such analysis the impacts of globalization on public health cannot be accurately assessed. This analysis will require new forms of collaborative enquiry—which transcend national and institutional boundaries. It will also require the re-orientation of the perspectives of donor agencies and national bodies responsible for international health (and research).

**10.** *Develop new (and additional) types of external assistance that provide incentives and payments to countries that contribute to the production and provision of global public goods.*

With the world's wealthiest quintile now 135 times more affluent than the lowest income quintile, a strong moral argument can be made for increased levels of official development assistance (ODA). In practice, levels are low\* and declining, despite the OECD's adoption of a broader definition of development assistance, which serves to conceal decreased donor support for development activities (Raffer, 1998). A number of areas have been indicated for which greater levels of development assistance are required to support public health in low- and middle-income countries, such as support for research, surveillance, and capacity development (Kaul et al., 1999). The logic is that the provision of aid to produce global public goods (and reduce public bad) should not be motivated by altruisim, but by a sense of enlightened self-interest—indeed, a common interest. Most global public goods—including global health—cannot be achieved unless efforts are made to address problems at their root source. In the case of health, this achievement requires strengthening of health services in low- and middle-income countries (Chen et al., 1999; Zacher, 1999). Yet to suggest that the provision of global public goods is dependent on external finance alone is to miss an important point: namely that their

---

\*At the same time, the DAC ODA/GNP ratio has fallen to around 0.25%, well below the 0.33% average maintained in the 1970s and 1980s. This is some $20 billion per annum less aid than would have been had the previous level of effort been maintained" (Faure, 2000).

provision is dependent upon the coordinated action of a multitude of actors, both public and private, national and international.

## CONCLUSION

New threats to global stability are increasingly in the areas of poverty and scarcity, uneven development, the environment, and health. Pirages (1995) asserts that "infectious diseases are potentially the largest threat to human security lurking in the post-cold war world" (p. 11). Pollution and epidemics have no respect for national borders and are exacerbated by the increased mobility of people and goods. Reinicke (1998) has rightly drawn attention to the fact that no community (the world is a global village) can be sustained on such high levels of inequality as we presently witness in the world. No fewer than 80 countries have a lower per capita income than they had in 1989. The recent Human Development Report from Thailand (the first of its kind) demonstrated that its economic progress has been accompanied by great social inequalities (39% of the population, mostly rural, were found to be living in deprivation) and at an unacceptable cost to the natural resource base. "When people's lives are insecure, individuals are unable to flourish and social cohesion breaks down . . . thus as we enter the twenty-first century the major challenge for world leaders and policy makers is to ensure that human security concerns are placed at the center of the globalization debate" (Brandon, 2000). Or, from a national perspective, as stated in the Thai report,

"Overall, livelihoods have become more uncertain and threatened, social capital is being eroded, vulnerable groups have become more vulnerable and women have lost ground. All these consequences provide genuine reason for concern" (UNDP, 1999b).

We can ill afford a nongoverned world or indeed one governed by narrow, short-term, excessively profit-oriented interests. Public health professionals should refuse to view health as separate from social justice. "Globalization is a process where all people are global, but some are more global than others" (Koivusalo & Ollila, 1998).

Health is now part of the security agenda, not just in relation to the potential threat posed by bioterrorism but more so as a major determinant of social instability. In January 2000 the UN security council for the first time in its history devoted a session to "the social and economic devastation wrought by AIDS in Africa" (UN Security Council, 2000). There exists a unique historic opportunity for public health to help shape the global commitment to social justice and better living conditions. The lessons we learned in the industrialized world for national public health now need to be applied on a global scale. Global civil society is ready to move in this direction—it remains to impress upon national and international policy makers the social and economic imperative of an expanded approach to public health. If medicine is a social science, as Rudolf Virchow said in 1848 (Ackerknecht, 1981), and politics nothing but medicine on a grand scale, let public health be the champion of a healthy world.

## DISCUSSION QUESTIONS

1. List five transnational factors that arise out of globalization and specify their possible impact on public health.
2. Describe how and to what extent national health sovereignty is affected by globalization and the manner in which this may differ among industrialized and low- and middle-income countries.
3. Define governance and describe the new forms of global health governance that are emerging, including a discussion of their strengths and weaknesses.
4. What are five ways in which public health should respond to an environment characterized by globalization?

## REFERENCE

Ackerknecht, E. (1981). *Rudolf Virchow*. New York: Arno Press.

Annan, K. (1999, June). United Nations Secretary General's address to the United States Chamber of Commerce. Washington, DC.

Antia, N.H., & Uplekar, N.W. (1997). Medicalizing health research to suit the market. *National Medical Journal of India, 10*(4), 155–157.

Barnet, R.J., & Cavanagh, J. (1994). *Global dreams: Imperial corporations and the new world order*. New York: Touchstone.

Beaglehole, R., & McMichael, A.J. (1999, July). The future of public health in a changing global context. Paper presented at *Reponses to globalization: Rethinking equity in health,* an International Roundtable organized by the Society of International Development, the World Health Organization, and the Rockefeller Foundation. Geneva, Switzerland.

Berlinguer, G. (1998, May). Indivisibility and globalization of health. In *The effects of globalization on health*. Report from a symposium held at the annual meeting of the NGO Forum for Health, Geneva, Switzerland. Uppsala, Sweden: Dag Hammerskjold Foundation.

Berlinguer, G. (1999). Health and equity as a primary global goal. *Development, 42*(4), 17–21.

Bond, P. (1999). Globalization, pharmaceutical pricing and South Africa health policy: Managing confrontation with U.S. firms and politicians. Draft paper. Johannesburg, South Africa: Witwatersrand.

Brandon, J. (2000, January 3). Raising the world's standard of living. *Christian Science Monitor*.

Brugha, R., & Zwi, A. (1998). Improving the quality of private sector delivery of public health services. *Health Policy and Planning, 13*(2), 107–120.

Brundtland, G.H. (1999a). A call for health development. In WHO "WHO Report on Infectious Diseases: Removing Obstacles to Healthy Development." http://www.who.org/infectious-diseases-report/pages/textonly.html. Accessed 17 January 2000.

Brundtland, G.H. (1999b, April 9). "Global Health into a New Century." Speech by the Director General of WHO. http://www.who.int/director-general/speeches/1999/english/19990409_acc.html. Accessed 17 January 2000.

Bruyere, J. (1999). MMV goes independent: it's a new world. *TDR News, 61*. http://www.who.int/tdr/kh/rres_link.html.

Bull, H. (1977). *The Anarchical Society*. New York: Columbia University Press.

Buse, K., & Gwin, C. (1998). The World Bank and global cooperation in health: The case of Bangladesh. *Lancet, 351*, 665–669.

Buse, K., & Walt, G. (in press-a). Global public-private partnerships: Part 1—a new development in health? *International Bulletin of the World Health Organization*.

Buse, K., & Walt, G. (in press-b). Global public-private partnerships: Part 2—what are the issues for global governance? *International Bulletin of the World Health Organization*.

Buse, K., & Walt, G. (in press-c). Globalization and multilateral public-private health partnerships: Issues for health governance. In K. Lee, K. Buse, & S. Fustukian (Eds.), *Crossing boundaries: Health policy in a globalising world*. Cambridge, England: Cambridge University Press.

Caldwell, J.C. (1986). Routes to low mortality in poor countries. *Population and Development Review, 12,* 171–220.

Cash, R.A., & Narasimhan, V. (1999, July). Impediments to global surveillance of infectious disease: Economic and social consequences of open reporting. Paper presented at *Reponses to globalization: Rethinking equity in health*, an International Roundtable organized by the Society of International Development, the World Health Organization, and The Rockefeller Foundation, Geneva, Switzerland.

Castells, M. (1998). *End of millennium*. Oxford, England: Blackwell.

Cattaui, M.S. (1999, March 15). Business community takes up Kofi Annan's challenge. Press Release. Paris: International Chamber of Commerce.

Charter 99. (1999). A Charter for global democracy. http://www.charter99.org.

Chen, L.C., Evans, T.G., & Cash, R.A. (1999). Health as a global public good. In I. Kaul, I. Grunber, & M. A. Stern (Eds.), *Global public goods: International cooperation in the 21st century* (pp. 284–304). New York: Oxford University Press.

Childers, E. (1997). The United Nations and global institutions: Discourse and reality. *Global Governance, 3,* 269–276.

Cohen, L. (1999). Where it hurts: Indian medical material for an ethics of organ transplantation. *Daedalus, 128*(4), 135–166.

Corporate European Observer (CEO). (2000). Citizen's compact on the United Nations and corporations. http://www.xswall.nl/~ceo/untnc/citcom.html. Posted on 27 January 2000.

Cukier, W., Chapdelaine, A., & Collins, C. (1999). Globalization and small/firearms: A public health perspective. *Development 42*(4), 40–44.

Daniels, N., Kennedy, B.P., & Kawachi, I. (1999). Why justice is good for our health: The social determinants of health inequalities. *Daedalus, 128*(4), 215–251.

Das, V. (1999). Public goods, ethics, and everyday life: Beyond the boundaries of bioethics. *Daedalus, 128*(4), 99–134.

Deacon, B. (1999). *Towards a socially responsible globalization* (Globalism and Social Policy Programme [GASSP] occasional papers 1). Helsinki, Finland: Stakes.

Deacon, B., Hulse, M., & Stubbs, P. (1997). *Global social policy*. London: Sage.

Deutsch, C.H. (1999, December 10). Unlikely allies join with the United Nations. *New York Times*.

Diamond, J. (1997). *Guns, germs, and steel: The fates of human societies*. New York: W.W. Norton.

Diaz, T. (1999). *Making a killing*. New York: New York University Press .

Evans, I. (1995). SAPping maternal health. *Lancet, 346*(8982), 1046.

Evans, R.G. (1996, June). Keynote at the WHO European Conference on Health Care Reforms, Ljubljana.

Faure, J.C. (2000). Development Co-operation Report 1999. *DAC Journal, 1*(1).

Fidler, D. (1996). Globalization, international law and emerging infectious diseases. *Emerging Infectious Diseases, 2,* 77–84.

Fidler, D. (1999). *International law and infectious diseases*. Oxford, England: Clarendon Press.

Finnemore, M. (1996). *National interests in international society*. Ithaca, NY: Cornell University Press.

Fox, G.H. (1997). New approaches to international human rights: The sovereign state revisited. In S.H. Hashmi (Ed.), *State sovereignty: Changes and persistence in international relations* (pp. 105–130). State College, PA: Pennsylvania State University Press.

Fox, J.A., & Brown, L.D. (Eds.). (1997) *The struggle for accountability: The World Bank, NGOs, and grassroots movements*. Cambridge, MA, and London: MIT Press.

Friedman, T.L. (1999). DOScapital. *Foreign Policy, 116,* 110–116.

Frost, L., & Reich, M. (1998). *Mectizan® donation program: Origins, experiences, and relationships with coordinating bodies for onchocerciasis control*. Department of Population and International Health. Boston: Harvard School of Public Health.

Giddens, A. (1999). Reith lectures. http://news.bbc.uk.

Gilpin, R. (1987). *The Political Economy of International Relations*. Princeton, NJ: Princeton University Press.

Graubard, S.R. (1999). Bioethics and beyond. *Daedalus, 128*(4), v-vi.

Hamlin, C. (1998). *Public health and social justice in the age of Chadwick Britain 1800–1854*. Cambridge, England: Cambridge University Press.

Hashmi, S.H. (Ed.). (1997). *State sovereignty: Changes and persistence in international relations*. State College, PA: Pennsylvania State University Press.

Held, D., McGre, A., Goldbatt, D., & Perraton, J. (1999). *Global transformations. politics, economics and culture*. Stanford, CA: Stanford University Press.

Hertzman, C. (1996). What's been said and what's been hid: Population health, global consumption and the role of national health data systems. In D. Blane, E. Brunner, & R. Wilkinson (Eds.), *Health and social organization*. London and New York: Routledge.

Jamison, D.T., Frenk, J., & Knaul, F. (1988). International collective action in health: Objectives, functions, and rationale. *Lancet, 351* (9101), 514–517.

Kaferstein, F.K., Motarjemi, R., & Bettcher, D.W. (1997). Foodborne infectious disease control: a transnational challenge. *Bulletin of the World Health Organization, 3*(4), 503–510.

Kaplan, R.D. (1999, September 27). Could this be the new world? [Op ed]. *The New York Times*, p. A23.

Kapstein, E.B. (1999). Distributive justice as an international public good: A historical perspective. In I. Kaul, I. Grunberg, & M.A. Stern (Eds.), *Global public goods* (pp. 88–115). New York: Oxford University Press.

Kaul, I., Grunberg, I., & Stern, M.A. (Eds.). (1999). *Global public goods*. New York: Oxford University Press.

Kearney, M. (1995). The local and the global: The anthropology of globalization and transnationalism, *Annual Review of Anthropology, 24*, 547–565.

Keating, D.P., and Hertzman, C. (1999). *Developmental health and the wealth of nations*. New York and London: The Guilford Press.

Keck, M.E., & Sikkink, K. (1998). *Activists beyond borders*. Ithaca, NY, and London: Cornell University Press.

Keohane, R.O., & Nye, J.S., Jr. (1987). Power and interdependence revisited. *International Organization 41* (4), 724–753.

Kickbusch, I. (1997). New players for a new era: Responding to the global public health challenges. *Journal of Public Health Medicine, 19*(2), 171–178.

Kickbusch, I. (1999). Global + local: glocal public health. *Journal of Epidemiology and Community Health, 53*, 451–452.

Kickbusch, I. (in press). The international health system: Accountability intact? *Social Science and Medicine*.

Kickbusch, I., & Quick, J. (1998). Partnerships for health in the 21st century. *World Health Statistics Quarterly, 51*(1), 68–74.

Knight, M., Loayza, N., & Villanueva, D. (1996), The peace dividend: Military spending cuts and economic growth (World Bank workpapers Wps 1577). http://www.worldbank.org/html/dec/Publications/Workpapers/wps1577.

Koivusalo, M., & Ollila, E. (1998). *Making a healthy world*. London: Zed Books.

Kolata, G. (1999). *Flu: The story of the great influenza pandemic of 1918 and the search for the virus that caused it*. New York: Farrar, Straus and Giroux.

Krasner, S.D. (Ed.). (1983). International Regimes. Ithaca, NY: Cornell University Press.

Kristof, N.D. (1997, April 13). Rwandans, once death's agents, now its victims. *New York Times*, p. I1.

Lang, T. (1999). Diet, health and globalization: Five questions. *Proceedings of the Nutrition Society, 58*, 335–343.

Lee, K. (1998). *Globalization and health policy*. (Discussion Paper No. 1). London: London School of Hygiene and Tropical Medicine.

Lee, K. (2000). Globalization and health policy: A review of the literature and proposed research and policy agenda. In Pan American Health Organization, *Health and human development in the new global economy*. Washington, DC: Author.

Lurie, P., Hintzen, P., & Lowe, R.A. (1995). Socioeconomic obstacles to HIV prevention and treatment in developing countries: The roles of the IMF and the World Bank. *AIDS, 9*, 531–46.

Magnier. (1995, April 12). WTO test case held goal in US-Korea flap. *Journal of Commerce*.

Mathews, J. (1989, Spring). Redefining security. *Foreign Affairs, 730*(3), 162–177.

McKeown, T. (1976). *The role of medicine–dream, mirage or nemesis*. London: Nuffield Provincial Hospital Trust.

McKinlay, J.B., & Marceau, L.D. (2000). To boldly go . . . . *American Journal of Public Health, 90*(1), 25–33.

Michaud, C., & Murray, C.J.L. (1994). External assistance to the health sector in developing countries: A detailed analysis, 1972–1990. Reprinted from *The Bulletin of the World Health Organization, 72*(4), 639–651.

Morabia, A. (2000). Worldwide surveillance of risk factors to promote public health. *American Journal of Public Health, 90*(1), 22–24.

Navarro, V. (1998). Comment: Whose globalization? *American Journal of Public Health, 88*(5), 742–743.

Navarro, V. (1999). Health and equity in the world in the era of globalization. *International Journal of Health Services, 29*(2), 215–226.

Naylor, C.D., Jha, P., Woods, J., & Shariff, A. (1999). A fine balance: Some options for private and public health care in urban India. World Bank Human Development Network. Washington, DC: World Bank.

The non-governmental order. (1999, December 11). *The Economist*, 20–22.

Pirages, D. (1995). Microsecurity: Disease organisms and human well-being. *Washington Quarterly, 18*(4), 11.

Plotkin, B., & Kimball, A. (1997). Designing an international policy and legal framework for the control of emerging infectious diseases. *Emerging Infectious Diseases, 3*, 1–9.

Popkin, B.M. (1994). The nutrition transition in low income countries: An emerging crisis. *Nutrition Reviews, 52*, 285–298.

Price, D., Pollock, A., & Shaoul, J. (1999, November 27). How the World Trade Organisation is shaping domestic policies in health care. *Lancet, 354*, 1889–1892.

Radcliffe-Richards, J. (1998). The case for allowing kidney sales. *Lancet, 351*(9120), 1950–1952.

Raffer, K. (1998). Looking a gift horse in the mouth: Analysing donor's aid statistics. *Zagreb International Review of Economics and Business, 1*(2), 1–20.

Ramonet, I. (1999). Let them eat big macs. *Foreign Policy, 116*, 125–127.

Reinhardt, U. (1999). Social ethics and the globalization of health reform. In D.E. Holmes (Ed.), *Reflections on Globalization and Health: Consequences of the 3rd Trilateral Conference*. Washington, DC: Association of Academic Health Centers.

Reinicke, W.H. (1998). *Global public policy: Governing with government?* Washington DC: Brookings Institution Press.

Reinicke, W.H. (1999, Winter). The other World Wide Web: Global public plicy networks. *Foreign Policy.*

Rittberger, V., & Bruehl, T. (1999). Global governance: Civil society and the UN. *The United Nations University Work in Progress, 15*(3).

Rockefeller Foundation. (1999). *A New Course of Action*. New York: Rockefeller Foundation.

Rosecrance, R. (1999). *The Rise of the Virtual State*. New York: Basic Books.

Rosenau, J.N. (1995). Governance in the twenty-first century. *Global Governance, 1*(1), 13–43.

Sachs, J. (1999, August 14). Helping the world's poorest. *The Economist.*

Sen, A. (1999). *Development as freedom*. New York: Knopf.

Shkolnikov, V. (1997). The population crisis and rising mortality in transnational Russia. Unpublished, quoted in M. Bobak et al. (1998). Socioeconomic factors, perceived control and self-reported health in Russia: A cross-sectional survey. *Social Science and Medicine, 47*(2), 269–279.

Sikkink, K. (1986). Codes of conduct for transnational corporations: The case of the WHO/UNICEF code. *International Organization 40*, 815–840.

Szreter, S. (1988). The importance of social intervention in Britain's mortality decline v. 1850–1914: A reinterpretation of the role of public health. *Social History of Medicine, 1*(1), 1–38.

Taylor, C.E., Cutts, F., & Taylor, M.E. (1997). Ethical dilemmas in current planning for polio eradication. *American Journal of Public Health, 87*(6), 922–925.

Turmen, T. (1999). Making globalization work for better health. *Development, 42*(4), 8–11.

United Nations Acquired Immune Deficiency Syndrome Programme (UNAIDS)/World Health Organization (WHO). (1999). AIDS Epidemic Update. Geneva, Switzerland.

United Nations Development Program. (1999a). *Human development report*. New York: Author.

United Nations Development Program (1999b). *Human development report of Thailand 1999*. New York: Author.

United Nations High Commissioner for Refugees. (1998). "State of the world's refugees 1997." http://www.unhcr.ch/sowr97/statsum.htm. Accessed 23 October 1998.

United Nations Research Institute for Social Development (UNRISD). (1995). *States of disarray. The social effects of globalization*. London: Banson.

United Nations Security Council (2000). Security Council resolution 1308. New York: Author.

United Nations World Population Prospects: 1990. (1991). New York.

U.S. Institute of Medicine, Board of Health. (1997). *America's vital interest in global health: Protecting our people, enhancing our economy, and advancing our international interests*. Washington, DC: National Academy Press.

U.S. Institute of Medicine, Committee for the Study of the Future of Public Health (1988). *The future of public health*. Washington, DC: National Academy Press.

U.S. Trade Representative, Executive Office of the President. (1998, March 2). USTR 1998 trade policy agenda and 1997 annual report outlines ambitious global trade agenda ahead. Washington, DC.

Velasquez, G., & Boulet, P. (1997). *Globalization and Access to Drugs: Implications of the WTO/TRIPS Agreement* (World Health Organization/DAP Series No. 7). Geneva, Switzerland: World Health Organization.

Waddell, S. (1999). The evolving strategic benefits for business in collaborations with nonprofits in civil society: a strategic resources, capabilities and competencies perspective. Unpublished.

Wallach, L., & Sforza, M. (1999). *Whose trade organization? Corporate globalization and the erosion of democracy*. Washington, DC: Public Citizen.

Walt, G. (1994). *Health Policy: An introduction to process and power*. London: Zed.

Walt, G. (1998). Globalization of international health. *Lancet, 351*, 434–437.

Wapner, P. (1997). Governance in global civil society. In O.R. Young (Ed.), *Global governance: Drawing insights from environmental experience* (pp. 65–84). Cambridge, MA: MIT Press.

Wilkinson, R.G. (1999). Putting the picture together: Prosperity, redistribution, health and welfare. In M. Marmot & R.G. Wilkinson (Eds.), *Social Determinants of Health* (pp. 256–274). Oxford, England: Oxford University Press.

World Bank. (1987). *Financing health services in developing countries: An agenda for reform*. (World Bank Policy Study). Washington, DC: Author.

World Bank. (1993). *World development report 1993: Investing in health*. New York: Oxford University Press.

World Bank. (1994). *Governance: The World Bank's experience*. Washington, DC: Author.

World Bank. (1997). *Health population and nutrition strategy*. Washington, DC: Author.

World Bank. (1999). *The world development report: Entering the 21st century*. New York: Oxford University Press.

World Health Organization. (1981). Global strategy for Health for All by the Year 2000. Geneva, Switzerland: WHO.

World Health Organization. (1997a). *The Jakarta Declaration on leading health promotion into the 21st century.* Health Promotion International, 12, 261–264.

World Health Organization. (1997b). *Health and environment for sustainable development: five years after the earth summit.* Geneva, Switzerland: Author.

World Health Organization. (1998a). *The world health report 1998: Life in the 21st century, a vision for all.* Geneva, Switzerland: Author.

World Health Organization. (1998b, January). *The revision of the international health regulations.* Geneva, Switzerland: Author.

World Health Organization. (1999a). *Removing obstacles to healthy development: Report on infectious diseases.* Geneva, Switzerland: Author.

World Health Organization. (1999b, June 24). *World Health Organization guidelines on collaboration and partnerships with commercial enterprises* (Draft discussion document). Geneva, Switzerland: Author.

World Health Organization. (1999c). *Framework convention on tobacco control: The framework convention/ protocol approach* (Technical Briefing Series Paper No. 1). Geneva, Switzerland: World Health Organization and TFI.

World Health Organization Commission on Health and Environment. (1992). *Our planet, our health.* Geneva, Switzerland: World Health Organization.

Yach, D., & Bettcher, D. (1998). The globalization of public health I and II. *American Journal of Public Health, 88,* 735–741.

Yach, D., & Bettcher, D. (1999, December). Globalization of tobacco marketing, research, and industry influence: perspectives, trends and impacts on human welfare. In *Reponses to globalization: Rethinking health and equity Development, 42*(4).

Young, O.R. (1997). Rights, rules and resources in world affairs. In O.R. Young (Ed.), *Global governance: Drawing insights from environmental experience* (pp. 1–24). Cambridge, MA: MIT Press.

Zacher, M.W. (1999). Global epidemiological surveillance: International cooperation to monitor infectious diseases. In I. Kaul, I. Grunber, & M.A. Stern (Eds.), *Global public goods: International cooperation in the 21st century* (pp. 266–283). New York: Oxford University Press.

Zielinski-Gutierrez, E.C., & Kendall, C. (2000). The globalization of health and disease: The health transition and global change. In G.L. Albrecht, R. Fitzpatrick, & S.C. Scrimshaw (Eds.), *Handbook of social studies in health and medicine.* London: Sage.

# Acronyms

**ACC** Administrative Committee on Coordination (United Nations)

**AIDS** acquired immune deficiency syndrome

**ALRI** acute lower respiratory infection

**ANM** auxiliary nurse midwife

**APA** American Psychiatric Association

**ARI** acute respiratory infection

**ASEAN** Association of Southeast Asian Nations

**AZT** zidovudine

**BBC** British Broadcasting Corporation

**BCG** bacillus Calmette-Guerin (vaccine)

**BDV** Borna disease virus

**BFHI** Baby Friendly Hospital Initiative

**BHW** basic health worker

**BMI** body mass index

**CDC** Centers for Disease Control and Prevention; communicable diseases control

**CDR** case disability ratio

**CEA** cost-effectiveness analysis

**CEO** chief executive officer

**CFR** case fatality rate

**CHD** coronary heart disease

**CHE** complex humanitarian emergency

**CHW** community health worker

**CIDI** composite international diagnostic interview

**CMR** crude mortality rate

**CNN** Cable News Network

**CNRT** Council of National Resistance in East Timor

**COPD** chronic obstructive pulmonary disease

**CPM** critical path method

**CQI** continuous quality improvement

**CSO** civil society organization

**CUA** cost-utility analysis

**CVD** cardiovascular disease

**CVI** childhood vaccine initiative

**DALY** disability-adjusted life year

**DDT** dichlorodiphenyltrichloroethane

**DFID** Department for International Development (United Kingdom)

**DHLL** days of healthy life lost

**DHS** demographic and health survey

**DIS** Diagnostic Interview Schedule

**DOSMD** determinants of outcome in severe mental disorders

**DOTS** directly observed treatment short-course strategy

**DPSEEA** Driving Forces, Pressure, State, Exposure, and Effort Model

**DPT** diphtheria, pertussis, and tetanus (vaccine)

**DRF** drug revolving fund

**DSM-II** *Diagnostic and Statistical Manual* of the American Psychiatric Association, second edition

**DSM-III** *Diagnostic and Statistical Manual* of the American Psychiatric Association, third edition

**DSM-III-R** *Diagnostic and Statistical Manual* of the American Psychiatric Association, third edition-revised

**DSM-IV** *Diagnostic and Statistical Manual* of the American Psychiatric Association, fourth edition

**EC** European Commission

**ECA** Epidemiological Catchment Area

**EHRA** environmental health risk assessment

**EIA** environmental impact assessment

**EMIC** explanatory model interview catalogue

**EMRO** Eastern Mediterranean Regional Office (WHO)

**EPI** expanded program of immunizations

**ERA** environmental risk assessment

**ERHI** employment-related health insurance

**ERR** economic rate of return

**ESOSOC** Economic and Social Council

**ETEC** enterotoxigenic *E. coli*

**ETS** environmental tobacco smoke

**EU** European Union

**FAO** Food and Agriculture Organization (United Nations)

**GATS** General Agreement on Trade in Services

**GATT** General Agreement on Trade and Tariffs

**GAVI** Global Alliance for Vaccines and Immunizations

**GBD** global burden of disease

**GDP** gross domestic product

**GNP** gross national product

**HAT** human African trypanosomiasis

**HAV** hepatitis A virus

**HBV** hepatitis B virus

**Hct** hematocrit

**HCV** hepatitis C virus

**HDI** Human Development Index

**HDP** health-damaging pollutant

**HDV** hepatitis D virus

**HeaLY** healthy life year

**HEV** hepatitis E virus

**HF** hemorrhagic fever

**HINAP** Health Information Network for Advanced Planning

**HIV** human immunodeficiency virus

**HIV/AIDS** human immunodeficiency virus/acquired immune deficiency syndrome

**HMIS** Health and Management Information System

**HMOs** health maintenance organizations

**HPI** Human Poverty Index

**HPV** human papillomavirus

**HRQOL** health-related quality of life

**IARC** International Agency for Research on Cancer

**ICC** International Chambers of Commerce

**ICCIDD** International Committee for the Control of Iodine Deficiency Disorders

**ICD** International Classification of Diseases (WHO)

**ICD-10** International Classification of Diseases, tenth revision

**ICIDH** International Classification of Impairments, Disabilities, and Handicaps (WHO)

**ICN** International Conference on Nutrition

**ICPD** International Conference on Population and Development

**ICRC** International Committee of the Red Cross

**IDD** iodine deficiency disorder

**IDDM** insulin-dependent diabetes mellitus

**IDP** internally displaced person

**IFI** international financial institution

**IHR** International Health Regulations

**ILO** International Labor Organization

**IMCI** Integrated Management of Childhood Illness

**IMF** International Monetary Fund

**IMR** infant mortality rate

**INCAP** Instituto Nutricional de Central America y Panama

**INTERFET** International Force in East Timor

**IOM** Institute of Medicine

**IPCC** Intergovernmental Panel on Climate Change

**IPSS** International Pilot Study of Schizophrenia (WHO)

**IPV** injectable polio vaccine

**IQ** intelligence quotient

**IU** international units

**IUD** intrauterine device

**LCL** lower control limit

**LNHO** League of Nations Health Office

**LQAS** lot quality acceptance sampling

**MISP** Minimum Initial Service Package

**MMWR** *Morbidity and Mortality Weekly Report*

**MOH** Ministry of Health

**MONICA** monitoring trends and determinants in cardiovascular disease

**MRDM** malnutrition-related diabetes mellitus

**MSA** medical savings account

**MSF** Medecins sans Frontieres (Doctors Without Borders)

**MT** metric ton

**MUAC** mid-upper arm circumference

**NASA** National Aeronautical and Space Administration

**NATO** North Atlantic Treaty Organization

**NCD** noncommunicable disease

**NCHS** National Center for Health Statistics

**NGO** nongovernmental organization

**NGT** nominal group technique

**NHA** National Health Account

**NIDDM** noninsulin-dependent diabetes mellitus

**NIMH** National Institutes of Mental Health

**NPV** net present value

**OCHA** Office for the Coordination of Humanitarian Affairs (United Nations)

**OCP**  Onchocerciasis Control Program

**ODA**  official development assistance

**OECD**  Organization for Economic Cooperation and Development

**OPV**  oral polio vaccine

**ORS**  oral rehydration solution

**ORT**  oral rehydration therapy

**PAHO**  Pan American Health Organization

**PCB**  polychlorinated biphenyls

**PEM**  protein-energy malnutrition

**PERT**  program evaluation and review technique

**PHC**  primary health care

**PM10**  particulate matter of less than 10 microns diameter

**ppm**  parts per million

**PRA**  probabilistic risk assessment

**PRC**  People's Republic of China

**PRECEDE**  Predisposing, Reinforcing and Enabling Causes in Educational Diagnosis and Evaluation

**PRICOR**  primary care operations research

**PSA**  prostate specific antigen

**PSE**  present state examination

**PSR**  Pressure-State-Response Model

**PTSD**  posttraumatic stress disorder

**PYLL**  potential years of life lost

**QA**  quality assurance

**QALY**  quality-adjusted life year

**RAP**  rapid assessment procedures

**RDA**  recommended dietary allowance

**RDC**  research diagnostic criteria

**RDR**  relative dose response

**RHU**  Refugee Health Unit

**SADCC**  Southern African Development Coordination Conference

**SADS**  schedule for affective disorders and schizophrenia

**SADS-L**  schedule for affective disorders and schizophrenia, lifetime version

**SCAN**  schedules for clinical assessment in neuropsychiatry

**SCN**  Subcommittee on Nutrition (United Nations)

**SD**  standard deviation

**SFP**  supplementary feeding program

**SIDA**  Swedish International Development Agency

**SIP**  sector investment program

**STI**  sexually transmitted infection

**SWAp**  sector wide approach program

**TBA**  traditional birth attendant

**TEA**  total exposure assessment

**TFP**  therapeutic feeding program

**TFR**  total fertility rate

**TGR**  total goiter rate

**TNC**  Transnational Corporation

**TNSM**  Transnational Social Movement

**TRIP**  Trade-Related Aspects of Intellectual Property

**TSH**  thyroid-stimulating hormone

**TT**  tetanus toxoid

**TTS**  temporary threshold shift

**UCL**  upper control limit

**UI**  urinary iodine

**UK**  United Kingdom

**UN** United Nations

**UNAIDS** United Nations Acquired Immune Deficiency Syndrome (Programme)

**UNCHR** United Nations Commission on Human Rights

**UNCTAD** United Nations Conference on Trade and Development

**UNDP** United Nations Development Programme

**UNESCO** United Nations Educational, Scientific and Cultural Organization

**UNFPA** United Nations Population Fund

**UNHCR** United Nations High Commissioner for Refugees

**UNICEF** United Nations Children's Fund

**US$** United States dollars

**USAID** United States Agency for International Development

**USCR** United States Committee for Refugees

**USI** universal salt iodization

**UV** ultraviolet

**UVR** ultraviolet irradiation

**VHC** village health committee

**WFP** World Food Programme

**WHA** World Health Assembly

**WHO** World Health Organization

**WPRO** Western Pacific Regional Office (WHO)

**WTO** World Trade Organization

**YLD** years lived with disability

**YLL** years of life lost

# Sources

## INTRODUCTION

**Exhibit I–1** Reprinted from B.J. Turnock, *Public Health: What it is and How it Works,* 2nd Edition, 2000, Aspen Publishers, Inc.

**Exhibit I–2** Reprinted with permission from H.V. Feinberg, Ethical Approaches to Health and Development, in *Ethical Dilemmas in Health and Development,* K. Aoki, ed., pp. 3–13, © 1994, Japan Science Society Press.

**Exhibit I–4** Reprinted with permission from Message from the Director General, *World Health Report,* pp. viii-xi, © 1999, World Health Organization.

## CHAPTER 1

**Exhibit 1–1** Reprinted with permission from *A Primary Health Care Strategy for Ghana,* © 1978, Ministry of Health, Republic of Ghana.

**Exhibit 1–2** Reprinted from *World Development Report,* © 1998, The World Bank, used with permission by Oxford University Press.

**Exhibit 1–5** Reprinted with permission from C.J.L. Murray, et al., *Summary Measures of Population: Health GPE Discussion Paper,* © 1999, World Health Organization.

**Figure 1–2** Reprinted with permission from A.A. Hyder, G. Rotlant, and R.H. Morrow, Measuring the Burden of Disease: Healthy Life Years, *American Journal of Public Health,* Vol. 88, pp. 196–202, © 1998.

**Figure 1–5** Reprinted from C.J.L. Murray and A.D. Lopez, eds., *The Global Burden of Disease and Injury 1990,* Tables 6–7, © 1996, World Health Organization, used with permission by the Harvard Center for Population and Development Studies.

**Figure 1–7** Reprinted with permission from *World Health Report 1999: Making a Difference,* Chapter 1, © 1999, World Health Organization.

**Figure 1–8** Reprinted with permission from *World Health Report 1999: Making a Difference,* Chapter 1, © 1999, World Health Organization.

**Table 1–1** Data from Ghana Health Assessment Team, A Quantatitive Method for Assessing the Health Impact of Different Diseases in Less Developed Countries, *International Journal of Epidemiology,* Vol. 10, pp. 73–80, © 1981 and C.J.L. Murray and A. Lopez, eds., *The Global Burden of Disease,* © 1996, World Health Organization.

**Table 1–2** Data from C.J.L. Murray and A. Lopez, eds., *Global Health Statistics 1990,* World Health Organization, © 1996.

**Table 1–3** Data from Ghana Health Assessment Team, A Quantatitive Method for Assessing the Health Impact of Different Diseases in Less Developed Countries, *International Journal of Epidemiology,* Vol. 10, pp. 73–80, © 1981.

**Table 1–8** Adapted with permission from United Nations Children's Fund, *State of the World's Children 1999,* © 1999, UNICEF.

**Table 1–9** Reprinted from C.J.L. Murray and A.D. Lopez, eds., *The Global Burden of Disease and Injury 1990,* Tables 6–7, © 1996, World Health Organization, used with permission by the Harvard Center for Population and Development Studies.

**Table 1–10** Reprinted from C.J.L. Murray and A.D. Lopez, eds., *The Global Burden of Disease and Injury 1990,* Tables 6–7, © 1996, World Health Organization, used with permission by the Harvard Center for Population and Development Studies.

**Table 1–11** Reprinted from C.J.L. Murray and A.D. Lopez, eds., *The Global Burden of Disease and Injury 1990,* Tables 6–7, © 1996, World Health Organization, used with permission by the Harvard Center for Population and Development Studies.

**Table 1–12** Reprinted from C.J.L. Murray and A.D. Lopez, eds., *The Global Burden of Disease and Injury 1990,* Tables 6–7, © 1996, World Health Organization, used with permission by the Harvard Center for Population and Development Studies.

**Table 1–13** Reprinted with permission from *World Health Report 1999: Making a Difference,* Chapter 1, © 1999, World Health Organization.

**Table 1–14** Reprinted with permission from *World Health Report 1999: Making a Difference,* Chapter 1, © 1999, World Health Organization.

**Table 1–15** Reprinted from C.J.L. Murray and A.D. Lopez, *The Global Burden of Disease and Injuries 1990,* Chapter 5, © 1996, World Health Organization, used with permission by Harvard Center for Population and Development Studies.

**CHAPTER 2**

**Exhibit 2–2** Reprinted with permission from S.C.M. Scrimshaw and E. Hurtado, *Rapid Assessment Procedures for Nutrtition and Primary Health Care: Anthropological Approaches to Improving Program Effectiveness (RAP),* p. 26, © 1987, UCLA Latin American Center.

**Exhibit 2–4** *The Relevance of Social Science for Medicine,* I. Eisenberg and A. Kleinman, eds., The Meaning of Symptoms: A Cultural Hermeneutic Model for Clinical Practice, B.J. Good and M.J.D. Good, © 1981, with kind permission of Kluwer Academic Publishers.

**Figure 2–1** Reprinted with permission from S.C.M. Scrimshaw and E. Hurtado, *Rapid Assessment Procedures for Nutrtition and Primary Health Care: Anthropological Approaches to Improving Program Effectiveness (RAP),* p. 26, © 1987, UCLA Latin American Center.

**CHAPTER 3**

**Exhibit 3–1** Data from *World Population Prospects: The 1998 Revision,* Volume 1, © 1998, United Nations.

**Exhibit 3–3** **Bar graph:** Data from J. Cleland, et al., *The Determinants of Reproductive Change in Bangladesh,* © 1994, The World Bank and Mitra, et al.,

**Exhibit 3–4** Adapted with permission from J. Cleland, et al., *The Determinants of Reproductive Change in Bangladesh,* pp. 105–110, © 1994, The World Bank.

**Exhibit 3–5** Adapted with permission from J. Cleland, et al., *The Determinants of Reproductive Change in Bangladesh,* pp. 111–112, © 1994, The World Bank.

**Exhibit 3–6** Adapted with permission from J. Cleland, et al., *The Determinants of Reproductive Change in Bangladesh,* pp. 111–112, © 1994, The World Bank.

**Figure 3–1** Data from *World Population Prospects: The 1998 Revision,* Volume 1, © 1998, United Nations.

**Figure 3–2** Data from *World Population Prospects: The 1998 Revision,* Volume 1, © 1998, United Nations.

**Figure 3–3** Data from *World Population Prospects: The 1998 Revision,* Volume 1, © 1998, United Nations.

**Figure 3–5** Edited by D.T. Jamison, et al., *Disease Control Priorities in Developing Countries,* Figure 17.1, Copyright 1993 The International Bank for Reconstruction and Development/The World Bank. Used by permission of Oxford University Press, Inc.

**Table 3–1** Data from *World Population Prospects: The 1998 Revision,* Volume 1, © 1998, United Nations.

**Table 3–2** Adapted with permission of the Population Council, from John Bongaarts, "The Fertility-Inhibiting Effects of the Intermediate Fertility Variables," *Studies in Family Planning,* Vol. 13, No. 6/7, (June/July 1982) pp. 182–183.

**Table 3–3** Adapted with permission of the Population Council, from John Stover, "Revising the Proximate Determinants of Fertility Framework: What Have We Learned in the Past 20 Years?, " *Studies in Family Planning,* Vol. 29, No. 3, (September 1998) p. 263.

**Table 3–4** Reprinted with permission from A.O. Tsui, J.N. Wasserheit, and J.G. Haaga, eds., *Reproductive Health in Developing Countries. Expanding Dimensions, Building Solutions,* Panel on Reproductive Health, Committee on Population, Commission on Behavioral and Social Sciences, and Education, Copyright 1997 by the National Research Council. Courtesy of the National Academy Press, Washington, D.C.

**Table 3–5** Reprinted with permission from A.O. Tsui, J.N. Wasserheit, and J.G. Haaga, eds., *Reproductive Health in Developing Countries. Expanding Dimensions, Building Solutions,* Panel on Reproductive Health, Committee on Population, Commission on Behavioral and Social Sciences, and Education, Copyright 1997 by the National Research Council. Courtesy of the National Academy Press, Washington, D.C.

**Table 3–6** Reprinted with permission from A.O. Tsui, J.N. Wasserheit, and J.G. Haaga, eds., *Reproductive Health in Developing Countries. Expanding Dimensions, Building Solutions,* Panel on Reproductive Health, Committee on Population, Commission on Behavioral and Social Sciences, and Education, Copyright 1997 by the National Research Council. Courtesy of the National Academy Press, Washington, D.C.

**Table 3–7** Reprinted with permission from A.O. Tsui, J.N. Wasserheit, and J.G. Haaga, eds., *Reproductive Health in Developing Countries. Expanding Dimensions, Building Solutions,* Panel on Reproductive Health, Committee on Population, Commission on Behavioral and Social Sciences, and Education, Copyright 1997 by the National Research Council. Courtesy of the National Academy Press, Washington, D.C.

**Table 3–8** Adapted with permission from R.A. Bulatao, *The Value of Family Planning Programs in Developing Countries,* Table 1, © 1998, RAND.

**Table 3–9** Adapted with permission from R.A. Bulatao, *The Value of Family Planning Programs in Developing Countries,* Table 2, © 1998, RAND.

**Table 3–10** Reprinted with permission from Population Division, Department of Economic and Social Affairs of the United National Secretariat (1999), *World Contraceptive Use 1998,* (United Nations, New York, Sales No. E.99.XIII.4), http://www.undp.org/popin/wdtrends/scu/scupwld.txt

**Table 3–11** Adapted with permission from Committee on Population, Working Group on Health Consequences of Contraceptive Use and Controlled Fertility, *Contraception and Reproduction. Health Consequences for Women and Children in the Developing World.* Copyright 1989 by the National Research Council. Courtesy of the National Academy Press, Washington, D.C.

**Table 3–12** Data from Committee on Population, Working Group on Health Consequences of Contraceptive Use and Controlled Fertility, *Contraception and Reproduction. Health Consequences for Women and Children in the Developing World.* Copyright 1989 by the National Research Council. Courtesy of the National Academy Press, Washington, D.C.; and J.N. Hobcraft, Does Family Planning Save Lives?, *International Conference on Better Health for Women and Children through Family Planning,* Nairobi, October 5–9.

**Table 3–13** Reprinted with permission from A.O. Tsui, J.N. Wasserheit, and J.G. Haaga, eds., *Reproductive Health in Developing Countries. Expanding, Dimensions, Building Solutions.* Panel on Reproductive Health, Committee on Population, Commission on Behavioral and Social Sciences, and Education, Copyright 1997 by the National Research Council. Courtesy of the National Academy Press, Washington, D.C.

**Table 3–14** Edited by D.T. Jamison, et al., *Disease Control Priorities in Developing Countries,* Table 17.3, Copyright 1993 The International Bank for Reconstruction and Development/The World Bank. Used by permission of Oxford University Press, Inc.

**Table 3–15** Adapted with permission from Committee on Population, Working Group on Health Consequences of Contraceptive Use and Controlled Fertility, *Contraception and Reproduction. Health Consequences for Women and Children in the Developing World.* Copyright 1989 by the National Research Council. Courtesy of the National Academy Press, Washington, D.C.

**Table 3–16** Adapted with permission from Committee on Population, Working Group on Health Consequences of Contraceptive Use and Controlled Fertility, *Contraception and Reproduction. Health Consequences for Women and Children in the Developing World.* Copyright 1989 by the National Research Council. Courtesy of the National Academy Press, Washington, D.C.

**Table 3–17** Adapted with permission from Committee on Population, Working Group on Health Consequences of Contraceptive Use and Controlled Fertility, *Contraception and Reproduction. Health Consequences for Women and Children in the Developing World.* Copyright 1989 by the National Research Council. Courtesy of the National Academy Press, Washington, D.C.

## CHAPTER 4

**Figure 4–1** Reprinted from Progress Toward Elimination of Neonatal Tetanus: Egypt, 1988–1994, *Morbidity and Mortality Weekly Report,* Vol. 45, pp. 89–92, 1996, the Centers for Disease Control and Prevention.

**Figure 4–2** Reprinted with permission from C. Bern, et al., The Magnitude of the Global Problem of Diarrhoeal Disease: A Ten Year Update, *Bulletin of the World Health Organization,* Vol. 70, No. 6, p. 707, © 1992, World Health Organization.

**Figure 4–3** Reprinted with permission from P.S. Moore, Meningococcal Meningitis in Sub-Saharan Africa: A Model for the Epidemic Process, *Clinical Infectious Diseases,* Vol. 14, pp. 515–525, © 1992, University of Chicago Press.

**Figure 4–4** Reprinted with permission from P.J. Dolin, M.C. Raviglione, and A. Kochi, Global Tuberculosis Incidence Mortality During 1990–2000, *Bulletin of the World Health Organization,* Vol. 72, No. 2, p. 218, © 1994, World Health Organization.

**Figure 4–5** Reprinted with permission from World Health Organization Expert Committee on Leprosy, *World Health Organization Technical Report Series, 874,* 1998, Figure 1, Prevalence of Leprosy in the World, © 1997, World Health Organization.

**Figure 4–6** Reprinted with permission from A.C. Gerbase, J.T. Rowley, and T.E. Mertens, Global Epidemiology of Sexually Transmitted Diseases, *The Lancet,* Vol. 351, pp. 2–4, © 1998, The Lancet Ltd.

**Figure 4–7** Reprinted with permission from Adults and Children Estimated to be Living with HIV/AIDS as of the end of 1998, World Health Organization UNAIDS website, www.unaids.org/highband/document/epidemio/index.html, © 1998, UNAIDS.

**Figure 4–8** Reprinted with permission from H.S. Margolis, M.J. Alter, and S.C. Hadler, Viral Hepatitis, in *Viral Infections of Humans: Epidemiology and Control,* 4th Edition, A.S. Evans and R.A. Kaslow, eds., pp. 363–418, © 1997, Plenum Publishing Corp.

**Figure 4–9** Reprinted with permission from Hepatitis C: Global Prevalence, *Weekly Epidemiology Record,* Vol. 72, p. 342, © 1997, World Health Organization.

**Figure 4–10** Reprinted with permission from Malaria Distribution and Problem Areas, *A Global Strategy for Malaria Control,* Figure 1, © 1993, World Health Organization.

**Figure 4–11** Reprinted with permission from J.G. Rigau-Perez, et al., Dengue and Dengue Haemorrhagic Fever, *The Lancet,* Vol. 352, pp. 971–977, © 1998, The Lancet Ltd.

**Table 4–2** Reprinted with permission from S. Gove, Integrated Management of Childhood Illness by Outpatient Health Workers: Technical Basis and Overview, *Bulletin of the World Health Organization,* Vol. 75, Supplement No. 1, pp. 7–24, © 1977, World Health Organization.

## CHAPTER 5

**Exhibit 5–3** Reprinted from B.S. Hetzel, J.T. Dunn, and J.B. Stanbury, eds., *The Prevention and Control of Iodine Deficiency Disorders,* pp. 7–31, © 1987.

**Exhibit 5–6** Reprinted with permission from *International Conference on Nutrition, World Declaration and Plan of Action for Nutrition, Food and Agricultural Organization of the United Nations and World Health Organization,* Rome, December 1992, World Health Organization.

**Figure 5–2** Reprinted from D.L. Pelletier, Nutritional Status: The Master Key to Child Survival, in *Scaling Up, Scaling Down, Overcoming Nutrition in Developing Countries,* T.J. Marchione, ed., p. 2:27, © 1999 by Overseas Publishers Association, N.V. Used with permission by Gordon and Breach Publishers.

**Figure 5–3** Reprinted from D.L. Pelletier, Nutritional Status: The Master Key to Child Survival, in *Scaling Up, Scaling Down, Overcoming Nutrition in Developing Countries,* T.J. Marchione, ed., p. 2:31, © 1999 by Overseas Publishers Association, N.V. Used with permission by Gordon and Breach Publishers.

**Figure 5–4** Reprinted with permission from *4th Report on the World Nutrition Situation,* © 2000, ACC/SCN and International Food Policy Research Institute.

**Figure 5–5** Reprinted with permission from *The State of the World's Children 1998,* p. 24, © 1998, UNICEF.

**Figure 5–6** Reprinted with permission from Physical Status: The Use and Interpretation of Anthropometry, in *World Health Organization Technical Report Series 854,* p. 5:220, © 1995, World Health Organization.

**Figure 5–8** Reprinted with permission from *The Global Prevalence of Vitamin A Deficiency,* © 1995, World Health Organization.

**Figure 5–9** Reprinted from A. Sommer and K.P. West, Jr., *Vitamin Deficiency: Health, Survival, and Vision,* p. 2:30, Copyright © 1996 by the Oxford University Press, Inc. Used with permission of Oxford University Press, Inc.

**Figure 5–10** Reprinted with permission from T.H. Bothwell and R.W. Charlton, *Iron Deficiency in Women,* Report for the International Nutritional Anemia Consultative Group (INAGC), p. 35, © 1981, The Nutrition Foundation.

**Figure 5–11** Reprinted with permission from *Global Prevalence of Iodine Deficiency Disorders,* Micronutrient Deficiency Information System, p. 17, © 1993, World Health Organization.

**Figure 5–12** Copyright © John Dunn, M.D.

**Figure 5–13** Reprinted with permission from Zinc Investigators' Collaborative Group: Z.A. Bhutta, et al., Prevention of Diarrhea and Pneumonia by Zinc Supplementation in Children in Developing Countries: Pooled Analysis of Randomized Controlled Trials, *Journal of Pediatrics,* Vol. 135, No. 6, p. 693, © 1999, Mosby, Inc.

**Figure 5–14** Reprinted with permission from K.H. Brown, et al., Effect of Zinc Supplementation on Children's Growth: A Meta-Analysis of Intervention Trials, *Bibl Nutr et Dieta,* Vol. 54, p. 79, © 1998, KARGER.

**Figure 5–16** Reprinted with permission from M.K. Fleischer, Value of Prolonged Breast-feeding, Letter to the Editor, *The Lancet,* Vol. 2, p. 788, © 1988, The Lancet Ltd.

**Figure 5–17** Reprinted with permission from T.G. Sanghvi and J. Murray, Improving Child Health Through Nutrition: The Nutrition Minimum Package, *BASICS,* p. 6, © 1997 Basic Support for Institutionalizing Child Survival.

**Table 5–1** From *Human Development Report 1999* by United Nations Development Programme, copyright © 1999 by the United Nations Development Programme. Used by permission of Oxford University Press, Inc.

**Table 5–2** Adapted with permission from M. de Onis, et al., The Worldwide Magnitude of Protein-Energy Malnutrition: An Overview From the World Health Organization Global Database on Child Growth, *Bulletin of the World Health Organization,* Vol. 71, pp. 703–712, © 1993, World Health Organization.

**Table 5–5** Adapted with permission from B. Torun and F. Chew, *Modern Nutrition in Health and Disease,* M.E. Shils, et al., eds., Lippincott Williams & Wilkins, © 1999.

**Table 5–6** Adapted with permission from A. Sommer, *Vitamin A Deficiency and Its Consequences: A Field Guide to Their Detection and Control, 3rd Edition,* © 1995, World Health Organization; and *Indicators for Assessing Vitamin A Deficiency and Their Application in Monitoring and Evaluating Intervention Programs,* © 1996, World Health Organization.

**Table 5–7** Adapted with permission from *Vitamin A Supplements: A Guide to Their Use in the Treatment and Prevention of Vitamin A Deficiency and Xerophthalmia, 2nd Edition,* © 1997, World Health Organization.

**Table 5–8** Reprinted with permission from Maternal Health and Safe Motherhood Programme, *The Prevalence of Anemia in Women: A Tabulation of Available Information, 2nd Edition,* © 1992, World Health Organization.

**Table 5–9** Data from *Iron Deficiency Anemia: Prevention, Assessment and Control,* Report of WHO/UNICEF/UN Consultation, © 1998, World Health Organization.

**Table 5–10** Reprinted with permission from R.L. Stoltzfus and M.L. Dreyfuss, *Guidelines for Use of Iron Supplements to Prevent and Treat Iron Deficiency Anemia,* International Nutrition Anemia Consultative Group/ World Health Organization/ United Nations Children's Fund, © 1998, ILSI Press.

**Table 5–11** Adapted with permission from *Indicators for Assessing Iodine Deficiency Disorders and Their Control Through Salt Iodization,* © 1994, World Health Organization.

**Table 5–12** Adapted with permission from *Indicators for Assessing Iodine Deficiency Disorders and Their Control Through Salt Iodization,* © 1994, World Health Organization.

## CHAPTER 6

**Figure 6–1** Reprinted from *British Medical Journal,* Vol. 318, pp. 933–936, © 1999, with permission from the BMJ Publishing Group.

**Figure 6–2** Reprinted from C.J.L. Murray and A. Lopez, eds., *The Global Burden of Disease,* © 1996, World Health Organization. Used with permission by Harvard University Press.

**Figure 6–3** Data from M. Karvonen, et al., A Review of the Recent Epidemiological Data on the Worldwide Incidence of Type 1 (insulin-dependent) Diabetes Mellitus, *Diabetologia,* Vol. 36, pp. 883–892, © 1993, World Health Organization DIAMOND Project Group.

**Figure 6–4** Adapted with permission from K.G. Manton, L. Corder, and E. Stallard, Chronic Disability Trends in Elderly United States Populations: 1982–1994, in *Procedures of the National Academy of Science 94,* pp. 2593–2598, Copyright 1997 National Academy of Sciences, U.S.A.

**Figure 6–5** Reprinted from C.J.L. Murray and A. Lopez, eds., *The Global Burden of Disease,* © 1996, World Health Organization. Used with permission by Harvard Center for Population and Development Studies.

**Figure 6–6** Reprinted with permission from M. McKenna, *The World Health Report 1997: Conquering Suffering Enriching Humanity,* © 1998, World Health Organization.

## CHAPTER 7

**Exhibit 7–2** Data from T.N.K. Raju, The Nobel Chronicles, *The Lancet,* Vol. 352, p. 1714, © 1998, The Lancet Ltd.

**Exhibit 7–3** Reprinted with permission from Swaminathan S. Anklesaria Aiyar, We Need More Slums, *Indian Express,* p. 8, © 1998.

**Exhibit 7–4** Copyright © V. Nelly Salgado de Snyder.

**Figure 7–1** Data from *World Health Report 1999,* Annex table 3, 1999, World Health Organization.

**Figure 7–2** Data from P. Cowley and R.J. W. Wyatt, Schizophrenia and Manic-Depressive Illness, in *Disease Control Priorities in Developing Countries,* D.T. Jamison, et al., eds., © 1993, Oxford University Press for World Bank.

**Figure 7–4** Reprinted with permission from *The Lancet,* Vol. 349, No. 3, pp. 115–135, © 1997, The Lancet Ltd.

**Table 7–1** Data from *The Global Burden of Disease,* Vol. 1, p. 271, © 1996, World Health Organization.

## CHAPTER 8

**Exhibit 8–3** Reprinted with permission from Smith, *Biofuels, Air Pollution, and Health: A Global Review,* © 1997, Plenum Publishing Corp.

**Exhibit 8–4** Data from K.R. Smith, *National Burden of Disease from Indoor Air Pollution in India,* © 1998, Indira Gandhi Institute of Development Research.

**Figure 8–1** Reprinted from C.J.L. Murray and A.D. Lopez, *The Global Burden of Disease and Injury,* © 1996, World Health Organization. Used with permission by Harvard Center for Population and Development Studies.

**Figure 8–2** Adapted with permission from S. Tong, et al., Lifetime Exposure to Environmental Lead and Children's Intelligence at 11–13 years: The Pt. Pine Cohort Study, *British Medical Journal,* Vol. 312, pp. 1569–1570, © 1996, BMJ Publishing Group.

**Figure 8–3** Reprinted with permission from Smith, *Biofuels, Air Pollution, and Health: A Global Review,* © 1997, Plenum Publishing Corp.

**Figure 8–6** Data from M. Bobak and D. Leon, Air Pollution and Infant Mortality in the Czech Republic 1968–1988, *The Lancet,* Vol. 340, pp. 1010–1014, © 1992, The Lancet Ltd.

**Figure 8–7** Adapted with permission from T. Kjellström and C. Corvalan, Framework for the Development of Environmental Health Indicators, *World Health Statistics Quarterly,* Vol. 48, pp. 144–154, © 1995, World Health Organization; and C. Corvalan, et al., Development of Environmental Health Indicators, in *Linkage Methods for Environment and Health Analysis,* World Health Organization.

**Figure 8–8** Adapted from D. Smith, Worldwide Trends in DDT Levels in Human Breast Milk, *International Journal of Epidemiology,* Vol. 28, pp. 179–188, Copyright © 1999 by Oxford University Press, Inc. Used by permission of Oxford University Press, Inc.

**Figure 8–9** Data from A.K.N. Reddy, R.H. Williams, and T.B. Johansson, *Energy After Rio: Prospects and Challenges,* p. 176, © 1997, United Nations Development Programme.

**Figure 8–10** Adapted from *Global Environmental Change,* Vol. 9, P. Martens, et al., Climate Change and Future Populations at Risk of Malaria, pp. S89–S107, Copyright 1999, with permission of Elsevier Science.

**Table 8–1** From *The Health of Adults in the Developing World,* edited by Richard Feachem, et al., copyright 1992 by © International Bank for Reconstruction and Development/The World Bank. Used by permission of Oxford University Press, Inc.

**CHAPTER 9**

**Exhibit 9–1** Data from M.J. Toole, A. Rodger, *The Impact of the Asian Financial Crisis on Health,* © 2000, Australian Agency for International Development.

**Exhibit 9–3** Data from Goma Epidemiology Group, Public Health Impact of Rwandan Refugee Crisis, What Happened in Goma, Zaire, in July 1994?, *The Lancet,* Vol. 349, pp. 339–344, © 1995, The Lancet Ltd.

**Exhibit 9–4** Data from Goma Epidemiology Group, Public Health Impact of Rwandan Refugee Crisis, What Happened in Goma, Zaire, in July 1994?, *The Lancet,* Vol. 349, pp. 339–344, © 1995, The Lancet Ltd.

**Figure 9–1** Data from P. Wallensteen and M. Sollenberg, Armed Conflict, 1989–1998, *Journal of Peace Research,* Vol. 36, No. 5, pp. 593–606, © 1999.

**Figure 9–2** Reprinted with permission from *Internally Disabled Persons: A Global Survey,* p. 28, © 1998 Norwegian Refugee Council.

**Figure 9–3** Data from Goma Epidemiology Group, Public Health Impact of Rwandan Refugee Crisis. What Happened in Goma, Zaire, in July 1994?, *The Lancet,* Vol. 345, pp. 339–344, © 1995, The Lancet Ltd.

**Figure 9–4** Reprinted with permission from Goma Epidemiology Group, Public Health Impact of Rwandan Refugee Crisis: What Happened in Goma, Zaire In July 1994?, *The Lancet,* Vol. 345, pp. 339–344, © 1995, The Lancet Ltd.

**Figure 9–5** Data from UNHCR/WFP Guidelines for Selective Feeding Programmes in Emergency Situations, © 1999, United Nations High Commissioner for Refugees and the World Food Programme.

**Figure 9–6** Data from Unher, CDC Famine Affected, Refugee, and Displaced Populations: Recommendations for Public Health Issues, *Morbidity and Mortality Weekly Report,* Vol.

41, RR13, 1992, the Centers for Disease Control.

**Table 9–1** Reprinted with permission from *Refugees by Numbers,* © 2000, United Nations High Commission for Refugees.

**Table 9–5** Data from The Sphere Project, *Humanitarian Charter and Minimum Standards in Disaster ,* © 1998, The Sphere Project Group.

## CHAPTER 10

**Exhibit 10–1** Reprinted with permission from *World Development Report 1998/99,* © 1998, The World Bank.

**Exhibit 10–2** Data from E. Bos, et al., *Health, Nutrition, and Population Indicators: A Statistical Handbook,* © 1998, The World Bank; *Las Cuentas Nacionales de Salud y el Financiamiento de los Servicios,* © 1994, Fundacion Mexicana para la Salud; *Health and the Economy: Proposals for the Progress in the Mexican Health System,* © 1995, Fundacion Mexicana para la Salud; and V. Tangcharoensathien, et al., National Health Accounts Development: Lessons from Thailand, *Health Policy and Planning,* Vol. 14, No. 4, pp. 342–353.

**Exhibit 10–3** Data from personal communication with Sally Lake and Miguel Betancourt.

**Exhibit 10–4** Data from *Zambia Health Sector Expenditure Review,* © 1995, University of Zambia and Swedish Institute for Health Economics; Berman, *Financing of Rural Health Care in India,* © 1995, International Workshop on Health Insurance in India; *Las Cuentas Nacionales de Salud y el Financiamiento de los Servicios,* © 1994, Fundacion Mexicana para la Salud; and V. Tangcharoensathien, et al., National Health Accounts Development: Lessons from Thailand, *Health Policy and Planning,* Vol. 14, No. 4, pp. 343–353, © 1999.

**Exhibit 10–5** Reprinted from *An Introduction to Health Economics for Eastern Europe and the Former Soviet Union,* S. Witter and T. Ensor, p. 83. Copyright John Wiley & Sons Limited. Reproduced with permission.

**Figure 10–1** Reprinted with permission from *Sector Strategy: Health Nutrition and Population,* 1997, The World Bank Group.

**Figure 10–2** From *National Health Systems of the World, Volume I: The Countries* by Milton I. Roemer, Copyright © 1991 by Oxford University Press, Inc. Used by permission of Oxford University Press, Inc.

**Figure 10–3** Reprinted with permission from A. Mills, Reforming Health Sectors: Fashions, Passions, and Common Sense, in *Reforming Health Sectors,* (in press) Kegan Paul International.

**Table 10–1** Reprinted with permission from C. Donaldson and K. Gerard, *Economics of Health Care Financing: The Visible Hand,* © 1993, MacMillan Press, Ltd.

**Table 10–2** Reprinted with permission from Bennet, et al., *Public and Private Roles in Health: A Review and Analysis of Experience in Sub-Saharan Africa,* Division of Strengthening of Health Services, © 1994, World Health Organization.

**Table 10–4** Reprinted from *World Development,* Vol. 26, No. 8, P. Berman, Rethinking Health Care Systems: Private Health Care Provision in India, p. 1467, Copyright 1998, with permission from Elsevier Science.

**Table 10–5** Reprinted with permission from S. Bennett, Health-care Markets: Defining Characteristics, in *Private Health Providers in Developing Countries,* S. Bennett, B. McPake, and A. Mills, eds., p. 92, © 1997, Zed Books.

**Table 10–6** Used with permission from *Hospital and Health Services Administration,* Vol. 35, pp. 25–42. (Chicago: Health Administration Press, © 1991.)

## CHAPTER 11

**Exhibit 11–4** Adapted with permission from *The Functional Analysis of Health Needs and Services,* p. 18, © 1976, William A. Reinke.

**Exhibit 11–5** Data from *The Functional Analysis of Health Needs and Services,* © 1976, William A. Reinke.

**Exhibit 11–12** Data from J.M. Hughes, Reducing Health Care Costs: A Case for Quality, *Physician Executive,* Vol. 18, No. 4, pp. 9–15, © 1992.

**Table 11–1** Adapted with permission from *The Functional Analysis of Health Needs and Services,* p. 197, © 1976, William A. Reinke.

**Table 11–2** Adapted with permission from *The Functional Analysis of Health Needs and Services,* p. 190, © 1976, William A. Reinke.

**CHAPTER 12**

**Exhibit 12–1** Reprinted from *Journal of Econometrics,* Vol. 77, A. Bhargava, Nutritional Status and the Allocation of Time in Rwandese Households, pp. 277–295, Copyright 1997, with permission from Elsevier Science.

**Exhibit 12–3** Reprinted with permission from R.H. Dholakia and ed. Joel Almeida, The Potential Economic Benefits of the DOTS Strategy against TB in India, *The Global TB Programme of the World Health Organization,* Research and Surveillance Unit, © 1997, World Health Organization.

**Figure 12–2** Reprinted with permission from *World Health Report 1999: Making a Difference,* p. 11, © 1999, World Health Organization.

**Figure 12–3** Adapted with permission from J. Leslie and D.T. Jamison, Health and Nutrition Considerations in Education Planning, 1. Educational Consequences of Health Problems Among School-Age Children, *Food and Nutrition Bulletin,* Vol. 12, No. 3, © 1990, Published by United Nations University Press.

**Figure 12–4** Reprinted with permission from *World Health Report 1999: Making a Difference,* p. 5, © 1999, World Health Organization.

**Figure 12–6** Reprinted with permission from *World Development Report 1980,* © 1980, The World Bank.

**Figure 12–7** Reprinted with permission from *World Development Report 1980,* © 1980, The World Bank.

**Figure 12–8** Reprinted with permission from *World Health Report 1999: Making a Difference,* p. 39, © 1999, World Health Organization.

**Figure 12–9 Panel A:** Reprinted with permission from *World Development Report 1980,* © 1980, The World Bank.

**Table 12–2** Adapted with permission from J. Leslie and D.T. Jamison, Health and Nutrition Considerations in Education Planning, 1. Educational Consequences of Health Problems Among School-Age Children, *Food and Nutrition Bulletin,* Vol. 12, No. 3, © 1990, Published by United Nations University Press.

**Table 12–3** Reprinted from *Health, Nutrition, and Population Indicators: A Statistical Handbook,* © 1999, The World Bank.

**Table 12–5** Reprinted from *Journal of Econometrics,* Vol. 77, P. Gertler and R. Sturm, Private Health Insurance and Public Expenditures in Jamaica, pp. 237–257, Copyright 1997, with permission from Elsevier Science.

**Table 12–6** Data from B.C. Madrian, Employment-Based Health Insurance and Job Mobility, *Quarterly Review of Economics,* Vol. 109, No. 1, pp. 27–54, © 1994; D. Holtz-Eakin, Health Insurance Provision and Labor Market Efficiency in the United States and Germany, in *Social Protection Versus Economic Flexibility,* R.M. Blank, ed., pp. 157–188, © 1994, University of Chicago Press; J. Gruber and B.C. Madrian, Health Insurance and Job Mobility, *Industrial and Labor Relations Review,* Vol. 48, No. 1, © 1994; A.C. Monheit and P.F. Cooper, Health Insurance and Job Mobility, *Industrial and Labor Relations Review,* Vol. 48, No. 1, © 1994; and T.C. Buchmueller and R. G. Valletta, The Effects of Employer-Provided Health Insurance on Worker Mobility, *Industrial and Labor Relations Review,* Vol. 49, No. 3, © 1996.

**Table 12–7** Reprinted with permission from S. Reddy and J. Vandemoortele, *User Financing of Basic Social Services: A Review of Theoretical Arguments and Empirical Evidence,* Office of Evaluation and Planning, UNICEF.

**Table 12–8** Reprinted with permission from *Health, Health Care and Health Economics: Perspectives on Distribution,* M.L. Barer, et al., eds., Copyright 1998, © John Wile & Sons Limited. Reproduced with permission.

## CHAPTER 13

**Exhibit 13–1** Reprinted with permission from K. Lee, S. Collinson, G. Walt, and L. Gilson, Who Should be Doing What in International Health: A Confusion of Mandates, *British Medical Journal,* Vol. 312, pp. 302–312, © 1996, BMJ Publishing Group.

**Exhibit 13–3** Reprinted with permission from P. Kanavos, M. McKee, and T. Richards, 1999 Editorial: Cross Border Health Care in Europe, *British Medical Journal,* Vol. 318, pp. 1157–1158, © 1999, BMJ Publishing Group.

**Exhibit 13–6** Adapted with permission from G. Walt, *Health Policy: An Introduction to Process and Power,* © 1994, Zed Books.

**Exhibit 13–7** Reprinted from *Health Policy,* Vol. 24, G. Walt, WHO Under Stress: Implications for Health Policy, pp. 125–144, Copyright 1993, with permission from Elsevier Science.

**Exhibit 13–8** Reprinted with permission from D. Jamison, J. Frenk, and F. Knaul, 1998 International Collective Action in Health: Objectives, Functions and Rationale, *The Lancet,*

Vol. 351, pp. 514–517, © 1998, The Lancet Ltd.

**Exhibit 13–10** From G. Walt, et al., Managing External Resources: Are There Lessons for SWAps?, *Health Policy and Planning,* Vol. 14, No. 3, Copyright © 1999 by Oxford University Press, Inc. Used by permission of Oxford University Press, Inc.

**Exhibit 13–11** Reprinted with permission from W. Muraskin, *The War Against Hepatitis B,* © 1995, University of Pennsylvania Press.

**Figure 13–2** Data from The State in a Changing World, *World Development Report,* © 1997, The World Bank.

**Table 13–1** Adapted with permission from A. Lucas, et al., *Cooperation for Development: The World Health Organization's Support to Programmes at Country Level,* Report for the Governments of Australia, Canada, Italy, Norway, Sweden, UK, p. 13, © 1997, London School of Hygiene and Tropical Medicine.

## CHAPTER 14

**Exhibit 14–2** From *Global Public Goods: International Cooperation in the 21st Century,* edited by Inge Kaul, et al., copyright © 1999 by the United Nations Development Programme. Used by permission of Oxford University Press, Inc.

**Figure 14–1** Reprinted with permission from *Removing Obstacles to Healthy Development: Report on Infectious Diseases,* p. 35, © 1999, World Health Organization.

**Table 14–1** From *Global Public Goods: International Cooperation in the 21st Century,* edited by Inge Kaul, et al., copyright © 1999 by the United Nations Development Programme. Used by permission of Oxford University Press, Inc.

# Index

## M